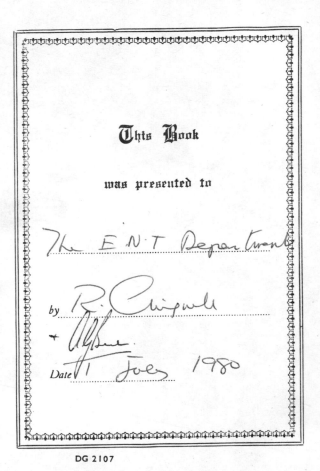

𝔗𝔥𝔦𝔰 𝔅𝔬𝔬𝔨

was presented to

The E.N.T Department

by R. Chipwell

+

Date 1 Joey 1980

DG 2107

Scott-Brown's
Diseases of the Ear, Nose and Throat

Volume 2
The Ear

Titles of other volumes

Scott-Brown's
Diseases of the Ear, Nose and Throat

Fourth Edition

Volume 2

The Ear

Editors

John Ballantyne, FRCS, HON FRCS (I)
Consultant Ear, Nose and Throat Surgeon,
The Royal Free Hospital and King Edward VII Hospital for Officers, London;
Civilian Consultant in Otolaryngology to the Army

John Groves, MB, BS, FRCS
Consultant Ear, Nose and Throat Surgeon,
The Royal Free Hospital, London

Butterworths
London Boston
Sydney Wellington Durban Toronto

| United Kingdom | **Butterworth & Co (Publishers) Ltd** |
| London | 88 Kingsway, WC2B 6AB |

Australia	**Butterworths Pty Ltd**
Sydney	586 Pacific Highway, Chatswood, NSW 2067
	Also at Melbourne, Brisbane, Adelaide and Perth

| Canada | **Butterworth & Co (Canada) Ltd** |
| Toronto | 2265 Midland Avenue, Scarborough, Ontario, M1P 4S1 |

| New Zealand | **Butterworths of New Zealand Ltd** |
| Wellington | T & W Young Building, 77–85 Customhouse Quay, 1, CPO Box 472 |

| South Africa | **Butterworth & Co (South Africa) (Pty) Ltd** |
| Durban | 152–154 Gale Street |

| USA | **Butterworth (Publishers) Inc** |
| Boston | 10 Tower Office Park, Woburn, Massachusetts 01801 |

First edition 1952
Second edition 1965
Reprinted 1967
Reprinted 1968
Third edition 1971
Reprinted 1977
Fourth edition 1979

© Butterworth & Co (Publishers) Ltd, 1979

ISBN 0 407 00148 4   Individual volume
ISBN 0 407 00143 3   Set of four volumes

British Library Cataloguing in Publication Data

Scott-Brown, Walter Graham
  Scott-Brown's diseases of the ear, nose and throat—4th ed.
  Vol. 2: The ear
  1. Otolaryngology
  I. Ballantyne, John II. Groves, John
  616.2'1   RF46   79–41008

  ISBN 0–407–00148–4
  ISBN 0–407–00143–3 Set of 4 vols

Typeset by CCC and printed and bound at
William Clowes & Sons Limited, Beccles and London

Introduction to the Fourth Edition

Some eight years after the last edition of this work appeared it may now seem to the practising clinician that the present decade has been a relatively quiet one in the history of our specialty. In fact, there has been a steady growth in the scientific foundations upon which an increasing amount of our practice is built, and it is therefore not surprising that the first volume, *Basic Sciences*, has now been considerably enlarged.

There has also been a steady expansion of clinical knowledge, and in planning this new edition we quickly became aware that no single volume from the last edition could stand without revision.

Sadly, the list of authors has been depleted by deaths and retirements of old friends and colleagues, whose contributions to British otolaryngology will never be forgotten. We thank sincerely all our colleagues, both old and new, who have spared no effort in preparing their manuscripts for this new presentation. The connoisseur will notice that a number of distinguished contributors from overseas have again been invited; we hope that this broadening of outlook will be welcomed by readers, and it is in keeping with the concepts of Mr W G Scott-Brown who originated the text nearly 30 years ago and who continues to flourish and to practice.

In some parts of the work, notably in Volume 2 (*The Ear*), advances in academic research have out-paced our ability to classify neatly a plethora of theories, facts (and sometimes fancies) for clinical application. Retaining the clinical approach as far as possible has compelled us, therefore, to commission chapters (for example in the field of sensorineural deafness) which overlap one another very considerably in content, while differing widely in emphasis. We hope that the reader will bear with this, and that the overall presentation will form a wider basis for learning than could be achieved by a more rigidly structured approach.

As far as we could we have used metric and SI units of measurement, even though a sense of humour is needed to accept some of the numerical absurdities which result. We are increasingly aware, too, that the SI system has brought upon us a hybrid and irrational system, heavily be-spattered with eponymously named units, at a time when eponyms are discouraged in the basic scientific disciplines. We are confident that the present generation will continue to honour Eustachius, Morgagni, Paget, Pott, Rosenmüller, and a hundred and one other great names, however the winds of pseudo-change may blow.

It is a great pleasure to thank and acknowledge all those who have helped so much in the preparation of this edition. We are grateful to those many colleagues who have lent us illustrations; to our registrars who have read proofs, criticized, advised and encouraged; and to those artists who have drawn new illustrations. Among the latter we thank especially Mr Frank Price for his unfailing generosity and technical skills. Equally we thank Mr Cedric Gilson and the Photographic Department of the Royal Free Hospital for their tremendous and willing efforts to provide so many of the new photographs.

Finally, our gratitude goes to our publishers, Butterworths, who have done so much to lighten our editorial tasks.

London, 1979
John Ballantyne
John Groves

Introduction to the Third Edition

A radical new departure is made in the presentation of this work in four separately available volumes. This has been done for two main reasons. First, there is a real need, we feel, to recognize the diverse requirements of different readers—the newcomer to the specialty who needs a compact presentation of the special anatomy, physiology and radiology (for preparation for the DLO Part I and Primary FRCS examinations), and the specialist who is more interested in, say, the ear than in the throat. Secondly, advances are more numerous and more rapid in some sub-divisions of the specialty than in others so that it will be advantageous in the future to revise one volume at a time. The reduction in bulk of the individual volumes results, we hope, in easier handling and more pleasant reading.

A consequence of this change in format and policy is that page and chapter cross-references between different volumes cannot be given, nor is it practicable any longer to compile the symptom index featured in the last edition. To offset the former disadvantage some overlapping of subject material has been deliberately introduced wherever it was felt that too frequent referral to another volume would otherwise be necessary. Each volume has its own Table of Contents and Index, the latter compiled on the basis of noun-entries only.

The text throughout has been comprehensively revised. As a matter of general editorial policy, for this and for any subsequent editions which may appear under our direction, we have invited contributions only from those of our colleagues who are still actively engaged in hospital, university or college practice; and it has been our pleasure to welcome several new contributors. By including several new chapters, we have been able to remedy some of the omissions from earlier editions (for example, 'Congenital Diseases of the Larynx'), and also to give due emphasis to such topics as 'Acoustic Trauma' and 'Acoustic Neuroma', each of which now demands a separate chapter. The weights and liquid measures of all drugs, as well as the measures of distance, are all given in the metric system.

We are grateful to all the authors for submitting their work on schedule so that the production can be uniformly up-to-date. We warmly appreciate the efforts and enthusiasm of the Publisher's Editorial Staff, and the kind help we have received from colleagues, artists, and many friends too numerous to be named. It has been a tremendous encouragement to have the continuing interest of Mr W G Scott-Brown,

CVO, MD, FRCS, who has read and contributed substantially to the editing of a large part of this edition. We wish to thank him for the honour of his invitation to join in the Editorship of this standard textbook, which was established solely by him in the First Edition of 1952. Although he has now handed over completely the pleasant duties of joint Editorship to us and our successors, it remains his book and it retains his name.

London, 1971
John Ballantyne
John Groves

Introduction to the Second Edition

The objects set out in the Introduction to the First Edition have been the guiding principles in the present work. In order to make this new edition authoritative and contemporary in outlook, I asked two of my colleagues to join me as co-editors and I have been most fortunate in having the help and inspiration of John Ballantyne and John Groves. We have together re-cast the main sections, sub-sections and chapters and have given more emphasis to those departments of the specialty which have undergone the greatest changes. We have also made great efforts to have all contributions written and despatched to the printer within one year of starting the project, in order that all the articles shall be finished at the same time and be up-to-date when published. This object has been achieved thanks to the cooperation of our contributors.

It will be seen that the sections on physiology have been extended and improved and the chapters on the ear have been considerably altered and enlarged to include the many fresh ideas and techniques associated with both infective and non-infective ear conditions. The sections on endoscopy have been re-arranged to make the subject as practical as possible for our speciality. It is hoped that the necessary curtailment has not given rise to any major omissions. Neoplasms of the larynx and pharynx have been separated and new chapters on voice and speech have been introduced.

The index has been completely revised, and an innovation in a textbook of this size is an additional index—a symptom index—which is complete for the whole work at the end of each volume. It is hoped that this may be particularly useful to candidates for higher examinations and to general practitioners looking for causes of particular symptoms.

It is a pleasure to acknowledge the generous help which has been given by all the contributors, a number of them new to this book, and to artists and friends, for their kindly and stimulating interest. It is not possible here to record individual acknowledgments, but a special word of thanks must be made to the Editorial Staff of the Publishers.

London, 1965
W G Scott-Brown

Introduction to the First Edition

This work has been compiled with the object of presenting a textbook on Diseases of the Ear, Nose and Throat which would include most of the subject matter required by students and post-graduates with sufficient detail for those taking the higher specialized qualifications. It should also be a suitable reference book for general practice.

To achieve this it was decided to ask a number of teachers, examiners and other well-recognized authorities in the specialty to contribute articles on this general plan while leaving them free to put forward their own views of the particular subject in their own way. This has in some cases meant the presentation of individual preferences, classifications or theories, but as far as possible these have been integrated with the more usual views to give a balanced appreciation of the subject. It is hoped that this individuality of articles will give a more stimulating approach to the subject in spite of some overlapping of subject matter and differences of opinion.

Each section is prefaced by its anatomy and physiology as an essential basis to the understanding of the subject, and also to include in a concise manner the material necessary for the examinee. Methods of examination on the other hand have been cut to a minimum as they can only be learnt by the practical examination of patients. After considerable deliberation it was decided to include a chapter on plastic surgery of the nose and ear which should set out what can be done rather than entering into details of technique which are largely the province of the plastic surgeon.

My thanks are due in the first place to all the contributors who have lightened the editorial burden: they have all been most cooperative and have given freely of their time, knowledge and, in many cases, helpful criticism. Acknowledgment is made in the text for opinions and illustrations used.

I must particularly thank the Publisher's team, all of whom have been not only helpful but also encouraging during the many unavoidable delays and difficulties in the production of a new work.

London, 1952
W G Scott-Brown

Colour plates in this volume

Contributors to this volume

Peter W Alberti, MB, PHD, FRCS, FRCS (C)
Otolaryngologist-in-Chief, Department of Otolaryngology, Mount Sinai Hospital, Toronto

John Ballantyne, FRCS, HON FRCS (I)
Consultant Ear, Nose and Throat Surgeon, The Royal Free Hospital and King Edward VII Hospital, London; Civilian Consultant in Otolaryngology to the Army

Philip H Beales, MB, BS, FRCS (ED)
Consultant Ear, Nose and Throat Surgeon, Royal Infirmary, Doncaster

J B Booth, FRCS
Consultant Ear, Nose and Throat Surgeon, The London Hospital

B H Colman, CHM, FRCS
Head, Department of Otolaryngology, Radcliffe Infirmary, Oxford; Consultant Ear, Nose and Throat Surgeon, Oxfordshire Area Health Authority (Teaching); Clinical Lecturer, University of Oxford

J D K Dawes, BSC, MD, BS, FRCS
Reader in Otolaryngology, University of Newcastle upon Tyne; Consultant Ear, Nose and Throat Surgeon, Newcastle Area Health Authority (Teaching)

R L G Dawson, MB, FRCS
Plastic Surgeon, The Mount Vernon Centre for Plastic Surgery, Northwood, Middlesex

Ellis Douek, FRCS
Consultant Ear, Nose and Throat Surgeon, Guy's Hospital, London

William G Edwards, MA, MB, BCH, FRCS, DLO
Senior Consultant Surgeon, Ear, Nose and Throat Department, King's College Hospital; Consultant Ear, Nose and Throat Surgeon, Hospital for Sick Children, Great Ormond Street, London

A G Gibb, MB, CHB, FRCS (ED), DLO
Consultant Ear, Nose and Throat Surgeon, Ninewells Hospital, Dundee; Head, Department of Otolaryngology, University of Dundee

W P R Gibson, MB, FRCS
Consultant Neuro-otologist, The National Hospital for Nervous Diseases, Queen Square, London; Consultant Ear, Nose and Throat Surgeon, Royal National Throat, Nose and Ear Hospital, London

John Groves, MB, BS, FRCS
Consultant Ear, Nose and Throat Surgeon, The Royal Free Hospital, London

Valentine Hammond FRCS
Consultant Ear, Nose and Throat Surgeon, St. Thomas's Hospital, London

John Hankinson, MB, BS, FRCS
Professor of Neurosurgery, University of Newcastle upon Tyne; Consultant Neurosurgeon, Regional Neurological Centre, Newcastle General Hospital and Royal Victoria Infirmary, Newcastle upon Tyne

J W P Hazell, FRCS
Honorary Consultant Neuro-otologist, University College Hospital, London; Research Fellow, Royal National Institute for the Deaf, London

John S Lewis, MD, FACS
Associate Professor in Otolaryngology, Columbia University; Chief, Ear, Nose and Throat Service, Roosevelt Hospital, New York; Associate Attending Surgeon, Head and Neck Service, Memorial Hospital, New York

H Ludman, FRCS
Consultant Ear, Nose and Throat Surgeon, King's College Hospital, London; Consultant Neuro-otologist, National Hospital for Nervous Diseases, Queen Square, London

M C Martin, OBE
Head of Scientific and Technical Department, The Royal National Institute for the Deaf, London

Stuart R Mawson, MB, FRCS, DLO
Senior Consultant Surgeon, Department of Otolaryngology, Kings College Hospital (including Belgrave Hospital for Children) London

Andrew W Morrison, MB, CHB, FRCS, DLO
Senior Otolaryngologist, The London Hospital; Lecturer in Otolaryngology at the University of London and Institute of Laryngology and Otology, London

K S Pegg, M PHIL, CTD
Head, Centre for the Deaf, City Literary Institute, London

P M Shenoi, CHM, FRCS, FRCS (ED), DLO
Consultant Ear, Nose and Throat Surgeon, Department of Otolaryngology and Oral Surgery, East Birmingham Hospital

James D Smith, MD
Department of Otolaryngology, School of Medicine, University of Oregon

Ian G Taylor, MD, DPH, FRCP
Ellis Llwyd Jones Professor of Audiology and Education of the Deaf; Honorary Consultant in Audiological Medicine at the Manchester Royal Infirmary, Royal Manchester Children's Hospital and Booth Hall Hospital

J L W Wright, FRCS
Consultant Ear, Nose and Throat Surgeon, St. Mary's Hospital, Paddington, London

Frank M Yatsu, MD
Department of Neurology, School of Medicine, University of Oregon

Contents

1 The physical and functional examination of the ear

W P R Gibson

The successful practice of otology must begin with confidence in reaching the correct diagnosis before any medical or surgical treatment is undertaken. The diagnosis can often be determined after evaluation of the patient's symptoms and physical signs, but in some instances the otologist also needs to obtain the results of functional investigations and tests. The purpose of this chapter is to give an outline of the methods involved. For descriptive purposes the subject has been separated into three main groups, although these groups often overlap in clinical practice.

(1) Inflammatory disorders: pain, discharge, irritation or blockage.
(2) Auditory disorders: hearing loss or tinnitus.
(3) Vestibular disorders: vertigo or imbalance.

Apart from purely cosmetic problems, virtually all the pathological conditions that affect the ear, including congenital and neoplastic conditions, present in at least one of the above groups. The investigation of vestibular disorders is described in the next chapter.

Inflammatory disorders

History

The commonest symptoms resulting from an inflammatory disorder are earache (otalgia) and discharge (otorrhoea). It is always necessary to enquire whether they have occurred on any previous occasion and whether there has been any surgery performed on the ear.

OTALGIA
Pain in and around the ear may either be due to local disease or may be referred from another structure which shares a common root innervation. The otologist should determine the manner of onset of the pain and its distribution, severity, character and periodicity. Factors which aggravate the pain or relieve it should be noted.

Local causes

Otalgia may be caused by almost any inflammatory disorder which affects the outer or middle ear. Itching or irritation is a common symptom of eczematous otitis externa. Acute diffuse otitis externa causes pain of variable severity (Senturia, 1973), and this depends on the amount of oedema tenting the tight, sensitive epithelial lining of the external acoustic meatus. The pain is often aggravated by moving the pinna or by biting or chewing. A furuncle (acute localized otitis externa) causes very severe pain. Intense pain may also be caused by herpes simplex or herpes zoster infection.

Otitis externa haemorrhagica or bullous myringitis (probably caused by a viral infection) is characterized by small purple blebs which appear on the surface of the tympanic membrane. It usually presents with severe pain.

Otitis media is one of the commonest paediatric problems encountered by general practitioners. Acute bacterial otitis media can give rise to considerable pain, particularly when the tympanic membrane is distended, but in the early stages of the condition, the young child may present merely with pyrexia and vomiting. Children with auditory tube dysfunction commonly experience pain within an hour of lying down at night. This is probably due to dependent oedema exacerbating the tubal dysfunction.

Referred otalgia

Pain referred to the ear is a common symptom and despite careful examination, no abnormality can be detected within the ear. The pain may be referred through the fifth, seventh, ninth and tenth cranial nerves, the upper cervical nerves and possibly through the sympathetic nerve supply. The commonest sources of referred otalgia are from carious or impacted molar teeth, from the posterior tongue, pharynx, tonsils and larynx. A carcinoma of the pyriform fossa often presents initially as otalgia. Mollison has been quoted as saying, 'a lump in the neck and a piece of cotton wool in the ear mean a carcinoma of the pharynx' (Watkyn-Thomas, 1953).

Dysfunction of the temporo-mandibular joint may produce otalgia amongst other symptoms (Costen, 1934). This dysfunction is often revealed by the presence of malocclusion (due to bruxism, worn dentures, etc.), by a 'clicking' on opening the mouth widely, or by spasms within the muscles of mastication.

Pain radiating along the glossopharyngeal nerve may result from an abnormally elongated styloid process (Moffat, Ramsden and Shaw, 1977). This may be detected by bimanual palpation and by radiography. Glossopharyngeal neuralgia is fortunately rare. It is characterized by severe spasms of pain which radiate from the throat into the tongue and ear, and the pain may begin after the stimulation of a 'trigger zone'.

Herpes zoster infection involving the lower cranial nerves or upper cervical nerves frequently causes severe otalgia which may precede the skin eruptions. This condition may be associated with facial paralysis (Ramsay Hunt syndrome). Indeed, idiopathic facial paralysis may be preceded by otalgia of variable severity and by disturbances of taste. Tenderness of the upper sterno-mastoid attachment and referred pain from fibrositis in the deep muscles may also present as otalgia.

OTORRHOEA

Otorrhoea is a frequent consequence of inflammatory ear conditions. The onset and duration of the discharge, its character, colour, amount and any odour should be noted.

A watery, odourless discharge commonly occurs in eczematous otitis externa. The colour of the discharge caused by bacterial otitis externa may suggest the pathogenic organism and aid the choice of the initial antibiotic. A copious, foul-smelling discharge is often suggestive of chronic otitis media; this may be secondary either to a 'safe' central perforation of the tympanic membrane and tubo-tympanic disease, or to 'dangerous' attic disease and cholesteatoma. Unduly copious discharge may be associated with coalescent mastoiditis. The discharge fills the concha and on mopping it away, the discharge rapidly reappears ('reservoir sign'). This sign is more commonly observed in recent times when the ear has been subject to radical mastoid surgery and the mastoid cavity has become grossly infected and full of pus.

Three conditions deserve special mention. Malignant neoplasms are rare, but when they do occur, they usually appear in ears affected by longstanding otorrhoea. Diabetic patients, and occasionally patients on immunosuppressive therapy may rarely develop malignant otitis externa which is due to a vicious invasion by *Pseudomonas aeruginosa*. These patients usually suffer from severe pain and there is a blue-green, pungent discharge. Unless radical treatment is instituted, multiple cranial nerve palsies occur and the outcome is invariably fatal. Another condition occasionally encountered is osteonecrosis of the bony portion of the external acoustic meatus following radiotherapy to lesions near the ear (Ramsden *et al.*, 1975).

OTHER ASSOCIATED SYMPTOMS

Headache
The association of otorrhoea and headache merits careful attention as it may indicate an intracranial extension of the disease process. Headache is one of the earliest symptoms and if its significance is overlooked, the patient may present at a more serious advanced stage with drowsiness, stupor or even coma.

Visual impairment
Papilloedema must be marked before there is any loss of visual acuity.

Aphasia
Nominal aphasia, in particular, suggests involvement of the temporal lobe. Temporal lobe lesions may also be accompanied by varying degrees of homonymous hemianopia.

Auditory and vestibular dysfunction
Hearing loss due to damage to the middle-ear mechanism or to the cochlea often occurs as a consequence of inflammatory conditions. Vestibular symptoms due to invasion of the otic capsule require urgent investigation and treatment. Labyrinthitis may easily lead to meningitis. These matters are mentioned in greater detail later in the next chapter.

Examination of the ear

The ear itself is only one item to be considered when examining a patient suffering from an inflammatory disorder. The minimum examination should include the nose and paranasal sinuses, the post-nasal space, the oropharynx and the facial nerve.

Whenever necessary, the examination has to be extended to include the larynx and other cranial nerves.

Both ears should always be examined. It is best to begin with the normal ear as this makes the transfer of infective debris from the inflamed ear to the healthy ear less likely. The examination of each ear begins with an inspection of the pinna and the surrounding scalp. Failure to detect a healed retro-auricular incision is an embarrassment for the clinician and a stumbling block for the examination candidate. Before insertion of an aural speculum, the pinna should be gently manipulated to detect any discomfort and to reveal the presence of any aural discharge. On inserting the speculum, the external meatus is straightened: in adults by gently pulling the pinna in an upward and backward direction; and in young children by traction in a horizontal and backward direction.

The technique used for holding an electric auriscope is important especially when dealing with young apprehensive children who may suddenly jerk their heads. *Figure 1.1a* shows a common but incorrect method of holding the instrument as any sudden head movement will cause the end of the speculum to dig painfully into the lining of

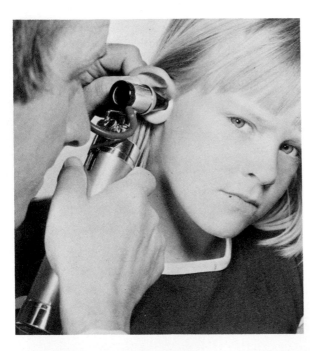

Figure 1.1   (a) The incorrect method

the external meatus. The correct method of holding the auriscope is shown in *Figure 1.1b*. The auriscope is held like a pen above the palm of the hand between the thumb and forefinger whilst the other fingers are gently held against the child's cheek. The advantage of this latter method is that whenever the child's head moves, the whole auriscope moves in unison.

The external acoustic meatus must be cleared of any debris. This is best accomplished using an aural speculum illuminated by a head mirror or operating microscope. Removal of all discharge is essential for the proper treatment of suppurating ear disease, but one should not forget to take a sample of the pus for bacteriological investigation. When clean, the external acoustic meatus may be examined. Bony overgrowths may be generalized (hyperostosis) or localized (exostosis), and their size and position should be noted. The meatus should also be examined for any areas of ulceration or soft tissue swelling. The postero–superior bony wall should be inspected carefully as it is easy to overlook erosion due to cholesteatoma or the opening in cases of poorly performed mastoid surgery.

Proper examination of the tympanic membrane requires both good illumination and optical magnification. The magnification may be provided by either the use of Siegle's speculum or an electric auriscope but the advantages of using the operating microscope cannot be over-stressed.

The normal tympanic membrane below the anterior and posterior malleolar folds presents a glistening light grey appearance. This larger part of the tympanic membrane is known as the pars tensa and it is composed of three separate layers with a total thickness of about 0.1 mm. The lateral layer is squamous epithelium, the middle layer is fibrous tissue and the innermost layer is the mucous membrane of the middle-ear cavity. An easily identifiable landmark is the handle of the malleus lying as the hand on a clock face. In the right ear it lies at 1 o'clock and in the left ear it lies

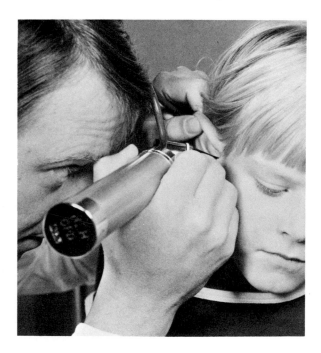

Figure 1.1 (b) The correct method

at 11 o'clock. The most inferior point of the malleus handle lies at the umbo, and from this point the light of the auriscope reflects from the pars tensa in a triangular area leading to the antero-inferior rim of the membrane (the so-called 'cone of light'). Above the anterior and posterior ligaments of the malleus marking the postero-superior border of the pars tensa lies that area of the tympanic membrane named the pars flaccida. This area of the tympanic membrane has a dull red appearance which resembles the colour of the meatal wall.

The tympanic membrane should be inspected for signs of inflammation. The normally light-grey pars tensa has an angry red appearance in acute otitis media and the tympanic membrane may be distended. Retraction of the tympanic membrane is often revealed by loss of the light reflex and by an indrawing of the malleus handle causing it to assume a more horizontal and seemingly foreshortened position. Occasionally, it is possible to detect air bubbles within a middle-ear effusion. Chronic infection may lead to heterotopic calcification, known as tympanosclerosis, within the fibrous layer of the tympanic membrane. The mobility of the membrane should be tested using Siegle's speculum or a pneumatic attachment to an electric auriscope. This often reveals thin atrophic areas and distinguishes them from perforations. It is not unusual today to find a grommet lurking at the medial end of the meatus.

The exact position of any perforation of the tympanic membrane should be noted and recorded by a simple drawing. It is particularly important to discover whether the perforation is marginal or central, and whether it involves the pars flaccida. Central perforations of the pars tensa are usually associated with tubo-tympanic disease and rarely cause serious complications, but perforations of the pars flaccida or attic region are frequently associated with cholesteatoma formation and may lead to dangerous complications. If there is a possibility of attic erosion, the effect of altering the pressure within the external acoustic meatus should be noted; a sensation of vertigo will be reported by the patient in cases when there is a fistula between the lateral semicircular canal and the middle-ear cavity.

When there is a 'safe' central perforation, it is usually possible to obtain some view of the middle-ear cavity. The state of the middle-ear mucosa should be noted as frequently it becomes hypertrophied and polypoidal. In some cases, large polyps may arise which fill the external acoustic meatus. The presence of the ossicles and the function of the incudostapedial joint can often be assessed. It is also advantageous to view the opening of the auditory (eustachian) tube and rarely a dehiscence in the bony facial canal is visible. All these findings may be of value for the planning of reconstructive surgery.

Examination of auditory tube function may be made by observing the tympanic membrane closely and noting any movement when the patient performs a Valsalva manoeuvre. In the past the Valsalva manoeuvre was followed if necessary by the use of Politzer's bag or the eustachian catheter, but with the introduction of impedance audiometry, these techniques are now seldom necessary (see later in this chapter).

Although the need to examine the nose and throat in every case has already been mentioned, it should be emphasized that a careful examination of the post-nasal space is essential whenever there is serous otitis media. It is often possible to visualize an adenoid pad in young children but, more importantly, the auditory tube orifices must be inspected in adult patients to exclude the possibility of a post-nasal neoplasm.

Investigations

When there is otorrhoea, bacteriological investigation of the discharge can be helpful in deciding the choice of antibiotic treatment. The possibility of a fungal infection should be considered, especially in diabetic or debilitated patients, and after the prolonged use of antibiotics. Fungal otitis externa is particularly common in tropical countries.

Haematological investigation is required for patients with persistent infection and for pre-operative assessment. The haemoglobin, white blood cell count and serological tests for syphilis are most commonly requested, but more specific haematological tests may be needed according to the individual patient's requirements.

Auditory and vestibular investigations are essential for many patients, especially when surgical treatment is contemplated. The pure-tone audiogram will provide an indication of the patient's hearing threshold and, in cases of conductive hearing loss, an estimate of the cochlear reserve. Impedance audiometry provides an excellent indication of middle-ear function. The details of these audiometric tests are described later in this chapter. Vestibular investigations are necessary whenever it is suspected that the inflammatory process has involved the labyrinthine structure.

Radiography is useful. Standard radiography of the middle-ear cleft and mastoid is confined mainly to demonstrating gross pathology such as lack of mastoid aeration, mastoid 'clouding', fractures and gross erosions. Tomography of the middle-ear cleft may reveal some of the finer details but as this technique delivers a high dose of irradiation to the eyes, there is some justification for seeking the combination of simple views which reveals the most anatomy (Parker, 1975). Radiography of the paranasal sinuses may reveal sinus infection requiring treatment before it is possible to treat the ear disease. Lateral views of the nasopharynx and the axial view of the skull are helpful in tubal disorders.

Computerized axial tomography (EMI scan) is of considerable value whenever an intracranial extension of the inflammatory process is suspected. This technique shows clearly extradural and intracerebral abcesses and it seems destined to become the first choice investigation rather than the more hazardous radiographic techniques such as arteriography.

Auditory disorders

Markides (1977) estimates that 3.3 million adults in the UK (population approximately 55 million) suffer from impaired hearing and half of these require hearing aid amplification. It is no surprise that auditory dysfunction is a common problem in otological practice. The usual symptoms of auditory dysfunction are hearing loss and tinnitus, but other symptoms include loss of discrimination, diplacusis and phonophobia.

Evaluation of auditory dysfunction depends on a careful history, examination and certain relevant investigations. There are today such a wealth of investigatory techniques that, in practice, the otologist has to select carefully the tests which are the most relevant for the individual case. There are some general guidelines. The younger the patient, the more thorough should be the clinical investigation. Patients with progressive hearing losses, especially progressive unilateral hearing losses, always merit careful attention. Patients aged over 70 years with bilateral high frequency hearing losses most commonly suffer from presbyacusis, and it is both impracticable and inhumane to submit these patients to extensive investigation.

History

The term 'deafness' should be reserved for total loss of auditory function and the term 'hearing loss' used for partial hypoacusis.

The history obtained from a patient with a hearing loss occurring after infancy obviously differs in emphasis from the history sought when a hearing loss is suspected in a baby. These two situations will therefore be considered separately.

HEARING LOSS AND DEAFNESS—ADULTS

Whether one or both ears are affected, the duration of the hearing loss, and the degree of handicap it imposes, should all be noted. The manner of the onset of the hearing loss is important; for instance, a sudden hearing loss requires urgent investigation and it is suggested that treatment is only effective if administered within a few days of the onset (Morrison and Booth, 1970). A gradually-progressing unilateral hearing loss may be the first symptom of a cerebello-pontine angle tumour. The aetiology of the hearing loss may be related to an event which occurred about the time of onset; some examples include the impaction of cerumen against the tympanic membrane after swimming, the presence of a middle-ear effusion after a severe head cold or an aeroplane journey and the severe sensory hearing loss (*see Table 1.5*) which may follow meningitis. The progression of the hearing loss can be a matter for concern, especially if there is rapid deterioration. Fluctuation in the level of hearing occurs in some conductive disorders, such as serous otitis media, wax, and in conditions associated with endolymphatic hydrops.

Table 1.1   Hearing loss—history (adults and older children)

Ears affected—right/left/if both, which is the 'better' ear?
History of present complaint—duration
        severity
        onset—sudden or gradual
          —any events related to onset
        progression—rapid or gradual
        fluctuations
Characteristics of the hearing loss—difficulties in hearing speech
        loudness discomfort
        paracusis
        diplacusis
Associated aural symptoms—tinnitus
        inflammatory disturbances
        vestibular disturbances
        pain (tension or fullness within the ear)
Associated general symptoms especially—headache
        visual disturbances
Past history—otological—past inflammatory disorders
        previous otological operations
        trauma
        excessive exposure to noise
        ototoxic antibiotics and other drugs and agents
      general—serious illnesses (especially meningitis, typhoid)
        severe childhood illnesses (measles, mumps, etc.)
        cardiovascular disease
        diabetes
Family history—hearing loss in relatives
Social history—alcohol
        tobacco
        occupation

The characteristics of the remaining hearing may indicate the site of the auditory dysfunction (*see Table 1.5*). Patients with sensorineural hearing losses have far more difficulty in understanding speech than patients with conductive disorders who usually maintain discrimination provided the speech intensity is raised. A characteristic of sensory damage is the phenomenon of recruitment and so patients with cochlear damage often find loud noises disagreeable. These patients may have considerable difficulty following conversation amongst background noise, whereas patients with stapedial fixation have an apparent *improvement* in hearing in background noise. Willis (1672) reported a woman who could only hear her husband speaking when he was beating a drum and the phenomenon of apparent increase in hearing amid background noise was named 'paracusis Willisii'. In fact, the hearing improves as the speaker has raised the intensity of his voice which is heard without distortion by the sufferer. Patients with neural disorders commonly have poor speech discrimination although they do not often suffer from recruitment. A patient with an eighth nerve tumour sometimes presents with difficulty following a telephone conversation using the affected ear. Diplacusis is the apparent difference in pitch of a pure tone between the normal and affected ear when the sound is presented binaurally. This phenomenon is usually noticed by musically-adept patients when they suffer from conditions causing endolymphatic hydrops.

The presence of any other aural symptoms other than hearing loss should be determined. Inflammatory disorders are often associated with conductive hearing loss. Tinnitus may accompany pathological conditions which affect all levels of the auditory system and the nature of the tinnitus may indicate the aetiology (*see Table 1.3*). Vestibular disorder accompanies several auditory disorders and may require detailed investigation. One symptom worth noting is the sensation of fullness or pressure within the ear; it commonly suggests dysfunction of the auditory tube but it is also noted by many patients suffering from Menière's disorder. A sensation of numbness around the affected ear may sometimes occur when there is a cerebello-pontine angle tumour.

Non-otological symptoms may be associated with the onset of the hearing loss. The patient should be carefully questioned about his general health. Some symptoms are especially important; for instance, headaches and visual disturbances may indicate an intracranial disturbance.

The past history which occurred before the hearing loss should be noted. The otological past history should include any past inflammatory conditions and any surgical operations. Important causes of cochlear damage include trauma, blast injuries, excessive noise exposure and ototoxic drugs. Head injuries may involve the middle-ear structures and cause a conductive hearing loss, or may involve the inner ear causing a severe sensory loss. Excessive noise exposure will lead to a loss of hair-cells especially within the basal turn of the cochlea. This noise may be impulse (impact) noise, or steady-state noise, or may be a mixture of both. People affected by impulse noise include gunners, riveters and the hunchback of Notre Dame. Hearing loss may result from exposure to steady-state noise of no more than 90 dB(A) if this is present for more than 8 h each day. People at risk include tractor drivers, machinists and pop musicians. The other important cause of hearing loss is ototoxic agents (Ballantyne, 1973). These agents may have been prescribed by a doctor or simply bought over the chemist's counter. Ototoxic drugs include salicylates, quinine, cytotoxic drugs, powerful diuretics and antibiotics. It is the aminoglycoside group of antibiotics (streptomycin, gentamicin, tobramycin, etc.) which is most prone to cause damage to the auditory system.

Serious illness, such as typhoid fever, cerebral malaria, meningitis and measles, may cause serious bilateral hearing problems. Mumps usually affects the hearing only in one ear. The presence of symptoms of generalized cardiovascular disease make it probable that a bilateral sensory, high-frequency hearing loss is due to the effects of bilateral cochlear ischaemia. Sudden vascular occlusion leading to hearing losses is commoner in diabetic patients than in other groups of patients.

The family history may reveal a hereditary cause for loss of hearing. Patients with otosclerosis commonly have a number of relatives affected by the same complaint. Finally, the patient's social history may prove helpful both in suggesting possible aetiological factors and in providing a guide to the most suitable form of therapy.

HEARING LOSS AND DEAFNESS—BABIES AND YOUNG CHILDREN

The history alters greatly in emphasis with a young child suspected of poor hearing. The history is usually obtained from the parents or from a guardian. A cardinal rule is never to disbelieve a mother who suspects her child of being deaf. The mother is seldom wrong. It is a grave misconception to believe that the assessment of a suspected

Table 1.2   Hearing loss—history (babies and infants)

Ears suspected—right/left/both
person suspecting the hearing loss
History of present complaint—when noticed
why noticed
any fluctuations
severity (does he hear mother's voice, footsteps, doorbell, loud noises, etc.?)
Past history—otological
—pre-natal—infections, especially rubella
contact with infectious disease
drugs
toxaemia and nephritis
metabolic state, diabetes, hypothyroidism
—natal—birthweight and gestational age
birth trauma
anoxia
jaundice
—post-natal—past inflammatory disorders
trauma
excessive noise exposure
ototoxic drugs and agents
—general—childhood infection (measles, mumps, etc.)
severe infections (especially meningitis)
state of general health
milestones of development
speech ability
Family history—siblings
possibility of congenital syndromes (draw family tree)
Social history—parent occupations
home situation
language or languages spoken at home
schooling difficulties

baby should be deferred until he reaches a certain age when testing becomes feasible. Nowadays it is possible to detect deafness even at birth and it seems logical to suppose that the sooner the deafness is detected, the sooner the family situation can be adjusted and the sooner remedial therapy can start.

As congenital deafness is discussed more fully in Chapter 16, only a brief outline of the history is shown in *Table 1.2* and only the more salient points will be discussed. The assessment of a child with a hearing loss requires the efforts of a specialist team (otologist, paediatrician, audiologist, speech therapist, psychologist, etc.) and only a preliminary examination is generally made by the ENT surgeon in his ordinary clinic.

It is customary to separate the aetiological causes of hearing loss in infants into genetic and non-genetic categories. There are several well-known genetic abnormalities which result in damage to the auditory system. The Scheibe type of sacculocochlear maldevelopment and syndromes such as Waardenburg's syndrome appear to be most commonly encountered. The non-genetic category may be divided into pre-natal, natal and post-natal causes. The commonest cause of pre-natal cochlear damage is undoubtably rubella and careful questioning of the mother may be necessary. Drugs taken by the mother during the first trimester are another important cause. Thalidomide is now fortunately of historic interest only but the possibility of further tragedies should not be overlooked. Any ototoxic drugs taken by the mother during this period may transfer to her child.

The natal history should include the birthweight and gestational age of the child. Premature babies are far more likely to suffer anoxic damage. Rhesus incompatibility between the mother and her baby results in haemolysis of the baby's blood and jaundice. If the jaundice is severe, the breakdown products of haemoglobin may damage the brainstem nuclei and cause deafness (kernicterus neonatorum). The history of the post-natal period covers essentially all the points relevant to the adult examination. Particular emphasis, however, is laid on the possibility of hearing loss resulting from an infectious illness such as measles or mumps.

TINNITUS—HISTORY

The absence of any specific treatment for most patients suffering from tinnitus may fill the clinician with despair when faced by a patient with tinnitus during a clinic. Tinnitus is however an important symptom of auditory dysfunction and may provide the earliest diagnostic clue to conditions which include otosclerosis and eighth nerve tumours. Tinnitus is discussed in detail in Chapter 3 and so only a brief outline of the history sought is shown in *Table 1.3* and only a few of the more relevant details will be discussed.

The patient may be able to lateralize his tinnitus to one or other ear, but sometimes both ears are affected or the tinnitus appears to arise centrally. The manner of the onset of the tinnitus may relate to the aetiology. A gradual onset is uncommon except in otosclerosis. If questioned carefully, the patient may be able to relate the onset of the tinnitus to an event such as an infection, trauma or a cardiovascular or psychological upset. Trauma may be due to excessive noise, an injury or to iatrogenic causes which are most commonly related to ear syringing or impedance audiometry. The tinnitus due to these causes generally settles over the ensuing days or weeks but occasionally the tinnitus may continue unabated for years. Any person who undertakes ear

Table 1.3   Tinnitus—history

Localization of tinnitus—right ear/left ear/both ears/inside head
History of present complaint—duration
                              onset—sudden or gradual
                                    any events related to onset
                              progression—getting better/same/worse
                              fluctuation
Characteristics of the tinnitus—subjective description
                              continuous, pulsatile, clicking, etc.
                              hissing noise, pure tone, etc.
                              pitch of tinnitus
                              severity
                        —aggravating factors
                              alcohol, exercise, neck twisting, etc.
                        —relieving factors
                              drugs, yawning, etc.
Associated aural symptoms—hearing disorder
                              vertigo
Associated general symptoms—especially—headache
                                            visual disturbances
Past history—otological—past inflammatory disorders
                              previous otological operations
                              trauma
                              excessive exposure to noise
                              ototoxic antibiotics and other drugs or agents
            —general—metabolic disturbances (e.g. thyroid disorders)
                              cardiovascular disease and hypertension
                              allergies
Family history—hearing loss (especially otosclerosis)
                              tinnitus
Psychiatric history
Social history—occupation
                              alcohol and tobacco

---

syringing or impedance audiometry should ensure that sudden pressure changes within the external acoustic meatus do not occur.

The characteristics of the tinnitus may indicate the aetiology. A pulsatile tinnitus may indicate a glomus tumour but more commonly it is related to some other cause of a conductive hearing loss. The patient hears his own pulse transmitted by bone conduction to the affected ear. A continuous tinnitus is more typical of a sensorineural condition. The pitch is often characteristic of the specific disorder (Douek and Reid, 1968). A low-pitched tinnitus is typical of Menière's disorder, a pure tone corresponding to the frequency showing the maximum loss on pure-tone audiometry is typical of acoustic trauma and a high-pitched hissing noise is common in patients with ischaemia affecting the cochlea. The description of the severity of the tinnitus is most subjective and varies considerably according to the tolerance of the sufferer. Most patients notice the tinnitus when there is no background noise to mask it. A description of very severe tinnitus is common in patients with syphilitic disorders and those with a total hearing loss especially when it follows a surgical procedure.

Occasionally some factor may be noticed by the patient which alters his tinnitus. Patients with auditory tube dysfunction may report tinnitus when their noses are congested. Workers subject to excessive noise levels may notice their tinnitus after finishing their work. Rarely a patient is encountered who can alter his tinnitus by twisting his neck into a certain position. More often patients will report that alcohol affects the intensity of their tinnitus.

It is important to detect any associated aural symptoms. A progressive hearing loss, especially when associated with imbalance, may suggest the presence of a tumour. The tinnitus of Menière's disorder is often louder before or during the vertiginous attacks. In Lermoyez's syndrome, a variant of Menière's disorder, the tinnitus actually decreases during the attacks. It is worth remembering that Menière's disorder is exceptionally rare in Negroes. Ashcroft *et al.* (1967) were unable to find a single native sufferer in Jamaica.

Past inflammatory ear disease and previous otological operations may be relevant to both the aetiology of tinnitus and to the interpretation of investigations. Occasionally patients with large mastoid cavities complain of a 'sea-shell' noise within the operated ear, and this noise can be altered by filling the mastoid bowl with ointment. Acoustic trauma and ototoxic drugs are important causes of tinnitus and may act synergistically together or with other factors which cause sensory (cochlear) damage. One third of all patients taking excessive doses of salicylates suffer from tinnitus. The tinnitus caused by salicylates is always reversible on stopping the drug, but the tinnitus caused by most other ototoxic drugs is irreversible.

The non-otological history should include general questions about the patient's health. Although no definite association is known, the presence of any allergies should be noted for occasionally a patient is encountered who develops tinnitus after eating certain foods.

The family history can be interesting. It may reveal the possibility of early otosclerosis. A peculiar objective whistling tinnitus can affect families of daschund dogs and a similar condition has been reported in man (Glanville, Coles and Sullivan, 1971). The whistling tinnitus in these patients could be heard clearly by an observer and was thought to have been transmitted down the cochlear duct from a valvular arteriovenous anastomosis.

A psychiatric history has to be obtained both because it may have an aetiological significance and because it may indicate a particular reason for the patient seeking advice. Some patients fear that they have developed a brain tumour and others fear that the tinnitus will drive them to insanity. Even if the clinician cannot ease the tinnitus, he may be able to reassure the patient. The history may also help the clinician to choose the most appropriate advice for the patient on how to cope with the condition should no treatment be available.

CLINICAL EXAMINATION

The examination of a young child suspected of hearing impairment cannot be undertaken properly during the usual busy adult clinic. The clinician may undertake a preliminary examination but usually needs to refer the child on to a specialized clinic. The examination of such a child is discussed in detail in Chapter 16.

Apart from examination of the ear itself, in the manner already described, the nose, throat and other parts of the body should be inspected. When a conductive hearing loss is suspected, it is important to examine the post-nasal space. In adults, particularly those of the Chinese race, hardwood workers and patients with a history of exposure to chemical irritants, careful examination of the post-nasal space may reveal a post-nasal carcinoma. Other parts of the body also merit examination: for example, conductive hearing loss may be associated with Paget's disease and patients with blue sclerae may suffer from osteogenesis imperfecta.

The examination of patients with a suspected sensorineural hearing loss varies according to the diagnosis suspected. Elderly patients with a bilateral sensory hearing loss should have their blood pressure checked but extensive investigations are probably unnecessary as the likely diagnosis is presbyacusis. Patients with a fluctuating hearing loss require a vestibular examination as Menière's disorder is a likely diagnosis. Occasionally a patient with Menière symptoms also suffers from interstitial keratitis and this makes a diagnosis of late-onset congenital syphilis probable. The patient with a progressing unilateral hearing loss always merits careful examination, as a cerebello-pontine angle tumour may be present. The eyes and cranial nerves should be examined. A large tumour may cause papilloedema but, except in gross cases, the patient will not notice any visual impairment. The eye movements should be inspected both with and without the use of Frenzel's glasses as the presence of any nystagmus is a most important sign. The function of the trigeminal nerve can be assessed and the testing of the corneal sensation provides a simple screening test. The facial nerve should always be examined in every patient with a hearing loss. The facial movements are observed during the course of clinical examination and can be tested by asking the patient to make certain facial movements. A minor degree of impairment is often manifested by an inability to bury the eyelashes equally on forced eye closure and by a delay on blinking. The lacrimation and taste may also be tested (*see* Chapter 27). Ninth, tenth and higher cranial nerve palsies only occur with massive cerebello-pontine angle tumours, but are common with glomus jugulare tumours.

When a patient is suffering from tinnitus, the clinician should listen to the ear using an aural stethoscope to determine if the tinnitus is objective. If the tinnitus is pulsatile, the presence of any carotid or skull bruits is important. In cases of a clicking tinnitus, there may also be a palatal myoclonus and a lesion of the dentate nucleus or of the brainstem pathways involved is likely. It is also useful to note if the tinnitus alters on occluding the external meatus on altering the pressure within the external meatus, or on compression of the carotid artery.

THE SIMPLE TESTS OF HEARING AND TUNING-FORK TESTS

The clinician himself should always make a simple assessment of the auditory function before selecting the audiometric investigations which he believes to be the most appropriate. Fifty years ago clinicians were skilful at using whisper and voice tests and at using a number of different tuning-fork tests but with the rapid development of more sophisticated audiometric tests, some of the tuning-fork tests have passed into obscurity.

Whisper and voice tests

In bygone days a standard method of assessing hearing was to measure the distance at which the patient could hear the examiner's voice, using either a whisper or a conversational voice. Such a method is inexact as variations in intensity occur unless the examiner maintains exactly the same voice intensity and performs the test in a quiet anechoic room. The concept of the examiner backing away from his patient and carefully measuring the distance between them is no longer tenable but a forced whisper test may still be used to gain a crude estimate of the patient's discrimination level. During such a test it is usual to mask the non-test ear by rustling the tragus with a finger.

Tuning-fork tests
Some of the tuning-fork tests are as essential today to the proper examination as in the past. The Rinne and Weber tests should always be performed and there are some cunning tests for detecting non-organic hearing losses.

The Rinne test   (*Figure 1.2a* and *b*)
Commonly a 512 Hz fork is selected but, when necessary, the test can be repeated using forks with frequencies ranging from 128 to 2048 Hz. The tuning fork is carefully struck to produce its sound without any distortions and its base is pressed against the patient's mastoid process. The examiner asks his patient to raise his hand as soon as he can no longer hear the fork, and at that moment, the fork is quickly transferred to a position 2 cm lateral to the external meatus. If the patient can then hear the fork, the Rinne test is *positive*. The test procedure is next reversed and if the patient hears the fork better by bone conduction, the Rinne test is *negative*. A patient with normal hearing is Rinne positive and a patient with a conductive loss of at least 20 dB (depending on the frequency of the tuning fork) is Rinne negative. A sensorineural dysfunction will reduce the hearing of both air and bone positions although the fork

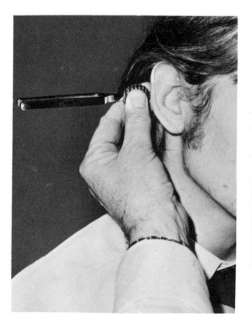 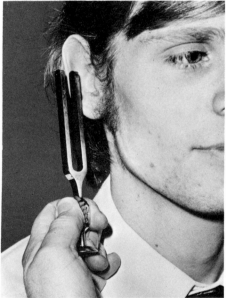

Figure 1.2   The Rinne Test: (a) bone conduction—the fork applied to the mastoid process; (b) air conduction—the orientation of the prongs of the fork, and its distance from the meatus (2 cm), are important

is heard better by air conduction (reduced Rinne positive). A severe sensorineural impairment may prevent the patient hearing the fork by bone conduction although he may still be able to hear it by air conduction (infinitely positive Rinne).
    The false Rinne negative may occur whenever a patient has a very severe sensorineural hearing loss and much better hearing in the non-test ear. Such a patient cannot hear the tuning fork using the affected ear by air conduction, but when the fork is pressed against the mastoid, the sound of the fork passes freely through the skull and is heard

by the non-test ear. As the patient may not be able to localize the sound, his report of hearing may be mistakenly construed as demonstrating a conductive hearing loss in the affected ear. The Weber test may lateralize and prevent this error or the mistake usually can be rectified by masking the non-test ear using a Bárány noise box so that the patient reports a marked change in his hearing of the tuning fork, but occasionally the mistake is not detected and the patient undergoes an unnecessary operation.

The Weber test (Figure 1.3)

This test involves pressing the base of a vibrating tuning fork (usually 256 or 512 Hz) against the midline of the skull either at the vertex or on the forehead. The test compares the bone conduction of the two ears and the patient is asked to point his finger to the site at which he hears the sound loudest. A subject with normal hearing

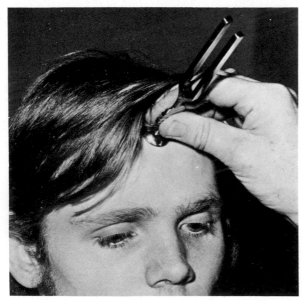

Figure 1.3   The Weber Test

Table 1.4   Classification of possible Rinne and Weber test results

		Rinne	
Auditory status	*Weber*	*Left ear*	*Right ear*
Normal hearing	↑	+	+
Left conductive loss	L←	−	+
Bilateral equal conductive loss	↑	−	−
Left moderate SN loss	→R	+ (reduced)	+
Bilateral moderate SN loss	↑	+ (reduced)	+ (reduced)
Bilateral severe SN loss	not heard	+ (infinite)	+ (infinite)
Left severe SN loss	→R	− (false)	+
(Normal hearing right ear)	(or ↑)		

(SN: sensorineural)

will hear the sound equally in both ears and usually points to the midline. Patients with bilateral symmetrical hearing losses will also point to the midline, providing they have sufficient hearing to hear the fork. When one ear has more hearing than the other, the patient usually localizes the sound to a particular ear. A patient with a sensorineural hearing loss hears the sound in the better hearing ear, while a patient with a conductive loss localizes the sound to the affected ear. In longstanding cases of unilateral sensorineural hearing loss, the Weber may fail to lateralize.

The following tuning-fork tests are now mainly of historic interest.

The Schwabach test compares the bone conduction of the patient with the bone conduction of a normally hearing person (usually the clinician). In this test the external meatus is not occluded and the test results are quantified as the number of seconds by which the patient's hearing differs from that of the normally hearing person.

The absolute bone conduction test is similar to the Schwabach test but avoids some pitfalls by comparing the bone conduction of the patient and the normal hearing person with the external meatus blocked in each case.

The Gellé test relies on the finding that altering the air pressure within the external acoustic meatus alters the bone conduction threshold in normal ears and in those affected by a sensorineural loss but produces no change when the stapes is immobilized as by otosclerosis. Huizing (1960) conducted several experiments and reported that, in normal ears, a 500 Hz tone decreased in loudness by a maximum of 15 dB after a positive change in air pressure of 60–80 cm (water).

The Escat test is a modification of the Gellé test. The patient is asked to auto-inflate his middle-ear cleft using the Valsalva method. In normal subjects with normal auditory tube function, the hearing for bone conduction is reduced during the period of increased intratympanic pressure. The test is not very reliable and has been replaced by acoustic impedance measurements.

The Bing test relies on the phenomenon of increased loudness for bone conducted sounds of less than 2 kHz when the external meatus of a normal ear is occluded. Bing (1891) noted that this effect was generally absent in patients with conductive hearing losses but present in patients with sensorineural impairments.

The Bonnier test. If a vibrating tuning fork of 256 Hz is held on the condyle of the humerus and the meatus is lightly occluded, a patient hearing the fork is said to have stapedial fixation! Actually the test is not reliable and is only mentioned because it is humorous.

Some comments on the bone conduction phenomena
It is an impossibility to attribute all the bone conduction phenomena outlined by these simple tuning-fork tests to a simple mechanism.

The Bing test reveals an improvement in low frequency bone conduction on occluding the meatus. The explanation cannot be wholly due to a reduction of ambient (masking) background noise as the effect is still noted in an anechoic, sound-proofed chamber. The main mechanism responsible appears to be the vibration of the walls of the external acoustic meatus and the radiation of sound energy into the canal. The external acoustic meatus, when open, acts as a highpass filter and, hence, when blocked produces a low frequency emphasis. Although this explanation accounts for the Bing test and for the Weber test lateralizing to the occluded ear in normal subjects, it does not explain the lateralization of the Weber response in middle-ear disorders such as otosclerosis.

The other major mechanisms of bone conduction (Tonndorf, 1966) are the inertial response of the middle-ear ossicles and inner-ear fluid, and the compressional responses of the inner-ear spaces. In the latter, the vibrating energy reaching the cochlea causes alternate compression and expansion of the cochlear shell. The cochlear fluid is incompressible but moves because the oval window is less compliant than the round window. This effect is, of course, enhanced in stapedial fixation. In a clinic, background noise will have a further effect in lateralizing sound to the unmasked ear.

Tuning-fork tests in non-organic hearing loss

There are several useful tuning-fork tests which can be quickly tried in the clinic whenever a non-organic hearing loss is suspected.

The Chimani-Moos test is a modification of the Weber test. If a malingerer states he cannot hear in one ear, he usually lateralizes the Weber test to the normal ear. The meatus of the good ear is then occluded and if the patient has a true hearing loss, he will continue to lateralize the Weber to the good ear. A malingerer may become uncertain as to which ear he should say he can hear the fork and may deny hearing it in either ear.

The Stenger test may be performed using tuning forks or using a pure-tone audiometer. This test relies on the phenomenon that if two sounds of identical frequency are presented simultaneously to both ears, the subject will only hear the louder of the two sounds. To perform this test it is best to blindfold the patient (or use Frenzel's glasses which make him less suspicious). A tuning fork (often 512 Hz) is struck and placed 20 cm from the good ear and the patient reports hearing the sound. The tuning fork is then transferred to the 'bad' ear and placed 4 cm from the ear and the patient denies hearing the fork. Finally, without allowing the patient to notice, a similar tuning fork is struck and placed 15 cm from the good ear whilst the other fork is sounding from 4 cm into the 'bad' ear. If the patient has a genuine loss, he will immediately report the sound of the fork in the good ear, but if he can hear the sound in the 'bad' ear and is denying this, he will be unable to hear the sound of the fork near his good ear.

Investigations

AUDIOMETRY

The most relevant investigations of auditory dysfunction involve audiometry. The term 'audiometry' is derived from the Latin 'audire' (to hear) and from the Greek 'metrios' (to measure), but nowadays audiometry is not merely confined to the measurement of hearing as it provides a sophisticated tool for otological diagnosis. Using audiometric tests, it is possible to classify hearing loss according to the anatomical site of the auditory dysfunction.

Audiometric tests are sometimes described as either subjective or objective. A subjective test involves a conscious or willing response on behalf of the subject. An objective test, in the audiometric context, involves only passive cooperation from the subject although some subjective judgement by the tester may be exercised. In actual fact, none of the objective audiometric tests (with the possible exception of contingent negative response and other 'late' responses) measure the entire hearing process, but they merely show the function of the audiometric pathway at a particular level.

PURE-TONE AUDIOMETRY (PTA)

The pure-tone threshold audiogram remains the most useful clinical test of auditory function. It is a measure of the minimum intensity of a pure-tone stimulus, presented

Table 1.5 Classification of auditory dysfunction according to anatomical sites

Site of dysfunction	Terminology
External or middle ear	Conductive HL
Sensory structure of cochlea	Sensory HL
Neural auditory pathways	Neural (or retrocochlear) HL
Either sensory or neural elements (or both)	Sensorineural HL
Both conductive and sensorineural	Mixed HL
Subdivision of retrocochlear hearing loss	
Eighth nerve	
Brainstem	
Auditory cortex and association areas	
No demonstrable site of dysfunction	Non-organic HL

(HL: hearing loss)

over 1–2 s, that is audible. The tones may be presented by air conduction (AC) by headphones, or by bone conduction (BC) using a vibrator placed over the ipsilateral mastoid. The frequencies measured usually range from 125 to 8000 Hz in regular steps.

The reference zero (0 dB) for pure-tone audiometers is determined by the normal hearing threshold and is, therefore, a biological specification. The normal value is a modal value determined by testing an adequately large number of otologically normal subjects within the age limits of 18–25 years of age. An otologically normal subject is a person in a normal state of health who is free from all signs or symptoms of ear disease and from wax in the external meatus and has no history of undue noise exposure. It is clearly impractible to calibrate every audiometer by testing large numbers of normal subjects and clinical audiometers are usually calibrated using an artificial coupler, or better an artificial ear, which has been designed to measure the exact amount of sound emitted by the particular earphone.

The first reference zero was established in the United States of America and was based on a study of normal ears in 1937. Fifteen years later the British established their reference zero using more modern equipment and as a consequence, the British standard (BSA) was approximately 10 dB more sensitive than the American standard (ASA). It was clearly undesirable that there should be two different standards and as a consequence an international standard was established in 1964 (ISO).

The 0 dB level on the PTA chart represents the standard agreed for each frequency as representing normal hearing thresholds. A change of 20 dB represents a tenfold alteration in sound pressure which is measured in pascals (dB $= 20 \log_{10} P_1/P_2$, where P_1 is the pressure of the sound presented and P_2 is the pressure of the reference sound).

Method

Headphones are used to measure the air conduction thresholds. These are placed comfortably over the subject's head. The subject should sit in a soundproof area and not be able to see the tester's hand operating the audiometer. The subject is asked to respond by pressing a switch whenever he can hear the sound, *no matter how faint*, and this switch activates a light on the audiometer. The tones are delivered for approximately 2 s intervals, starting at a level which is clearly audible to the subject. It is usual to test the better ear first using a 1000 Hz tone and to decrease the intensity by 10 dB steps until the patient no longer hears the sound and fails to signal. The intensity is then raised by 5 dB steps until the subject responds. The intensity may then be lowered again and when the tester is sure that the subject is accurately responding, the lowest intensity at which the sound was heard is recorded. The same routine is then repeated for other test frequencies and after completing the chart it is usual to recheck one or two frequencies.

The PTA for the deafer ear is recorded next. If there is a loss of 50 dB or more at any frequency, masking of the non-test ear is required. After completing the air conduction thresholds, the bone conduction thresholds are *sometimes* required. Accurate bone conduction thresholds require skilful testing and time. It is pointless to request bone conduction thresholds for every patient and much better to reserve this test for cases in which the bone conduction (cochlear reserve) must be known accurately (usually pre-operative patients). Impedance audiometry can give more information during a shorter test period in the majority of patients.

Notes on masking.

Everyone concerned with audiometric tests must know that under certain circumstances the sound intended for one ear can cross the head and be heard by the opposite ear. This phenomenon is known as cross-over and it may lead to serious misinterpretation of audiometric results.

Masking involves delivering noise to the non-test ear so that the cochlea hears the noise rather than the test sound intended for the test ear. The rationale for such a concept is that masking is essentially an ipsilateral phenomenon and this implies that one sound can only have an effect on the hearing of another sound in as much as it stimulates the same cochlea. This hypothesis is not entirely true as intense masking noise can affect the opposite ear (cross masking) but it still provides a useful guide. An amusing example of this hypothesis concerns the use of a telephone in a busy place. Many people try to improve the telephone reception by blocking the opposite ear, but this has little effect as it is the background noise, picked up by the telephone mouthpiece and carried to the earphone, which masks the conversation. A considerable improvement in speech reception can be achieved by covering the telephone mouthpiece.

The masking of a pure tone is best accomplished by using a narrow band noise centred on the test frequency. The choice of the correct level of masking is complex but there are some practical guidelines for when masking is required:

(1) Masking for air conduction (AC) is necessary whenever the hearing loss of the tested ear exceeds 50 dB.
(2) Masking for bone conduction (BC) is *always necessary*, except:
    (a) when the BC thresholds for the test ear are more sensitive than the BC thresholds for the non-test ear;

(b) when no BC response is obtained using the maximum output of the audiometer.

SELECTION OF THE CORRECT MASKING LEVEL

Air conduction

When measuring the AC threshold for an ear, the threshold is first obtained without masking. If the unmasked threshold is worse than 50 dB, a relatively low level of masking noise (40 dB) is introduced to the non-test ear. If this results in a threshold shift of 10 dB or more, the masking is increased by 10 dB steps until the threshold stabilizes (plateau method). This technique reduces the risk of over-masking (*Figure 1.4*). If the better-hearing ear has a sensorineural hearing loss, the initial choice of masking level should be high enough to ensure a significant threshold shift.

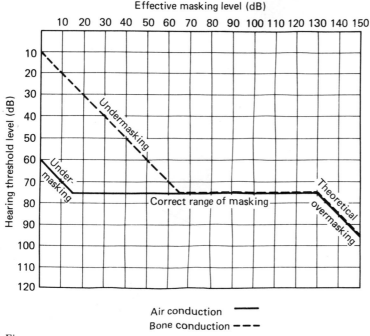

Figure 1.4

Bone conduction

The masking technique is similar to that for AC but has to be performed in virtually every case. The BC threshold is first obtained without masking. Next masking noise of the appropriate band is introduced to the non-test ear and if this results in a shift of the BC threshold of more than 10 dB, the masking is increased by 10 dB steps until the threshold 'plateau' is reached. Further increments of masking noise will cause the BC threshold to fall due to excessive masking and this is known as the 'change-over' point.

Excessive masking

Too much masking noise will adversely effect the threshold of the test ear. There are two main causes. Firstly, the masking noise may leak around the head to affect the cochlea of the test ear (over-masking). Secondly, 'central masking' may occur. This is best described as a threshold shift in one ear caused by the presentation of a masking sound to the other ear at an intensity which is too low to cause over-masking. Central masking occurs because the two ears are not isolated neurologically (Ward, 1973) and may involve the efferent auditory pathways.

THE CLINICAL RESULTS (*Figure 1.5*)

Most clinicians will accept a loss of 0–20 dB as unimportant and as the age of the patient increases, further losses especially in the higher frequency range can be

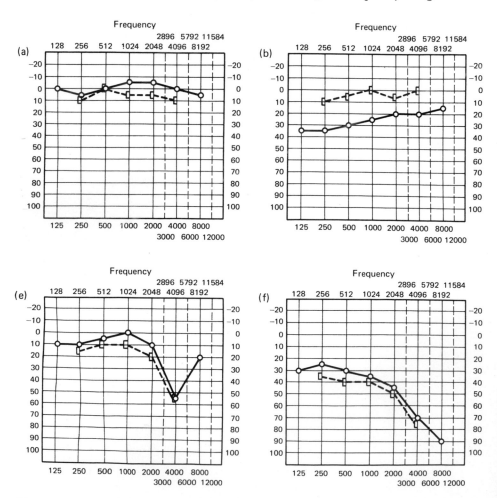

Figure 1.5 Examples of pure-tone audiograms. (a): Normal ear; (b): seromucinous otitis media; (c): otosclerosis; (d): Menière's disorder; (e): noise-induced hearing loss; (f): presbyacusis; (g): Waardenburg's syndrome; (h): congenital rubella

accepted. A conductive loss, as caused by serous otitis media, usually shows a maximum AC loss at low frequencies due to the greater impedance for these sounds (*Figure 1.5b*). In otosclerosis, the BC threshold may show a 'dip' at 2 kHz, the Carhart notch, which usually recovers after successful stapedectomy. This notch is due to loss of the ossicular inertial component which determines a resonant frequency and contributes to BC hearing (*Figure 1.5c*).

Patients with Menière's disorder have a fluctuating low frequency sensory loss, due to the increased impedance of the distended cochlear fluids, and a variable but permanent high frequency sensory loss due to hair-cell damage (*Figure 1.5d*). Noise trauma tends to cause a specific loss of hair-cells in the basal turn of the cochlea and this results in a notch in the audiogram at around 4 kHz (*Figure 1.5e*). Patients with presbyacusis usually have a bilateral high frequency sensory loss as the ischaemia tends to damage the basal portion of the cochlea more than the higher turns. In

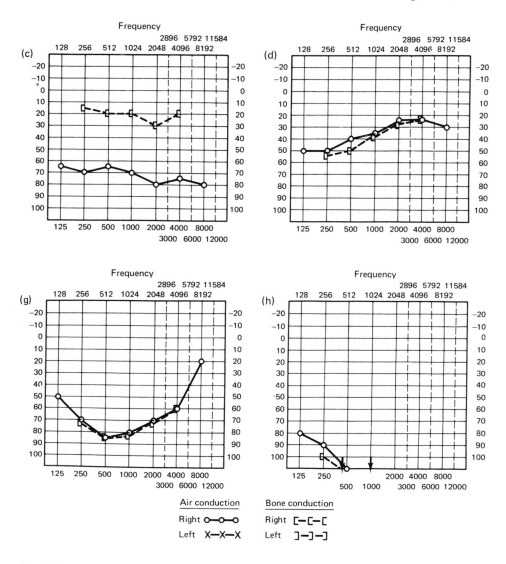

familial syndromes, such as Waardenburg's syndrome, the audiogram may be 'U-shaped' (*Figure 1.5f*), while after cochlear damage caused by intra-uterine infection, the audiogram often shows only a small island of residual hearing in the lowest audiometric frequencies (*Figure 1.5g*).

An eighth nerve tumour causes a hearing loss which has several different audiometric patterns. Johnson (1968) reported the audiometric patterns in 200 patients with acoustic neuroma. He found that no audiometric thresholds were obtained in 16 per cent. Of the remainder, 64 per cent had a downward-sloping curve, 20 per cent had a flat curve, 8 per cent had an ascending curve and 8 per cent had a 'U-shaped' audiometric curve.

THE RAINVILLE AND SAL TECHNIQUES

In 1955, Rainville suggested a novel method of measuring BC. Instead of measuring the threshold for bone conducted pure tones while masking the non-test ear with AC noise, he reversed the procedure. He measured the alteration of the AC threshold on introducing BC noise. A simplified version of his test was introduced by Jerger and Tillman (1960), called the SAL test.

The SAL test is performed by measuring the AC threshold for a pure tone, first without any masking and then after introducing a known level of narrow-band BC noise. The noise is delivered from a bone vibrator placed on the midline of the skull. The difference in dB between the thresholds obtained is compared with the difference produced by the same noise in a normal ear.

On testing a normal ear, the AC threshold will be found to deteriorate linearly with increasing (BC) noise intensity after a certain initial noise level has been reached (*x* dB) (*Figure 1.6*). In a pure BC hearing loss, the AC threshold will begin to deteriorate after the same intensity of noise (*x* dB) has been introduced. In a pure sensorineural hearing loss, the AC threshold will not be affected until the BC noise reaches an intensity equal to *x* dB plus the loss due to the sensorineural loss. The sensorineural

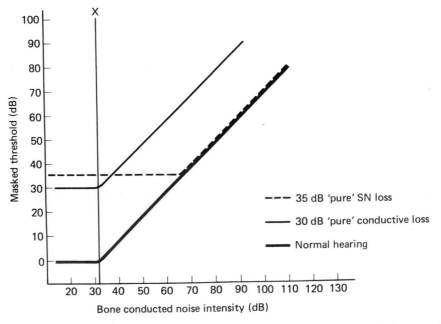

Figure 1.6   Diagram of SAL procedure (X marks the level, 32 dB, at which the normal threshold alters with further increases of the intensity of the bone conducted noise)

level (SAL) is calculated by subtracting *x* dB from the intensity of bone conducted noise at which the AC threshold altered.

Unfortunately there are several pitfalls. For instance, the BC threshold is altered in normal ears when the ear canal is occluded (see Bing test), and the effect of wearing earphones is difficult to judge (Tillman, 1963). Nevertheless, the SAL procedure can be very useful for assessing difficult cases as over-masking cannot occur.

SPEECH AUDIOMETRY

Speech audiometry gives a measure of the practical consequences, in terms of the ability to communicate, of a hearing loss. In most countries, the speech audiogram is charted using phonetically-balanced monosyllabic words (e.g. cat, den). Sometimes only a single measure is recorded, the speech reception threshold (SRT), which is the intensity at which the patient is able to correctly repeat 50 per cent of the words he hears. The speech detection threshold (SDT) is the intensity at which the subject can hear 50 per cent of the words without understanding them. The SDT is remarkably stable in normal ears and provides an easy method of calibrating speech material (Hood and Poole, 1977).

Speech audiometry may be accomplished by two different techniques. The commonest method is to present a list of 25 words at each intensity and to score the percentage repeated correctly. Another method is to present 10 words at each intensity (often the Boothroyd lists are used) and to write down the patient's reply. The percentage of phonemes repeated correctly is scored, e.g. cat for cat scores 3, cap scores 2, cop scores 1 and pig scores nil. Hood and Poole (1977) investigated the reliability of both methods and found the 95 per cent confidence limits to be ± 12.7 per cent for words and ± 9.5 per cent for phonemes. In the clinical situation it seems unlikely that the extra work involved in scoring phonemes is justified.

The normal speech curve has a sigmoid shape and reaches 100 per cent discrimination at intensities of less than 50 dB HL (*Figure 1.7*). A conductive hearing loss produces a similar curve but it is shifted to the right of the chart as higher intensities are required to reach 100 per cent discrimination scores. The graph for the patient with sensory impairment does not reach 100 per cent as recruitment causes

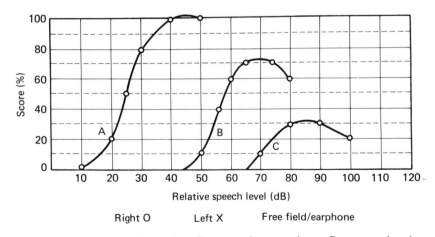

Figure 1.7   Examples of speech audiograms. A: normal ear; B: sensory hearing loss; C: neural hearing loss

deterioration of speech reception at higher intensities. Classically, a retrocochlear lesion causes far worse speech discrimination than would be expected from the pure-tone audiogram, and maximum scores of less than 20 per cent are not uncommon.

Speech tests for central 'hearing loss'

Bocca *et al.* (1955) first showed that a defect in speech understanding can be demonstrated in the ear contralateral to a temporal lobe lesion. Subsequent work has shown that such patients ordinarily show no significant 'hearing loss' on pure-tone audiometry and that it is speech intelligibility tasks involving binaural, non-coherent signals that are especially affected by temporal lobe lesions.

Morales-Garcia and Poole (1972) have devised a simple test which can be accomplished using the normally-available clinical apparatus. They measured the speech intelligibility in the presence of ipsilateral broad-band masking noise. Patients with brainstem lesions showed significantly lower masked speech scores than normal subjects although they could not predict which ear would be affected. Patients with temporal lobe lesions consistently gave lower masked speech scores from the ear contralateral to the lesion than those from the ipsilateral ear.

There are many other tests devised to detect central auditory dysfunction but these are not included in this chapter as they usually need special apparatus. Interested readers should refer to Jerger (1973).

MEASUREMENTS OF LOUDNESS RECRUITMENT

Loudness recruitment is the phenomenon whereby the loudness of sounds presented to an affected ear increases more rapidly with increasing sound intensity than in a normal ear. This phenomenon is usually associated with destruction of sensory elements, especially the outer hair-cells, within the cochlea. It is therefore an important localizing sign. The physiological explanation for recruitment is described by Evans (1975) and represents the loss of neural tuning within the cochlea, sometimes called the 'second filter mechanism'. There are many audiometric tests which demonstrate the presence of recruitment and those based on pure-tone psychoacoustic measurements will now be described.

Alternate binaural loudness balance (Fowler's test)

This test compares intensities that give equal loudness in the impaired ear and the corresponding normal or near normal ear. The more normal ear must be used as the reference (Hood, 1977). The loudness is first compared at the threshold value and then at 10 dB increments (*Figure 1.8*). The results of the test can be classified as follows:

(1) Complete recruitment: The sensation of loudness in the impaired ear grows to equal that of the other ear at high intensity levels.
(2) Incomplete recruitment: The sensation of loudness approaches but does not equal that of the other ear at high intensity levels.
(3) Over-recruitment: The sensation of loudness in the affected ear exceeds that of the other ear at high intensity levels. This commonly occurs in Menière's disorder but rarely occurs in noise-induced hearing loss.
(4) Absence of recruitment: The growth of loudness parallels the increase in loudness of the other ear; this finding usually indicates either a conductive or a retrocochlear disorder.

(5) Loudness-reversal: The sensation of loudness in the impaired ear grows more slowly than in the other ear; this finding is almost pathognomonic of a retrocochlear disorder.

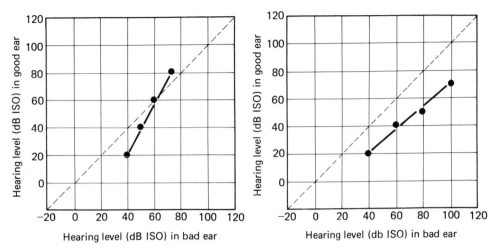

Figure 1.8 Examples of the alternate binaural loudness balance procedure: left: over-recruitment due to Menière's disorder, right: loudness reversal due to an acoustic neuroma

Monoaural loudness balance (Reger's) test
This test compares intensities of sounds of different frequencies that give an equal sensation of loudness within the same ear. Both the patient and the tester find this task difficult and so the test has lost favour.

The short increment sensitivity index (SISI) test
This test measures the suprathreshold intensity difference limen. A 'recruiting' ear is more sensitive than a normal ear to small increments of sound. Jerger (1973) suggested presenting a pure tone continuously at 20 dB above threshold and modulating the intensity by 1 dB increments of 200 ms duration every 5 s. The patient is asked to identify each increment and the percentage of increments correctly identified is scored. The results can be grouped as follows:

0–20 per cent—normal hearing, conductive and retrocochlear hearing loss.
20–60 per cent—'recruiting' sensory hearing loss.

There are so many pitfalls to this test, such as patient cooperation and abnormal adaptation, that the test cannot be recommended for routine clinical work.

The loudness discomfort level (LDL)
This is a most useful monaural test for recruitment and it was popularized by Hood and Poole (1966). It measures the threshold of uncomfortable loudness using pure tones, and it only takes a few seconds to add these data when performing a pure-tone audiogram. Normal subjects and those with conductive or retrocochlear disorders find sounds of 90 dB or more above their hearing threshold uncomfortable. Patients with recruiting forms of hearing loss find much smaller differences uncomfortable; such a

patient may have a pure-tone threshold of 50 dB and a LDL of 90 dB—a gap of only 40 dB. Sometimes in severe cases, the gap may be as little as 10 dB.

Some workers prefer to use the most comfortable level of loudness but this can be difficult to define especially during a busy clinic.

MEASUREMENTS OF ABNORMAL AUDITORY ADAPTATION

Abnormal auditory adaptation is sometimes called *tone decay*, but this term is inappropriate as the frequency does not decay, it is the loudness that changes. Abnormal adaptation usually indicates a lesion affecting the first or second order cochlear neurones. Measurement may either be taken close to the hearing threshold (Carhart's test, Owen's test) or at suprathreshold levels.

The modified Carhart test

A tone is presented at 5 dB above the measured threshold (Rosen modification) for 60 s. If the patient ceases to hear the tone during this period, it is increased without a break, by 5 dB steps. The test is continued either until the patient hears a particular intensity for 30 s or until 3 min have elapsed from the beginning of the test. The amounts of auditory adaptation found in this test can be grouped as follows:

0–15 dB—normal ears and conductive disorders.

0–20 dB—cochlear dysfunction. The larger amounts of auditory adaptation occur at higher frequencies (above 2 kHz).

Over 20 dB—suggestive of a retrocochlear lesion, especially of over 20 dB at 500 Hz or 1 kHz.

Owen's test of abnormal auditory adaptation

This test follows essentially the same procedure as the modified Carhart test, but a recovery period of 20 s is allowed after each increment of 5 dB. A maximum number of 4 increments are given and the test results relate to the period that each increment was heard. The only advantage of this test is that it is easier for those patients with severe tinnitus or when a high masking intensity is being delivered to the non-test ear.

Suprathreshold tests for abnormal auditory adaptation

The better tests involve the use of Békésy audiometry or measurement of the acoustic reflex.

A simple method of using the pure-tone audiometer has been suggested by Jerger and Jerger (1975). They presented a pure tone at 110 dB (SPL) for 60 s and if the patient ceased to hear the tone during this period, the test was regarded as positive. The authors reported that only 4 per cent of patients with known retrocochlear disorders failed to give a positive result at 500, 1000 or 2000 Hz. Unfortunately, the test raised a false alarm in 45 per cent of patients with purely cochlear pathology.

BÉKÉSY AUDIOMETRY

This is a form of audiometry in which the patient traces out his own threshold to both a continuous and a pulsed stimulus (Békésy, 1947). There are two basic techniques.

Sweep frequency Békésy audiometry

In this test, the signal frequencies are swept from low to high over a period of about 10 min while the intensity is maintained at a just audible level by the patient, himself, operating a switch. The resulting traces give a measure of threshold, recruitment and abnormal auditory adaptation. Recruitment causes the width of the tracing to decrease as the patient becomes more sensitive to small changes in loudness. The presence of abnormal auditory adaptation is shown when the tracing to the continuous signal falls below the tracing to pulsed signals. Jerger (1960) analysed several hundred tracings and suggested classfying them into four main groups. Later, Jerger and Herer (1961) added a fifth group which they noted frequently when a non-organic hearing loss was present. The types described are as follows:

Type I: The continuous and pulsed tracings overlap throughout the recording. This type is commonly encountered in testing normal ears and those with conductive hearing disorders (*Figure 1.9a*).

Type II: The continuous and pulsed tracings overlap at lower frequencies but at around 1000 Hz, the continuous tracing falls below the pulsed tracing. This fall is due to small amounts of auditory adaptation and commonly occurs in sensory hearing losses (*Figure 1.9b*).

Type III: The continuous tracing drops abruptly away from the pulsed tracing, the break occurring before 500 Hz. This finding indicates massive abnormal auditory adaptation and is almost pathognomonic of a retrocochlear hearing loss (*Figure 1.9c*).

Type IV: The continuous tracing stays below the pulsed tracing throughout the recording, showing some abnormal auditory adaptation even at the lower frequencies. This is commoner when there is a retrocochlear rather than a sensory lesion (*Figure 1.9d*).

Type V: The continuous tracing lies above the pulsed tracing at some point of the recording. This strongly suggests the presence of a non-organic hearing loss (*Figure 1.9e*).

Fixed frequency Békésy audiometry

This test provides an elegant method of measuring abnormal auditory adaptation. The patient is presented with a signal of fixed frequency, usually 500 Hz or 4 kHz, and controls the intensity so that the sound remains just audible. The signal is delivered continuously and then as pulses (2/s). The difference between the tracings to the two types of signal are measured after a known period of testing; for example, if the continuous trace lies more than 40 dB below the pulsed trace after 60 s, the presence of a retrocochlear lesion should be suspected.

ACOUSTIC IMPEDANCE MEASUREMENTS

Acoustic impedance measurements provide one of the most important diagnostic aids available to otologists. The earliest measurements were made with mechanical devices (Metz, 1946; Zwislocki, 1963) but it was the introduction of the electro-acoustic bridge (Terkildsen and Nielson, 1960) that provided the simplicity and ease of operation that allowed its widespread clinical acceptance.

Theory of acoustic impedance

Sound travels in waves rather like the ripples caused by dropping a stone into water. Three factors impede the flow of sound into the ear: *stiffness*, mainly provided by the tympanic membrane and the ossicles; *mass or inertia*, mainly due to the bulk of the ossicles, and *resistance or friction*. The effects of stiffness and mass act in opposite directions, tending to cancel each other, and together comprise one vector of

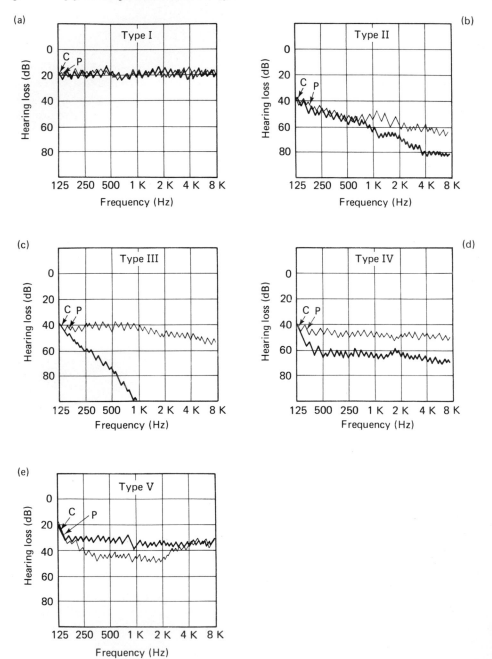

Figure 1.9   Békésy audiometry: the typical patterns

impedance known as reactance. The other vector is provided by the effect of resistance and it acts at a right angle to the reactance vector.

Acoustic impedance is therefore the complex ratio of two vector forces. The concept of vector quantities is simple. Imagine being asked to calculate the distance travelled in 1 h by a man rowing a boat at 4 km/h over a lake which had a water current flowing at 3 km/h. If the water is flowing at right angles to the direction in which the man is rowing, he will travel 5 km in 1 h. In a similar manner, the acoustic impedance can be calculated from the Pythagorus theorem if the resistance and reactance values are known (*Figure 1.10*). Acoustic impedance is measured in ohms.

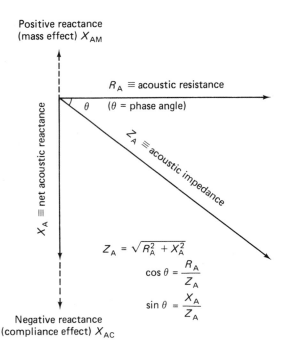

Figure 1.10 The vectors of acoustic impedance

An alternative approach is to measure the flow of sound which enters the ear or the acoustic admittance. Admittance is the reciprocal value to impedance. Admittance is also a complex ratio of vector forces. The

$$\text{admittance (flow)} = \frac{1}{\text{impedance}}$$

Impedance vectors of resistance and reactance find their admittance counterparts as conductance (G) and susceptance (B) respectively. The unit of admittance is the mho (ohm spelt backwards).

The acoustic impedance when a low frequency sound of under 350 Hz enters the ear is mainly determined by the stiffness of the middle-ear system. Most clinical equipment measures *compliance* alone and uses a probe tone of around 220 Hz. (Compliance is the reciprocal of stiffness.)

The basic theory of an electro-acoustic bridge
An electro-acoustic impedance meter may be regarded as having the following basic parts (*Figure 1.11*):

(A) An audiometer which is connected to an earphone to provide an acoustic stimulus for eliciting the acoustic reflex.

(B) A section for measuring the acoustic compliance.

(C) A pressure system comprising a pump and a manometer so that the pressure within the sealed external acoustic meatus can be altered.

The probe tone, usually 220 Hz, is delivered through a probe which is inserted into the external acoustic meatus in an airtight fashion. There are three openings in the probe tip. One channel conveys the probe tone, another is connected to the pressure system and the third allows a microphone to monitor the sound pressure within the meatus.

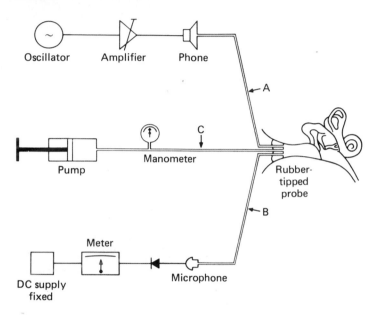

Figure 1.11   A block diagram of an acoustic impedance meter

A common method of measurement is to control the probe-tone intensity until the microphone records a pre-determined intensity level (e.g. 95 dB SPL). The older machines use a balance meter connected to a DC bridge to achieve a high degree of sensitivity, but modern technology has overcome this requirement. It would be quite acceptable merely to measure the probe-tone intensity using a decibel scale, but it has become usual practice to measure the loss of intensity between the probe and microphone in terms of the compliance of an equivalent volume of air (ml). The smaller a volume of air within a sealed container, the less it can be compressed, the lower its compliance value and the less the loss of sound within the container.

Clinical applications

MEASUREMENT OF STATIC COMPLIANCE

Static compliance measurements can be made without altering the air pressure within the external acoustic meatus. If the equipment is properly calibrated, it is possible to compare the compliance of the ear to an equivalent volume of air. The distribution of maximum static compliance in normal subjects and in patients with certain types of middle-ear dysfunction are shown in *Table 1.6*.

The problem of using static measurements clinically is that although the median values separate certain pathological groups in a predictable manner, the range of values for each condition is so wide as to make diagnosis in an individual case hazardous.

Table 1.6   The distribution of maximum static compliance (after Jerger *et al.*, 1974a)

Group	N		Compliance values (ml)		
	Subjects	Ears	Percentiles		
			10	50	90
Normal	825	—	0.39	0.67	1.30
Otosclerosis	60	95	0.10	0.35	1.01
Otitis media	62	118	0.06	0.29	0.81
Cholesteatoma	20	30	0.04	0.16	0.44
Scarred or thickened tympanic membrane	12	20	0.04	0.37	2.83
Ossicular discontinuity	18	19	0.76	1.93	3.66

TYMPANOMETRY

The tympanogram is constructed by recording the range of compliance on altering the air pressure within the external acoustic meatus from $+200$ mmH$_2$O to -600 mmH$_2$O ($+2$ kPa to -6 kPa). The measured compliance reaches a maximum when the pressure in the external acoustic meatus equals that within the middle-ear cavity, and so the peak of the tympanogram provides a good indication of the middle-ear pressure. As the pressure in the external meatus changes away from the middle-ear pressure, the tympanic membrane is stretched outwards or inwards and stiffens, causing the compliance value to fall. At the extremes of the tympanogram, the compliance value indicates the volume of air sealed within the external acoustic meatus. Characteristic tympanograms are seen in different middle-ear conditions.

(a) Normal ears
Ninety five per cent of normal ears in children have a range of compliance varying from 0.35 to 1.4 ml, and the middle-ear pressure varies from -100 mmH$_2$O to $+50$ mmH$_2$O (Brooks, 1969) (*Figure 1.12a*).

(b) Seromucinous otitis media
The tympanogram usually shows a negative middle-ear pressure $(-300$ mmH$_2$O) and there is a very small range of compliance. The tympanogram almost appears as a flat slope (*Figure 1.12b*).

(c) Otosclerosis
Early stages of otosclerosis provide a tympanogram that is within the lower range of normal values. As the otosclerosis advances, the range of compliance diminishes. If the compliance range is greater than 0.6 mm, a thick otosclerotic footplate (Types III or IV) is unlikely to be encountered during surgery.

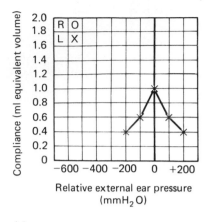

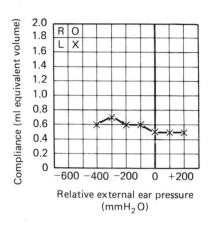

(a)

(b)

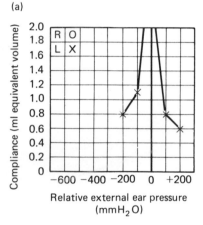

(c)

Figure 1.12   Examples of tympanograms. (a): normal ear; (b): seromucinous otitis media; (c): ossicular disconnection

(d) Ossicular disconnection

An increased range of compliance is usual. The peak of the tympanogram may exceed 3 ml (*Figure 1.12c*).

EFFECT OF ALTERING THE PROBE-TONE FREQUENCY

At low frequencies, such as 220 Hz, the contribution of mass to the net reactance is minimal compared with that of stiffness, and the tympanogram is displayed peaking in a positive direction. As the frequency of the probe tone increases, the contribution of mass increases and the contribution of stiffness decreases until at a certain resonant point, they act equally in opposite directions. At this point the net reactance becomes zero and the compliance tympanogram suddenly dips. The compliance tympanogram has a notched form at or just above the resonant frequency because when the pressure alters to stiffen the drum, the compliance begins to dominate again. If the frequency of the probe tone is raised further, the mass component begins to predominate and the tympanogram changes to a negative form (*Figure 1.13*).

The practical value of tympanometry using different probe tones is that drum-loosening pathologies, such as ossicular disconnection and healed perforations lower the resonant frequency, while drum-stiffening pathologies, such as otosclerosis or tympanosclerosis, raise the resonant frequency. For this reason some clinical equipment is supplied with a 660 Hz probe tone in addition to a 220 Hz probe tone. It is possible to detect any drum-loosening pathology by noting the presence of a notched tympanogram using the 660 Hz probe tone.

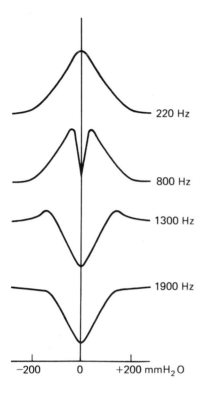

220 Hz

800 Hz

1300 Hz

1900 Hz

−200   0   +200 mmH₂O

Figure 1.13 The effect of altering the probe-tone frequency on the pattern of the normal tympanogram

ASSESSMENT OF GROMMET PATENCY AND THE DETECTION OF SMALL DRUM PERFORATIONS
Impedance testing can help decide whether a grommet has remained patent. If the grommet is blocked, either a normal tympanogram or a tympanogram typical of seromucinous otitis media is obtained. If the grommet is patent, the tympanogram has a base value of over 2 ml as the compliance of the whole middle-ear cleft is measured. When the auditory tube is patent, no pressure seal can be obtained. Similar results are obtained when a small tympanic perforation has passed unnoticed.

Early diagnosis of a glomus tumour
Whenever a patient has a pulsatile tinnitus, impedance testing should be performed as this may provide early diagnosis of a glomus tumour. The compliance needle is seen to oscillate at maximum sensitivity in time with the pulse, and if the ipsilateral carotid is compressed, these oscillations are damped.

Measurements of auditory (eustachian) tube function

When the tympanic membrane is perforate, the manometer portion of the impedance meter is used alone, but it the tympanic membrane is intact, it is necessary to begin with tympanometry and to find the resting middle-ear pressure. A resting middle-ear pressure outside the range -100 to $+50$ mmH$_2$O indicates abnormal tube function. Once the middle-ear pressure is known, a number of tests of tube function can be undertaken.

Patulous tubal dysfunction

If the auditory tube fails to close during respiration, the patient may experience a sensation of fullness or discomfort within the ear. The condition is common during pregnancy. The diagnosis is made by noting acoustic impedance fluctuations in time with the respiration.

Inflation–deflation tests

The pressure is decreased in the external meatus and the patient is asked to swallow. Swallowing should alter the middle-ear pressure and cause a change in the compliance value.

Toynbee's test

The effect of nasal obstruction on auditory tube function is simulated by having the patient swallow while his nose is held closed. Normally, the middle-ear pressure increases momentarily and then decreases. A positive test indicates the tube is patent and sufficiently stiff to withstand nasopharyngeal negative pressure.

Valsalva's test

The effect of high positive nasopharyngeal pressure is evaluated by the Valsalva test. The test is positive if the middle ear can be inflated by forced expiration when the mouth and nose are closed. A positive test indicates a distensible auditory tube.

Intra-aural muscle reflex measurements

The stapedius muscle and the tensor tympani muscle both contract to a number of different stimuli. Fear of a loud sound and anxiety will cause both muscles to contract spontaneously. Both muscles contract reflexly just before vocalization and this probably helps one to hear external sounds whilst talking. Touching the skin in either external acoustic meatus or on the ipsilateral side of the face below the eye causes both muscles, but mainly the stapedius, to contract.

Obviously, it would be ideal to have a means of stimulating each muscle independently. The stapedius muscle, in man, contracts alone to sound unless it is of sufficient intensity to cause a startle reaction. Lifting the upper eyelids or blowing a jet of air across the cornea causes the tensor tympani to contract but usually the stapedius muscle contracts as well. Bosatra, Russulo and Semeraro (1975) have suggested that electrical stimulation of the tongue causes the tensor tympani muscle to contract alone.

The acoustic (stapedius) reflex

The stapedius reflex can be noted by measuring the small change of compliance which occurs when the tympanic membrane is stiffened by contraction of the stapedius muscle. The reflex may be elicited either by stimulation of the opposite ear (contralateral reflex) or by stimulation of the same ear (ipsilateral reflex). It is often wrongly stated that the reflex is bilateral and consensual, but the ipsilateral reflex is 15 dB (on average) more sensitive than the contralateral reflex. The minimum sound intensity needed to evoke a noticeable reflex is known as the acoustic reflex threshold (ART). The ART lies at a characteristic level in various conditions.

Normal ears

The normal values for the contralateral ART are reported by Chiveralls *et al.* (1976) (*Table 1.7*). The mean contralateral ART for noise is 62 dB SL. The median values for the ipsilateral reflex are: 59 dB (SL) at 0.5 kHz; 62.5 dB at 1 kHz; 67 dB at 2 kHz and 67 dB at 4 kHz (Reker, 1977).

It can be seen that the difference between the pure-tone threshold and the contralateral ART lies within the range of 75–95 dB in most normal cases.

Table 1.7 Contralateral acoustic reflex thresholds in a normal population. Span in dB (Chiveralls *et al.*, 1976)

Frequency (Hz)	250	500	1 k	1.5 k	2 k	3 k	4 k
Mean	78.4	77.2	82.4	84.5	81.9	84.2	84.2
Standard deviation	11.7	12.1	11.5	12.2	12.1	14.8	16.4
Number of subjects	100	128	128	100	128	100	100

CONDUCTIVE HEARING DISORDERS

Often the reflex cannot be measured using impedance equipment as the pathology prevents the movement of the tympanic membrane. When the reflex is obtained, albeit at a reduced amplitude, the ART lies at a similar level with respect to the hearing threshold as in normal ears. Two conditions deserve special mention.

(1) Otosclerosis

In early stages of otosclerosis, the acoustic reflex may have a diphasic pattern in contrast to the monophasic increase observed in normal ears (Flottorp and Djupesland, 1970). As the condition advances, the acoustic reflex is no longer obtained but the tensor tympani reflex may show a diphasic pattern. Finally, at late stages, neither middle-ear muscle reflex can be obtained.

(2) Ossicular disconnection

The acoustic reflex is not obtained but the tensor tympani reflex has an abnormally large amplitude.

RECRUITING HEARING DISORDERS

The difference between the ART and the hearing threshold narrows and is a good measure of the amount of recruitment (Metz, 1946). A patient with such a hearing loss may have a pure-tone threshold of 55 dB and an ART of 85 dB, which is a difference of only 30 dB. In normal ears, the loudness discomfort level (LDL) is 15 dB greater than the ART, but this difference decreases considerably in recruiting ears so that the ART can be used confidently to estimate the LDL. This can be useful as a guide to suitable hearing aids for children and very elderly patients.

Neural hearing losses

Often the ART is not obtained using the maximum output of the audiometer as the ART lies at or above the normal range. If the reflex is present it should be examined for abnormal adaptation (decay).

Brainstem hearing loss

Occasionally, the reflex may be absent in either the contralateral ear or ipsilateral ear on stimulating the affected ear but present in both ears on stimulating the normal ear. It is thought that this may be due to interruption of the reflex arc within the brainstem. The rise time of the reflex may be abnormal in multiple sclerosis (Colletti, 1975).

Facial paralysis

If the facial nerve is damaged proximal to the branch supplying the stapedius muscle, the reflex is not obtained. It has therefore a topodiagnostic value in conditions such as traumatic facial paralysis. In idiopathic facial paralysis (Bell's palsy), the reflex may be used to verify the completeness of the palsy or to search for early signs of re-innervation.

ACOUSTIC REFLEX ADAPTATION (DECAY)

If a sound is presented continuously, the amplitude of the stapedius reflex contraction may eventually decrease or decay due to adaptation. The rates of reflex decay to 50 per cent of a maximum amplitude using stimuli of 10 dB above the ART are reported by Chiveralls *et al.* (1976), *Table 1.8*.

Table 1.8   Results of prolonged stimulation on the acoustic reflex (Chiveralls *et al.*, 1976)

Frequency (Hz)		*50% decrement times at 10 dB above the reflex threshold*			
		500	*1 k*	*2 k*	*4 k*
Normal ears	Mean	No decay	32.0	14.5	7.4
	SD	—	6.5	5.0	2.1
	Range	—	12.5–60	2.3–34	1.5–12.5
	Number of ears	106	106	107	101
Sensory loss	Mean	No decay	18.1	10.2	5.5
	SD	—	12.9	8.3	4.9
	Range	—	0.5–52.0	0.5–34.5	0.5–17.5
	Number of ears	58	58	59	39

In normal ears, there is no noticeable decay using wide band noise and this may be useful for assessing patients who do not yield a reflex using pure tones.

The presence of acoustic reflex decay using 500 Hz, 1 kHz or wide band noise stimulation is most suggestive of a retrocochlear disorder (Anderson, Barr and Wedenburg, 1970). Classically, the reflex amplitude is halved within 5 s. Reflex decay at 2 kHz and 4 kHz has no special pathological significance.

ESTIMATION OF PURE-TONE HEARING THRESHOLDS

The ART for pure tones cannot be used to estimate the pure-tone hearing threshold (PTT) as the difference between the ART and the PTT varies, especially in recruiting forms of hearing loss. Niemeyer and Sesterhenn (1974) have devised a simple method of overcoming this difficulty by comparing the ART for pure tones (ART_1) with the ART for wide band noise (ART_2). They have suggested the following formula:

$$PTT = ART_1 - 2.5\,(ART_1 - ART_2)$$

Where PTT is the average threshold for pure tones (0.5–4 kHz), ART_1 is the average acoustic reflex threshold for pure tones (0.5–4 kHz) and ART_2 is the acoustic reflex threshold for wide band noise. This test was validated by Jerger *et al.* (1974b) and found to be reliable with serious errors only occurring in 4 per cent of 1156 patients tested. They also introduced the use of high pass and low pass noise so that the slope of the audiogram could be estimated.

ELECTRIC RESPONSE AUDIOMETRY (ERA)

ERA involves the measurement of bio-electric signals produced by the body in response to sound stimulation. These signals are so minute that they are easily swamped by larger random potentials generated from other parts of the body. Electronic techniques allow the retrieval of ERA potentials by the processes of summation and averaging (*Figure 1.14*). The summating technique involves storing the sound-evoked electrical activity produced over a certain time period, and then adding it to the activity evoked by successive sound stimuli. The ERA response tends

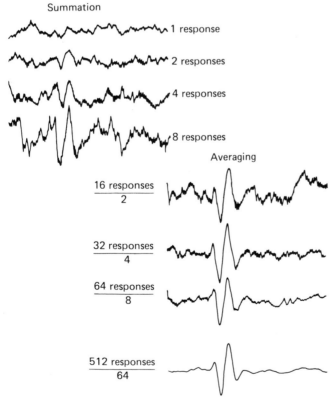

Figure 1.14 An example of summation and averaging techniques. (Gibson, 1978, by permission Churchill Livingston Ltd., Edinburgh)

to occur at the same point in time on each separate recording and so adds while the background potentials being random in nature tend to cancel each other. The averaging technique merely involves dividing the final recording by a known factor. This reduces the background noise to produce a smooth baseline but also reduces the ERA response.

Cortical electric response audiometry (CERA)

Changes in EEG activity in response to sounds may be detected more easily using averaging techniques. The activity is best recorded by an active electrode placed on the vertex of the head with a reference electrode placed on the mastoid. The potentials are definitely generated from the cortex of the brain but not necessarily from primary auditory areas. A typical CERA response consists of a small inconsistent positive (with respect to the vertex) peak (P1) at 50–60 ms after the stimulus onset, a large negative peak (N1) at about 100 ms, and a large positive peak (P2) at about 175 ms. Usually this is followed by a second low negative peak (N2) at 200–250 ms which may be especially large in children, and a late positive peak (P3) at around 300 ms which is larger when the subject is certain that he has correctly performed a task cued by the sound stimulus.

CERA gives an accurate estimate of the pure-tone audiometric thresholds in adults and older children. The CERA potentials get smaller as the sound intensity diminishes until they become unidentifiable close to the audiometric threshold (*Figure 1.15*).

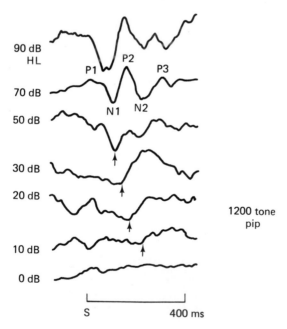

Figure 1.15 Cortical electrical response audiometry (CERA). (Adapted from Gibson, 1978)

Passive cooperation is essential as movements cause artefacts which obliterate the response. As a comprehensive test takes 1 h, many young children cannot be satisfactorily tested. Unfortunately, sedation tends to make response interpretation hazardous. The initial optimism which greeted the use of CERA has faded, since many of the children untestable by behavioural methods have also proved untestable by CERA.

Currently the use of CERA is restricted to adults and older children. It provides an excellent method of assessing non-organic hearing loss. It has no value, when used alone, as a method of neuro-otological diagnosis.

The middle latency responses

The earlier components of the cortical response are stable during sedation and have a potential use for estimating children's hearing thresholds. The characteristic response has a positive wave at 13 ms (Po), a negative wave at 22 ms (Na), a positive wave at 34 ms (Pa) and a negative wave at 44 ms (Nb). The response has not been found to be entirely reliable for estimating hearing thresholds (Davis and Hirsch, 1975). Recently Robinson and Rudge (1977) have suggested that it may have a value in the detection of multiple sclerosis.

The myogenic (sonomotor) responses

Apart from the muscles within the ear, other muscles of the body react to sound, but usually they do so in an inconsistent fashion. The scalp muscles, and in particular those behind the ear respond even to sounds of low intensity. The post-auricular sonomotor response may be recorded bilaterally and simultaneously from behind both ears and has been clinically named the *crossed acoustic response* (Douek, Gibson and Humphries, 1973). Postauricular responses can provide a crude indication of the hearing level in young children without the need for sedation. They may also have a use in confirming the integrity of the neural pathway involved.

ELECTROCOCHLEOGRAPHY (*ECochG*)

ECochG gives a direct measure of the electrical activity within the cochlea after acoustic stimulation. It provides the otologist with a clinical tool comparable with the use of electrocardiography by cardiologists. The cochlear activity is recorded from a fine needle electrode which is inserted through the tympanic membrane so that its point lies on the promontory close to the round window niche (*Figure 1.16*). The ECochG procedure appears to be very safe and a comprehensive review of 1500 tests failed to report any serious complications (Crowley, Davis and Beagley, 1975). Three types of cochlear activity can be measured (*Figure 1.17*).

(a) The action potential (AP)

The AP recorded from near the round window membrane represents an integral of the combined activity of many individual nerve action potentials firing in a manner determined by their position along the cochlear partition and by the nature of the travelling wave. The fibres in the basal turn fire in close unison and contribute to the major component of the click-evoked AP. Stimuli of low frequency content (below 1 kHz) only evoke a poorly synchronized AP which is difficult to identify. The stimulus intensity at which the AP is deemed unidentifiable (usually a criterion voltage level of 0.1 or 0.2μV) is known as the AP threshold. The AP threshold may be used confidently to estimate hearing in the higher audiometric range in any subject even during general anaesthesia.

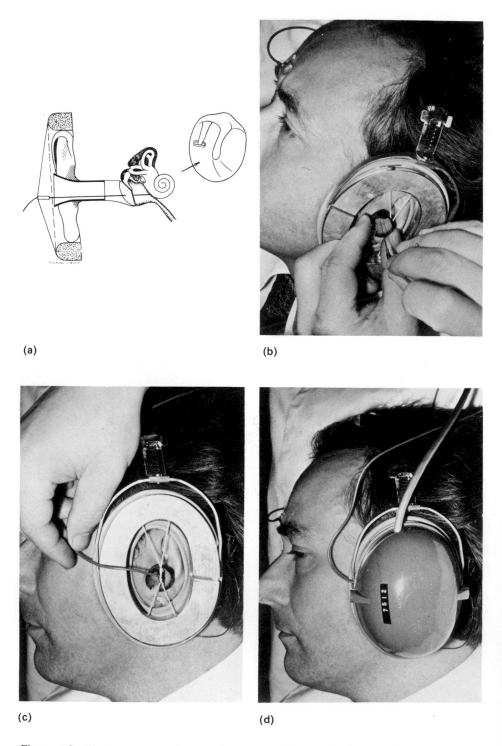

(a)

(b)

(c)

(d)

Figure 1.16 The technique of electrode insertion and fixation in electrocochleography

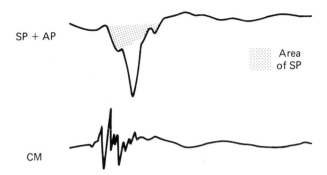

Figure 1.17   The normal electrocochleogram (ECochG) potentials

(b) The cochlear microphonic (CM)

The CM is an alternating potential originating from the cuticular surface of hair-cells. The electrical waveform of the CM so closely resembles the electrical waveform of the stimulus that care has to be taken not to confuse it with electrical artefacts. The CM recorded by the transtympanic electrode varies considerably depending on the exact position of the needle and only measures activity from hair-cells lying within a few millimetres of the round window membrane. The CM threshold is not related in any consistent manner to the hearing threshold.

(c) The summating potential (SP)

The SP is a multicomponent potential arising from non-linear sources within the cochlea. The major source results from the asymmetrical vibration of the basilar membrane, which is particulary marked at higher stimulus intensities, causing the CM to be generated unequally with a preponderance towards one electrical polarity.

As an objective audiometric test, ECochG has many advantages. It is extremely reliable and the responses are easy to identify. No masking of the non-test ear is required and sedatives do not affect the potentials. ECochG also shows promise as a means of identifying and investigating causes of hearing impairment. Characteristic findings occur in certain conditions.

Normal ears (Figure 1.18a)

The AP is characteristically monophasic at high intensities and, as the stimulus intensity decreases, it diminishes in amplitude and the latency increases. At threshold the AP latency is 4–6 ms. The SP is much smaller than the AP. The CM has a 0.1 μV threshold at around 60 dB HL.

Conductive hearing loss

The ECochG resembles the normal ECochG providing the same stimulus intensity in dB relative to the subject's hearing threshold is used. The AP for a conductive loss of 40 dB HL has a monophasic waveform at 120 dB HL, the SP is relatively very small and the CM threshold lies at around 100 dB HL. At threshold the AP latency is 4–6 ms.

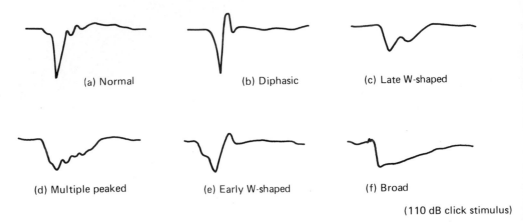

(a) Normal   (b) Diphasic   (c) Late W-shaped

(d) Multiple peaked   (e) Early W-shaped   (f) Broad

(110 dB click stimulus)

Figure 1.18   Typical patterns of ECochG responses

Hair-cell loss (Figure 1.18b)
The ECochG shows many interesting changes: the AP has a diphasic waveform at high intensities, the latency at threshold is little changed from that at higher intensities (2–3 ms), the CM threshold is usually around 90 dB HL and the SP is often unidentifiable.

Selective hair-cell loss due to acoustic trauma (Figure 1.18c)
The click-evoked AP often has a characteristic late W form due to an attenuation of the synchronized basal coil activity which normally contributes so generously to the AP waveform. The SP and CM are usually minute.

Menière's disorder (Figure 1.18d)
In the majority of 'true' cases the ECochG reveals a massive SP which swamps a small diphasic AP (Gibson, Moffat and Ramsden, 1977). This SP almost certainly represents the manner in which the endolymphatic hydrops distorts the basilar membrane. The CM is small.

Syphilitic hearing loss (Figure 1.18e)
This condition causes endolymphatic hydrops but unlike Menière's disorder, there is extensive hair-cell damage and neural degeneration. The ECochG usually shows an enhanced SP, but rarely does this affect the upgoing limb of the AP. As a result a characteristic 'early W' shape is seen. The CM is minute (Ramsden, Moffat and Gibson, 1977).

Acoustic neuroma (Figure 1.18f)
The ECochG usually shows a broad waveform similar to that encountered in Menière's disorder. In many cases, the onset of the broad waveform does not coincide with the onset of the CM showing that this is not an enhanced SP but the result of disordered neural activity. Often the CM is large and it may be larger than that measured from the normal ear. Even when no AP can be recorded, the CM may have a 0.1 μV threshold at normal levels. The more medially-placed tumours may spare

some of the nerve fibres within the cochlea with the result that the AP threshold is better than the subject's hearing threshold.

Brainstem tumours
Brainstem tumours do not often affect the ECochG so that a completely normal ECochG may be obtained despite subjective deafness. The brainstem electrical responses should be performed to localize the lesion further.

Brainstem electrical responses (BER)
The electricity generated by various parts of the auditory tract can be measured using surface electrodes. The active electrodes are often placed on the forehead immediately below the hairline and over the ipsilateral mastoid. An interesting series of waves is obtained (*Figure 1.19*). The first wave is generated by the first order cochlear fibres, the second by the cochlear nucleus, the third by the superior olive, the fourth and fifth from the region of the lateral lemniscus and inferior colliculus. Sometimes a sixth wave and even a seventh wave are visible.

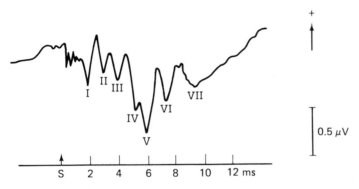

Figure 1.19   The normal configuration of the brainstem electrical response (BER) (90 dB HL, 4 kHz stimulus; polarity with respect to mastoid; bandpass 3.2 Hz–3.2 kHz)

BER offers an excellent method of estimating the hearing threshold. The waves are not affected by sedatives and the fourth and fifth waves provide a good measure of the threshold (*Figure 1.20*). It is possible to test premature infants of as little as 34 weeks gestational age (Schulman-Galambos and Galambos, 1975). The response is more frequency-specific than the electrocochleogram as it provides better low frequency information.

BER also provides an excellent neuro-otological tool. Selters and Brackmann (1977) investigated 100 patients with tumours. Tumours that pressed on the auditory nerve often caused a latency delay that was best seen by comparing the fifth wave latencies of the two ears. The normal interaural latency difference is less than 0.2 ms, but in over 90 per cent of the tumour cases the delay exceeded 0.4 ms. They also noted that the larger tumours caused a latency delay between the third and fifth waves.

Robinson and Rudge (1977) have shown a latency delay of the fifth wave in 79 per cent of patients suffering from multiple sclerosis. None of the patients had a subjective hearing loss and even in a group of patients without any other brainstem signs, they noted the latency delay in 51 per cent of cases. BER may also be used to localize brainstem tumours by noting the absence of response components (Starr and Hamilton, 1976).

OTHER INVESTIGATIONS OF AUDITORY DYSFUNCTION

Apart from audiometric tests, the vestibular tests described in the next chapter can be invaluable in reaching the correct diagnosis in conditions such as Menière's disorder and acoustic neuroma. An absent caloric response helps in the diagnosis of a completely 'dead' ear as sometimes it is difficult to exclude the possibility of bone conducted hearing.

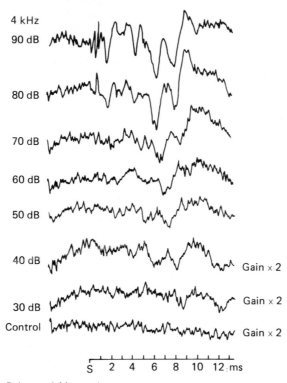

Baby aged 11 months
Epileptic fits

Figure 1.20 The BER used to estimate the hearing threshold of a small baby

When an acoustic neuroma is suspected, it is important to investigate the function of other cranial nerves, especially in the facial nerve. Schirmer's test may show diminished lacrimation, electrogustometry may show some loss of taste sensation on the ipsilateral two-thirds of the tongue and nerve conduction studies may show a conduction delay.

Serological tests for syphilis are important and must not be forgotten. Congenital syphilis usually presents in middle age and it is often associated with interstitial keratitis. Even when interstitial keratitis is not readily apparent, ophthalmological examination may reveal 'ghost vessels' within the cornea. Congenital syphilis is difficult to detect on routine (WR and VDRL) testing and 25 per cent of patients are not diagnosed unless the fluorescent treponemal antibody test (FTA) is done.

Radiological examination is often indicated. In congenital hearing loss, the absence of the cochlea or part of it may be noted, or a bony atresia of the external acoustic meatus visualized. Radiological examination of the middle ear, antrum and mastoid air-cell system may indicate the cause of a conductive impairment. In sensorineural hearing impairment, radiology of the internal acoustic meatuses will reveal the rare acoustic neuroma when present with an accuracy of 84.6 per cent (Olivecrona, 1967). The specialized techniques required (including tomography and EMI scan or CAT scan) and more detail of the diagnostic potential of radiography are described in Volume 1.

References

Anderson, H., Barr, B. and Wedenburg, E. (1970) *Acta Otolaryngologica, suppl,* **263**, 232

Ashcroft, M. T., Cruickshank, E. K., Hinchcliffe, R., Jones, W. I., Miall, W. E. and Wallace, J. (1967) *West Indian Medical Journal,* **16**, 223

Ballantyne, J. C. (1973) *Recent Advances in Otolaryngology,* Chapter 10. Edinburgh; Churchill Livingston

Békésy, G. Von (1947) *Acta Otolaryngologica,* **35**, 411

Bing, A. (1891) *Wein Med. Blatter,* **41**

Bocca, E., Calearo, C., Cassinari, V. and Migliavacca, F. (1955) *Acta Otolaryngologica,* **45**, 289

Bosatra, A., Russulo, M. and Semeraro, A. (1975) *Acta Otolaryngologica,* **79**, 334

Brooks, D. N. (1969) *International Audiology,* **8**, 563

Chiveralls, K., FitzSimmons, R., Beck, G. B. and Kernohan, H. (1976) *Audiology,* **10**, 122

Colletti, V. (1975) *Audiology,* **14**, 63

Costen, J. B. (1934) *Annals of Otology,* **43**, 1

Crowley, D. E., Davis, H. and Beagley, H. A. (1975) *Annals of Otology,* **84**, 1

Davis, H. and Hirsh, S. K. (1975) Paper read at IIIrd Symposium of I.E.R.A.S.G., Bordeaux

Dix, M. R., Hallpike, C. S. and Hood, J. D. (1948) *Journal of Laryngology,* **62**, 671

Douek, E. E., Gibson, W. P. R. and Humphries, K. N. (1973) *Journal of Laryngology,* **87**, 711

Douek, E. E. and Reid, J. (1968) *Journal of Laryngology,* **82**, 1039

Evans, E. F. (1975) *Sound Reception in Mammals,* p. 133. London; Academic Press

Flottorp, G. and Djupesland, G. (1970) *Acta Otolaryngologica, suppl.,* **263**, 200

Gibson, W. P. R. (1978) *Essentials of Clinical Electric Response Audiometry,* Edinburgh; Churchill Livingstone

Gibson, W. P. R., Moffat, D. A. and Ramsden, R. T. (1977) *Audiology,* **16**, 389

Glanville, J. D., Coles, R. R. A. and Sullivan, B. M. (1971) *Journal of Laryngology,* **85**, 1

Hood, J. D. (1962) *International Audiology,* **1**, 174

Hood, J. D. (1977) *Audiology,* **16**, 215

Hood, J. D. and Poole, J. P. (1966) *Journal of the Acoustical Society of America,* **40**, 47

Hood, J. D. and Poole, J. P. (1977) *British Journal of Audiology,* **11**, 93

Huizing, E. H. (1960) *Acta Otolaryngologica, suppl.,* **155**

Jerger, J. (1960) *Journal of Speech and Hearing Research,* **3**, 275

Jerger, J. (1973) *Modern Developments in Audiology,* Chapter 3. New York; Academic Press

Jerger, J., Anthony, L., Jerger, S. and Maudlin, C. (1974a) *Archives of Otolaryngology,* **99**, 165

Jerger, J., Burnley, P., Maudlin, L. and Crump, B. (1974b) *Journal of Speech and Hearing Disorders.,* **39**, 11

Jerger, J. and Herer, G. (1961) *Journal of Speech and Hearing Disorders,* **26**, 390

Jerger, J. and Jerger, S. (1975) *Archives of Otolarynyology,* **101**, 403

Jerger, J., Shedd, J. L. and Harford, E. (1959) *Archives of Otolaryngology,* **69**, 200

Jerger, J. and Tillman, T. (1960) *Archives of Otolaryngology,* **71**, 948

Johnson, E. W. (1968) *Archives of Otolaryngology,* **8**, 598

Markides, A. (1977) *British Journal of Audiology, suppl.,* **1**

Metz, O. (1946) *Acta Otolaryngologica, suppl.,* **63**

Moffat, D. A., Ramsden, R. T. and Shaw, H. J. (1977) *Journal of Laryngology,* **91**, 279

Morales-Garcia, C. and Poole, J. P. (1972) *Acta Otolaryngologica,* **74**, 307

Morrison, A. W. and Booth, J. B. (1970) *British Journal of Hospital Medicine,* **4**, 287

Niemeyer, W. and Sesterhenn, G. (1974) *Audiology,* **13**, 421

Olivecrona, H. (1967) *Journal of Neurosurgery,* **26**, 6

Parker, R. (1975) *Journal of Laryngology,* **89**, 151

Rainville, M. J. (1955) *Journal français de Otolaryngologie* **4**, 851

Ramsden, R. T., Bulman, C. H. and Lorigan, B. P. (1975) *Journal of Laryngology,* **89**, 941

Ramsden, R. T., Moffat, D. A. and Gibson, W. P. R. (1977) *Annals of Otology*

Reker, U. (1977) *Archives of Otorhinolaryngology,* **215**, 25

Robinson, K. and Rudge, P. (1977) *Brain*, **100**, 19

Schulman-Galambos, C. and Galambos, R. (1975) *Journal of Speech and Hearing Research*, **18**, 456

Selters, W. A. and Brackmann, D. (1977) *Annals of Otology*, **103**, 181

Senturia, B. H. (1973) *Annals of Otology*, **82**

Starr, A. and Hamilton, A. E. (1976) *Electroencephalography and Clinical Neurophysiology*, **41**, 595

Terkildsen, K. and Nielsen, S. (1960) *Archives of Otolaryngology*, **72**, 339

Tillman, T. W. (1963) *Archives of Otolaryngology*, **78**, 20

Tonndorf, J. (1966) *Acta Otolaryngologica, suppl.* **213**

Ward, W. D. (1973) *Modern Developments in Audiology*, Chapter 9. New York; Academic Press

Watkyn-Thomas, F. W. (1953) *Diseases of the Throat, Nose and Ear*, London; Lewis

Willis, T. (1672) *De Anima Brutorum*, London

Zwislocki, J. (1963) *Journal of Speech and Hearing Research*, **6**, 303

2 The functional and physical examination of the vestibular system

W P R Gibson

Vertigo is the primary symptom of a vestibular disorder. In many cases the site of dysfunction lies within the ear and within the realm of the otologist. The evaluation of a patient presenting with vertigo encompasses the history, examination and investigations outlined in Chapter 1 and then involves the further history, examination and investigations necessary to diagnose the cause of the vestibular disorder. A properly conducted investigation of vertigo takes longer than 1 h and so it is small wonder that the busy otologist may experience a slight decline in spirit when confronted by such a patient, especially as the understanding and treatment of many of the causes is still inadequate. Nevertheless successful management of a patient with vertigo is most rewarding. This chapter emphasizes the importance of a clear history and a competent examination for reaching a correct diagnosis, and describes methods of examination which are of value to the clinician.

The vestibular system provides an essential input to the central nervous system (CNS) feeding the mechanisms which maintain body posture and equilibrium. Other sensory inputs arise from the eyes and from the proprioceptor systems. The vestibular system may be functionally separated into left and right halves and each half acts independently within the brainstem so that a disturbance affecting one part tends to cause a sensation of abnormal body movement. The visual and proprioceptor systems act mainly in a bilateral manner within the brainstem and dysfunction tends to cause a feeling of general instability.

The three sensory inputs are modified by interaction between themselves and by activity arising from the cerebellum, cerebral cortex and reticular system. The cerebellum is intimately associated with the function of the vestibular system and with the proprioceptor system. The cerebellum integrates the sensory information to maintain spatial orientation and equilibrium; it sends efferent fibres to the vestibular nuclei, to the basal ganglia to influence muscle tone, and to the cerebral cortex. The primary afferent cortical area is not known for certain in man but, in monkey, it is located in the posterior part of the post-central gyrus at the base of the intraparietal sulcus between the first and second somatosensory fields, Brodman's area 2 (Fredrickson *et al.*, 1966). It appears that the cerebellum and these posterior areas of the temporal lobes exert primarily an inhibitory influence upon the vestibular nuclei. The symptoms resulting from disorder of the cerebellum or temporal lobes or the associated neural pathways may be explained by a release of activity within the vestibular nuclei. Lesions of these structures may, therefore, cause a vestibular disorder.

The vestibular system may be separated into two parts on an anatomical basis; the peripheral vestibular system and the central vestibular system. The peripheral system consists of the vestibular end-organs, Scarpa's ganglia and the vestibular nerves. The central system consists of the vestibular nuclei within the brainstem and their connecting central pathways. Each vestibular end-organ includes three semicircular canals, the utricle, saccule and endolymphatic sac. The cristae in the ampulla of each semicircular canal respond to angular acceleration. The maculae of the utricle respond to linear acceleration. The function of the saccule is not clear; it may be concerned with hearing very low frequencies or with vertical acceleration or with both. The anatomy and physiology of the vestibular system are described in greater detail in Volume I.

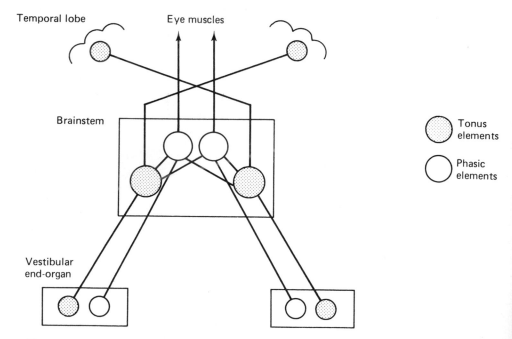

Figure 2.1   A diagram of the localization of phasic and tonus elements

The vestibular system may also be separated into two elements on a functional basis; the phasic elements and the tonus elements. The phasic elements are determined by alterations of sensory inputs, for instance canal stimulation evokes increased phasic activity as shown by the induced nystagmus. The tonus elements represent continuous on-going activity within the vestibular system and in normal circumstances, the tonus elements on the left and right sides are balanced. Loss of tonus on one side upsets this balance and may result in nystagmus directed towards the normal side. In resolving or less severe lesions there is no spontaneous nystagmus, and the tonus imbalance is only evident on inducing nystagmus by caloric stimulation, when the exaggerated nystagmus towards the normal side is known as a directional preponderance (DP).

There is evidence to suggest that the utricle has an important role in maintaining gaze deviation and that destructive lesions involving only the utricle produce a DP towards the opposite side (Owada, Shiizu and Kimura, 1960). The utricle is likely to be the important peripheral site for tonus.

Carmichael, Dix and Hallpike (1965) argue that the tonus elements project to the most caudal regions of the vestibular nuclei below the cochlear nuclei, i.e. the descending nucleus and the most caudal portion of the medial nucleus. The phasic elements which are peripherally situated mainly in the canals project to more rostral areas of the vestibular nuclei. It is also known that a lesion affecting the posterior part of the temporal lobe may result in an ipsilateral directional preponderance (Carmichael, Dix and Hallpike, 1954). A diagram of the arrangement of phasic and tonus elements is shown in *Figure 2.1*.

A simple analogy is to compare the tonus element of each side of the vestibular system to the engines on each wing of an aircraft. If one engine fails, the plane veers to the affected side. In a similar fashion the patient will veer or fall to the affected side and his eyes will drift slowly towards this side until the CNS detects this drift and quickly jerks the eyes back towards their starting position (nystagmus). If the pilot has sufficient time and skill, he adjusts the controls of the plane to make it fly straight again. He does this by adjusting the plane to veer to the side and so counteract the drift to the affected side (analogy with directional preponderance). This analogy is simplistic but nevertheless provides a useful guide to the events described later in this chapter.

History

A careful history is of immense value in the diagnosis of the cause of vertigo. As many people have difficulty describing their symptoms, the clinician must be patient and help the patient without projecting any of his own opinions. Some workers have suggested a proforma which the patient can complete before his consultation and so help the clinician to choose the most relevant line of questioning. It is not wise for the clinician to spend his time together with the patient completing a proforma. The objection is that a proforma is too rigid and that the clinician must act like a detective and follow the most relevant clues to reach a correct diagnosis. A rough scheme of questioning is shown in *Table 2.1* which shows the trails normally pursued.

It is best to begin taking the history by allowing the patient to describe the symptoms without interruption. A few patients give a clear description but many require some gentle prompting. The clinician should then fill in any missing details with specific questioning. It is very helpful to try to decide from the outset whether the patient is suffering from light-headedness or from true vertigo.

Light-headedness is often experienced by patients suffering from syncope, fever, hypoglycaemia, anxiety states and after immobilization for prolonged periods following systemic diseases.

True vertigo involves a hallucination of movement, which may consist of a feeling of rotation, swaying, falling or tilting—of the outside world or of the patient's own body. True vertigo occurs only with lesions of the peripheral or central vestibular system.

A lesion affecting the vestibular end-organ usually causes rotational vertigo of sudden onset. Often the vertigo is intense and episodic. The vertigo may last a few seconds or a maximum of 24 h. Lesions of Scarpa's ganglion may, however, result in vertigo lasting several days. Changing the head position usually alters the vertigo. Falls are common and these tend to be towards the side of the lesion. Loss of consciousness is exceptionally rare.

Table 2.1   History (outlines)

The patient's own description of the vertigo	
Specific questioning	Date of onset
	Manner of onset: gradual or sudden
	Events related to onset: injuries, infections, drugs, etc.
	Periodicity: episodic or continuous
if episodic	—description of first attack
	—if rotational —direction of rotation
	duration of actual rotation
	duration and nature of after-effects
	severity (was first attack the worst?)
	—if fall or a sensation —direction of fall or sensation
	of falling any warning symptoms
	any loss of consciousness (? any epileptic
	features)
	—if possible drop attack ask for symptoms of transient ischaemic
	attacks
	Description of subsequent attacks and periodicity
if continuous	—description of the sensation, e.g. light-headed, woozy, etc.
	any loss of stability
	effect of darkness and eye closure
	direction of any falling sensation
Aggravating factors	—head movements, suddenly standing, etc.
Relieving factors	—drugs, bed rest, etc.
Associated symptoms	—Does the patient note any associated symptoms?
Otological	—suppuration
	hearing loss: character, onset, relation to vertigo, etc.
	tinnitus: pitch, onset, relation to vertigo, etc.
	otalgia: character, distribution, relation to vertigo, etc.
Autonomic	—nausea, vomiting, palpitations, sweating, hyperventilation,
	etc.
Visual	—disturbances of vision, diplopia, oscillopsia, etc.
Headaches	—character, distribution, relation to vertigo, etc.
	—any features of migraine
Cervical	—pain or restriction of head movements
Nose and throat	—rhinitis, bleeding, hoarseness, dysphagia, etc.
Present medication	
Past medication	especially at onset of vertigo
	ototoxic drugs
Past history	
Otological	—suppuration, operations, acoustic trauma, etc.
Non-otological	—serious illnesses, operations, head injuries,
	cardiovascular disease, epilepsy, etc.
Family history	
Psychiatric history	
Social history	Does the disability prevent normal working?
	Alcohol intake and any relation to vertigo
	Any smoking?
	Occupation

A tumour affecting the vestibular nerve usually affects the vestibular system so gradually that central compensation occurs without any violent attacks of vertigo. Occasionally a vascular disaster, secondary to the tumour, causes an acute labyrinthine attack but generally the patient only notices imbalance in the dark when he may stumble towards the affected side.

Central tumours also cause an insidious loss of balance and only occasionally sudden, episodic attacks of vertigo. The symptoms are mild and progressive. The duration of imbalance may last several months or years and altering the head position has little effect. Central vascular disorders act in a quite different manner. For instance, vertebrobasilar insufficiency causes transient ischaemic attacks (TIA) and suddenly sitting up or extending the neck may precipitate a sudden attack of vertigo. Drop attacks occur quite commonly but complete loss of consciousness is rare. Details of vertebrobasilar insufficiency and other vascular disorders affecting balance are described in Chapter 26.

Psychogenic disorders often produce light-headedness which the patient may find difficult to describe. Often a sensation of floating or swimming is given, and the symptoms are not aggravated by head movements. Sometimes the sensation is worse in crowds or 'attacks' only occur in the presence of a sympathetic audience. It is necessary to discover whether there is any underlying anxiety or depression.

Examination

The general condition of the patient during the examination should be noted not only because it is important diagnostically, but because it may force the clinician to modify his approach. The general outline of a typical neuro-otological examination is shown in *Table 2.2*, and this discussion is limited to only a few of the relevant areas.

Before the patient is seen by the clinician, it is useful to ask the nurse to record the blood pressure both standing and lying, to weigh the patient and to perform routine screening tests on the patient's urine.

The examination for spontaneous nystagmus

It is essential to examine the eye movements properly. The fundi, visual fields, and pupillary reflexes should be included as appropriate. The physical sign of paramount importance is the presence of spontaneous nystagmus. It may only be excluded after careful examination of the eyes in all fields of gaze both with and without optic fixation. Optic fixation can be reduced adequately for all clinical purposes by using Frenzel's glasses (Frenzel, 1928). Alternative techniques involve an infrared viewer or electronystagmography.

The examination for nystagmus must be conducted under good diffuse lighting. The patient's spectacles must be removed. It may help to use a source of magnification and even a simple magnifying glass can help. The eyes are observed with the patient's gaze directed straight ahead and deviated to the right and left just within the limits of binocular vision. A rough guide to this is when the limbus and the caruncle of the adducting eye just meet. Nystagmus within these limits is pathological. Nystagmus

Table 2.2   Examination (outline)

Blood pressure (standing and lying) and pulses		
Patient's condition during examination		Date
State of mucous membranes (anaemia, jaundice, etc.)		
Any enlarged lymph nodes in the neck? Any vascular bruits?		
Nose and throat examination	Nose	
	Mouth	
	Post-nasal space	
	Indirect laryngoscopy	
Examination of the ears	Appearance, fistula test, tests of hearing, etc.	
Cranial nerves	I ⎱ examine whenever	
	II Fundi, visual fields ⎰ appropriate	
	Pupillary reflexes	
	III, IV, VI—eye movements, spontaneous	
	nystagmus ($\pm$ Frenzel's glasses).	
	command, convergence/divergence	
	V corneal reflexes, sensation V_1, V_2 and V_3	
	VII any palsy or spasms (can patient bury eyelashes	
	equally?)	
	Acoustic, reflex, lacrymation, taste	
	IX Sensation on and above each tonsil	
	X Gag reflex, palate movements, vocal cord	
	movements	
	XI Sternomastoid contractions	
	XII Movement of tongue	
Cerebellar tests (see Table 2.4)		
Tests of body posture and gait	Romberg	
	Unterberger	
	Gait	
Cervical posture test		
Positional tests		
Optokinetic nystagmus		
Doll's head eye movements		

outside these limits commonly occurs in normal subjects as they have difficulty maintaining the muscular movement required (endstellungsnystagmus or end-point nystagmus). Nystagmus can be classified into two main categories, vestibular nystagmus and non-vestibular nystagmus.

VESTIBULAR NYSTAGMUS

Vestibular nystagmus has a characteristic saw-tooth character. The eyes slowly deviate towards the side of a paralytic lesion and then quickly jerk back towards their starting position. The direction of the nystagmus is named after the direction of the fast component. Vestibular nystagmus like torture occurs in three degrees and third degree nystagmus is the worst. According to Alexander's classification; left nystagmus is first degree when it only occurs on left gaze, it is second degree when it is also present on straight ahead gaze, and it is third degree when it is present, in addition, on right gaze.

To return to the aeroplane analogy, the plane drifts in the direction of the failing engine before the pilot notices the error and quickly realigns the plane. In man, the eyes slowly drift towards the affected side before the CNS quickly jerks them back towards the original position. Usually, the patient feels the room is turning in the direction of the fast component or that his body is turning in the direction of the slow component. The nystagmus is worse on looking away from the side of the paralytic lesion, and if one observes a patient after labyrinthectomy, he lies on the normal side to avoid having to look in this direction.

Spontaneous vestibular nystagmus may be due either to a peripheral lesion or to a centrally-placed lesion. The relevant features are shown in *Table 2.3*. The effect of removing optic fixation varies in an orderly manner according to the site of the lesion and this is discussed later under electronystagmography.

Table 2.3 Characteristics of spontaneous vestibular nystagmus

	Peripheral type	*Central type*
Duration	Temporary—maximum 3 weeks	Permanent
Direction	One direction only	May be bidirectional
Character	Conjugate (allow for squints)	May be dissociated or deranged
Effect of removing optic fixation*	Enhanced	Unchanged or inhibited

*See Table 2.7

Dissociated nystagmus

Internuclear ophthalmoplegia is the commonest form of dissociated nystagmus. It is due to a lesion affecting the medial longitudinal bundle between the III and VI nuclei and is most commonly associated with multiple sclerosis. The nystagmus is more pronounced or entirely confined to the abducting eye, and in advanced cases incomplete adduction of the adducting eye occurs.

In early cases, only slowing of the adduction of the affected eye occurs which is not visible on direct examination and the nystagmus may not have developed. Dual channel electronystagmography can reveal a difference between the relative velocities of the two eyes in executing saccadic movements or in the fast phase of optokinetically induced nystagmus. A vascular lesion in the brainstem may cause an ipsilateral slowing of adduction but bilateral defects are highly pathognomic of multiple sclerosis.

Vertical nystagmus

Vertical nystagmus indicates a bilateral midline involvement of the vestibular pathways within the brainstem. Up-beating nystagmus is caused by high-placed lesions, while down-beating nystagmus suggests a lesion of the caudal brainstem or upper cervical region.

Rotatory nystagmus

Torsional or rotatory eye movements are almost exclusively controlled by the labyrinths and rotatory nystagmus indicates a lesion of the vestibular system, most commonly of the vestibular nuclei in the floor of the fourth ventricle.

Bidirectional (Bruyn's) nystagmus
Large extrinsic tumours which compress the brainstem at the level of the vestibular nuclei may cause bidirectional nystagmus. For instance, a large left eighth nerve tumour initially causes a first degree nystagmus directed to the right side, but when the tumour enlarges and compresses the inferior cerebellar peduncle, the patient will, in addition, develop a coarse nystagmus to the left.

Rebound nystagmus (Hood, Kayan and Leech, 1973)
Rebound spontaneous nystagmus, as distinct from rebound positional nystagmus, often occurs in chronic cerebellar disorders. Initially there is no nystagmus on straight ahead gaze. On lateral gaze deviation, a fatiguing nystagmus occurs. After the lateral nystagmus has faded, the eyes are brought swiftly back to the midline and now a fatiguing nystagmus in the opposite direction is seen. This nystagmus has a similar basic mechanism to ocular dysmetria.

NON-VESTIBULAR NYSTAGMUS
With the exception of optokinetic nystagmus, non-vestibular nystagmus is easily recognized as it does not have a saw-tooth character.

Pendular nystagmus
This is almost without exception congenital. The most striking feature is that despite a very obvious nystagmus, the patient's vision is unaffected. Unlike vestibular nystagmus, it has a jelly-like character, both components of the nystagmus having the same velocity. Pendular nystagmus is due to a lesion affecting the efferent neural mechanism controlling optic fixation which lies in the upper brainstem. Pendular nystagmus is associated less commonly with the following conditions:

Neoplasms
These rarely cause pendular nystagmus and are usually associated with other signs of brainstem involvement.

Absence of central vision
If this occurs in infants under the age of two, fixation reflexes do not develop.

Spasmus nutans

Peripheral ocular defects

Miner's nystagmus
In the past, miners worked long hours in near darkness and on surfacing exhibited a pendular nystagmus.

Nystagmus retractorius
This is characterized by irregular jerks of the eye backwards into the orbit and often indicated a tumour in the region of the pineal stalk. It is best seen when, during testing for optokinetic nystagmus, the patient is asked to look upwards at a drum rotating downwards.

Convergent nystagmus
Rarely, both eyes perform rapid converging movements which are associated with lesions involving the superior colliculi or Perlia's nucleus.

See-saw nystagmus
Again very rare. Viewed from a distance, one pupil appears to rise while the other appears to fall. This type of nystagmus is associated with tumours in the region of the optic chiasma, such as pituitary tumours.

(The clinical examination for spontaneous nystagmus may be augmented by the use of electronystagmographic investigations which are outlined later in this chapter.)

Examination of other cranial nerves

After careful examination of the eyes, the function of the other cranial nerves is noted. A great deal of topodiagnostic information can be gleaned by careful examination of the facial nerve; in addition to the motor functions (including stapedius muscle contraction), the parasympathetic function (lacrimation, salivation and the special somatosensory function of taste) should be tested (*see* Chapter 27).

CEREBELLAR TESTS
After testing the cranial nerves and examining the ear, it is convenient to consider the cerebellar system. The signs of cerebellar disorder vary according to whether the cerebellar hemisphere, the cerebellar vermis, or both are affected (*Table 2.4*).

Table 2.4   Signs of cerebellar dysfunction

Neurological
   Cerebellar hemisphere dysfunction (non-equilibratory)
     1. Asynergia or dissociated movements
     2. Dysmetria or past pointing
     3. Dysdiadochokinesis
     4. Rebound
   Midline cerebellar dysfunction (equilibratory)
     1. Truncal ataxia
     2. Wide-based gait
     3. Falling in any direction and inability to make sudden turns
Neuro-otological
   Spontaneous nystagmus
     1. Coarse vestibular nystagmus, if present
     2. Vertical nystagmus with cerebellar compression into foramen magnum
   Induced nystagmus
     1. Atypical positional nystagmus
     2. Enhanced caloric responses
     3. Often directional preponderance to affected side
     4. Optokinetic responses may be deranged or broken up
Following responses may be deranged
Electronystagmography
     1. Saccades
     2. Failure to maintain gaze position or drifting on eye closure or darkness
     3. Dysmetria
     4. Rebound nystagmus
     5. Centripetal nystagmus on eye closure or in darkness

Tests for cerebellar hemisphere function can mainly be performed with the patient sitting. Asynergia is noted by getting the patient to pat the back of each hand rapidly. Dysmetria is usually assessed by the finger-to-nose-to-finger test. The patient is asked to touch his own nose quickly with his index finger and then to touch the finger of the examiner. The examiner moves his finger each time so that the patient has a different target on each occasion. Failure to hit consistently the target indicates cerebellar dysfunction but the manner in which the patient misses is probably not a good localizing sign. Dysdiadochokinesia is noted by making the patient rapidly flip his hands from dorsal surface upwards to palmar surface upwards; and a difference between the two hands may be noticed. Rebound can be tested by forcibly restraining a patient's limb in one position while the patient is asked to push against the resistance. On suddenly releasing the limb, the patient is asked to try not to move the limb at all.

Midline cerebellar function is assessed partly during the sitting part of the examination and partly while testing the patient's standing and gait.

TESTS OF BODY POSTURE, EQUILIBRIUM AND GAIT

The Romberg test
The patient is asked to stand to attention with his legs together and arms down at his sides. If he is stable, he is then asked to close his eyes. Patients with paralytic vestibular disorders fall or sway towards the side of the lesion, although the localizing value in subacute or chronic conditions is not always clear-cut. Patients with central disorders often sway in different directions on repeated testing. Falling straight backwards like a wooden soldier is almost pathognomonic of hysteria. As an alternative to Romberg's test, Ruttick's modification involves the patient holding his arms outstretched in front of himself.

Unterberger's test
If the patient is fairly stable on Romberg testing, further information can sometimes be gained by using Unterberger's test. The patient is asked to clasp the palms of both hands together and to stretch his arms out in front of him. He then is asked to step up and down on the same spot with his eyes closed. This test appears to give better localization than Romberg testing and it can be quantified by measuring the number of degrees of deviation over a period of time.

Gait tests
The patient is asked to walk a straight line quickly between two points, first with eyes open and then with his eyes closed. Patients with paralytic vestibular lesions tend to deviate towards the affected side. The test must be properly supervised so that the patient does not fall and injure himself. If the patient is stable, the test can be increased in sensitivity, by asking the patient to walk with one hand outstretched over a distance of 3–4 m and touch a target with his eyes closed, or by asking the patient to walk across a mattress. Patients with bilateral vestibular loss due to antibiotic intoxication are able to walk easily with their eyes open but become very unstable on eye closure.

The cervical posture test
It is the author's practice always to perform cervical posture tests before proceeding to positional testing. The test involves extending the patient's neck in different

positions. This test warns when there may be a risk of injuring a patient with cervical spine problems by performing the positional test too vigorously. It also has the advantage of identifying any cervical nystagmogenic factors. Patients with transient ischaemic attacks (TIA) due to atheroma within the vertebral arteries, perhaps aggravated by neck problems, can often be identified.

The head shaking test

This test has many similarities to the positional test except that it is performed in the plane of the lateral semicircular canals. The patient's head is shaken rapidly from side to side about 20 times. Patients suffering from vestibular lesions causing loss of the lateral canal responses on caloric testing often develop nystagmus which fatigues readily and is directed towards the opposite side. The test is not routinely employed as it has dangers, especially in the elderly and in patients with raised intracranial pressure or retinal detachment.

The positional test (Dix and Hallpike, 1952)

This test is performed by sitting the patient upright on a couch and then briskly taking his head backwards until it is positioned 30–45° to one side with the head extended 30° over the back of the couch (*Figure 2.2*). The patient's spectacles must be removed if these are worn. The patient is told not to close his eyes and to keep his gaze centred on the examiner's forehead. It can be much easier to see any nystagmus and to detect its direction if the patient wears Frenzel's glasses. If there is no nystagmus after 15 s have elapsed, the glasses should be removed as central nystagmus may be inhibited by the reduction in optic fixation.

   The positional test measures at least three nystagmogenic factors: the cervical factor, the movement factor and the positional factor.

The significance of positional nystagmus

There are two main categories of positional nystagmus, benign positional nystagmus (BPN) and central positional nystagmus (CPN). The main points of difference between the two are summarized in *Table 2.5*. There is also a third category, atypical positional nystagmus (APN) which resembles BPN but has some atypical features.

Benign positional nystagmus (BPN)

This is relatively common. It commonly occurs after head injuries. Barber (1964) found that 47 per cent of patients had persistent BPN after longitudinal fractures which affected the temporal bone. BPN may even occur after relatively mild head injuries. Less commonly BPN occurs as a consequence of infection or vascular occlusion. The patient notices the vertigo on stooping, looking up, or turning over in bed. Careful questioning will reveal that there is a critical head position which is related to subjective vertigo. The condition is usually self-limiting and gradually resolves after several months. Often there are recurrences which may be related to further episodes of head injury. Neuro-otological examination reveals normal bithermal caloric responses and there are no central nervous system abnormalities. The positional test is always associated with subjective vertigo; typically the patient cries out in horror. The nystagmus occurs after a brief latent period and is directed towards the downmost ear. The amplitude of the nystagmus is enhanced by the use of Frenzel's glasses. After a period of less than 30 s, the nystagmus ceases and the patient

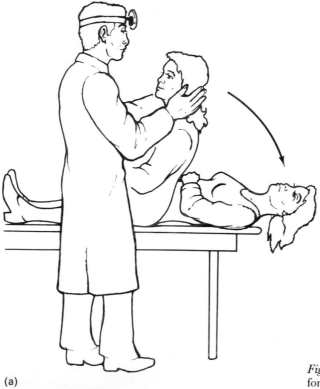

(a)

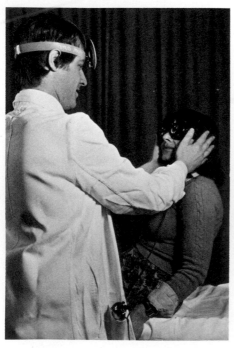

(b)

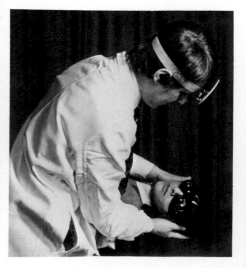

(c)

Figure 2.2   The test procedure for positional nystagmus

is no longer vertiginous even though the head position has not changed. On assuming the upright position again, the patient may experience some rebound positional nystagmus and vertigo. Some care has to be taken to differentiate rebound positional vertigo from transient cerebral ischaemia; patients receiving hypotensive drugs, for example, often experience vertigo if they rise too quickly from a lying position.

There is some dispute over the exact site of the lesion causing BPN. Bárány (1921) implicated the otolith organ and in histological studies Dix and Hallpike (1952) demonstrated pathological changes within the otolith organ. In their specimens, the subepithelial tissues were thickened with new bone formation, there was disappearance of the otolith membrane, fibrosis and irregular cell infiltrations. This picture suggests chronic inflammatory changes which could follow injury, vascular accident or circumscribed labyrinthitis.

The argument against the otolith organ being the primary site of dysfunction is that the vertigo is rotatory. A lesion of the otolith organ would be expected to cause a sensation of linear acceleration. Schuknecht (1962) believes that the dysfunction lies in the ampulla of the ipsilateral posterior semicircular canal. This does seem likely as the vertigo appears in the plane of that canal and would represent a recovery nystagmus like that seen on head shaking testing after a lateral semicircular canal lesion. A possible theory is that particles become detached from the otolith organ and float into the ampulla of the posterior semicircular canal affecting the function of the crista. Alternatively, a primary lesion of the crista may be postulated.

Central positional nystagmus (CPN)

This is by contrast with BPN relatively rare and often associated with the presence of intracranial tumours, multiple sclerosis or vascular disease. The striking features are the usual absence of any sensation of vertigo, the immediate onset of the nystagmus without any latent period, and the lack of any adaptation of the nystagmus. Occasionally CPN is the only sign of a posterior fossa tumour but generally other localizing signs can be detected. Commonly the tumour is a metastasis which has a primary elsewhere in the body, typically the bronchus. The responsible lesion is believed to involve the nervous pathways between the cerebellar roof nuclei and the medial vestibular nuclei.

Table 2.5 Differences between benign positional nystagmus (BPN) and central positional nystagmus (CPN)

	BPN	CPN
Latent period	2–10 s	None
Adaptation	Within 30 s	Persists
Fatiguability	Disappears on repetition	Persists
Vertigo	Present and may be severe	Usually absent or very mild
Direction of nystagmus	Towards downmost ear and enhanced by removing optic fixation	Variable
Incidence	Common	Rare

Atypical positional nystagmus (APN) resembles BPN but has atypical features, e.g. nystagmus is directed to uppermost ear, there is no latent period, or there is no adaptation. Patients suffering from vertebrobasilar insufficiency experience no significant vertigo in the head-down positions but some subjective vertigo on sitting up abruptly.

Atypical positional nystagmus (APN)

Although BPN and CPN are generally easily distinguished by their typical features, sometimes positional nystagmus is encountered which does not readily match either category. This type is associated with subjective vertigo but often there is no latent period, or no adaptation, or the nystagmus is not directed towards the downmost ear. The responsible lesion probably involves the neural pathways in the cerebellum which connect the nodulus to the otolith apparatus. Riesco McClure (1957) has reported APN in patients with tumours affecting the cerebellar vermis. APN may also be associated with plaques of multiple sclerosis.

Doll's head eye movements

The patient is asked to focus his eyes on an object (the lower edge of the optokinetic drum provides a suitable fixation point) and then his head is twisted up and down and from side to side. Loss of doll's head eye movements only occurs with extensive lesions of the brainstem, for instance after massive infarcts. Patients with tumours affecting the basal ganglia or anterior midbrain retain normal doll's head eye movements although they may be unable to move their eyes in a vertical direction on command or when following an optokinetic drum.

Optokinetic nystagmus

Optokinetic nystagmus is a normal phenomenon which may be observed on watching a train passenger's eyes when he is looking out of the window at the telegraph poles as they flash by. The passenger's eyes track each pole before returning quickly to focus on the next one.

Optokinetic nystagmus is more conveniently observed clinically by watching or recording with electronystagmography the patient's eye movements as he follows the black stripes on a revolving drum (*Figure 2.3*). The optokinetic nystagmus occurs in the opposite direction to that of the rotation of the drum (the exception is in patients with congenital nystagmus who often exhibit reversed optokinetic nystagmus).

The deviation of the eyes occurs in the direction of the slow component of the nystagmus when the subject is actively following the stripes on the drum. The direction of eye deviation is, however, in the direction of the fast component when the subject is merely gazing at the drum and not trying to follow the passing stripes (Hood and Leech, 1974).

Optokinetic nystagmus has a similar character to vestibular nystagmus as it is saw-toothed, and this gave rise to the original belief that the two reflexes involved a common neurological mechanism. In fact, the pathways subserving optokinetic nystagmus are entirely independent of those subserving the slow component of vestibular nystagmus. There are, nevertheless, common neurological pathways subserving conjugate voluntary gaze, the fast components of optokinetic nystagmus and vestibular nystagmus. These are thought to occupy the general region of the excitatory or activating reticular system. There is no doubt that the neural pathway of optokinetic nystagmus in man is complex and it is possible that more than one subcortical route exists (Hood, 1967). The abnormalities observed on testing patients with lesions at different levels in the nervous system are however a useful aid to neuro-otological diagnosis.

A directional preponderance towards the side of the lesion occurs with cortical and subcortical lesions. Carmichael, Dix and Hallpike (1954) showed that discrete lesions in a small area overlapping the occipital and parietal lobes affected the mechanism of optokinetic nystagmus because such lesions often extend deeply to involve the optic pathways. Lesions at lower levels within the brainstem tend to affect both the right and left optomotor pathways so that the responses tend to be absent, sluggish or broken up. The optokinetic directional preponderance may occur in the opposite direction to the bithermal caloric directional preponderance. Rarely, the optokinetic nystagmus may be reversed. In peripheral vestibular lesions, optokinetic nystagmus summates with the vestibular nystagmus and the directional preponderance tends to occur towards the normal ear.

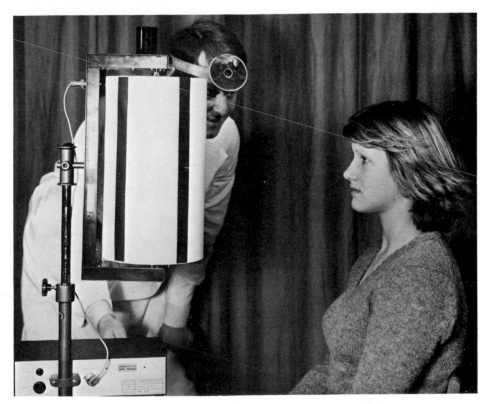

Figure 2.3   The test procedure for optokinetic nystagmus

Investigations

Investigation of disordered vestibular function includes audiometric tests. The usual audiometric tests are outlined in *Table 2.6* and these have been discussed in some detail in the preceding chapter. This discussion is mainly confined to the vestibular investigations.

Investigations of vestibular function

The vestibular tests included in the examination are usually performed by the clinician within the clinic. The investigations now described are often performed in a separate room and, perhaps, during a specially reserved time away from the rush of a busy clinic.

Table 2.6 Investigations (outline)

Audiometry	Pure-tone audiogram (including bone conduction thresholds if necessary)
	Loudness discomfort levels
	Tympanometry
	Acoustic reflex levels
	Acoustic reflex decay
if indicated	Loudness balance
	Tone decay
	Speech audiometry
if indicated	(Békésy audiometry)
	Electrocochleography
	Brainstem electrical responses (BER) (plus visual evoked responses if needed)
Vestibular tests	Bithermal caloric tests
	Electronystagmography
if indicated	Sono-ocular test
	Assessment of horizontal and vertical rotation testing
	(galvanic tests)
Radiographic investigations	Skull and neck
	Plain views of mastoids and IAMs
	Chest
if indicated	Paranasal sinuses
if indicated	Tomography of internal acoustic meatuses (IAM)
if indicated	Computerized axial tomography
if indicated	Contrast radiography
	Air studies
	Vertebral angiography
Blood investigations	Full blood picture (Hb, WBC, ESR)
	Serology including FTA abs.
in some instances	Barbiturate levels
	Other specific tests as indicated
Sundry investigations	Gamma scanning
	Electroencephalogram (EEG)
	Cerebrospinal fluid examination (CSF)

THE CALORIC TESTS

The caloric tests are the most useful tests of vestibular function in the absence of spontaneous nystagmus. They allow the vestibular function of each ear to be assessed independently.

The theory of the caloric test can be explained by considering the effect of irrigating the external acoustic meatus with cold water. The patient's head is first positioned so that the lateral semicircular canal (SCC) lies in a vertical plane (*Figure 2.4*). The cold water cools the bone around the lateral SCC as this is placed near to the tympanic membrane. The cooling causes a convection current within the labyrinthine fluid which falls away (ampullo-fugal) from the cristae of the lateral SCC. This bends the cristae downwards and so mimics a paralytic lesion by reducing the resting tonus. The result is nystagmus directed towards the opposite ear. Warm water has the contrary effect and causes nystagmus towards the same ear. Hence the mnemonic COWS (cold-opposite, warm-same).

If *both meatuses* are irrigated *simultaneously* with cold water, under normal circumstances the effect within both lateral SCC is equal and self-cancelling. Eventually, the cold water stimulates the vertical canals and causes a downward deflection of the eyes with an up-beating vertical nystagmus (CUD, cold-upward nystagmus).

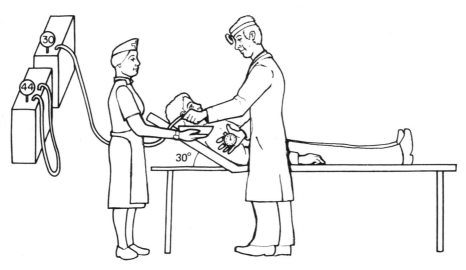

Figure 2.4 The test procedure for bithermal caloric testing

Many different methods of performing caloric tests have been described but the bithermal caloric test described by Fitzgerald and Hallpike (1942) has the advantage of quantification.

The Hallpike–Fitzgerald bithermal caloric test

This test is performed with the patient lying supine with his head raised by 30 degrees so that the lateral semicircular canal lies in the vertical plane (*Figure 2.4*). Each ear is irrigated in turn with water at 7° above or 7° below normal body temperature (30° or 44 °C) for periods of 40 s. It is essential that the ears are correctly irrigated. The meatus should be free of any cerumen; it may then be straightened and the water introduced. Then 250–500 ml of water should collect into the receiver. When in doubt the tympanic membrane is inspected after warm (44 °C) irrigation to check the presence of a red flush upon its surface.

There are several advantages in starting the test on the affected ear and using the warm water first. If the patient becomes nauseated, the test may have to be abandoned and this method ensures that the maximum amount of information possible has been obtained. If the test is abandoned after only cold water (30 °C), a canal paresis that is associated with a directional preponderance towards the opposite ear can be missed (*see Figure 2.5*).

It is important to ensure optic fixation before the onset of the nystagmus. The patient is asked to keep his eyes open and to gaze intently at a fixed point. The irrigation should continue for the full 40 s unless the patient becomes very nauseated. A severe caloric reaction may occur in the presence of a central lesion, and if the results of the previous examination have suggested this possibility, then special care should be taken. If after 20 s, the patient has developed nystagmus, the irrigation period should be limited to 30 s.

If there is no visible nystagmus in the presence of optic fixation, then fixation should be abolished by placing Frenzel's glasses on the patient or by observing the patient's eyes using an infrared viewer in total darkness. A comparison of the duration of nystagmus with and without optic fixation is known as the 'fixation index' and this has important diagnostic implications (*see below*).

The results of bithermal caloric testing in the presence of optic fixation are categorized in *Figure 2.5*. A normal reaction provides nystagmus which is no longer visible between 90 s and 140 s after the onset of the irrigation. In a normal subject the responses from each ear and at each temperature have durations within 20 s of each other.

A complete loss of labyrinthine function in one ear is shown by the total absence of nystagmus even in the absence of optic fixation. The test should be repeated using colder water (20 °C for 60 s) to ensure that there is indeed no reaction. Iced water should never be used as it is painful. It is rare to encounter total loss of vestibular function unless there is also total loss of cochlear function (a 'dead' ear).

A canal paresis of varying severity is due to a lesion of the phasic sensory vestibular elements and may be due to conditions affecting the labyrinths, the vestibular nerve or the vestibular nuclei within the brainstem. A directional preponderance is due to loss of tonus elements and commonly this occurs towards the unaffected ear. A right directional preponderance may indicate either left peripheral vestibular dysfunction or a central disorder, but if a left canal paresis is also evident, the cause lies either peripherally or at the vestibular nucleus. If optokinetic nystagmus reveals dissociated responses, the cause lies within the brainstem. When the caloric responses are enhanced, a directional preponderance most commonly indicates an ipsilateral lesion of the cerebellum or posterior temporal lobe or of the tracts which connect these structures to the vestibular nuclei. In recovering end-organ lesions, a slight directional preponderance may be directed towards the normal ear. Longstanding end-organ lesions may result in absence of any directional preponderance or even a directional preponderance directed towards the affected ear.

A very marked caloric response will occur if the ear is irrigated and the water passes into the middle-ear cavity. If the clinician overlooks a mastoid cavity, he will be

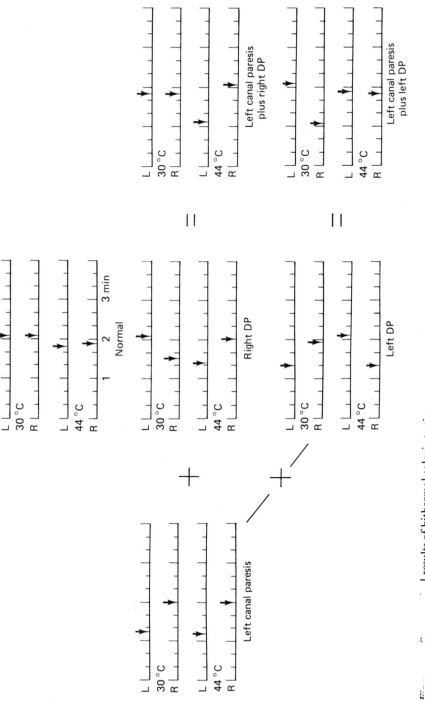

Figure ... Schematic results of bithermal caloric testing

horrified by the nystagmus he elicits by performing a water caloric test. The presence of any residual caloric function must be assessed in such patients by using an air caloric test. Enhanced caloric responses are also encountered in lesions involving the efferent vestibular fibres, multiple sclerosis, lesions affecting the cerebellum or temporal lobes in cases of raised intracranial pressure and in numerous other intracranial conditions.

Bilateral decreased caloric responses may indicate bilateral vestibular impairment (e.g. neurosyphilis). Alternatively decreased or absent responses may be due to habituation. For example, professional acrobats, ice-skaters, ballet dancers, etc., can suppress vestibular nystagmus by increasing their mechanism for optic fixation—so-called vestibular habituation. Anxious patients with longstanding vestibular impairments may also learn to suppress their vestibular responses. The situation is revealed by removing optic fixation and testing the patients with Frenzel's glasses, infrared light or electronystagmography.

The significance of optic fixation during caloric testing

Normally, the nystagmus induced by caloric testing is increased both in amplitude and in duration by the removal of optic fixation. There are several methods of abolishing optic fixation. These include the use of Frenzel's glasses in darkness (Frenzel's glasses in light reduce but do not abolish fixation), an infrared viewer in darkness, and the use of electronystagmography either with eye closure or in darkness.

The duration of the nystagmus in the absence of optic fixation is, in normal subjects, 2 min 40 s to 3 min 30 s and the mean duration is approximately 3 min. One problem is that the endpoint of the nystagmus is more difficult to detect with certainty than when there is optic fixation. It may seem strange that by increasing the sensitivity of the method, one is making the endpoint less certain but this can be explained on simple theoretical grounds. The response of the cupula to a caloric stimulus depends on its mechanical deflection which builds slowly and, after stimulation ceases, returns gradually under its own elastic forces (*Figure 2.6*). The neural activity which reaches the vestibular nuclei will follow a similar time course. At a point of time X, the neural activity is insufficient to evoke nystagmus in the presence of optic fixation and, as the cupula is moving relatively quickly at this point, the range of uncertainty is small (± 5 s). Later, at a point of time Y, the nystagmus ceases to be evident even in the absence of optic fixation and, as at this time the cupula is nearing its resting position, the cupula movement is relatively slow and the range of the endpoint of the nystagmus is large (± 15 s).

Electronystagmographic recordings of the caloric responses have many problems. It is difficult to detect the endpoint of the nystagmus either with or without optic fixation, and often the appearance of the first square wave or saccade is taken as the endpoint. Recording the caloric nystagmus with the eyes closed has several pitfalls. In many subjects, the eyes roll upwards and this movement inhibits the nystagmus (Bell's phenomenon). Often the eyes deviate towards the side of the slow component and this also inhibits the nystagmus. Even using DC recordings, these eye movements may be difficult to detect. The electronystagmographic recordings must be taken with the eyes open in darkness or with optic fixation. If darkness is preferred, the subject must undergo a period of dark adaptation before recordings are taken, as the corneo-retinal potential does not reach a constant figure for about 10 min. This requirement has disadvantages in a busy clinic. Naked eye observation has the advantage that the endpoint of the nystagmus can be estimated more reliably both with and without optic fixation, and also, that abnormalities in the character of the nystagmus, such as rotatory movements or movements in the vertical plane can easily be detected.

To overcome these problems, many workers have investigated other electronystagmographic measures of caloric nystagmus and these include the amplitude, the inter-beat interval and the velocity of the slow or fast phase. None of these measures have proved reliable. Henriksson (1956) made a direct comparison of the maximum slow component velocity and the durations of the four caloric responses in 25 normal subjects. He found that whereas the durations were relatively stable, the slow component velocities in any one subject showed considerable variations. Hood (1977) also found that the test/retest unreliability of the slow component velocity was unacceptably high. If experts have difficulties using slow component velocity measures, the clinician surely will obtain better results by using the simple duration measures with optic fixation and with optic fixation abolished by the use of Frenzel's glasses in darkness.

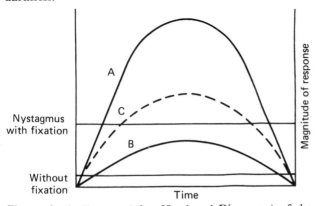

Figure 2.6 A diagram (after Hood and Dix, 1973) of the mechanical and neural responses of the cupula following thermal stimulation. *C* represents the time course of the mechanical cupula deflection which is similar when the vestibular nerve is functionally normal and when the nerve is damaged. *A* is the normal time course of the nystagmus when the nerve is normal and the amplitude of the nystagmus is sufficient to render it visible in the presence of optic fixation. *B* is the time course of the nystagmus when the nerve is damaged and the amplitude of the nystagmus is not sufficient to render it visible in the presence of optic fixation; note, however, that the duration of nystagmus measured without optic fixation is very similar to that of the normally-functioning nerve

The diagnostic importance of the fixation index

The duration of the caloric nystagmus may be recorded first with optic fixation and, secondly, without optic fixation. The difference between these two measures is known as the fixation index. The optic fixation index is useful in helping to place the actual site of a vestibular lesion (*Figure 2.7*).

(1) Lesions affecting cupula movement

Rarely do pathological conditions actually affect the movement of the cupula itself. More often they affect the nerve terminals or the nerve itself. One possible exception is Menière's disorder. Gibson, Moffatt and Hazell (1978) report that in 90 per cent of patients with Menière's disorder, the duration of the vestibular response in the affected ear is reduced *both with and without* optic fixation. The induced nystagmus is conjugate and enhanced when the patient looks in the direction of the fast phase. On removal of optic fixation, the nystagmus reappears with the same characteristics but the duration is less than 2 min 45 s.

(2) Lesions affecting the vestibular nerve, vestibular ganglion or vestibular nuclei
If there is total loss of nervous function, then there is no induced nystagmus either with or without optic fixation. If some residual function remains, the time course of cupula

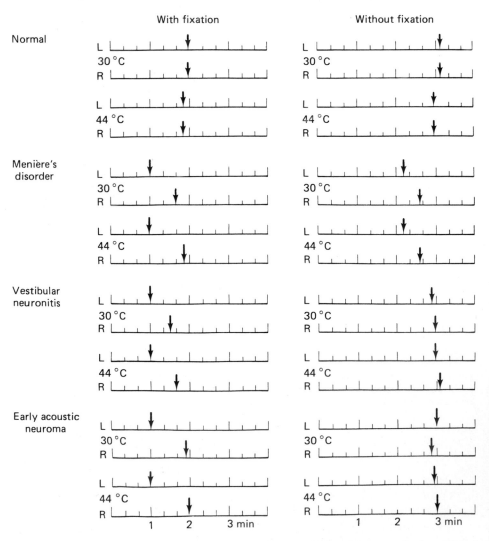

Figure 2.7   A comparison of the results of bithermal caloric testing in some typical peripheral vestibular lesions. The duration of the visible induced nystagmus both with optic fixation and without optic fixation (Frenzel's glasses in darkness) are shown. Note the diagnostic value of the optic fixation index, and note that measuring the duration of nystagmus with reduced optic fixation alone (Frenzel's glasses in light) produces almost valueless information

movement being normal, the duration of the nystagmus in the absence of optic fixation is virtually identical to that of the normal response. It is only the duration of the response with optic fixation that is reduced (see *Figure 2.6*). It is difficult to detect the caloric abnormality due to an early acoustic neuroma if the testing is performed in darkness or with eye closure. Even using Frenzel's glasses in the light may lead to misdiagnosis.

(3) Cerebellar and brainstem lesions

The caloric response may be exaggerated in these patients either in amplitude or duration or both. The removal of optic fixation does not influence the nystagmus so that, if the eyes are examined with Frenzel's glasses in darkness after the nystagmus is no longer evident with optic fixation, there appears to be no nystagmus visible.

(4) Temporal lobe lesions

The direction of the nystagmus may reverse on removal of optic fixation.

OTHER METHODS OF CALORIC TESTING

The Kobrak method

This involves irrigating the external meatus with 10–50 ml of iced water and observing the nystagmus through Frenzel's glasses. The disadvantages include absence of quantification, failure to detect the relatively common presence of a canal paresis associated with a contralateral directional preponderance and the loss of the clear endpoint given by optic fixation. This test can never detect the presence of an early acoustic neuroma.

The hot caloric test

This is probably the best caloric screening test (Barber, Wright and DeManuele, 1971). If use is made of the optic fixation index, many of the abnormalities present on bithermal testing can be detected and the clinician can save valuable time. Mistakes may be made in longstanding cases of vestibular dysfunction.

The minimal caloric test

This has some use as a screening test but only in the identification of a 'dead ear'. The patient sits and extends his neck backwards by 60 degrees. The meatus is filled with 10 ml of cold tap water and any nystagmus is observed through Frenzel's glasses. Usually nystagmus is observed without the patient experiencing any vertigo. The advantage is that the test can be used as a very quick office procedure which does not upset the patient. Obviously there are many disadvantages and in addition to those outlined in describing the Kobrak technique, the extension of the neck could produce nystagmus due to vertebral artery compression.

The air caloric test

This may have the advantage of not soaking the patient should the irrigation be performed carelessly and of being applicable to patients with tympanic membrane perforations. There are two problems. Firstly, the temperature of the air in the external meatus must be known accurately as air cools rapidly. This difficulty is overcome by modern technology as the air temperature can be accurately monitored at the probe tip. Secondly, the specific heat of air is much lower than that of water, which means that a greater temperature difference is needed to alter the temperature within the labyrinth by the same amount compared to water. Coats, Herbert and Atwood (1976) advise a flow rate of 13 litre/min through a 3 mm probe tip. An air temperature of 45.5 °C corresponds with a water irrigation of 44 °C, and an air temperature of 17.5 °C corresponds with a water temperature of 30 °C, but the air irrigation must last 100 s compared with the 40 s of water irrigation. There are further difficulties as the amount of bone lying over the lateral canal varies between subjects. The other major disadvantage lies with the high cost of the equipment which is many times that of a douche can.

Dundas Grant air caloric test

Here is the most convenient means of excluding a 'dead ear' in the presence of a tympanic perforation or mastoid cavity, unless there is sophisticated air caloric equipment available. Ethyl chloride is sprayed onto a coiled copper tube while air is pumped through the tube into the external meatus. If the patient develops vertigo and nystagmus, some residual labyrinthine function is present. It is not possible to quantify this test.

ELECTRONYSTAGMOGRAPHY (ENG)

In theory, this test should be named 'electro-oculography' to conform with the nomenclature of other tests, e.g. electrocochleography, electrocardiography, etc., but as the term 'electronystagmography' has already been widely accepted, it is used in this text. There are two methods of recording the eye movements electrically which are commonly used.

The photoelectric method

A beam of light is focused onto the sclera of the subject and the reflection is measured. This method is often difficult to use as random eye movements may seriously interfere with the test. The other disadvantage is that the nystagmus cannot be recorded with the eyes closed. The only real use of the photoelectric method is during galvanic testing.

The corneo-retinal potential method

Each eye acts as an electrical dipole; an electric field exists between the cornea (electrically-positive) and the retina (electrically-negative). ENG detects movements of these electrical fields and records them onto a continuous tracing. The polarity of the recording is arranged so that a deflection of the eye to the left causes a downward deflection of the pen, and a deflection of the eye to the right causes an upward deflection of the pen. The electrodes are placed lateral to each eye and on the forehead between the eyes. A single channel ENG machine summates the movements of both eyes onto the same trace. A two channel ENG machine records the movement of each eye separately and provides a sensitive means of detecting dissociated eye movements. A four channel machine, in addition, records the vertical movements of each eye and allows a separate assesment of the vertical components of nystagmus.

There is dispute in the literature over the relative merits of AC and DC ENG machines. An AC machine does not reveal the exact position of the eyes and slow eye movements are not detected. The AC machine will provide a tracing in the centre of the paper even if the eyes are twisted to one side. At Queen Square, it is felt that AC recordings are unsatisfactory in clinical neuro-otology for the following reasons: the eyes tend to deviate towards the slow component when the lids are closed, causing suppression of nystagmus; there are difficulties in recording the pendulum swing test; and the failure of gaze deviation maintenance is an important sign of cerebellar disease. The only advantage of an AC machine is that it is much easier to obtain electrode stability. Casual testing with dirty electrodes and poorly applied leads renders DC techniques unreadable.

Calibrating the ENG tracing
The patient is asked to look towards a mark 3 m directly in front of him, and then to look at marks 30 degrees to either side. The ENG records this known amount of eye movement and so it is possible to measure the absolute amplitude of any eye movements which occur (*Figure 2.8*).

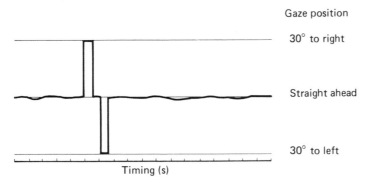

Figure 2.8 Calibration of electronystagmographic tracings

Measuring the nystagmus
The amplitude of any nystagmus is simply measured with reference to the calibration. The interbeat interval is measured using the time base—usually a marker indicates the passing of each second. The most useful measure is probably the velocity of the slow component. This can be simply measured by extending a line along the axis of the slow component until it covers the period of 1 s and by measuring its amplitude, e.g. 15 degrees/s (*Figure 2.9*).

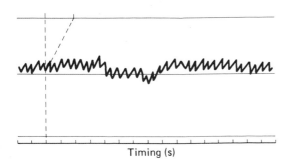

Figure 2.9 Measurement of the velocity of the slow component of a right spontaneous nystagmus

Table 2.7   Effects of abolishing optic fixation upon spontaneous nystagmus

Lesion	Darkness	Eye closure
Labyrinthine or eighth nerve	Nystagmus enhanced if present or made manifest if not	Nystagmus enhanced if present or made manifest if not
At or about the level of the vestibular nuclei	Nystagmus alters little in amplitude but the velocity of the slow component decreases	Nystagmus abolished
Above the level of the vestibular nuclei in the brainstem	Nystagmus abolished	Nystagmus abolished
Posterior temporal lobe or subcortical level	Nystagmus abolished or even reversed in direction	Nystagmus abolished

The clinical results

The main advantage of ENG is that some patients reveal nystagmus which is not readily visible on naked eye examination. ENG recordings also allow for quantification and the provision of a permanent record of the nystagmus. The clinical application is best considered by mentioning the findings under various circumstances (*Table 2.7*).

(1) Peripheral vestibular disorders

These may not cause nystagmus in the presence of optic fixation but the nystagmus is revealed or increased in amplitude on eye closure and in darkness. The eye movements are conjugate. The nystagmus is unidirectional with the largest amplitude on lateral gaze towards the direction of the fast component (*Figure 2.10*).

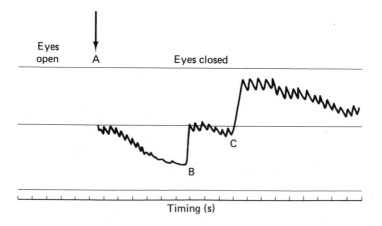

Figure 2.10   ENG in a peripheral vestibular disorder

(2) Lesions affecting the vestibular nuclei (nuclear lesions)

These are lesions such as a medially-placed eighth nerve tumour, and they provide nystagmus which is reduced or abolished by eye-closure. In darkness, the amplitude of the nystagmus may hardly alter but the velocity of the slow phase may be decreased. Often the nystagmus is bidirectional.

(3) Lesions of brainstem above the vestibular nuclei (supranuclear lesions)
These lesions may exhibit a nystagmus which is reduced or more often abolished both by eye closure and by darkness. The nystagmus may be disassociated. Optokinetic ENG recording usually reveals broken up, sluggish responses.

(4) Lesions of the cortex and subcortical levels (supratentorial lesions)
Spontaneous nystagmus is uncommon. Eye closure and darkness suppress the nystagmus and may even reverse its direction.

(5) Congenital nystagmus
This generally has a pendular character although saw-toothed (similar to vestibular) nystagmus may be supra-added on lateral gaze. Congenital nystagmus is usually unaffected by removal of optic fixation. The optokinetic responses are always abnormal and are often reversed.

(6) Cerebellar disorders
These may be revealed by the presence of multiple saccades or square waves (*Figure 2.11*). Another highly characteristic abnormality which can only be detected in DC ENG recordings is the failure to maintain lateral gaze either in darkness or with eye-closure, and slow drifting movements of the eyes in the absence of fixation (Leech *et al.*, 1977). Centripetal nystagmus, in which the fast phase of the nystagmus beats

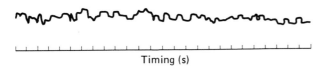

Timing (s)

Figure 2.11   ENG in a cerebellar disorder (saccades)

towards the position of primary gaze on eye-closure or in darkness, and rebound nystagmus (Hood, Kayan and Leech, 1973) are common in cerebellar disease but are also encountered in a variety of other conditions including peripheral vestibular disorders, drug intoxication and congenital abnormalities. Rebound nystagmus is best explained by describing a typical example: nystagmus to the right is evident on gaze deviation to the right, but unlike brainstem nystagmus it is transitory and only persists for some 20 s. If at the end of this period the eyes are returned to the primary position of gaze, then a transitory nystagmus to the left, not present initially, makes its appearance. Next gaze deviation to the left brings about transitory nystagmus to the left, and on returning the eyes to the primary position a nystagmus now beating to the right is produced.

   Patients with cerebellar disease may also have difficulties in executing command saccadic eye movements. When they are asked to turn their gaze laterally quickly, they overshoot the target. This abnormality is known as ocular dysmetria (Orzechowski, 1927). If present, it may be easily detected on ENG recordings.

The early detection of internuclear ophthalmoplegia

ENG can provide an early diagnosis of internuclear ophthalmoplegia. This condition manifests itself as a weakness or slowing of adduction on lateral deviation of the eyes on command or when executing the fast movement of optokinetic nystagmus. Bilateral internuclear ophthalmoplegia is pathognomonic of multiple sclerosis and indicates a high pontine lesion.

The ENG recordings are taken from both eyes separately (dual channel recording) using DC coupling. Normal eye velocities fall within the range 450–600 degrees/s and in general adduction is faster than abduction.

The pendulum eye-tracking test

The patient is asked to follow the movement of a pendulum as it swings from side to side about 0.5 m before his eyes. Normally the eyes follow the path of the pendulum smoothly and exactly (*Figure 2.12a*). Patients with mild peripheral vestibular disorders either have normal eye-tracking movements or occasional slight non-nystagmic deviations (*Figure 2.12b*). Patients with spontaneous nystagmus may show evidence of the nystagmus superimposed on the tracing (*Figure 2.12c*), particularly when they gaze in the direction of the fast nystagmic component. Patients with central disorders often show superimposed saccadic eye movements. Ataxic eye-tracking movements are pathognomonic of brainstem involvement (*Figure 2.12d*).

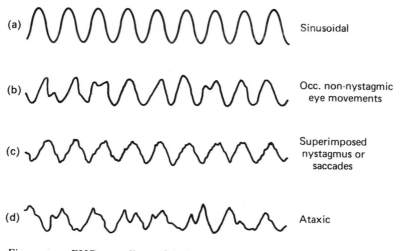

(a) Sinusoidal

(b) Occ. non-nystagmic eye movements

(c) Superimposed nystagmus or saccades

(d) Ataxic

Figure 2.12   ENG recordings of the pendulum swing test

ROTATIONAL TESTS

The rotational tests are performed by sitting the patient on a revolving chair which moves with high precision at angular acceleration of known duration and magnitude.

The advantage of rotational testing is that the precise physical force applied to the labyrinths can be calculated. The disadvantage is that both labyrinths are stimulated simultaneously and it is difficult to interpret the responses with respect to one particular labyrinth. Rotational tests provide an overall picture of labyrinthine function which may be helpful in determining bilateral labyrinthine damage, as follows streptomycin intoxication, or in demonstrating a directional preponderance.

The rotational testing is performed either with the eyes focused on a point which revolves with the patient (optic fixation) or in darkness (without optic fixation). The difference between the two measures provides a 'fixation index'.

Two types of rotational response can be demonstrated.

(1) Responses to angular acceleration

The cupulae of the semicircular canals respond to angular acceleration (increasing speed of rotation). The normal subjective threshold for the sensation of turning is about 0.5 degree/s^2. The threshold for recordable nystagmus is more sensitive than the threshold for subjective sensation. The induced nystagmus occurs in the direction of rotation of the chair, and the nystagmus threshold varies considerably in normal subjects according to whether optic fixation is present or absent. (The threshold is that angular acceleration which, when maintained for 20 s, is sufficient to evoke a just-recordable nystagmus.) The normal threshold in the absence of optic fixation is 0.15 degree/s^2, which is well below the subjective threshold for sensation and so provides a remarkably sensitive indication of labyrinthine function. With optic fixation, the nystagmus threshold is raised and is normally about 1 degree/s^2. In ballet dancers and in other 'vestibular acrobats', the threshold with optic fixation is even higher, sometimes reaching 7 degree/s^2, but the nystagmus threshold in darkness is quite normal. This clearly demonstrates that the mechanism for vestibular habituation in these subjects is due to an enhancement of the optic fixation mechanism. Sometimes a similar vestibular habituation is encountered on testing patients suffering from anxiety states.

(2) Responses to impulsive stimuli

Commonly the rotational chair is used to demonstrate the nystagmus resulting from impulsive stimuli. These stimuli result from suddenly starting the chair from a stationary position until it reaches a constant angular velocity, or suddenly stopping the chair from a constant angular velocity. These impulsive stimuli normally produce a nystagmus which may last for 30 s or more.

Impulsive stimuli can be used to demonstrate a directional preponderance. For example, a left directional preponderance is shown by a greater response on arresting the chair moving to the right (inducing a left nystagmus), than on arresting the chair moving to the left. This can be useful in the detection of cerebral lesions as, in darkness, the directional preponderance is either abolished or reversed in direction.

GALVANIC STIMULATION

This test has limited clinical value because its mechanism is unknown and the interpretation of the results is controversial. The usual technique is to fix surface electrodes over each mastoid process and to apply a DC current. Normally, a current of 1–2 mA induces a nystagmus directed towards the negative electrode. On switching off the current, the induced nystagmus usually reverses its direction for a short while.

The galvanic test gives a normal result in all vestibular end-organ disorders unless these have existed for many years with the consequence of neural degeneration. The galvanic response is typically absent with eighth nerve disorders including Schwannoma. Brainstem vestibular lesions do not produce any real change in the galvanic responses.

THE SONO-OCULAR TEST

The test is based on the Tullio phenomenon which relates to the induction of vertigo in certain pathological conditions on hearing very loud sounds. Classically, the Tullio phenomenon occurs if there is more than one mobile window on the vestibular side of the vestibular membrane and it was commonly noted in the days of fenestration operations. The phenomenon also occurs in other conditions such as congenital hearing loss, direct vestibular trauma, endolymphatic hydrops and after stapedectomy (Stephens and Ballam, 1974).

The sono-ocular test is an attempt to quantify the Tullio phenomenon. Loud sounds are introduced into the ear (usually 2 pulses/s at 110 dB HL at frequencies between 500 and 4000 Hz, and at 120 dB at 250 Hz). Any resulting nystagmus is measured using electronystagmography.

The practical value of the test is that it identifies end-organ vestibular dysfunction with certainty.

JUDGEMENT OF THE VISUAL VERTICAL AND HORIZONTAL (Friedmann, 1970)

For this test, the subject is seated and from a distance of 2 m he views a blackboard which bears an illuminated rod 0.5 m in length. The patient can rotate the rod by operating a control. Initially he judges the horizontal and vertical with the lights switched on, and then he repeats the test several times in darkness. The typical findings are:

Normal subjects can judge the horizontal and vertical with an error of less than 2 degrees.

Patients with peripheral and end-organ vestibular disorders and even most patients after unilateral labyrinthectomy can judge the horizontal and vertical within normal limits. A few patients immediately after labyrinthectomy show abnormal judgement in that they misplace the vertical towards the side of the lesion.

No abnormality can be detected in most patients with cerebellar and cortical lesions.

Patients with large eighth nerve tumours which are compressing the brainstem often deviate in their judgement of the vertical towards the side of the lesion.

The group of patients which does show marked deviations from normal is the group with unilateral brainstem damage. Marked deviations from normal are common in patients with multiple sclerosis.

Final remarks and acknowledgements

This brief account of a complex subject has inevitably left several fields unmentioned but it has attempted to concentrate on those details which are most likely to be important for the practising otologist. The methods described have often been developed at The National Hospital, Queen Square, and this account relates closely to the current clinical assessment routinely used at this hospital. There are several differences between these techniques and those practised elsewhere, particularly in the United States. In this respect the author has tried to present a reasoned approach so that the reader can reach his own conclusions.

The differential diagnosis of the pathological conditions causing vertigo may be classified into peripheral vestibular disorders and central vestibular disorders. A description of the neurological causes is to be found in Chapter 26, and the peripheral causes are mentioned in separate chapters (Menière's disease, Chapter 25, Eighth nerve tumours, Chapter 13)

Finally, I would like to thank my colleagues at The National Hospital, Queen Square, for their help and advice concerning this chapter. In particular, I would like to thank Dr Margaret Dix as she has been most helpful and kind.

References

Aschan, G. (1961) 'The pathogenesis of positional nystagmus', *Acta Otolaryngologica, suppl.,* **159,** 90

Bárány, R. (1921) 'Diagnose von krankheitserscheinungen im bereiche des otolithenapparates', *Acta Otolaryngologica,* **2,** 434

Barber, H. O. (1964) 'Positional nystagmus, especially after head injury', *Laryngoscope,* **74,** 891

Barber, H. O., Wright, G. and DeManuele, F. (1971) 'The hot caloric test as a clinical screening device', *Archives of Otolarngology,* **94,** 335

Carmichael, E. A., Dix, M. R. and Hallpike, C. S. (1954) 'Lesions of the cerebral hemispheres and their effects upon optokinetic and caloric nystagmus', *Brain,* **77,** 345

Carmichael, E. A., Dix, M. R. and Hallpike, C. S. (1965) 'Observations upon the neurological mechanism of directional preponderance of caloric nystagmus resulting from vascular lesions of the brainstem', *Brain,* **88,** 51

Coats, A. C., Herbert, F. and Atwood, G. R. (1976) 'The air caloric test', *Archives of Otolaryngology,* **102,** 343

Dix, M. R. and Hallpike, C. S. (1952) 'The pathology, symptomatology and diagnosis of certain common disorders of the vestibular system', *Proceedings of the Royal Society of Medicine,* **45,** 341

Dix, M. R. and Hallpike, C. S. (1966) 'Observations on the clinical features and neurological mechanism of spontaneous nystagmus resulting from unilateral acoustic neurofibromata', *Acta Otolaryngologica,* **61,** 1

FitzGerald, G. and Hallpike, C. S. (1942) 'Observations on the directional preponderance of caloric nystagmus resulting from cerebral lesions', *Brain,* **65,** 115

Frederickson, J. M., Figge, U., Scheid, P. and Kornhuber, H. H. (1966) 'Vestibular nerve projection to the cerebral cortex of the rhesus monkey', *Experimental Brain Research,* **2,** 318

Frenzel, H. (1928) 'Der nachweis von schwachem bei gewöhnlicher beobachtung nicht sichtbarem spontannystagmus', *Klinische Wochemschrift.,* **41,** 461

Friedmann, G. (1970) 'The judgement of the visual vertical and horizontal with peripheral and central vestibular lesions', *Brain,* **93,** 313

Gibson, W. P. R., Moffat, D. A. and Hazell, J. W. P. (1978) 'Human electrophysiology in the diagnosis and understanding of Menière's disorder'. Paper read at Summer meeting of sections of Laryngology and Otology of the Royal Society of Medicine, July 1978, Cranwell, England

Henriksson, N. G. (1956) 'Speed of the slow component and duration in caloric nystagmus', *Acta Otolaryngologica, suppl.* **125,** 1

Hood, J. D. (1967) 'Observations upon the neurological mechanism of optokinetic nystagmus with special reference to the contribution of peripheral vision', *Acta Otolaryngologica,* **63,** 208

Hood, J. D. (1977) 'Whither vestibular tests? (Editorial)' *Proceedings of the Royal Society of Medicine,* **70,** 675

Hood, J. D. and Dix, M. R. (1973) 'The significance of optic fixation in tests of vestibular function', *Equilibrium Research,* **3,** 95

Hood, J. D., Kayan, A. and Leech, J. (1973) 'Rebound nystagmus', *Brain,* **96,** 483

Hood, J. D. and Leech, J. (1974) 'The significance of peripheral vision in the perception of movement', *Acta Otolaryngologica,* **77,** 72

Leech, J., Gresty, M., Hess, K. and Rudge, P. (1977) 'Gaze failure, drifting eye movements and centripetal nystagmus in cerebellar disease', *British Journal of Ophthalmology,* **61,** 774

Orzechowski, C. (1927) 'De l'ataxie dysmetrique des yeux', *Neurologie,* **35,** 1

Owada, K., Shiizu, S. and Kimura, K. (1960) 'The influence of the utricle on nystagmus', *Acta Otolaryngologica,* **52,** 215

Riesco McClure, J. S. (1957) 'Es el vertigo aural de origen exclusivamente periferico?' *Review of Otorhinolaryngology,* **17,** 42

Schuknecht, H. F. (1962) 'Positional vertigo; clinical and experimental observations', *Transactions of the American Academy of Ophthalmology and Otology,* **66,** 319

Stephens, S. D. G. and Ballam, H. M. (1974) 'The sono-ocular test', *Journal of Laryngology,* **88,** 1049

3 Tinnitus
J W P Hazell

Tinnitus aurium (L. tinnire, to ring, tinkle) is the sensation of sound when there is no relevant external auditory stimulus present. *Subjective* tinnitus is audible only to the sufferer and usually indicates an abnormality in the auditory system. *Objective* tinnitus is an interesting rarity by comparison; it can be heard by others, and is often due to pathology outside the ear.

Objective tinnitus

Politzer first described palatal myoclonus in 1878, and this is the commonest cause of objective tinnitus. An irregular clicking sound may be heard in either or both ears and synchronous myoclonic contractions of the palate are often seen on indirect nasopharyngoscopy (MacKinnon, 1968). The condition is probably psychogenic and analogous to a nervous tic (Leventon, Mau and Floru, 1968); conscious suppression is often possible. However there is some evidence that neurological abnormalities may exist in the inferior olive (Weinstein and Bender, 1943; Bolrovnikova and Grigoriev, 1974) or in the olivo-dentate pathways (Herrmann, Crandall and Fang, 1957). Myoclonic tinnitus may be detected with an auscultation tube or by acoustic impedance testing (Coles, Snashall and Stephens, 1975). The condition is very resistant to treatment although insertion of a grommet in the affected ear may give temporary relief. Less often clicking tinnitus is due to myoclonus of the stapedius or tensor tympani muscles (Watanabe, Kumagami and Tsuda, 1974).

Pulsatile tinnitus due to vascular abnormalities are sometimes audible (Frank and Horak, 1976) and examination should always include auscultation of the head and neck with a stethoscope. A glomus jugulare tumour may present in this way (House and Glasscock, 1968). Aneurysms or arterio-venous fistulae (Tewfik, 1974) may cause tinnitus. The occipital artery (Arenberg and McCreary, 1971), superficial temporal artery (Zakrzewski, Kruk-zagajewska and Konopacki, 1971) and aortic arch (Schechter and Brownson, 1970) have been implicated; tinnitus often ceases on surgical correction of the defect. Cases of high-tone objective tinnitus have been described (Glanville and Coles, 1971; Huizing and Spoor, 1973) and are thought to be due to fibrous strands vibrating in the sigmoid or jugular blood flow.

Other physiological sounds may cause complaint, especially if conductive deafness is present. The commonest are the popping or crackling noises of eustachian tube obstruction or clicking sounds from the temporo-mandibular joint.

Occasionally infestation of the external meatus may present as objective tinnitus. Earwigs, cockroaches (Coles, Snashall and Stephens, 1975) and silverfish (Burgers, 1971) have been among the offenders.

Subjective tinnitus

Subjective tinnitus is extremely common, yet the patient seeking medical advice seldom gets much sympathy or help. A change in attitude is needed.

Incidence

The American National Health Survey in 1968 found 36 million American adults (approx 20 per cent of the population) suffered from tinnitus, which was 'severe' in 7.2 million (4 per cent). Almost everyone can hear some tinnitus (usully white noise) provided the environmental masking noise is removed by listening in a sound proofed room (Heller and Bergmann, 1953). In addition there is the common experience of transitory tonal tinnitus lasting only a few seconds, and of which some people are more aware than others. These types of physiological noise in the auditory system may well distort surveys based on questionnaires.

Age

The commonest age of onset is 50–60 years (Venters, 1953; Reed, 1960; Hinchcliffe, 1961). *Figure 3.1* shows the ages of cases presenting primarily with tinnitus at the Royal National Institute for the Deaf, London in 1975 and 1976. Nodar in 1972 investigated tinnitus in school children in New York over three years and found an overall incidence of 15 per cent which rose to 58 per cent in the group which failed auditory screening. Tinnitus is extremely rare in severe congenital deafness; auditory experience seems to be a prerequisite. However it may occur where there is a moderate congenital loss with a progressive element. There is a slight predominance of the symptom among women, but this could reflect variation in environmental noise.

Predisposing factors

The fact that tinnitus is often completely absent in sensorineural deafness (36 per cent in a recent random survey among deaf patients) is perhaps more suprising than finding sufferers amongst the normal hearing population (Kimura, 1974). When it occurs in conjunction with deafness, many attempts have been made to use it diagnostically. Douek and Reid in 1968 showed remarkable correlation between the pitch of tinnitus and the Clinical diagnosis. Correlation in two groups supported by clinical experience were the acoustic trauma group with high-tonal tinnitus and the Menière's group with low frequency tinnitus. Other authors, especially Reid (1960) in his analysis of 200 cases, found no correlation between any of the parameters that were measured.

There would appear to be a clear causal relationship between acoustic trauma and tinnitus although the onset may be years after the exposure. Salmivalli (1967) described tinnitus after gunfire in army personnel. Short duration tinnitus induced by noise was investigated by Loeb and Smith (1967) and Hempstock and Atherley (1970) who pointed out the relationship with temporary threshold shift.

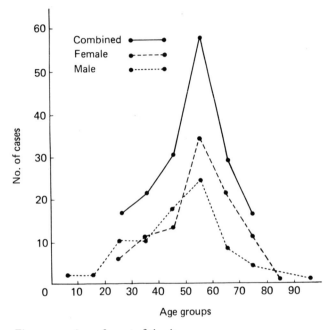

Figure 3.1 Age of onset of tinnitus

All the ototoxic drugs may cause tinnitus although this is usually associated with severe sensory damage. Aspirin is unique and interesting in this context in that tinnitus is often the first symptom of high dosage and is used by rheumatologists as a means of controlling blood levels (Myers and Bernstein, 1965; Morgan *et al.*, 1973; Mitchell *et al.*, 1973; McPherson and Miller, 1974). Hearing almost always returns to normal and the tinnitus disappears on withdrawing the aspirin. Unilateral tinnitus is the presenting symptom in acoustic neuroma in 8–10 per cent of cases (Ellis and Wright, 1974; Thomsen and Terkildsen, 1975).

Just occasionally patients present with tinnitus as a symptom of other systemic disease such as anaemia, Pagets disease (Gibson, 1973) or disseminated sclerosis. It is worth remembering in the enthusiasm of operating to correct otosclerotic deafness, that one of the most severe forms of tinnitus follows failed stapedectomy. In the surgery of otosclerosis with tinnitus, closure of the air-bone gap is not always accompanied by relief of tinnitus, especially when high frequency sensory loss pre-exists. A small number of patients with tinnitus have middle-ear effusions, but impacted wax is more often a result of poking down the ear in an attempt to obtain relief.

Aetiology of idiopathic subjective tinnitus

In the majority of cases, where a precise clinical diagnosis cannot be made it is a matter of conjecture where and what the causative lesion is. It is tempting to think of tonal unilateral tinnitus being produced by the cochlea (Fowler, 1939) but this may not be so. Cochlear nerve section, or the introduction of local anaesthetic into the cochlea may not abolish the tinnitus. Kemp and Martin (1976) however, showed that the 'microstructure' of the pure-tone audiogram contains many areas of increased sensitivity. These sometimes coincide with the pitch of tinnitus and it is tempting to postulate that neural resonators exist at these points.

It is much more likely that many different pathologies can exist. These may include small areas of demyelination in the acoustic pathway, or non-functioning nerve fibres causing an absence of spontaneous discharge. Pulsatile and some 'white noise' tinnitus is likely to be due to abnormalities in the microcirculation of the cochlea especially in view of the proximity of the stria vascularis to the organ of Corti. It is naive to expect that these microscopic abnormalities will necessarily relate to specific clinical diagnoses and as a result treatment based on these premises is unlikely to be successful.

Measurement of tinnitus

Assessment of the severity of tinnitus or its response to treatment is normally left to the patient's subjective report. This is notoriously unreliable and relates as much to the individual's personality and mood, as to the actual loudness of the tinnitus. The major efforts of investigators are summarized in *Table 3.1*.

Table 3.1   Tinnitus measurement

Masking by pure tones	Wegel (1931)
Measurement by loudness balance	Fowler (1939)
Free field matching of tinnitus	Mortimer (1940)
Masking in 'central' and 'peripheral' tinnitus	Fowler (1944)
Identification using taped sound effects	Goodhill (1952)
Audiometric study of 200 cases	Reed (1960)
Diagnostic value of tinnitus pitch	Douek and Reid (1968)
Classification of tinnitus by masking behaviour	Feldman (1971)

Feldman's technique uses the narrow band masking of a clinical audiometer. Slowly increasing levels of noise are presented through headphones until the tinnitus is no longer audible. The point of masking of the tinnitus is measured for different frequencies and a masking audiogram is produced (*Figure 3.2*). Sometimes residual inhibition occurs and the tinnitus disappears for a period after the masking noise is switched off.

The commonest types of subjective tinnitus are like pure tones or bands of white noise. However it is quite common for multiple sounds to be heard in different parts of the head. They can be very complex and bizarre, defying description.

Attempts to identify the frequency and spectrum of tinnitus by a matching technique very often produces spurious results. This indicates the limitations of an

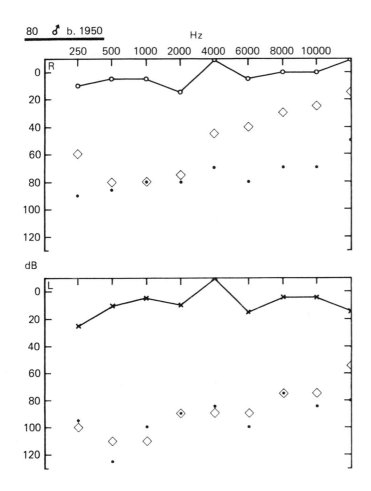

Masking: narrow band ◇   pure tone •

Figure 3.2   Masking audiogram

audiometer in providing comparison sounds. The author has used a commercially available music synthesizer (*see Figure 3.3*) which is theoretically capable of infinite variation and which often can produce an exact match for subjective tinnitus. Apart from being able to match cases of multiple and bizarre tinnitus, pulsatile signals can be presented for the correct identification of haemodynamic abnormalities. Although it may take a considerable time to achieve a good 'match' with this technique it is clear that many forms of tinnitus simply described as 'pure tone' are in fact more complex.

Attempts to measure the loudness of tinnitus by a loudness balance technique often appear to show severe tinnitus as relatively quiet. Fowler used this fact to reassure his patients that they were worrying over nothing. However this technique does not take into account the difficulties of comparing the loudness of a pure tone with a complex sound, or the reduced dynamic range that may be present in an ear with recruitment. If only ordinary acoustic equipment is available Feldman's tests are probably the most useful and repeatable.

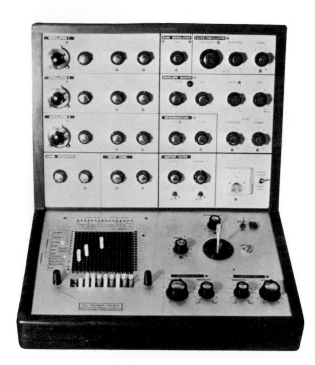

Figure 3.3   Apparatus used for tinnitus synthesis

In tonal tinnitus a 'dip' may be seen on the pure-tone audiogram at the frequency of the tinnitus (Sedlacek, 1948; Douek and Reid, 1968). Whether this is due to 'masking' of the stimulus tone by tinnitus or reduction of the threshold as part of the pathology is not clear. Some patients have no change in their speech discrimination, despite loud tinnitus. Others complain bitterly that they can hear nothing because of it.

Management

Goodhill wrote in 1954 'The treatment of tinnitus as a disease is an illogical dream, but the management of the patient with tinnitus is an everyday necessity'. Many efforts have been made over the centuries to 'cure' tinnitus and these are summarized in *Table 3.2*.

It is important to keep in mind the treatable causes, and apart from a thorough examination of the ears, nose and throat with pure-tone audiometry, tests should include haemoglobin and serological tests for syphilis. Most busy ENT departments will be unable to perform full neuro-otological examinations in all cases of tinnitus, neither is this desirable. However unilateral cases should at least be kept under review.

(1) Menière's disease

The tinnitus of Menière's disease is usually fluctuant and may well respond to drug therapy or surgery, especially if the other symptoms also respond. However tinnitus

Table 3.2   Some treatments used in tinnitus

Medical	
Antidepressants	Yasuda, Nishida and Ikeda (1975)
Cocaine (topical)	Cristiani and Lovino (1948)
Cortisone (topical)	Schroer (1955)
Dimethyl sulphoxide	Caro (1975)
Ergot	Tanner (1955)
Heparin	Breu (1956)
Hydergin	Tanner (1955)
Lignocaine (intravenous)	Lewy (1937); Englesson, Larsson and Lindquist (1976); Rahm *et al.* (1962)
Meprobamate	Carrara (1957)
Nicotinic acid	Wilms (1975); Flottorp (1955)
Nucleic acid	Makishima, Yasuda and Miyahara (1971)
Prostigmine	Judge (1942)
Thiamine	Shambaugh (1942)
Tranquillizers	Seltzer (1947)
Vitamin A	Anderson (1950); Lobel (1951)
Surgical	
Stellate ganglion block	Adlington (1971)
Tympano-sympathectomy	Lempert (1946); Portmann (1948)
Labyrinthectomy	Pedersen and Sorensen (1970); Pulec (1974)
Eighth nerve section	Antoli-Candela, Alvares de Cozar and Antoli-Candela (1975); Malmros, Ellrand and Andersen (1966)
Pre-frontal leucotomy	Elithorn and Beck (1955) Beard (1965)
Chorda tympani section	Rosen (1952)
Other	
Biofeedback	House, Miller and House (1977)
Electro-therapy	Halton, Elrukar and Rosenberg (1960); Gerkin and Hughes (1974)
Masking devices	Vernon (1977); Hazell (1977)
Hypnosis	Marlowe (1973)

is often not the worst of the presenting symptoms, and patients usually complain more strongly about their vertigo and deafness.

(2) Masking techniques

Hippocrates in 400 B.C. wrote 'Why is it that buzzing in the ears ceases if one makes a sound? Is it because the greater sound drives out the less?' Masking devices have been tried in many different situations. Often patients discover for themselves that radios, running water, etc., will mask their tinnitus and find these controllable noise sources preferable to their own relentless tinnitus. Recently a patient was seen who had purchased a number of old fan heaters and had one going noisily in each room of his house.

Ear level masking devices have been in use in the USA for some years now (Vernon, 1977) and a high degree of sophistication has been reached in adjusting the masking noise to the user's requirements. Very high frequency tonal tinnitus is very difficult to mask at all. In the UK a similar but simpler masking device is available through the Royal National Institute for the Deaf, London. Early results are encouraging but long-term evaluation is needed.

Many authors have written about the value of hearing aids in masking tinnitus, as well as improving discrimination in deafness (Saltzman and Ersner, 1947). Vernon in the USA has even combined a hearing aid and masking device with good effect in some cases.

(3) Ablative surgical treatment

It is often tempting to counter the desperate tinnitus sufferer with an offer of ablative surgery. Although no figures are available for this indication alone, labyrinthectomy or acoustic nerve section probably results in relief or improvement in about 50 per cent of cases. Unfortunately some cases are actually made worse, and others are quite unchanged, showing how little is known about the aetiology of this condition. Useful hearing must not be destroyed and proper vestibular analysis is essential, especially in the elderly, to make sure that contralateral peripheral vestibular function is adequate. In the really suicidal tinnitus patient it is often justified to take such extreme measures. However some of these patients have pre-existing depressive illness, and are only using the symptom as a lever to extract support. As a diagnostic procedure local anaesthetics may be introduced into the middle ear to produce temporary anaesthesia of the cochlea (Mitani and Tanaka, 1975). We use this technique with iontophoresis for added control. If tinnitus is not abolished despite temporary vestibular and facial paresis, destructive surgery is unlikely to be helpful.

It is interesting that House (1976) reporting on 13 patients with cochlear implantation showed that 11 had marked improvement of their tinnitus. In five of these the improvement occurred *only* after 1 month of electrical stimulation.

The effect of electrical stimulation was first reported by Volta (1800), but suppression of tinnitus only occurs during passage of the current (usually DC) (Graham and Hazell, 1977). It is possible that for some cases continuous stimulation with an implanted electrode, on the round window for instance, may provide an answer.

(4) Psychotherapy

Information and reassurance remain the mainstay of management in idiopathic subjective tinnitus. Many patients are convinced that the sudden onset of horrendous noise inside the head heralds haemorrhage, neoplasia or insanity, and who can blame them? Proper reassurance takes time and needs to be supported by proper examination. In the busy clinic we have found a specially prepared 'hand out' of explanation a great help. Patients must be encouraged to avoid listening intently for small changes in pitch and intensity, but to involve themselves as much as possible in extrovert activity. The great majority of patients will, within a year, learn to accept tinnitus as part of their 'environment' and will not seek further advice.

When anxiety or depression co-exist these should be treated, but it should be made clear that any therapeutic agents prescribed will not affect the level of tinnitus itself.

We are opposed to the widespread practice of prescribing unproven drugs for idiopathic subjective tinnitus. False hopes are raised of a 'cure' and some patients embark on long pilgrimages in search of 'the drug that will work'. What is needed is frank explanation of our present state of knowledge of this condition. Many patients have great difficulty getting to sleep and a mild hypnotic in this situation is very valuable. Tinnitus rarely, if ever, wakes the patient once asleep.

With the more complex forms of tinnitus patients may sometimes identify tunes or melodies and even put names to them. It is important to realize that this is not necessarily auditory hallucination. Only when sounds become more highly organized, e.g. recognizable speech, should one confidently diagnose primary psychiatric disturbance.

References

Adlington, P. (1971) 'Stellate ganglion block in the management of tinnitus', *Journal of Laryngology*, **85**, 159

Anderson, J. R. (1950) 'Treatment of deafness and tinnitus with parenteral Vitamin A in massive doses', *Eye, Ear, Nose and Throat Monthly*, **29**, 75

Antoli-Candela F. Jr., Alvares de Cozar, F. and Antoli-Candela, F. (1975) Transvestibular approach to the internal auditory canal', *Annals of Otology*, **84**, 145

Arenberg, I. K. and McCreary, H. S. (1971) 'Objective tinnitus aurium and dural arterio venous malformations of the posterior fossa, *Annals of Otology*, **80**, 111

Beard, A. W. (1965) Results of leucotomy operations for tinnitus', *Journal of Psychiatric Research*, **9**, 29

Bjork, H. (1954) 'Objective tinnitus due to clonus of the soft palate', *Acta Otolaryngologica, Suppl.*, **16**, 39

Bolrovnikova, T. I. and Grigoriev, G. N. (1974) 'Vibratory tinnitus caused by myoclonia of the soft palate', *Vestnik Otorinolaryngologii*, **36**, 61

Breu, H. (1956) 'Heparin therapy for tinnitus'. *Archiv für Ohren Nasen- und Kehlkopfheilkunde*, **169**, 342

Burgers, N. R. H. (1971) 'Aural infestation by thysamura', *Royal Society of Tropical Medicine and Hygiene*, **65**, 405

Caro, A. Z. (1975) 'Dimethyl sulfoxide therapy in subjective tinnitus of unknown origin', *Annals of New York Academy of Sciences*, **243**, 468

Carrara, (1957) 'Meprobamate in symptomatic therapy of tinnitus', *Ospedale Maggiore (Milano)*, **45**, 236

Coles, R. R. A., Snashall, S. F. and Stephens, S. D. G. (1975) 'Some varieties of objective tinnitus', *British Journal of Audiology*, **9**, 1

Cristiani, M. and Lovino, M. (1948) 'Possible tympanic origin of various forms of auricular noises, the cocaine test', *Minerva Medica*, **1**, 436

Douek, E. and Reid, J. (1968) 'The diagnostic value of tinnitus pitch', *Journal of Laryngology*, **82**, 1039

Elithorn, A. and Beck, E. (1955) 'Pre-frontal leukotomy in a patient with tinnitus and hypochondriasis', *Lancet* (Jan.), 23

Ellis, P. D. M. and Wright, J. L. W. (1974) 'Acoustic neuroma. A plea for early diagnosis and treatment', *Journal of Laryngology*, **88**, 1095

Englesson, S., Larsson, B. and Lindquist, N. G. (1976) 'Accumulation of 14C-lidocaine in the inner ear. Preliminary clinical experience utilizing intravenous lidocaine in the treatment of severe tinnitus', *Acta Otolaryngologica*, **82**, 297

Feldman, H. (1971) 'Homolateral and contralateral masking of tinnitus by noise bands and pure tones', *Audiology (Basel)*, **10**, 138

Flottorp, G. (1955) 'Nicotinic acid treatment to tinnitus', *Acta Otorhinolaryngologica belgica (suppl.)*, **118**, 85

Fowler, E. P. (1939) 'Use of threshold and louder sounds in clinical diagnosis', *Laryngoscope*, **48**, 572

Fowler, E. P. (1944) 'Head noises in normal and disordered ears', *Archives of Otolaryngology*, **39**, 498

Frank, F. and Horak, K. (1976) 'Analysis of objectifiable ear noises', *Laryngologie, Rhinologie, Otologie*, **55**, 518

Gerkin, G. M. and Hughes, E. C. (1974) 'Transdermal electrostimulation therapy', *Archives of Otolaryngology*, **100**, 96

Gibson, R. (1973) 'Tinnitus in Paget's disease', *Journal of Laryngology*, **87**, 299

Glanville, J. D. and Coles, R. R. A. (1971) 'A family with high-tonal objective tinnitus', *Journal of Laryngology*, **85**, 1

Goodhill, V. (1952) 'A tinnitus identification test', *Annals of Otology*, **61**, 778

Goodhill, V. (1954) 'Tinnitus. Otologic aspects', *Transactions of American Academy of Ophthalmology and Otolaryngology*, **58**, 529

Graham, J. M. and Hazell, J. W. P. (1977) 'Electrical stimulation of the human cochlea using a transtympanic electrode', *British Journal of Audiology*, **11**, 59

Halton, D. S., Erulkar, S. D. and Rosenberg, P. E. (1960). 'Some preliminary observations of the effect of galvanic current on tinnitus aurium', *Laryngoscope*, **70**, 123

Hazell, J. W. P. (1977) 'A tinnitus masker', *Hearing*, **32**, 147

Heller, M. F. and Bergmann, M. (1953) 'Tinnitus in normally hearing persons', *Annals of Otology*, **62**, 73

Hempstock, T. I. and Atherley, G. R. C. (1970) 'Tinnitus and noise induced tinnitus'. Proceedings of a Conference held at National Physical Laboratory Teddington; British Acoustical Soc., Special Vol. No. 1

Hermann, C. Jr, Crandall, P. H. and Fang, H. C. H. (1957) 'Palatal myoclonus. A new approach to the understanding of its production', *Neurology (Minneapolis)*, **7**, 37

Hinchcliffe, R. (1961) 'Prevalence of the commoner ENT conditions in the adult rural population of G.B. A study by direct examination of 2 random samples', *British Journal of Preventive and Social Medicine*, **15**, 128

Hippocrates (c400 B.C.) Book XXXII, 961a

House, W. F. (1976) 'Cochlear implants', *Annals of Otology Suppl.*, 27

House, J. W., Miller, L. and House, P. R. (1977) 'Severe tinnitus treatment with biofeedback training', *Transactions of the American Academy of Ophthalmology and Otolaryngology*, **84**, 697

House, W. and Glasscock, M. (1968) 'Glomus tympanicum tumors', *Archives of Otolaryngology*, **87**, 550

Huizing, E. H. and Spoor, A. (1973) 'An unusual type of tinnitus', *Archives of Otolaryngology*, **98**, 134

Judge, A. F. (1942) 'Prostigmine in the treatment of chronic deafness and tinnitus aurium', *Military Surgeon*, **90**, 177

Kemp, D. T. and Martin, J. A. M. (1976) 'Active resonance phenomena in audition'. Abstracts of 13th International Congress on Audiology

Kimura, Y. (1974) 'Tinnitus without hearing loss', *Otolaryngology (Tokyo)*, **46**, 819

Lempert, J. (1946) 'Surgical relief: tympano sympathectomy', *Acta Otolaryngologica*, **43**, 199

Leventon, G., Mau, A. and Floru, S. (1968) 'Isolated psychogenic palatal myoclonus as a cause of objective tinnitus', *Acta Otolaryngologica*, **65**, 391

Lewy, R. (1937) 'Treatment of tinnitus aurium by the intravenous use of local anaesthetic', *Archives of Otolaryngology*, **25**, 178

Lobel, M. H. (1951) 'Is hearing loss due to nutritional disorder', *Archives of Otolaryngology*, **53**, 515

Loeb, M. and Smith, R. P. (1967) 'Relation of induced tinnitus to physical characteristics of the inducing stimuli', *Journal of the Acoustical Society of America*, **42**, 453

MacKinnon, D. M. (1968) 'Objective tinnitus due to palatal myoclonus', *Journal of Laryngology*, **82**, 369

McPherson, D. L. and Miller, J. M. (1974) 'Choline salicylate effects on cochlear function', *Archives of Otolaryngology*, **99**, 304

Makishima, K., Yasuda, K. and Miyahara, T. (1971) 'Treatment of sensory-neural deafness and tinnitus with a nucleic acid derivative', *Arzneimittel-Forschung*, **21**, 9

Malmros, R., Elbrond, O. and Andersen, H. C. (1966) 'Results of partial or tonal nerve section in patients with Menière's disease', *Acta Otolaryngologica, Suppl.*, **244**, 76

Marlowe, F. (1973) 'Effective treatment of tinnitus through hypnotherapy', *American Journal of Clinical Hypnosis*, **15**, 162

Mitani, N. and Tanaka, M. (1975) 'Local anaesthesia in the inner ear for diagnosis and treatment of vertigo', *Bulletin of the Yamaguchi Medical School*, **22**, 535

Mitchell, C., Brummett, R., Himes, D. and Vernon, J. (1973) 'Electrophysiological study of the effect of sodium salicylate upon the cochlea', *Archives of Otolaryngology*, **98**, 297

Morgan, E., Kelly, P., Nies K., Porter W. W. and Porter H. E. (1973) 'Tinnitus as an indication of therapeutic serum salicylate levels', *Journal of the American Medical Association*, **226**, 142

Mortimer, H. (1940) 'Clinical method of localisation and measurement of its loudness level', *Transactions of the American Laryngological, Rhinological and Otological Society*, **46**, 15

Myers, E. N. and Bernstein, J. M. (1956) 'Salicylate ototoxicity', *Archives of Otolaryngology*, **82**, 485

Nodar, R. H. (1972) 'Tinnitus arium in school age children. A Survey', *Auditory Research*, **12**, 133

Pedersen, C. B. and Sorensen, H. (1970) 'Clinical effect of labyrinthectomy', *Archives of Otolaryngology*, **92**, 307

Politzer, A. (1878) 'Palatal myoclonus', Lehurbuch der Ohrenheil-kunde (Stuttgart)

Portman, M. (1948) 'Treatment by tympanic sympathectomy', *Acta Otorhinolaryngologica Belgica, Suppl.*, **78**, 137

Pulec, J. L. (1974) 'Labyrinthectomy: indications, technique and results', *Laryngoscope*, **84**, 1552

Rahm, W. E., Strother, W. F., Crump, J. F. *et al.* (1962) 'The effects of anaesthetics upon the ear', *Annals of Otology*, **71**, 116

Reed, G. (1960) 'An audiometric study of two hundred cases of subjective tinnitus', *Archives of Otolaryngologica*, **71**, 84

Rosen, S. (1952) 'Surgery and neurology of Menière's disease. 1. Role of the chorda tympani nerve in tinnitus, vertigo and deafness', *Archives of Otolaryngology*, **56**, 152

Salmivalli, A. (1967) 'Acoustic trauma in regular army personnel', *Acta Otolaryngologica, Suppl.*, **222**

Saltzmann, M. and Ersner, M. S. (1947) 'A hearing aid for the relief of tinnitus aurium', *Larynogoscope*, **57**, 358

Schechter, G. L. and Brownson, R. J. (1970) 'Aortic arch aneurysm and vertigo', *Annals of Otology*, **79**, 187

Schroer, R. (1955) 'Therapy of ear noises by pertubal administration of cortisone', *Archiv für Ohren-, Nassen- und Kehlkopfheilkund*, **167**, 617

Sedlacek, K. (1948) 'Effect of subjective tinnitus and of noise on audiogram', *Časopis lékařů českých*, **87**, 1094

Seltzer, A. (1947) 'The problems of tinnitus in the practice of otology', *Laryngoscope*, **57**, 623

Shambaugh, G. E. (1942) 'Therapy of nerve deafness and tinnitus aurium; use of large doses of thiamine . . . source of possible error in interpretation of improvement', *Archives of Otolaryngologica*, **35**, 513

Tanner, K. (1955) 'Treatment of tinnitus aurium accompanied by nerve deafness with hydergin', *Schweizerische Medizinische Wochenschrift*, **85**, 1100

Tewfik, S. (1974) 'Phonocephalography. An objective diagnosis of tinnitus', *Journal of Laryngology*, **88**, 869

Thomsen, J. and Terkildsen, K. (1975) 'Audiological findings in 125 cases of acoustic neuromas', *Acta Otolaryngologica*, **80**, 353

US Department of Health, Education and Welfare (1968) 'Hearing status and ear examination. Findings among adults, United States 1960–1962', *Vital and Health Statistics* **11**, No. 32

Venters, R. S. (1953) 'Discussion of tinnitus aurium', *Proceedings of the Royal Society of Medicine*, **46**, 826

Vernon, J. (1977) 'Attempts to relieve tinnitus', *Journal of the American Audiological Society*, **2**, 124

Volta, A. (1800) 'On the electricity excited by mere contact of the conducting substances of different kinds', *Transactions of the Royal Society, Philosophy*, **90**, 403

Watanabe, I., Kumagami, H. and Tsuda, Y. (1974) 'Tinnitus due to abnormal contraction of the stapedius muscle', *O. R. L.*, **36**, 217

Wegel, R. L. (1931) 'A study of tinnitus', *Archives of Otolaryngology*, **14**, 158

Weinstein, L. and Bender, M. B. (1943) 'Integrated facial patterns elicited by stimulation of the brain stem', *Archives of Neurology and Psychiatry, Chicago*, **50**, 34

Wilms, R. (1975) 'Effect of a delayed action formulation of dimenhydrinate plus nicotinic acid and pyridoxine in patients with vertigo and tinnitus', *Medizinische Welt*, **26**, 785

Yasuda, J., Nishida, Y. and Ikeda, Y. (1975) 'Application of anti depressants for patients with tinnitus and vertigo', *Otologia (Fukuoka)*, **21**, 658

Zakrazewski, A., Kruk-zagajewska, A. and Konopacki, K. (1971) 'Traumatic aneurysms of the superficial temporal artery', *Materia Medica, Poland*, **3**, 8

4 Affections of the external ear
Valentine Hammond

The auricle

The auricle is formed from mesenchyme in the region of the first branchial cleft. The tragus is derived from the first arch and the remainder from the second. In the young embryo the ears are below the region which will become the mandible and meet in the mid-line. With development they move laterally and rotate through 90° (Potter and Craig, 1975). Total failure of this migration due to arrested development results in the auricles being joined beneath the mandible (synotia). This is associated with hypoplasia of the mandible, buccal cavity and tongue. Less severe degrees of arrested development result in the caudoventral displacement of the ears (melotia), an anomaly often associated with hypoplasia of the mandible. Abnormally low-set ears may be associated with congenital anomalies elsewhere.

Many minor variations in the shape of the pinna occur. These cannot really be regarded as anomalies but rather variations of the normal. Some of these variations are constant enough to warrant description. Darwin's tubercle is seen as a small elevation on the postero-superior part of the helix. This tubercle is homologous with the tip of the mammalian ear. This is usually an inherited condition.

The antihelix is sometimes more prominent than the the helix (Wildermuth's ear) and when this raised antihelix joins the helix the appearance is known as Mozart's ear. Potter (1966) has described an anteverted cup-shaped pinna occurring in otherwise normal individuals as an autosomal dominant inheritance.

The lobule may be absent, adherent or rarely bifid (Wilson, 1959). Failure of the lobule to separate from the side of the head is more common in females and may occur in all females in a family (Potter and Craig, 1975). The upper part of the auricle is occasionally adherent to the head. In females and the young the auricle is covered by very fine vellus hairs but in older males coarse hair may appear on the upper margin of the helix. Hypertrichosis of the auricle, a marked growth of hair arising from the margin of the helix and only occurring in males, is an inherited trait. Genetically this is a Y-linked inheritance present in all male members of the affected family. An excessive growth of hair may also occur on the tragus—the so-called harbula hirci (Montagna and Giocometti, 1969).

Bat ears

This not uncommon deformity may have a familial basis in some cases. It is sometimes associated with congenital disorders of the genito-urinary tract. In these subjects asymmetry of the auricular deformity is often noted. The deformity of bat ears consists of abnormal protrusion of the pinna with reduction or absence of the antihelix. Minor degrees of bat ear require no treatment but if very pronounced the deformity may be corrected surgically (*see* Chapter 5, Plastic Surgery of Ear).

Congenital malformations of the auricle

Malformations may have genetic or chromosomal origin: This is passed on by a parent who carries the appropriate gene because of either previous inheritance or mutation. In a dominant inheritance genes from one parent may cause the abnormality. Recessive inheritance requires similar genes from both parents.

Certain chromosomal abnormalities have been recognized and malformations of the pinna may form part of the resulting syndrome (Potter and Craig, 1975). In Trisomy 21 (Down's syndrome) the pinna tends to be small and rounded in contour with a poorly developed lobule. The postero-superior part of the helix may be folded. In Trisomy E16–18, the ears stand out and are less upright than usual and tend to be misshapen. The ring chromosome in the 1–5 position produces microcephalic dwarfs with low set pinnae.

Malformations of the pinna are often associated with other malformations of the auditory apparatus and face. Very rarely the pinna is totally absent (anotia). An abnormally small and deformed auricle (microtia) may occur as an isolated anomaly (*Figure 4.1*) but is frequently associated with atresia of the external auditory meatus and anomalies of the middle ear. The degree of abnormality of the middle ear tends to be proportional to the external deformity (Jafek *et al.*, 1975). In the Treacher–Collins syndrome (mandibular-facial dysostosis) microtia is frequently present and

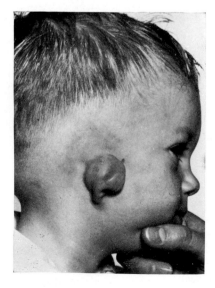

Figure 4.1   Congenital deformity of the right pinna. There was no meatal atresia present in this case. (Reproduced by permission of Mr. R. V. Battle)

usually accompanied by a meatal atresia and middle-ear anomalies. This is an inherited condition.

Abnormally large auricle (macrotia) is rare. The condition is usually bilateral. Very rarely the auricle may be divided into two by a congenital fissure. Both vertical and transverse fissures have been described.

The auricle and malformations of the genito-urinary tract

In 1946 Potter described the large low set ears with relatively little cartilage which occur in association with renal agenesis (*Figure 4.2*). Hilson (1957) drew attention to the association between malformations of the auricle, particularly when asymmetrical,

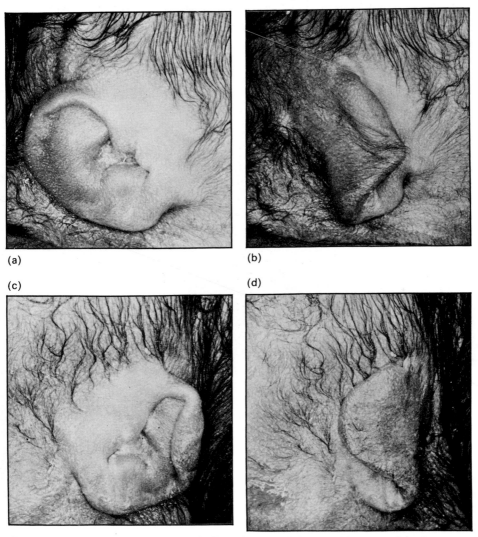

(a)   (b)

(c)   (d)

Figure 4.2   The auricle in renal agenesis (Potter's ear). It is large and low set and can be readily folded forward due to the lack of cartilage. (Reproduced by permission of Mr. Shawky El Serafy)

and anomalies of the genito-urinary tract. The ears in this syndrome tend to be folded over with squaring of the upper margin, folded forward and cup-shaped like a cockle shell or pointed and elfin in appearance. There may be marked asymmetry between the two ears. The genito-urinary anomalies recorded include agenesis, absence of one kidney and double ureter. The condition is thought to be genetically determined but not sex-linked.

Accessory auricles

Accessory auricles occur as small firm elevations of skin often containing a bar of elastic cartilage. They may be single or multiple. They most commonly occur just anterior to the tragus or ascending crus of the helix. They may also be found on the cheek along a line extending from the tragus to the angle of the mouth. When found in this situation they are frequently associated with other first arch anomalies. Accessory auricles may be excised but it must be remembered that they may contain bars of elastic cartilage extending deeply into the underlying soft tissues.

Congenital fistula

Congenital aural fistulas are blind tracks lined by squamous epithelium occurring in the region of the auricle. The majority open along the ascending crus of the helix (*Figure 4.3*). Others open along a line extending from the lower border of the helix to the angle of the mouth. In this situation they are often associated with congenital marks on the face. *Collaural fistulas* have an upper opening in the floor of the external auditory meatus and a lower one at the anterior border of the sternomastoid behind the angle of the jaw.

There is an association between pre-auricular pits, branchial fistula and deafness. This syndrome was first described by Heusinger in 1864 and has subsequently been well documented (Fitch *et al.*, 1976; Melnick, 1975). Both conductive and sensorineural deafness may occur, the former being due to malformations of the ossicular chain and

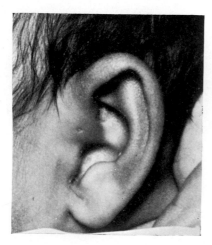

Figure 4.3   Pre-auricular fistula in a six-week-old infant. A similar lesion was present on the other side

the latter to impaired development of the cochlea. Other abnormalities including deformities of the auricle, blocked lacrimal ducts and facial palsy may occur. Anomalies of the genito-urinary tract have been described in the same subjects. This syndrome is due to a dominant inheritance.

If congenital fistulas are causing no symptoms they do not require any treatment. However, they may become infected, leading to a persistent discharge from the track and sometimes to abscess formation. When this occurs they must be completely excised. The operation requires great care as the track may extend deeply into the soft tissues and be closely related to branches of the facial nerve.

Congenital malformations of extrinsic origin

Not all congenital malformations of the auricle have a genetic basis. Some are produced as a result of external factors affecting the fetus during development. These factors are:

(1) Drugs (thalidomide, aminopterin) etc.
(2) X-rays and radioactivity.
(3) Viruses.

Microtia may occur in thalidomide embryopathy and is often associated with meatal atresia. There may also be abnormalities of the middle and inner ear. Ear anomalies occur when the drug is administered during the first 30–40 days of pregnancy (Takemori, Ishii and Suzuki, 1976). Aminopterin has been used in the past to produce therapeutic abortion and some infants born following the administration of this drug have had low set ears. Radiation to the maternal pelvis and viral infections during pregnancy both lead to a higher incidence of congenital malformations of the ear (Jafek *et al.*, 1975). Cosmetic plastic surgery of these malformations is described in Chapter 5. Associated middle-ear defects are considered in Chapter 6.

Congenital tumours

Haemangioma and lymphangioma may be encountered involving the auricle.

Dermoid cysts occasionally occur in relation to the pinna, usually just anterior to the helix.

Haematoma auris

This condition results from trauma to the pinna. It is frequently seen in boxers and rugby football players. An extravasation of blood occurs between the cartilage and the perichondrium producing a soft doughy swelling of the pinna. If untreated the blood clot may become organized, resulting in the deformity of cauliflower ear (*see Plate 1a, facing p. 108*).

Treatment

Cases seen shortly after the injury has occurred may be treated by aspiration through a wide bore needle using aseptic precautions. Cases of longer standing will require incision and evacuation of the clot. The incision is placed along the margin of the helix and any clot present is sucked out. Full aseptic precautions are essential for, if infection is introduced, perichondritis may occur. Following either aspiration or incision a firm dressing must be applied to the pinna to prevent a recurrence of the haematoma. It is useful to incorporate a mould of dental stent into the dressing. Repeated aspiration may be necessary.

Infections of the skin of the auricle

IMPETIGO

This is an infection of the superficial layers of the skin by staphylococci. Vesicles filled with serum arise on a reddish purple base. Later the vesicles burst to exude serum which dries to form semi-adherent amber crusts. The condition is most commonly seen in young children and may be secondary to the otorrhoea of a middle-ear infection.

Although the impetigo may involve the whole auricle it does not extend into the external auditory meatus. Commonly the neck and face are also involved.

Treatment

The crusts are removed by bathing with warm sterile saline. The area is then dried and neomycin cream applied. The treatment may have to be repeated daily for several days. If there is an otitis media or externa present this must be treated to prevent re-infection of the skin.

ERYSIPELAS

This is a streptococcal infection of the skin producing a raised red oedematous eruption with a characteristically well-defined edge. The auricle becomes intensely red and swollen and the infection spreads into the adjoining skin of the face. There is usually a marked systemic upset with a high temperature and rapid pulse.

Treatment

The infection usually responds rapidly to penicillin by injection.

Many generalized skin disorders may involve the pinna but require no separate description.

PERICHONDRITIS (see Plate 1b, facing p. 108)

Infection of the perichondrium of the auricle most commonly occurs when the cartilage is exposed either by a laceration or by surgery. The cartilage may also be exposed as a result of frostbite or burns. Infection may be introduced during the aspiration or incision of a haematoma auris. Sometimes superficial infections of the meatus or pinna spread deeply to involve the perichondrium.

In the early stages of the infection the pinna becomes red and tender. This is followed by a generalized swelling of the pinna and eventually by the formation of subperichondrial abscesses. The pus collects between the perichondrium and the underlying cartilage. The cartilage, deprived of its blood supply, may die. Extensive cartilage necrosis results in a marked deformity of the pinna.

Treatment
Cases of perichondritis should be treated promptly with a broad spectrum antibiotic as the infecting organism is rarely sensitive to penicillin.

Bacillus pyocyaneus is not uncommonly found in these cases. If there is any discharge coming from the ear a swab should be taken for culture and the determination of sensitivities. In the absence of definite information regarding the sensitivity of the organism, a broad spectrum antibiotic such as ampicillin should be administered. Pyopen and Colistin are antibiotics with a high degree of activity against many strains of *B. pyocyaneus* and their use may be indicated by sensitivity studies.

If subperichondrial abscesses form they should be incised and drained. Incision should be delayed until definite fluctuation can be elicited, as premature incision may result in a further spread of the infection.

In relatively rare instances, pain and suppuration may continue despite these measures and gross deformity is inevitable. In such cases, the whole of the auricular cartilage (except that of the helix) must be excised, through a wide incision on the anterolateral aspect of the auricle.

Chondrodermatitis nodularis chronicis helicis

This is the name given to small painful nodular lesions which occur on the upper free margin of the pinna. More common in men than women, the condition is thought to be brought about by exposure to low temperatures resulting in a local vasoconstriction.

Treatment
Local excision including a small wedge of the underlying cartilage results in cure.

Tophi

Small subperichondrial deposits of sodium biurate crystals may occur on the pinna in cases of gout. Although rarely troublesome they may occasionally become superficially ulcerated.

Treatment is that of the underlying condition.

Tumours of the auricle

Neoplasms of the auricle are uncommon. Benign tumours such as papilloma, fibroma and chondroma do occur but need no special description.

SQUAMOUS CELL CARCINOMA
The clinical diagnosis of an epithelioma does not usually present any difficulty. Typically the lesion presents as an indurated ulcer with everted margins (*Figure 4.4*). The diagnosis is confirmed by biopsy.

The regional lymph nodes may be involved but this is not usually an early occurrence in tumours confined to the auricle.

Treatment

Small lesions on the upper half of the auricle can be removed by a wedge incision with a wide margin of healthy tissue and the edges of the defect sutured together. Large lesions and those involving the lower half of the auricle require total excision of the pinna.

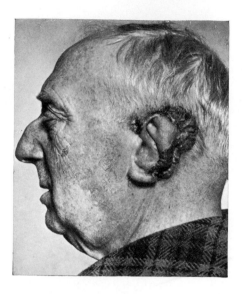

Figure 4.4   An extensive epithelioma of the pinna. (Reproduced by permission of Mr. R. V. Battle)

Lesions occurring on the upper half of the auricle carry a far better prognosis than those in the lower half.

BASAL CELL CARCINOMA (*rodent ulcer*)

Common sites for the discovery of these basal cell growths are the tragus, the border of the helix and the meatal entrance. There is at first the typical raised plaque with a rolled-over edge and tendency to central crusting. Bleeding takes place when the central crust is removed. In late cases the whole auricle may be destroyed whilst the underlying bone and parotid may be infiltrated.

Cystic forms are sometimes encountered (*Figure 4.5*). In appearance they are smooth, often pigmented tumours without any crusting or ulceration and when small may be confused with naevi.

The regional lymph nodes are not involved.

Treatment

Rodent ulcers of the pinna are best treated surgically, the lesion being excised together with a margin of healthy tissue.

Very small superficial lesions may be successfully treated with radiotherapy.

Advanced cases with infiltration of the underlying bone and soft tissues require wide excision and post-operative radiotherapy.

With adequate excision small rodent ulcers carry a very good prognosis. When extensive infiltration of the deep tissues has occurred it may be impossible to eradicate the tumour. The patient will eventually succumb although the progress of the disease is usually very slow.

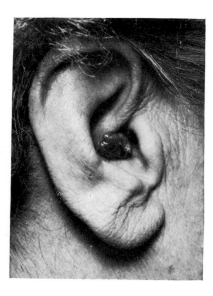

Figure 4.5   A cystic type of basal cell carcinoma. (Reproduced by permission of Mr. R. V. Battle)

MALIGNANT MELANOMA

The auricle is rarely affected by this form of malignancy. When it occurs it is seen as a nodular pigmented lesion which tends to enlarge rapidly and eventually to ulcerate. Involvement of the regional lymph nodes and distant metastasis may occur when the primary lesion is still quite small.

Treatment

Radical excision of the lesion offers the only prospect of cure. This may involve complete excision of the pinna and an *en bloc* dissection of the regional nodes. Even with early lesions the prognosis is poor.

The external auditory meatus

Atresia

Meatal atresia may be congenital or acquired. Congenital meatal atresia is discussed in detail in Chapter 6.

ACQUIRED ATRESIA AND STENOSIS

Acquired atresia is more common than the congenital variety. It may arise from many different causes such as lacerations, mastoid surgery, the introduction of corrosives and chronic otitis externa.

Both the site and the extent of the atresia will depend upon the cause. Burns, lacerations and mastoid surgery usually produce a narrowing of the outer part of the meatus. Chronic otitis externa may result in a generalized narrowing of the meatus due to thickening of the meatal skin. Occasionally localized webs are seen in the deep meatus following a severe otitis externa.

Treatment

In minor cases, acquired atresia may be successfully treated by dilatation with rubber or plastic tubing in increasing sizes, especially in traumatic cases; but if the atresia is causing deafness or rendering the control of an external- or middle-ear infection difficult it should be treated surgically. This is done by opening the meatus through a post-auricular incision and excising the scar tissue or thickened meatal skin. It is essential to enlarge the bony meatus. The enlarged meatus is packed and allowed to re-epithelialize spontaneously. This is preferable to the use of split thickness skin grafts.

Cerumen

The skin lining the cartilaginous portions of the external auditory meatus contains two types of glands, sebaceous glands and modified apocrine sweat glands or ceruminous glands. Both types of gland contribute to the formation of cerumen.

The quantity of wax produced varies greatly from individual to individual. In the majority of people the wax dries and separates as small flakes which fall out of the meatus. However, wax may accumulate and cause deafness by blocking the meatus.

Treatment

Wax may be removed by syringing but this method should not be used if there is a past history of ear trouble. In these cases the wax should be removed under direct vision using a ring-ended probe or a blunt hook and aural dressing forceps.

If syringing is undertaken normal saline at 38 °C is used as the irrigating solution. Any marked variation from body temperature may cause vertigo due to labyrinthine stimulation. Either a metal syringe or a Higginson's syringe attached to a curved metal canula may be used for syringing.

Metal syringes should be kept well greased so that they have a smooth action. When in use the nozzle of the syringe should be supported by the hand holding the patient's pinna to prevent a sudden head movement forcing the nozzle deeply into the meatus. If these precautions are taken the metal syringe may be used with safety.

Before syringing an ear the pinna should be pulled upwards and backwards in adults and directly backwards in children in order to straighten the meatus. The stream of lotion should be directed along the roof of the meatus. Syringing directly onto a mass of wax will only tend to impact it more deeply in the meatus.

When the wax is very hard it cannot be removed by syringing until it has first been softened. The patient should be advised to instil a few drops of olive oil into the ear twice a day for a week before syringing.

Keratosis obturans

In this condition a cholesteatoma-like mass is found filling the deep meatus. The mass consists of desquamated squamous epithelium. Typically the mass has a pearly white surface but this may be obscured by overlying wax.

Keratosis obturans can produce erosion of the bony meatus so that when the epithelial mass is removed a marked expansion of the deep meatus may be found. The tympanic membrane is usually intact but perforations may occur as a result of pressure necrosis. The cartilaginous meatus is not involved but granulations may occur at the junction of the eroded bony meatus and the cartilaginous meatus.

Keratosis obturans appears to arise as the result of abnormal desquamation of epithelium in the deep meatus. Unlike other skin, that in the deep meatus does not normally shed the superficial layer of cells from its surface. There is a constant migration of cells from the surface of the tympanic membrane along the deep meatus (Alberti, 1964). It would seem probable that migration fails to occur in keratosis obturans and so a mass of desquamated epithelium accumulates in the deep meatus.

There is a not uncommon association between chronic sinusitis, bronchiectasis and keratosis obturans. Harpman (1953) has suggested that in these cases there is an inborn abnormality of both the respiratory mucosa and the meatal skin.

Morrison (1956) attributed the keratosis obturans to an excessive secretion of wax which blocks the meatus and leads to an accumulation of desquamated epithelium in the deep meatus. It is postulated that in bronchiectasis there is a stimulation of the efferent vagal nerve endings in the bronchi, producing a reflex secretion of wax in the meatus.

Munro Black (1964), while supporting the theory of excessive wax secretion, regards the sinusitis as the primary lesion.

Treatment

Patients with keratosis obturans usually present with either pain or deafness in the affected ear. The treatment consists of removing the mass from the deep meatus. This may be very difficult to achieve, especially if there is also some otitis externa present. Syringing is best avoided as it rarely succeeds in shifting the mass and may increase the patient's discomfort. If difficulty is experienced in separating the mass from the meatal wall it is advisable to complete the removal under general anaesthesia.

After the meatus has been cleared the patient should be kept under observation, as the keratosis tends to re-form. Local applications do not appear to be of any value in preventing recurrence.

Benign necrotizing osteitis of the meatus

This usually presents as a small ulcer in the floor of the deep meatus. Careful examination reveals an area of bare bone exposed in the floor of the ulcer.

The symptoms are variable and may consist of discomfort, aching or a sensation of blockage in the ear. Scanty otorrhoea is often present but may not be noticed by the patient.

The ulceration tends to persist for several months but eventually heals, often after a small flake of dead bone has separated. Rarely, extensive bone necrosis may occur involving a large part of the tympanic plate.

Although trauma and infection have been suggested as possible causative factors the aetiology of the condition is unknown.

Foreign bodies

A great variety of foreign bodies may be encountered in the external auditory meatus. Insects may enter the meatus accidentally but most foreign bodies are introduced by the patient. Children and the mentally retarded account for the majority of cases.

Otitis externa is often encountered in association with meatal foreign bodies. This may be secondary to the presence of the foreign body or induced by traumatic attempts at removal. Sometimes a foreign body such as cotton-wool or a piece of matchstick is introduced into the ear by the patient in an attempt to relieve the irritation of a pre-existing otitis externa.

Treatment

Insects should first be killed by instilling spirit into the external auditory meatus.

Small objects are most easily removed by syringing but this method must not be used if the foreign body closely fits the meatus as it may become more deeply impacted.

Vegetable foreign bodies may be hygroscopic and swell if syringed with saline. They should either be removed with small forceps or syringing should be performed with alcohol.

Large foreign bodies should be removed under direct vision with small forceps or a blunt hook, but forceps should never be used for smooth, rounded objects. It is essential that the patient remains completely still during the procedure. General anaesthesia is generally desirable in children and may be indicated in very nervous adults.

When a foreign body is impacted in the deep meatus it may be necessary to open the meatus via a post-auricular incision and remove some bone from the posterior wall of the bony meatus in order to facilitate removal.

Otitis externa

Otitis externa may arise primarily in the meatus or may be a manifestation of a generalized skin condition.

When considering lesions confined to the meatus it is usual to classify the disease on the basis of its gross appearance:

(1) Circumscribed otitis externa (furunculosis).
(2) Diffuse otitis externa.

Perhaps a more useful classification is that adopted by Mawson (1967) which defines two main groups of cases:

(1) Infective: (*a*) bacterial; (*b*) fungal; (*c*) viral.
(2) Reactive: (*a*) eczema; (*b*) seborrhoeic dermatitis; (*c*) neurodermatitis.

Peterkin (1974) has classified the possible predisposing factors as:

(1) Genetic—narrow canal, excessive wax, inherited tendency to eczema.
(2) Environmental—heat, humidity and swimming.
(3) Traumatic—matchsticks and hairgrips.
(4) Infective.

Morrison and Mackay (1976) found a high incidence of excessive negative middle-ear pressure in patients suffering from recurrent otitis externa. They have postulated that impaired eustachian tube function may be a factor in causing otitis externa. It is suggested that the negative pressure in the middle ear may cause discomfort inducing the sufferer to probe the ears to relieve it and so traumatizing the meatal skin. Another possible explanation is that the negative pressure interferes with normal migration of epithelium along the external auditory meatus leading to a build up of epithelial debris in the canal. In any individual case many factors may contribute to the clinical picture. Several predisposing factors may be present and the situation may be further complicated by the development of secondary infection or eczematous reactions to the applications being used in treatment.

FURUNCULOSIS

A furuncle arises as a staphylococcal infection of a hair follicle. The condition occurs only in the cartilaginous meatus as hair follicles are not found in the skin of the bony meatus. The lesions may be multiple and recur over long periods.

The early symptoms of a furuncle are tenderness in the meatus and pain which is aggravated by movements of the jaw. As the condition progresses the pain becomes more severe and the meatus may become occluded by the swelling causing deafness. In severe cases the oedema may spread to the post-auricular sulcus producing forward displacement of the auricle. Eventually the furuncle discharges and unless there are multiple lesions present, the condition rapidly resolves.

Diagnosis

Examination reveals a tender red swelling in the cartilaginous portion of the meatus with a normal deep meatus and tympanic membrane beyond it. Pain is produced on pressing the tragus and on pulling the pinna upwards and backwards. There may be enlarged, tender lymph nodes palpable, anterior to the tragus, over the mastoid process and below the lobule of the ear.

Difficulties in diagnosis arise when there is gross meatal swelling preventing an examination of the tympanic membrane. As swelling and tenderness may also occur in the post-auricular region the condition must be distinguished from an acute mastoiditis. The main points of distinction are shown in *Table 4.1*

Table 4.1

Sign	Furunculosis	Acute mastoiditis
Post-auricular tenderness	Diffuse	Maximal over mastoid antrum
Displacement of pinna	Forwards	Typically forwards and downwards
Enlarged lymph nodes	Present	Absent
Pressure on tragus and moving the pinna	Pain	No pain
Mastoid x-rays	Mastoid air-cells clear	Mastoid air-cells cloudy

Treatment

When a furuncle is developing, local heat is helpful in reducing the pain and accelerating the inflammatory process. Heat may be applied by means of a covered hot water bottle, electric pad or as short-wave diathermy.

In the early stages local dressings are painful to apply and of no therapeutic value. Incision should be avoided as there is a danger of spreading the infection, especially to the cartilage.

When a furuncle has begun to discharge, the pus should be carefully mopped away. A wick soaked in glycerine may then be inserted. This dressing should be changed daily until the lesion is dry.

Systemic antibiotics are indicated when there is marked oedema or adenitis present or in cases with multiple furuncles. Penicillin is usually the antibiotic of choice, although an increasing number of penicillin resistant staphyloccal infections are encountered. A swab should always be taken for culture and sensitivity tests, and penicillin started pending the results.

RECURRENT FURUNCLES

The above methods of treatment are used in recurrent furunculosis but steps must also be taken to eliminate the staphylococci from the external auditory meati. The organisms are often carried in the nasal vestibules in these cases and this site also needs attention. A cream containing an antiseptic such as Vioform or Hibitane should be applied to both the meatus and the nasal vestibules twice a day.

The urine should always be tested to exclude diabetes mellitus.

DIFFUSE OTITIS EXTERNA

The condition has received a variety of names in the past, emphasizing its frequent occurrence in hot and humid climates, for example 'tropical' ear, Singapore ear. However, diffuse otitis externa is widely encountered in all climatic conditions. Although heat, humidity and bathing are aggravating factors in some cases, the most important factor is local trauma. Scratching the ears, vigorous drying of the meatus with a dirty towel and unskilled syringing are some of the ways in which minor abrasions of the meatal skin may be produced. These abrasions provide access for the causative organisms.

Some cases are secondary to an underlying chronic suppurative otitis media and this possibility should always be borne in mind and excluded by careful examination of the tympanic membrane.

The organisms most commonly found in diffuse otitis externa are *B. pyocyaneus, B. proteus* and *Staph. aureus.*

The condition is seen in two stages, acute and chronic.

The acute stage

The symptom of the acute stage is discomfort developing into pain in and around the ear. The pain is aggravated by movements of the jaw. In severe cases there may be swelling of the surrounding soft tissues and outward displacement of the pinna.

On examination the meatal skin is red, swollen and very tender. Pus is found in the meatus and, as the disease progresses, the meatal epithelium desquamates, forming a mass of cheesy debris in the deep meatus. The tympanic membrane is often dull and injected in appearance.

Treatment

The most important part of treatment is the meticulous cleaning of the meatus. Particular attention must be paid to the deep antero-inferior meatal recess where pus and debris tend to accumulate. A swab should be taken and cultured.

After cleaning, the meatus is packed with 12 mm ribbon gauze impregnated with an antiseptic and hydrocortisone cream such as Vioform and hydrocortisone. Neomycin with hydrocortisone is an alternative preparation which is widely used and gentamicin has proved valuable particularly when *B. pyocyaneus* is present but topical antibiotics must be used with caution as sensitization of the skin may occur and they may also encourage the development of fungal infections.

The patient must keep the ear dry and should be forbidden to rub or scratch it.

The chronic stage

The chief symptoms of the chronic stage are irritation and discharge. Deafness may occur due to the accumulation of debris in the meatus.

There is no tenderness but there may be thickening of the meatal skin with a reduced meatal lumen. Pus and debris are found in the meatus. There may be small granulations on the surface of the tympanic membrane denoting a loss of epithelium.

Treatment

As in the acute phase careful cleaning of the meatus with clearance of the deep meatal recess is the essential part of treatment. If there is marked meatal swelling this can be reduced by packing the meatus daily with 12 mm gauze wicks impregnated with an antiseptic and hydrocortisone cream (for example, Vioform and hydrocortisone cream). Preparations of this type are also useful in controlling the irritation. When there is no appreciable meatal swelling the antiseptic and hydrocortisone cream may be applied to the meatus. Ear drops of neomycin or gentamicin and hydrocortisone are often effective in clearing up the infection at this stage but may produce a sensitivity reaction in some individuals. This may be difficult to recognize as it may be masked by the presence of hydrocortisone in the preparation. In cases which fail to respond to treatment the reasons may be:

(1) Underlying chronic suppurative otitis media.
(2) Fungal infection.
(3) Sensitization of the skin to the topical application being used.

'MALIGNANT' OTITIS EXTERNA (see *Plate 1c, facing p. 108*)

Chandler (1968) first adopted this term to describe a severe progressive form of otitis externa usually occurring in elderly diabetic patients. Zaky *et al.* (1976) in an extensive review of the literature found 91 per cent of patients suffering from the condition to be over the age of 55 and 93 per cent to be diabetic. Joachims (1976) has described two cases occurring in childhood. Neither were diabetic but both suffered from malnutrition and anaemia.

The onset of the condition is insidious with the development of a purulent discharge from the ear and increasing pain. The infection may spread to the soft tissues of the neck and into the parotid region and may involve the temporo-mandibular joint. Periosteum and cortical bone are initially resistant to the spread of the infection but later may become involved leading to mastoiditis, osteomyelitis of the temporal bone and a spreading osteomyelitis of the base of the skull. The tympanic membrane tends to remain intact but may be obscured by granulation tissue. Seventh nerve palsy when it occurs is generally held to be a bad prognostic sign. This is usually caused by the involvement of the seventh nerve by the soft tissue infection in the region of the stylomastoid foramen. Spreading osteomyelitis of the base of the skull may result in other cranial nerve palsies and meningitis may occur. The condition carries a high mortality. Of the cases reviewed by Zaky 53 per cent died of the condition. The causative organism is always *B. pyocyaneus*. The infection starting in the meatal skin spreads through the cartilage of the meatal floor via the Clefts of Santorini—naturally occurring fissures in the cartilage normally filled by blood vessels and nerves. By this route the soft tissues of the neck and parotid become infected and the cartilage is involved at the same time. The patient, usually elderly and diabetic, will present with a painful, discharging ear. Examination reveals a purulent discharge coming from the meatus with a variable amount of surrounding soft tissue swelling and marked localized tenderness. Granulation tissue is found in the meatus arising from the floor at the junction of the cartilagenous and bony canals. Careful probing of the meatal floor may reveal exposed bone and a cavity extending inferiorly into the soft tissues. In more advanced cases widespread soft tissue swelling and cranial nerve palsies may be present. The diagnosis is made on the basis of the clinical picture and the culture of *B. pyocyaneus* from the aural discharge. Radiological examination is not helpful in the early stages. Examination of the blood shows a normal or slightly raised white blood cell count but the ESR will be raised. Blood tests and urine examination to determine the presence and severity of diabetes should be carried out.

Treatment

In early cases local aural toilet and topical gentamicin combined with systemic antibiotics may control the condition. For systemic use a combination of carbenicillin and gentamicin intravenously is usually recommended. It must be remembered that gentamicin is nephrotoxic as well as ototoxic and its use must be carefully monitored.

When the infection is more advanced and there is obvious cartilagenous or soft tissue involvement wide excision of the infected cartilage and adjacent soft tissues is indicated. In some cases where there is bone involvement a radical mastoidectomy may also be necessary.

OTOMYCOSIS

Fungal infection of the external auditory meatus has long been recognized as a fairly common cause of otitis externa in tropical climates. It is only in the last few years that the importance of fungi as pathogens in otitis externa in temperate climates has been generally appreciated. It would seem that the incidence of otomycosis is increasing. A greater awareness of the condition on the part of clinicians would partly explain this but there seems little doubt that fungus infection is, in fact, becoming more common as the result of widespread use of topical antibiotic preparations in the treatment of otitis externa.

The fungi most frequently found in otomycosis are *Aspergillus niger* and *Candida albicans*.

Symptomatically the condition may be indistinguishable from bacterial otitis

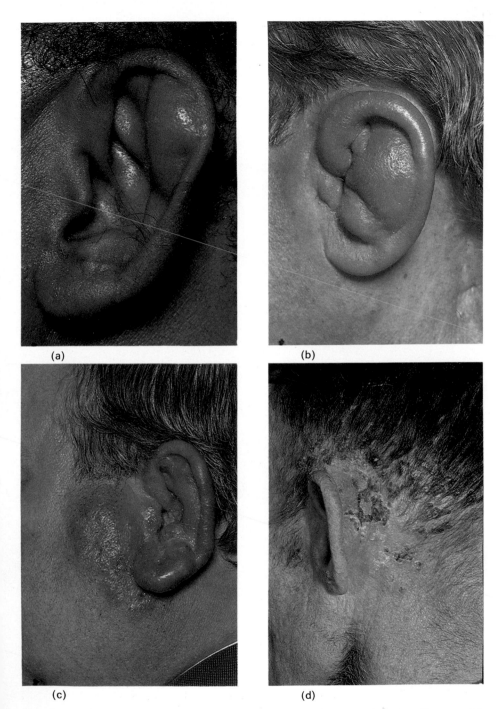

(a)

(b)

(c)

(d)

Plate 1   (a) Haematoma of the auricle; (b) perichondritis of the auricle; (c) malignant otitis externa; (d) herpes oticus

externa although the irritation is usually more marked in fungal infections. Occasionally severe pain in the ear is the presenting symptom.

On examination a mass of greyish white debris, resembling wet blotting paper, may be seen filling the meatus. In *Aspergillus niger* infection the conidiophores may be seen as black specks in the debris.

The typical appearances are not always present and in any case of otitis externa which fails to respond to treatment the possibility of a fungus infection must be considered. The diagnosis can be confirmed by microscopical examination of the debris or by culture.

Treatment

Fungi thrive in moist conditions and in the presence of epithelial debris. It is therefore essential to remove all the debris and discharge from the meatus. A specific anti-fungal agent can then be applied. Of these the most widely used is Nystatin. This may be applied as a powder, as an ointment or as drops. Its greatest activity is against monilia but it is also extremely useful in treating other fungus infections.

Amphotericin B (Fungilin) is another effective topical anti-fungal agent which exhibits greater *in vitro* activity against monilia than Nystatin and appears to be at least as effective as Nystatin in clinical use.

Ear drops of 2 per cent salicylic acid in alcohol may prove effective but can cause marked discomfort if the meatal skin is very inflamed. If there is a perforation present, they should not be used.

Treatment should be continued for at least a week after the condition has apparently cleared up clinically.

OTITIS EXTERNA HAEMORRHAGICA (BULLOUS MYRINGITIS)

This condition is characterized by the formation of purple blebs on the tympanic membrane and the skin of the deep meatus. The purple colour is due to the haemorrhagic effusion filling the vesicles.

Pain, often severe, is the first symptom and serosanguineous discharge may occur within 12 h as a result of bursting of the blebs. The pain is not relieved by the onset of the discharge. In uncomplicated cases the middle ear is not involved so the hearing remains normal.

The aetiology of the condition is uncertain but it is thought to be due to a virus infection. In some influenza epidemics many cases of otitis externa haemorrhagica are seen and there does appear to be an association between the two conditions.

Treatment consists of prescribing analgesics for the pain and keeping the ear clean and dry.

Antibiotics have no influence on the course of the disease. The blebs should not be incised as this is of no value in relieving the symptoms and may only introduce secondary infection.

HERPES ZOSTER OTICUS (*see Plate 1d, facing p. 108*)

Herpes zoster of the geniculate ganglion may give rise to skin lesions with or without involvement of either the seventh or eighth cranial nerves. The herpetic eruption occurs on the meatal skin, tympanic membrane and the auricle, particularly in the conchal region. Initially the rash consists of small tense blisters with surrounding erythema. Lesions may also be found on the buccal mucosa and the hard palate. The blisters gradually dry up, leaving adherent crusts which usually persist for a week to ten days.

The appearance of the rash is often preceded by pain in the ear for several days. Apart from keeping the ear dry no local treatment is indicated.

HERPES SIMPLEX

Herpes simplex occurs most commonly on the lips as the so-called 'cold sore'. Occasionally the skin of the auricle and meatus are affected. The eruption at first consists of a crop of small vesicles which dry up after a few days leaving the skin red and scaly.

There is no specific treatment, and apart from keeping the ear dry no local treatment is necessary.

SEBORRHOEIC DERMATITIS

The main feature of this disease is a scaly condition of the scalp usually referred to as dandruff or scurf. This is often associated with scaling in the external auditory meatus, post-auricular sulcus and below the lobe of the auricle.

The aetiology of the condition is unknown.

When the ear is involved, secondary infection may be introduced by scratching, leading to a diffuse otitis externa.

Treatment

The scalp condition always requires attention. Regular washing with a cetrimide shampoo is an effective method of keeping the dandruff under control.

In uncomplicated cases there may be a tendency for debris to accumulate in the meatus. This may require regular removal. The patient should be advised to avoid getting water in the ears and to refrain from attempting to remove the waxy debris with hair pins or matchsticks.

ECZEMA

The eczematous reaction occurs as the result of sensitization of the skin cells. This sensitization may be produced by an infecting organism or by contact with an allergenic material. Of the latter group, the substances which most commonly evoke this response are the antibiotics. Neomycin is by far the most troublesome in this respect. The topical application of any antibiotic may result in a sensitivity reaction.

Clinically the eczematous reaction is characterized by the formation of vesicles. When the vesicles burst, serous discharge exudes from the raw surface.

The eruption is usually accompanied by intense irritation.

Treatment

When the eczematous dermatitis is secondary to an infective process the condition is best treated by cleaning the meatus and applying a cream containing Vioform and hydrocortisone.

In cases resulting from the topical application of an antibiotic, the preparation responsible for the trouble must be withdrawn. The ear should be kept dry and either a cream or lotion containing hydrocortisone 1 per cent applied. In severe cases fluocinoline acetonide cream (Synalar) is often more effective than hydrocortisone.

NEURODERMATITIS

In some cases of otitis externa there is an underlying psychosomatic disturbance which not only initiates the condition but also makes it difficult to clear up.

In these patients the initial symptom is irritation in the ears. At this stage the skin is normal in appearance. Constant scratching may lead to lichenification of the skin or secondary infection may be introduced, causing a diffuse otitis externa.

Treatment

Local treatment consists of clearing up any secondary infection and attempting to alleviate the irritation with topical hydrocortisone or fluocinolone acetonide (Synalar) cream. In severe cases it may be necessary to bandage the ears to prevent scratching. In management due attention must be paid to the psychological aspect of the problem.

Benign tumours of the external auditory meatus

Papilloma, fibroma, chondroma and angioma may occur in the external auditory meatus but require no special description.

Teratoid tumours attached to the wall of the osseous canal have been described (Adams and Gilmour, 1930).

ADENOMA

There are two types of gland in the skin of the external auditory meatus and both may give rise to adenomas.

(1) *Sebaceous adenoma.* This tumour arises in the sebaceous glands of the meatus. It is seen as a smooth, painless, skin-covered swelling in the outer part of the meatus. It may be treated by local excision.

(2) *Ceruminoma.* This is a rare tumour arising from the ceruminous glands of the meatal skin. The ceruminous glands are modified apocrine sweat glands and histologically a ceruminoma closely resembles the sweat gland tumours seen elsewhere in the skin. For this reason some authors (Johnstone, Lennox and Watson, 1957; O'Neill and Parker, 1957) prefer the term hidradenoma of the meatus to ceruminoma.

Clinically the tumour presents as a firm skin-covered mass in the cartilaginous meatus. Both sessile and polypoid forms have been described (O'Neill and Parker, 1957; Juby, 1957; Arora, 1964). There are no symptoms until the mass enlarges sufficiently to cause a feeling of obstruction in the ear.

Treatment

Ceruminomas show a marked tendency to local recurrence after removal and may become frankly malignant adenocarcinomas. In view of this, treatment should consist of wide excision including a margin of healthy skin. Should the lesion prove to be an adenocarcinoma histologically, post-operative radiotherapy is indicated.

OSTEOMA

The solitary cancellous osteoma occurs as a smooth, rounded pedunculated tumour attached to the outer part of the bony meatus. It arises from the region of either the tympanosquamous suture or the tympanomastoid suture.

These tumours can be readily removed by fracturing through their narrow attachment to the meatal wall.

EXOSTOSES

Exostoses produce smooth hemispherical elevations in the deep part of the bony meatus adjacent to the tympanic membrane. The lesions are usually multiple and the condition is commonly bilateral. The exostoses consist of dense ivory bone covered by a thin layer of normal meatal skin.

Although their aetiology is not certain there appears to be a definite relationship between bathing in cold water and the formation of meatal exostoses. Fowler and Osman (1942), working with guinea-pigs, were able to demonstrate the formation of new bone on the inner surface of the tympanic bulla following irrigation of the external canal with cold water.

Harrison (1962) carried out similar experiments with guinea-pigs and found histological evidence of new bone formation in the deep meatus after prolonged irrigation with cold water.

Meatal exostoses do not cause any symptoms when they are small and so are usually discovered incidentally during examination of the ears. When large they may completely block the meatus or so greatly reduce the lumen that it is readily blocked by small amounts of wax or epithelial debris. When this occurs the patient will complain of deafness.

Treatment

When exostoses are small they require no treatment. If they are large enough to be causing deafness or impede the treatment of a chronic middle-ear infection they should be removed.

Exostoses consist of dense ivory bone and attempts to remove them with a hammer and gouge may produce fractures in the surrounding bone, possibly resulting in facial palsy. Removal should be undertaken with a high speed drill and a cutting burr. The overlying meatal skin is elevated and the exostoses reduced with the burr until an adequate meatus has been formed.

Malignant tumours of the external auditory meatus

SQUAMOUS CELL CARCINOMA

The meatus is a rare site for the development of an epithelioma. Although the disease may occur in otherwise healthy ears it is more commonly seen in ears which have been subject to long-standing chronic otorrhoea.

The presenting symptoms are bleeding from the ear or bloodstaining of a pre-existing otorrhoea, and pain.

The clinical appearance varies from a small ulcer on the meatal wall in early cases to a large friable mass filling the meatus in more advanced cases.

Local spread of the tumour involves the underlying bone of the meatus and the middle ear. The facial nerve is commonly involved as the disease progresses.

Involvement of the regional lymph nodes tends to be a relatively early occurrence in the course of the disease. The pre-auricular, post-auricular or superficial cervical nodes are usually the first to be affected and later the upper deep cervical nodes may become involved. Distant metastasis is very rare.

Treatment

Wide excision of the tumour by means of an extended radical mastoidectomy followed by post-operative radiotherapy offers the best prospect of cure. However, with the possible exception of very early lesions, the prognosis is extremely poor.

BASAL CELL CARCINOMA

Although rodent ulcers are not uncommon on the auricle, they are rarely seen arising in the meatal skin.

Clinically the lesion is difficult to distinguish from an epithelioma and the diagnosis depends upon the histological findings following biopsy.

As with epitheliomata treatment consists of radical excision combined with post-operative radiotherapy.

ADENOCARCINOMA

An adenocarcinoma may arise primarily from the glands of the meatal skin or as the result of malignant change in either a sebaceous adenoma or a ceruminoma. Clinically these tumours resemble other malignant lesions in the meatus and the diagnosis depends on the biopsy. Treatment consists of radical surgery combined with post-operative radiotherapy.

References

Adams, J. and Gilmour, M. D. (1930) *Journal of Laryngology*, **45**, 550

Alberti, P. W. R. M. (1964) *Journal of Laryngology*, **78**, 908

Altmann, F. (1951) *Archives of Otolaryngology*, **54**, 115

Arora, Y. R. (1964) *Journal of Laryngology*, **78**, 569

Chandler, J. R. (1968) *Laryngoscope*, **78**, 1257

Chandler, J. R. (1972) *Annals of Otology*, **81**, 648

Fitch *et al.* (1976) *Annals of Otology, Rhinology and Laryngology*, **85**, 268

Fowler, E. P. Jnr. and Osman, P. M. (1942) *Archives of Otolaryngology*, **36**, 455

Harpman, J. A. (1953) *Journal of Laryngology*, **67**, 189

Harrison, D. F. N. (1962) *Annals of the Royal College of Surgeons of England*, **31**, 187

Heusinger, C. F. (1864) *Virchows Archiv für pathologische Anatomie und Physiologie und für Klinische Medizin*, **29**, 358

Hilson, D. (1957) *British Medical Journal*, **2**, 785

Jafek, B. W., *et al.* (1975) *Translations of the American Academy of Ophthalmology and Otalaryngology*, **80**, 588

Joachims, H. Z. (1976) *Archives of Otolaryngology*, **102**(4), 236

Johnstone, J. M., Lennox, B. and Watson, A. J. (1957) *Journal of Pathology and Bacteriology*, **73**, 421

Juby, H. B. (1957) *Journal of Laryngology*, **71**, 832

Mawson, S. R. (1967) *Diseases of the Ear*. London; Edward Arnold

Melnick, M. (1975) *Birth Defects*, **11**(5), 121

Montagna, W. and Giocometti, L. (1969) *Archives of Dermatology*, **99**, 757

Morrison, A. W. (1956) *Journal of Laryngology*, **70**, 317

Morrison, A. W. and Mackay, I. S. (1976) *Journal of Laryngology*, **15**, 495

Munro Black, J. I. (1964) *Journal of Laryngology*, **78**, 785

O'Neill, P. B. and Parker, R. A. (1957) *Journal of Laryngology*, **71**, 824

Peterkin, G. A. G. (1974) *Journal of Laryngology*, **88**, 15

Potter, E. L. (1946) *Journal of Paediatrics*, **29**, 68

Potter, E. L. (1966) *Anales del Desarrollo (Granada)*, **13**, 307

Potter, E. L. and Craig, J. M. (1975) *Pathology of the Fetus and the Infant*, 3rd edn, New York; Year Book Publishers

Takemori, S., Ishii, T. and Suzuki, J. (1976) *Archives of Otolaryngology*, **102**, 425

Wilson, T. G. (1959) *Journal of Laryngology*, **73**, 439

Wilson, T. G. (1962) *Diseases of the Ear, Nose and Throat in Children*, 2nd edn, London; Heinemann

Zaky, D. A. *et al.* (1976) *American Journal of Medicine*, **61**(2), 298

5 Plastic surgery of the ear
R L G Dawson

The plastic surgeon is concerned with congenital and acquired deformities of the external ear.

Congenital deformities

Bat ears

These are by far the commonest of the congenital deformities. They tend to be familial. The deformity is not influenced by any form of external bandage while the child is a baby. When severe, the boy is open to ridicule by his fellow schoolboys while girls ask for treatment when they start putting their hair back. Boys, therefore, come for treatment earlier than girls. The degree of prominence of the ears varies considerably, but basically the deformity can be classified into (a) the conchal type; and (b) the conchoscaphoid type.

The conchal type has a reasonably well-formed antihelix and fossa of the antihelix but has a very prominent and large conchal cartilage standing out at 90 degrees from the skull. The conchoscaphoid type not only has a large and prominent conchal cartilage, but also has an absent antihelix fold and an absent fossa of the antihelix. The lobe of the ear also in these cases tends to be more prominent than normal.

The ears should not be operated upon until such time as the cartilage is stiff and in severe conchoscaphoid types one may have to wait until the child is seven or eight years old before enough stiffening of the cartilage has developed.

The basic treatment is an operation, preferably under general anaesthetic, when, with the head suitably draped, both ears are cleaned well with 1 per cent Savlon and spirit, and an ellipse of skin is marked out on the posterior aspect of the ear. The ear is also turned backwards so that the antihelix prominence becomes obvious. This is then marked with ink from the external aspect and three Hagedorn needles tipped with Bonney's blue pierce all layers of the ear in the line of the new antihelix fold. When the needles have appeared on the posterior aspect, more ink is applied to the points and they are withdrawn, thus marking the cartilage of the ear on the posterior aspect with three blue dots. The posterior and anterior aspects of the ear are then infiltrated with 0.5 per cent lignocaine with 1 : 200 000 adrenaline using approximately 4 ml for each ear. This not only achieves haemostasis to a very large degree, but also allows separation of the cartilage from the skin more easily. The ellipse of skin marked out on the posterior aspect of the ear is then removed and the cartilage incised from the posterior aspect along the whole length of the predetermined antihelix in line with

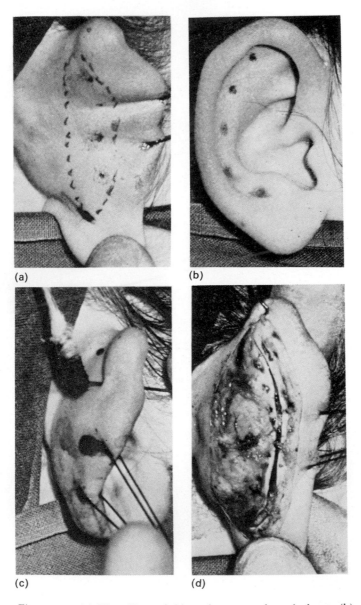

Figure 5.1 (a) The ellipse of skin to be removed marked out; (b) line of the new antihelix is marked; (c) Hagedorn needles bearing ink are used to mark the actual cartilage; (d) the incision in the cartilage along the ink marks

the blue dots. This incision passes downwards medially through the conchal cartilage in the actual concha of the ear. The perichondrium and skin of the *outer* aspect of the ear is then dissected off the cartilage with blunt-ended curved scissors and the cartilage itself held firmly in forceps and riberated in close parallel cuts from the outer surface. In this way, as the cuts progress, the previously stiff conchal cartilage turns over on itself, with the convexity outwards hinged on the perichondrium of the posterior

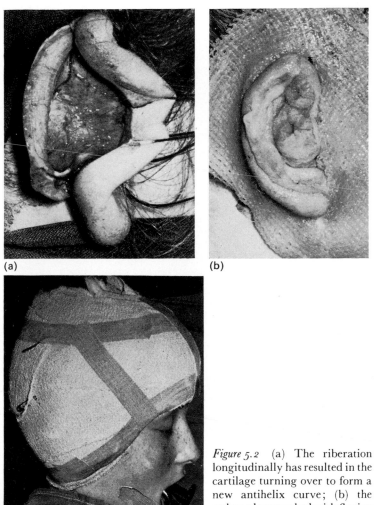

(a)

(b)

(c)

Figure 5.2 (a) The riberation longitudinally has resulted in the cartilage turning over to form a new antihelix curve; (b) the reshaped ear packed with flavine wool; (c) a firm pressure dressing is applied

aspect of the ear. Transverse small cuts are made in line with the lower limb of the antihelix, so that the fossa of the antihelix can be defined and the excess cartilage in the lower part is trimmed down so that it will not project into the concha. For a satisfactory curve of the cartilage the actual spring of the upper part of the ear is broken. Complete haemostatis is secured and then the lips of the posterior excision approximated with a subcuticular 3/0 catgut tied over a small dressing.

As the subcuticular suture is tightened, the ear comes back towards the side of the skull and the new antihelix becomes prominent. Paraffin-flavine wool is then packed into the concha and the fossa of the antihelix and the fossa of the helix to define the cavities and convexities of the ear. A dry dressing and wool are applied and when the opposite side has also been remodelled, a firm, but not tight, 7.5 cm crêpe bandage is applied as a figure-of-eight held in place with 2.5 cm Elastoplast.

Post-operatively the patient is sat up when he is conscious, and he remains in hospital for two days. Routine prophylactic erythromycin is given for five days. At the end of two weeks the patient attends, his dressing is removed, and his new ears are unpacked. The parent is then given a 7.5 cm crêpe bandage to apply at night only for the next two weeks, after which time no further protection is needed.

The above method of correction is only one of many. It was shown to the author by Dr. Murray of Toronto 17 years ago and he has used it ever since, and has found it a method which, in his opinion, has provided him with more consistently good results than others.

COMPLICATIONS

Bleeding
This rarely occurs if proper packing has been maintained. When it does occur it is usually from a vessel on the skin edge which has not been picked up with the subcuticular suture. If bleeding does occur, or if there is an excessive amount of pain, the dressings must be removed, and where haematoma is present with gross swelling of the ear, a further anaesthetic has to be given, the haematoma evacuated, bleeding stopped and the ear repacked. Bleeding from the skin edge can usually be caught with further sutures.

Infection
This is fortunately a very rare complication. When it does occur urgent steps must be taken to combat the infection, otherwise a chondritis will set in with severe loss of cartilage support and subsequent severe ear deformity. The wound must be opened up, any pus allowed to escape and an antibiotic appropriate to the infection prescribed. The ear must be inspected daily and if chondritis does occur as revealed by increasing pain, local tenderness, local oedema and thickening of the affected part of the ear, this area must be opened up and the affected cartilage removed before the stripping of the perichondrium progresses to a disastrous degree.

Keloid formation in the posterior scar
This occasionally happens and in such cases large thick red scars occur in the post-auricular sulcus. Where true keloid forms, shaving of the keloid with the application of a thin split skin graft will ultimately be needed. Radiotherapy is not advised for fear of chondritis. Steroid injections are not efficacious. When the thickened scar is hypertrophic it will settle and soften down in time; therefore if this does occur, the utmost patience must be exercised by all concerned.

Lop ears

These ears are a more severe variant of bat ears. Usually they are small and the upper half of the auricle falls over the lower half covering its external aspect. There is a severe conchal deformity with absence of a good antihelix. The cartilage is soft, has a permanent bend, and the skin on the outer aspect of the ear is short, while that on the posterior aspect is relatively redundant. In principle, therefore, the redundant skin must be removed from the back of the ear and applied to the outer aspect whilst the cartilage is divided along its principal bend and also in the line of the predetermined antihelix. This division is performed in the same way as for the usual bat ear but where a severe lop-ear deformity occurs with an actual skin-shortening on the outer side, an incision has to be made on the outer aspect to allow a defect to be created into which redundant skin from the posterior aspect can be fitted. Dressings and packing of the cavities and convexities, and the post-operative treatment are the same as for bat ears.

Buried ears

This deformity is the opposite of the lop ear, and one finds the upper half of the auricle buried beneath a fold of skin of the scalp. The cartilage in this case has bent slightly with the convexity outwards and it is the helix that lies beneath the scalp fold. There is no post-auricular sulcus in the upper half of the ear, therefore there is shortness of skin in this area, whereas there is a relative excess of skin on the outer aspect of the ear. This therefore means that the procedure used for 'lop ear' must be reversed and after the sulcus has been made and the spring of the cartilage reversed by suitable longitudinal cuts, from the posterior aspect in this case, the excess skin on the outer aspect of the ear is transposed over to the defect in the post-auricular sulcus. The same dressings and the same post-operative treatment are used.

Darwinian tubercles

These small atavistic appendages are noticed in many patients and when they are large removal is requested. Simple longitudinal excision is performed along the outer margin of the helix with skin coaptation.

Pre-auricular remnants

These are very common and vary considerably in size from minute nodules to large pedunculated lumps. They contain elements of cartilage which can be traced in continuity with the main auricular mass in large deformed appendages associated with ears showing a slight deformity. Sometimes the appendages are so small and so well pedunculated that the midwife or parent will tie a small piece of cotton thread round them to allow them to drop off by necrosis. At other times surgical excision under local anaesthetic can be performed in a small baby. The larger ones usually need a short general anaesthetic as the cartilage remnants may be quite large beneath the skin. It has been noted that the pre-auricular remnants are significant of a first arch deformity, and in the more severe cases may be associated with mandibular maldevelopment, a shortness of the mandibular body and absent mandibular condyle on the same side; but even mild discrepancies of mandibular development do occur, and these patients must be watched carefully for some years after removal of the remnants.

Absent or partially absent external ear

This may occur unilaterally or bilaterally and is usually associated with a stenosis or absence of the external auditory meatus. Where bilateral absence of the ears occurs, subnormal hearing may also be present and the ear, nose and throat surgeon has usually fashioned a meatus to improve the air conduction. The middle ear is usually present. Total absence is rare. A forward displaced lower third or one-quarter of the auricle which is also displaced too far downwards is the usual condition. There is a very frequent association of mandibular maldevelopment with this condition.

Operative treatment is performed in stages and I quote the method of Barinka

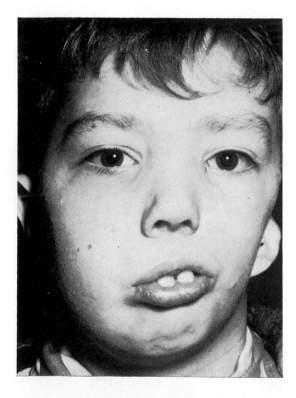

Figure 5.3 A first arch deformity involving the ear and the skeletal and soft tissues of the face

(1966) modified from the methods of Tanzer (1959) and Converse (1964) as the most acceptable. The operation is not performed before the age of ten years because an adequate amount of costal cartilage must be present. The seventh, eighth and ninth costal cartilages are removed *en bloc* and the wound closed in layers with drainage. The cartilage is then finely carved to the shape of the auricle (most average about 2.5 mm in thickness except at the rim) and is perforated by numerous small punch holes (*Figure 5.4a*). The skin over the mastoid process and neighbouring scalp is undermined in the predetermined position, and the cartilage inserted, abutting onto the auricular remnants. A firm dressing is applied. After not less than 3–4 weeks a second operation

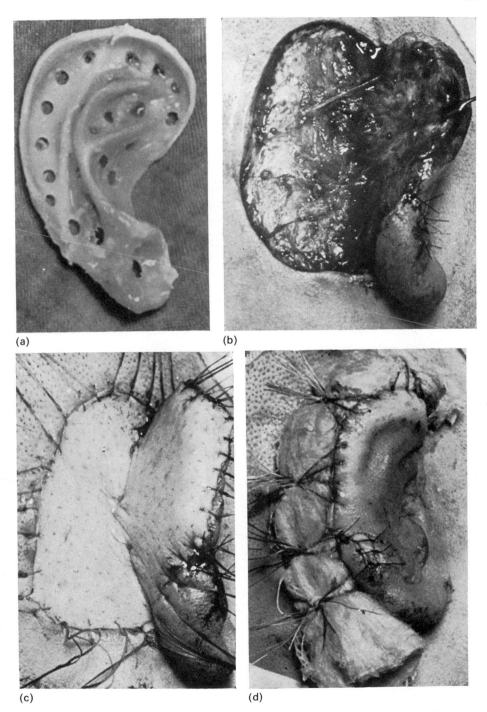

(a) (b)

(c) (d)

Figure 5.4   (a) Costal cartilage modelled to form the framework of the new pinna; (b) implanted cartilage and overlying skin raised to form post-auricular sulcus; (c) raw sulcus re-surfaced with thick-skin graft; (d) pressure dressing secured with tie-over sutures. (Reproduced by courtesy of Dr. L. Barinka)

transfers the auricular remnants posteriorly to form the lobule, and part of the remnants may be used to form a false meatus as atresia is common. Four months later the new auricle, which is lying close to the skull, is lifted away by an incision along the border of the new helix to define a post-auricular sulcus (*Figure 5.4b*). Care must be taken not to expose the cartilage at all; a layer of soft tissue must cover it. A thick-skin graft removed from the thigh, is then sutured on to the raw area on the mastoid process, and on the back of the new auricle, fixed in place with tie-over sutures. A pressure dressing is maintained for seven days (*Figures 5.4c* and *5.4d*).

Pre-auricular sinus

This sinus, frequently bilateral, often fills up with sebaceous material which becomes infected when an abscess needs to be opened. Chronic discharging pre-auricular sinuses have to be tracked by a pre-auricular exposure downwards to the post-mandibular region. Very rarely they pass as a track between the bifurcating carotid arteries into the pharynx, but much more frequently the sinuses end behind the angle of the jaw. Care must be taken in their dissection so that the facial nerve is not injured. They travel superficial to the facial nerve. It is advisable to put a small drain into this incision for two days, with a pressure dressing. Occasionally the sinuses pass posteriorly into the substance of the external ear itself, in which case the sinus has to be unroofed by incision of the skin and cartilage of the ear and it is necessary to clear out all epithelial remnants otherwise they will recur.

Acquired deformities

Traumatic

The collection of a haematoma beneath the perichondrium with subsequent liquefaction followed by fibrous tissue replacement forms a so-called 'cauliflower ear'. If the haematoma is encountered soon after the trauma, it is best to make a small incision over the swelling, evacuate all haematoma and pack with paraffin–flavine wool and apply a very firm crêpe bandage dressing. This should be maintained for at least a week before being changed to avoid a reforming of the swelling. After several days, if the haematoma has not been evacuated, it may develop into a seroma in which case aspiration is indicated every day followed by packing and a firm bandage or an incision followed by packing and bandaging, for one week, to prevent further swelling. Once fibrosis has occurred there is a thickened ear deformity and the only way to correct this is to lift the skin off the mass of fibrous tissue and shave down the fibrous tissue until suitable folds of the external ear have been achieved again. The skin is then laid back over these folds and the folds and concavities are preserved by packing with paraffin–flavine wool and a pressure dressing applied for two weeks.

Tissue loss

This can occur as a result of many forms of accident and is most common through windshield injuries and dog-bites. If the ear has been severely lacerated but is still

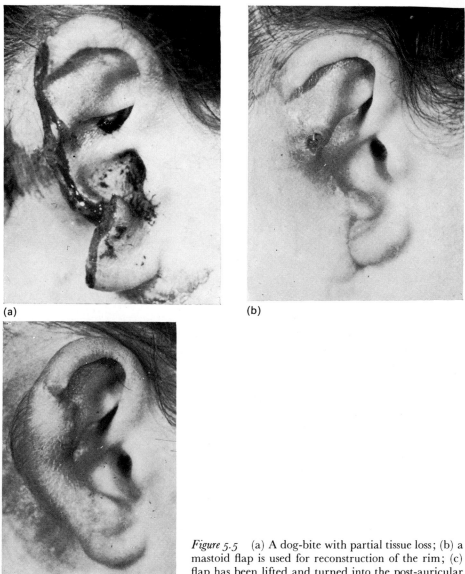

(a)

(b)

(c)

Figure 5.5 (a) A dog-bite with partial tissue loss; (b) a mastoid flap is used for reconstruction of the rim; (c) flap has been lifted and turned into the post-auricular sulcus. A skin graft covers the mastoid area

hanging on even by the smallest attachment, it must be sutured back into place and a firm bulky dressing applied which should not be disturbed for a week. It sometimes happens that the ear is brought up in a bag from the scene of the accident, in which case do not be tempted to suture the ear back on immediately. Take the skin off the cartilage, preserve the cartilage by burying it in the abdominal wall and use whatever of the auricular skin you need to make good the defect on the scalp. Subsequently the cartilage can be buried underneath scalp and auricular skin when the area has been well healed for about six months and can subsequently be brought outwards by incision along its upper border and a free skin graft inlaid posteriorly. If the auricle has been cleanly cut off, and is not crushed (as for example in a windscreen accident), and if the detached auricle has been rescued early, packed in ice, and accompanies the patient to a plastic surgery centre, the micro-surgical reattachment is, nowadays, a possibility. This will require the anastomosis of one principle artery, and preferably two veins. Light packing and bandaging is indicated. For partial loss of the auricle, the post-auricular skin can be used to form the external layer of lost skin with the base of the flap over the mastoid process. A subsequent operation after six weeks allows the mastoid skin to be lifted, still attached to the ear, and it can be then turned to form the post-auricular layer, with a free skin graft to the defect on the mastoid process. At the second operation it may be advisable to tie sutures through the rim of the ear from external to internal surface to fashion a helix rim and keep the two layers of the flap together. Only use one or two sutures, because if too many are used the distal part of the flap, that is the part lying on the post-auricular region, may be killed. Subsequently, if the flap lacks suitable support, a small portion of conchal cartilage can be removed from the opposite ear and inserted as a strut.

Contracted meatal opening

This may occur as a result of surgery or a direct trauma, in which case the opening can be enlarged and scar tissue excised and if it is a ring contracture a small flap of ear skin can be sutured into the meatus as a Z-plasty. If it is a large defect a thick skin graft on a gutta percha mould can be put in place. The gutta percha mould can be subsequently replaced by clear acrylic with a small hole down the centre of it to allow air to enter the inner part of the meatus. This mould must be worn for at least six months or further skin graft contracture will occur.

Infective

Chondritis occurs most frequently as a result of burns, dog-bites or human bites on the ear. Where established chondritis is present there is a very painful and swollen 'boggy' helix and concha. The ear must be split around the helix margin and opened out into its external and posterior skin layers. The infected cartilage will then be seen and all infected cartilage must be removed, otherwise the perichondrial stripping will progress until all cartilage has necrosed and the external ear finishes as a small crumpled-up piece of skin. The two leaves of auricular skin must then be packed open with daily quarter-strength Eusol dressings and after a bacteriological swab has shown the sensitivity of the organisms, the appropriate antibiotic must be given. systemically. If prompt treatment is performed, a large amount of the subsequent deformity of the ear can be prevented in this way.

Neoplastic conditions

It is often said that basal cell carcinoma of the ear is rare, but in the author's experience it is not uncommon. Basal cell carcinoma and squamous cell carcinoma occur at about the same frequency, but the squamous cell carcinoma tends to be more frequent on the exposed rim of the ear whereas the basal cell carcinoma is most

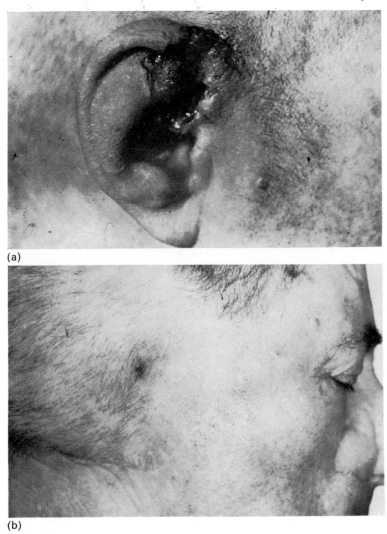

(a)

(b)

Figure 5.6 (a) A squamous carcinoma of the ear needing wide resection and scalp flap cover of the bare bone; (b) the scalp flap in place

frequent in the conchal region itself abutting on the external meatus or in the post-auricular fold in its lower part, and it is this area that has the worst prognosis because the mastoid is very near, bone invasion occurs relatively soon, and treatment is often delayed through the patient reporting late. With small neoplasms in the conchal region it is advisable to excise with a clear margin, taking the conchal cartilage. A very good vascular bed is thereby provided to receive a post-auricular Wolfe graft from the same ear sutured in place using long tie-over sutures to fix a small dressing of flavine wool over the graft. The concha is packed and a pressure dressing applied. For lesions of the periphery of the pinna a wedge excision is indicated, but this wedge must be staggered, a quadrilateral piece being removed from the helix and the fossa of the helix. A vertical incision is used along the line of the antihelix, a subsequent staggered triangle being removed from the concha. In this way when the pinna is sutured in its posterior and external layers, a Z-type of incision and scar occurs which prevents notching and also avoids too much 'cockling' of the pinna. Small lesions on the rim of the helix can be removed in line with the helix with advancement of the post-auricular skin upwards and direct closure. New growths in the post-auricular

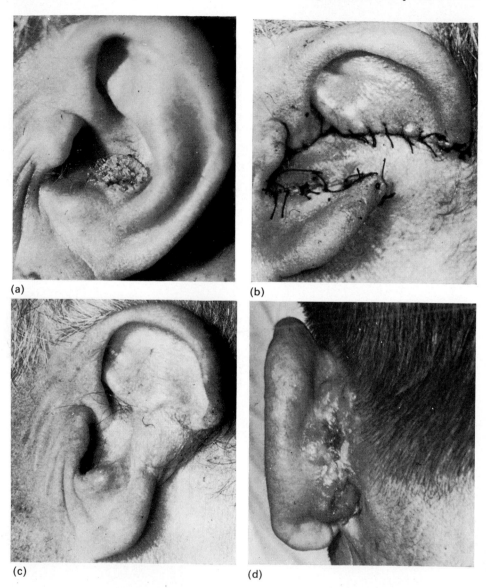

(a)   (b)

(c)   (d)

Figure 5.7   (a) A basal cell carcinoma involving cartilage; (b) excision and a post-auricular flap repair; (c) a new sulcus has been made; (d) a post-auricular sulcus basal celled carcinoma needing a total ear excision and split-skin graft

sulcus should be removed widely and a free skin graft, usually removed from the thigh, sutured into place and packed in with flavine wool and a pressure dressing. Lesions in the concha itself, passing through all layers of the ear, must be excised with a good margin of normal tissue and then the post-auricular skin and that skin over the mastoid can be advanced in to form the external layer of auricular skin. A small buttonhole remains which subsequently is closed in a secondary procedure.

Perichondritis nodularis helicis chronica

This curious condition, by some authorities regarded as due to arteriovenous fistulae, occurs in the rim of the ear and was seen very frequently among ex-soldiers who had spent the severe winter of the first year of the war in northern Europe. Clinically, the condition shows itself as a small painful nodule on the helix or in the fossa of the helix, the nodule being about the size of a split pea with a small amount of scaling from the epithelium over it. It is painful on pressure and therefore the patient always tends to lie on the opposite side. Excision under local anaesthesia and direct closure of the defect by post-auricular skin advancement usually cures this affliction.

References

Barinka, L. (1966). *Acta chirurgica plastica*, **8**, 1 (Czechoslovakia)

Converse, J. M. (1964). *Reconstructive Plastic Surgery*. London; Saunders

Tanzer, R. C. (1959). *Plastic reconstructive Surgery*, **23**, 1

6 Congenital conditions of the middle-ear cleft

William G Edwards

Introduction

Exploration of the middle ear by tympanotomy in cases of conductive deafness has revealed a wide range of congenital anomalies within the tympanic cavity which have been previously of little clinical significance. Many of these anomalies are now of considerable surgical importance as, in many cases, incomplete development or malformation is found to be the primary cause of deafness. When this is so, conductive deafness is due to functional disjunction of the ossicular chain by incomplete development or to fixation of the chain at some point to the walls of the tympanic cavity. In addition to the more obvious congenital meatal atresia, this chapter discusses those congenital middle-ear anomalies which cause a significant deafness but lie deep to an apparently normal tympanic membrane.

The term congenital meatal atresia will be used to describe those abnormalities of the pinna and external auditory meatus most commonly associated with middle-ear malformation; the visible atresia or microtia is but one aspect of the total clinical problem which is better expressed by the term *congenital aplasia of the ear*. In general the severity of the outer ear deformity suggests a parallel severe dislocation of the middle-ear structures but there is no close or even consistent relationship and the state of the middle-ear development cannot be assessed from the external appearance.

Although both outer and middle ear are deformed, the inner ear may remain unaffected. This is because the outer and middle ears have different embryological origins and develop independently of the inner ear. The outer- and middle-ear structures are formed from the tissues at the dorsal ends of the first and second branchial arches enclosing the first branchial cleft—the primitive eustachian tube; the inner ear develops from an outgrowth of the hind brain which becomes encapsulated as the otocyst, later differentiating into the membranous labyrinth. These primordia come together very early and their interrelationship is established by the sixth week of fetal life.

Anomalies of other regions derived from the first and second branchial arches may be associated with aplasia of the ear to a varying degree. The clinical expression of this is seen most typically in the syndrome of mandibulofacial dysostosis (Treacher–Collins, Franceschetti–Zwahlen) in which congenital meatal atresia is coupled with extensive malformation of the facial bones and soft tissues. But less severe deformity is the more common and the practising otologist must look for slight asymmetry of the face or especially of the mandible as a clue to the existence of a middle-ear deformity even in the absence of a visible atresia (Edwards, 1974).

In clinical practice, therefore, one can recognize congenital aplasia of the ear in the following presentations:

(1) *Complete atresia*, unilateral or bilateral, usually associated with microtia but without any other apparent malformation.

(2) *Atresia and often microtia*, associated with other facial, cervical or cranial malformation, as in the syndrome of mandibulofacial dysostosis and other rare conditions.

(3) *Congenital conductive deafness* in relation to a patent external auditory meatus terminated by a functional tympanic membrane.

(a) Many of these cases are diagnosed in retrospect at tympanotomy for presumed otosclerosis when a congenital middle-ear lesion is found.

(b) Some cases may be diagnosed before operation if minor anomalies of the facial features, mandible or pinna are present or if a history of deafness since very early childhood is realized to be valid—the 'minor aplasias' (Ombredanne, 1968).

In uncomplicated meatal atresia the developmental anomaly is centred on the atresia plate, malleus and incus—the *lateral* components of the sound conduction system deriving largely from first branchial arch elements—whilst the inner face of the tympanic cavity is relatively spared. The promontory, oval window and stapes are often found functionally normal and a good hearing result can be anticipated from surgery if a stable external meatus is created. In congenital conductive deafness with a patent meatus and intact tympanic membrane the oval window niche and stapes are most often primarily included in the developmental distortion of the *medial* tympanic cavity: the anatomical situation in many cases may be highly unfavourable for sophisticated stapes surgery which could involve unacceptable risk to cochlear function in these circumstances. By reason of these patterns of developmental defect the overall prospect of hearing improvement is greater in congenital aural atresia, although major surgical problems of reconstruction are presented, than in the apparently simpler deformity seen in congenital conductive deafness.

The independent development of the inner ear results in a normal labyrinth in the majority of these cases even though the middle ear and external ear may be grossly deformed. In every case of congenital aplasia of the ear the surgeon must satisfy himself that adequate cochlear function is present before undertaking a difficult surgical exploration. He must be certain that a reasonable—if not a fully normal—potential hearing level exists which may be brought forth by successful surgery.

Pre-natal anatomical development of the ear

The development of the middle ear and its associated structures is largely established within the first trimester of pregnancy. From that period on the major events concern the extension of the tympanic cavity and remodelling of anatomical structure by resorption of cartilage and bone: some clinical anomalies will arise from aberrations in this process. Early development involves the interaction between ectoderm and endoderm around the first pharyngeal pouch which gives rise to the mucosa lining the tympanic cleft; the tympanic membrane itself derives from all three elements (Bowden, 1977). Encircling these structures the squamous temporal, tympanic ring and petrous temporal components begin ossification from multiple centres: it is the growth of the petrous bone in its long axis which elevates the pinna and reduces the obliquity of the primitive external meatus and tympanic membrane. Downward extension of abnormal ossification into mesenchyme at this stage may give rise to the typical atresia plate as it escapes the organizing influence of the tympanic ring primordium (Wright, Phelps and Fraser, 1977).

The external ear

The pinna arises from a series of six hillocks which appear encircling the primitive meatus during the sixth week of intrauterine life. One of these, destined to form the tragus, is indubitably of first branchial arch origin whilst the others variously arise from tissues of both first and second arches. The pinna rises to its normal position by the fourth fetal month but does not reach adult size until the age of nine. The external auditory meatus is not finally formed until late in gestation—at eight weeks a solid epithelial cord grows inwards from the primitive meatus but these cells do not undergo dissolution until the seventh month. This process of canalization begins medially, forming the outer surface of the tympanic membrane, and proceeds outwards to reach the surface at the end of the seventh month.

The middle ear

The tympanic membrane forms at the 28th week as the deep meatus becomes canalized; its fibrous middle layer derives from mesenchyme at the upper end of Meckel's cartilage (first arch) which may explain the frequent presence of a dense bony plate in this position in cases of atresia. The tympanic cavity extends in the middle fetal months with dissolution of the spongy mesenchymal tissue which originally fills the potential space; the antrum appears at 23 weeks and pneumatization of the mastoid is about to begin at term.

The ossicles develop much earlier than this—they are identified and continuous in the six-week embryo. The ossicular chain is formed and beginning to ossify by the 12th week and the ossicles are of adult size at birth.

The continuity of the ossicular chain is established as a consequence of complex interrelationships between the tissue primordia at the dorsal ends of the first and second branchial arches, as a result of which the part of the ossicular chain *superior* to the facial nerve is derived from tissues of first arch origin and the lower part from second arch tissues. This view of a complex origin is surgically significant for it is not uncommon for the otologist to find malformation of the lower half of the ossicular chain (the manubrium of the malleus and the long process of the incus) in conjunction with marked stapedial anomalies; this would correspond with defective development from second arch tissues. (A congenital failure of formation of the incudostapedial articulation in isolation is not described.)

The bodies of the malleus and incus are formed from first branchial arch tissues: the respective manubrium and long process originate from mesenchyme located around the second arch. The stapes also has a double origin: the main structure derives from the second branchial arch but the inner (vestibular) aspect of the footplate differentiates from the otic capsule itself—this area is termed the lamina stapedialis. As development proceeds the cells immediately adjacent to this lamina will normally form the annular ligament and the lamina becomes incorporated into the footplate of the stapes. Histiocyte remodelling of the stapes superstructure in close relation to the stapedial artery causes the sacrifice of a large fraction of its initial mass in the middle phase of fetal life (Richards and Gibbin, 1977).

The internal ear

The cochlea is identifiable at the sixth week.

The organ of Corti is fully differentiated at 20 weeks and the labyrinth is of adult size at the 24th week.

Aetiology

There is little direct evidence reported as to the incidence of aplasias of the ear other than that of Sullivan, McAskile and Smith (1959) who quote the figure of eight cases of atresia arising amongst 30 000 live births examined in the neonatal period. They suggest that the true incidence of atresia may well be greater than this in view of the difficulties of early examination; even so this figure could not include congenital middle-ear lesions found in later life. Also in the previous decade the natural incidence of ear malformations has been greatly increased by the maternal use of the drug thalidomide, as a sedative, during early pregnancy when congenital atresia may be induced. Jafek and his colleagues (1975) report a series of 241 cases of congenital aural atresia in which the influence of thalidomide was excluded by North American legislation: 29 per cent of referred cases were bilateral with a distinct preponderance in the whole series to the male child in 61 per cent and to the right side in 56 per cent of referrals. In 14 per cent of all patients a definite family history of similar malformation existed whilst no fewer than 56 per cent of the children had some associated handicap. Radiological evidence of inner-ear anomaly was demonstrated in 11 per cent of the series.

In any review of congenital atresia it is unusual for any pattern of genetic transmission to emerge except in truly hereditary cases of mandibulofacial dysostosis (Nevin, 1977). In almost the majority of cases no specific cause is recognizable. Neither is there evidence of genetic relationship to congenital perceptive deafness; although the author has operated for aplasia on a child of perceptively deaf parents, this case is only mentioned to emphasize the point that deafness in the young child must not too easily be presumed to be perceptive when bone conduction audiometry can confirm its true nature.

The factors which may cause congenital aplasia are (1) genetic; and (2) teratogenic, such as virus infections or toxic chemical factors operating *in utero* during the early months of pregnancy. Only in very occasional cases is it possible to link directly the deformity produced to the period of development in which the embryo was damaged. In practice it is very difficult to know the exact age of the fetus, or the date when the damage was incurred. *Figure 6.1* is of interest as all the details are known. It shows a baby with bilateral congenital meatal atresia whose mother took thalidomide. The date of conception is known, and the date, dosage and duration of administration of the drug are also known (total—150 mg thalidomide from the 43rd to the 45th day). This evidence is circumstantial rather than directly conclusive but it does indicate the potent teratogenic effect which the drug may exert and also the severity of the defect induced by dislocation or arrest of development at this early stage. An experimental animal model of the induction of mandibulo-facial dysostosis had been presented by Poswillo (1975) in the offspring of Wistar rats given large amounts of vitamin A on the eighth day of embryonic development. The mechanism of malformation begins as a destructive effect, possibly by focal haemorrhage, upon the neural crest cells of the facial and auditory primordia; hypoplasia of these regions results in compensatory migration of the otic vesicle as the combined basis of the final deformity.

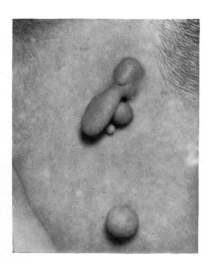 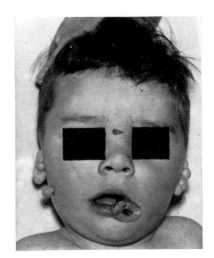

Figure 6.1   Case of the late Mr. Gavin Livingstone

When development is arrested after the third month, the pinna and middle ear may be normal but the external auditory meatus may have failed to reopen, leaving a fibrous atresia. The bony meatus may be partially formed and its deep part found patent adjacent to a partially differentiated tympanic membrane.

Surgical pathology

A wide range of malformations have been described in these cases and it is common to find more than one anomaly in combination as a cause of deafness. The pattern of combined defects broadly corresponds to the embryological development already described but classification is more easily based on anatomical subdivisions.

The external ear

ABNORMALITIES OF THE PINNA

(1) Total absence.
(2) Microtia.
(3) Accessory auricles.
(4) Pre-auricular sinus (*see* p. 122).
(5) Congenital aural fistula.
(6) Minor anomalies of contour.

In congenital aplasia the pinna is rarely entirely normal; a bizarre range of malformation is seen as regards size and contour but the position of the pinna is consistently lower down on the head and placed further forward than is normal (Gill, 1969). The presence of an identifiable tragus suggests that the external auditory meatus is partially formed and indicates a rather better prospect of successful surgical exploration.

ABNORMALITIES OF THE EXTERNAL AUDITORY MEATUS

(1) Complete atresia.
(2) Shallow blind depression.

In both conditions the potential external canal is usually dense bone, but there may be cartilaginous remnants. The middle ear will usually be abnormal, and in severe cases the middle-ear cleft may be completely absent. When the lumen of the canal is replaced by dense fibrous tissue alone the pinna is not usually affected.

(3) Stenosis associated with accentuated curvature of the canal in both horizontal and
    vertical planes corresponding to the downward and forward displacement of the
    pinna. The narrowed, arched meatus often renders the tympanic membrane
    impossible to see in its entirety. The membrane itself may be only partly developed
    and is usually smaller than normal.

The middle ear

ABNORMALITIES OF THE OSSICLES

The malleus
This is the most frequently malformed ossicle and is often fused to the body of the incus with obliteration of the normal articulation. It may be fixed by bone to the walls of the epitympanum, especially in the region of the short process and the superior face of the malleus head. The manubrium is usually shortened and incurved; it is frequently confluent with the dense bone of the inferior part of an atresia plate replacing the lower anterior portion of the tympanic membrane.

The incus
This is often fused with the malleus as a compound bony mass. The incus body may be adherent to the medial wall of the epitympanum and is usually rather reduced in

size. The long process of an abnormal incus is almost always deformed—either it is grossly foreshortened and lies medially ending on the facial nerve sheath; or a long, thin fibrous process extends to the head of the stapes. This is ineffective in sound transmission but represents continuity of the chain during development—congenital separation of a normal long process from the stapes head is not described.

The stapes

In isolated congenital fixation of the stapes the superstructure of the ossicle is typically normal and little change may be apparent in the footplate excepting that it is circumferentially fixed, blending into the bone of the surrounding otic capsule without a definable annular ligament although there is not the overgrowth of bone seen in active otosclerosis.

Absence of the stapedius tendon is found in 1 per cent of cases explored by tympanotomy and is thus a fairly common anomaly but apparently of no consequence to sound transmission. In cases of aplasia the stapes arch may be distorted, the crura attenuated and the capitellum small. In some cases the whole bone is hypoplastic, assuming an embryonic form in severe malformations (*Figure 6.2*) when the oval window niche may have failed to differentiate. If the stapes is totally absent there may be no depression or other indication of the site of the vestibular window. A variation occasionally seen is a truly monopodal stapes as in *Figure 6.2* which illustrates well the hypoplastic footplate generally found associated with any severe anomaly of the ossicle. Fixation of such a footplate must be noted as a feature of the greatest surgical importance and is frequently found at exploration.

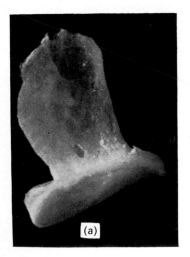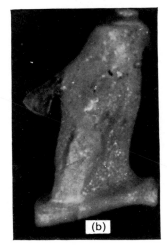

(a)   (b)

Figure 6.2 Monopodal malformation of stapes: from two cases of Treacher–Collins syndrome without atresia

Bennett (1966) discussing subarachnoid—tympanic fistulae illustrates the rare anomaly of a central defect in the stapes footplate in two cases associated with recurrent meningitis and cerebrospinal tympanic effusion. This observation has been expanded in many subsequent reports—thus Hipskind *et al.* (1976) vividly describe the presentation of a perilymph 'gusher' in such a congenitally deformed footplate.

Richards and Gibbin (1977) review the developmental origin of the stapes footplate and its possible relation to cochlear dysplasia and raised intralabyrinthine pressure. Clinical investigation in cases of congenital conductive deafness should include detailed tomography as a distended vestibular sac is characteristically seen as a dilated bony vestibular capsule sometimes associated with Mondini type cochlear dysplasia (*Figure 6.3*).

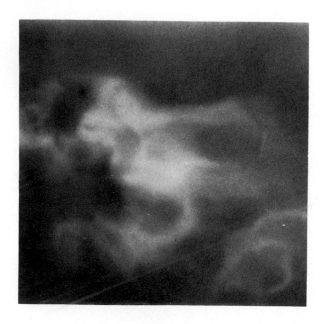

Figure 6.3 Detail of polytome 'vestibular cut' of the right ear. Significant dilatation of the vestibule is shown. This young woman had a profuse perilymph 'gusher' at stapedectomy

THE OVAL WINDOW

Congenital occlusion or absence of the oval window is a rare finding at tympanotomy— in these cases a rudimentary stapes fragment, the 'banana' stapes (*Figure 6.6*)—hangs freely above an undifferentiated oval window niche and the facial nerve may be exposed or displaced downwards crossing the occluded window or the promontory. Jahrsdoerfer (1977) has reviewed his own experience and 39 cases in the literature commenting that in these cases the risk/benefit ratio of attempted oval window fenestration is highly unfavourable.

THE ROUND WINDOW

Total occlusion of the round window niche may occur but is very rare (Ombredanne, 1968). The normal variation in contour of the round window niche is such that it is difficult to recognize true congenital anomaly but on several occasions the author has noted an enlargement of the fenestra, and in one case its replacement by a thin leaking perilymphatic cyst. The cochlear coils were not present on pre-operative tomography in this patient.

THE FACIAL NERVE

Congenital dehiscence of the bony facial canal in the region of the oval window is a very common finding at tympanotomy and was present at 31 per cent of normal temporal bones examined by Leonard and Alexander (1968). Bulging of the nerve sheath sufficient to obscure the oval window may create great difficulty in reconstructive surgery, but is not likely to cause deafness in isolation.

The great fear in undertaking exploration of a congenital atresia is that the facial nerve is likely to pursue an entirely abnormal course which may not be recognized. In 1965 Livingstone, widely respected as the pioneer of surgery for aural atresia in this country, found the nerve displaced only rarely in his series and felt that this fear was probably exaggerated. The current surgical experience is more cautious in that an abnormal course of the facial nerve may be anticipated in at least one third of cases (Crabtree, 1974). The surgeon must aim to identify the facial nerve at the earliest practicable stage of his exploration: the most constant anatomical course is far forward in the horizontal segment as it enters the anterior tympanic cavity. In the gradation of arrested development encountered, the facial nerve trunk tends to be foreshortened, taking a more acute angle at the external genu to rise superficially in the region of the posterior annulus; this course will restrict surgical access to the stapes and oval window and places the nerve at great risk of damage in this region.

An anomalous course of the facial nerve is most often an inferior displacement so that it runs unprotected across the promontory below the oval window (Dickinson, Srisomboon and Kamerer, 1968); or the main trunk may be bifid, with one section taking this anomalous route. Only extremely rarely will such an anomaly directly obstruct sound transmission but the author has successfully explored a child in whom the facial nerve trunk covered the footplate and pierced the anterior crus, which itself was fixed to the promontory (*see also* Butler, 1968).

Vascular abnormalities

A congenital defect of the posterior and inferior bony walls of the middle ear may allow extensive herniation of the jugular bulb into the tympanic cavity. This can be an alarming discovery during a tympanotomy and, although it is not usually a cause of deafness, the author has explored cases in which this anomaly appeared responsible for the hearing loss, presumably because the venous sinus overlay the round window and in one case pressed upon the stapedial arch (Moretti, 1976; Graham, 1975).

The stapedial artery is important embryologically as the residual artery of the second branchial arch: in rare cases it persists as a moderately large vessel crossing the anterior stapes footplate (Hough, 1963). In this instance the aberrant vessel was associated with otosclerotic stapes fixation and its position posed exceptional technical problems in stapedectomy. Seventeen cases of a persistent stapedial artery are reviewed by Steffen (1968) in addition to other anomalies of the jugular bulb and internal carotid artery appearing within the tympanic cavity. An aberrant or aneurysmal internal carotid artery may be demonstrated by contrast arteriography (Goldman, Singleton and Holly, 1971).

Congenital haemangiomas may be seen in the middle-ear cleft but do not appear as a cause of deafness, although theoretically deafness could arise from involvement of either window region or the ossicular chain by a haemangioma.

Congenital tumours

Several cases are recorded of a rare choristoma of salivary gland origin in the middle ear (Abadir and Pease, 1978). These arise from a 'christa' of normal tissue displaced in embryonic development and may be associated with ossicular chain defects. Though of great interest, true congenital cholesteatoma is extremely rare but has been described deep to a congenital atresia plate (Schuknecht, 1974).

Abnormalities induced by thalidomide

Thalidomide was introduced around 1958 as a sedative and hypnotic drug: in November 1961 Lenz, a German paediatrician, noted an increasing number of children born with severe malformations, usually associated with fetal damage between the fourth and seventh weeks of intrauterine development, and he suspected the relationship of these to ingestion of thalidomide by the mother. The most common deformities were a severe hypoplasia or total absence of a limb whilst congenital astresia of the ear is also relatively common (Livingstone, 1965); some 150 cases of congenital aplasia are estimated in a total of around 450 thalidomide-affected children in this country.

Detailed tomography of the temporal bone in these cases often reveals extensive combined dysplasia of both inner- and middle-ear regions which, though ordinarily rare, are frequent in this group. The inner-ear involvement in the dysplasia is strikingly high, at least 25 per cent of cases (Livingstone, 1965) although these are not of any specific character, nor fundamentally different types of deformity (Mondini, Sibermann, Michel) from those seen in other cases (Mundnich, 1974). In the middle ear multiple anomalies of the ossicles are usually present whilst the atresia of the meatus is often associated with branchial fistulae. Although many of these children have a congenital facial nerve paresis no particular anomaly of the course or appearance of the nerve is described and the paresis is ascribed to a central nuclear aplasia.

The prospect of successful middle-ear surgery is less good in these cases of thalidomide-induced atresia, and the decision for operation must be taken with full consideration of the other handicaps many of these children suffer whilst realizing that their hearing loss may be their greatest handicap to educational progress. In these children temporal bone tomography is essential in their pre-operative assessment, as evidence of cochlear aplasia would normally be an absolute contraindication to operation on that ear.

Congenital atresia in association with other malformations

The syndrome of mandibulofacial dysostosis—Treacher–Collins syndrome; Franceschetti–Zwahlen syndrome—is the most common combined malformation; it primarily affects the facial structures deriving from the first branchial arch but also, especially the ear, involves second arch structures. The severity of the deformity varies from the complete form with severe bilateral distortion of the facial features and bilateral microtia with atresia to incomplete, even unilateral, forms with little disfigurement and solely middle-ear malformation (Edwards, 1964). The clinical features in the complete form (*Figures 6.4* and *6.5*) are:

(1) The ocular characteristics.
Antimongoloid inclination of the palpebral fissures.
Notching of the *lower* eyelid in its lateral part.
Atrophic lid margins and deficient eyelashes medial to this coloboma.
(2) Hypoplasia of the middle third of the face.
The peculiar hypoplasia of the malar prominence.
A more generalized hypoplasia of the maxilla.
(3) Hypoplasia of the mandible.
(4) Congenital atresia of the ear with microtia.

The dysplasia of the middle and outer ears in the complete forms of this syndrome is severe and in many cases an aerated middle-ear space has failed to develop—over 40 per cent were noted by Livingstone (1965) to show a diminished middle-ear space and of his total cases 25 per cent had radiological deformity of the labyrinth. The chance of successful middle-ear exploration in these severe forms of the syndrome is poor and Gill (1969) considers that severe facial deformity of this type with microtia and radiological doubt as to the presence of a middle-ear cleft is a contraindication to operation.

Other first arch syndromes are recognized especially in the paediatric literature; malformation of the ear may be associated with these and children with features of a first branchial arch malformation must be suspected of a congenital deafness until this is definitely excluded. A cleft palate is the common deformity resulting from defective

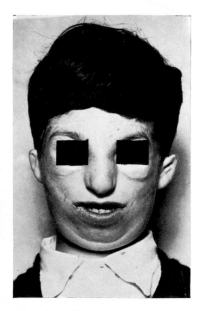 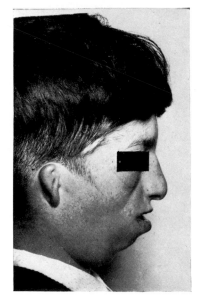

Figure 6.4   Treacher–Collins syndrome

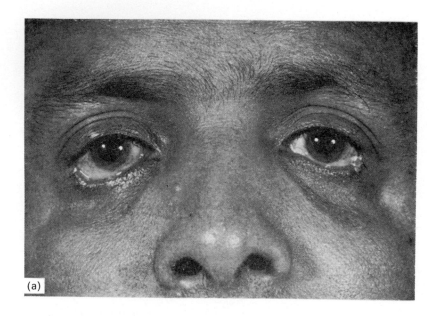

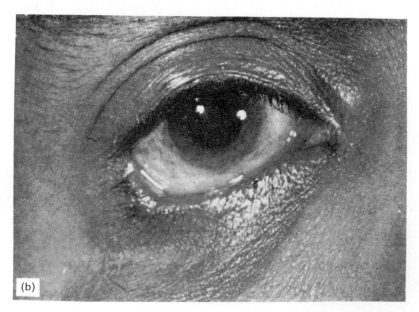

Figure 6.5 The ocular features of Treacher–Collins syndrome (mandibulo-facial dysostosis)

fusion of the maxillary processes in the midline; this congenital defect does not appear to be associated with middle-ear malformation either in general experience of paediatric otology or in the literature, except when the palatal cleft is but part of a more severe deformity (for example mandibulofacial dysostosis). Middle-ear deafness is frequent in children who have had a successful palatal repair and is almost invariably due to the presence of effusion (Young, 1968). A rare otopalatodigital syndrome has been described with anomalies of the stapes.

The Klippel–Feil syndrome of malformation of the cervical vertebrae resulting in a short, webbed neck, is occasionally associated with congenital anomalies of the ear. A perceptive deafness is more common in this syndrome and cases of atresia may show a combined hearing loss.

Some cases of atresia of the ear, especially those induced by thalidomide, show certain congenital ophthalmic anomalies (Livingstone and Delahunty, 1968). Among these syndromes are:

(1) Duane's syndrome—a congenital paresis of the horizontally-acting external ocular muscles; most often the lateral rectus is involved with absent lateral abduction of either eye.

(2) Moebius' syndrome of facial diplegia with aplasia of other brainstem nuclei affecting the external ocular muscles. It is possible that the cochlear nuclei may be involved but a perceptive hearing loss can also arise from labyrinthine malformation. Congenital bilateral abducens palsy is a similar condition which may be associated with atresia.

(3) Goldenhar's syndrome of congenital eyelid dermoids, notching of the upper eyelids and various first arch facial anomalies (Singh and Gaudi, 1977). Vertebral anomalies are described in the original description of this ocular–auriculovertebral syndrome.

Another group of rare associations of congenital atresia comprise various

Table 6.1 **Surgical and histological findings at operation or post mortem in the common clinical syndromes associated with congenital conductive hearing loss. There are frequently associated sensorineural hearing losses also**

	Pinna	Meatus	Malleus and incus	Stapes	Facial nerve
Mandibulofacial dysostosis	Deformed	Atretic	Fused and fixed	Deformed	Anomalous
Crouzon deformity	Low	Atretic	Fixed	Deformed	Normal
Marfan's syndrome	Collapsed	Narrow	Normal	Normal	Normal
Klippel–Feil syndrome	Deformed	Atretic	Deformed	Deformed	Normal
Trisomy D & E	Deformed	Absent	Deformed	Absent	Anomalous
Cretinism	Normal	Normal	Fixed	Fixed	Normal
Osteogenesis imperfecta	Normal	Normal	Normal	Fixed	Normal
Osteopetrosis	Normal	Normal	Cartilage	Fixed	Normal
Thalidomide	Absent	Atretic	Deformed	Absent	Anomalous
Rubella	Normal	Normal	Normal	Fixed	Normal

(From Wright, Phelps and Fraser, 1977 reproduced by courtesy of the authors and *Proceedings of the Royal Society of Medicine*)

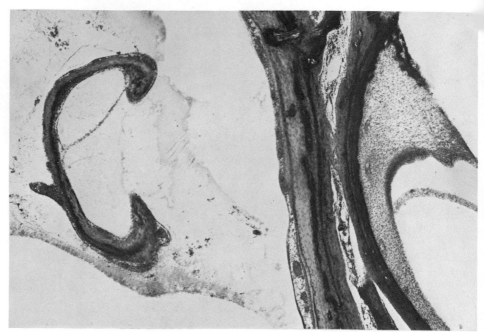

Figure 6.6   Histological section showing a rudimentary banana-shaped stapes superstructure. There was no footplate differentiation (×24). (From Wright, Phelps and Fraser (1977), *Proceedings of the Royal Society of Medicine*, **70**, 816 by permission of the authors)

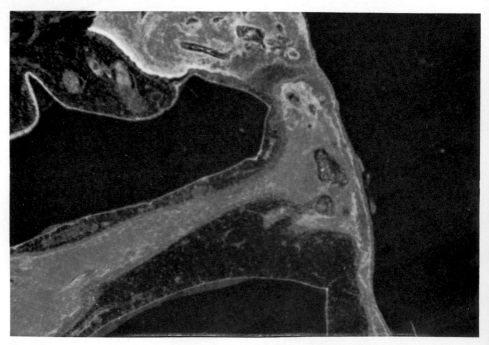

Figure 6.7   Shows a columella stapes which is fixed by a cartilaginous bar. M = middle ear, V = vestibule (×80). (From Wright, Phelps and Fraser (1977), *Proceedings of the Royal Society of Medicine*, **70**, 816 by permission of the authors)

malformations of the renal tract, especially reduplications and agenesis (Winter *et al.*, 1968). A very extensive literature exists on rare individual syndromes involving congenital atresia and other ear anomalies (Sando and Wood, 1971) whilst the known pathology of the ear in these syndromes is authoritatively recorded by Schuknecht (1974).

All cases of facial anomaly or cervical spine malformation present one feature of outstanding clinical importance—the combination of deformities renders endotracheal intubation difficult and in some cases even the most experienced will be unable to expose the larynx adequately. General anaesthesia, even for investigations such as tomography, must be carefully induced and the *anaesthetist warned of probable difficulty.*

Radiological investigation

To judge the prospects of surgical exploration it is essential to have some knowledge of the situation that lies beyond the atresia and this may be revealed with considerable accuracy by fine section tomography of the temporal bone. Conventional radiological views are of value when pneumatization of the mastoid and middle-ear cleft is shown but tomography is needed to delineate the detailed anatomy of the tympanic plate, ossicular chain and tympanic cavity of the middle ear and, equally important, the anatomy of the bony labyrinth, as deformity of this is presumptive evidence of cochlear malformation with sensorineural deafness (Phelps and Wright, 1976).

As many radiologists use the Massiot polytome with a polycyclic motion during exposure this technique is often termed polytomography; but du Boulay and Bostik (1969) show the excellent films which may be obtained using more standard cranial linear tomography if careful attention is paid to details. Tomography in the antero-posterior plane in the supine position is most usual, as the simultaneous exposure of both ears both greatly shortens the procedure and allows for easier identification of structures as well as comparison of the two ears. (The time factor may be important when examining small children under general anaesthesia.) Details of the ossicular chain and oval window can be better demonstrated in this position with the head turned 20 degrees towards the side to be examined (the semi-axial view). Tomography in the lateral plane is of value in showing the ossicles and the position of the descending portion of the facial nerve canal. In the antero–posterior plane two tomographic sections are of fundamental value (Phelps, Sheldon and Lloyd, 1976).

(1) The 'vestibular cut' showing the incus, lateral semicircular canal and vestibule, oval window leading into the basal turn of the cochlea and the internal auditory meatus.

(2) The 'cochlear cut'—some millimetres anterior to the vestibule passing through the malleus head and showing the coil of the cochlea around its central bony spiral (the modiolus).

Demonstration of inner-ear deformity will give an indication of the probable severity of sensorineural loss although both interpretation and correlation are not clear cut (Phelps, Lloyd and Sheldon, 1975; Phelps, Sheldon and Lloyd, 1976). The outline and size of the internal auditory meatus may be conclusive as narrowing below a corrected diameter of 3 mm or tapering of its vestibular end is associated with severe sensorineural loss. A solitary labyrinthine sac—the Michel deformity—indicates a total deafness in that ear but some cochlear function is retained in limited labyrinthine dysplasia such as dilatation or partial absence of the semicircular canals. In the Mondini deformity the central bony spiral (modiolus) of the cochlea is absent and the distal one and a half coils of the cochlea are replaced by an 'empty sac' appearance. Although some hearing may be retained its quality and value is uncertain and these children are very deaf. Slight deformity of the bony labyrinth, with a normal internal auditory canal, is usually associated with normal cochlear hearing. Dilatation of the vestibule may however indicate the possibility of cerebrospinal fluid fistula through the oval window either spontaneous in origin or as a consequence of surgery (*Figure 6.3*).

The wide range of congenital deformities of the middle and external ears are well demonstrated radiologically (Phelps, Lloyd and Sheldon, 1977); the anatomical plan shown guides the decision on surgical feasibility (*Figure 6.8*).

(1) The external auditory meatus is shown in outline, enhanced if wished by coating with contrast medium to demonstrate the character of the fibrous or bony atresia and the dimensions of the atretic tympanic plate. This usually lies external to the tympanic cavity with the malleus handle confluent with its inner face but rarely an atresia plate may lie medial to a rudimentary tympanic cavity in the position of the promontory (Reisner, 1969).

(2) The tympanic cavity is normally well pneumatized in cases of unilateral atresia but encroachment by the atresia plate, a high jugular bulb or descent of the tegmen superiorly may be visible. Total aplasia with absence of any tympanic cavity is rare but a minimal distorted 'air space' is a contraindication to surgery as this is often not aerated but filled with radiolucent mucus or mesenchymal tissue. Thin bony septa may divide the middle-ear cavity and confuse the surgeon if he is unaware of this possibility.

(3) The major ossicles will normally be seen within the upper tympanic cavity; in the lateral view the malleus and incus present the classic 'molar tooth' outline as an articulated or fused mass. Fixation and discontinuity of the chain are not demonstrable within the normal limits of resolution.

(4) Occlusion of the oval window or displacement from normal position can be shown with good technique although the stapes itself is not normally defined.

(5) The facial nerve canal is identifiable and any suspected displacement should be studied more closely in the lateral projection for the descending portion which may take a more direct anterior and superficial route potentially hazardous at surgery.

Polytomography of the temporal bone is of greatest value in complete atresia but in aplasias where the tympanic membrane is visible, although the details of middle-ear anatomy may be more definitely revealed by surgical tympanotomy, these techniques can demonstrate unsuspected malformation of the inner ear. In thalidomide-induced atresia, and in severe mandibulofacial dysostosis, tomography is invaluable as the incidence of inner-ear involvement in these cases is strikingly high. In all cases the tomograms provide the best information on which to base the choice of ear for initial exploration in the young child.

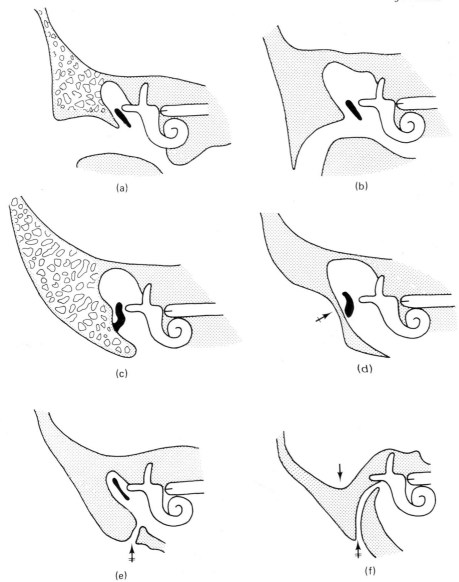

Figure 6.8 Six line drawings to illustrate typical congenital deformities of the middle and external ears. (a) Normal ear; (b) curved EAM running upwards; (c) thick pneumatized atretic plate with S-shaped ossicular mass; (d) thin atretic plate (arrow) and an ossicular mass; (e) slit attic with 'spindly' ossicles. The facial nerve (arrow) passes out laterally through the floor of the middle ear; (f) descent of the tegmen (plain arrow). There is a slit middle-ear cavity, no ossicles or oval window and an anteriorly situated facial nerve canal. (From Phelps, Lloyd and Sheldon (1977), *British Journal of Radiology*, **50**, 714 by permission of the authors)

Repeated tomography, or an extended study involving a large number of exposures may be unwise in the young child and in all cases the limitation of the total irradition should be carefully considered.

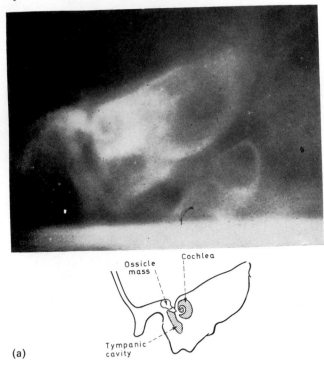

(a)

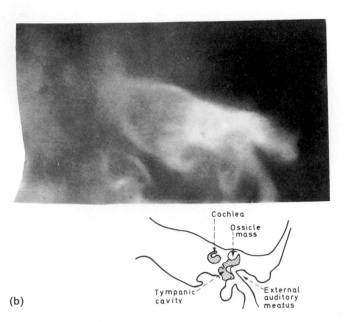

(b)

Figure 6.9 **Tomo**graphs of an adult case of mandibulofacial dysostosis wit**h** ***bila***teral atresia; in (a) a bony external meatus is visible—this is **absen**t in (b)

Congenital conductive deafness without atresia

Diagnosis

The recognition of these cases in the adult and the pre-operative distinction from clinical otosclerosis rests primarily on the realization of a deafness dating from childhood and the absence of typical features of otosclerosis in the clinical history. Hough (1963) suggests the following observations as an indication that a middle-ear malformation may be present.

(1) A history of hearing loss since birth or since the earliest recollection of childhood.
(2) Deafness present with a malformation is usually greater than that seen in the usual acquired cases of deafness.
(3) If any other anomaly is present in the branchial arch regions one should suspect a middle-ear malformation.
(4) A patient with unilateral conductive deafness is more likely to have a congenital lesion of the middle ear.
(5) Audiometrically a congenital conductive deafness tends to produce a more severe conductive loss, around 70 dB, than that seen in the usual acquired cases of deafness. The air conduction curve tends to be flat through the speech frequencies, while the bone conduction is on the 'top line' with Carhart's notch not present in the graph.

House, House and Hildyard (1958), describing congenital fixation of the stapes footplate, stress the non-progressive character of the conductive deafness and comment upon similar audiometric features. Other indications which may be observed at clinical examination include anomalies of the face, mandible or pinna whilst the external auditory canal is often narrow and arch-like as it curves sharply forward. The tympanic membrane is often lustreless, apparently small and lacking in mobility; the malleus handle may appear foreshortened and distorted.

The essential investigation of these cases is the precise audiometric confirmation of a conductive hearing loss, especially in cases of unilateral deafness, and the detailed examination of the tympanic membrane under the microscope as deformity or fixation of the malleus may be confirmed and in some cases the outline of the long process of the incus may be seen. In children a middle-ear effusion is a far more common cause of deafness and the tympanic changes due to this will be visible. Wide variation in the contour of the tympanogram curve is demonstrated by impedance audiometry which may indicate, for example, ossicular discontinuity in the lateral components of the ossicular chain. In most cases the presence of conductive loss will prevent elicitation of the ipsilateral stapes reflex but in unilateral cases the crossed reflex may exist, demonstrating stapes mobility in the affected ear as a favourable indication for exploratory tympanotomy. Pre-operative temporal bone tomography should be available primarily to exclude abnormalities of the cochlear anatomy and labyrinthine features which could be associated with a perilymph gusher were stapedectomy attempted. Normal tomographic definition gives less information on middle-ear anatomy as significant details of ossicular fixation, fibrous replacement, or anomalous position of the facial nerve canal are unlikely to be revealed. In practice, then, the surgeon advises exploratory tympanotomy on the evidence of a conductive deafness associated with an intact and mobile tympanic membrane, suspecting a congenital anomaly which can only be confirmed at operation when the middle ear is opened.

The contour of the meatus in these cases very often limits access through a permeatal tympanotomy and an endaural tympanoplasty approach should always be considered; the incision may incidentally allow for a meatoplasty to ensure later access to the tympanic membrane (Edwards, 1974). Early identification of the course followed by the facial nerve is of the greatest importance; the ossicular chain, and oval and round windows are inspected, and the mobility of the stapes is carefully assessed. When the stapes is mobile, sound transmission into the vestibule may be established by any appropriate ossiculoplasty technique having due consideration of the long-term stability of the reconstruction achieved. Scheer (1967) advocates stapedectomy in all cases as a remnant of malleus handle is always present for reconstruction using a suitable prosthesis. Many surgeons would prefer tympanoplastic transposition or interposition techniques, using homografts in some cases, whenever the footplate is mobile, as removal of the stapes carries a greater risk of sensorineural deafness— perhaps especially so in these anomalies—and contraindicates similar surgery on the other ear (Sale, 1969). However, in some cases a far better result will be achieved by stapedectomy as the often small, fragile stapes is particularly difficult to link effectively to the malleus handle. In isolated congenital stapes fixation classic mobilization of the stapes can be expected to give long-term hearing gain when the stapes mobilizes readily as refixation is unlikely (Linthicum, 1971). If stapedectomy is considered the initial approach should be a fine needle puncture or trephine of the fixed footplate to observe any excessive flow of perilymph; if this is encountered the small hole may be closed with a supported graft as for a fistula in view of the increased cochlear risk associated with stapedectomy in these circumstances. From the literature and personal experience it seems likely that the initial hearing gain achieved by fenestration of an abnormal oval window tends to relapse in the longer term and the surgeon must remain cautious in view of the *immediate cochlear risk and the diminished long-term expectation from stapedectomy for congenital anomaly.*

Plastic reconstruction of the pinna

In this country this is the field of the specialist plastic surgeon to whom the reconstruction is one of great difficulty and challenge to produce an acceptable pinna (Batstone, 1974). This difficulty is increased by the need, when operating on a child, to allow for the fact that the reconstructed appendage does not grow and that a reconstruction must be initially oversize to allow for correct relative proportion in the older child: also in unilateral cases there are the problems of matching level, contour and colour to the unaffected side. All techniques implant cartilage or Silastic which may necrose or be rejected in the presence of any chronic infection, such as could persist in a poorly-healed external meatus following middle-ear surgery. The plastic surgeon therefore prefers an untouched ear and two main types of technique are available to him:

(1) A sculpted implant of rib cartilage ('Tanzer') which involves a series of at least five stages begun at the age of four years.

(2) A Silastic implant contoured as for a normal pinna inserted beneath skin pedicles. This technique, giving a more natural contour and pliable consistency may supplant the cartilage implant when problems of local necrosis have been overcome. It seems that a later age—perhaps 8–9 years—is preferable when Silastic is used and this leaves the problem of the early years at school to be met by a prosthesis.

The appearance of a prosthesis may be excellent, and preferable to that of a plastic reconstruction, but psychologically it is natural for a child to prefer his own ear, firmly attached and partly hidden by hair, to one which is stuck on. Especially important is the value a reconstructed pinna may be in supporting an ear level aid as, despite a successful surgical result, many of these children will still need amplification in normal school conditions.

Plastic surgeons consider the final appearance of the pinna is improved by the formation of a meatal aperture into the mastoid cells. This technique is indefensible— the reconstruction and formation of an external auditory meatus should be carried out by the otologist as an integral part of his middle-ear reconstruction (Edgerton, 1969).

Congenital atresia of the ear

The normal baby develops comprehensive hearing with location of and interest in sound at six months when he is 'ready to listen' and this response progresses to the emergence of speech beginning at the end of the first year and continuing throughout the second year, during which time he is 'ready to speak'. By the age of four years the normal child speaks fluently and has a wide range of expression—i.e. he has learnt the concepts of language as a means of communication. He has the greatest facility for learning to speak during the first three years, and for initiation of interest in listening during the first year. In order to give a deaf child his optimum chance of speaking well he must be exposed to as much correct sound as possible during these early critical years.

The management of children with atresia is governed by one overriding criterion— *whether the atresia is unilateral or bilateral.* The newborn with bilateral atresia is immediately recognized as having a severe congenital deafness which will limit acquisition of speech and language throughout infancy and will later affect his whole education. Cases of unilateral atresia, provided the other ear has normal hearing, will acquire speech and language as a normal child, and although this development should be supervised in the early years there is not the urgent need of amplification and auditory training that exists when the atresia is bilateral. However, the apparently normal ear must not be presumed to have normal hearing as many of these children have a lesser anomaly with a purely middle-ear malformation on the 'good side' and, despite appearances, this ear may be as deaf as its counterpart with obvious atresia. In unilateral atresia normal hearing in the unaffected ear must be confirmed by repeated examination from 6–24 months of age; if an overall loss is suspected at this time an air-conduction aid should be fitted in the normal meatus and auditory training continued until the hearing level can be definitely established.

Bilateral atresia

Livingstone was the first to advocate early surgical exploration of the middle ear in cases of bilateral atresia as there is a good hope of establishing an adequate hearing level for the early acquisition of speech. He regarded the optimum period for initial exploration of the more suitable ear as from 18 months to 2 years as this closely corresponds to the natural timing for acquisition of speech. There are several surgical arguments in favour of this period also:

(1) The labyrinth is already fully developed at birth.
(2) The ossicles are of adult size at birth and by two years the middle-ear cleft is well pneumatized in the majority of cases.
(3) By this age the presence of adequate cochlear function will have been demonstrated by the response to louder sounds and in the effective, even though difficult, use of a bone transducer hearing aid.
(4) Radiology, and in particular tomography, may be of greater definition and value before the temporal bone has become completely ossified.
(5) A reconstructed meatus will allow fitting of an air-conduction aid, either by insert or circumaural earphone, and more effective auditory training can be continued until the definitive hearing result is apparent.

Early surgery in this age group has been undertaken by many surgeons; difficulties in post-operative management have been largely overcome and are not reasons for postponing surgery. Although temporal bone surgery is advocated at this early age in these cases the plastic reconstruction of the pinna is commenced much later—usually when the child is four or five years old. Most plastic surgeons prefer to operate on an untouched ear, and in bilateral cases if hearing becomes adequate the second ear may not be explored until the pinna has been reconstructed.

Unilateral atresia

Where the hearing of the unaffected ear is poor the developmental problem is the same as if the child had a bilateral atresia: an insert aid is fitted to the ear with the normal pinna and meatus and auditory training begun at six months. The hearing results with this aid are compared with that of a bone transducer aid to afford some confirmation of the degree of conductive deafness present and an early decision made with a view to early surgical exploration of the atretic middle ear at 18 months of age.

Where the hearing of the unaffected ear is normal the timing of both plastic surgery to the pinna and middle-ear surgery is a matter of election. The hearing results following reconstruction for unilateral atresia have been disappointing to some surgeons, often comparing unfavourably with the normal ear and the hoped-for stereophonic hearing is not truly achieved. On the other hand exploration offers the only hope of a useful hearing gain, and present, and future, techniques may well show considerable improvement on past results. Unless tomographs show unfavourable limited development of the middle ear or an inner-ear anomaly, exploration of the middle-ear cleft is well-justified in these unilateral cases and should be carried out at any convenient stage of the child's school career after full discussion of all that is involved *with the child and his parents.*

Infection of the middle-ear cleft in congenital atresia

Acute otitis media does not appear to be a problem in these children, and only Gill (1969) discusses chronic infective changes discovered during surgical exploration. In his series he found such changes in 53 per cent of the ears explored; these changes were of varying severity but included some cases of extensive disease, even one of subdural abscess, in which there had been no pre-operative indication of infection. Three other cases were explored on urgent clinical signs of acute mastoiditis, facial paralysis and acute labyrinthitis respectively; in these cases a radical mastoidectomy was completed but in the more quiescent infective changes an appropriate tympanoplastic reconstruction was performed. In the world literature Peron and Schuknecht (1975) have found 20 recorded cases of congenital cholesteatoma deep to a bony atresia plate.

Aims of surgery

(1) To open and inspect the middle-ear cleft.
(2) To reconstruct the hearing mechanism of the middle ear.
(3) To create an external meatus and line it with stable epithelium.
(4) To prevent stenosis of the new meatus.

In approaching surgery, the total problem of the child's deafness must be reviewed and the concept of the dominant ear understood in its educational significance. This is the 'better ear'—on which an aid is consistently preferred and in the older child the ear which gives better speech discrimination and educational comprehension; this ear must be respected surgically and techniques which may cause perceptive loss avoided as far as is reasonable. The conversion of a purely conductive deafness into a combined sensorineural loss with impaired discrimination, even though a pure-tone threshold gain has been achieved, may represent an overall educational loss and may have an effect on the quality of speech. Therefore, radiological anatomy being favourable, the deafer ear is by preference first explored; unless this is remarkably successful subsequent reconstruction in the better ear is more wisely restricted to techniques which do not open the labyrinth. In many cases of congenital atresia the stapes and oval window region are grossly abnormal and the risk to the inner ear may be much higher than in stapedectomy for otosclerosis; also long-term deterioration may be an as yet unknown problem following stapes removal in young children. The author considers bilateral surgery which involves opening into the inner ear is *never* justified in these children. The otologist must be prepared to do nothing in cases where there is no real hope of hearing improvement, or if the only possibility lies in opening the labyrinth at operation on the second side.

TO EXPLORE THE MIDDLE-EAR CLEFT
Small isolated cartilaginous remnants should be removed, and if possible a lobe of the ear should be created in the correct position.

Usually the external remnants of the ear are of little use in indicating where the middle ear is situated and, unless there are indications of where the meatus should be, the shape of the incision should be discussed with the plastic surgeon. In every case he should decide which tissue he wishes to be preserved or discarded.

A high post-auricular incision placed well behind the pinna will provide for some elevation and retroposition of a formed pinna as an essential provision against soft-tissue collapse and possible stenosis of the reconstructed meatal entry. The meatal reconstruction itself will involve an appropriate endaural incision with creation of a meatus by wide excision of cartilage and soft tissues. In cases with a well-placed normal pinna an extended endaural incision alone may be used to expose the temporal bone. There are two main methods of approach to the middle ear.

(1) Through the antrum and then forwards towards the tympanic cavity.
   The antrum is approached down the sinodural angle following the tegmen tympani anteriorly; this cavity is extended within the bone to leave a thin posterior bony wall to the temporo-mandibular joint and downwards to locate the ossicles and middle-ear cleft. This new meatal cavity may be seriously limited by an anteriorly placed lateral sinus in the unpneumatized temporal bone.
(2) Directly down to the middle ear through the attic. This approach leaves a much neater round meatus and should be used where possible (Lund and Phelps, 1978).

When the middle-ear cleft is opened as much mucosa as possible should be preserved and the entry of bone dust into the middle ear minimized. As the superior aspect of the fused middle-ear mass is exposed great care must be taken to avoid direct contact with the drill—a fine diamond burr at this stage—since contact will transmit acoustic and mechanical trauma to the cochlea resulting in sensorineural loss. Some surgeons advocate early dislocation of the ossicle mass from the stapes to lessen this risk but inevitably much dense bone has to be removed before the incudo–stapedial joint can be separated under direct vision. Below, lateral and running forward from the ossicle mass lies the atresia plate, most often composed of dense bone fixing the malleus as the manubrium becomes confluent with its inner face. Removal of the atresia plate is a time consuming process using a soft diamond burr under high magnification and irrigation: as the upper edge is thinned the anterior horizontal segment of the facial nerve must be identified and its course to the region of the posterior annulus slowly exposed. Gradual advance will lead to exposure of the whole ossicular chain and oval window unless sharp curving forward of an anomalous facial nerve prohibits full removal of the atresia plate. The development of the oval window and of the stapes itself are the crucial factors determining reconstruction of a hearing mechanism and no decision can be taken until this region is well seen.

TO RECONSTRUCT THE HEARING MECHANISM OF THE MIDDLE EAR

Malformation of the stapes or oval window in congenital atresia presents peculiar difficulty in successful surgical reconstruction; not only is there no stabilized malleus or incus for attachment of a homocraft ossicle or prosthesis but the facial nerve may be involved in the deformity and severely restrict access to the oval window. Fenestration of the lateral semicircular canal may be considered but few surgeons report success in these circumstances; the risks of stapedectomy, deferred to a second stage operation when the meatus is healed and free from infection, remain high even when the situation is anatomically favourable. A miniscule deformed stapes, even though itself mobile, may not prove capable of linkage into an ossiculoplasty technique and any natural connection to the ossicle should be carefully utilized.

Tympanoplasty techniques are adapted to meet the problem of each individual case; in principle a full-depth tympanic cavity should be created to form a stable, aerated space and minimize long-term intratympanic adhesion and fixation. The tympanic membrane is reconstructed by a sheet of temporalis fascia (or periosteum) large enough to line the whole inner face of the operative cavity and to cover any homograft membrane which has been utilized. Deep to this the mobile stapes will be connected through the undisturbed ossicular mass, or this may be removed and sculpted into a more stable 'crown' fitting over the capitellum of the stapes; alternatively a homograft ossicle may be shaped and fitted in an ossiculoplasty. Marquet (1970) has achieved considerable success using a homograft membrane with attached malleus which he rotates into position on the head of the stapes.

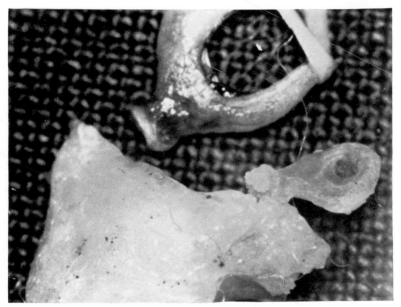

Figure 6.10 (Top) A normal stapes. (Bottom) Embryonic stapes attached to a fixed mass of malleus and incus; from a child aged two years

TO LINE THE NEW MEATUS WITH EPITHELIUM

The long-term complications that may arise in the reconstructed external auditory meatus are broadly of three groups:

(1) *Infection* Many reconstructions are intermittently unstable as is generally true of otological cavities in children: others are permanently infected and Colman (1974) quotes a minimum figure of 18 per cent in the Oxford series. On the other hand many of these split skin reconstructions have remained patent and dry for years with wax-secreting glands developing in the new meatus.

(2) *Stenosis* This complication has arisen with all techniques and is frequently associated with chronic infection; Colman found that 24 per cent of 181 ears explored at Oxford had restenosed at a late review. An important factor in prevention of stenosis is the full excision of soft tissue at the site of the new meatus

and the proper elevation and repositioning of the pinna in relation to it. Stenosis may be minimized by the attachment of the skin graft to overlap the cut external skin edge by 2–3 mm or by turning a local pedicle flap into one segment of the new meatus.

(3) *Lateralization* of the tympanic graft associated with fibrous occlusion of the deep meatus when the fascial layer moves apart from the ossicular mass with loss of continuity and no effective hearing gain.

These complications must be considered in choice of the most appropriate technique of meatal reconstruction from three broad options available.

(1) Thick split-thickness skin graft measuring 7.5 cm × 2.5 cm is taken from the upper thigh and sewn into the shape of a bag with the raw surfaces together (Livingstone, 1959). The bag is turned inside out and then it is packed and stitched around the skin edges of the new meatus. The bag is packed with pledgets of plastic sponge soaked in antibiotic solution so that it approximates on to the ossicular chain and to the bony wall of the new meatal cavity: the meatal entry should be over 1 cm in diameter. Gelfoam or blood-clot may be used to support the ossicles and prevent the bag pressing unduly into the middle ear.

(2) Full-thickness skin may be taken from the post-auricular or clavicular area and inserted in a spiral form to line the new meatus. Friedberg (1977) describes success with this technique using a superiorly-based long pedicle flap of post-auricular skin but personal experience suggests that contraction of full-thickness skin tends to draw upon the tympanic graft with lateralization and subsequent deep canal stenosis. A similar flap is used by Lund and Phelps (1978) to line the operative cavity following an extended conservative radical mastoidectomy technique, their aim being early healing of a stable meatus and a dry cavity in which an aid can be inserted without breakdown.

(3) Pracy (1977) describes a two-stage operative technique. At the first exploratory operation the tympanoplasty is completed and a split-thickness skin graft laid upon the myringoplasty graft to line the whole meatal cavity This is held in position by pieces of sterile plastic sponge and the outer edges of the skin graft are turned epithelial side inward to complete a 'cyst' enclosing the plastic sponge. The post-aural incision is closed without drainage. Three to four months later the incision is reopened to remove the packing material, the skin lining the cavity is inspected and freed for suture into one limb of an extended Z-plasty to form a new meatus. The other limbs of the incision are used to position the pinna below and posterior to this meatal opening. This technique would seem to minimize the three major complications discussed and does protect the middle-ear reconstruction from initial disturbance or infection in the young child.

Post-operative management

After the operation the ear is not touched for 14 days. Any stitches and plastic sponge are then removed and replaced with loose BIPP ribbon gauze. This is changed weekly for a further three weeks.

In young children, the wound dressing should be kept in position by a plaster of paris bandage round the head. This will prevent the child interfering with the ear. After the first dressing a further plaster bandage is applied.

The child should later be fitted with an insert or appropriate hearing aid. Holding the aid in position is always a problem as the insert alone will not be efficient and may damage the new epithelial lining.

An aid should be worn until an audiogram can be taken and the hearing can be accurately assessed.

Auditory training should be recommenced when the ear has healed.

Parent guidance

It is important to see the parents during the child's first year. Reassurance can then be given and a detailed scheme and timetable of rehabilitation can be discussed between them, the plastic surgeon and the otologist. Parent guidance over auditory training should be given by a teacher of the deaf.

A rough timetable for bilateral cases can be given as follows. At one year, x-ray investigation under general anaesthetic. At two years, one ear should be explored and an attempt be made to restore the sound-conducting mechanism. At four or five years, plastic surgery to construct new pinnas may begin. The parents should be told that several operations will be required for the plastic reconstruction and that the operations will be spaced over two years. On completion of the plastic surgery, the second ear can be opened to form a new meatus and, if it is thought advisable, an attempt can be made to restore the sound conducting mechanism in this ear.

Results

Hearing improvement results are difficult to assess, as operation often takes place before it is possible to obtain an audiogram. However, the children operated on usually develop normal language. Sometimes this occurs without operation if the child is given sufficient auditory stimulation and the parents cooperate in auditory training.

Past results have been reviewed by Lund and Phelps (1978) in the phrase; 'Hearing improvement is poor, meatuses tend to stenose and frequently become wet and infected, with the final answer still being awaited'. The current emphasis in bilateral atresia is on early operation to create a stable meatus on which a miniature aid can be worn while opinion is reserved on the value of surgery for unilateral atresia. Although congenital aural aplasia presents as the most difficult otological reconstruction, in a series of congenital abnormalities of all types, operated on as adults or during childhood, Pulec and Freedman (1978) report that 55 per cent were improved to adequate levels of hearing without the use of a hearing aid.

References

Abadir, W. F. and Pease, W. S. (1978). 'Salivary gland choristoma of the middle ear', *Journal of Laryngology and Otology*, **92**, 247

Batstone, J. H. F. (1974). 'Surgery of agenesis of the external ear', *Proceedings of the Royal Society of Medicine*, **67**, 1199

Bennett, R. J. (1966). 'On subarachnoid–tympanic fistulae', *Journal of Laryngology and Otology*, **80**, 1242

du Boulay, G. and Bostik, T. (1969). 'Linear tomography in congenital abnormalities of the ear', *British Journal of Radiology*, **42**, 161

Bowden, R. E. M. (1977). 'Development of the middle and external ear in man', *Proceedings of the Royal Society of Medicine*, **70**, 807

Butler, G. E. (1968). 'Transtapedial congenital malposition of the facial nerve', *Archives of Otolaryngology*, **88**, 268

Colman, B. H. (1974). 'Congenital atresia—the otological problem', *Proceedings of the Royal Society of Medicine*, **67**, 1203

Crabtree, J. A. (1974). 'The facial nerve in congenital ear surgery', *Otolaryngologic Clinics of North America*, **7**, 2, 505

Dickinson, J. T., Srisomboon, P. and Kamerer, D. B. (1968). 'Congenital anomaly of the facial nerve', *Archives of Otolaryngology*, **88**, 367

Edgerton, M. T. (1969). 'Ear construction in children with congenital artesia', *Journal of plastic and reconstructive surgery*, **43**, 373

Edwards, W. G. (1964). 'Congenital middle-ear deafness with anomalies of the face', *Journal of Laryngology and Otology*, **78**, 152

Edwards, W. G. (1974). 'Congenital middle-ear deafness', *Proceedings of the Royal Society of Medicine*, **67**, 1205

Friedburg, J. (1977). 'Correction of congenital meatal atresia', *Journal of Otolaryngology*, **6**, 1, 5

Gill, N. W. (1969). 'Congenital atresia of the ear', *Journal of Laryngology*, **83**, 551

Goldenhar, M. (1952). 'Association malformatives de l'oeil et de l'oreille', *Journal de génétique humaine*, **1**, 243.

Goldman, N. C., Singleton, G. T. and Holly, E. H. (1971). 'Aberrant internal carotid artery', *Archives of Otolaryngology*, **94**, 269

Graham, M. D. (1975). 'The jugular bulb', *Archives of Otolaryngology*, **101**, 560

Hipskind, M. M., Lindsay, J. R., Jones, T. D. and Valvassori, G. E. (1976). 'Recurrent meningitis and labyrinthine gusher', *Laryngoscope*, **86** (5), 682

Hough, J. V. D. (1963). 'Congenital malformation of the middle ear', *Archives of Otolaryngology*, **78**, 335

House, H. P., House, W. F. and Hildyard, V. H. (1958). 'Congenital stapes footplate fixation', *Laryngoscope*, **68**, 1389

Jafek, B. W., Nager, G. T., Strife, J. and Gayler, R. W. (1975). 'Congenital aural atresia—analysis of 311 cases', *Transactions of the American Academy of Ophthalmology and Otolaryngology*, **80** (6), ORL 588

Jahrsdoerfer, R. A. (1977). 'Congenital absence of the round window', *Transactions of the American Academy of Ophthalmology and Otolaryngology*, **84** (5), ORL 904

Leonard, J. R. and Alexander, D. A. (1968). 'Anatomic variations in the area of the oval window', *Archives of Otolaryngology*, **87**, 48

Linthicum, F. H. (1971). 'Surgery of congenital deafness', *Otolaryngology, Clinics of North America*, **4** (2), 401

Livingstone, G. H. (1959). 'Sound conduction in congenital deformities of the external ear', *Journal of Laryngology*, **73**, 223

Livingstone, G. H. (1965). 'Congenital ear abnormalities due to thalidomide', *Proceedings of the Royal Society of Medicine*, **58**, 493

Livingstone, G. H. and Delahunty, J. E. (1968). 'Malformation of the ear associated with congenital ophthalmic and other conditions', *Journal of Laryngology and Otology*, **82**, 495

Lund, W. S. and Phelps, P. D. (1978) 'The surgery of congenital deafness', *Journal of Laryngology and Otology*, **92**, 561

Marquet, J. (1970). 'Problemes particuliers se rapportant aux homograffes tympano-ossiculaires'. *Acta oto-rhino-laryngologie, belgique*, **24**, 99

Moretti, J. A. (1976). 'Highly placed jugular bulb and conductive deafness', *Archives of Otolaryngology*, **102**, 430

Mundnich, K. (1974). 'The dysplasias of the middle and inner ears', *Proceedings of the Royal Society of Medicine*, **67**, 1197

Nevin, N. C. (1977). 'Hereditary deafness associated with external ear malformation', *Journal of Laryngology and Otology*, **91**, 717

Ombredanne, M. (1968). 'Absence congenitale de fenêtre ronde', *Annals of Otolaryngology*, **85**, 369

Peet, E. W. (1971).*Congenital absence of the ear.* (Monograph). Edinburgh; Churchill Livingstone

Peron, D. L. and Schuknecht, H. F. (1975). 'Congenital cholesteatoma with other anomalies', *Archives of Otolaryngology*, **101**, 499

Phelps, P. D., Lloyd, G. A. S. and Sheldon P. W. E. (1975). 'Deformity of the labyrinth and internal auditory meatus in congenital deafness', *British Journal of Radiology*, **48**, 973

Phelps, P. D., Sheldon, P. W. E. and Lloyd, G. A. S. (1976). 'Hearing in patients with congenital deformity of the inner ear', *Clinical Otolaryngology*, **1**, 31

Phelps, P. D. and Wright, J. L. W. (1976). 'Coils of the cochlea', *Clinical Radiology*, **27**, 415

Phelps, P. D., Lloyd, G. A. S. and Sheldon, P. W. E. (1977). 'Congenital deformities of the middle and external ear', *British Journal of Radiology*, **50**, 714

Poswillo, D. (1975). 'Causal mechanisms of craniofacial deformity', *British Medical Bulletin*, **31** (2), 101

Pracy, R. (1977). 'Surgery for congenital conductive deafness', *Proceedings of the Royal Society of Medicine*, **70**, 823

Pulec, J. L. and Freedman, H. M. (1978). 'Management of congenital ear abnormalities', *Laryngoscope*, **88**, 420

Reisner, K. (1969). 'Tomography in inner and middle-ear malformations', *Radiology*, **92**, 11

Richards, S. H. and Gibbin, K. P. (1977). 'Recurrent meningitis due to congenital fistula of the stapedial footplate', *Journal of Laryngology and Otology*, **91**, 1063

Sale, C. (1969). 'Bilateral deafness due to stapes surgery', *Archives of Otolaryngology*, **90**, 467

Sando, I. and Wood, R. P. (1971). 'Congenital middle-ear anomalies', *Otolaryngologic Clinics of North America*, **4** (2), 291

Scheer, A. A. (1967). 'Correction of congenital middle-ear deformities', *Archives of Otolaryngology*, **85**, 269

Schuknecht, H. F. (1974). *Pathology of the Ear*, Chapter 4, 'Developmental defects'. Harvard University Press

Singh, H. B. and Gaudi, S. L. (1977). 'Goldenhar Syndrome', *Journal of Laryngology and Otology*, **91**, 1101

Steele, B. C. (1969). 'Congenital fixation of the stapes footplate', *Acta otolaryngologica Stockholm*, Suppl. 245

Steffen, T. N. (1968). 'Vascular anomalies of the middle ear', *Laryngoscope*, **78**, 171

Sullivan, J. A., McAskile, K. and Smith, B. (1959). 'Surgical Management of Congenital Atresia of the Ear', *Journal of Laryngology*, **73**, 201

Valvassori, G. E. and Buckingham, R. A. (1975). *Tomography and cross sections of the ear*. Stuttgart; Thieme

Winter, J. S. D., Kohn, Gertrude, Mellman, W. J. and Bergner, S. (1968). 'A familial syndrome of renal, genital and middle-ear anomalies', *Journal of Pediatrics*, **72**, 88

Wright, J. L. W., Phelps, P. D. and Fraser, I. (1977). 'Anatomical findings in congenital conductive deafness', *Proceedings of the Royal Society of Medicine*, **70**, 816

Young, A. (1968). 'The state of the ears in children with a cleft palate deformity', *Journal of Laryngology*, **82**, 707

7 Traumatic conductive deafness

John Ballantyne

For many years otologists have recognized and reported a variety of traumatic lesions of the sound-conducting apparatus, but renewed interest in the effects upon the ear of changes in pressure has been aroused by the greatly increased use of air travel, both in war and in peace. Even more recently the rapid development of microsurgical techniques has focused our attention more and more upon closed injuries to the structures within the middle ear itself (especially to the ossicles), which occur with greater frequency as the numbers of road accidents grow, and with them the number of head injuries. According to Hough (1973), about three-quarters of all road traffic accidents involve the head, and when the head is severely injured, the ear is the most frequently damaged sensory organ.

Conductive deafness may be caused by occlusion of the external auditory canal, by foreign bodies; by the effects of compression on the tympanic membrane, either directly through the external auditory canal or indirectly through the eustachian tube; by rupture of the tympanic membrane, from compression or blast, from fractures of the skull, or from direct injury by foreign bodies or by attempts to remove them; by the collection of blood or other fluids within the middle-ear cavity; or by disruption of the ossicular chain, usually following severe head injuries accompanied by fractures of the skull base.

Foreign bodies of the ear

A surprisingly wide range of foreign bodies may be inserted into the ear, and indeed practically any object that is small enough to be pushed into the external auditory canal must have found its way there at some time or other. Some of them are very hard, some soft; some are metallic, others non-metallic; and many of the vegetable foreign bodies are hygroscopic.

A foreign body in the external meatus will produce a conductive deafness when it is large enough to occlude the meatus completely; when it is hygroscopic and swells up to produce complete occlusion; or when, especially in the case of a vegetable foreign body, it gives rise to an inflammatory reaction in the canal walls, with subsequent swelling and closure.

Most foreign bodies can be removed fairly easily with crocodile forceps or syringe, but an exception must always be made with a smooth rounded foreign body which is more than likely to be pushed further inwards by these instruments, sometimes far enough to rupture the tympanic membrane and even, on occasions, to enter the middle ear.

Traumatic rupture of the tympanic membrane will also, of course, cause some deafness which must, by its definition, be conductive in nature; and this may be due not only to penetration and perforation by the foreign body itself (especially in the case of long slim objects such as matches, hair clips or knitting needles) but also to unskilled attempts to remove a foreign body (particularly the smooth round variety) from the meatus. In children, as also in many adults, this should never be attempted without a general anaesthetic, except in the rather rare instances when the foreign body is very superficial. The removal of such objects is effected most safely with a simple right-angled hook. When the foreign body has entered the middle ear it will usually be possible to remove it through a permeatal tympanotomy.

Barotraumatic otitis media

This condition, alternatively known as aero-otitis or otitic barotrauma, may be defined as a non-infective inflammatory reaction produced in the middle-ear cleft when the air pressure within it is considerably lower than that of the surrounding atmosphere. It occurs particularly when flying, during loss of height, but also in diving or in compression in a decompression chamber.

Barotraumatic otitis media assumed particular importance during the Second World War, especially in aircrew and naval divers, but this importance has grown into the days of peace with the rapid expansion of civilian air travel, and it must present considerable problems in space flight. It may also occur in patients who are being treated by radiotherapy under hyperbaric oxygen unless precautions are taken to prevent its effects by the creation of controlled perforations, with grommets inserted through small myringotomies.

Aetiology

Otitic barotrauma is caused by failure or inability to open the eustachian tube, when a large alteration in atmospheric pressure occurs.

The tube is normally opened by muscular action, and this allows the air pressure within the middle-ear cleft to be raised to that of the surrounding atmosphere. When the tube cannot be so opened, it is said to be 'locked'.

As the extratympanic pressure decreases during *ascent* in aircraft or during decompression in a chamber, the egress of air from the middle ear through the eustachian tube is easy and automatic. Conversely, during loss of height in aircraft during *descent*, or compression in a chamber, the tube behaves in an entirely different way, for the normal tube does not open passively and air does not enter the tympanic cavity without the intervention of muscular action or of therapeutic inflation. Consequently a positive pressure develops extratympanically and this pushes the tympanic membrane inwards and invaginates it around the contents of the middle ear.

According to McGibbon (1947), the difference between the extratympanic and intratympanic pressures depends not only upon the amount of height lost but also upon the altitudes at which the loss of height occurs. Thus, for example, with a loss of 3048 m from 9144 m to 6096 m, a difference of pressure of 123.6 mmHg is developed; whilst with a similar loss of 3048 m, but from 3657.6 m to 609.6 m, a difference of pressure of 223.4 mmHg is brought about; that is, for any given height loss, the pressure differential is much greater at a low altitude than at a high one.

Armstrong and Heim (1937) found that the muscles which normally open the eustachian tube are unable to do so when the pressure differential exceeds 90 mmHg, that is, 'locking' occurs at this 'critical pressure difference'.

'Locking' occurs at a lower pressure differential when the tubal lining is oedematous; it is prevented by a perforation of the drumhead made either by nature or by surgery.

Pathology

The tympanic membrane retracts inwards with the relative decrease of pressure in the cleft.

Vascular engorgement occurs throughout the cleft lining and is followed by oedema, ecchymosis and transudation of fluid, which may become sanguineous in severe cases.

With sudden and intense pressure changes, the membrane may split.

Clinical features

The most constant feature of barotraumatic otitis media is deafness, which may amount to no more than a feeling of 'woolliness' in the ear or ears, but may be quite severe subjectively. The deafness may be accompanied by autophony or by a sensation of fluid in the ear; and it may occur during descent or after landing, sometimes several hours or even a few days after landing.

Increasing discomfort and pain are common symptoms and the pain may be intense; fortunately, it usually disappears within a few hours. Tinnitus, usually short-lived, occurs commonly; vertigo occurs occasionally.

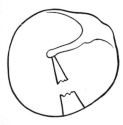

Figure 7.1   'Indrawn' right tympanic membrane

The tympanic membrane is red soon after the onset, and it usually becomes invaginated (*Figure 7.1*). There may be solitary or multiple interstitial haemorrhages into the drumhead, and effusions may form in the middle ear, with the appearance of a meniscus or bubbles, sometimes foam-like, through the membrane. Bleeding into the middle ear may produce a haemotympanum, and in severe acute cases a rupture may occur, usually in an anterior central position.

Treatment

'UNLOCKING'

A return to the height (that is, the pressure) at which the tube 'locked' will often allow it to be opened but this of course is rarely practicable.

Subsequent descent should be slow, and auto-inflation (by Valsalva's manoeuvre) should be performed frequently. This treatment is unlikely to be effective if the tube has been 'locked' for more than an hour.

Eustachian catheterization will usually cure the condition when fluid is absent.

Myringotomy is necessary if fluid is present, and Canfield and Bateman (1944) recommend that the incision be made postero-inferiorly, half-way between the umbo and the meatal wall; they point out that it serves the double purpose of letting fluid out and letting air in.

Evacuation of the fluid may be assisted by suction with Siegle's speculum, followed by gentle and—if necessary—repeated inflation of the tube by politzerization or catheterization. In very resistant cases, a grommet should be inserted through the incision and left in position until the condition has subsided completely, usually after about one month.

An appropriate systemic antibiotic is necessary if secondary infection supervenes.

Prevention

Most aircraft today are pressurized, but even with the most effective pressurization (which is rarely equivalent to less than 1828.8 m at a height of 9144 m), otitic barotrauma is still a fairly common condition. It is more likely to occur if there is a mechanical obstruction in the nose, such as deviation of the septum or polypi.

Ideally, nobody should fly with an upper respiratory infection, and passengers should be discouraged from sleeping during descent, as the eustachian tubes are not opened by swallowing during sleep.

Vasoconstrictors, in the form of either nasal sprays or oral preparations or both, may facilitate the opening of the tubes, and they should be used half an hour to one hour before the anticipated time of descent. Some commercial airlines provide boiled sweets or chewing gum, to encourage swallowing during flight, and auto-inflation by Valsalva's method should be performed regularly as the atmospheric pressure rises.

In those who are suspectible to recurrences of barotraumatic otitis media, special attention must be paid to obstructive conditions in the nose and nasopharynx, and to allergic or infective conditions of the nose, throat and sinuses. In more resistant cases a grommet should be inserted through a myringotomy and, in those who do much flying, left in position for as long as it will remain there.

Traumatic rupture of the tympanic membrane

The tympanic membrane may be ruptured by the penetration of a foreign body or surgical instrument; in severe cases of barotraumatic otitis media; by extension from a fracture of the skull base (*see below*); or by a variety of factors which produce sudden compression of the tympanic membrane, either through the eustachian tube (as in forceful inflation by politzerization or catheterization) or through the external auditory canal (as in boxing, hand-slap or forceful syringing, or a blow on the ear when the canal is filled with water, as in water polo or in high diving).

It is doubtful whether the membrane is ever perforated by inflation, tympanometry or syringing unless it is already weakened by previous disease or injury.

Blast rupture is a rather special form of traumatic rupture, in that there are two phases of the so-called blast-wave; a primary wave of positive pressure producing a percussion effect; and a secondary wave of negative pressure producing a suction effect. It is not known which is the more important factor in producing aural damage.

Boyes Korkis (1946) made a special study of blast injuries of the ear in military base hospitals in the Middle Eastern and Italian campaigns of 1939–45. He found that rupture of the drumhead was most likely to be caused by high-explosive shells; that it was unilateral in about three-quarters of the cases; and that in unilateral cases (as one would expect), the ear nearer the source of the explosion was the one usually affected, bilateral rupture being more common when the injury took place in a confined space.

Blast rupture always affects the pars tensa, never the pars flaccida; the perforation may be of any shape—most commonly reniform; and of any size—not often large; and it may occur in any part of the pars tensa—most of the cases in Korkis' series occurring anteriorly, and mainly in the lower half of the membrane. This author confirmed the findings of Negus (1940) that, in uninfected cases, these perforations have a clean-cut edge and present the appearance of being punched out (*Figure 7.2*), in contrast with other traumatic perforations which usually have a ragged edge, often haemorrhagic.

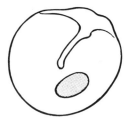

Figure 7.2   Blast rupture of right tympanic membrane

Deafness and tinnitus occurring together constituted by far the most common presenting symptoms—in 99 of 167 cases; pain was surprisingly uncommon, occurring in only eight of these cases altogether, either alone or in combination with other symptoms. This finding contrasted with that of Collier (1940), who recorded that during the Spanish Civil War traumatic rupture was usually accompanied by sharp pain in the affected ear.

Although the deafness is conductive in type in most cases of traumatic perforation, Korkis emphasized that it was 'mixed' in most cases of true blast injury.

Tinnitus and vertigo are usually transient. Bleeding from the ear is an important sign, always to be looked for carefully in head injuries, especially in those where a basal fracture is suspected. The main treatment of traumatic rupture is to leave the ear strictly alone, never syringing, discouraging the patient from allowing anything to enter the ear until healing has taken place, and reserving the use of systemic antibiotics for those cases in which infection threatens or supervenes. However, if the patient is seen early enough and his general condition permits, the edges of the perforation may sometimes be replaced surgically, through the operating microscope, especially when the lesion is associated with a longitudinal fracture of the temporal bone (Guerrier, De Jean and Serrou, 1967) or with blast injury (Gapany-Gapanavičius, Brama and Chisin, 1977). On the other hand, Kerr and Byrne (1975) find it difficult to justify surgical intervention in view of the very high rate of spontaneous healing.

Conductive deafness associated with basal skull fractures

As head injuries from road accidents become more common, so also do fractures of the skull base, and the temporal bone is not uncommonly involved; approximately 75 per cent of these injuries affect male patients; 80 per cent of temporal bone fractures are of the longitudinal type, the line of fracture occurring in the long axis of its petrous portion (*Figure 7.3*, B–B) and it is this type of injury that may implicate the sound-conducting apparatus, thus causing conductive deafness.

Longitudinal fractures of the petrous bone are usually caused by blows to the temporal or parietal areas rather than to the occipital or frontal areas (Proctor, Gurdjian and Webster, 1956; McHugh, 1959). When the fracture line spreads into the thin tegmen tympani, bleeding may occur into the tympanic cavity, giving the appearance of a 'blue drum' (haemotympanum) on otoscopic examination. If the tympanic membrane is torn, bleeding will occur also into the external meatus, and indeed bleeding from or into the ear is one of the signs which must always be looked for in any severe head injury, and it always suggests a longitudinal fracture. Such fractures, however, may not be discernible in x-rays of the skull. Ecchymosis over the mastoid area is often indicative of bleeding into the pneumatic spaces of the temporal bone (Guerrier, De Jean and Serrou, 1967).

In either of these relatively minor injuries—otologically speaking—full recovery of hearing is to be expected in practically every case, providing that the ear is left well alone and any threat of secondary infection is treated promptly and energetically with systemic antibiotics.

In unilateral cases, which most of these injuries are, it is fair to say that the demonstration of a conductive deafness is usually a good prognostic sign, distinguishing these recoverable lesions from the untreatable perceptive deafness which results from bleeding into the labyrinth in the less common transverse fractures of the petrous temporal bone (*Figure 7.3*, A–A) due primarily to blows in the occipital area, or in mixed fractures (Hough and Stuart, 1968).

Nevertheless, conductive deafness due to head injuries does not always recover, and more and more cases are now being reported which tell us that, in most instances, persistence of such deafness is due to disruption of the ossicular chain.

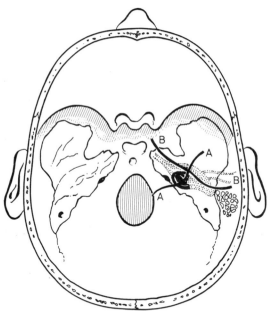

Figure 7.3 Base of skull, showing the two types of fracture of the petrous temporal bone which may implicate the ear and hearing. A–A: transverse fracture; B–B: longitudinal fracture

Traumatic disruption of the ossicular chain

Traumatic disruption of the ossicular chain, although most often due to accidental trauma, may also result occasionally from surgical injury. The incus is the ossicle most frequently affected but the malleus and stapes are not immune from injury. Of all the injuries of this type, the most common is a disruption of the incudostapedial joint.

More than a hundred years ago, Toynbee (1866), in the last paper he ever wrote, realized that the long process of the incus could be separated from the head of the stapes by a blow on the head, and he called the condition 'disconnexion of the ossicles'. Keleman (1944) examined serial sections of temporal bones removed from persons who had died after head injuries; and he found several instances of disruption of the incudostapedial and malleoincudal joints. But it was not until the operating microscope had been in regular use for several years that Thorburn (1957) reported the first case of a traumatic ossicular lesion in which the hearing had been improved by the application of the original tympanoplastic principles. This patient had had a head injury in 1941 and there had been bleeding from the left ear. When he was first seen by Thorburn in 1955, the left tympanic membrane was normal but tuning-fork tests demonstrated a conductive deafness. The ear was explored in the following year, 15 years after injury. The head of the malleus was fixed by ossification inside the attic, and the incus projected beyond the stapes without making contact with it; the stapes was intact and mobile. The incus and the head of the malleus were removed, and the tympanic membrane was pushed inwards to make contact with the head of the stapes, producing the 'columellar effect' of Wüllstein's type III tympanoplasty (myringosta-pediopexy). Post-operatively the hearing was practically normal.

A similar method was successfully employed by Bauer in 1958, and in the following year Freeman reported a case in which he was able to reposition an incus which had been dislocated 16 years earlier during the course of a simple cortical mastoid operation, performed when the patient was only five months old. This resulted in an improvement of hearing by air conduction of no less than 60 dB.

Many such cases have now been reported in the literature, the largest series being that of Hough (1969) who has personally seen and treated at least 35 cases. In all of them, there had been loss of consciousness and bleeding from the affected ear at the time of the accident; in many there had been a transient facial palsy, which occurs in approximately 20 per cent of patients with longitudinal fractures (Hough, 1973); and in two of his earlier cases (1964), the lesion had been caused by lightning. Two other large personal series have been reported by Marquet (1965) and Cremin (1969).

These traumatic lesions of the ossicles are rather uncommon, the one most frequently affected being the incus. That this should be so is not surprising for, apart from the rather flimsy incudal ligament which connects its short process to the fossa incudis, it lacks any really firm anchorage. By contrast, the stapes is fixed in the oval window by the annular ligament and is further secured by the insertion into its neck of the stapedius tendon; whilst the malleus is attached to the tegmen tympani by a superior ligament, to the margins of the notch of Rivinus by a lateral ligament which passes from its short process, and to the tympanic membrane itself. Furthermore, it is suspended by an anterior ligament and receives further stabilizing support from the insertion of the tensor tympani tendon into the upper part of the handle. As would be expected the malleus is the ossicle least often disturbed by trauma.

Of all these rare but fascinating lesions, the commonest is a simple subluxation or dislocation of the incudostapedial joint; other lesions of the incus have been reported but rarely.

The crura of the stapes may be fractured, and the stapes superstructure may come to lie freely in the middle ear, save for its attachment to the stapedius tendon; rarely, stapedial fractures may be accompanied by depression of the footplate into the oval window. This latter lesion tends to be followed by severe sensorineural hearing loss.

In one unique case seen recently by the present author the stapes and long process of the incus, still partially attached to one another by the joint capsule, were seen to lie in the external auditory meatus. The patient, a boy of nine, had been pushed into a bush by his friends, and a twig had entered his ear. Overcome by violent giddiness he withdrew his head immediately and the twig, whose end was shaped like a crochet hook, penetrated the drumhead and must have hooked itself round the long process of the incus; as the boy's head was withdrawn the stapes was pulled out of the oval window and 'delivered' into the meatus still tenuously attached to the lenticular process. Apart from some high-frequency loss, sensorineural function was saved in this case by early sealing of the oval window by a small plug of fat.

Least frequently of all, the malleus may be displaced and may even be torn away from its attachments to the tympanic membrane and incus; or it may become fixed in the attic by bone or fibrous tissue. These ossicular lesions may be multiple.

Hough (1959) suggested three possible mechanisms for the production of these lesions: (i) a severe vibratory reaction to an impact sufficient to produce a fracture of the skull may cause momentary separation and weakening of the joint tissues; (ii) inertial strains may be accountable, as when the head in motion strikes a stationary object, or when the head is struck by a moving object. In such cases the movable objects inside the head, including the ossicles, react in a physical way to acceleration and deceleration; (iii) severe head injuries may give rise to a sudden tetanic contraction of the intratympanic muscles, with an abrupt change in the axis of rotation of the ossicles. In all such cases, a severe conductive deafness persists after a head injury.

Although most of these traumatic lesions have followed severe head injuries, one of Sadé's cases followed a stab in the ear with a paint-brush, and total dislocation of the incus has more commonly followed operations for cortical mastoidectomy. Such cases have been reported by Schuknecht and Trupiano (1957), Hough (1959) and Freeman (1959). More recently Anklesaria (1963) recorded such a case and the present author has seen one following head injury, and two following previous surgery, in early childhood.

These injuries are usually unilateral, but bilateral cases of traumatic subluxation of the incudostapedial joint have been described by Gisselsson (1958) and by Flisberg and Floberg (1960).

Diagnosis

The diagnosis of these injuries depends upon the detection, after the drumhead has healed, of a persistent conductive deafness after trauma, usually accidental but occasionally surgical. The tuning-fork tests show a reference of bone-conducted sound to the affected ear in the Weber test, and a true negative Rinne response on that side. This latter must be distinguished from the false negative response which may be found in those rare cases of sensorineural deafness which may also follow head injuries.

When there is total functional disruption of the ossicular chain, the loss of air conduction by pure-tone audiometry usually exceeds 50 dB, the hearing by bone conduction remaining normal; and the bone conduction audiograph is approximately parallel to the air conduction audiograph. Bauer (1958) has pointed out that Carhart's notch is usually absent.

A history of head injury will usually distinguish traumatic ossicular disruption from otosclerosis, but such evidence may not be available in every case. In such instances Bauer believes that, if the bone conduction audiograph does *not* show Carhart's notch, the oval window is unlikely to be blocked by stapes fixation. It must be remembered, however, that traumatic ossicular lesions may co-exist with otosclerosis (Bicknell, 1966; Hammond, 1964; Hough and Stuart, 1968; Jackson, 1976).

Acoustic impedance measurements are helpful, the tensor tympani reflex being increased, and the tympanogram producing a W-shaped curve, in disruptive lesions. Compliance is increased, and the stapedius reflex response abolished.

The final confirmation of the diagnosis is dependent upon the direct inspection of the middle ear through the operating microscope, by way of a permeatal tympanotomy.

Treatment

These traumatic lesions of the auditory ossicles may be corrected, usually with complete closure of the air–bone gap, by a variety of ossiculoplastic procedures which make use of the principles and practice of tympanoplasty or stapes surgery. Some cases are suitable for the use of various artificial prostheses; others are more suitable for the use of natural materials, such as cortical bone or connective tissue. Alternatively incus autografts or homografts may be employed; but a growing body of otological opinion is tending to favour the use of natural, rather than foreign, materials.

In cases of subluxation of the incudostapedial joint (*Figure 7.4a*), it may be possible to restore hearing simply by repositioning the tip of the incus on to the head of the

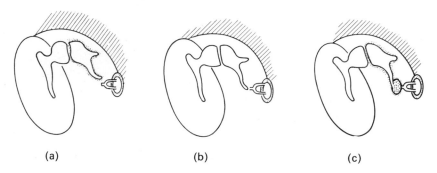

(a)   (b)   (c)

Figure 7.4   Subluxation of the incudostapedial joint: (a) the lesion (Ballantyne; Brown Kelly; Cremin; Does and Bottema; Flisberg and Floberg; Gisselssen; Hammond; Hough; Marquet; Robinson; Sadé); (b) simple repositioning (Brown Kelly; Hough); (c) interposition of bone or connective tissue between lenticular process of incus and head of stapes (Anderson, Jepsen and Ratjen; Ballantyne; Hough; Irvine and Taylor; Rosen, cited by Brown Kelly)

stapes (*Figure 7.4b*); however, when this is not possible, a piece of bone or connective tissue may be interposed between the lenticular process of the incus and the head of the stapes (*Figure 7.4c*). The same technique (*Figure 7.5b*) may be applied when there is erosion of the long process of the incus, with wider separation of the incudostapedial joint (*Figure 7.5a*); alternatively, a piece of polythene tubing may be interposed between the incus and the stapes (*Figure 7.5c and d*); or a prosthesis may be placed between the incus and the stapedial footplate (if it is mobile) or, after stapedectomy, the oval window (*Figure 7.5e*).

Brownlie Smith (1965) describes one case in which the long process of the incus had become impacted between the crura of the stapes (*Figure 7.6a*); unable to reposition it, he removed the stapes and put in a piston (*Figure 7.6b*).

Marquet (1965) has treated two fractures of the long process of the incus (*Figure 7.7a*) by immobilization of the fragments with bone struts secured by polythene rings (*Figure 7.7b*).

Dislocation of the body of the incus from the head of the malleus (*Figure 7.8a*) is a rare lesion, but Wilmot (1966) has treated two such cases successfully by simple repositioning (*Figure 7.8b*). Total dislocation of the incus (*Figure 7.9a*) can be treated by repositioning (*Figure 7.9b*); or by removal and interposition of the incus between the malleus and the head (*Figure 7.9c*) or footplate (*Figure 7.9d*) of the mobile stapes.

Total absence of the incus (*Figure 7.10a*) is a difficult lesion to treat, but it is of considerable historical interest, as one such was the first traumatic ossicular lesion to be treated successfully by surgery, when Thorburn (1957) performed a myringostapediopexy (*Figure 7.10b*) after removal of the incus. Does and Bottema (1965) were the first otologists to describe cases in which hearing was improved by the interposition of polythene tubing between the neck of the malleus and the head (*Figure 7.10c*) or footplate (*Figure 7.10d*) of the stapes. Hough (1969) has treated such cases with incus homografts (*Figure 7.10e*)—probably the most satisfactory method now available.

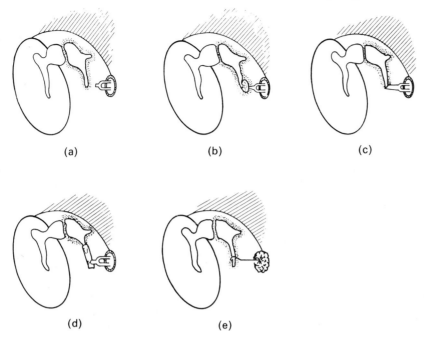

(a)   (b)   (c)

(d)   (e)

Figure 7.5 Separation of the incudostapedial joint, with erosion of the long process of the incus: (a) the lesion (Ballantyne; Cremin; Hough; Ransome; Rosen, cited by Brown Kelly; Russell; Sooy; Stewart); (b) interposition of bone or connective tissue between long process of incus and head of stapes (Anderson, Jepsen and Ratjen; Ballantyne; Hough; Irvine and Taylor; Rosen, cited by Brown Kelly); (c) interposition of polythene between long process of incus and head of stapes (Ballantyne; Cremin; Hammond; Ransome; Stewart); (d) interposition of polythene between eroded long process of incus and head of stapes (Russell; Sooy); (e) prosthesis between incus and oval window, after stapedectomy (Ballantyne; Cremin; Robinson; Sadé)

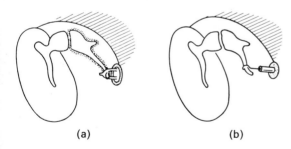

(a)   (b)

Figure 7.6 Impaction of long process of incus between stapedial crura: (a) the lesion (Brownlie Smith); (b) prosthesis between incus and oval window, after stapedectomy (Brownlie Smith)

Alternatively, good results have been obtained by inserting a prosthesis between the malleus and the stapedial footplate (*Figure 7.10f*) or, after stapedectomy, the oval window (*Figure 7.10g*).

With simple fracture of the stapedial crura (*Figure 7.11a*), the hearing has been improved by the interposition of connective tissue or gel-foam between the fragments (*Figure 7.11b*); when the superstructure has been grossly displaced (*Figure 7.12a*), good results are to be expected from the insertion of a prosthesis between the incus and the mobile footplate (*Figure 7.12b*); if the footplate is depressed into the oval window (*Figure 7.13a*) the whole stapes must be removed immediately and a prosthesis put between the incus and oval window (*Figure 7.13b*). Arragg and Paparella (1964) have

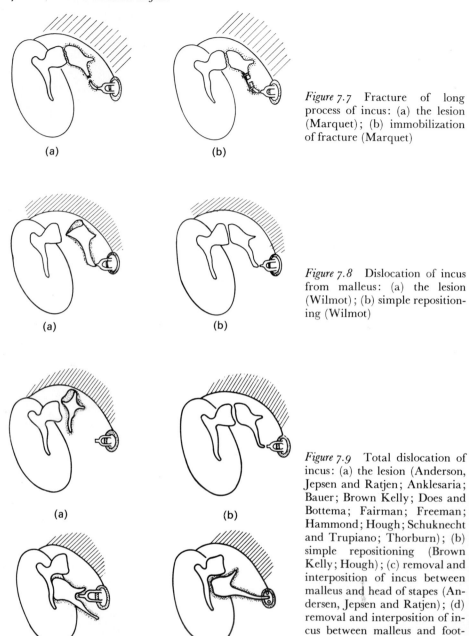

Figure 7.7 Fracture of long process of incus: (a) the lesion (Marquet); (b) immobilization of fracture (Marquet)

Figure 7.8 Dislocation of incus from malleus: (a) the lesion (Wilmot); (b) simple repositioning (Wilmot)

Figure 7.9 Total dislocation of incus: (a) the lesion (Anderson, Jepsen and Ratjen; Anklesaria; Bauer; Brown Kelly; Does and Bottema; Fairman; Freeman; Hammond; Hough; Schuknecht and Trupiano; Thorburn); (b) simple repositioning (Brown Kelly; Hough); (c) removal and interposition of incus between malleus and head of stapes (Andersen, Jepsen and Ratjen); (d) removal and interposition of incus between malleus and footplate of stapes (Hough)

suggested that some at least of the hearing may be salvaged by this procedure, even though the loss tends to be mainly sensorineural. An open oval window must be sealed off as a matter of urgency, preferably by some form of connective tissue, and any reconstructive procedure is undertaken at a later date.

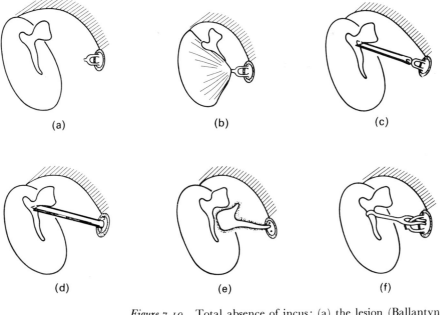

Figure 7.10 Total absence of incus: (a) the lesion (Ballantyne; Brown Kelly; Cremin; Does and Bottema; Marquet; Oppenheimer and Harrison; Ransome); (b) myringostapediopexy (Bauer; Brown Kelly; Cremin; Thorburn); (c) interposition of polythene between neck of malleus and head of stapes (Does and Bottema; Ransome); (d) interposition of polythene between neck of malleus and footplate of stapes (Does and Bottema; Ransome); (e) incus homograft (Hough); (f) Smyth 'clothes-peg' prosthesis between handle of malleus and footplate of stapes (Marquet); (g) piston between handle of malleus and oval window, after stapedectomy (Ballantyne; Cremin; Oppenheimer and Harrison)

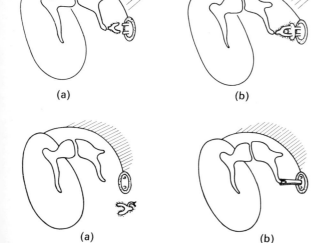

Figure 7.11 Fracture of stapedial crura: (a) the lesion (Cremin; Does and Bottema; Irvine and Tylor; Robinson; Sadé); (b) interposition of bone or connective tissue between fragments (Does and Bottema)

Figure 7.12 Fracture-dislocation of stapes superstructure: (a) the lesion (Does and Bottema; Hammond; Irvine and Taylor; Ransome); (b) interposition of polythene between incus and footplate of stapes (Does and Bottema; Ransome)

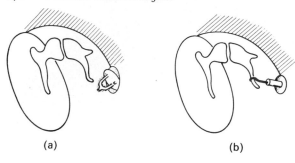

Figure 7.13 Fracture of stapedial crura with depression of footplate into oval window; (a) the lesion (Arragg and Paparella; Irvine and Taylor); (b) prosthesis between incus and oval window, after stapedectomy (Arragg and Paparella; Irvine and Taylor)

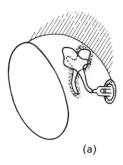 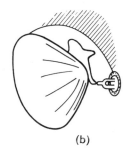 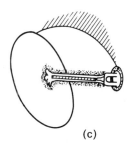

Figure 7.14 Dislocation of malleus: (a) the lesion (Cremin; Groves; Hammond; Marquet); (b) myringo-incudopexy (Groves; Hammond); (c) interposition of bone strut and vein sleeve between tympanic membrane and head of stapes (Marquet)

The most difficult of these lesions to treat is a dislocation of the malleus (*Figure 7.14a*), but moderately successful results have been obtained by myringo-incudopexy (*Figure 7.14b*), or by the interposition of a bony strut and vein sleeve between the tympanic membrane and the head of the stapes (*Figure 7.14c*). It is possible that in the future this rare lesion may be more satisfactorily treated by the use of a 'membrane–plus–malleus' homograft.

Summary

When a head injury is followed by conductive deafness, this is most likely to be due to haemotympanum or traumatic perforation of the tympanic membrane, and in such cases complete recovery is to be expected provided that infection does not supervene. However, if the hearing has not recovered after all the blood has been resorbed and the drumhead has healed, disruption of the ossicular chain must be suspected and the middle ear should be explored through a permeatal tympanotomy. In such instances the hearing can usually be restored to normal or near-normal by the application of ossiculoplastic techniques. It is therefore desirable that every case of head injury should be referred to the otologist.

References

Andersen, H. G., Jepsen, O. and Ratjen, E. (1962) *Acta otolaryngologica*, **54**, 393

Anklesaria, D. M. (1963) *Journal of Laryngology*, **77**, 528

Armstrong, H. G. and Heim, J. W. (1937) *Journal of the American Medical Association*, **109**, 417

Arragg, F. G. and Paparella, M. M. (1964) *Laryngoscope, St. Louis*, **74**, 1329

Ballantyne, J. C. (1962) *Journal of Laryngology*, **76**, 661

Ballantyne, J. C. (1966) *Proceedings of the Royal Society of Medicine*, **59**, 535

Bauer, F. (1958) *Journal of Laryngology*, **72**, 676

Bauer, F. (1964) *Journal of Laryngology*, **78**, 408

Bicknell, P. R. (1966) *Journal of Laryngology*, **80**, 748

Brown Kelly, H. D. (1966) Personal communication

Brownlie Smith, A. (1965) Personal communication

Brownlie Smith, A. (1966) *Proceedings of the Royal Society of Medicine*, **59**, 549

Canfield, N. C. and Bateman, G. H. (1944) *Journal of Aviation Medicine*, **15**, 340

Carhart, R. (1959) *Journal of Laryngology*, **73**, 196

Collier, J. (1940) *Proceedings of the Royal Society of Medicine*, **34**, 10

Cremin, M. D. (1969) *Journal of Laryngology*, **83**, 845

Does, I. E. S. and Bottema, T. (1965) *Archives of Otolaryngology*, **82**, 331

Fairman, H. D. (1966) Personal communication

Flisberg, K. and Floberg, L. E. (1960) *Archives of Otolaryngology*, **51**, 467

Freeman, J. (1959) *Journal of Laryngology*, **73**, 196

Gapany-Gapanavičius, B., Brama, I. and Chisin, R. (1977) *Journal of Laryngology*, **91**, 565

Gisselsson, L. (1958) *Journal of Laryngology*, **72**, 329

Groves, J. (1965) Personal communication

Guerrier, Y., DeJean, Y. and Serrou, B. (1967) *Montpellier Chirugical*, **7** (4), 483

Hammond, V. T. (1964) *Journal of Laryngology*, **78**, 837

Hough, J. V. D. (1959) *Laryngoscope*, **69**, 644

Hough, J. V. D. (1964) Personal communication

Hough, J. V. D. (1969) *Annals of Otology, Rhinology and Laryngology*, **78**, 210

Hough, J. V. D. (1973). In *Otolaryngology*, Vol. 2, p. 241. Ed. by Paperella and Shumrick. London, Philadelphia and Toronto; W. B. Saunders Company

Hough, J. V. D. and Stuart, W. D. (1968) *Laryngoscope*, **78**, 899

Irvine, G. and Taylor, L. R. S. (1966) Personal communication

Jackson, P. D. (1976) *Journal of Laryngology*, **90**, 707

Keleman, G. (1944) *Archives of Otolaryngology*, **40**, 333

Kerr, A. G. and Byrne, J. E. T. (1975) *Journal of Laryngology*, **89**, 131

Korkis, F. B. (1946) 'Effect of blast on the human ear', *British Medical Journal*, **1**, 198

Korkis, F. B. (1946) 'Rupture of the tympanic membrane of blast origin', *Journal of Laryngology*, **61**, 367

McGibbon, J. E. G. (1947) In *Contributions to Aviation Otolaryngology*. Ed. by Dalziel Dickson, E. D. London: Headley

McHugh, H. E. (1959) *Annals of Otolaryngology*, **68**, 855

Marquet, J. (1965) *Acta oto-rhino-laryngologica belgica*, **20**, 5

Negus, V. E. (1940) *Proceedings of the Royal Society of Medicine*, **10**, 47

Oppenheimer, P. and Harrison, W. H. (1963) *Archives of Otolaryngology*, **78**, 143

Proctor, B., Gurdjian, E. S. and Webster, J. E. (1965) *Laryngoscope*, **66**, 16

Ransome, J. (1962) *Royal Free Hospital Journal*, **25**, 91

Ransome, J. (1969) Personal communication

Robinson, M. (1961) *Laryngoscope*, **71**, 181

Russell, T. S. (1966) Personal communication

Sadé, J. (1964) *Archives of Otolaryngology*, **80**, 258

Schuknecht, H. E. and Trupiano, S. (1957) *Laryngoscope*, **67**, 396

Sooy, F. A. (1960) *Annals of Otology, Rhinology and Laryngology*, **69**, 650

Stewart, D. N. (1966) Personal communication

Thorburn, I. B. (1957) *Journal of Laryngology*, **71**, 542

Toynbee, J. (1866) *Med.-chir Transactions*, **49**, 147

Toynbee, J. (1866) *Medical Times Gazette*, **1**, 646

Wilmot, T. J. (1966) Personal communication

8 Acute inflammation of the middle-ear cleft

Stuart Mawson

Introduction

The middle-ear cleft consists of the eustachian (auditory) tube, tympanic cavity and the petrous portion of the temporal bone containing the mastoid antrum and air-cells. Acute inflammation of this area is usually a complication of an upper respiratory infection. Acute otitis media is inflammation confined to the mucoperiosteal lining of the middle-ear cavity (epi-, meso- or hypotympanum). Spread of infection to mastoid or petrous air-cells results in acute mastoiditis or petrositis. The symptoms vary according to the type of infecting organism, the anatomy of the ear, the extent of infection and the age of the patient.

Acute otitis media

Aetiology

Acute otitis media is nearly always a sequel to upper respiratory infection, and is seen most commonly in childhood with a peak incidence in the 5–6 age group. Organisms reach the middle ear via the eustachian tube. Exceptions to this are entry through a perforated drumhead due either to previous disease, trauma or tympanotomy. It is possible that viral infections following exanthemas and influenza are blood-borne.

In infants, where the tube is relatively wide and straight, milk or vomit can enter the middle ear if the child is fed lying down and vomits. In older children forcible nose blowing may have the same effect. Should the nasopharyngeal end of the eustachian tube become closed by swollen peritubal lymphoid tissue, the natural absorption of the active gases in the cleft will create a lowered intratympanic pressure, thus facilitating the movement of infected mucus up the tube into the middle ear.

Common infecting organisms are *Streptococcus pneumoniae*, *Haemophilus influenzae* and *Staphylococcus pyogenes*. It is probable that virus diseases, for example measles, prepare the ground for secondary invasion of the middle ear by these bacteria, when acute otitis media complicates the exanthemas.

NATURAL HISTORY

Early infections involve only the mucosal and submucosal layers of the middle ear. The bone is not affected. In childhood both ears are commonly involved. This results in mucosal oedema, paralysis of ciliary action and blockage of the eustachian tube. There is increase in goblet cells. The absorption of the active gases (oxygen and carbon dioxide) produces a negative pressure in the middle ear. This both retracts the tympanic membrane and promotes a fluid exudate.

Oedema of all structures interferes with function and results in increasing deafness. As the volume of exudate increases, fluid pressure will rise in the middle ear. This will cause increasing pain; absorption of toxins will lead to pyrexia and malaise.

If no treatment is given the increasing intratympanic pressure will interfere with the blood supply to the tympanic membrane. That portion which is under the greatest tension will suffer pressure necrosis, capillary thrombosis and rupture. Pus at first blood-stained, runs out of the ear, and pain is at once relieved. The temperature will quickly fall to normal. Otorrhoea will continue until the inflammation in the middle ear has settled, after which the tympanic membrane will usually heal with a fibrous scar, and hearing will return to normal.

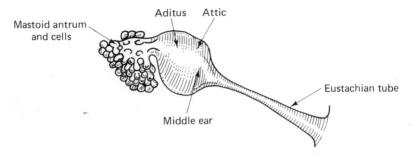

Figure 8.1   Middle-ear cleft. (From Mawson's *Diseases of the Ear*, reproduced by courtesy of Edward Arnold)

When the infecting organism is more virulent, or the patient debilitated, infection may progress, with increasing deafness. The discharge will become more creamy yellow in colour and smelly. This change is due to pressure necrosis in the mastoid air-cells causing destruction of the cell walls. Ultimately the mastoid antrum and air-cells coalesce into one cavity filled with pus and granulation tissue. At this stage, the temperature will rise again, and pain will return with considerable general toxic reaction. In the untreated case this process takes at least a week. The skin over the abscess cavity will become oedematous and later red, pushing the pinna forwards. There will, of course, be tenderness on pressure over this area. If still untreated, further complications will arise.

In general, an acute otitis media will give rise to a temperature of about 37·8–40 °C which settles after rupture of the drumhead. An acute mastoiditis causes a second rise, up to about 38 °C, and any further complication to temperatures up to 38.3–40 °C or even higher.

Where antibiotic treatment is given the course of the disease will be modified at every stage. When adequate treatment is given early, the whole attack will be aborted and hearing and health restored quickly to normal. Adequate treatment may also include the release of pus by incision of a membrane under tension (myringotomy, *see* p. 183).

Where inadequate chemotherapy is given for a short time, the disease is halted temporarily but will recur in 1–3 weeks' time. This may give rise to erroneous histories of repeated attacks of otitis media at weekly intervals. This does not happen but the latent disease re-appears. Antibiotics can only overcome bacteria in their active phase of life. The quiescent period may last 2–3 days. Adequate treatment must thus ensure a constant high blood level of antibiotic for at least five days. In recurrent or relapsing cases courses may need to be extended to ten days or even three weeks. Relapses should also alert the otologist to the possible presence of fluid in the middle ear or latent mastoid air-cell infection.

REACTION TO INFECTION

The more common type of mastoid, well-pneumatized, will react in the manner described under 'Natural History' (p. 176).

The non-pneumatized mastoid will often give a proliferative reaction. This may give rise to an acute polypus presenting through a perforation in Shrapnell's membrane or simply to a painful congestion in the attic region with considerable deafness.

ACUTE OTITIS HAEMORRHAGICA (ACUTE INFLUENZAL OTITIS)—SEE 'MYRINGITIS BULLOSA HAEMORRHAGICA,' p. 191.

The middle ear occasionally is invaded from haemorrhagic external otitis (about 10 per cent of cases).

Diagnosis

The diagnosis of acute middle-ear disease can only be made by an adequate history and by inspection of the tympanic membranes. It is essential that both membranes should be completely seen. External auditory canals are of many shapes, and the presence of osteomata may convey a false impression. All wax, debris and discharge must therefore be removed.

HISTORY OF ILLNESS

An accurate history of the time of onset, symptoms and previous treatment is essential. It is an advantage if both parents, as well as the family doctor, are present when a child is examined.

It is important to find whether the present illness is the first earache experienced. If not the interval elapsed since the previous attack can be important. Inadequate antibiotic treatment can mask a latent infection for up to four weeks before a flare-up becomes apparent.

Acute otitis media can recur in a patient who has a dry perforation of the tympanic membrane either as a complication of a 'cold' or by introduction of water into the middle ear down the external auditory canal from hair washing, swimming or aural syringing. Jumping into water may force water up the eustachian tube via the nose.

Traumatic rupture of the drumhead will not by itself cause otitis media but infection of the middle ear is frequently brought about by well-intentioned use of aural drops or aural toilet. The traumatized tympanic membrane should be left severely alone.

Tympanotomy may be followed by acute otitis media particularly if the operation is performed when the patient has an upper respiratory infection.

At every age acute inflammation of the middle-ear cleft will produce the classic symptoms and signs of inflammation.

SYMPTOMS

A very young child will be ill and off his food. There will probably be a purulent nasal discharge. The temperature will be about 38–39 °C and there may be bowel disturbances. The ear drum may be red and bulging.

If the child is seen early or if the attack is a mild one, the drumhead may be pink and the redness may appear only after the child has been crying (*see* 'Differential Diagnosis', p. 181). Both ears are usually affected.

In older children there will often be signs of a recent upper respiratory infection. Findings will be as above but one ear may be noticeably worse than the other. Older children will be able to cooperate with tuning-fork tests. Rinne's test will often be negative on both sides, and Weber's test will be referred to the worse affected ear.

In adults, commonly, only one ear is affected. This has often been the site of previous infection. Examination of the nasopharynx may show scarring around the appropriate eustachian cushion or there may be an obvious concurrent maxillary antral infection on that side, with pus in the nasopharynx around the eustachian cushion.

When there has been previous infection the membrane may bulge irregularly, the greatest prominence being through an old scar.

When infection has been introduced through a perforation pain will be severe but of short duration due to congestion of the mucosa. As soon as pus forms the pain will diminish.

When otitis media follows traumatic rupture of the drumhead there will be blood clots in the external canal and the membrane will be seen only with difficulty.

The above description covers the common modes of presentation of acute otitis media in the patient with a well-pneumatized mastoid; *Figures 8.2* to *8.5* show this. The red appearance of the drumhead is frequently hidden by a thin layer of desquamatory epithelium overlying it. This cannot be moved because to do so would be very painful, but it is easily recognized.

Patients with non-pneumatized mastoids may react differently. The stage of injection involves the upper part of the membrana tensa and attic more than the lower part (*Figures 8.6* and *8.7*). Shrapnell's membrane may bulge considerably (*Figure 8.8*) and may be the site of a perforation producing a localized crust (*Figure 8.9*). This may be difficult to differentiate from an acute-on-chronic infection.

Treatment in children and adults

The patient should be in bed so that he or she can be maintained in an atmosphere of steady temperature and humidity. This will rest the upper respiratory system as far as possible. Bedroom windows should be kept shut at night and in winter, and humidity maintained particularly if central heating is on.

Treatment is directed towards curing the infection and restoring hearing to normal.

Infection is generally introduced to the middle ear up the eustachian tube. The

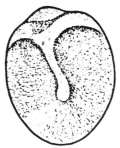

Figure 8.2 Normal
tympanic membrane

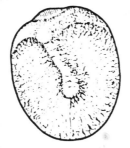

Figure 8.3 Early otitis
media showing injection
of the membrane

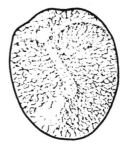

Figure 8.4 Otitis media;
intense vascular injection

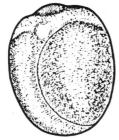

Figure 8.5 Otitis media;
red bulging membrane

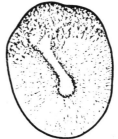

Figure 8.6 Early acute
epitympanitis. Intense
injection of Shrapnell's
membrane

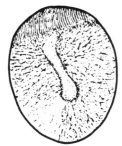

Figure 8.7 Acute
epitympanitis. Injection
and slight bulge of
Shrapnell's membrane

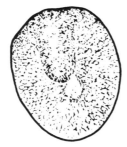

Figure 8.8 Otitis media;
localized bulge of
Shrapnell's membrane

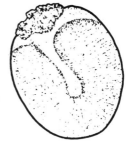

Figure 8.9 Epitympan-
itis; crust obscuring
perforation through
Shrapnell's membrane

natural drainage by ciliary movement of the middle-ear system is down this tube.
Congestion of the nose and nasopharynx by sinus infection, enlarged adenoid tissue
and peritubal lymphoid tissue will perpetuate eustachian tube obstruction.

In the early stages of acute otitis media when the tympanic membrane is injected
and retracted, antibiotics should be withheld for 24 h. Drainage of the eustachian tube
by the use of nasal decongestants (0.25, 0.5 or 1 per cent adrenaline in normal saline
in an atomizer, or as nose drops, given four-hourly followed 10 min later by steam
inhalations with Vap.menth.co. or tinct.benz.co. for 5–10 min) will often relieve early
cases. Warm olive oil ear drops may relieve pain but no ear drops can pass through the

intact stratified squamous epithelium of the tympanic membrane. Analgesics may be required.

If there is no improvement and the drumhead becomes full and red, systemic antibiotic treatment must be started at once. It is most important that once the treatment has been started it shall be continued for at least seven days in such a manner that an adequate blood level of antibiotic is maintained throughout each 24 h. This may cause difficulties when the patient is being treated at home but the danger of inadequate or improper treatment must be explained to the parents. The use of daily or twice-daily injections of antibiotics has much to recommend it. The so-called psychological upsets caused by this method are often used to cover up the administrative difficulties of the daily injection. Not only may inadequate oral treatment result in masking of the infection but it may also induce drug sensitivity. Nevertheless there remains an inherent dislike of injection treatment by general practitioners and patients, and in practice it is more usual to prescribe an oral preparation. Of those currently available amoxycillin 250 mg (adjusted to age) eight-hourly is useful as avoiding the necessity to disturb sleep for administration and as being effective against the common causal organisms.

When the patient is first seen with a painful, red, bulging drumhead there is no doubt that the treatment of choice is myringotomy under general anaesthesia. The membrane is incised at the point of maximum bulge and the single incision is made from below upwards. If a double incision is used, a permanent perforation may result because the blood supply of the drumhead is by end-arteries (*Figure 8.10*).

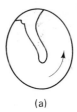 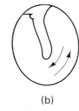

(a)   (b)

Figure 8.10   Myringotomy incision:
(a) correct; (b) incorrect

As soon as the patient awakes, the pain has gone. The otorrhoea will continue until the middle-ear infection has settled down, after which the drumhead will heal and hearing return to normal. Antibiotics should be given for at least seven days supported by nasal decongestants.

If the otalgia is not too severe and can be controlled by analgesics, it is justifiable to treat the patient medically by full and regular antibiotics but the progress of the patient must be followed closely by an otologist. If there is not a steady clinical improvement, the middle ear should be drained.

When the patient is first seen after the tympanic membrane has ruptured no myringotomy will be necessary. Nasal decongestants and a full course of antibiotic treatment will hasten recovery.

As soon as drainage of the middle ear through the membrane has been established aural toilet to the ear is started. This consists in dry mopping the ear down to the drumhead. With adequate illumination the pneumatic speculum may be used gently to suck mucopus from the middle ear and mastoid cells. In a fully equipped otological clinic evacuation of discharge with an electric sucker under an operating microscope will be preferred. Ideally this treatment is carried out on alternate days until the ear is dry. The majority of ears become dry after two or three visits.

When otitis media has entered through a previous perforation or through a ruptured tympanic membrane, a complete course of systemic antibiotics and nasal decongestants will prove effective. Once again aural toilet will hasten resolution.

In some small children, aural toilet may not be possible by mopping and suction. Gentle syringing using warm sterile normal saline or bicarbonate followed by drying of the canal as far as possible is an adequate substitute.

The removal of the discharge will not only encourage drainage but will also prevent secondary infection and hasten resolution and healing. When the ear has become dry there is still a need for observation, to ensure return of the ear and hearing to normal. Failure of the membrane to heal will be accompanied by persistent conductive deafness and risk of reinfection. Surgical repair of the defect may need to come under consideration.

Differential diagnosis

INFANTS

Acute otitis media in infants must be differentiated from referred otalgia and sympathetic injection of the tympanic membrane produced by teething. The baby will frequently be crying when examined and this, of course, will increase the tympanic injection. The fact that the baby is teething and is not very ill, although the temperature may be raised one or two degrees by the effort of crying, will help. The tympanic membrane will not bulge but often appears retracted. If treatment is withheld for 24 h the membrane of the child with otitis media will show marked changes whereas the membrane of the teething child will be unaltered. If the speculum is warmed it may be possible to examine the baby's ears whilst he is asleep.

CHILDREN

In children with enlarged adenoids there may be conductive deafness with an upper respiratory infection but the absence of pain will exclude otitis media (unless antibiotics have been adminstered for the 'cold').

Teething again may cause some confusion, but observation over 24 h will clarify the diagnosis.

In older children and young adults the presence of a mal-erupting lower wisdom tooth will produce otalgia; mild injection of the drumhead, particularly along the handle of the malleus; and a feeling of fullness and possibly tinnitus, but no conductive deafness. The pain will vary, being worse on lying down. Inspection of the mouth and possibly x-ray of the lower molar regions will confirm the diagnosis.

ADULTS

Adults and older children are subject to aural furunculosis. This is the most important differential diagnosis from otitis media. The presenting symptoms of a boil are pain and, later, discharge with some deafness. Tenderness behind the ear is at first not marked, whereas movement of the pinna or tragus increases the pain. Later the post-auricular lymph glands will become enlarged and tender. In otitis media pain is present, with marked deafness. Pain is severe unless the drumhead has ruptured; movement of the pinna or tragus is not painful (*see* 'Acute Mastoiditis', p. 185).

Acute otitis media in infants

Acute otitis can arise as the result of spread of infection from the nasopharynx or milk inhalation through the eustachian tube, by blood-borne infection, or by infection from the external auditory meatus through a previously perforated tympanic membrane. The great majority of cases are caused by spread up the eustachian tube which, in infants, is shorter and more nearly horizontal than in adults, spread of infection being thereby facilitated. Acute otitis media is therefore a common condition in infants. The tympanic membrane is relatively tough and otorrhoea is therefore often a late symptom. The other two cardinal symptoms, earache and deafness, being subjective, cannot be noticed by the parents. The baby with otitis media is therefore presented to the doctor as an ill and restless baby, and only rarely is the doctor's attention drawn to the ears by the mother. The diagnosis of acute otitis media is made on the appearance of the tympanic membrane, and the ears of an infant should always be examined when the child has a pyrexial illness. In no other way can the diagnosis be made.

AETIOLOGY

Feeding

This condition is more common in bottle-fed babies than it is in breast-fed babies. There are various possible causes of this. The position of the baby while taking food is thought to have an important influence on the causation of acute otitis media. To suckle at the breast the baby is held in a partially upright position so that there is little tendency for regurgitated milk to remain in the nasopharynx. With the bottle, the baby is often fed lying on its back and when it regurgitates the milk may lie in the nasopharynx; then, with swallowing, milk may be forced up the eustachian tube into the middle ear.

Milk in the bottle is more likely to be infected than breast milk and this may be an additional cause of the greater frequency of acute otitis media in bottle-fed babies.

The most likely factor, however, is that the breast-fed baby is, on average, healthier than the bottle-fed baby and is therefore better able to resist infection by the pathogenic organisms to which its upper respiratory tract is, from time to time, exposed. It is probable that all infants are liable to aspirate some fluid from the nasopharynx into the ear, but in the majority of cases this does not lead to an otitis media. The cilia in the eustachian tube are able to expel the fluid.

Teething

Acute otitis media is particularly common in infants when they are teething. This causes diagnostic difficulties, for the symptoms of the two conditions are very similar; it is only by examining the ears that otitis media can be excluded. The reasons for this association between cutting teeth and otitis media are unknown, although many suggestions have been made. These suggestions are purely speculative and there is no real evidence to support any of them. It is possible that the general upset caused by painful teething lowers the resistance of the child to the organisms to which he is exposed and thus upper respiratory infections and their complications, such as otitis media, are likely to occur. This is clearly not a complete explanation because children are seen who get otitis with the eruption of each tooth, whereas other children who are seriously disturbed by teething do not get otitis media.

SYMPTOMS AND SIGNS

General disturbance

The symptoms are almost exclusively those of a general disturbance. The child is clearly in pain but there may be nothing to suggest that the pain is in the head and only rarely is there anything to suggest that the pain is in the ear. The child is very restless and does not sleep well. He takes his feeds badly and frequently vomits. There may also be diarrhoea, but a severe attack of diarrhoea and vomiting when not due to gastroenteritis suggests that the acute otitis has progressed to acute mastoiditis even though there are no local superficial physical signs of mastoid infection. This fact suggests that acute otitis media in infants may be entirely free of local symptoms which would indicate the true nature of the infant's ill health. This is particularly true of so-called delicate children in whom indifferent health is common; for an attack of acute otitis may at first be thought to be yet another 'bilious attack' and it is only when the attack has lasted rather longer than usual that the child is examined to find the cause, and the presence of otitis media is revealed.

Occasionally the child gives obvious evidence from the first of pain in the head, for example, pulling or rubbing the ear, or banging its head against a wall or cot, and it is usual in these cases for the diagnosis to be made early, as the ear is an obvious place to examine.

Tympanic membrane

The appearance of the tympanic membrane in otitis media can be very confusing. The diagnosis is difficult even with the best equipment, and can be impossible with a poor auriscope. The meatus may be very small and therefore a small speculum must be used. This means that the light must be accurately centred or it will not be projected beyond the end of the speculum. The membrane may be red and bulging but this is less common than a dull, lustreless and full membrane. It may even be difficult to detect any change except loss of the light reflex, yet on myringotomy pus may be evacuated. Acute otitis media in infants is often associated with diarrhoea and vomiting and with acute lung infections which do not respond normally to appropriate therapy. It is this failure of response which leads to examination of the ears.

TREATMENT

Myringotomy

If it is suspected that the middle ear contains infected material, pus or fluid, and there has been no improvement in the infant's condition with medical treatment serious consideration must be given to the operation of myringotomy. This should be carried out under general anaesthesia. It is sometimes said that the infant is not fit for a general anaesthetic and that the operation is better performed without anaesthesia. This view surely exaggerates the danger of modern anaesthesia. Only a very few moments of peace are required to do an operation which is very difficult to perform on a moving subject. Furthermore, it is difficult to hold a child absolutely still and the smallness of many meatuses makes myringotomy difficult even in the best circumstances. Adequate incision of the membrane is essential. This membrane in infants is sometimes surprisingly thick and thus under poor conditions attempts at myringotomy succeed only in scratching the surface of the membrane and fail to perforate it. More harm results from such failure to drain the middle ear than from the administration of a general anaesthetic. Once adequate drainage has been established the infant's general condition should rapidly improve.

Persistence of the general symptoms and signs, such as diarrhoea and vomiting, particularly associated with profuse drainage from the ear, should raise the question of mastoiditis and the necessity for simple mastoidectomy (*see* p. 185).

Myringotomy may be withheld in cases in which the surgeon considers that there is no fluid in the middle ear. This is always a difficult decision to make and in cases of doubt myringotomy should be performed. Occasionally a case is seen where there is injection of the membrane which still retains its lustre and light reflex. This may reasonably be watched, particularly as an infant can cause injection of the membranes by the violence of its crying. Thus unilateral injection is of more significance than bilateral injection. This is another reason for examining both ears in every case of suspected ear disease. It is, however, much more common for a surgeon to regret not performing a myringotomy than to regret performing one. The incision into a healthy membrane rapidly heals and it is extremely rare for it to cause any lasting disability.

If it is thought that there is no pus in the middle ear either chemotherapy or antibiotics, or both, may be given in adequate dosage, but an undrained ear must be very carefully watched until the hearing is absolutely normal. These drugs may mask the signs of infection very effectively so that a severe recurrence may occur a few days or up to four weeks after the drugs are discontinued. This is further discussed under the treatment of latent otitis media (*see* p. 190).

The dosage of the drugs depends on the body weight of the infant. It should be emphasized that the dosage should be adequate and maintained for a sufficiently long period to be effective. It should be maintained for at least 48 h after the temperature has become normal.

Local treatment

This consists in local toilet and the maintenance of a healthy state of the skin of the pinna and meatus. The toilet of the ear and meatus and the avoidance of a stagnant pool of pus in the meatus are the really important factors in local treatment. This toilet can be done by mopping out the meatus with sterile cottonwool on a wool carrier and must be done with adequate illumination such as a headlight or mirror. After the deep meatus has been mopped dry, the middle ear and mastoid-cell system are emptied of pus by gentle use of suction. Several suckings and moppings will be necessary, so that adequate treatment of an ear will take 10 min. Ideally this treatment is carried out on alternate days until the ear is dry. As an alternative in children who do not tolerate mopping *gentle* syringing with saline and bicarbonate solution can be useful. It permits initial cleansing of a stagnant meatus but is potentially hazardous and must never be done by personnel lacking specialized training.

Ear drops selected according to laboratory reports on pus cultured for organisms and sensitivities may be helpful but must be inserted properly. The ear dropper is filled two-thirds full and the fluid is worked into the external canal a few drops at a time. Moving the jaw and pumping the drops in, using the tragus as a pump lever, forces drops in through the perforation.

Normally the ear will become dry a week or so after the otorrhoea commences but no anxiety need be felt if it continues for two weeks. Continuance after this should lead to a review of the condition and its treatment. If purulent otorrhoea persists for four weeks despite adequate aural toilet, drainage of the mastoid may have to be considered.

PREVENTION OF FURTHER ATTACKS OF OTITIS MEDIA
Blockage of the nasopharyngeal end of the eustachian tube by enlarged adenoids is a common cause of recurring otitis media. Adenoidectomy is the first and most important step to be taken in preventing recurrences. It is very rarely necessary before the age of three years and is better postponed until the child is four or five save in exceptional circumstances. When the adenoids are removed at a younger age there is a likelihood of further lymphoid tissue developing. Moreover, as the space is very small, there is increased risk of scarring the eustachian cushions and producing adhesions between them and the nasopharyngeal walls.

If a child or young adult who has previously had his tonsils and adenoids removed develops a series of attacks of otitis media, adhesions may be seen with a post-nasal mirror or further adenoid tissue may be noted around the eustachian cushions. This should be dealt with under general anaesthesia. When the infection enters the middle ear through a perforation of the membrane, myringoplasty may be considered.

Acute mastoiditis

Although it is nowadays relatively rare, the most common complication of acute otitis media is persistent purulent otorrhoea associated with disease in the mastoid antrum and air-cells. Congestion and oedema of their mucosa will cause thrombosis of arterioles and venules resulting in necrosis of the cell linings. Otorrhoea will become more profuse, creamier and offensive at this stage. The production of pus will exceed the rate of discharge through the ear. Pain will return in the ear; deafness will increase. There may be persistence of low-grade pyrexia due to toxic absorption. Oedema over the mastoid area will obliterate the post-auricular sulcus and push forwards the pinna. Movement of the pinna will not be painful but pressure over Macewen's triangle will hurt. There may be some generalized reddening over the area. There will be reddening and oedema in the attic region of the deep meatus.

A radiograph of the mastoids will show clouding of the whole system on the affected side with decalcification and loss of cellular outlines. The semicircular canals may be clearly visible on occasions.

TREATMENT
The patient must be admitted to hospital and the treatment is always surgical. A simple mastoidectomy (Schwartze) is performed (*Figure 8.11*). The purpose of the operation is to drain the mastoid abscess completely, to make sure that there has been no further spread of infection to adjacent structures and to restore normal hearing. The hair is shaved for 5 cm round the ear; under a general anaesthetic a curved incision is made 1.25 cm behind the pinna from the lower border of the temporal muscle to the lower edge of the mastoid tip. An assistant controls bleeding by digital pressure, one thumb pressing in front of the mastoid tip and one holding the pinna forwards. The periosteum is incised throughout the length of the incision exposing

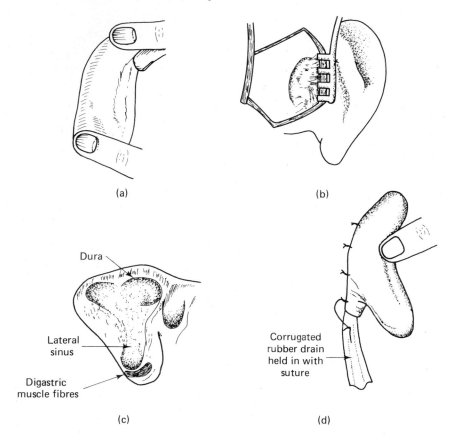

(a)   (b)

Dura

Lateral
sinus

Digastric
muscle fibres

Corrugated
rubber drain
held in with
suture

(c)   (d)

Figure 8.11   Simple (Schwartze's) Mastoidectomy: (a) Incision 1.25 cm behind ear
from root to mastoid tip; (b) Mollison's retractor in position showing increased
vascular marking over Macewen's triangle; (c) horizontal fibres of posterior belly of
digastric (landmarks exposed); (d) final result

Macewen's triangle in the centre of the incision. A 1-cm cut backwards and at right
angles to the incision in the periosteum, will allow good exposure of bone by a rugine.
Care must be taken not to detach the periosteum from the bony external canal
otherwise post-operative stenosis may occur. Exposure of the mastoid antrum is
obtained by using an electric drill. The approach is made by entering the bone over
Macewen's triangle. When the cavity is entered, Lempert's bone scoops will prove
useful in removing soft bone. If pus is found in the antrum, this is sent for culture and
sensitivity tests, and granulation tissue is sent for examination to exclude tuberculous
infection or even a malignant granuloma or glomus tumour. The operation is complete
when four landmarks are visible: above, the tegmen tympani; behind, the lateral
sinus plate; anteriorly, the posterior end of the horizontal semicircular canal; and
below, the horizontal fibres of the posterior belly of the digastric muscle, which lies
deep to the mastoid tip. The dura is exposed by removing a small piece of the tegmen
tympani to exclude the presence of an extradural abscess and a small piece of the sinus
plate is removed to exclude perisinus abscess or lateral sinus thrombosis. If abnormal
dura is discovered further bone must be removed until normal dura is exposed all

round the area of disease. If there is any doubt about the condition of the lateral sinus, this is explored with a needle and syringe (*see* 'Complications of Infections of the Middle Ear', Chapter 12. Finally, the cavity is saucerized as far as practicable.

The wound is then closed with interrupted sutures, after a dusting with antibiotic powder. A corrugated rubber drain is stitched into the lower end of the wound for 24 h to lessen the chance of haematoma formation. A pressure dressing is then applied to the wound in an effort to obliterate the cavity as far as possible. If the bony canal periosteum has been stripped up far it is wise lightly to pack the meatus for 24 h with 6-mm ribbon gauze to prevent a haematoma from narrowing the deep meatus. A full seven-day course of antibiotic is given. The patient should be fit to leave hospital after the stitches are removed at the end of a week.

When infection has been virulent, particularly from some strains of haemolytic streptococci or pneumococcus type III, there may have been spread of disease before operation to nearby structures.

Subperiosteal abscesses may form by pus tracking through Macewen's triangle and presenting under the skin (relatively common) or into the bony canal (rare); or the pus may track down the sternomastoid muscle presenting as a swelling in the posterior triangle of the neck (Bezold's abscess). Treatment of these is by simple mastoidectomy, although a Bezold's abscess may require separate additional dependent stab drainage. On rare occasions the pus tracks forward above the pinna if there are zygomatic air-cells present and this will present as a swelling in front of the ear in the region of the zygoma. It is treated by simple mastoidectomy carrying the incision further forwards than usual above the ear.

The osteitis caused by the infection causes local venous thrombosis. This may enable pus to track through the tegmen tympani or the lateral sinus plate, forming extradural and perisinus abscesses, respectively.

Treatment here too is by simple mastoidectomy. At the end of the operation the dura or lateral sinus must be widely exposed until healthy tissue is seen surrounding the granulations of the abscess cavity. Dural granulations should never be removed. The lateral sinus must be carefully examined and if there is any question of thrombosis then it must be opened.

DIFFERENTIAL DIAGNOSIS

Scalp lesions
Superficially enlarged post-auricular lymph nodes from scalp infections will resemble acute mastoiditis. The finding of lice or skin lesions will prove helpful in the diagnosis. The patient will have no deafness.

Furunculosis
Aural furunculosis may prove a difficult differential diagnosis. The enlarged post-auricular node will push the ear forwards. There may be intense pain in the ear and later there will be purulent discharge. However, movement of the pinna or tragus will be very painful and there will be little deafness. X-ray will show a normal mastoid cell system, but soft-tissue swelling may cause blurring.

Swellings around the ear include sebaceous cysts, which may suppurate; enlarged lymphatic nodes due to tuberculosis, Hodgkin's disease or the other reticuloses; mixed salivary tumours, neurofibromatosis, carcinoma of the outer or middle ear, or even trauma. These conditions should all be diagnosed on history and examination. Costen's syndrome may present difficulty at times because nipping of the temporomandibular joint cartilage can be very painful but there is no related deafness and the irregular dentition and jaw movements should point to the diagnosis.

Acute petrositis

The cells surrounding the cochlea, semicircular canals and internal auditory meatus and the cells in the petrous apex (*Figure 8.12*) may develop a purulent infection following acute otitis media.

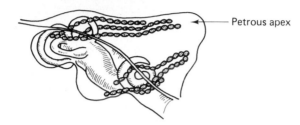

— Petrous apex

Figure 8.12 Schema showing cell chains between middle ear and petrous apex. (From Mawson's *Diseases of the Ear*, reproduced by courtesy of Edward Arnold)

The intrapetrosal stage of infection is overshadowed by the symptoms of acute mastoiditis. Petrositis is therefore diagnosed 7–10 days after the mastoid has been drained by persistence of thick purulent otorrhoea, pain or even the development of Gradenigo's syndrome. Fistulous tracks may be found on four sites:

(1) Behind the semicircular canals.
(2) Under the arch of the superior semicircular canal.
(3) Below the cochlea (hypotympanic cells).
(4) In front of the cochlea near the eustachian tube.

SYMPTOMS
Pain is referred to around the homolateral eye. At first it is intermittent, but later it becomes persistent. It often starts at night and is due to involvement of the first branch of the trigeminal nerve.

Temperature is only slightly raised and white cell counts are not markedly increased.

There is occasional photophobia and the palpebral fissure may be narrowed.

Otorrhoea will increase again, after having diminished following mastoidectomy.

A few days later the sixth cranial nerve may become paralysed, causing diplopia and on rare occasions facial palsy develops. Gradenigo's syndrome is paralysis of the sixth cranial nerve and pain in the area supplied by the fifth nerve due to the infection affecting the area of the petrous apex. Vestibular nystagmus may be sometimes found.

DIAGNOSIS
Acute apical petrositis is suspected when there is an increase in purulent otorrhoea with periorbital pain, in a patient who has recently undergone simple mastoidectomy.

X-ray will show decalcification in the petrous area of the affected ear compared with the normal side. Townes' and Stenvers' views will be of great assistance in the diagnosis.

DIFFERENTIAL DIAGNOSIS

It may be difficult to differentiate this condition from acute labyrinthitis. In the latter there will be a cochlear deafness, whereas in apical petrositis the deafness is conductive in type.

TREATMENT

Once apical petrositis has been diagnosed, the treatment is by surgical drainage.

Extrapetrosal drainage

The simple mastoidectomy field is reopened. Any fistulous tracks found must be followed. If pus appears to come from the middle-ear region in front of the cochlea, the operation must be converted into a radical mastoidectomy. Tracks may then be found which lead towards the apex from the hypotympanum (near the eustachian tube) or from the attic region.

Various routes for a deeper exploration are described (*Figure 8.13*).

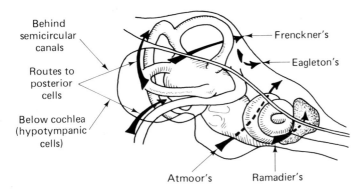

Figure 8.13   Routes to the petrous apex (after Mawson)

Eagleton's operation

A wide exposure of the dura of the middle fossa is made by removal of the tegmen, the base of the zygoma and part of the squamous temporal bone. The dura of the middle fossa is gently elevated towards the petrous apex.

Intrapetrosal drainage

A radical mastoidectomy must be performed.

Almoor's operation

The petrous apex is approached through a triangle bounded by the tegmen tympani above, the carotid artery anteriorly and the cochlea posteriorly.

Ramadier's operation

Here the petrous apex is approached more widely. The tympanic plate of the external auditory canal, posterior to the base of the glenoid fossa suture line, is removed. The carotid artery is lifted forward by a gauze sling. The petrous apex may then be explored through the posterior wall of the bony carotid canal.

Frenckner's operation

Sometimes a group of cells runs under the arch of the superior semicircular canal. This would always be the best approach to the petrous apex except for the fact that the hypotympanic areas cannot be reached.

Latent otitis media and its complications

Latent otitis media is the most common complication of acute otitis media since the introduction of antibiotic therapy. It is the result of inadequate treatment.

Typically a patient is said to have had two, three or four attacks of acute otitis media in as many weeks; this is impossible. The apparent response to treatment is merely the result of a reduction in the number of active bacteria in the area. These patients must be treated very seriously, ideally under hospital supervision. Parenteral antibiotics are ideal for five days but if this is impossible then strictly supervised oral treatment at the correct times should suffice. The patient must then be kept under the observation of a competent otologist for at least four weeks to make sure that no latent infection remains. Hearing should have returned almost to normal by this time if the disease is extinct.

Latent mastoiditis

Patients with latent otitis media have, of course, also latent mastoiditis. If a case is first seen with pain, pyrexia and a pink drumhead, observation in hospital with full antibiotic treatment is justifiable. If, however, there is oedema and reddening of the deep bony meatus, and some obliterative periostitis over Macewen's triangle, simple mastoidectomy is the treatment of choice. For these signs to appear there must be pus and granulations in the middle ear and mastoid cavity.

Even if resolution does occur with antibiotic treatment a permanent conductive deafness may result from the organization of middle-ear exudate. Thorough surgical drainage of the middle ear and mastoid in these cases offers a much better prospect of eventual restoration of hearing.

Masked infection in the mastoid is a highly treacherous condition, and mastoidectomy must be readily undertaken if intracranial complications are to be averted.

Myringitis bullosa haemorrhagica (Acute influenzal otitis, Otitis externa haemorrhagica)

AETIOLOGY

This condition is associated with viral infection in the body. The commonest infection is influenza, but the condition is also found in patients with measles, mumps, chicken pox, pertussis, acute coryza, bronchitis, sinusitis, and infectious mononucleosis. It mainly affects the age group below 30.

SYMPTOMS AND SIGNS

The patient presents with serous or haemorrhagic bullae on the tympanic membrane or in the external auditory meatus. Characteristically there is a sudden onset of excruciating pain in the ear with relatively little constitutional disturbance. The severity of the pain is most striking. It is centred in the ear but may radiate to the mastoid tip, or occiput, or temporomandibular joint. The discomfort usually lasts up to three days, but some cases lasting up to six weeks have been reported. Crops of bullae appear. There is no deafness unless the condition becomes complicated by otitis media. When the bullae rupture there will be a serosanguineous otorrhoea. When the condition is resolving about 10 per cent of patients develop an otitis media. Tetracyclines appear to prolong the course of the disease and tend to result in serous otitis. After the bullae have ruptured, dry black crusts will be seen on the tympanic membrane.

DIFFERENTIAL DIAGNOSIS

The condition must be differentiated from acute otitis externa, in which there is usually marked oedema of the soft tissues of the external auditory canal, and frequently a history of getting water into the ear or eczematous dermatitis.

It must be differentiated from acute otitis media, in which the onset of pain is more gradual, there are more severe constitutional symptoms, and there is a marked conductive hearing loss. The tympanic membrane is reddened more or less uniformly without bullae.

There is a rare condition in which a solitary bleb occurs at the umbo of the malleus due to a lipoid degeneration. It produces no symptoms and is a chance finding on routine examination.

The Ramsay Hunt syndrome must be borne in mind too when this condition is met. The differential diagnosis becomes clear with the onset of facial palsy. The vesicles in this condition are usually smaller and not so vividly coloured.

COMPLICATIONS

Ten per cent of these patients have a secondary otitis media or a serous otitis media; on rare occasions, labyrinthitis or sensorineural hearing loss may follow.

Dawes has reported two patients who developed encephalitis following haemorrhagic bullous myringitis. But it must be borne in mind that this condition is associated with childhood diseases, and the complications often follow the initial disease rather than the myringitis.

PROGNOSIS

The prognosis is excellent in uncomplicated cases; in those developing secondary suppuration, adequate treatment by antibiotics should suffice.

When facial palsies or vestibular or acoustic nerve lesions occur, these recover quickly and completely.

TREATMENT

Treatment is entirely symptomatic. Pain may be relieved with topical anaesthetic ear drops. There is no evidence that prophylactic antibiotics are of the least help. Incision of vesicles does not relieve the pain, and should be discouraged. Incision only encourages secondary bacteria. It has been suggested that pain can be relieved by the use of local anaesthetics such as those employed when doing a tympanotomy under local anaesthetic. It is important to prevent secondary infection, so that the ears must be protected from the entry of water when washing. It is also wise to keep these patients in bed for a few days in order to forestall any possible rare complication.

9 Non-suppurative otitis media
A G Gibb

Introduction

The term non-suppurative otitis media is used here to embrace a group of conditions affecting the middle ear, which are generally considered to be of inflammatory origin but which present no evidence of suppuration. The group includes secretory otitis media, atelectasis, adhesive otitis media and tympanosclerosis. These conditions are probably interrelated and possibly represent different stages of the same pathological process: however, each may occur as a separate entity.

The inflammatory nature of all these conditions is by no means certain, the multiplicity of synonyms applied to secretory otitis media being an indication of the uncertainty surrounding its cause and underlying pathology. Some middle-ear effusions are of non-inflammatory origin, for example those occurring in barotrauma and carcinoma of the nasopharynx, but these represent a small percentage of the total and are included under the title secretory otitis media to complete the classification. The changes in the middle ear in atelectasis are commonly regarded as an end result of prolonged negative pressure but this in turn is probably secondary to an inflammatory process in most cases. Tympanosclerosis and adhesive otitis media are thought to represent the end stage of severe middle-ear infection possibly of a suppurative nature, but, if this is so, the active phase of the condition has long since disappeared by the time they become evident. Their exact relationship to secretory otitis media has yet to be clarified.

Greater attention has been focused on non-suppurative otitis media in the last two decades partly because of the widening potential of micro-surgery in its treatment but also because of a possibly increased incidence consequent on the widespread use of antibiotic drugs in the treatment of middle-ear infections.

Secretory otitis media

(Synonyms: exudative otitis media: serous otitis media: sero-mucinous otitis media: tubotympanic catarrh: catarrhal otitis media: middle-ear effusion: hydrotympanum: tympanic hydrops: glue ear.)

Definition and terminology

Secretory otitis media is characterized by the presence of non-purulent fluid in the middle ear. The fluid may be of watery or viscous consistency and may arise as a transudate, exudate or glandular secretion, hence the multiplicity of titles applied to this condition. The viscosity of the fluid is generally greater in children so that the middle-ear contents frequently have a thick glue-like consistency to which the term 'glue ear' has been applied.

For the sake of clarity and to avoid confusion the various terms employed in relation to fluid in the middle ear are defined as follows:

Effusion —the escape of fluid into a part or tissue.
Transudate—fluid formed as a result of hydrostatic imbalance between intravascular and extravascular compartments despite normal permeability.
Exudate —a fluid which leaks from blood vessels as a result of increased vascular permeability.
Secretion —fluid produced by specialized glandular organs.

It is evident from these definitions that a transudate might arise as a result of pressure changes in the middle ear whereas exudates and secretions would tend to occur in inflammatory states.

History

The first detailed description of secretory otitis media is ascribed to Politzer (1867) but both Wathen (1756) and Cooper (1801) appear to have recognized the condition much earlier than this. In 1874 Hinton, of Guy's Hospital, described the detailed otoscopic appearances encountered in secretory otitis media with remarkable accuracy indicating that the middle-ear fluid could be either serous or viscid. By the turn of the century the condition was widely recognized and detailed descriptions appeared in the standard textbooks of ear diseases. The term 'glue ear' was introduced shortly after the end of the Second World War by Jordan (1949) and a few years later the whole pattern of treatment became altered following the introduction of the first effective ventilation tube by Armstrong (1954).

Incidence and epidemiology

There is much evidence to suggest that during the last two decades the incidence of secretory otitis media has become greater. This increase may, to some extent, be apparent rather than real in that more accurate diagnosis, aided by the introduction of the Zeiss microscope together with a greater awareness of the condition has led to its more frequent recognition. However, there may also be a true increased incidence possibly as a side effect of antibiotic therapy. The latter has doubtless been responsible for a greater prevalence of viral infections in the community, certain of which may well cause secretory otitis media. In addition, many cases which in the past developed frank middle-ear suppuration now have the infection 'damped down', but not necessarily cured, by antibiotic treatment so that suppuration and tympanic membrane rupture may be replaced by a mucous or serous effusion behind an intact tympanic membrane.

In a survey of hearing-impaired children Watson (1969) found chronic secretory otitis media to be the cause in 81 per cent of cases. Litton and McCabe (1962) carried out an extensive investigation of 9543 healthy children and detected middle-ear effusions in more than 10 per cent. Shah (1975) found a similar proportion of young children to be affected. Malcomson (1963) reported a 10 per cent incidence of middle-ear effusion, proved by myringotomy, in 522 children admitted for routine tonsil and adenoid removals.

All observers are agreed that the commonest age group to be affected is the first decade (Kersley and Wickham, 1966; Watson, 1969). Shah (1975) reported that over 85 per cent of his cases occurred between the ages of five and nine but Howie (1975) found the condition to be commonest in babies, 67 per cent of his cases having the initial otitic episode below the age of two years. Secretory otitis media in its chronic form is much less common in adults but acute effusions occur not infrequently in association with upper respiratory tract infections and also in allergic states, while barotrauma and malignant neoplasms of the post-nasal space also account for occasional cases. The condition occurs more frequently in males than in females and tends to affect the poorer social classes of the community (Robinson *et al.*, 1967; Kersley and Wickham, 1966; Harvey, 1975). The incidence is higher during the winter months than in summer.

Aetiology

While the exact mode of production of the effusion in secretory otitis media remains the subject of controversy there is universal agreement that malfunction of the eustachian tube is the essential underlying cause. In his anatomical studies Holborow (1962) demonstrated that whereas in the adult the slit-like lumen of the eustachian tube is placed vertically, in the infant it lies on a horizontal plane parallel to the base of skull—a situation which detracts from the efficiency of the muscles responsible for opening the tube. After the age of five years the plane of the lumen begins to alter and muscular action becomes more effective so that by the time adult life is reached maximum efficiency in tubal opening is already established. It is not surprising therefore that secretory otitis media is commonest in young children and that the incidence gradually diminishes as age increases. The cause of eustachian malfunction which is normally located in the nose or throat may be obvious in some cases but in others, and especially in adult patients, the aetiology may be obscure.

The following are the most important causes of tubal malfunction leading to secretory otitis media.

(a) UPPER RESPIRATORY TRACT INFECTION
An acute infection of viral or bacterial origin frequently precedes the onset of secretory otitis media, influenza being a common cause. Shah (1975) reported that 40 per cent of his cases presented with an upper respiratory tract infection and 18 per cent with tonsillitis. Viruses have been cultured from time to time from middle-ear effusions and

the same virus has on some occasions been cultured from the throat. The fact that viruses have been isolated relatively infrequently is possibly due partly to the technical problems concerning virus culture from middle-ear effusions and partly to the tendency of viruses to be present only in the early stages of infections before the patient seeks advice. Chronic rhinitis, sinusitis, nasal polypi and septal deviations may also predispose to secretory otitis media since they frequently impair eustachian tube patency.

(b)   ADENOID AND TONSIL HYPERTROPHY

In children enlargement of the adenoids and tonsils are important causes of secretory otitis media especially if there is associated infection. Tumarkin (1961) expressed the opinion that mechanical blockage of the eustachian tube could occur in some cases where the bulk of the adenoid mass was very large but more often tubal patency is compromised by inflammatory oedema due to an ascending salpingitis arising from recurrent or chronic tonsil and adenoid infections. Dawes (1970), Mawson and Fagan (1972) and others considered that the importance of the adenoids and tonsils in the causation of secretory otitis media was exaggerated and pointed out that the condition is commonly found in children in whom the tonsils and adenoids are very small or have previously been removed. It is the experience of most otologists, however, that the adenoids (and to a much lesser extent, the tonsils) play a significant aetiological role, at least in a proportion of cases, the dramatic cure or improvement which not infrequently follows their removal affording strong supporting evidence that this is so.

(c)   ALLERGY

Clinical opinion is sharply divided regarding the importance of allergy as a cause of secretory otitis media. Proetz (1931) although unable to find eosinophils in the middle-ear fluids firmly believed that effusions arose and recurred in allergic subjects following exposure to specific allergens. Wright and Kapadia (1969) were also unable to detect eosinophils in a series of middle-ear effusions. Senturia, Gessert and Baumann (1958), after studying the cytology of over 100 effusions, concluded that the eosinophil count did not justify the diagnosis of allergy, while Stevens (1958) also reported a low incidence of allergy in secretory otitis media. Dohlman (1943) on the other hand, in a series of 125 cases, found pronounced eosinophilia in the secretions of 28 of these, while Koch (1947) found large numbers of eosinophilic cells in mucoid secretions in 41 out of 222 patients, many of whom suffered from nasal allergy. In a review of 111 cases of secretory otitis media, Jordan (1952) came to the conclusion that no fewer than 87 per cent were allergic in origin and other observers have also stressed the importance of allergy in the causation of the condition (Lecks 1962; Draper 1967).

The immunoglobulin studies of Lim *et al.* (1976) and Mogi *et al.* (1974) of the IgE levels in the serum and middle-ear fluids tended to disprove the concept of an allergic aetiology. Both sets of workers concluded that atopic allergy played no significant role in secretory otitis media. On the other hand Friedmann (1974), basing his judgment on histological studies, considered that the metaplastic respiratory-type epithelium encountered in the middle ear in established cases of secretory otitis media might be expected to react to allergens in a similar fashion to nasal and sinus mucosa and thus produce secretions of high viscosity in the tympanic cavity.

In conclusion it can be stated that the importance of allergy as a cause of secretory otitis media is still controversial. While it is accepted that a proportion of middle-ear effusions are allergic in origin it does not necessarily follow that this is inevitably the case in every subject with an allergic diathesis.

(d) CLEFT PALATE

In cleft palate cases there is gross disturbance of eustachian function. The mechanism of the problem was explained by Holborow (1962) who pointed out that in this condition the eustachian tube failed to open on swallowing due mainly to limitation of the action of the tensor palati muscle: this in turn was partly related to muscular hypoplasia but mainly to lack of a solid anchorage for the muscle at its midline insertion in the soft palate without which effective contraction cannot take place. Even after surgical repair of the palate the problem may continue or may even be aggravated if the palatal muscles have been traumatized or if fracture of the hamular process has been deliberately carried out. The incidence of secretory otitis media in cleft palate cases is very high especially in childhood when tubal problems tend to be accentuated: according to the findings of Paradise, Bluestone and Felder (1969) virtually all cleft palate infants under 20 months suffer from otitis media, frequently in its secretory form.

(e) OTITIC BAROTRAUMA

Middle-ear effusions may result from sudden changes of barometric pressure. These occur most frequently during flying or deep sea diving especially if an upper respiratory infection is present. They result from a failure of the eustachian tube to compensate for changes (increases) in the atmospheric pressure. A marked negative pressure develops in the middle ear and this is followed by a transudation of serous fluid from the lining epithelium. The effusion is frequently blood-stained due to rupture of small vessels in the mucosa.

(f) TUMOURS OF NASOPHARYNX

Tumours of the nasopharynx, especially of malignant type, are an important cause of secretory otitis media in the adult. Most cases arise initially because of tubal blockage due to local congestion in the vicinity of the tumour but later on the tumour may invade the eustachian tube or even the tympanic cavity. Conductive deafness is often the first indication of the presence of a nasopharyngeal carcinoma. All cases of secretory otitis media in adults, especially if unilateral, require careful examination of the nasopharynx.

(g) RADIATION THERAPY

Middle-ear effusion commonly occurs after radiotherapy in the vicinity of the base of skull. The effusion is generally serous in type and is believed to result from an inflammatory reaction of the middle ear and eustachian tube with impaired lymphatic drainage leading to secondary eustachian obstruction (Dias, 1966).

(h) ANTIBIOTIC-SUPPRESSED OTITIS MEDIA

The possible role of inadequate antibiotic therapy in cases of acute otitis media as a cause of middle-ear effusion was highlighted by Laff (1962), Walsh (1963) and Mawson (1964). While the antibiotic drugs are of unquestionable value in the management of acute infections of the upper respiratory tract and ears, inadequate therapy may lead to incomplete resolution of the infection, with a residual exudate in the middle ear. Failure of antibiotics may be the result of several factors such as: (a) inadequate dosage or too short a prescribed course; (b) discontinuance of the drug before the course is completed following dramatic symptomatic improvement; (c) resistance to taking medicines on the part of the child, often combined with lack of parental discipline; (d) inappropriate choice of antibiotic without bacteriological control; (e) reliance on antibiotic therapy alone in cases manifestly meriting myringotomy; and (f) failure of follow-up to ensure complete middle-ear resolution.

(i) SYSTEMIC DISEASES

Occasionally secretory otitis media is associated with immunological, metabolic or other systemic disorders. The relationship to allergy has already been discussed, and the condition is also known to occur in hypothyroidism. Hypogammaglobulinaemia is a rare but important cause and should always be excluded in recurrent cases.

Histopathology

The epithelium lining the normal middle-ear cleft shows considerable variation in different areas. The posterior parts of the tympanic cavity and the mastoid are covered with a flat or cuboidal epithelium with only very few ciliated and goblet cells. In other areas, notably around the eustachian tube, the hypotympanum and the promontory, the epithelium changes to a stratified columnar or cuboidal type and contains numerous mucus secreting elements and cilia. In an ultrastructural study of the epithelium in the anterior part of the middle ear Hentzer (1976) identified five types of cells—non-ciliated cells (with and without secretory granules), ciliated cells, intermediate cells and basal cells. He believed that a basal cell, via an intermediate cell, could differentiate into either a ciliated cell or a secretory (goblet) cell. Sadé (1966) concluded that the middle-ear lining was a true mucosa capable of secreting mucus both from the surface epithelium and from mucosal gland-like structures.

In secretory otitis media marked changes occur, the lining epithelium becoming considerably thickened and transformed into a pseudo-stratified columnar type with numerous cilia and a striking increase in glandular elements so that it comes to resemble the respiratory mucosa of the nose (Friedmann, 1963) (*Figure 9.1*). In some cases gross thickening occurs and the epithelium may appear polypoidal. Similar changes may also be observed in the mastoid antrum and air-cells.

Types of effusion

Effusions differ widely in their colour, viscosity and content.

(a) SEROUS

In serous effusions the fluid is generally watery, crystal clear and of a pale yellow colour. The viscosity is low and no mucous strands are present. The liquid clots within a few minutes of removal on exposure to air. The protein content is higher than in mucous effusions (Senturia, 1970). Such an effusion may be produced either by transudation or exudation.

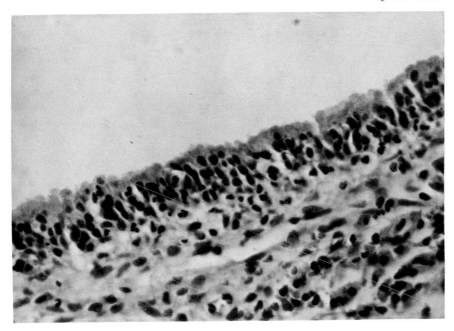

Figure 9.1 Pseudo-stratified columnar epithelium from the middle ear in secretory otitis media. (From Friedmann, *Pathology of the Ear*. Blackwells. By courtesy of the author and publishers)

(b) MUCOUS

Mucous effusions are common in children and consist of greyish or yellowish cloudy exudates of high viscosity; mucous strands are present. Sometimes the effusion is so tenacious as to resemble glue. Thick effusions consist essentially of glandular secretions but in less viscous effusions there may be an element of exudation.

Mucous effusions contain large quantities of mucopolysaccharides which may be demonstrated by staining with the periodic acid Schiff reagent or with alcian blue. A number of cells shed from the lining of the middle ear and eustachian tube are also present. These commonly take the form of lymphocytes and polymorphonuclear leucocytes, and less frequently monocytes and phagocytes. The protein content is lower than in serous effusions.

(c) HAEMORRHAGIC

Haemorrhagic effusions may occur in chronic secretory otitis media but are more commonly associated with the condition of idiopathic haemotympanum (blue drum) which is probably a variant of the former condition. It seems likely that the pathogenesis is basically the same in both conditions in that sub-epithelial vascular leakage occurs as a result of infection or changes in pressure. However, whereas in secretory otitis media the vessel wall generally remains intact allowing only plasma to escape, rupture occurs in idiopathic haemotympanum due either to severe pressure alterations or to infection, allowing blood to extravasate initially into the submucosal space and later into the tympanic cavity and mastoid. The latter condition was first described under the title of 'blue drum membrane' by Shambaugh in 1929, the term 'idiopathic haemotympanum' being used by O'Donnell in 1941. Ranger (1949) drew attention to the fact that the altered blood in the middle ear was also frequently present in the mastoid air-cells. The effusion in this condition is generally dark brown in colour and consists of altered blood, debris and epithelial cells. It is sterile on culture and the Van den Bergh reaction is positive. The tympanic membrane is dark in colour usually assuming a gun-metal blue appearance—hence the term 'blue drum'. Idiopathic haemotympanum is often associated with cholesterol granuloma. The latter however, as Friedmann (1974) has pointed out, is a non-specific condition which may occur in association with any form of chronic otitis media where haemorrhage takes place into the tissues. Cholesterol which is an insoluble constituent of blood tends to crystallize out and act as a tissue irritant thereby provoking an active granulomatous response with large numbers of foreign body giant cells. The tissue has a brownish colour due to the presence of granules of haemosiderin and numerous cholesterol clefts are visible on microscopy.

Microbiology

The majority of otologists have for many years assumed that middle-ear effusions are sterile. The findings of Jordan (1949) and of Tönder and Gundersen (1971) who reported negative cultures seemed to support this belief. Evidence however is growing that this is not always the case since micro-organisms can be isolated and cultured from effusions in a significant percentage of cases. Yoshie (1955) isolated the influenza (A) virus from the middle-ear exudate in 16 cases and the Coxsackie, para-influenza and adenoviruses have also been cultured from middle-ear effusions. Klein and Teele (1976) investigated the middle-ear fluids from 663 patients; and he succeeded in isolating viruses, mainly the respiratory syncytial virus, in 29 of these (4.4 per cent). He also cultured *Mycoplasma pneumoniae* in one case. In many instances the same virus was cultured from the subject's throat. Commenting on the relative infrequency of positive cultures he stressed the problems surrounding virus isolation from middle-ear effusions.

Bacteria have also been isolated from middle-ear fluids. Liu *et al.* (1975) found bacteria in smears of 77 per cent of effusions and 52 per cent yielded positive bacterial cultures. Only half of these bacteria were pathogenic. Bacterial contamination of specimens, although possible, was considered unlikely especially in view of the fact that the immunoglobulin levels were in inverse proportion to the number of bacteria present, suggesting an effective immune response to the infection on the part of the host: the high proportion of non-pathogenic organisms obtained from the cultures might be explained on the grounds that following antibiotic treatment with elimination of pathogens these organisms act as opportunists producing a hypovirulent infection with a sustained inflammatory response. The presence of bacteria in middle-ear effusions has also been reported by a number of other workers including Senturia, Gessert and Baumann (1958), Silverstein, Miller and Lindeman (1966) and Bernstein and Hayes (1971). The most common bacteria detected were *Haemophilus influenzae*, streptococcus, diphtheroids, *Staphylococcus albus* and pneumococcus. The foregoing evidence suggests that positive bacterial cultures were confined mainly to cases of antibiotic suppressed acute otitis media.

In conclusion it seems likely that a significant percentage of effusions do contain micro-organisms at the onset, especially if this is associated with an upper respiratory infection. Failure to isolate and identify these is frequently related to shortcomings in present laboratory techniques.

Immunology

Siirala and Lahikainen (1952) were the first to demonstrate that middle-ear fluids possessed bacteriostatic and virus inhibiting properties. Recent studies add further support to the concept that the middle ear is protected by an immunological defence system. Liu *et al.* (1975) using the radial immunodiffusion technique demonstrated the presence of IgA and IgG in middle-ear effusions in higher concentrations than in the corresponding sera. Secretory lysozyme has also been found in effusions in large quantities (Veltri and Sprinkle, 1973). The immunoglobulin system of the middle ear matures with age and is more active in mucoid type effusions where increased secretory activity occurs (Liu *et al.*, 1975). Large numbers of tissue and wandering macrophages can be found in the mucosa and effusions indicating that the middle ear is capable of efficient phagocytosis.

Bernstein (1976) on the other hand reported the presence of certain factors in middle-ear effusions which he described as mediators of inflammation. He suggested that the role of these was the maintenance of inflammation in the middle-ear cleft. The mediators comprised chemotactic and macrophage inhibition factors, activated complement and prostaglandins. The last-named cause increased capillary permeability which in turn may result in persistence of the effusion. Their presence, however, may have additional significance in that prostaglandins have been shown to stimulate bone resorption in tissue cultures. A similar action in the middle ear might be a factor in the frequent and often unexplained tendency to incus resorption in otitis media.

Pathogenesis

It was formerly thought that middle-ear effusions arose as a result of negative middle-ear pressure—hydrops ex vacuo. This resulted primarily from a failure of the eustachian tube to open on swallowing so that the air in the middle ear became hermetically sealed off from the atmospheric air. If this happens there is a continuous absorption of gases from the middle ear which is not compensated by the normal mechanism of intermittent tubal ventilation. The sum of the partial pressures of gases in the tympanic air—101.080 kPa (760 mmHg) is higher than that in the surrounding tissues—93.100 kPa (700 mmHg)—so that there is a diffusion gradient of about 7.980 kPa (60 mmHg) between the middle ear and the tissues. Oxygen, carbon dioxide and nitrogen may all diffuse into the tissues in this way (Elner, 1976). An increasing negative pressure develops in the rigid chamber of the tympanic cavity, initially minimized by retraction of the tympanic membrane, and when the pressure reaches a certain limit transudation occurs. If the tube is blocked for long enough the whole tympanic cavity will ultimately become filled with transudate.

The validity of this theory in secretory otitis media has been questioned on the grounds that although a negative pressure is known to exist it is considered to be insufficient, except in barotrauma, to cause transudation (Van Dishoeck, 1948). Other observers maintain that the eustachian tube is hardly ever completely blocked in this condition thus rendering the theory invalid (Brieger, 1914; Sadé, 1966). In addition Zöllner (1942) and Sadé (1966) did not regard retraction of the tympanic membrane as a feature of the disease. Further doubts were cast on the hydrops ex vacuo theory as evidence accumulated in favour of the theory of infection.

It has already been pointed out that middle-ear epithelium normally contains mucus-producing elements so that some secretory activity is to be expected: the resultant mucus, however, is never evident clinically in the normal ear and is presumably evacuated continuously by ciliary action via the eustachian tube. In secretory otitis media the hypertrophic changes which occur in the epithelium together with the dramatic increase in glandular structures and increased mucus production are typical of a local response to infection. If at the same time the mucus clearance system becomes inefficient partly because the cilia cannot cope with the sticky secretion and partly because the negative pressure renders evacuation more difficult the middle ear will fill up with mucous secretion. If this theory is accepted the middle-ear effusion must be regarded as a reaction to inflammation resulting partly from exudation due to increased capillary permeability and partly from increased glandular secretion. Analysis of the contents of the middle-ear fluid supports this hypothesis. Palva, Raunio and Nousiainen (1974) in a biochemical study of mucous effusions in children found that the mean protein level was higher than that in the corresponding serum indicating that the fluid could not be a simple transudate from the serum but must be locally secreted. The isolation of both viruses and bacteria from middle-ear effusions adds support to the infective theory. The low percentage of positive cultures does not seriously invalidate this concept in view of the difficulties of viral isolation already mentioned. Furthermore, it has been pointed out that viruses are obligatory cell parasites which are normally present in the epithelium rather than in the effused fluid (Bauer, 1975). The high concentrations of IgA and other immunoglobulins reported by Liu *et al.* (1975) and the high titres of lysozyme noted by Veltri and Sprinkle (1973) also suggest a local response to infection. IgA covers the surface of the mucosa as a thin film protecting it from bacteria while lysozyme is bactericidal in the presence of immunoglobulins and complement components. According to Liu *et al.* (1975) and other observers the levels of IgA, IgG and lysozyme are higher in middle-ear fluids than in the corresponding sera suggesting that they are secreted locally in response to infection. Further evidence of the theory of infection is derived from the fact that bacteria are found in inverse proportions to the IgA, IgG and lysozyme levels in the effusions suggesting a local immune response. The fact that the immunological system matures with age accords well with the diminishing incidence of secretory otitis media in older children. Veltri and Sprinkle (1976) regarded the condition as an immune-mediated disease process.

In conclusion it can be stated that much of the recent evidence suggests that secretory otitis media is a response to infection rather than a hydrops ex vacuo. Nevertheless negative pressure does appear to play some part in the aetiology. It is remarkable how a middle ear secreting large amounts of mucus appears to stop producing this fluid immediately after ventilation is established. This finding is difficult to equate with the infective theory alone since the production of mucus might be expected to continue undiminished until the mucous membrane had sufficient time to return to normal. The only immediate consequence of ventilation is the relief of the negative pressure which must be assumed to be the reason for the apparent reduction in secretion: whether this is due to diminished fluid production (transudation) or merely to improved ciliary clearance, as suggested by Bauer (1975), is not proven. Doubtless different varieties of secretory otitis media exist in which the relative importance of negative pressure and of infection vary according to type.

Diagnosis

Secretory otitis media falls into two clinical types—an acute condition in which deafness usually develops during the course of an acute upper respiratory infection and a chronic form which may result either from an untreated acute condition or develop insidiously, sometimes remaining undetected for a considerable period.

HISTORY

(a) Acute secretory otitis media

In the acute form the onset of deafness may or may not be accompanied by pain during the course of an upper respiratory infection. Sometimes the condition is recurrent and there is a history of repeated episodes of otalgia each followed by deafness which clears up slowly and may eventually persist indefinitely and enter a chronic phase. In other instances the patient is referred to the otologist with a history of pain in the ear, several days previously, treated with antibiotics: the pain has disappeared but the deafness persists. When the otologist sees the patient there is no evidence of acute inflammation, the appearances of the tympanic membrane being indicative of secretory otitis media. There is little doubt, however, that in such a case an acute inflammatory condition existed which was controlled but not cured by the antibiotic. In this type of case positive bacteriological or viral culture from the middle-ear secretion is a distinct possibility.

The diagnosis of secretory otitis media is often easy if the patient can give an adequate history. The presence of upper respiratory disease in association with the onset of deafness should alert the doctor to the possible presence of the condition. In addition, an adult patient is usually able to give an accurate description of the hearing loss. This is often described as 'stuffiness', or a 'muffled' or 'cotton wool' feeling rather than a true deafness. Tinnitus is frequently present, usually taking the form of crackling or bubbling noises. Autophony is also a feature, the patient frequently complaining of sounds echoing in the ear. If the exudate is serous, as is often the case in adults, the hearing may alter with changes in position due to movement of the fluid within the tympanic cavity.

(b) Chronic secretory otitis media

In the chronic form of secretory otitis media pain is not a feature, the only symptom being deafness which in the child may remain undetected for a long period. The deafness is often fluctuating in type and may eventually be suspected by the parents or the school teacher or its discovery may result from a routine screening test. In severe cases retardation of speech, language, or educational development may point to the presence of the deafness. A significant lowering of verbal intelligence was noted by Holm and Kunze (1969) and Kaplan et al. (1973). The description of the deafness may be similar to that in the acute condition but some modification of the picture is inevitable since the fluid is usually mucoid rather than serous and the condition is commonest in children from whom a detailed history is usually unobtainable.

Examination

OTOSCOPIC DIAGNOSIS

The otoscopic diagnosis in both the acute and chronic forms may be easy or extremely difficult.

Alteration of the colour of the tympanic membrane is the most obvious feature of this condition and change from the normal lustrous grey membrane to a glistening syrupy or amber colour is common. In some instances the tympanic membrane assumes a plum colour while in others it has a dull grey ground-glass appearance: less frequently the colour may alter to gun-metal blue or even black indicating the presence of blood pigments in the effusion, while a bright green appearance has been observed in severe congenital biliary cirrhosis (Ballantyne, 1977). As a result of the altered background colour the ossicles tend to appear whiter than usual. In some cases, especially those in which pain has been a feature, there may be injection of the radial blood vessels and the general appearance of the tympanic membrane tends to be rather dull.

Retraction of the tympanic membrane is often a feature and is sometimes severe. Secretory otitis media is closely related to middle-ear atelectasis where gross retraction of the tympanic membrane is frequently accompanied by a middle-ear effusion.

If the effusion is of serous type a *fluid level* may be present which can usually be recognized by the presence of crescentic black hairlines, concave upwards, one anterior and one posterior to the handle of malleus: above these menisci the tympanic membrane is of normal appearance whereas the inferior part of the tympanic membrane exhibits the colour changes typical of intratympanic effusion.

Air bubbles may also be visible and if several are present they may produce a mosaic pattern, the circumference of the air bubbles appearing as dark spherical lines (*Figure 9.2*). In some cases the alterations in the tympanic membrane appearance are minimal; indeed a normal otoscopic appearance may be observed but in these circumstances reduced elasticity of the membrane can sometimes be recognized by the presence of diminished mobility on examination with a pneumatic speculum.

It must be stressed that the detection of fluid may be extremely difficult by otoscopy alone and examination with the microscope under high power may prove invaluable. In some cases however it may still be difficult to decide whether fluid is present or not even when using a magnification of 16 × for the examination. Furthermore the problems of detection are greatly increased if the tympanic membrane is thickened or tympanosclerotic. In cases where all investigations are inconclusive it may be necessary to carry out exploratory myringotomy or even tympanotomy to exclude the presence of fluid.

GENERAL EXAMINATION

The examination must always include a careful inspection of the nose and throat, special attention being paid to the detection of enlarged adenoids, sinusitis, nasal polypi, deviated septum and nasopharyngeal neoplasm in adult cases. A general examination is also necessary to exclude systemic disease.

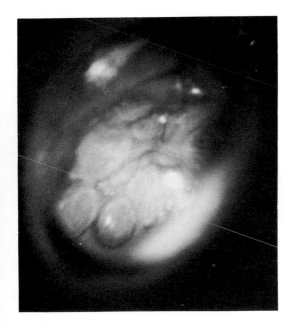

Figure 9.2   Air bubbles in the middle ear in secretory otitis media

EUSTACHIAN TUBE FUNCTION

Examination of the eustachian tubes by the conventional methods of Valsalva, Toynbee and Politzer and by eustachian catheter, may provide useful information concerning tubal patency and function. For example, the knowledge that the eustachian tubes open on swallowing during the Toynbee test is invaluable in assessing prognosis, while the ability to perform Valsalva's inflation successfully may suggest the possibility of incorporating this manoeuvre in the treatment. Additional information regarding tubal function can be obtained from tympanometry.

VOICE AND TUNING-FORK TESTS

The hearing loss in secretory otitis media is often so slight that testing by whispered voice may be misleading. Even if a whispered voice is readily heard the examiner should not assume that the hearing is normal. Audiometric testing of all cases, apart from very young children, is essential. The hearing loss is conductive in type but is seldom of sufficient severity to reverse the Rinne test which in most cases remains positive or equivocal. In unilateral hearing loss the employment of the Weber test is more helpful. This is a much more sensitive test than the Rinne and even in minor degrees of hearing loss lateralization to the affected ear occurs.

AUDIOMETRY

Audiometry is invaluable and the audiogram typically shows a conductive hearing loss with a flat graph and an air–bone gap. The average loss is often in the region of 20 dB but in severe cases of glue ear this may be increased to around 40 dB.

Occasionally there is an additional sensorineural component in the deafness.

TYMPANOMETRY

Tympanometry has proved a valuable and reliable method of detecting the presence of fluid in the middle ear (Brooks, 1973). It is useful in both the diagnosis and management of secretory otitis media and is employed extensively in many paediatric otological clinics. It is a simple procedure well tolerated even by a young child and provides useful information regarding the state of the middle ear and eustachian tube. A mobile tympanic membrane is important for the investigation as thickening or fixation will invalidate the results. In secretory otitis media a negative middle-ear pressure is recorded and the presence of fluid is recognized by a reduction in compliance. The resulting tympanogram shows a flat tracing which climbs slowly to 399.0 kPa (300 mmH$_2$O) or 532.0 kPa (400 mmH$_2$O) of water but does not come to an actual peak. Alterations in middle-ear pressure resulting from swallowing or the Valsalva manoeuvre can readily be detected and recorded, thus giving an indication of eustachian function. The patency of ventilation tubes can also be checked by tympanometry. If the middle ear communicates with the meatus indicating that the ventilation tube is patent the normal peak in the tympanogram is absent and replaced by a horizontal straight line. Conversely, the presence of a normal peak indicates that the ventilation tube is blocked or has been extruded.

RADIOGRAPHS

X-rays provide useful information regarding the development and state of the mastoid air-cell system. The information may be highly relevant to the management of difficult cases of secretory otitis media in which mastoid involvement has occurred. The presence of an effusion is indicated by loss of definition of the mastoid air-cells on x-ray: in many cases the air-cell system is poorly pneumatized. The radiological changes may be more marked if cholesterol granuloma is present. X-rays of the nasopharynx and sinuses may be helpful in detecting hypertrophy of the adenoids, sinusitis and neoplasms of the post-nasal space.

Differential diagnosis

Secretory otitis media must be distinguished from other forms of conductive deafness of congenital, traumatic, inflammatory or otosclerotic origin. The diagnosis is reached after a complete assessment of the otoscopic, audiometric and tympanometric findings. In cases of doubt it may be necessary to carry out exploratory tympanotomy.

It is important also to distinguish an effusion arising from secretory otitis media from that due to other causes. These include the following:

(1) Cerebrospinal otorrhoea. An effusion of clear fluid resulting from leakage of cerobrospinal fluid may follow fractures of the temporal bone. The diagnosis is made on the history, radiographic examination including polytomography and if necessary exploratory tympanotomy.
(2) Perilymph fistula. Leakage of perilymph usually from the regions of the oval or round windows may follow trauma (including surgical trauma, e.g. stapedectomy) or sudden changes of pressure. The latter may result from heavy weight-lifting or barotrauma as in deep sea diving. A detailed history may be extremely helpful in arriving at a diagnosis but tympanotomy with careful examination of both labyrinthine windows under high magnification is essential to confirm the presence of a fistula.
(3) Salivary gland choristoma. A clear effusion may be associated with the occurrence

of salivary gland tissue in the middle ear (Abadir and Pease, 1978). This may take the form of an embryological choristoma or, less commonly, a salivary gland tumour, for example, cylindroma. The resulting effusion consists of saliva. The diagnosis of this rare condition is generally made after tympanotomy and biopsy.

HAEMORRHAGIC EFFUSIONS
Bleeding may take place into the middle-ear cleft in a variety of conditions including temporal bone fractures, epistaxis (especially after nasal or post-nasal packing), tumours of the ear (for example glomus jugulare) and bleeding dyscrasias such as leukaemia. These conditions are generally easily distinguished from idiopathic haemotympanum and other blood-stained effusions by the history and examination.

Treatment

The principal aim of treatment is the restoration of normal eustachian tube function.

(a) ACUTE SECRETORY OTITIS MEDIA
In acute secretory otitis media it is likely that the eustachian disturbance is of a temporary nature being related as a rule to an acute upper respiratory infection, an acute allergic attack or sometimes to air travel or deep sea diving. Spontaneous restoration of tubal function can be anticipated when the acute disturbance subsides and this is likely to be followed by a rapid disappearance of the effusion, which in most instances is serous in type.

Treatment is therefore of a conservative nature and is directed to the nose, nasopharynx and eustachian tube to assist and accelerate recovery. Decongestants are often of value especially those administered systemically. Oral preparations combining an ephedrine derivative with an antihistamine are effective in clearing the nasal airway and improving tubal patency. Local decongestant preparations such as nasal drops, sprays or inhalations are less likely to prove effective owing to their limited access to the eustachian tube. After the acute stage of the respiratory infection is past auto-inflation by Valsalva's method should be carried out. If this procedure cannot be performed effectively Politzerization or inflation by catheter may assist recovery. Myringotomy may be required to enable the effusion to be evacuated by aspiration but the insertion of ventilation tubes is seldom required in the acute disease and is reserved for cases showing no response to other treatments. In adults a short course of steroids may clear up the condition in resistant cases. Prednisolone is advised in high dosage (80 mg) daily for five days with progressive reduction of dosage thereafter, the total course seldom exceeding ten days.

(b) CHRONIC SECRETORY OTITIS MEDIA
In the management of chronic or recurrent secretory otitis media it should be remembered that the condition cannot be considered as cured until the epithelium of the middle ear, which is often grossly hypertrophic, has reverted to its normal state. This reversal normally occurs spontaneously if adequate middle-ear ventilation is achieved.

The first objective in treatment therefore is to attempt to restore ventilation, if possible by the normal eustachian route, by eliminating any primary source of infection or obstruction in the nose, nasopharynx or pharynx. Thus vasomotor rhinitis, allergy, sinusitis and nasal obstruction from any cause including (very rarely) malignant disease of the nasopharynx, should receive appropriate treatment. In children, consideration must be given to removal of the adenoids and in selected cases the tonsils also. Adenoid removal is frequently associated with a dramatic improvement in the ear condition, especially if gross adenoidal hypertrophy is present. Improvement may also occur in cases where the adenoids are relatively small, the benefit presumably resulting from elimination of the source of ascending tubal infection. For similar reasons the removal of infected tonsils may also prove beneficial. Doubt has been cast on the validity of these procedures in this condition by Mawson and Fagan (1972), Dawes (1970) and others who in their surveys found no convincing evidence of their overall usefulness. Mawson came to the conclusion that adenoidectomy should not be employed as a primary treatment of this condition. The present author considers that adenoidectomy with or without tonsillectomy should not be regarded as a panacea in secretory otitis media but in selected cases the procedure may prove very effective.

The next line of treatment is directed to the eustachian tube itself. Regular inflation by Valsalva's method, by Politzer bag or by catheter may assist in re-establishing or maintaining tubal patency. If Valsalva's auto-inflation is unsuccessful initially the administration of decongestant drugs may render the manoeuvre possible. In subjects in which Valsalva's inflation can be carried out regularly and effectively the prognosis is generally good. Politzerization is generally reserved for cases in which auto-inflation is not possible. Although this treatment is normally performed in the clinic the author can recall occasional cases resistant to other treatments where success was achieved by giving the patient or parent a Politzer bag with instructions regarding its use at home. Hunt-Williams (1968) pointed out that in young children active ventilation of the middle ear is generally impossible by auto-inflation and unpleasant by Politzerization. He therefore recommended the insertion of a carnival blower into one nostril which the child is instructed to inflate while the mouth is kept closed and the other nostril is occluded. Most children cooperate readily, regarding the performance of this procedure as an acceptable 'game'. During the course of the manoeuvre the nasopharyngeal pressure rises sufficiently to overcome the resistance of the eustachian tube which is forced open and ventilation of the middle ear results. If tubal opening does not occur higher pressures can be achieved by substituting a balloon for the carnival blower with a suitable nozzle attachment to fit the nostril.

Myringotomy and aspiration of the middle-ear effusion is reserved for those cases which do not clear up on the treatments already mentioned. This procedure is frequently performed in conjunction with adenoidectomy in children. The author as a rule performs myringotomy at the same time as adenoidectomy in cases of painless effusion suspected to be of a mucoid type, but omits the myringotomy in obvious serous effusions, in patients with recurrent otalgia and in cases of gross adenoidal hypertrophy. In the latter groups the ear condition frequently resolves spontaneously after adenoidectomy alone. If myringotomy is employed for aspiration purposes only and a ventilation tube is not inserted the incision normally heals in 24–48 h. The size and situation of the myringotomy incision differs from that employed in acute suppurative otitis media. A much smaller incision is adequate and this is placed radially to minimize subsequent scarring of the tympanic membrane. If an effusion is very thick aspiration may prove difficult. This is partly due to the gluey nature of the exudate and partly to the difficulties inherent in aspirating a solution through a single small opening from a cavity in which a negative pressure is present. In problem cases a second or 'relief' incision in another part of the tympanic membrane is used to eliminate the vacuum effect and facilitate the aspiration of secretions. A variety of local preparations have been injected into the middle ear to help liquefy the glue in order to facilitate its removal (*Figure 9.3*). Litton and McCabe (1962) made use of alpha-chymotrypsin while Bauer (1975) advocated a fresh solution of urea which he found to be a powerful mucolytic agent causing viscid effusions to liquefy within a few minutes. Aspiration is usually carried out through a fine needle connected to a powerful electric suction pump and is best performed under the operating microscope.

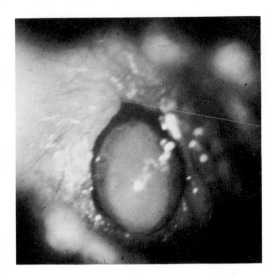

Figure 9.3   Glue exuding from middle ear following myringotomy

Such equipment may not always be available and under these circumstances some of the following older methods of evacuating effusions may be successfully employed. In serous effusions myringotomy followed by suction with Siegle's pneumatic speculum may be successful. The fluid collects in the meatus from which it can be readily mopped. Alternatively the pneumatic speculum can be used as a pump to blow the fluid or glue down the eustachian tube into the nose from which the patient can evacuate it. As an alternative, Politzerization can be used in conjunction with myringotomy to blow the fluid out through the drumhead incision into the external auditory meatus from which it can then be removed. Reverse Politzerization has also been practised by a number of otologists but has come to be recognized as a dangerous procedure. Ahren and Thulin (1965) reported a death with lethal intracranial complications following paracentesis and inflation with a Politzer bag placed in the external auditory meatus. The patient had a congenital dehiscence of the tegmen tympani and the procedure caused detachment of the overlying dura mater with vascular damage and extradural haematoma together with diffuse and severe brain damage due to a sudden increase in intracranial pressure. Later the authors examined 94 autopsies selected at random and found defects in the tegmen tympani in approximately 6 per cent. Myringotomy is sometimes performed without anaesthesia in cooperative adults but it is preferable to use some form of anaesthetic, especially if a grommet is inserted, and general anaesthesia is mandatory in all children. Surface anaesthetic agents are only partially effective on account of poor tissue penetration.

Bonain's solution, in which the main active agent is phenol, has been used since the last century. Recently a more efficient method of surface anaesthesia has been introduced (Comeau, Brummett and Vernon, 1973; Ramsden, Gibson and Moffat, 1977) employing the technique of iontophoresis in conjunction with a Xylocaine 2 per cent and adrenaline 1:2000 solution in the ear canal. The author has for many years employed infiltration anaesthesia for grommet insertion using the same technique as that employed in stapedectomy.

The potential benefits to be derived from prolonged ventilation were recognized more than 100 years ago by Politzer (1867) and Hinton (1869) who attempted to create a permanent perforation by burning a hole in the tympanic membrane with galvano-cautery and inserting some foreign material such as catgut or a silver cannula to maintain patency. Unfortunately, these efforts met with little success and it was not until 1954 that the first real advance was made in this direction when Armstrong succeeded in maintaining a plastic tube in position. This resulted in immediate hearing improvement which was maintained as long as the tube remained patent. The method was widely publicized and rapidly adopted by otologists all over the world. Armstrong later coined the term 'tympanostomy tube'. It is now recognized that the primary function of the tube is ventilation rather than drainage. In the course of the last two decades numerous designs of tubes have been produced. These for the most part resemble hollow collar studs or grommets. The latter term has been widely applied to many of these models, the Shepard grommet being the design favoured by most otologists in the UK.

Ventilation tubes act as temporary substitutes for the eustachian tube. The rationale for their use is related not only to the immediate hearing improvement which follows insertion but also to the fact that with improved ventilation the epithelium of the middle ear gradually reverts to normal, glandular activity being reduced and ciliary action restored. In chronic cases epithelial recovery may take weeks or even months. While ventilation is being maintained the otologist must never lose sight of his main objective, namely the restoration of normal eustachian function, as failure to achieve this will inevitably result in recurrence of the effusion when the ventilation tube ceases to function. However, as Holborow (1962) pointed out, time is on the side of the otologist when dealing with secretory otitis media in children since spontaneous improvement in eustachian function can be anticipated from the age of five years onwards. Long-term ventilation via the tympanic membrane presents problems as most tubes are extruded after about six months. This occurrence is related to the unique behaviour of the squamous epithelium on the surface of the tympanic membrane and deep meatal walls. In 1882 Blake noted that patches of glazed paper placed on the surface of the tympanic membrane migrate from the umbo outwards, usually towards the postero–superior canal wall, whence they progress to the wax-bearing area of the meatus. This migratory movement, later confirmed by Stinson (1936), Litton (1963) and Alberti (1964), has an important bearing on the behaviour of ventilation tubes in that their extrusion is directly related to epithelium migration. After a grommet has been in position for several months the surrounding epithelium appears to grow beneath it gradually displacing the grommet outwards and sealing off the underlying myringotomy opening. Sometimes this state of affairs can be recognized on otoscopy by the fact that the grommet, although apparently in its original situation is now lying more superficially on the surface of the tympanic membrane. Confirmation that the original perforation has sealed off may be obtained by using a

Siegle's pneumatic speculum or by tympanometry to demonstrate the presence of mobility of the tympanic membrane. If the grommet is then picked off the drum surface the latter often shows a circular indentation with a mound in the centre corresponding to the original position of the grommet. If extrusion is allowed to proceed without interference, healing of the tympanic membrane invariably occurs before the grommet moves from its original site. Eventually the grommet is carried by epithelial migration off the tympanic membrane altogether and along the meatal wall towards the exterior and frequently in this process it becomes embedded in desquamated epithelium and wax.

Alberti (1964), while observing the direction of movement of ink spots applied to the drum head was able at the same time, to estimate the rates of epithelial migration. It became clear that the migration was slowest at the umbo and over the handle of malleus but the rate increased towards the periphery. In a comparison of the four standard quadrants of the drum head it appeared that migration was slower in the antero–superior quadrant than elsewhere. It may thus be concluded that extrusion is likely to be slowest if grommets are placed in this area, i.e. immediately anterior to the handle of malleus.

Other methods have been developed in an effort to extend the functional 'life' of ventilation tubes. These have resulted in the design of many different patterns of tubes and the use of different materials. A tube with a side clip of stainless steel which fitted over the handle of the malleus was designed by Silverstein (1966) to prevent extrusion. Silverstein (1970) later approached this problem in a different way by drilling a narrow tunnel in the posterior bony meatal wall through which he introduced a flanged silicone rubber tube to the region of the facial recess or failing this to the mastoid antrum. The present author considers that such a procedure even in expert hands carries a considerable risk of damage to the facial nerve and for this reason does not recommend the technique. Goode (1973) introduced a silicone-rubber T-tube as a means of preventing extrusion. The horizontal arms of this tube lie in the middle ear and collapse readily during insertion and removal. In 1969 Per-Lee designed a plastic tube with a wide flexible round flange at the inner end (*Figure 9.4*). The tube is clumsy

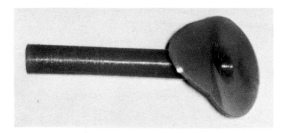

Figure 9.4 Per-Lee (wide flange) ventilation tube

to insert, although it can be trimmed if necessary, but it has proved successful in overcoming the problem of extrusion. Per-Lee reported a rejection rate of only 2.5 per cent in 80 ears. The author has personal experience of this tube and has so far had no problems of extrusion despite the fact that some tubes have been functioning for over six years.

If the use of a wide-flanged tube is contemplated it is necessary to balance the disadvantages of the larger myringotomy incision necessary for its insertion against the scarring likely to result from repeated replacement of an ordinary grommet. The author reserves the use of Per-Lee tubes for severe glue ears in which long-term ventilation is likely to be required. In less severe cases ventilation by a standard grommet is preferred. Kilby, Richards and Hart (1972) reported on the results of treatment by grommets, in a controlled two-year trial in 54 children with bilateral secretory otitis media in which only one ear was treated, the other being used as the control. The hearing results at the end of this period were approximately the same in both groups but there was a significant increase in scarring and tympanosclerosis of the tympanic membranes of the treated ears. The authors concluded that ventilation did not confer any long-term hearing benefits but merely resulted in middle-ear scarring.

If, however, ventilation is not undertaken other measures would be essential to overcome the problem of deafness, especially during the formative years of childhood when language development and education may be retarded. Some otologists have argued that a hearing aid might be used as a temporary measure in the belief that eventually, and usually by adolescence, the condition will resolve spontaneously. This practice is not recommended since it is considered that middle-ear effusions should not be left untreated because of the potential sequelae of atelectasis and adhesive otitis media.

Technique of grommet insertion

Grommet tubes should be inserted atraumatically under the operating microscope, using general or local anaesthesia. The following method is advised. A radial myringotomy incision slightly shorter in length than the diameter of the grommet is made with a sharp myringotome: blunt myringotomes such as are often supplied in disposable packs should be discarded as they tend to tear rather than incise the tympanic membrane. The grommet is next placed alongside the incision and using a right-angled pick the edge of the grommet is insinuated under the upper margin of the slit (*Figure 9.5*). Gentle pressure is then applied with the side of the pick to the lower surface of the grommet which should readily snap into position. Clumsy insertion with too large an opening may result in premature extrusion while haemorrhage at the time of insertion may occlude the lumen and prevent ventilation. Blockage of the grommet by glue secretion is uncommon but does occur: the author has experience of

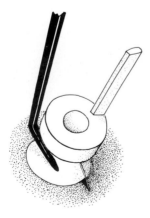

Figure 9.5   Insertion of Shepard's grommet

an adult patient with bilateral disease where the secretions were so tenacious that every ventilation tube, including a Per-Lee tube, became blocked within 48 h of insertion.

There is no universal agreement as to how long ventilation tubes should be left in position. The author considers removal unnecessary in view of the rapid extrusion rate. One of the arguments advanced in favour of removal is to enable the patient to swim without fear of water entering the middle ear. It has been the practice at the University Clinic in Nijmegen to remove grommets in children during the summer months and re-insert them if necessary the following winter. The child is thus able to swim without risk during the summer season. It is probable that the dangers of bathing in the presence of grommets are exaggerated and the author now permits swimming provided that cotton wool smeared with vaseline is inserted in the concha and a tight bathing cap is used, believing that with these precautions the risks of water entering the middle ear are minimal. Occasionally a grommet remains functional for much longer than six months and the otologist may be tempted to remove it. This is not always advisable. The author can recall the case of a teenage boy whose grommet was still functioning over a year after insertion. His decision to remove the grommet proved unwise as secretory otitis media recurred rapidly after its removal.

Certain cases are resistant to conventional methods of treatment and in these the otologist should always suspect the possibility of a co-existing secretory mastoiditis. Mucus secreting epithelium has been demonstrated within the mastoid, aditus, antrum and air-cells (Lim, Shimada and Yoder, 1973) so that there is every likelihood that the mastoid air-cell system will be involved at the same time as the middle ear. Ventilation of the mesotympanum via the tympanic membrane is unlikely to have much beneficial effect on the mastoid disease unless there is free communication through the aditus. Frequently the epithelium in this area is so swollen that aeration of the mastoid is not possible and the air-cells fill up with fluid like a reservoir, the secretions occasionally spilling over into the middle ear.

In such cases a cortical mastoidectomy operation with exenteration of the air-cell system is necessary. The air-cells are generally found to be filled with typical gluey secretion: a grommet is inserted in the tympanic membrane at the time of operation and it may also be prudent to leave a plastic tube in the post-auricular wound for ventilation and drainage of the mastoid. Unfortunately, this method of treatment may fail, presumably because it is not always possible to exenterate every mastoid air-cell and the effusion may recur in both the middle ear and the mastoid. Palva (1977) therefore advocates a more radical approach to the problem. The mastoid air-cells are exenterated as thoroughly as possible and a muscular flap based on the posterior meatal wall is then turned into the cavity and draped like a curtain over the aditus to seal off the mastoid from the middle ear: the remainder of the mastoid cavity is then obliterated, partly by the muscle flap and partly by bone dust. The long-term results of this procedure are not yet available nor have the indications for operation been clearly defined but the technique is worthy of consideration in the management of problem cases. A modified radical mastoid operation with the creation of an 'open' mastoid cavity may have to be considered in cases where the mastoid is acellular or where other treatments fail. Mastoidectomy is always required in cases of cholesterol granuloma. Careful exenteration of the diseased area, is carried out in conjunction with the operative techniques already described.

While the main aim of treatment is the restoration of normal hearing, the otologist must at the same time recognize the need for rehabilitation in cases where communication problems already exist. This applies particularly to children with severe long-standing secretory otitis media in whom speech and language development is retarded or educational progress is slow. In these cases it may be necessary to enlist the help of the teacher of the deaf, the speech therapist and the educational psychologist to assist with the rehabilitation.

Sequelae

Long-standing untreated cases of secretory otitis media are prone to develop permanent deafness due to atelectasis, adhesive otitis media or chronic suppurative otitis media. Tympanosclerosis may also be connected with unresolved secretory otitis media although the exact relationship between these conditions has yet to be defined.

Chronic suppurative otitis media, usually with cholesteatoma formation, is liable to develop as a result of collapse of the tympanic membrane. Prolonged negative pressure in the middle ear and mastoid predisposes to the formation of retraction pockets especially in the postero–superior segment. Keratin tends to accumulate in the pockets due to interference with epithelial migration and the nucleus of a cholesteatoma sac is thus formed. Infection may follow, often with the formation of granulation tissue.

Middle-ear atelectasis

(Synonym: atelectatic middle ear.)

Definition and description

The term middle-ear atelectasis signifies collapse of the tympanic membrane so that it becomes displaced inwards towards the promontory.

The condition occurs in association with eustachian malfunction which leads to inadequate ventilation of the middle-ear cleft. Thus it is closely related to chronic secretory otitis media and adhesive otitis media. According to Sadé and Berco (1976) four degrees of atelectasis can be defined as:

(1) Retraction of the tympanic membrane.
(2) Severe retraction of the tympanic membrane with draping against the incus or stapes.
(3) Collapse of the membrane on to the promontory (plastering).
(4) Collapse with adherence of the membrane to the promontory (adhesion).

The stage of adhesion however would be more correctly classified under adhesive otitis media.

Tympanic membrane retraction may be generalized or localized to a particular area, notably the posterior half of the membrane, the postero–superior quadrant, the central area or the antero–superior quadrant.

Aetiology

The condition is intimately associated with eustachian dysfunction and according to Sadé and Berco (1976) the majority of cases follow either secretory or suppurative otitis media.

Diagnosis

The diagnosis is made on the appearances of the tympanic membrane. More than half the cases are bilateral. The degree of retraction and mobility of the tympanic membrane can be determined by otoscopy performed in conjunction with a Siegle pneumatic speculum. Examination under the microscope while employing a Siegle speculum with a plain lens, is useful not only as a means of confirming the otoscopic diagnosis but also to help the otologist to determine if fluid is present in the middle ear and to assess the state of the ossicular chain. Frequently the tympanic membrane is extremely thin, transparent and atrophic—a situation which facilitates the examination of the middle-ear contents (*Figure 9.6*). Incus necrosis is relatively common and

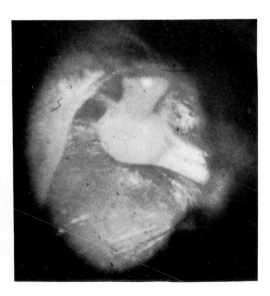

Figure 9.6   Atelectasis of the left tympanic membrane with atrophic 'collapse' posteriorly. The lower end of the long process of the incus has lost its normal contour. (From Harrison and Watson (1969), reproduced by courtesy of the Editor of *Proceedings of the Royal Society of Medicine*)

occasionally the stapes crura are also necrosed. The necrotic areas in the ossicular chain may be surrounded with granulation tissue. Granulations may also occur along the posterior rim of the annulus (Sadé and Berco, 1976) which tends to stand out as a sharp ridge as a result of collapse of the adjacent tympanic membrane into the sinus tympani. Tuning-fork tests and audiometry typically show a conductive hearing loss while tympanometry shows a markedly negative middle-ear pressure with an average impedance (Sadé and Berco, 1976). Tympanometric recording carried out before and after tests of eustachian patency, such as the Valsalva and Toynbee manoeuvres, may be useful as a means of recognizing alterations in middle-ear pressure which indicate that opening of the eustachian tube has taken place.

RADIOGRAPHIC EXAMINATION

Atelectasis is associated with arrested development of the mastoid air-cell system so that the mastoid process is generally poorly pneumatized.

Differential diagnosis

Adhesive otitis media closely resembles atelectasis. Indeed, as has already been suggested it may represent the end stage of the atelectatic ear. The author, however, agrees with Buckingham's (1969) contention that the two conditions although closely allied should be regarded as separate entities. Careful otoscopic examination with a Seigle's speculum should be sufficient to differentiate an atelectatic tympanic membrane collapsed against the promontory from an adherent tympanic membrane which is characteristic of adhesive otitis media.

Treatment

Restoration of middle-ear ventilation forms the basis of treatment and every effort should be made to remedy causes of eustachian dysfunction in the nose or nasopharynx, as outlined in the section on secretory otitis media. If this is not possible ventilation may be achieved by the insertion of a grommet in the tympanic membrane. This minor procedure may present difficulties in severe atelectasis since it may be difficult to find an air space where a ventilation tube can be inserted if the tympanic membrane is plastered against the medial tympanic wall. In these circumstances Wright (1969) has suggested preliminary Politzerization to aerate the middle ear and re-expand the collapsed membrane. A very thin atrophic tympanic membrane is liable to tear when the myringotomy is made and the ventilation tube is inserted. Following insertion of the grommet aeration and re-expansion of the collapsed tympanic membrane normally occurs accompanied by an immediate improvement in middle-ear function. However, the atelectasis will certainly recur after extrusion of the grommet if the eustachian dysfunction has not been corrected. Re-insertion of the grommet is likely to cause further scarring of the already atrophic tympanic membrane so that long-term ventilation using a Per-Lee tube should be considered as an alternative method of management.

The passage of bougies or the insertion of plastic tubing along the eustachian tube, as described by Zöllner (1963), are not recommended as they are liable to result in scarring and stricture formation. Various operations on the eustachian tube itself designed to overcome severe obstruction have been described. House, Glasscock and Miles (1969) introduced a tuboplasty technique using a middle-fossa approach in which the tubal obstruction was removed and the stenosed lining of the tube was excised. A rolled up Silastic sheet was then inserted to form a matrix around which the regenerating epithelium might extend to form the new tube. Although the authors reported encouraging early results the value of this procedure has never been established.

Tympanoplastic operations are useless in the presence of a poorly functioning eustachian tube and should only be considered if normal tubal function can be restored.

Adhesive otitis media

(Synonyms: chronic middle-ear catarrh; adhesive process; fibrotic otitis media.)

Definition and aetiology

The term adhesive otitis media is applied to the condition where fibrous adhesions are present in the middle ear as a result of previous inflammation. It thus represents the final stage of a past inflammatory process resulting from any form of otitis media—acute or chronic, suppurative or non-suppurative. Many authorities, however, exclude cases caused by overt middle-ear suppuration under this title. The author considers such a classification to be artificial and unpractical since it is usually difficult or impossible to distinguish the sequelae of a suppurative from those of a non-suppurative process. Adhesive otitis media due to any type of inflammation is therefore included under this heading provided the tympanic membrane is intact: cases with a residual perforation are excluded. Middle-ear adhesions due to other causes such as surgical damage to the mucosa or reactions to irritant implanted foreign materials do not strictly come within this title although their pathology and surgical treatment are essentially the same.

Pathology

The adhesive changes may affect the tympanic membrane, the middle-ear cavity, the ossicular chain and the mastoid air-cells. In the mildest cases only a few adhesions may be present and these may well be compatible with normal hearing.

In more advanced cases the adhesions are more numerous while in the most severe cases the middle-ear cavity is virtually replaced by masses of scar tissue so that the air space becomes more or less obliterated. Adhesions are commonest in the posterior part of the mesotympanum and in the attic. Frequently the tympanic membrane becomes thickened and bound down to the inner tympanic wall in the region of the promontory. The ossicles and window areas are often involved and the adhesions may pass from one ossicle to another or bind the ossicles to the tympanic membrane or to the bony walls of the tympanic cavity. Sometimes the oval window area is filled with a mass of fibrous tissue in which the stapes and long process of the incus are buried. The round window niche may be partially or completely obliterated. On histological examination the adhesions consist of dense mature fibrous tissue covered by an intact investing epithelium. According to some of the early observers calcification and ossification of the scar tissue may supervene but this occurrence is much less common than in tympanosclerosis and it seems possible that the two conditions have at times been confused. Bone absorption may occur and affect parts of the ossicular chain.

Pathogenesis

Politzer (1926) considered that there was a close connection between the exudative catarrhs of the middle ear and adhesive processes making it difficult to draw a sharp line of demarcation between them. Ojala (1953) also recognized an association with exudative middle-ear disease and suggested the following three stages in the development of the terminal adhesive condition.

(1) An acute stage of otosalpingitis with eustachian tube obstruction and inflammatory reaction throughout the entire middle-ear cleft resulting in mucosal damage and the production of a fibrinous exudate.

(2) An intermediate stage characterized by organization of the exudate and the formation of adhesions. In this stage the mucosal lining of the middle ear and mastoid air-cells is oedematous and there is a residual exudate sometimes containing cholesterol crystals. The mastoid air-cells become filled with connective tissue and there is some surrounding bone sclerosis.

(3) The terminal stage in which mature fibrous adhesions are present together with diminished aeration of the mastoid air-cells. In addition to the mucosal changes there may be evidence of bone absorption especially affecting the long process of the incus. The eustachian tube, which was blocked in the initial stage, may be patent.

Ojala considered that the above concept adequately explained why adhesions form most frequently in certain areas unfavourably located for the drainage of exudates via the eustachian tube—the apical mastoid cells, the small cells round the antrum and the inner parts of the tympanum such as the window niches, Prussak's space and around the ossicular chain.

MacNaughtan (1956) while supporting Ojala's view pointed out that adhesions will develop only if the inflammatory process is severe enough to cause mucosal damage and the fibrinous exudate remains in the middle ear long enough to allow organization to take place. He considered that reliance on antibiotic therapy alone in the treatment of acute middle-ear infections without establishing adequate drainage was an important factor in the development of adhesive otitis media. This view was shared by Siirala (1960) who stressed the importance of careful follow-up after acute middle-ear infection to ensure that complete hearing recovery occurred and to guard against the hazards of persisting middle-ear effusion and latent mastoiditis. He stressed the importance of re-establishing adequate middle-ear ventilation, if need be by employing Politzerization. Ojala (1953) went as far as to suggest that the widespread employment of chemotherapeutic treatment in middle-ear infections might lead to a virtual replacement of chronic suppurative otitis media by adhesive otitis media.

Buckingham (1969) stressed the importance of malfunction of the eustachian tube in the development of adhesive otitis media and considered the condition to be closely allied to middle-ear atelectasis. On the other hand Lumio (1951) in a study of 185 cases of adhesive otitis media expressed the opinion that severe tympanic sepsis following specific fevers predisposed to the condition.

Clinical features

The main symptom is deafness which is often bilateral (Lumio, 1951). Frequently there is a history of previous ear trouble with or without suppuration. Tinnitus is commonly present but paracusis and vertigo are relatively rare.

The tympanic membrane is intact and occasionally looks relatively normal but more commonly it has a dull appearance and variable degrees of thickening may be present. Mobility is commonly reduced or absent. Atrophic areas, scarring or chalk patches may be present. Retraction is common and may be severe and sometimes the tympanic membrane becomes adherent to the promontory. The eustachian tube is frequently patent on inflation.

The deafness is essentially conductive in type although a sensorineural element is not uncommon (Siirala, 1960). Tuning-fork and audiometric tests are important in arriving at a diagnosis and also in assessing the chances of hearing improvement by surgery. Tympanometry is seldom helpful since the tympanic membrane is frequently grossly abnormal.

Radiological examination of the mastoid process commonly reveals reduced cellularity with blurring of the cell outlines. The semicircular canals are usually sharply defined (Hutchison, 1955).

Differential diagnosis

OTOSCLEROSIS
In otosclerosis, where there is also a conductive deafness, there is often a family history of deafness and normally no history of past otitis media. The tympanic membranes and middle-ear pressures are normal, and the eustachian tubes are patent in otosclerosis while the mastoid air-cell structure is radiologically normal.

TYMPANOSCLEROSIS
Adhesive otitis media and tympanosclerosis may resemble each other closely and often the diagnosis cannot be established without tympanotomy. The presence of chalk patches in either tympanic membrane is suggestive of intratympanic tympanosclerosis.

Treatment

The treatment of adhesive otitis media is unsatisfactory as once the middle ear is enveloped in masses of scar tissue the situation from a surgical point of view is unfavourable or even hopeless. The main aim of the otologist should therefore be to prevent the occurrence of the condition by more effective treatment of secretory and suppurative otitis media, special attention being focused on the drainage of exudates.

Before undertaking surgical treatment in the established condition it is essential to ensure that eustachian function is satisfactory otherwise any operation is doomed to eventual failure. If tubal function is abnormal further major surgery is contraindicated unless normal ventilation can be re-established. A ventilation tube may be inserted in an effort to achieve this. If surgery is decided upon the author advises a preliminary permeatal tympanotomy to assess the state of the middle ear and plan any further surgical measures. If it is decided to proceed with surgery the adhesions are carefully divided and scar tissue masses excised to re-create an adequate tympanic air space; if the tympanic membrane is adherent to the promontory particular care must be taken to avoid tearing the membrane during separation. After dividing all the adhesions a sheet of Silastic or Gelfilm should be placed in the middle ear to prevent further adhesion formation during the healing phase. A cortisone solution may also be instilled locally with the same aim in view. The state of the ossicular chain is carefully assessed and any areas of ossicular fixation or erosion noted. Operations on the ossicular chain are usually better deferred to a second stage when the middle ear is free of adhesions. A delay of at least six months between operative stages is advisable. At the second operation the middle ear is re-opened; if Silastic was previously inserted it is removed and the state of the middle ear mucosa is noted. If tubal function is satisfactory and adhesions have been successfully eliminated treatment follows the lines described under tympanosclerosis, ossiculoplasty or stapedectomy being undertaken depending on the pathology encountered. In considering the advisability of these procedures the risk of sensorineural degeneration following surgery should always be kept in mind in view of its fairly common association with adhesive otitis media. Fenestration of the lateral semicircular canal may also be considered as a means of bypassing the adhesive process but the results of this procedure have been rather variable. Cawthorne (1956) stressed the necessity of confirming the presence of stapes fixation before proceeding with this operation in view of the risk of producing the Tullio phenomenon (giddiness on exposure to noise) if a new fenestra is created in the presence of a mobile stapes.

In conclusion the key to success in the management of adhesive otitis media lies in prevention rather than cure as the results of surgery in the established condition are unsatisfactory. The provision of a suitable hearing aid may provide the best solution to this intractable condition.

Tympanosclerosis

(Synonyms: hyalinization; hyalinosis.)

Definition and description

Tympanosclerosis is an abnormal condition of the middle ear characterized by the local deposition of plaques of collagen beneath the lining epithelium. Plaques may be laid down in the substance of the tympanic membrane where they are often referred to as 'chalk patches' or 'calcareous deposits', but they are also found in the tympanic cavity and occasionally in the mastoid. Frequently the tympanosclerosis is confined to the tympanic membrane or less commonly to the middle ear, but in severe cases both areas are involved.

Deposits may be small and clinically unimportant but in some instances they occupy large areas of the tympanic cavity, frequently forming a layer resembling thick cream or cement around the ossicles. These plaques typically occur in certain sites of election (*see Figure 9.7*), the commonest being the stapes–oval window area, the sub-fallopian groove and the upper promontory (*Figure 9.8*). Adjacent structures such as the long process of incus (*Figure 9.9*), stapedius tendon and fallopian canal (horizontal portion) are also frequently involved. Deposits are common in the epitympanum and in relation to the malleus but tympanosclerosis in the eustachian tube area, the hypotympanum and the round window niche is rare, while deposits in

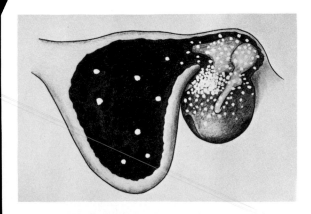

Figure 9.7 Diagram to show distribution of plaques in intratympanic tympanosclerosis

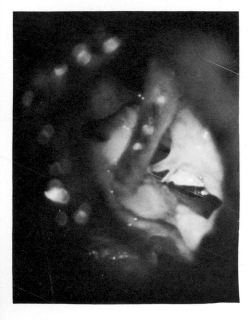

Figure 9.8 Calcified intra-tympanic tympanosclerosis involving oval window area and stapedius tendon

the mastoid are also uncommon. A severe conductive hearing loss may result from impaired ossicular movement caused by plaque formation or from ossicular disruption which is often encountered in association with tympanosclerosis. Erosion of the long process of the incus and the stapes crura are the commonest causes of discontinuity (Gibb, 1976).

History

Tympanic membrane chalk patches were recognized in the eighteenth century by Cassebohm (1734) in his anatomical studies of the ear but the first comprehensive description of tympanosclerosis within the tympanic cavity is attributed to Von Tröltsch (1869) of Würzburg who observed the thickened inelastic epithelial lining and referred to it as 'sclerosis'. Further descriptions followed shortly after this by Politzer (1883), Habermann (1892) and Walb (1893) but little attention was paid to

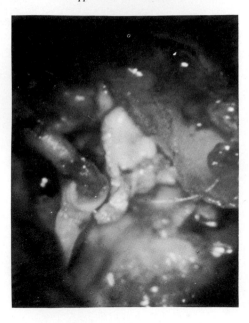

Figure 9.9   Intra-tympanic tympanosclerosis
with erosion of the long process of incus

tympanosclerosis until the middle of the present century when a paper by Zöllner and
Beck (1955) in which they described in detail the appearances under the operating
microscope led to a revival of interest in the condition.

Classification

Tympanosclerosis is classified into closed and open varieties, depending on the
integrity, or otherwise, of the tympanic membrane (Gibb, 1971).

Aetiology

It is widely accepted that tympanosclerosis represents the end product of past otitis
media in which an unusual healing response has occurred. Evidence of previous
inflammation is frequently obvious in the form of tympanic membrane perforation or
scarring. There is normally no active disease present although the diagnosis does not
necessarily preclude this. In most instances the initial infection appears to have taken
place many years previously and tympanosclerosis represents the ultimate scar of the
burnt-out disease process. The reason for the excessive collagen production is obscure:
the author considers that the original inflammatory episode may initiate the release of
a collagen stimulating factor but the reason why this should occur is unknown. There
appears to be no relationship between tympanosclerosis and other recognized
connective tissue disorders and although the histological appearances are similar to
those encountered in keloid there is no other obvious link with this condition. As far
as is known the predisposing inflammatory condition is not due to allergy or to any
specific virus or bacterium although the long time lag between the initial infection
and the final healed process makes this difficult to confirm.

Histopathology

Tympanosclerosis is of mesodermal origin and affects mainly connective soft tissues but changes may also occur in the underlying bone. The plaques are located either in the stratum fibrosum of the tympanic membrane or between the lining epithelium and periosteum elsewhere in the middle ear. On naked-eye examination the plaques appear as white patches in the tympanic membrane or as raised white masses in the tympanic cavity. It is possible under the operating microscope to recognize two distinct types of plaque—(1) a softer, creamy type with a rubbery or cartilaginous texture which on removal tends to peel off in onion layers; (2) a pure white, extremely hard, dense plaque, frequently firmly adherent to the surrounding bone, which may fracture when the plaque is removed.

On histological examination the tissue is seen to consist of masses of hyaline material almost totally devoid of cells and blood vessels, covered by an extremely thin, flattened epithelium. The hyaline substance is bi-refringent to polarized light and consists of masses of collagen fibres; the latter are mainly arranged in bundles exhibiting an irregular fibrillar appearance but in some areas the bundles are replaced by an amorphous hyaline mass. Deposition of calcium is common and areas of new bone may be distinguished: this occurs most frequently in the hard white type of plaque (*Figures 9.10* and *9.11*).

Ossicles adjacent to tympanosclerotic tissue, especially the incus, frequently appear 'moth-eaten', porous and demineralized when viewed under the operating microscope (*Figure 9.12*). Histological sections confirm the presence of bone absorption with replacement by tympanosclerotic tissue. Bone destruction is not uncommon and may result in ossicular discontinuity.

Harris (1961) believed that two types of tympanosclerosis could be distinguished histologically: (1) a non-invasive superficial form which he called sclerosing mucositis, in which the adjacent mucosa and periosteum remain intact; and (2) a deeper invasive type to which he gave the name osteoclastic mucoperiostitis in which there is invasion and destruction of the underlying bone. The present author, however, considers the existence of this invasive type to be extremely doubtful.

It is unlikely that the bone destruction observed in association with tympanosclerosis is due to the tympanosclerotic process itself: in all probability it relates to the primary inflammatory precursor which initiated the unusual healing response (House and Sheehy, 1960). It is possible however that the bony changes in the ossicles may in part be related to a reduction in blood supply caused by the possible strangling effect of the surrounding sheath of dense avascular tympanosclerotic tissue. The histological appearances suggest that, in general, tympanosclerosis is essentially an inactive process and does not invade adjacent structures.

On electron microscopic examination the most striking feature is a mass of collagen fibres with a periodicity of around 340 nm. The ultrastructural findings have been described in detail by Wong Chang (1969) who noted the following additional features:

(1) Marked proliferation of collagen fibres in the extracellular space, and electron-dense materials within or close to collagen bundles suggesting degeneration of collagen fibres with early calcium deposition.

(2) Degeneration of cytoplasm with fusion to the cell membrane to form an amorphous granular opaque mass.

(3) Electron-dense masses within the matrix of mitochondria of the fibrocyte-like cells, in the membrane-bound fragment, in the 'autophaged lysosomes' or in the collagen fibres indicating destruction of the fibrocyte-like cell.

(4) Shrinkage and increased density of nuclear chromatin.

The author has also noted the presence of mast cell granules and fat-like globules.

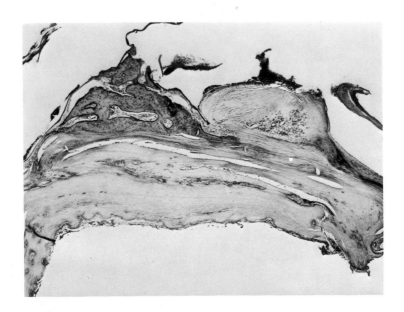

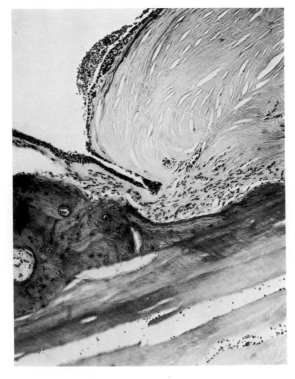

Figure 9.10 Photomicrograph of mucosa of middle ear showing marked thickening by a tympanosclerotic plaque. Note bone formation on the left and hyaline collagenous tissue to the right immediately beneath the epithelium. Deep to these areas there is a long narrow zone of calcified collagen. (By courtesy of Professor L. Michaels)

Figure 9.11 High power of *Figure 9.10*

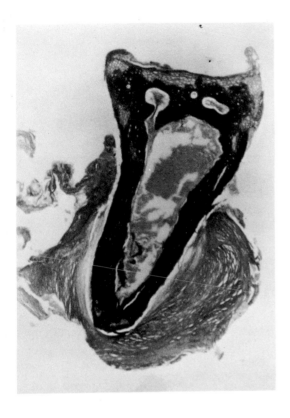

Figure 9.12 Low power section of tympanosclerosis surrounding an ossicle

Biochemical analysis of plaques

The molecular structure of tympanosclerotic deposits may be examined by the x-ray diffraction technique or by infrared spectroscopy. The latter method is particularly sensitive for detecting phosphate and oxalate compounds. The absorption spectrum of the tympanosclerotic material derived from plaques typically shows a broad absorption band centred at 1000 cm^{-1}, which is a region of phosphate compound absorption frequencies. The principal absorption bands indicating carbonate groups appear at approximately 1410 cm^{-1} and 1450 cm^{-1} while additional evidence of the presence of these groups may be visible at approximately 1520 cm^{-1} and 870 cm^{-1}. The presence of calcium can be confirmed by atomic absorption or scanning electron microscopy analysis.

The above findings indicate that the tympanosclerotic material exhibits all the characteristics of carbonate apatite (Gibb, 1976).

Pathogenesis

In an analysis of 138 cases of tympanosclerosis involving the tympanic membrane and/or the middle-ear cleft the author made the following observations—(1) there was invariably a history of past otitis media; (2) the ears were dry in a high percentage of patients (83 per cent); (3) the perforations were large in the vast majority of cases

(84 per cent); and (4) all the perforations were confined to the pars tensa (Gibb, 1976).

These features in general are atypical of the clinical findings encountered in chronic otitis media but are characteristic of the picture which might be expected after acute necrotizing otitis media which frequently used to occur in association with the acute infectious fevers of childhood. These observations suggest that the precursor of tympanosclerosis may be a severe acute otitis media of viral or bacterial origin rather than chronic middle-ear infection. It is important to realize that the association between tympanosclerosis and chronic ear disease is relatively uncommon and certainly less so than might be expected in a condition characterized by the presence of large perforations of the tympanic membrane in a high proportion of cases. The co-existence of tympanosclerosis and cholesteatoma in the author's experience is not common; indeed he agrees with Plester (1972) that the association of the two conditions is no more than accidental.

The author (Gibb, 1976) also studied and analysed the unusual and highly characteristic distribution of the plaques throughout the middle ear and mastoid (*see* Definition and Description) demonstrating that these occur (a) in the areas where the gland population is lowest (Sadé, 1966; Tos and Bak-Pedersen, 1974) and (b) in areas where cilia are scanty (Sadé, 1966). The gland population of the tympanic mucosa in tympanosclerosis was compared to that in chronic secretory otitis, adhesive otitis and granulating otitis by Tos and Bak-Pedersen (1974). These studies clearly demonstrated that there is considerably less mucosal secretory activity in tympanosclerosis than in the other conditions; not only was the mean gland density low but practically all the existing glands were devoid of secretory function.

From these findings it can be deduced that tympanosclerotic deposits tend to form mainly in narrow or cul-de-sac areas where inflammatory exudates are liable to be trapped during the course of infections: they also favour conditions and sites where glandular activity is virtually absent. The absence of effective ciliary function together with a reduction in glandular secretion doubtless compromises the elimination of the exudates from these narrow spaces so that they may become organized and possibly converted later into tympanosclerotic plaques. While this sequence of events could well be initiated by an episode of acute otitis media a similar situation might also arise in chronic secretory otitis media where the same difficulties would apply to the elimination of secretions of high viscosity with their inherent tendency to cling to the ossicles and especially around the crura of the stapes where tympanosclerotic deposits are most common. Indeed Sadé (1966) expressed this view when he stated 'viscous fluid in the attic and region of the stapes . . . would be evacuated with difficulty as these areas are usually very poor in cilia'. The theory that plaques arise from organization of exudates presupposes that mucosal destruction also occurs, which is less likely in glue ear than in acute necrotizing otitis media. On the other hand the characteristic lamellated structure of the plaques suggests repeated deposition of collagen over a long period which would fit in well with the concept of a chronic secretory condition with repeated minor episodes of acute infection causing mucosal damage and further exudation and collagen deposition.

In summary it appears probable that tympanosclerosis is a post-inflammatory condition of the middle ear arising from the organization of fibrinous exudates, and in general the evidence suggests that the precursor is a severe acute otitis rather than a chronic condition. It should be appreciated, however, that all degrees of tympanosclerosis are encountered ranging from a solitary insignificant plaque to massive and widespread deposits; and whereas the most severe cases may be precipitated by an acute necrotizing otitis media lesser degrees of tympanosclerosis may result from chronic disease (possibly with repeated acute episodes) so that a close relationship could well exist between the development of tympanosclerotic plaques and the organization of untreated effusions in chronic secretory otitis media.

Clinical picture

SYMPTOMS

The only symptom normally complained of is deafness although tinnitus may occasionally be present. There is generally a history of past otitis media. The condition is frequently bilateral.

EXAMINATION

Otoscopy

The diagnosis may be easy if the characteristic white chalk patches are present in the tympanic membrane or can be detected through a perforation, in open tympanosclerosis. Plaques in the tympanic membrane always occur in the pars tensa, varying in size from insignificant deposits of no clinical importance to very large plaques covering extensive areas of the tympanic membrane. In the latter instance mobility of the membrane may be reduced or may even disappear completely if the plaque is adherent to the bony annulus or the handle of the malleus, or makes contact with the promontory. A typical large plaque often involves the whole anterior half of the tympanic membrane and is fixed to the bony annulus in front and the handle of the malleus behind: such a plaque not only affects the mobility of the tympanic membrane but causes fixation of the ossicular chain at the same time.

Perforations of the tympanic membrane are present in roughly two-thirds of tympanosclerotic cases (Gibb, 1976): they are invariably confined to the pars tensa, are generally large and non-infected and are seldom associated with chronic suppuration or cholesteatoma. In some cases plaques on the promontory or around the stapes area may be visible through a perforation (*Figure 9.13*). Although plaques usually have a fairly typical appearance on naked eye examination, magnification with the microscope is generally desirable to avoid errors in diagnosis.

Hearing assessment

Tuning-fork tests, full audiometric investigations and tympanometry are important aids in arriving at the correct diagnosis. The deafness is normally conductive in type with a typical air–bone gap. Tympanometry is only of value if the tympanic membrane is uninvolved: the usual findings are a normal middle-ear pressure and a tympanogram showing flattening of the normal peak due to the presence of a stiffness factor.

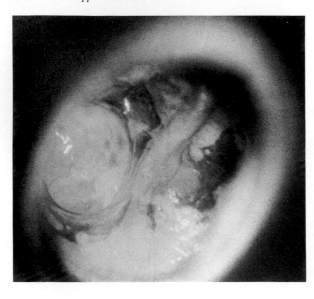

Figure 9.13 Tympanosclerosis of the tympanic membrane showing additional plaques on the promontory, visible through a perforation

Radiographic examination
In cases of tympanosclerosis the mastoid process generally shows poor cell development and bone sclerosis.

Differential diagnosis

Accurate diagnosis is extremely important. Tympanosclerosis is more difficult to treat than most other middle-ear conditions. If misdiagnosis occurs an inexperienced otologist may find difficulty in coping with the complicated surgical problem which confronts him. Failure to diagnose tympanosclerosis is possible in the following types of situation:

(1) in closed tympanosclerosis where the tympanic membrane is normal;
(2) in instances where plaques are mistaken for some other abnormality;
(3) in cases of other middle-ear pathology where the co-existence of tympanosclerosis is not recognized.

OTOSCLEROSIS (and other types of conductive deafness)
Tympanosclerosis of the closed variety may easily be confused with otosclerosis or conductive deafness due to other causes but should always be suspected if (a) there is no family history of deafness, (b) the conductive deafness is non-progressive, (c) there is a history of previous otitis media, (d) chalk patches are visible in either ear, (e) the tympanic membrane shows evidence of scarring, or (f) the mastoid is radiologically acellular.

CHOLESTEATOMA
Intratympanic plaques, by virtue of their whitish colour may be mistaken for a localized mass of cholesteatoma. The latter, however lacks the glistening appearance

of a tympanosclerotic plaque and is softer to the touch. Magnification using the microscope will generally solve the problem. The otologist should keep in mind that both conditions may co-exist even although this is a relatively infrequent occurrence. Radiological examination may be helpful and is essential in cases of doubt.

Treatment

The primary objective of treatment is the relief of deafness. Surgical treatment in tympanosclerosis may be difficult and complicated and should only be undertaken by a highly experienced and competent aural micro-surgeon. Since it is seldom possible to assess the exact extent and severity of the disease process pre-operatively the otologist must have the skill and the necessary equipment to cope with any situation which may arise at operation. Virtually every recognized technique employed in the surgery of the middle ear may be required. Treatment is based on the premise that tympanosclerosis is essentially a non-active, non-invasive condition with little or no tendency towards recurrence after removal. The surgical methods employed aim at the restoration of normal mobility to affected structures, the repair of defects of the tympanic membrane and ossicular chain and in cases where these methods are unsuitable or inappropriate a bypass may be created to circumvent the affected area.

The author normally adopts the following procedure. The initial operation (which

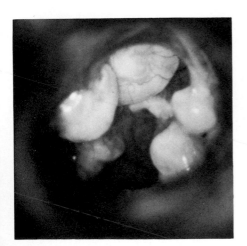 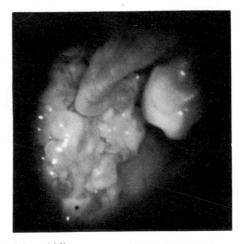

Figure 9.14 Two examples of tympanosclerosis of the middle ear as seen at tympanotomy

may be the only one), is primarily concerned with problems relating to the tympanic membrane such as plaque removal or perforation repair. In addition, however, the operation provides the opportunity to assess the extent and severity of any intratympanic tympanosclerosis (*see Figure 9.14 a, b*). If this is absent or can be treated forthwith a second operation becomes unnecessary but in many instances a two-stage procedure is required. In the latter event the second stage should be planned as far as possible at the time of the initial tympanotomy, the surgeon deciding on the most appropriate approach to the middle ear and method of repair to be adopted.

Myringoplasty and stapedectomy should not be performed at the same operation because of the risk of labyrinthitis. If, at the first operation, removal of plaques results in a considerable loss of epithelium it may be advisable to insert silastic sheeting to prevent adhesions and promote mucosal regeneration: the silastic implant is removed at the subsequent operation.

APPROACH TO THE MIDDLE EAR

The author normally uses a permeatal approach and raises a tympanomeatal flap as in stapedectomy. If wider access is desired an endaural or post-auricular incision may be utilized and the mastoid opened as required. In this event a closed type of mastoid operation is advised, there being no necessity to create an open mastoid cavity. A combined approach technique with posterior tympanotomy gives excellent access to the plaque-bearing areas and has much to commend it in epitympanic tympanosclerosis. The exploration of the mastoid and attic may sometimes prove advantageous in that unsuspected cholesteatoma may be discovered. The author has also occasionally employed atticotomy and attic inspection window techniques in selected cases of epitympanic tympanosclerosis. Retraction pockets seldom develop after tympanosclerosis surgery.

The general principles of treatment employed in tympanosclerosis will now be outlined but the technical details of many of the procedures are more fully described elsewhere. Special consideration, however, will be given to techniques which relate specifically to tympanosclerosis.

SURGERY OF THE TYMPANIC MEMBRANE

Plaque removal
Plaque removal should be undertaken if sound transmission is impaired. Small plaques not interfering with the mobility of the tympanic membrane are normally left alone. If removal is carried out preservation of the epithelium overlying the plaque is frequently possible if scrupulous care is exercised and high magnification ($\times$ 16) is employed.

Technique (Figure 9.15)
The plaque is approached from the medial aspect of the tympanic membrane either through an existing perforation or failing this by elevating a tympanomeatal flap. A fine angled elevator of Marquet type or a Hough 'whirlybird' is inserted between the plaque and the outer epithelial layer of the tympanic membrane and the former is dissected free as far as possible, taking care at the same time to avoid creating a perforation. The plaque is then displaced medially using the flat surface of the elevator until it is completely freed from all its attachments and it is then extracted from the middle ear.

Myringoplasty
The success rate from myringoplasty in cases where plaques involve the drum remnant is roughly the same as that achieved in tympanic membrane repair where no evidence of tympanosclerosis exists (Gibb, 1976). The removal of plaques prior to grafting is not always advisable. Plaques contiguous with a perforation and not interfering with drum mobility may be retained, since grafts applied over these survive in surprising

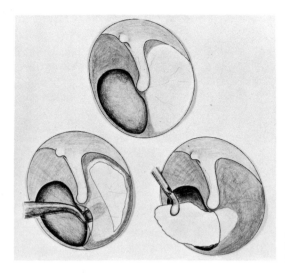

Figure 9.15   Technique of removal of a tympanosclerotic plaque from the tympanic membrane

fashion: furthermore, plaque removal in this situation carries a risk of enlarging the perforation either as a result of epithelial reaction or occasionally from tearing of the tympanic remnant if it is very attenuated. If plaques are removed by the technique already described the medial surface of the tympanic membrane is automatically de-epithelialized thus creating an ideal bed for a graft. For this reason the author regards the underlay grafting technique particularly suitable in tympanosclerosis.

SURGERY OF THE OSSICULAR CHAIN

Plaque removal

In mild or moderately severe cases of tympanosclerosis removal of plaques around the ossicles to restore full mobility may be worthwhile in selected cases. Great care must always be exercised during this procedure especially in removing plaques adherent to the stapes. The possibility of causing severe commotion of the labyrinthine fluids from transmitted vibrations with resultant sensorineural hearing loss must be constantly kept in mind. In other cases an initial hearing improvement after plaque removal may be short lived as fibrous scarring at the operation site can lead to hearing regression of conductive type. For this reason the role of plaque removal as a means of restoring mobility to the ossicular chain is somewhat limited and in severe cases of tympanosclerosis more radical techniques such as stapedectomy or ossiculoplasty are more likely to produce lasting hearing improvement.

Stapedectomy

The operation differs from that carried out for otosclerosis in the following respects. (1) Although tympanosclerosis may invade the annular ligament and thereby cause true footplate fixation (Habermann, 1892), stapes immobility in this condition is more often due to the splinting effect of a surface layer of collagen of variable thickness spread over the footplate and surrounding bone. In the latter event removal of the collagenous tissue usually restores footplate mobility and if the stapes superstructure has already been removed there is an ever present risk of creating a floating footplate with all its concomitant risks and sequelae. Great care must therefore be taken to avoid such an occurrence. (2) The long process of the incus is frequently devitalized in tympanosclerosis and is thus unsuitable for the attachment of a prosthesis because of the increased liability to incus necrosis: alternative techniques such as attaching the prosthesis to the handle of the malleus may have to be employed. (3) The existence of increased cochlear fragility has been suspected in tympanosclerosis because of a higher incidence of post-stapedectomy 'dead ears' than in otosclerosis. However, there is as yet no definite proof that the cochlea is unduly sensitive in this condition. The author believes that the increased post-operative failure rate may be related to the high incidence of multiple operations in the treatment of tympanosclerosis, stapedectomy often being carried out as the final surgical procedure in an ear already 'sensitized' by previous operation(s).

Ossiculoplasty

This procedure is employed either in epitympanic fixation of the ossicular chain or for the repair of ossicular discontinuity. Tympanosclerosis affecting the attic frequently causes severe fixation of both the malleus and the incus especially if the deposits become calcified or ossified. Indeed in any case of 'fixed malleus syndrome' tympanosclerosis should be suspected as the possible cause. The problem can be managed by two different methods, either by fully exposing the epitympanum and removing the obstructing plaques to restore mobility or by carrying out an ossiculoplasty to bypass the attic. If the former technique is employed plaques or new bone are removed until the ossicular chain becomes fully mobile: Silastic sheeting or a similar material is then inserted to prevent the redevelopment of adhesions with ossicular refixation. The author prefers the latter alternative as being the more likely to result in lasting hearing improvement. The ossiculoplasty can readily be carried out by a stapedectomy approach. The incus and the head of the malleus are removed and either of these bones, according to preference, is re-positioned between the handle of the malleus or the adjacent tympanic membrane and the capitulum of the stapes. If the stapes superstructure has been destroyed the remains of the removed incus or, failing this a homograft malleus, can be carefully placed between the handle of the malleus and the stapes footplate.

Additional techniques

In more complicated and extensive cases of tympanosclerosis a combination of the foregoing methods may be employed but in some circumstances additional techniques are required. If, for example, all three ossicles are firmly fixed a standard stapedectomy would be ineffective because of the immobility of the malleus–incus complex. In such cases a malleus–oval window bypass is carried out using the following method. A subperiosteal pocket is created in the soft tissues just below the short process of the malleus to permit the fitting of a prosthesis around the malleus handle. The head of the malleus is then amputated and the incus and head of malleus are removed. The stapes is then extracted and a wire or piston prosthesis of appropriate length is fitted between the handle of the malleus and the oval window.

A possible alternative is fenestration of the horizontal semicircular canal, a technique which is now seldom used since the advent of the stapedectomy operation in the surgery of otosclerosis. This procedure provides a satisfactory bypass of the diseased area but has two main disadvantages, namely that an open mastoid cavity is created and closure of the air–bone gap cannot be achieved. The author therefore tends to reserve this technique for cases of extensive tympanosclerosis where gross plaque formation affects the tympanic membrane in addition to the ossicular chain, in which the operation probably provides the best chance of achieving socially adequate hearing in adverse circumstances (Gibb, 1976). Monoblock transplants of tympanic membrane and ossicles may also be utilized in severe tympanosclerosis but the value of this technique in relation to long-term hearing improvement has yet to be established.

Finally it must be emphasized that the results of multiple surgical procedures in severely damaged middle ears are seldom comparable to those achieved in lesser forms of disease. Extensive or repeated operations are liable to cause cochlear damage with consequent sensorineural hearing loss. For these reasons the otologist should weigh up the patient's chances very carefully before deciding to operate. If the prospects of a successful surgical result are considered doubtful it is generally preferable to fit a hearing aid.

References

Abadir, W. F. and Pease, W. S. (1978). 'Salivary gland choristoma of the middle ear', *Journal of Laryngology*, **92**, 247

Ahren, C. and Thulin, C. A. (1965). 'Lethal intracranial complication following inflation in the external auditory canal in treatment of serous otitis media and due to defects in the petrous bone', *Acta Otolaryngologica Stockholm*, **60**, 407

Alberti, P. W. R. M. (1964). 'Epithelial Migration on the Tympanic Membrane', *Journal of Laryngology*, **78**, 808

Armstrong, B. W. (1954). 'A new treatment for chronic secretory otitis media', *Archives of Otolaryngology*, **59**, 653

Ballantyne, J. C. (1977). Personal communication

Bauer, F. (1975). 'Tubal function in the glue ear. Urea for glue ears', *Journal of Laryngology*, **89**, 63

Bernstein, J. M. (1976). 'Biological Mediators of Inflammation in middle ear effusions', *Annals of Otology*, **85**, Suppl. 25, 90

Bernstein, J. M. and Hayes, E. R. (1971). 'Middle ear mucosa in health and disease', *Archives of Otolaryngology*, **94**, 30

Blake, C. J. (1882). 'The progressive growth of the dermoid coat of the membrana tympani', *American Journal of Otology*, **4**, 266

Brieger, O. (1914). Cited by Hussl. B. (1973b). 'Der chronische sekretorische Mittelohrkatarrh im Kindesalter', *Monatsschrift fur Ohrenheilkunde u. Laryngo-Rhinologie*, **107**, 141

Brooks, D. N. (1973). 'Hearing screening—a comparative study of an impedance method and pure tone screening', *Scandinavian Audiology*, **2**, 67

Buckingham, R. A. (1969). In Round Table on 'Management of Atelectatic Middle Ear', *Archives of Otolaryngology*, **89**, 199

Cassebohm, I. F. (1734). *Tractatus quatuor anatomici de aure humana*. Halae Magdeburgicae

Cawthorne, T. (1956). 'Chronic Adhesive Otitis', *Journal of Laryngology*, **70**, 559

Comeau, M., Brummett, R. and Vernon, J. (1973). 'Local Anaesthesia of the Ear by Iontophoresis', *Archives of Otolaryngology*, **98**, 114

Cooper, A. (1801). 'Further observations on the effects which take place from the destruction of the membrana tympani of the ear with an account of an operation for the removal of particular species of deafness', *Philosophical Transactions*, **91**, 435

Dawes, J. D. K. (1970). 'The aetiology and sequelae of exudative otitis media', *Journal of Laryngology*, **84**, 583

Dias, A. (1966). 'Effects on the hearing of patients treated by irradiation in the head and neck area', *Journal of Laryngology*, **80**, 276

Dishoeck, H. A. E. Van (1948). 'Hydrotympanum in the different clinical aspects of tubotympanical catarrh', *Acta Otolaryngologica Stockholm*, **36**, 429

Dohlman, G. (1943). 'Allergiska processer i mellanorat', *Nordisk medicin*, **17**, 224

Draper, L. W. (1967). 'Secretory otitis media in children. A study of 540 children', *Laryngoscope*, **77**, 636

Elner, A. (1976). 'Normal Gas Exchange in the Human Middle Ear', *Annals of Otology*, **85**, Suppl. 25, 161

Friedmann, I. (1963). 'The Pathology of Secretory Otitis Media', *Proceedings of the Royal Society of Medicine*, **56**, 695

Friedmann, I. (1974). In *Pathology of the Ear*, p. 82. Oxford; Blackwell

Friedmann, I. (1974). In *Pathology of the Ear*, p. 103. Oxford; Blackwell

Gibb, A. G. (1971). 'Tympanosclerosis', *Acta Oto-rhino-laryngologica belgica*, **25**, 956

Gibb, A. G. (1976). 'Tympanosclerosis', *Proceedings of the Royal Society of Medicine*, **69**, 3, 155

Goode, R. L. (1973). 'T-Tube for Middle Ear Ventilation', *Archives of Otolaryngology*, **97**, 402

Habermann, J. (1892). In *Schwartzes Handbuch der Ohrenheilkunde. Leipzig* **1**, 243

Harris, I. (1961). 'Tympanosclerosis: A revived clinicopathologic entity', *Laryngoscope*, **71**, 1488

Harvey, R. M. (1975). 'Environmental factors in glue ear', *Journal of Laryngology*, **89**, 73

Hentzer, E. (1976). 'Ultrastructure of the middle ear mucosa', *Annals of Otology*, **85**, Suppl. 25, 30

Hinton, J. (1869). *Guy's Hospital Report*, **29**, 149

Hinton, J. (1874). 'On the diagnosis of diseases of the ear', *Guy's Hospital Report*, 3rd series, **19**, 267

Holborow, C. A. (1962). 'Deafness associated with cleft palate', *Journal of Laryngology*, **76**, 762

Holm, V. A. and Kunze, L. H. (1969). 'Effect of chronic otitis media on language and speech development', *Pediatrics*, **43**, 833

House, W. F. and Sheehy, J. L. (1960). 'Tympanosclerosis', *Archives of Otolaryngology*, **72**, 308

House, W. F., Glasscock, M. E. and Miles, J. (1969). 'Eustachian Tuboplasty', *Laryngoscope*, **79**, 1765

Howie, V. M. (1975). 'Natural history of otitis media', *Annals of Otology*, **84**, Suppl. 19, 67

Hunt-Williams, R. (1968). 'A Method for Maintaining Middle-Ear Ventilation in Children', *Journal of Laryngology*, **82**, 921

Hutchison, C. A. (1955). 'Radiography as an aid to differential diagnosis between otosclerosis and chronic adhesive process', *Journal of Laryngology*, **69**, 617

Jordan, R. (1949). 'Chronic secretory otitis media', *Laryngoscope*, **59**, 1002

Jordan, R. (1952). 'Role of allergy in otology', *Archives of Otolaryngology*, **55**, 363

Kaplan, G. J., Fleshman, J. K., Bender, D. R., Baum, C. and Clark, P. S. (1973). 'Long-term effects of otitis media', *Pediatrics*, **52**, 577

Kersley, J. A. and Wickham, H. (1966). 'Exudative Otitis Media in Children', *Journal of Laryngology*, **80**, 26

Kilby, D., Richards, S. H. and Hart, G. (1972). 'Grommets and glue ears: two year results', *Journal of Laryngology*, **86**, 881

Klein, J. O. and Teele, D. W. (1976). 'Isolation of viruses and mycoplasmas from middle-ear effusions. A review', *Annals of Otology*, **85**, Suppl. 25, 140

Koch, H. (1947). 'Allergical Investigations of Chronic Otitis' (Thesis) University of Lund, *Acta Otolaryngologica Stockholm*, Suppl. 62

Laff, H. I. (1962). 'What can be done for conductive hearing losses in children', *Clinic Pediatrica*, **1**, 11

Lecks, H. I. (1961). 'Allergic aspects in serous otitis media in childhood', *NY State Journal of Medicine*, **61**, ii, 2737

Lim, D. J., Shimada, T. and Yoder, M. (1973). 'Distribution of Mucus-Secreting Cells in Normal Middle Ear Mucosa', *Archives of Otolaryngology*, **98**, 2

Lim, D. J., Liu, Y. S., Schram, J. and Birch, H. G. (1976). 'Immunoglobulin E in Chronic Middle Ear Effusions', *Annals of Otology*, **85**, Suppl. 25, 117

Litton, W. B. (1963). 'Epithelial Migration over Tympanic Membrane and External Canal', *Acta Otolaryngologica, Stockholm*, Suppl. 240

Litton, W. B. and McCabe, B. F. (1962). 'Chymotrypsin—A useful adjunct to the management of "glue ear"', *Laryngoscope*, **72**, 182

Liu, Y. S., Lim, D. J., Lang, R. W. and Birch, W. L. (1975). 'Chronic Middle Ear Effusions', *Archives of Otolaryngology*, **101**, 278

Lumio, J. S. (1951). 'Contribution to the knowledge of chronic adhesive otitis: the diagnosis', *Acta Otolaryngologica, Stockholm*, **39**, 196

MacNaughtan, I. P. J. (1956). 'Chronic Adhesive Otitis Media', *Journal of Laryngology*, **70**, 549

Malcomson, K. G. (1963). In 'Symposium "Secretory Otitis Media"', *Proceedings of the Royal Society of Medicine*, **56**, 701

Mawson, S. R. (1964). 'Tympanotomy for "Glue" Ears', *Journal of Laryngology*, **78**, 853

Mawson, S. R. and Fagan, P. (1972). 'Tympanic effusions in children', *Journal of Laryngology*, **86**, 105

Mogi, G., Honjo, S., Maeda, S., Yoshida, T. and Watanabe, N. (1974). 'Immunoglobulin E (IgE) in middle ear effusions', *Annals of Otology*, **83**, 393

O'Donnell, J. H. (1941). '"Blue Drum" or Idiopathic Hemotympanum in children', *British Medical Journal*, **2**, 86

Ojala, L. (1953). 'Pathogenesis and Histopathology of Chronic Adhesive Otitis', *Archives of Otolaryngology*, **57**, 378

Palva, T., Raunio, V. and Nousiainen, R. (1974). 'Secretory otitis media, protein and enzyme analyses', *Annals of Otology*, **83**, Suppl. 11, 35

Palva, T. (1977). Personal communication

Paradise, J. L., Bluestone, C. D. and Felder, H. (1969). 'The Universality of otitis media in 50 infants with cleft palate', *Pediatrics*, **44**, 35

Per-Lee, J. (1969). 'Experience with a "permanent" wide flange middle ear ventilation tube', *Laryngoscope*, **79**, 581

Plester, D. (1972). 'European Trends in Tympanoplasty', *Journal of the Oto-laryngological Society of Australia*, **3**, 320

Politzer, A. (1867). *Wiener medizinische Wochenschrift*, **17**, 244

Politzer, A. (1883). In *Textbook of Diseases of the Ear and Adjacent Organs*. Translat. and ed. by J. P. Cassells, London; Bailliere, Tindal & Cox

Politzer, A. (1926). In *Diseases of the Ear*. London; Bailliere, Tindal & Cox

Proetz, A. W. (1931). 'Allergy in the middle and internal ear', *Annals of Otology*, **40**, 67

Ramsden, R. T., Gibson, W. P. R. and Moffat, D. A. (1977). 'Anaesthesia of the tympanic membrane using iontophoresis', *Journal of Laryngology*, **91**, 779

Ranger, D. (1949). 'Idiopathic Hemotympanum', *Journal of Laryngology*, **63**, 672

Robinson, G. C., Anderson, D. O., Moghadam, H. K., Cambon, K. G. and Murray, A. B. (1967). 'A survey of hearing loss in Vancouver school children. I. Methodology and prevalence', *Canadian Medical Association Journal*, **97**, ii, 1199

Sadé, J. (1966). 'Middle ear mucosa', *Archives of Otolaryngology*, **84**, 137

Sadé, J. and Berco, E. (1976). 'Atelectasis and Secretory Otitis Media,' *Annals of Otology*, **85**, Suppl. 25, 66

Senturia, B. H. (1970). 'Classification of middle ear effusions', *Annals of Otology*, **79**, 358

Senturia, B. H., Gessert, C. F. and Baumann, E. S. (1958). 'Studies concerned with Tubotympanitis', *Annals of Otology*, **67**, 440

Shah, N. (1975). 'Glue ear: Diagnosis and management', *Proceeding of The Royal Society of Medicine*, **68**, (1), 37

Shambaugh, G. E. (1929). 'The Blue Drum Membrane', *Archives of Otolaryngology*, **10**, 238

Siirala, U. (1960). 'Adhesive Otitis', *Acta Otolaryngologica*, **158**, 301

Siirala, U. and Lahikainen, E. A. (1952). 'Some observations on the bacteriostatic effect of the exudate on otitis media', *Acta Otolaryngologica, Stockholm*, Suppl. **100**, 20

Silverstein, H. (1966). '"Malleus Clip" Tube for long-term equalisation of middle ear pressure', *Trans-American Academy of Ophthalmology and Otolaryngology*, **70**, 640

Silverstein, H. (1970), 'Permanent Middle Ear Aeration', *Archives of Otolaryngology*, **91**, 313

Silverstein, H., Miller, G. F. and Lindeman, R. C. (1966). 'Eustachian tube dysfunction as a cause for chronic secretory otitis in children', *Laryngoscope*, **76**, 259

Stevens, D. (1958). 'Serous Otitis as a cause of catarrhal deafness in childhood', *Lancet*, **2**, 22

Stinson, W. D. (1936). 'Reparative processes in the Membrana Tympani', *Archives of Otolaryngology*, **24**, 600

Tönder, O. and Gundersen, T. (1971). 'Nature of the fluid in serous otitis media', *Archives of Otolaryngology*, **93**, 473

Tos, M. and Bak-Pedersen, K. (1974). 'Middle-ear mucosa in tympanosclerosis', *Journal of Laryngology*, **88**, 119

Tröltsch, A. Von (1869). In *Lehrbuch der Ohrenheilkunde*. Leipzig

Tumarkin, A. (1961). 'Pre-epidermosis', *Journal of Laryngology*, **75**, 487

Veltri, R. W. and Sprinkle, P. M. (1973). 'Serous otitis media—immunoglobulin and lysozyme levels in middle ear fluids and serum', *Annals of Otology*, **82**, 297

Veltri, R. W. and Sprinkle, P. M. (1976). 'Secretory Otitis Media', *Annals of Otology*, **85**, Suppl. 25, 135

Walb, H. (1893). In *Schwartzes Handbuch der Ohrenheilkunde*. **2**, 195. Leipzig

Walsh, T. (1963). In 'Symposium "Deafness in Children"', *Journal of Laryngology*, **77**, 858

Watson, T. J. (1969). 'Long-term follow-up of chronic exudative otitis media', *Proceedings of the Royal Society of Medicine*, **62**, 455

Wathen, J. (1756). 'A method proposed to restore the hearing when injured from an obstruction of the tuba Eustachian', *Philosophical Transactions of the Royal Society of London*, **49**, 213

Won Chang, I. (1969). 'Tympanosclerosis', *Acta Otolaryngologica, Stockholm*, **68**, 62

Wright, W. K. (1969). 'Round Table on "Management of Atelectatic Middle Ear"', *Archives of Otolaryngology*, **89**, 199

Wright, I. and Kapadia, R. (1969). 'The cytology of "glue ear"', *Journal of Laryngology*, **83**, 367

Yoshie, C. (1955). 'On the isolation of influenza virus from mid-ear discharge of influenza otitis media', *Japanese Journal of Medicine, Science and Biology*, **8**, 373

Zöllner, F. (1942). *Anatomie, Physiologie und Klinik der Ohrtrompete*. Berlin; Springer-Verlag

Zöllner, F. (1963). 'Therapy of the eustachian Tube', *Archives of Otolaryngology*, **78**, 394

Zöllner, F. and Beck, C. (1955). 'Die Paukensklerose', *Zeitschrift für Laryngologie, Rhinologie, Otologie und ihre Grenzgebiete*, **34**, 137

10 Chronic suppurative otitis media— assessment

Philip H Beales

Introduction

The assessment and management of chronic suppurative otitis media presents many challenging and fascinating problems. The state of an individual ear involved in chronic disease represents the balance established at a particular time between the progression of the disease process on the one hand and the healing response within the middle-ear cleft on the other. Accordingly the manifestations of chronic suppurative otitis media are extremely variable and there may be any lesion from a small healed deformity of the tympanic membrane, to a cholesteatoma infiltrating widely throughout the temporal bone.

The pathological changes associated with acute and chronic otitis media are essentially different. In acute otitis media, with appropriate treatment, a return to normality is usually to be expected. It is true that in the pre-antibiotic era chronic disease which followed an acute necrotizing otitis media was a common sequel to the exanthemata in childhood; fortunately this acute–chronic sequence is now relatively uncommon. A few acute infections leave disabilities or deformities which may affect the course or development of a subsequent chronic lesion. For example in recent years a high incidence of exudative otitis media has been observed in children of early school age. Many of these cases resolve but some may leave a legacy of mucosal disease, intratympanic negative pressure and deformities of the tympanic membrane which may influence the development or course of a subsequent chronic suppurative otitis media (Thomas, 1967).

Any or all of the following physiopathological features may have a direct or indirect influence upon the development and behaviour of chronic disease of the middle-ear cleft:

(1) Disorder of ventilation.
(2) Reactions of the mucoperiosteal lining (mucosal factor).
(3) Infiltration by keratinizing stratified squamous epithelium (keratinizing factor or cholesteatoma).
(4) Secondary infection by saphrophytic or pyogenic organisms.
(5) Bone reactions—erosion, necrosis or sclerosis.

The clinical study of cholesteatoma indicates that this type of disease usually has an insidious onset and tends to be well established before the patient presents with symptoms. In this disease spontaneous healing may occur and it is not uncommon to find evidence of healed chronic disease of which the patient is genuinely unaware.

The classic symptoms of uncomplicated chronic suppurative otitis media are quite simply, otorrhoea and deafness. The close relationship of the middle-ear cleft to the facial nerve, the auditory labyrinth, the lateral sinus and the middle and posterior cranial fossae, make it all too easy for complications to develop. A patient may often disregard his initial deafness and slight otorrhoea and first seek advice because of pain, facial paralysis, vertigo or headache. It is important to realize that these are not symptoms of the chronic ear disease but of an impending or developed complication of that disease.

Classification

It is usual to divide chronic otitis media into two varieties, 'tubotympanic' and 'attico–antral' disease.

In tubotympanic disease the mucosal factor is the important feature and in attico–antral disease the long-standing erosion of bone by cholesteatoma is the significant factor. Serious complications may result from attico–antral disease whilst tubotympanic varieties are seldom dangerous to life.

Tubotympanic disease

Two main clinical varieties of tubotympanic disease will be described:

(1) The permanent perforation syndrome.
(2) Persistent mucosal disease.

Pathogenesis of tubotympanic disease – the mucosal factor

Two types of mucous membrane are found in the tympanic cavity, attic and mastoid.

The eustachian tube, hypotympanum and anterior mesotympanum are lined by a ciliated columnar epithelium with mucus-secreting cells. In the posterior tympanum, attic and mastoid, the lining is a cuboidal epithelium (Sadé, 1966). During the embryological development of the middle-ear cleft, the mucous membrane encloses all the elements—ossicles, nerves and ligaments and thus many folds and potential or actual pockets remain and these are subject to considerable variations (Proctor, 1964; Sammut, 1968). The surface epithelium is bound to the underlying areolar submucous tissues by oxytalin fibres which form the basement membrane and within this submucous layer are capillaries, blood vessels and glands. The deepest layer in contact with bone is the periosteum (Dawes, 1970).

Infection reaches the middle ear by travelling to it from the nasopharynx along the eustachian tube or directly from the external meatus through a perforation of the tympanic membrane. An inflammatory reaction occurs and if a purulent exudate forms, it may become trapped in a mucosal pocket. Prompt and adequate treatment with restoration of normal ventilation of the middle ear will usually lead to complete resolution with return to a normal mucous membrane. The mucous membrane can be seriously damaged by repeated infections or uncontrolled infections by organisms resistant to antibiotics. The terms 'reversible' and 'irreversible' change have been used to describe middle-ear mucous membrane affected by chronic infection. Although localized areas may show the presence of granulation tissue or polypi that require to be removed before resolution occurs and although pockets of infection may become walled off in a developmental fold or a mucosal pocket, a chronic irreversible change in the mucous membrane of the middle ear is uncommon and it has a remarkable power of recovery. Hyaline degeneration is seen in the submucous layer, particularly in long-standing chronic ear disease with large perforations of the tympanic membrane. The exposure of the mucous membrane to the drying effects of air is thought to be a factor in the production of this condition which is known as tympanosclerosis, and it will cause deafness if the deposits encroach on the oval or round window areas.

CHOLESTEROL GRANULOMA

If there is obstruction to ventilation of the middle-ear cleft from an inadequately functioning eustachian tube, a mucoid exudate may form (exudative, serous otitis media or 'glue ear') and with an inflammatory reaction, capillary haemorrhage occurs and cholesterol crystals are deposited and blood pigments set free. The tympanic membrane may appear to be 'blue' in colour and the mastoid air-cells may contain swollen mucous membrane showing the typical microscopic appearance of cholesterol granuloma (*Figure 10.1*). The essential histopathological features of cholesterol granuloma are as follows: the presence of cholesterol crystals, surrounded

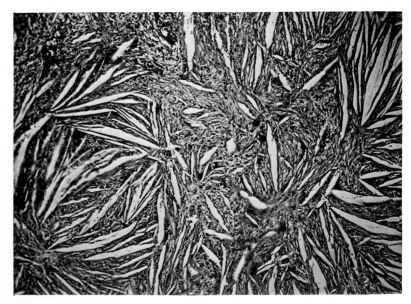

Figure 10.1 Cholesterol granuloma. Note the presence of cholesterol crystals and foreign body giant cells embedded in fibrous granulation tissue. (Reproduced by courtesy of Professor I. Friedmann)

by foreign-body giant cells, embedded in fibrous granulation tissue. Blood pigment (haemosiderin) is usually present and in the surface epithelium, mucin granules may be visible. Cholesterol granuloma occurs where there is stasis and haemorrhage and there is no evidence that it is a precursor of cholesteatoma.

The permanent perforation

In this condition there is a defect of the pars tensa of the tympanic membrane, exposing the mucous membrane of the tympanic cavity to the possibility of repeated recurrent infections. The infection may spread to the middle ear from the nasopharynx along the eustachian tube as a result of respiratory tract infections or it reaches the middle ear by travelling along the external auditory canal, usually carried by water, often from swimming pools. If no infection is present, the mucous membrane of the medial tympanic wall is thin, pale pink or grey. There are no foci of granulations or keratinization and the membrane is barely moist. Areas of hyaline degeneration in the submucous layer—tympanosclerosis—may be visible without infection and the drying effect of the air may be a factor in the production of this condition.

Infection can occur at any time, although some patients rarely develop it and are unaware that they have a defect in the tympanic membrane. Swimming in contaminated pools, syringing, unclean habits, poking pieces of wool in the ear and upper respiratory tract infections may give rise to infection characterized by a swollen mucous membrane, a mucoid or mucopurulent discharge and pulsation close to the eustachian tube. Pain is seldom a feature but there may be a diminution of hearing or even improved hearing. In neglected cases, a secondary otitis externa develops, making the diagnosis more difficult. Treatment by aural toilet and appropriate local

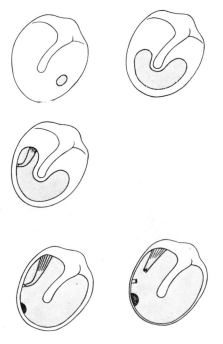

Figure 10.2 Different types of perforation of the tympanic membrane associated with tubo-tympanic disease. Usually the hearing loss increases in proportion to the posterior extent of the perforation

antibiotics leads to a rapid resolution of the infection but long-standing perforations seldom heal as there is a fibrous ring at the junction of the mucous membrane and outer layer of the tympanic membrane. Repeated infections lead to slowly progressive cochlear degeneration over the years and these changes are irreversible.

This type of perforation is confined to the pars tensa of the tympanic membrane and does not involve the fibrous annulus. The healed edge is clearly defined as it is fibrous tissue. They vary in size from pinhead perforations to large kidney-shaped defects. The long process of the incus is often damaged and occasionally the handle of the malleus is destroyed (*Figure 10.2*).

The loss of hearing is variable and may be small with an anterior perforation but greater with a posterior one, due to the loss of protection of the round window. There is characteristically a conductive deafness, but in addition there may be a sensorineural hearing loss if there have been repeated attacks of infection. If the ossicular chain is intact, the degree of hearing loss varies between 25 and 40 dB for the speech frequencies. The patient may state that when the ear is discharging the hearing improves and this is due to a closure of the defect by a film of mucus or a loading of the round window. If there is a hearing loss of over 45 dB, it indicates that there may be additional lesions present such as tympanosclerosis causing ossicular fixation or ankylosis of the malleo–incudial joint. A complete interruption of the chain from destruction of part of the long process of the incus may produce a 60-dB hearing loss. Fixation of the stapes footplate by otosclerotic or tympanosclerotic deposits may be present and should be considered when there is a severe hearing loss and the ossicular chain appears normal.

A useful clinical test that can be carried out in the clinic or consulting room is to close the defect temporarily with a patch and to observe if there is any hearing improvement. A small piece of Silastic film is applied to cover the defect after a drop of liquid paraffin has been placed on it. This is easily carried out under microscopic control and will give some indication of the pathology and the anticipated result of a simple myringoplasty operation.

IMMEDIATE MANAGEMENT

It is essential to see the perforation clearly and wax and debris must be removed with forceps, probe or suction tip. An operating microscope makes this procedure easier and allows the surgeon to examine the mucous membrane more accurately and such an instrument must be regarded as essential in all otological clinics today.

The patient with a dry ear must be instructed to keep it dry, to use no ear drops and to protect the ear with wool and vaseline when washing or showering. Swimming, especially in pools, should not be permitted.

If the ear is discharging when first seen, culture and sensitivity tests are carried out and appropriate aural toilet instituted.

LONG-TERM MANAGEMENT

With suitable precautions, care and cleanliness, it is often possible to keep the ear free of infection and in older patients this may be acceptable. Most younger patients will not tolerate restrictions such as the absence of swimming. They will need periodic visits to hospital and they will be barred from certain occupations such as service in the armed forces and the mining industry. Surgical closure of the perforation by the operation of myringoplasty is often advised.

Advantages of myringoplasty
Control of recurrent otitis media   If reinfection is occurring along the external ear canal, myringoplasty will prevent it but if reinfection is coming from the eustachian tube, it is essential to eliminate disease, such as chronic sinusitis or enlarged adenoids, in the nose or nasopharynx before myringoplasty is contemplated.

Prevention of cochlear degeneration
Repeated attacks of infection will slowly lead to cochlear loss. The closure of a tympanic membrane defect is a protection from sensorineural deafness that can result from recurrent middle-ear infections.

Prevention of tympanosclerosis
The drying effect of air on the mucous membrane of the middle ear may be a factor leading to tympanosclerosis.

Improvement of hearing
Myringoplasty, either the simple closure of a defect in the tympanic membrane or ossicular chain repair, will improve hearing.

Hearing-aid inserts
The wearing of a hearing-aid insert in the external canal in an ear with a defect of the tympanic membrane often leads to ear discharge and myringoplasty will prevent such infection.

Necessity in certain occupations
Candidates for the armed forces and certain occupations such as mining are not accepted with a defect of the tympanic membranes.

PREVENTION OF VERTIGO
Some patients with a defect of the tympanic membrane experience vertigo in climates with cold winds. Closure of the defect will eliminate this symptom.

The operation of myringoplasty with modern techniques is an excellent procedure and can be confidently recommended except for young children (when breakdown is more common) and for those over 65 years of age (when there is a slight risk of sensorineural deafness resulting from the operation). Each case must be judged on its merits and hard-and-fast rules cannot be laid down.

Persistent mucosal disease

DIAGNOSTIC FEATURES
In this condition, the mucous membrane lining the whole of the middle-ear cleft is involved to a greater or lesser extent. A large central or anterior perforation is seen and there is a purulent discharge in the external-ear canal which may produce a secondary otitis externa. Tubal, tympanic and tympanomastoid types of disease may be differentiated and are not usually dangerous but mastoiditis may occur in the tympanomastoid varieties. The classification is not always clear-cut but is useful in the understanding of the pathology.

TUBAL TYPE

Typically this is seen in the 'catarrhal child' from the lower socioeconomic section of the community. The perforation is anterior and a profuse mucopurulent discharge is present which suggests chronic infection of the eustachian tube and of the peritubal and hypotympanic cells. Treatment is directed to dealing with any obvious sources of infection such as chronic sinusitis and enlarged adenoids. Measures to improve the general health of the patient such as an adequate diet, fresh air and rest are advised together with aural toilet which may have to be repeated frequently. Often a stay in hospital with really adequate treatment is helpful in very resistant cases. With improvement in the health of schoolchildren, this type of chronic otitis media should become less common. As the child grows up, the perforation may heal; if not, myringoplasty can be advised after puberty.

TYMPANIC TYPE

In this type of chronic suppurative otitis media there is a large defect of the membrana tensa with retraction of the handle of the malleus. The exposed mucous membrane is hyperplastic and oedematous and an aural polyp may form, which, as it increases in size, can fill the meatus. The polyp is insensitive and smooth in outline, and a probe can be passed round it, between it and the meatal wall. It should be mentioned that polypi can be produced by bone necrosis or osteitis and if this involves the oval or round windows, removal of the polyp could provoke a labyrinthitis.

The history of this type of otitis media is that of a persistent or recurrent otitis media. Flare-ups may occur with upper respiratory tract infections and swimming in infected pools may convert the discharge to a profuse mucopurulent one. An aural polyp prevents drainage and until it is removed, aural toilet will be ineffective. A history of severe deafness or vertigo makes one suspect that the aural polyp may involve the labyrinth.

TYMPANOMASTOID TYPE

This type of otitis media represents an extension of the tympanic type to the mastoid air-cells which are usually well developed. Secondary acquired cholesteatoma may occur and lead to bone destruction.

Clinically there is a purulent pulsating discharge in the upper and posterior part of the tympanum and this becomes foul smelling if cholesteatoma has developed. There is a marked degree of conductive deafness and poor response to aural toilet as the disease has extended to the mastoid air-cells.

Conservative treatment of tubotympanic disease

The basis of treatment is to eradicate infection and produce a dry ear by means of aural toilet. The discharge is cultured and sensitivity tests are performed. The presence or otherwise of enlarged adenoids and sinusitis is determined.

AURAL TOILET—METHODS

Dry mopping

The ear is cleaned with a sterile cotton-tipped probe. This is best carried out in the clinic but a relative of the patient may at times be taught how to perform this procedure. It is important for the toilet to be carried out efficiently each day and following the toilet, an antibiotic powder may be insufflated.

Wet toilet

The ear is syringed to remove pus and debris and this is followed by dry mopping and powder insufflation. Although this is an efficient method of cleaning the ear, it can spread infection to other areas of the tympanum and mastoid and so is used less often. It should be emphasized that the prolonged use of antibiotic powders must be avoided as skin sensitivity problems can arise. The use of antiseptic powders such as boracic acid with 1 per cent iodine is of value and can be used after a period of treatment with antibiotic powders.

Suction toilet

This method, first described by Verhoeven of Antwerp and introduced to this country by McGuckin of Newcastle upon Tyne, is of value for two reasons. Firstly, the ear is examined by a microscope and suction with fine cannulae enables a precise assessment of the extent of the disease to be made. Secondly, removal of areas of proliferative mucous membrane and polypoid mucous membrane breaks down pockets of infection and allows drainage and resolution of the infective process to take place. Small encysted cholesteatomas may be removed or the presence of an unsuspected cholesteatoma revealed. A general anaesthetic is necessary for children but suction toilet may be performed in the clinic without anaesthesia in cooperative adults.

Zinc ionization and radiotherapy

These methods are not indicated today. Zinc ionization is not as effective as careful aural toilet and radiotherapy in the treatment of tubotympanic infections associated with lymphoid hyperplasia of the nasopharynx is dangerous because of the now-recognized radiation hazard.

Indications for surgery

SURGERY IN CHRONIC MUCOSAL DISEASE

Conservative treatment as outlined above may take a great deal of time and patience but is especially worthwhile in children with persistent peritubal infection, since the underlying nasal catarrhal trouble becomes less active as they grow older. Most of these children have already had their tonsils and adenoids removed, but if not this operation may be indicated, as also may be washout of the maxillary sinuses. Revision operation for removal of adenoid remnants around the eustachian tube is best done by a method of 'direct' adenoidectomy; fortunately residual adenoid tissue tends to shrink spontaneously at puberty.

Aural polypus

An aural polyp may prevent drainage and must be removed. This should always be carried out under general anaesthesia using the otomicroscope. Precise removal of the aural polyp using fine suction tips and small forceps is necessary. Naked-eye removal with a snare is not recommended as the polyp may be in close relationship with the oval or round window or the facial nerve may be abnormal or lying free in the middle ear. Damage to the ossicular chain and increased deafness can be caused by a snare used without proper visualization of the middle ear.

Myringoplasty and tympanoplasty

Tympanosclerosis is a relatively common condition and it is important to prevent it as surgical treatment of the deafness caused by the encroachment of tympanosclerotic deposits in the oval and round window areas is rarely successful. It is probable that an open middle ear and recurrent infection are the important factors in the production of this condition and so operations to close the tympanic membrane defect, with tympanoplasty as a second stage operation in some cases with a disrupted ossicular chain are valuable once the infection is under control. Myringoplasty is possible in the presence of infection if antibiotics are used but the results are usually better in a dry ear.

Mastoidectomy

Cortical mastoidectomy   This operation may be of value in patients with a tympanic disease that has spread to the mastoid air-cells. If there is failure to respond to adequate aural toilet and an x-ray of the mastoid air-cells shows cloudiness, the operation should be considered.

Radical operations

If vertigo is present or cholesteatoma is revealed, some form of radical operation may be necessary. An open mastoid cavity is essential if cholesteatoma is found and tympanoplasty may be possible as a second stage procedure at a later time.

Combined approach tympanoplasty is contraindicated in the presence of cholesteatoma but is of value in some cases of chronic mucosal disease where investigation suggests a disruption of the ossicular chain as this approach enables accurate reconstruction of a disrupted ossicular chain to be performed. A further advantage of combined approach tympanoplasty is that it avoids the open mastoid cavity and there is no post-operative healing problem. However, it is possible to eradicate cholesteatoma and exteriorize the mastoid cavity without producing a large cavity. This is a safe operation in the long term and there is seldom any healing problem with the small mastoid cavity.

Attico–antral disease

Cholesteatoma

The term 'cholesteatoma' is long established and although it is not an accurate description as it is not a tumour and does not always contain cholesterin, it is useful to remember that it behaves as a 'tumour' in the temporal bone because it expands and destroys bone.

The characteristic feature of cholesteatoma is the presence within the middle-ear cleft of keratinizing stratified squamous epithelium. This epithelium forms a matrix which continuously desquamates and the sheets of desquamated epithelium (keratin) form the bulk of the cholesteatoma. Cholesteatosis (Young, 1950), epidermosis (Tumarkin, 1961), keratosis (McGuckin, 1960, 1963), are terms used to describe the same entity according to the authors' ideas of aetiology.

The simplest definition of cholesteatoma is that it is 'skin in the wrong place' (Gray,

1964). Normal skin has a thin surface epidermis composed of a keratinizing stratified squamous epithelium and a thick deeper layer, the corium, composed of fibrous and elastic tissue and containing blood vessels, sebaceous glands and hair follicles. The surface desquamation is not usually allowed to collect since it gets rubbed off or washed away. The external auditory meatus is the only part of the body where the skin is not truly superficial. It has adapted itself to this special environment in a variety of ways. The epithelium covering the inner two-thirds of the bony external auditory meatus and over the surface of the tympanic membrane is extremely thin; it has no corium and rests directly on the periosteum of the bony meatus and on the middle layer of the tympanic membrane. It contains no glands or hair follicles, the wax-secreting glands being confined to the outer one-third of the meatus. The growth of the epithelium appears to be faster at the centre of the tympanic membrane and slower towards the periphery so that a continuous thin keratinizing layer migrates outwards over the surface of the meatus until it becomes dissolved in the cerumen and periodically discarded. It is this specialized skin covering the deep meatus and the surface of the tympanic membrane which is the source of cholesteatoma according to the more popular immigration theories.

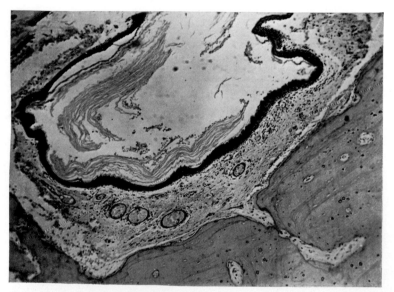

Figure 10.3   Cholesteatoma. A mastoid cell is seen lined by granulation tissue, keratinizing stratified squamous epithelium (matrix) and filled with sheets of desquamated epithelium (keratin). (Reproduced by courtesy of Professor I. Friedmann)

To assist discussion of the pathogenesis of cholesteatoma the clinical distinction is made between primary and secondary acquired cholesteatoma, as advocated by Shambaugh (1967). Primary acquired cholesteatoma refers to disease arising in the attic or in the posterosuperior part of the tympanum where there has been no apparent predisposing chronic suppurative otitis media. Secondary acquired cholesteatoma occurs in ears known to have had previous active or inactive chronic disease, usually with substantial defects of the tympanic membrane.

THEORIES OF PATHOGENESIS

Congenital

Cawthorne (1963) supported McKenzie (1931) in the belief that cholesteatoma has an embryonic origin. Cawthorne refers to 25 cases, 13 personal and 12 in the literature, of primary epidermoid tumours of the petrous bone which closely resemble cholesteatoma. Without necessarily involving the middle-ear cleft these epidermoid tumours may cause extensive bone erosion, usually with loss of cochleovestibular function and facial paralysis. He believes that attic cholesteatoma, like the deeper petrous collection, may originate as an embryonic rest which eats away bone until it breaks through the outer attic wall. Most otologists, however, regard the congenital origin of cholesteatoma as a possible but very rare cause of the commonly experienced attic cholesteatoma.

Immigration

Ruedi, Tumarkin and McGuckin share the view that cholesteatoma is derived by immigration from the deep meatal and tympanic epithelium, but disagree with regard to the precise mechanism.

Ruedi (1963), from the study of extensive animal experimental and human histological material, has reached the following conclusions concerning the pathogenesis of acquired cholesteatoma in the middle ear:

There are two *predisposing factors*: (a) the special growth potential (wachsum potenz) of the basal cells in the stratum germinativum in a circumscribed zone of the meatal skin adjoining the upper margin of the tympanic membrane; (b) the persistence of a submucous connective tissue layer in the middle-ear spaces associated with incomplete pneumatization of the preformed bony spaces.

As the causative factor he suggests an inflammatory stimulus; two main types are stressed: (a) necrotizing otitis media (secondary acquired cholesteatoma); and (b) recurrent acute otitis media in infancy (primary acquired cholesteatoma).

In the development of all types of acquired cholesteatoma there is: (a) an active phase of growth. In response to the inflammatory stimulus the epidermoid basal cells penetrate the submucous connective tissue or newly formed granulation tissue within the middle ear, with simultaneous deposition of sclerosing new bone in the submucous connective tissue. Proliferation of basal cells ceases when available connective or granulation tissue, or both, have been used up. (b) A passive phase of growth. This is characterized by enlargement of the cholesteatoma sac according to the degree of surface desquamation of horny lamellae from the matrix and at the expense of osteoclastic bone destruction.

Tumarkin (1961) has been influenced by Friedmann (1959) to abandon his earlier support for metaplasia in favour of immigration. He elaborates a comprehensive theory to explain hypocellularity, exudative otitis media, cholesterol granuloma and cholesteatoma. All are traced to recurrent upper respiratory virus infections in infancy and childhood, with associated eustachian obstruction and intratympanic vacuum. Tumarkin clearly differentiates between cholesteatoma and cholesterol granuloma. Since the presence of cholesterin crystals is not an essential feature of cholesteatoma, he wants to discard the term cholesteatoma and substitute 'epidermosis'. The keynote of his theory is its emphasis on the preceding collapse of a part or the whole of the tympanic membrane—this he calls 'pre-epidermosis'. During this inactive stage, which can last many years or indefinitely, there may be invagination of Shrapnell's membrane into the attic or of a thin posterior segment of the tympanic membrane into the sinus tympani. The 'threat' of cholesteatoma arises only when the epidermic sac accumulates keratin; when this becomes activated by secondary infection the patient presents with the typical clinical appearances of attico–antral cholesteatoma; then in a period of weeks bone erosion and granulation tissue can arise. It is stressed that in the early stage of keratin accumulation careful treatment, for example by suction clearance, can restore the ear to the state of inactive 'pre-epidermosis'.

Table 10.1   Summary of Tumarkin's comprehensive theory of the pathogenesis of chronic disease of the middle-ear cleft

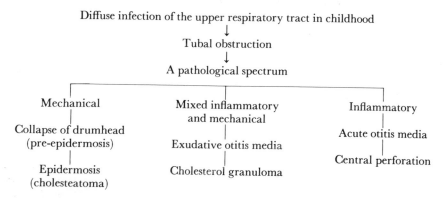

Diffuse infection of the upper respiratory tract in childhood
↓
Tubal obstruction
↓
A pathological spectrum

Mechanical	Mixed inflammatory and mechanical	Inflammatory
Collapse of drumhead (pre-epidermosis)		Acute otitis media
	Exudative otitis media	
Epidermosis (cholesteatoma)	Cholesterol granuloma	Central perforation

Tumarkin's theory is plausible, ingenious and comprehensive and has gained wide acceptance amongst otologists. However, this chapter follows the general practice in preferring the term cholesteatoma to epidermosis although the two are regarded as synonymous.

McGuckin (1960, 1963) would like to discard the terms 'chronic otitis media' and 'cholesteatoma' and substitute 'non-malignant destructive ear disease' as the descriptive title of a silent hyperkeratotic disease, of as yet unknown aetiology, starting always in the unique skin of the deep bony canal and outer layer of the tympanic membrane.

Based upon the otomicroscopic study of very extensive clinical material he is unable to agree that either intratympanic negative pressure or infection are initially significant factors in activating the disease. He also emphasizes that pressure by keratin (cholesteatoma) is not the cause of bone dissolution; he suggests that there may be chemical or enzymal factors derived from the breakdown of the keratin but is prepared to admit that the precise mechanism of soft tissue and bone erosion is not yet properly understood.

McGuckin stresses that in the management of chronic ear disease, particular attention must be paid to the tympanic mucous membrane, which retains extraordinary resistance to penetration by disease and a remarkable healing potential once the keratin is removed by microscopic suction clearance.

Metaplasia

Squamous metaplasia of the flattened epithelium lining the middle-ear cleft has been supported as a possible cause of cholesteatoma since it was originally proposed by Wendt in 1873. Friedmann has demonstrated that columnar metaplasia occurs in chronic otitis media, and Birrell (1958) found squamous metaplasia of the attic and mastoid mucosa in cases of enclosed cholesterol granuloma but remarks on the absence of prickle cells. He found only true cholesteatoma with prickle cells when there was a perforation in the posterosuperior quadrant or in Shrapnell's membrane, potentiating the immigration of squamous epithelium.

Squamous metaplasia is known to be provoked by chronic infection in the ciliated mucous membrane of the nose in atrophic rhinitis and of the bronchi in bronchiectasis. Prior chronic infection of the middle-ear cleft is now admitted only as a predisposing factor in secondary acquired cholesteatoma. Here squamous metaplasia is possible but so also is the marginal immigration of squamous epithelium from the meatus.

In short the possibility of squamous metaplasia has to be admitted but it is only an acceptable explanation in the ear with prolonged irritation.

PATHOGENESIS OF CHOLESTEATOMA–CLINICAL FEATURES

Whatever the pathogenesis, once cholesteatoma becomes established in the middle-ear cleft, the following features are noteworthy (Thorburn, 1968):

(1) The 'focal area' is Shrapnell's membrane, the posterosuperior part of the membrana tensa and the adjacent skin of the deep external auditory meatus (*Figure 10.4*).

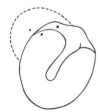

Figure 10.4   Focal areas from which cholesteatoma may arise

(2) Expansion from the focal area into the middle-ear cleft may be influenced by anatomical factors: (a) the pneumatization of the mastoid, which is usually but not necessarily hypocellular; and (b) the distribution of mucosal ligaments, folds or adhesions, especially around the malleus, incus and chorda tympani.

These features all have a bearing upon the 'ventilation anatomy' of the middle-ear cleft and determine its ultimate size and shape. The eustachian tube is responsible for maintaining the ventilation of the whole middle-ear cleft and also the balance of the tympanic membrane. In the hypocellular or acellular mastoid, ventilation beyond the mesotympanum is entirely dependent upon the tympanic isthmuses (*Figure 10.5*) (Proctor, 1964). If either of the isthmuses or the aditus

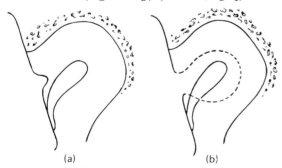

(a)   (b)

Figure 10.5   (a) Dimple in Shrapnell's membrane.
(b) Formation of cholesteatoma sac

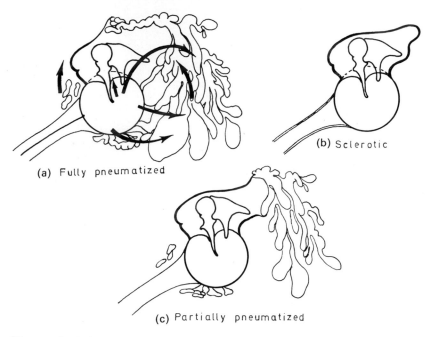

(a) Fully pneumatized

(b) Sclerotic

(c) Partially pneumatized

Figure 10.6   Different types of pneumatization. Note that in a fully pneumatized mastoid there may be a communication between the hypotympanum or posterior tympanum and the mastoid independent of the attic and aditus. (From Dawes (1970), reproduced by courtesy of the Editor of *Journal of Laryngology and Otology*)

itself becomes obstructed, the middle-ear cleft may be divided into compartments which no longer communicate with the eustachian tube. However, in a well pneumatized bone, there is usually an additional communication between the posterior mesotympanum and the mastoid (*Figure 10.6*).

(3) Following simple eustachian tubal obstruction oxygen is soon absorbed by the rich mucosal capillary blood circulation; this produces a relative intratympanic vacuum, so that the tympanic membrane is retracted, with rotation of the ossicular chain and narrowing of the isthmuses. Transudation or exudation of fluid occurs and is often the most troublesome feature of this syndrome, for the familiar 'glue ear' may persist when the tubal obstruction is relieved. This 'glue' has a tremendous surface tension and must surely grip the under surface of the drumhead, increasing retraction and affecting the nutrition of the membrane so that it may lose its middle fibrous layer.

(4) Retraction pockets. Under these stresses something has to give way—indeed a perforation of the tympanic membrane may be the simple solution. The whole tympanic membrane may become thinned, retracted against the promontory and recessed beyond the annulus into the hypotympanum and sinus tympani. A more common result of intratympanic negative pressure is the formation of retraction pockets involving the attic or the posterior tympanic segment. It is likely that the retraction site is determined by the localization of the vacuum. For example, limited retraction of Shrapnell's membrane may be due to obstruction to the

ventilation of Prussak's space; or, if both isthmuses are obstructed, the vacuum which develops in the mastoid and attic produces a much larger attic pocket. Meanwhile the mesotympanum may have recovered normal tubal function.

Another commonly observed deformity is retraction of a thin posterior segment of the membrana tensa behind the handle of the malleus; this resembles an expanding posterior marginal perforation and is only differentiated by very careful examination. This thin retracted membrane becomes adherent to the promontory, wrapped round the long process of incus (which is often eroded) in contact with the head of stapes and deeply invaginated under the annulus into the sinus tympani. *Figure 10.7* indicates how this deformity may arise by transmission

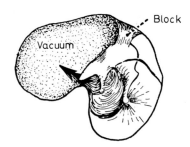

Figure 10.7 Retraction of posterior segment. Transmission of negative pressure from mastoid cavity to the posterior segment of tympanic membrane via the isthmus tympani posticus. (From Thorburn (1968), reproduced by courtesy of the Editor of *Proceedings of the Royal Society of Medicine*)

of negative pressure from the mastoid along the isthmus tympani posticus to the thin posterior segment. The converse of this retraction is seen when such an ear is examined under nitrous oxide and oxygen anaesthesia. Through capillary diffusion of nitrous oxide into the middle-ear cleft the previously retracted posterior segment becomes grossly distended, unless it is already bound down by adhesions. Buckingham and Ferrer (1966) have demonstrated by serial microphotography, that such a deformed drum can be restored to its normal level by air venting with a grommet in the anterior part of the tympanic membrane.

(5) Migration. Successful outward migration may keep these retraction pockets free of keratin for many years or indefinitely. If keratin collects in a pocket it soon becomes moist, swollen and an ideal medium for the growth of proteolytic bacteria, for example *Proteus*. Next, ulceration of the epidermis lining the pocket occurs proceeding to osteitis with bone absorption; this is signalled by the appearance of granulation tissue growing from the sinus tympani or from the attic (epitympanic polypus). The long process of the incus or the head and crura of the stapes are frequently destroyed in this way. Further expansion of the disease into the mastoid or attic may be effectively resisted by mucosal swelling within the isthmuses and around the ossicles. Resolution of this localized disease may occur by spontaneous healing, possibly assisted by microscopic suction toilet leaving a slight thinning and retraction deformity of the tympanic membrane whose epithelial surface migrates normally.

(6) Expansion of cholesteatoma. In the less fortunate cases there is a quiet expansion of the epidermis-lined retraction pocket with failure of migration and infection. If part of the pocket is shut off this fills with keratin and expands within the middle-ear cleft. The expansion may be contained by mucous membrane giving the resulting cholesteatoma an encysted appearance as though it were herniating into the tympanum or mastoid. If the mucosal barrier fails a rapid expansion

occurs so that the cholesteatoma infiltrates every part of the middle-ear cleft; this diffuse type is commonly seen in children. Exceptionally a cholesteatoma inside an intact tympanic membrane is encountered; it does not necessarily follow that this is congenital in origin since, either the original 'neck' of the retraction pocket may have healed across, or Ruedi's theory of over-activity and invasion from the stratum germinativum may apply.

Figure 10.8 shows that the direction of spread of cholesteatoma from the attic is backwards into the aditus and mastoid antrum, downwards on either side of the body and long process of incus and anteriorly under the head and neck of the malleus towards the mesotympanum. Often the mesotympanum is isolated from

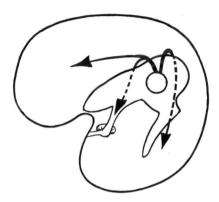

Figure 10.8   Directions of spread of cholesteatoma from the attic

the attic by mucosal folds. These used to be regarded as a protective reaction limiting the spread of disease but a more acceptable argument may be that they caused the initial failure of ventilation with consequent attic retraction and cholesteatoma formation.

Figure 10.9 indicates that spread of cholesteatoma from the posterior tympanic segment is from the upper end of the sinus tympani along the isthmus tympani

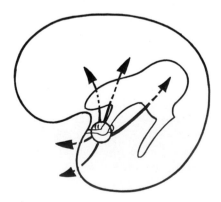

Figure 10.9   Directions of spread of cholesteatoma from the posterior segment of the tympanic membrane

posticus under the body of the incus; or under the neck of the malleus along the isthmus tympani anticus to the attic. According to Alberti (1963) the long process of the incus has a poor blood supply along the shaft in 4 per cent of cases but in the healthy state the incus has an excellent blood supply from the anastomotic vessels on its surface. Presumably in many cases the destruction of the long process of the incus and the stapes superstructure is a result of a low grade osteitis accompanying the preceding exudative otitis media or the cholesteatoma itself.

Strangely, this loss of the long process need not impair hearing since the disease can still act as an efficient sound conductor. The expansion of an infected cholesteatoma into the middle-ear cleft is, to some extent, relieved by the fact that there is usually some communication with the outer ear which allows escape of discharge and broken-down keratin. Thus there is no positive pressure within the cholesteatoma pocket to cause pain or to explain the bone erosion, which is the characteristic and dangerous feature of this disease.

(7) Cholesterol granuloma. An expanding cholesteatoma must sooner or later obstruct the ventilation and drainage of the mastoid antrum and air-cells. The resultant negative pressure in the mastoid induces a simple mucosal oedema but there may be additional minor inflammatory episodes with fluid exudation and small haemorrhages. It is therefore understandable that cholesterol granuloma, usually black or dark green in colour, is a common association. This is also referred to as 'black cellular cholesteatosis' (Birrell, 1956).

(8) Healing responses. A failure of resistance to cholesteatoma results in a diffuse chronic suppurative otitis media with mucosal oedema, possibly osteitis and granulation tissue or polypus formation. Successful healing responses have as their main objective the limitation and extrusion of the disease and many ears show evidence of spontaneous healing. Where there is a defect in the tympanic membrane this may close by mucosal growth. Epithelium then readily grows over the outer surface of the mucous membrane. However, if epithelial and mucosal growth coincide before the defect is bridged, a permanent perforation of the membrane results. The peculiar thin 'false membrane' formed by this type of healing has no middle fibrous layer.

Since active cholesteatoma originates in the epitympanic segment, healing is often most effective in excluding disease from the antero-inferior part of the tympanum, here a small functioning tympanic cavity may form with the physiological mechanism of type 3 or type 4 tympanoplasty. Furthermore the cholesteatoma itself may absorb bone from the outer attic or deep posterior meatal wall sufficient to make room for its own extrusion, as happens in a so-called 'natural' modified radical mastoidectomy.

(9) Tympanosclerosis. Tympanosclerosis is another type of healing response and may be seen in any form of chronic suppurative otitis media. It is characterized by hyaline deposit through degeneration of fibrous tissue elements in the subepithelial layer of the mucous membrane, in the lamina propria of the tympanic membrane and in organized granulation tissue. In advanced cases hyaline is laid down in layers, the less mature layer being next to the surface of the mucous membrane; mature hyaline may become calcified or even ossified. Hyaline has a firm tough consistence and a white glistening appearance and so is easily distinguished from the diffused keratinizing surface of cholesteatoma.

The external auditory meatus may itself be involved in the healing responses of chronic suppurative otitis media. A 'false fundus' is a thin membrane, partial or complete, present at the isthmus of the external auditory meatus. The impression is given that a deformed tympanic membrane lies nearer to the eye of the observer than does the normal drumhead. In such an ear extensive tympanosclerotic deformity may be expected. An allied feature is a failure of epithelial growth over the surface of the meatus deep to the isthmus; here it may be replaced by a simple cuboidal epithelium or by a thin layer of granulation tissue. This failure of epithelial growth may produce a deep meatal stenosis and must prejudice healing if a tympanoplasty operation is carried out.

CLINICAL ASSESSMENT OF ATTICO–ANTRAL DISEASE AND CHOLESTEATOMA

Symptoms and signs
(1) Uncomplicated disease   In the absence of complications, there are three symptoms. These are otorrhoea, hearing loss which may be associated with tinnitus and occasional bleeding from granulation tissue.

The discharge is usually scanty and is malodorous. The musty smell of the discharge may be noticed by the patient or by others and is often the reason for seeking advice. It is surprising how tolerant some patients are of a discharging ear, believing that if an ear is discharging, it is safe. Loss of hearing is usually present and if it is unilateral and slowly progressive, it may escape the patient's notice. Hearing may be only slightly impaired in advanced cholesteatoma as the disease can transmit sound to the oval window or bridge a gap in the ossicular chain (*Figure 10.10*).

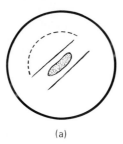
(a)

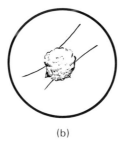
(b)

Figure 10.10 (a) Fistula in lateral semi-circular canal produced by cholesteatoma. (b) Cholesteatoma bridging gap between incus and stapes

(2) Complicated disease   Earache, vertigo and headache are important symptoms suggesting a complication of the primary ear disease (*Figure 10.10*).

Examination and differential diagnosis
While much can be learned about the probable condition of an ear from a carefully taken case history, a correct diagnosis depends upon accurate (and if necessary repeated) examination. Even if only one ear is affected, both ears should always be examined since the condition of the opposite ear often yields valuable clues about the pathology of the affected ear. In uncomplicated chronic otitis media there is no urgency about reaching a final diagnosis.

When the patient first presents, the ear is usually full of discharge and debris. The otologist has the advantage that with good illumination from a forehead mirror, he can carry out a thorough controlled aural toilet, preferably with suction. Following aural toilet, examination with a Siegle's pneumatic speculum often yields valuable information as it gives a twofold magnification, demonstrates the mobility of the remains of the tympanic membrane and reveals pus or moist cholesteatomatous debris in a hidden attic or marginal defect. A good electric auriscope gives an excellent magnified view of the tympanum but the pneumatic attachment is seldom satisfactory.

In all cases, and certainly in any ear presenting difficult diagnostic features, examination with the otomicroscope is of the utmost value; controlled palpation with a fine probe and the use of suction usually resolve doubtful features.

The appearances should be recorded and sketched. The following observations may be relevant to the differential diagnosis.

(1) The precise situation, size and shape of any deformity, recession or perforation of the tympanic membrane (*Figure 10.11*).
(2) The presence and location of cholesteatoma, granulations or discharge.
(3) The presence of pulsation—a sign of activity and loculation of infection.
(4) The odour of the discharge which, if foetid, suggests saprophytic infection of a cholesteatoma and bone necrosis.
(5) Inflation by Valsalva's method or by politzerization may show that part of the tympanum is shut off from disease but remains in communication with the eustachian tube. The use of inflation or the pneumatic speculum will also distinguish between granulating myringitis, and chronic otitis media in which the perforation is hidden by granulations.
(6) If a small scab is present over the attic or upper annulus this must be removed, since it may hide attic or posterosuperior marginal disease (*Figure 10.11*).

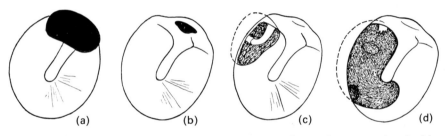

Figure 10.11   Deformities or perforations of the tympanic membrane associated with attico–antral disease

(7) Aural polypi (*see* p. 244) and granulations must be distinguished from malignant disease and it is a wise precaution to submit all doubtful tissue for histological examination. Granulations and polypi originate from chronic disease within the middle-ear cleft and should be distinguished from a glomus jugulare tumour. Granulations may arise from ulceration of the meatal wall caused by keratosis obturans. A malignant neoplasm is indurated and friable, bleeds easily and, unlike a polypus, is attached to the meatal wall so that a probe cannot pass all the way round it.
(8) With the otomicroscope it may be possible to assess the condition of the ossicles, labyrinthine windows and exposed tympanic mucosa. An apparently small attic cholesteatoma may be seen to invaginate deeply underneath an intact membrana tensa, giving a dull white firm shadow outline, convex downwards, on one or both sides of the handle of the malleus.
(9) The differential diagnosis between otitis externa and chronic otitis media often presents a difficult problem. The infected discharge from chronic otitis media itself may be the cause of a persistent dermatitis or of recurrent furunculosis. Fungus infection, especially with *Aspergillus niger*, can be confusing but the

diagnosis is readily established by microscopic examination of the debris, demonstrating the characteristic mycelia and spores.

A frequent cause of otitis externa in cases of chronic otitis media is, paradoxically, the use of antibiotic drops for the treatment of the condition. Chloromycetin and neomycin are common offenders and can provoke an acute sensitization eczema which may well be responsible for the patient seeking specialist advice. The presence of an otitis externa therefore by no means excludes a diagnosis of chronic otitis media. Stenosis of the meatus by soft tissue swelling or the presence of an exostosis of the deep bony meatus, can make it very difficult to obtain a satisfactory view of the drumhead. In these cases suction toilet and the introduction of a fine aural speculum should relieve the deafness, giving tentative re-assurance that there is no active middle-ear disease.

Hearing assessment

After thorough aural toilet normal routine hearing tests are carried out and any difference of hearing, before and after tubal inflation, is noted. Speech tests include the hearing for a light whisper and a monitored conversational voice using numbers and spondee words. Tuning-fork tests (Rinne, Weber and Schwabach) and an air and bone conduction audiograph usually show a mainly conductive hearing loss. The bone conduction threshold is a useful indicator of the residual cochlear function. Cochlear degeneration may develop very insidiously in chronic otitis media and should be carefully noted since it discourages any non-essential operative treatment. Weber's test is of value when both ears are very deaf, since the tuning forks are lateralized to the ear with the better cochlear function. Before the hearing response can be accepted as genuine in an ear with severe deafness, it is essential that the opposite ear be adequately masked with a Bárány noise box or with a white noise generator.

Although the drumhead, ossicular chain and labyrinthine windows are often hidden from view by disease, the degree of hearing loss usually reflects the extent of interference with their mobility and integrity. Therefore, when an operation is necessary the knowledge that useful hearing is present offers both encouragement and a challenge to the otologist. The physiological mechanism naturally established by the healing response of the tympanum must be uncovered and retained, provided this course is consistent with complete excision of the disease.

Bacteriology

Knowledge about the bacterial flora and antibiotic sensitivity is only of practical therapeutic value in chronic otitis media when there is an acute exacerbation of infection with pyogenic organisms. Moist disintegrating keratin provides a suitable nidus for the growth of *B. proteus*, *Ps. aeruginosa* and *Ps. pyocyaneus*, but the elimination of these organisms depends upon the eradication of the cholesteatoma and not on treatment with an antibiotic to which they show an '*in vitro*' sensitivity.

Radiography

Routine radiography is of little value in the diagnosis and assessment of attico–antral disease. However, it should always be carried out to demonstrate the cellularity of the mastoid and the position of the lateral sinus and the middle fossa. The degree of bone destruction by cholesteatoma is not accurately detected by simple techniques and these x-rays can be misleading. Modern tomographic techniques available in specialized centres are able to show detail in the temporal bone and are of great value. The application and interpretations of these sophisticated methods require close collaboration between the otologist and the radiologist with a special interest in the subject.

Tuberculosis of the middle-ear cleft

In adults, tuberculosis of the ear usually appears in those suffering from advanced pulmonary tuberculosis. In children it may occur in the relatively healthy. The elimination of bovine tuberculosis has greatly reduced the incidence of the disease in the very young. With modern treatment advanced phthisis has decreased, and therefore tuberculous otitis media has become rare.

Symptoms and signs

The condition is painless and the hearing is always severely impaired. Middle-ear tuberculosis is mainly a benign lesion and, according to Blegvad (1951), its earliest features are:

(1) Marked protrusion of the posterior part of the tympanic membrane.
(2) Characteristic diffuse colouring of the tympanic membrane which is at first rosy pink and later yellowish-white.
(3) Pronounced dilatation of the vessels in the anterior part of the tympanic membrane, which persists for a long time and is pathognomonic of middle-ear tuberculosis.

Later, the swelling extends to the anterior part of the membrane which becomes more yellow in colour, but the tortuous vessels persist. One, two or even three perforations develop and the membrane becomes grossly thickened. Ultimately the perforations may coalesce and produce a total defect of the pars tensa. In some cases there is no perforation and the membrane is covered by a whitish exudate from which tubercle bacilli can be grown. Once a total defect of the pars tensa has developed, the tympanic appearances are not characteristic of tuberculosis. If granulations appear they recur rapidly after removal and demonstrate histologically tuberculous features. Radiologically the mastoid process is usually well pneumatized, often with opacity of the cells, but bone destruction is seen only when there is clinical evidence of a mastoid complication. This is less common in adults than in children and the associated post-aural swelling is relatively painless and is a typical 'cold abscess'. Other complications occasionally encountered are facial paralysis, labyrinthine fistulae, necrosis of the malleus or incus and, rarely, tuberculous meningitis.

Management

Once the disease is recognized, routine treatment with streptomycin, isoniazid and para-aminosalicylic acid is instituted. Under this chemotherapeutic cover it should be safe to carry out mastoid surgery where specifically indicated. At operation there may be several fistulae through the cortex. Bone destruction is more extensive than in an ordinary mastoiditis. There is an unusual amount of pale granulation tissue filling the mastoid, and tubercles may be seen macroscopically. A cortical operation or a radical mastoidectomy may be required, according to the extent of the disease.

References

Alberti, P. W. R. M. (1963). *Laryngoscope*, **73,** 605

Birrell, J. F. (1956). *Journal of Laryngology*, **70,** 260

Birrell, J. F. (1958). *Journal of Laryngology*, **72,** 620

Blegvad, N. R. L. (1951). *Proceedings of the Fourth International Congress of Otolaryngology*, 1949

Buckingham, R. A. and Ferrer, J. L. (1966). *Laryngoscope*, **76,** 993

Cawthorne, T. (1963). *Archives of Otolaryngology*, **78,** 248

Dawes, J. D. K. (1970). *Journal of Laryngology*, **84,** 583

Friedmann, I. (1959). *Annals of Otology*, **68,** 57

Gray, J. D. (1964). *Proceedings of the Royal Society of Medicine*, **57,** 9

Holmquist, J. R. (1976). 'Auditory tubal function', *Scientific Foundations of Otolaryngology*, p 252. London; William Heinemann Medical Books Ltd

James, J. Angell (1963). *Journal of Laryngology*, **77,** 752

McGuckin, F. (1960). *Postgraduate Medical Journal*, **36,** 256

McGuckin, F. (1963). *Archives of Otolaryngology*, **78,** 358

McKenzie, D. (1931). *Journal of Laryngology*, **46,** 163

Mawson, S. R. (1974). *Diseases of the Ear*, London; Edward Arnold

Proctor, B. (1964). *Journal of Laryngology*, **78,** 631

Ruedi, L. (1963). *Archives of Otolaryngology*, **78,** 252

Sadé, J. (1966). *Archives of Otolaryngology*, **84,** 137; **84,** 267

Sadé, J. (1967). *Archives of Otolaryngology*, **86,** 22

Sammut, J. J. (1968). *Journal of Laryngology*, **82,** 283

Shambaugh, G. E. Jnr. (1967). *Surgery of the Ear*. Philadelphia; Saunders

Thomas, R. (1967). *Journal of Laryngology*, **81,** 1071

Thorburn, I. B. (1968). *Proceedings of the Royal Society of Medicine*, **61,** 395

Tumarkin, A. (1961). *Journal of Laryngology*, **75,** 487

Wendt, H. (1873). *Archiv fur Ohrenheilkunde*, **14,** 428

Young, G. (1950). *Proceedings of the Royal Society of Medicine*, **43,** 75

11 Management of chronic suppurative otitis media
Philip H Beales

Introduction

In the early part of this century, the otologist was concerned with producing a safe ear and preventing the development of intracranial complications. Surgery was concerned with the elimination of disease, usually at the expense of useful hearing. The introduction of antibiotics, the operating microscope and modern anaesthetic techniques directed at producing a dry operation field have radically changed this outlook. Modern otological techniques aim to produce a safe ear with improvement of hearing. Wullstein and Zollner in 1955 laid down the principles of this new kind of surgery which they called tympanoplasty, and the five basic types of tympanic physiology described by Wullstein are references to explain how hearing is possible with various tympanic deformities. Many developments have taken place since Wullstein's original concept and the emphasis today is the direct reconstruction of the sound conducting mechanism after removal of disease. These methods include ossicular autografts, homografts, and prostheses of plastic and wire materials, and will be described in detail in this chapter.

Surgical anatomy

The normal anatomy of the middle-ear cleft is described in Volume I. The trainee otologist will be well advised to develop his micro-surgical technique and become thoroughly familiar with the normal anatomical landmarks by dissecting as many temporal bones as possible. Unfortunately, in chronic ear disease the bony outline of the middle-ear cleft may be modified by sclerosis or erosion and filled with granulation tissue, oedematous mucosa and cholesteatoma. Accordingly important landmarks are obscured or destroyed so that vital structures may be exposed and liable to injury. In such difficult circumstances certain anatomical concepts relative to pneumatization, mastoid outline and the tympanic cavity may be of value.

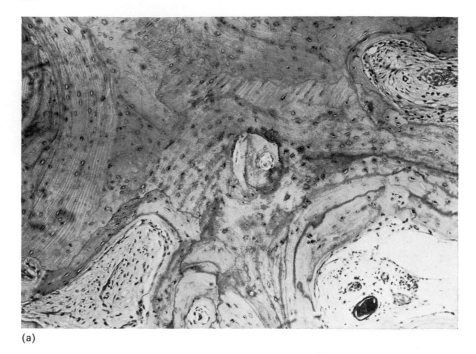

(a)

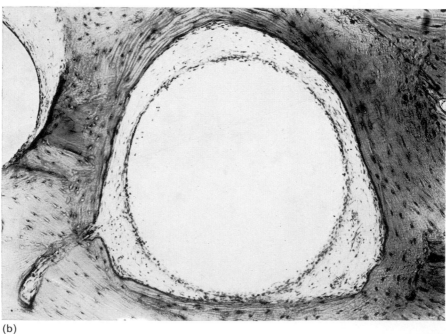

(b)

Figure 11.1 (a) Chronic mastoiditis. Note irregularity of cement lines and lines of apposition. In right bottom corner mastoid cell containing some fibrous tissue and gland containing mucus (× 130, reduced to three-quarters on reproduction); (b) mastoid air-cell, lined by moderately thickened fibrotic mucosa. The cell is surrounded by lamellar bone (× 140, reduced to three-quarters on reproduction). (Reproduced by courtesy of Professor I. Friedmann)

Pneumatization

The extent of pneumatization of the mastoid or of the petrous temporal bone determines the outline of the middle-ear cleft. It has long been recognized that in the vast majority of ears with active chronic disease the mastoid is sclerosed, hypocellular or acellular. Opinions differ as to cause and effect. Friedmann (1956, 1957) considers that the infantile mastoid process normally becomes pneumatized. If pneumatization fails the bone remains diploetic and may be converted into compact bone; the result is an acellular mastoid. If there is invasion of the pneumatized mastoid by chronic disease, absorption of normal bone and deposition of scerotic bone occurs. This is easily distinguished microscopically since sclerotic bone shows irregularity of cement lines (*Figure 11.1a*), whereas compact bone is lamellar bone (*Figure 11.1b*), laid down in marrow spaces.

Mastoid outline

The mastoid outline (*Figure 11.2*) is a useful anatomical concept which removes most of the uncertainty and danger from exploration of the mastoid in chronic ear disease. This outline is determined in each temporal bone by the extent of pneumatization. Rarely is there an acellar mastoid with only a small antrum and aditus connected with the epitympanum. It is safer to enter such a small antrum by exploring directly through the posterior canal wall. Usually there is some degree of pneumatization beyond the antrum, and the mastoid is explored from the cortex inwards until the healthy bony walls of the mastoid outline, together with the antrum and aditus, are defined. The anterior wall of the mastoid outline is the posterior aspect of the external auditory meatus and is in line with the descending part of the facial nerve. The

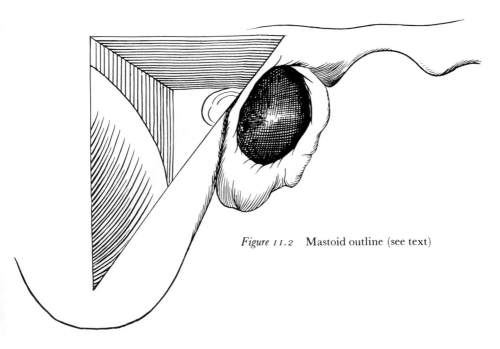

Figure 11.2   Mastoid outline (see text)

superior wall is the tegmen, formed by compact bone following the concavo–convex outline of the middle cranial fossa. The posteromedial wall is formed, from before backwards, by the osseous vestibular labyrinth, the compact bone over the posterior fossa (Trautmann's triangle) and the lateral sinus. The tip of the mastoid is a variable inferior expansion which comes into relatationship with the digastric groove. Superficially there is the mastoid cortex which is continuous with the outer table of the skull. Three angles in the mastoid outline are important, and if these angles are fully dissected no diseased cells should be overlooked.

(1) The anterior wall meets the tegmen at an acute angle which leads into any zygomatic extension of cells.
(2) The superior and posteromedial walls meet at the sinodural angle; when fully dissected this should form a right angle with the superior petrosal sinus at its apex.
(3) The solid angle is the space outlined by dissection of the posterior aspect of the three bony semicircular canals. This space lies behind the prominence of the lateral semicircular canal; since it is also at the medial end of the sinodural angle the tegmen lies above and Trautmann's triangle behind. A complete dissection of the solid angle is often necessary in chronic otitis media since it contains perilabyrinthine cells which may be infiltrated by disease.

Tympanic cavity

The surgical landmarks of the tympanic cavity are often altered or hidden by cholesteatoma or granulation tissue. In such conditions prelimary exploration of the mastoid gives an extra bearing on the tympanic anatomy and the most useful landmark is the prominence of the lateral semicircular canal. Once this is defined the horizontal portion of the facial canal is readily found. When extensive disease has destroyed the lateral semicircular canal, it is possible to find the horizontal portion of the fallopian canal by dissecting downwards from the tegmen in the region of the attic. Great care must be taken in this dissection, for the facial nerve may be exposed and vulnerable.

The incus and malleus are useful landmarks when present, but since they are commonly eroded or destroyed they cannot always be relied upon for reference. Since dislocation or removal of the stapes in chronic ear disease may be catastrophic to labyrinthine function, it is important that its situation be carefully defined. A useful guide is the horizontal portion of the fallopian canal, or the stapedius tendon when intact.

Sinus tympani and facial recess

The sinus tympani and the facial recess (suprapyramidal recess) lie deep to the posterior tympanic sulcus and fibrous annulus and immediately behind the labyrinthine windows. This region is commonly infiltrated by keratinizing disease associated with retraction of the posterior segment of the tympanic membrane. As shown in *Figure 11.3*, the facial recess lies superficial to the sinus tympani and is separated from it by the descending portion of the facial nerve and the processus

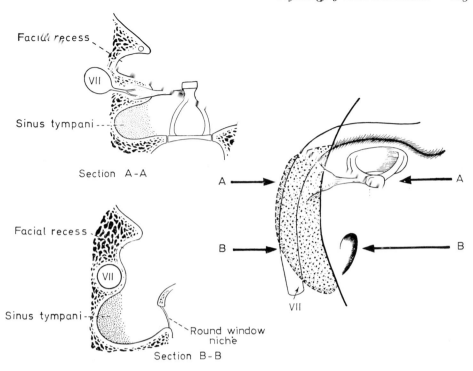

Facial recess
VII
Sinus tympani
Section A-A

Facial recess
VII
Sinus tympani
Round window niche
Section B-B

A   A

B   B

VII

Figure 11.3   The sinus tympani and the facial recess. The correct anatomical description of the sinus tympani is that it starts above at the oval window niche; it occupies a groove deep to the descending portion of the facial nerve and to the pyramid and passes behind the round window niche to the hypotympanum. The facial recess is a term not yet accepted by anatomists: it is an alternative name for the suprapyramidal recess (Sheehy and Patterson, 1967). The facial recess may be entered from the mastoid by opening up small cells usually present between the fossa incudis, the deep posterior bony canal and the descending portion of the facial nerve. (From Thorburn (1968), reproduced by courtesy of the Editor of *Proceedings of the Royal Society of Medicine*)

pyramidalis. Accordingly, access from the mastoid to the sinus tympani is restricted by the facial nerve. Adequate access to the sinus tympani may be obtained by taking down the deep posterior meatal wall anterior to the descending portion of the facial nerve. To do this safely the horizontal part of the facial canal should be clearly seen. The sinus tympani cannot be clearly viewed during intact canal-wall tympanoplasty, and so there is a danger that cholesteatoma may be left *in situ* with this technique.

Physiology of sound transmission (*see* Volume 1)

Attention has been drawn to the fact that the tympanic membrane, with the ossicular chain, is an efficient mechanism for transmitting and augmenting acoustic energy from the larger tympanic membrane to the smaller stapes footplate, where the sound waves are transmitted to the labyrinthine fluids. The normal mechanism for conduction of sound by the middle ear depends upon the following three factors:

(1) An intact and freely mobile tympanic membrance and ossicular chain.
(2) A functioning eustachian tube able to maintain an equal pressure on both sides of the tympanic membrane.
(3) The two labyrinthine windows, one on either side of the scala media of the cochlea, must be freely mobile. As the movement of the stapedial footplate stimulates fluid inside the labyrinth, the round window membrane must be free to compensate for the pressure changes. It is therefore essential that the round window receives sound waves in a different phase from the oval window. To achieve this the round window must be protected by an air-containing tympanic baffle.

In chronic ear disease, whether active or healed, there is generally some abnormality of the conducting mechanism. Wullstein (*Figure 11.4*) has classified the more

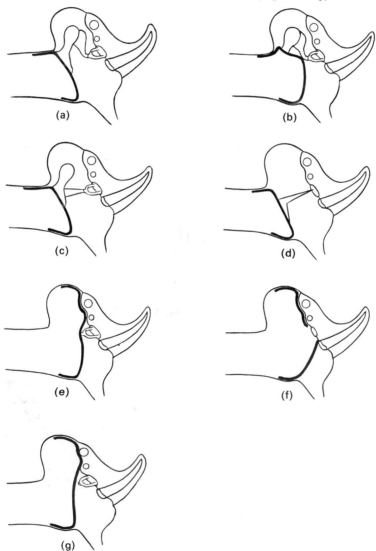

Figure 11.4   Tympanic physiology: (a) Type 1; (b) Type 2a; (c) Type 2b; (d) Type 2c; (e) Type 3; (f) Type 4; (g) Type 5 (after Wullstein)

commonly encountered abnormal patterns of sound transmission into five types. It is convenient to refer to these mechanisms when assessing an existing defect of the tympanum or when describing a planned tympanoplastic reconstruction.

Type 1 defines the normal middle ear with an intact mobile ossicular chain.

Type 2 originally referred to sound transmission through a deformed but functioning ossicular chain (*Type 2a*). It is proposed also to include any reformed mechanism joining the tympanic membrane with the stapes footplate which retains a lever advantage. This may be either a malleus–stapes assembly (*Type 2b*), or a new construction independent of the malleus (*Type 2c*).

Type 3 (also known as the columella effect) transmits sound directly through a mobile stapes. When the head of the stapes does not project far enough beyond the fallopian canal, it may have to be built up to bring it into contact with the drumhead. Alternatively, by removing the posterior canal wall and the bridge, the tympanic cavity is made shallow or flat so that the membrane comes into contact with the head of the stapes.

Type 4 (also known as the baffle effect) leaves the oval window with mobile footplate exposed; a small middle-ear cavity in continuity with the eustachian tube provides sound protection (a baffle) for the round window.

Type 5 (fenestration) has a fixed stapes, and sound enters the labyrinth by a fistula or fenestra of the lateral semicircular canal which is on the side of the scala media opposite to the round window. An intact tympanic membrane forms a flat middle-ear cavity and provides sound protection for the round window.

Sound inversion (Garcia-Ibanez, 1961) (*Figure 11.5*). The round window is left exposed to the direct impact of the sound wave and a mobile stapes footplate is protected by a small tympanic air space in continuity with the eustachian tube.

Although the above classification is of value in enabling us to understand abnormalities of the conducting mechanism, the actual techniques of reconstruction of the middle ear have advanced in the last few years. Modern methods of reconstruction of the middle ear are concerned with the *direct* reconstruction of the sound conducting mechanism as the hearing results are superior. The type 3 tympanoplasty (or columella effect) is, however, still a most useful procedure, especially in the hands of the less expert, and can give socially acceptable hearing a little above the 25 dB level for the speech frequencies. The type 4 and type 5 tympanoplasty operations give uncertain results and are seldom performed today.

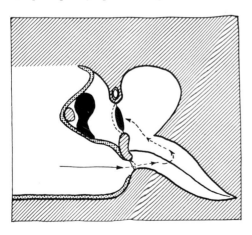

Figure 11.5 Sound inversion. The round window receives the direct impact of the sound wave and the oval window is protected by a tympanic air space in continuity with the eustachian tube. (Reproduced by courtesy of Dr. L. Garcia-Ibanez)

Technique of temporal bone surgery

The essentials of a good technique in temporal bone surgery are good illumination with a clear view of the operation area, a bloodless or relatively bloodless field and the ability to use fine precision instruments.

Although a good headlight combined with a binocular loupe giving 2–2.5 diameters of magnification is of value in the preliminary steps of the operation, an operating microscope is absolutely essential for all the detailed work in the mastoid cavity and tympanum. The surgeon must be comfortably seated for precision work and it is important to choose an operating table that can be lowered sufficiently for this to be done. Many operating tables are not low enough as they are designed for general surgery. The Zeiss Otoscope was the first operating microscope to provide the essential features needed for micro-surgery of the ear. These are:

(1) The height of the microscope and the angle of the microscope head must be easily adjustable.
(2) The built-in light of the microscope must be centred with the visual axis of the microscope.
(3) There must be stereoscopic vision with a choice of magnification.
(4) It must be possible to attach a camera or cine camera or videotape recorder. The attachment of a colour television camera is of great value for teaching purposes.
(5) It must be possible to attach a viewing tube so that assistants can view all stages of the operation. This is essential for teaching purposes.

The colour television camera and monitor should be regarded as necessary items of equipment for all larger centres. Not only do they enable students and assistants to observe details of the operation but they are of value in enhancing the interest of nursing staff, and the anaesthetist is able to observe the operating field and control haemostasis.

Two methods of temporal bone surgery are available; the older mallet and gouge technique and the modern drill technique. Modern precision surgery demands a drill technique and this has superseded the hammer and gouge method. Bone nibbling forceps and curettes may be used with the drill technique. The modern electric drill should rotate to at least 12 000 r/min, possess a good torque and have an adjustable foot-pedal speed control. The motor is small and the drill handle attaches directly to it, and a long drive cable is avoided. Straight and angled handpieces such as the 'Kavo' should be available, with a selection of cutting and diamond paste burrs of different sizes. The air drill is a useful instrument for preliminary bone work in sclerotic mastoids as it is very powerful and cuts extremely dense bone rapidly.

Rules for the use of a drill in temporal bone surgery

There must be:

(1) Proper sterilization and lubrication of the drill handpiece and spare sterile handpieces must be available in case of seizure or breakdown. The surgeon must be comfortably seated at the correct height and the handpiece is held like a pen whilst the fifth finger or hypothenar eminence rests lightly on the patient's head.
(2) Major bone removal is effected by long-shanked straight cutting burrs as the

larger burr is less liable to damage the dura or lateral sinus. Diamond paste burrs are of value in polishing bone or controlling bleeding from bone. They should be used when vital structures such as the facial nerve are close.

(3) The burr must never be used blindly. It is essential to obtain a clear view at all times and so the mastoid outline is followed, keeping the cavity bevelled towards the periphery. A cutting burr rotating in a clockwise direction tends to run off to the right side and it is advisable in a delicate situation when one is close to the facial nerve to stroke from right to left using little pressure. The direction of a diamond drill may be reversed.

(4) There must be continuous irrigation with warm normal saline to avoid overheating of the bone and clogging of the teeth of the burr. The assistant controls the irrigation with a syringe whilst the surgeon, using a suction cannula in his free hand, removes the excess fluid. Combined suction–irrigation cannulae of various sizes are available. Suction is essential in tympano–mastoid surgery but it must be used discreetly as it has a cooling effect on the labyrinth with resulting vertigo, nausea and sickness after operation. Loss of labyrinthine function can occur if suction is transmitted directly or indirectly to the perilymph. Strong suction must not be applied close to a fistula or to the labyrinthine windows and fine suction ends must be substituted for the suction tip in these circumstances.

Operative surgical terminology

The name given to a particular operation on the middle-ear cleft should, as far as possible, be accurately descriptive in three respects:

(1) Soft tissue approach, whether post-aural, endaural or permeatal.
(2) Surgical exposure of bone, indicating the manner of access to disease in the mastoid and tympanic cavities: for example atticotomy; attico–antrostomy; cortical mastoidectomy; posterior tympanotomy; conservative or modified radical mastoidectomy; radical mastoidectomy. A *transcanal* (or a *transmeatal*) tympanotomy or tympanoplasty implies a bone exposure limited by an intact bony canal wall where the soft tissue approach may yet be either permeatal or endaural.
(3) Functional conservation or reconstruction attempted relative to the different types of tympanic physiology described in *Figures 11.4* and *11.5*.

Soft tissue approaches

Surgical access to chronic disease of the middle-ear cleft is considerably influenced by the soft tissue approach. Pre-operative assessment of the disease should determine a choice of soft tissue approach which provides not only adequate exposure of bone but also access to temporal fascia or even to deal with a suspected complication. A permeatal approach would only be chosen where the disease appears to be limited to the tympanic and attic regions. If the disease is found to be more extensive than expected, then there should be no hesitation in changing to an endaural or post-aural approach.

PERMEATAL

This refers to the limited but direct view of the deep meatus and tympanic cavity obtained through a suitably chosen aural speculum. Tumarkin's slotted speculum permits an instrument—for example, a gouge or curette—to be introduced through the slot and used under clear visual control. Since the speculum takes advantage of the mobility of the outer cartilaginous meatus and auricle, considerable variation in the angle of view is possible. The otomicroscope has greatly enhanced appreciation, both of the usefulness and of the limitations of the permeatal approach.

ENDAURAL

Lempert was mainly responsible for popularizing the endaural approach to the middle-ear cleft. He also emphasized that to exploit this approach to the full an otologist should have a competent drill technique for temporal bone surgery. The recommended endaural incision is in two parts, both extracartilaginous (*Figure 11.6*).

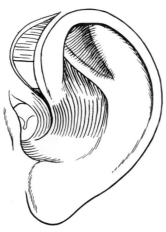 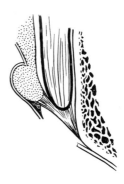

Figure 11.6   Endaural incision (see text)

A special endaural dilating speculum opens up the space between tragus and concha and later spreads the incision as it develops. The first part is a curved incision down to bone between the outer margin of the posterior meatal wall and the anterior edge of the conchal cartilage. The upper end of this incision should reach half way round the superior meatal wall. The second part of the incision extends the first part upwards through the skin and fibrous tissue, separating tragus from helix, and continues along the anterior margin of the helix. The incision is deepened to expose temporal fascia but is kept superficial to it. The inner aspect of the auricular cartilage is attached by strong fibrous bands to the aponeurosis between temporal fascia and mastoid periosteum. These fibrous bands are deliberately cut in the plane of the temporal fascia so that the auricle is mobilized and easily retracted when the mastoid periosteum is elevated. Perichondritis can result from cartilage trauma and ischaemia caused by prolonged forceful retraction. Self-retaining retractors should therefore spread the cartilaginous margins of the incision gently, and if more room is required the incision can easily be extended.

POST-AURAL

The classic approach to the mastoid is by a post-aural incision. This gives excellent access and should certainly be preferred to the permeatal or endaural approach where there is a suspected complication of mastoid disease or it is desired to have free access to the lateral sinus and posterior fossa. An incision made over or just behind the retro-auricular skin fold is cosmetically acceptable. In the adult the incision may safely be extended upwards beyond the zygoma or downwards over the tip of the mastoid. If an exceptional amount of room is required, for example when there is an extensive lateral sinus thrombosis, an additional incision backwards at a right angle may be made. In infants the mastoid tip is small, and the facial nerve and stylomastoid foramen superficial; accordingly the incision should not reach below the middle of the retro-auricular fold.

Ordinarily the skin incision continues through the periosteum which is elevated to expose the cortex of the mastoid. According to Jako (1967) and Smyth and Kerr (1969) a periosteal flap should be dissected separately. The initial incision only goes through the skin and subcutaneous tissues; then the posterior skin edge is retracted and undercut widely to expose periosteum over and beyond the mastoid. This periosteum is now incised on a wide posterior circumference and elevated as a flap pedicled either on the auricle or on the temporal muscle and fascia. The flap is made large if there is an intention to use it for obliteration of the mastoid cavity; if the osseous canal wall and the mastoid cavity are to be preserved a smaller flap is cut and is resutured in position at the completion of the operation. Jako considers that this replaced flap prevents the growth of unwanted granulation tissue into the mastoid cavity and helps to form new bone over the cortex of the mastoid. It also avoids post-operative retro-auricular depression which may collect dirt and make the wearing of spectacles uncomfortable.

MEATAL SKIN FLAPS

The most valuable part of the meatal skin is the thin skin lining the inner two-thirds of the external auditory meatus; this may be used in a variety of ways. In a permeatal approach a small postero–superior meatal or tympano–meatal flap is elevated and later replaced, providing adequate access for tympanotomy or atticotomy operations. In limited myringoplasty operations using an endaural incision, the meatal skin may be elevated either as pedicled flaps, or as a free graft dissected from without inwards under microscopic control. Where there is an anterior bony canal wall overhang its removal is essential so that there is a clear view down to the annulus and to eliminate a narrow angle between the anterior canal wall and the drumhead. The skin of the superior meatal wall should if possible be conserved since it has a rich blood supply and will assist healing and epithelialization. It is referred to as the 'cutis strip' (House, 1960) and the 'vascular strip' (Plester, 1963) (*Figure 11.7*). Many surgeons using endaural or post-aural incisions tend initially to preserve the meatal skin as an intact cuff until the bone dissection is complete. However, especially with an endaural approach, it will greatly improve access if the meatal skin flap is dissected at an early stage and displaced to lie in a position where it is not liable to instrumental trauma. Such a meatal skin flap may be pedicled inferiorly (*Figure 11.8*), or superiorly, or on the tympanic membrane as in a Lempert tympano–meatal flap. The author has usually preferred an inferior pedicled flap and at the end of a wide access operation the meatal skin is easily placed over and behind the facial ridge to partly cover the medial wall and floor of the mastoid cavity.

In a post-aural radical mastoidectomy similar meatal skin flaps may be used.

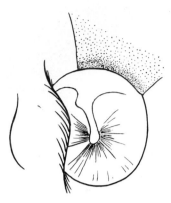

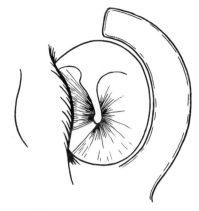

Figure 11.7   Vascular   strip
(after House and Plester)

Figure 11.8   Inferior   pedicled
posterior meatal skin flap

However two alternative methods, taught by the old Vienna school, are worthy of mention. In Körner's meatoplasty (*Figure 11.9*) part of the conchal cartilage is removed and a wide ribbon of posterior meatal skin is cut and stitched inside the

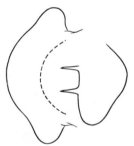

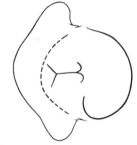

Figure 11.9   Körner's
meatoplasty

Figure 11.10   Siebenmann's
meatoplasty

auricle to help line the outer aspect of the mastoid cavity. In Siebenmann's meatoplasty (*Figure 11.10*) a Y-shaped incision splits the posterior aspect of the meatal skin cuff xtending into the conchal part of the auricle.

ırgical exposure of bone

ccess adequate for the assessment and repair of limited defects in the tympanic mbrane, ossicular chain and mesotympanum may be provided by a transcanal npanotomy in which the outline of the bony canal wall is preserved. If wider access the middle-ear cleft is necessary one of the following three ways may be selected:

A graduated removal of bone from the posterosuperior annulus and outer attic wall backwards to expose the attic and aditus (atticotomy), the mastoid antrum (attico–antrostomy) and, if necessary, the whole mastoid outline (modified radical mastoidectomy). The advantage of this technique is that the surgeon is working from the site of the disease, for example cholesteatoma, and may be able to remove it without the creation of a large cavity that can prove difficult to heal.

(2) First explore the whole mastoid outline, then work forwards to open up the aditus and expose the epitympanum, retaining the whole posterior meatal wall (cortical mastoidectomy); access to the mesotympanum may be provided by dissection of the facial recess (posterior tympanotomy) (*see* p. 262).

(3) Remove the outer part of the posterior canal wall and fully explore the rest of the mastoid outline; the deep posterior meatal and outer attic walls are retained initially as a protective 'bridge'. Then, using the microscope, the condition of the tympanum is assessed and the bridge is removed so that dissection of disease proceeds under clear visual control (modified radical or radical mastoidectomy).

The term radical mastoidectomy is applied here to an operation in which free access is provided to the mastoid and tympanic cavities, the intervening posterior canal wall having been removed almost to the level of the descending portion of the facial nerve. All cells in the mastoid are opened up until the mastoid outline is defined by healthy bone. In the tympanum a methodical microdissection is carried out with excision of any contents which are judged to have undergone irreversible pathological changes. This dissection may include remnants of the tympanic membrane, malleus, incus and fibrous annulus; the pyramid with stapedius muscle and the tensor tympani muscle and its bony semicanal. Special care is taken with the stapes; usually only the footplate survives and if healthy it is retained to protect the integrity of the labyrinth. Labyrinthine function may suffer severely if there is a fracture or a partial dislocation of the footplate. For this reason the oval window region is left until dissection elsewhere is complete and bleeding controlled. Then, with fine suction tips, needles and forceps, the stapes is cleared of matrix, hyaline or granulations. Should dissection of disease in the oval window niche appear hazardous, limited disease may be left and kept under observation. If there is a defect it may be safer, very rarely, to remove the footplate, clean the niche and close the oval window with a plug of fat, vein or fascial graft. Even with such a complete radical mastoidectomy some form of reconstructive tympanoplasty may be attempted. In a modified (or conservative) radical mastoidectomy care is taken, when excising irreversible pathology, to define and preserve any existing hearing mechanism. Thus the preservation of the stapes and of any surviving healthy mucous membrane between the eustachian tube and the labyrinthine windows makes a tympanoplasty operation easier to perform. Accordingly, although the terms 'modified radical' or 'conservative radical' may appear contradictory, the idea which this tries to convey is that the operation is radical with regard to access and excision of disease but conservative with regard to function. This seems acceptable provided that the type of functional conservation or reconstruction is defined.

Functional reconstruction

Tympanoplasty is a deliberate exploration of the middle-ear cleft; firstly to eliminate disease; secondly to assess the functions of the eustachian tube, the ossicular chain and the labyrinthine windows, and to relate these to the known state of hearing by air and bone conduction; and thirdly either to conserve a good functional hearing response or to reconstruct the tympanum according to a type of physiology which must be clearly stated (*see Figure 11.4*). In practice a properly executed myringoplasty is difficult to differentiate from a type 1 or type 2 tympanoplasty.

Accurate nominal description of a particular operation should now be possible, referring to the soft tissue approach, the bone exposure and the tympanic physiology. When surgical improvization is necessary to deal with unusual findings or when exploration is restricted because of the need to conserve good hearing, precise labelling may not be possible.

Tympanoplasty

It is proposed initially to discuss the repair of mechanical or functional defects of the tympanum assuming that irreversible mucosal disease and cholesteatoma are absent. Ideally the ear should have been observed to be free of infection for several months prior to operation.

The prerequisites for a tympanoplasty are that:

(1) Audiometry and tuning-fork tests show hearing to be better by bone conduction than by air conduction.
(2) Adequate cochlear function is present; that is, the hearing threshold by bone conduction averages 30 dB or better over the speech frequencies.
(3) The eustachian tube should be patent. However it is not possible pre-operatively to assess the post-operative function of the tube.
(4) The functional state of the ossicular chain, of the individual ossicles and of the labyrinthine windows has been assessed.
(5) The tympanic mucous membrane appears healthy enough to be safely enclosed inside a new tympanic cavity. It is difficult to estimate the condition of the mucous membrane in the tympanic cavity at operation as it has remarkable powers of recovery and the surgeon must adopt a conservative attitude and not excise mucous membrane in a radical fashion.

Technique in tympanoplasty

Since chronic ear disease is so varied in its manifestations, the technique employed in its surgical management must be adaptable. These techniques are very dependent upon individual and cumulative experience, especially when choosing graft materials for the repair of the tympanic membrane and the ossicular chain. In the discussion of graft materials which follows, an attempt is made to define the general principles which may determine their successful application in a wide variety of tympanoplastic techniques.

Graft materials

AUTOGRAFTS
A considerable variety of fresh autograft material has been used in tympanoplasty:
(a) for the repair of *soft tissue defects*—mucous membrane from the nose and mouth,

conjunctiva, vein, fascia, perichondrium, periosteum, fat and connective tissue; and (b) for the repair of *defects in the ossicular chain* or bony meatal wall—cartilage from rib, nasal septum or auricle, bone from the mastoid or iliac crest—and 'reassembly' of the patient's own ossicles.

In their original tympanoplasty techniques Wullstein and Zöllner employed skin to rebuild the tympanum. Wullstein preferred full thickness skin taken from behind the ear and Zöllner used split thickness skin from the upper arm. Experience has shown that extrameatal skin has several faults:

(1) Although with careful technique free skin grafts will take initially in the tympanum and mastoid, the end result is usually unsatisfactory. The grafts usually become chronically infected and glandular elements in the dermis hypertrophy, giving the graft the appearance of 'peau d'orange' (Thorburn, 1960).

(2) Graft cholesteatoma may occur.

(3) Surface keratin collects on the graft as the normal 'self-cleansing' mechanism of the tympanic membrane is no longer present.

(4) The skin graft may be replaced by granulation tissue and there is a high incidence of breakdown and perforation.

The use of extrameatal skin in the middle ear or mastoid cavity should be avoided if at all possible. The only condition where it is still used is in the repair of developmental defects of the middle ear. The results of these operations are not very satisfactory but there may be no alternative.

Temporal fascia

This is the graft material now preferred by the majority of otologists for tympanoplasty. It has a low metabolic rate and consequently a good survival prospect. Fascia is readily available via an endaural, post-aural or independent incision; it should be taken as high as possible over the surface of the temporal muscle where it is thin and of good quality. It is spread on a hard surface and any redundant fat or connective tissue is scraped away with a sharp knife edge. It may be kept moist and used in its natural state. The common practice is to allow the fascia to dry or even to compress it in a special clamp. In this dry parchment-like state it is easily cut to size and accurately applied in the repair of a tympanic membrane defect. It soon absorbs tissue fluids and recovers a normal appearance.

It is not advisable to dry temporalis fascia grafts by heat as is sometimes recommended as the graft may be devitalized in parts, leading to a higher incidence of graft failure.

Bone and cartilage

A small defect between the tip of the long process of the incus and the head of the stapes may occasionally be repaired with a small bone chip. Usually with erosion of the long process of the incus it is necessary to remove the incus and remodel it so that it fits snugly between the head of the stapes and the handle of the malleus. If the incus is not available the head of the malleus may be used in this way. In the presence of cholesteatoma it may be unwise to use an autograft ossicle since it may carry the seeds of residual disease.

Cartilage from the auricle, tragus or nasal septum has been used for ossicular reconstruction. The results are not always satisfactory in the long term as the material is too soft and pliable and easily becomes displaced or sometimes obsorbed. The strengthening of the cartilage by the introduction of a metal splint has also not proved to be entirely satisfactory in the long term.

HOMOGRAFTS

Homograft materials are being used increasingly for tympanoplasty. It is convenient to have septal cartilage and ossicles readily available in bottles preserved either in 70 per cent alcohol (Smyth) or Cialit 1 in 5000 (Marquet) at ± 3 °C. If preserved in alcohol they are taken from the refrigerator and washed in saline for 1 h before use. Jansen (1963) embeds septal cartilage, sterile, in a special hard plastic material (Palacos).

Homograft perichondrium is preferred by Jansen to fascia for tympanic membrane repair. The material used is really subperichondrial membrane which is stripped from the surface of the preserved cartilage by sharp dissection; the true perichondrium remains with the mucous membrane.

Homograft varicose veins, kept in deep-freeze conditions, have been used successfully for tympanoplasty by King (1964).

Homograft ossicles or tympanic membranes. The temporal bones must be removed from the refrigerated cadaver within 12 h of death. The bones are kept in the deep-freeze until it is convenient to dissect them. If a tympano-ossicular homograft is required it is removed 24 h beforehand under sterile conditions, with the malleus and incus attached, and preserved in Cialit solution. If only the ossicles are wanted these are removed in the course of an ordinary temporal bone dissection and preserved in alcohol or Cialit solution.

Tympanic response to homografts

Homografts in the ear are used for a structural rather than a functional purpose and they seem to be well tolerated so that rejection is not a problem. According to Marquet (1968) the tympanic membrane transplant acts as a temporary scaffolding which is soon replaced by host connective tissue. The fate of incus autografts and homografts in the cat has been reported by Wilson, Pulec and Van Vliet (1966) and by Smyth, Kerr and Jones (1967). The formation of viable sclerotic new bone was observed replacing the enchondral bone of the graft. This was also seen in the incus graft denatured by preservation in absolute alcohol for two weeks.

Smyth and Kerr (1970) reported further on human revision operations where homograft ossicles preserved in alcohol had been used. The ossicles remain as dead bone but they soon acquire a covering of mucous membrane; fibroblasts followed by blood capillaries infiltrate the surface of the dead bone and the actual haversian canals. These fibroblasts seem to function as osteoblasts and gradually dense bone is laid down. Therefore instead of being absorbed as might have been expected, a homograft incus becomes reossified and develops a normal appearance microscopically. An autograft incus behaves in the same way but the process is faster. Homograft nasal cartilage in the ear does not alter its histological appearance. It acquires a mucosal covering and simply remains as inert 'dead' cartilage.

Van den Broek (1968) reports on the fate of incus grafts in rats. He finds an almost identical behaviour in the repositioned autograft and the freshly transplanted homograft incudes. Histological study at intervals of up to two years after operation, shows a varying degree of cellular death quickly followed by formation of new bone around the incus. This bone regeneration is most evident in the long and short processes of the incus, the body being the least viable part. When an incus is denatured by boiling or by preservation in alcohol, no revitalization of bone tissue is observed. The bone remains dead yet it is covered by normal mucoperiosteum. Similar behaviour is observed where the incus is left exposed to the atmosphere for more than 30 min. It seems that in the rat revitalization of the incus depends upon cell survival in the graft. An ossicle transplanted into the middle ear behaves differently from orthotopic bone transplants elsewhere. Incudes transplanted into muscle are resorbed, the autograft more slowly than the homograft or denatured ossicle, and the histological features suggest a transplantion reaction, a feature not observed in the middle ear.

HETEROGRAFTS

Tissue membranes from other animal species, particularly the calf, have been employed successfully in tympanoplasty but their use is still in the experimental stage.

INERT MATERIALS

Metals, for example stainless steel and tantalum wire, and plastics, for example polyvinylchloride (polythene), polytetrafluorethylene (Teflon) and silicone rubber (Silastic), have been used extensively in reconstructive ear surgery. On the whole these have been well accepted provided that contact with the tympanic membrane is avoided. However, it seems reasonable that body tissues, autograft or homograft, should where possible be preferred to metal or plastics. There is a place for the use of stainless steel wire in the operation of ossicular chain repair as greater accuracy in placement and hence better hearing results can be obtained. Incus autografts or homografts are difficult to shape and place exactly in the right position.

Management of small perforations or tears of the tympanic membrane

A small non-marginal perforation of the tympanic membrane usually heals if the outer epithelium is removed, scarified or cauterized a few times with trichloracetic acid for about 2 mm around the circumference of the perforation. Mucosal growth is now possible from the inner aspect of the perforation and is assisted if the perforation is temporarily closed with connective tissue, fat or gel-foam soaked in blood. A traumatic perforation or tear of the tympanic membrane, whether central or marginal, will readily heal if the ear is kept dry and is protected.

Transcanal tympanoplasty

Myringoplasty simply means the repair of a defect or perforation of the tympanic membrane. Wullstein (1963) stressed that myringoplasty should never be an independent operation but always part of a transcanal tympanoplasty. He has in mind that it is important to assess the condition of the mucous membrane, the eustachian tube, the ossicular chain and the labyrinthine windows. Accordingly, any defect in the ossicular chain should be repaired and, if keratinizing epithelium or a small cholesteatoma is uncovered, then it is excised with great care since none must be enclosed.

INDICATIONS

Transcanal tympanoplasty is usually reserved for dry ears. Within the limitations of access imposed by the transcanal technique, perforations of the tympanic membrane and some defects in the ossicular chain may be successfully repaired. This technique may be appropriate for the ear which has the active disease successfully treated by microscopic suction clearance but still has a defect in the tympanic membrane or ossicular chain.

CONTRAINDICATIONS

The presence of active or inaccessible disease. Such disease may be controlled by further treatment; otherwise a wide access technique should be employed.

Technique

PERMEATAL

If the external auditory meatus is reasonably wide and has no anterior overhang, it is possible to repair the tympanic membrane defect without an endaural incision.

A transverse incision is made over the temporal region just above the pinna and the temporalis fascia is exposed and a graft is taken. The incision which will be above the hair line is then sutured.

The tympanic membrane is then visualized with speculum and microscope and the fibrous tissue lining the inside of the defect is excised with a sharp sickle knife. An incision is then made between the thinner skin of the deep meatus and the thicker skin of the outer meatus. The flap of thin skin is then carefully elevated from the posterior meatal wall in continuity with the tympanic membrane. The tympanum and ossicular chain are examined and if all is in order, the fascial graft is insinuated to lie beneath the meatal flap and extend beneath the tympanic membrane. The use of suction with a footswitch that can interrupt vacuum greatly facilitates this procedure. If the perforation is a large one, gelatin foam may be placed beneath the graft to support it provided that the mucous membrane of the middle ear has not been damaged. Small pieces of thin silastic film can be placed on the surface of the graft overlapping the remnants of the tympanic membrane. They hold the graft in position and act as a splint. A dressing of gelatin foam is placed on top of the silastic and a final dressing of gauze soaked in 'BIPP' paste is put in the external meatus.

ENDAURAL

Myringoplasty is usually performed with an endaural incision as this gives better access.

An incision about 3 cm in length is made anterior to the tragus, starting at the meatal opening. The skin and subcutaneous tissues are incised and the fascia over the temporalis muscle is exposed. A self-retaining retractor is inserted and a piece of temporalis fascia is removed for the graft. The graft is scraped to remove muscle and fat and is left to dry in the air.

The retractor is loosened and the incision is carried over the posterior meatal wall at the junction of the thick skin of the outer third of the external auditory meatus with the thin meatal wall skin lining the inner two thirds of the meatus. The posterior meatal wall skin is elevated and held in the posterior jaw of the retractor which is now reintroduced. Occasionally, if there is a very narrow external canal or if there is an overhang of bone anteriorly, it is necessary to raise a flap of meatal skin anteriorly and then enlarge the bony canal with a drill and burr. It is essential for the anterior aspect of the ear canal to be seen completely.

The remainder of the operation follows the description of the permeatal operation. If the mobility of the tympanic membrane is impaired by hyaline plaques, they must be removed. The mobility of the ossicular chain is tested and the round window reflex observed if possible. The graft is placed beneath thin meatal wall skin and extends anteriorly beneath the defect and the handle of the malleus. It is fixed in position as previously described.

This technique has many advantages over the onlay technique as it is easier to perform and the incidence of post-operative perforation is less. The risk of enclosing epithelial elements is much less as the graft is beneath the epithelium.

POST-AURAL

The post-aural route gives good exposure of an anterior perforation and drilling of the anterior meatal wall is seldom required with this approach. A posterior meatal wall flap is raised and the technique is on similar lines to the one described for the endaural route.

AFTER-CARE

Antibiotic cover is provided for five days when any sutures are removed. The gel-foam is left undisturbed and removed by suction after two to three weeks, when the drumhead should be healed. Any granulations outside the plane of epithelial growth are removed with forceps rather then by use of caustic agents. If there is normal eustachian tubal function, post-operative inflation is not necessary. Otherwise the patient is taught Valsalva's manoeuvre, or gentle politzerization is practised from two weeks after operation.

Modifications

(1) Where some degree of tympanic mucosal infection is present Plester (1963) advocates drainage by the provision of an antrostomy opening made with a drill from the cortex of the mastoid. A polythene tube is inserted and is removed a few days after any discharge has settled. In such a case, if the mucosal infection is diffuse, a cortical mastoidectomy may be preferable.

(2) Marquet (1966, 1968) has evolved a technique of myringoplasty by eardrum transplantation. A bank of cadaver tympanic membranes is established preserved in Cialit solution 1 in 5000. The outer epithelium of the transplant eardrum is discarded and only the mesodermic elements are retained; these comprise the middle fibrous layer, the mucous membrane, the fibrous annulus, possibly the malleus itself and sometimes the periosteum adjacent to the fibrous annulus. For a limited repair only a segment of the transplant drum is used.

Marquet employs a very conservative permeatal technique. The fibrous rim of the perforation is removed and the surface epithelium of the tympanic membrane is dissected from within outwards. For a small central or segmental perforation this dissection to prepare a bed for the graft stops at the annulus; for a large perforation the deep meatal skin is also elevated as several flaps radiating beyond the level of the annulus and in this case the meatal periosteum is included with the transplant. Marquet says that since the homograft tympanic membrane retains the fibrous annulus, it fits perfectly and does not need any support within the tympanum. In healed conditions favourable for myringoplasty he obtains good results by this technique in over 90 per cent of cases. This acceptance rate is encouraging although the results are no better than those obtained with fascia in transcanal myringoplasty operations. However, an interesting application may be the use of a homograft tympanic membrane with malleus attached where there is a defect in the tympanic membrane together with loss of the malleus and incus. The transplant membrane should be rotated so that the head of the malleus makes contact with the head of the stapes.

Special technical problems in tympanoplasty

CICATRIZATION OF THE MUCOUS MEMBRANE AND TYMPANOSCLEROSIS

Small deposits of hyaline may be ignored but large plaques impair the mobility of the ossicles and of the tympanic membrane. Removal of the plaque involves the loss of some healthy mucous membrane so that scars or adhesions will result. Should the tympanic mucous membrane be badly deficient steps must be taken to encourage its regeneration otherwise grafts become fixed in scar tissue. Paraffin wax has been used for this purpose but necessitates a staged technique (Rambo, 1958, 1965). Silicone sheet and Teflon film were introduced by House and Sheehy (1963) and Supramid by Sheehy (1970) to encourage mucosal regeneration and to prevent cicatrization and adhesion between the fascial graft and the medial tympanic wall. Silicone sheet 0.125 mm thick, is tailored to lie flat on the medial tympanic wall extending from the eustachian tube to the labyrinthine windows. It is well tolerated and need not be removed. These refinements of technique should try to make provision for the ventilation of any part of the middle-ear cleft enclosed by the tympanoplasty.

In advanced tympanosclerosis, the stapes may be buried in the deposits. It is possible to dissect the plaques away from the stapes in some cases and to free it. It is, however, a difficult procedure and if the oval window is opened and perilymph escapes, a sensorineural deafness may result. The deposits tend to recur and fix the stapes again and the long-term results of this procedure are poor. Because of the poor results of this method, some surgeons (Gibb, 1976) advocate stapedectomy with a Teflon piston. It is the author's experience that this procedure in tympanosclerosis may give good immediate results but the long-term hearing results are poor as senorineural deafness will develop in a high proportion of patients after such an operation. Closure of the perforation and the provision of a hearing aid is a safer method of treatment in many cases of tympanosclerosis.

REPAIR OF DEFECTS IN THE OSSSICULAR CHAIN

The determination of the precise cause of an ossicular fixation or defect requires careful microscopic examination and palpation with a fine probe. Transmission from the malleus, incus or stapes through the labyrinthine fluids to the round window is an interesting observation but should be done gently lest it cause a fracture of the ossicles or a hydraulic injury to the labyrinth. Where there is healthy tympanic mucosa an immediate repair of the ossicular defect may be attempted. In the presence of cicatrization or mucosal loss this repair must be combined with the measures already described to prevent a recurrence of adhesions. Management will be discussed relative to the particular defects involving the ossicular chain:

(1) Fixation of the malleus/incus complex may occur by mucosal hyperplasia, hyaline or bone within the confined space of an intact canal or outer attic wall. By careful microdissection it may be possible to free the ossicles. Where mucosa, hyaline or bone is removed refixation will readily occur; this possibility is minimized by placing silicone sheet or Teflon film between apposing bone surfaces where there is no protective mucous membrane.

(2) Incus. The long process of the incus has a precarious blood supply (Alberti, 1963) and is commonly eroded in chronic ear disease. Rarely a small defect between the tip of the long process and the head of the stapes may be bridged with a bone chip. In the absence of disease a substantial defect is best corrected by 'incus version' (malleus-stapes assembly). The incus is removed and shaped so that it fits over the head of the stapes and makes stable contact with the malleus; alternatively the short process may be directed to fit under the handle of the malleus. If the incus is deficient the head of the malleus, or a homograft incus, may be used in a similar way.

(3) Stapes. (a) Fixation of the stapes by hyaline (tympanosclerosis) is common; even where this involvement is diffuse successful dissection is possible but refixation readily occurs. Fixation by hyaline limited to the stapedius tendon is easily corrected. (b) Fixation limited to the footplate, caused either by otosclerosis or tympanosclerosis, may occur along with a simple perforation of the tympanic membrane. If the incus and malleus are intact and mobile the perforation is repaired; limited stapes mobilization may be attempted and if unsuccessful a stapedectomy operation performed subsequently. (c) Loss of the head and crura of the stapes is often associated with collapse or perforation of the posterior segment of the tympanic membrane. With a mobile footplate an attempt should be made to bridge the gap between the footplate and the malleus or tympanic membrane. An autograft incus is not really long enough unless the long process has survived. Marquet recommends the use of a homograft incus with the tip of the long process centred on the footplate and the body and short process under the handle of the malleus. Jansen (1963, 1968) prefers to fashion an L- or T-shaped prosthesis made from homograft septal cartilage reinforced with stainless steel wire to connect the footplate with the tympanic membrane or malleus. These and other ingenious techniques devised for this purpose are illustrated in *Figure 11.11*. Details of two of these techniques, incus transposition and homograft malleus, are illustrated in *Figures 11.12* and *11.13* respectively.

The disadvantages of homograft tympanoplasty is that it is a time-consuming method involving the obtaining and preparing of the homograft and meticulous surgery in a bloodless field. Repair of tympanic membrane defects by fascial grafts and modern ossicular chain reconstruction techniques give satisfactory healing and functional results and will be the choice of most surgeons today.

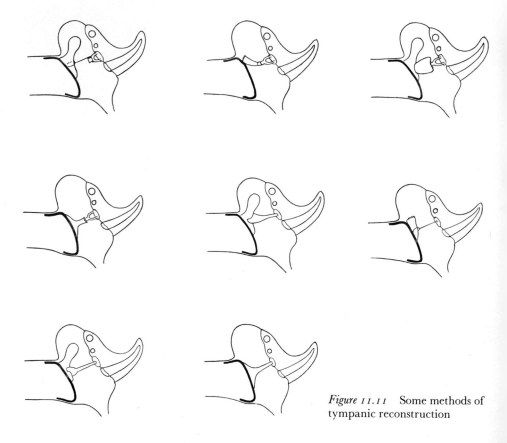

Figure 11.11   Some methods of tympanic reconstruction

(4) For a major reconstruction involving the tympanic membrane and ossicles it may be convenient to use a transplant membrane with malleus and incus attached—a tympano-ossicular homograft. By the selection of ears which are free of active disease for this operation, Marquet obtained satisfactory healing and good functional results in 78 per cent. Where this reconstruction was carried out in the presence of active chronic disease, House, Glasscock and Sheehy (1969) obtained satisfactory healing in 75 per cent but the immediate functional results were poor. Smyth and Kerr (1969) report 65 per cent satisfactory healing in a small controlled series with active disease; they compared this with 98 per cent successful healing using fascia and ossicular reconstruction techniques as described in combined approach tympanoplasty.

(5) Schiller (1970) has described a method of reconstruction of the ossicular chain when the malleus is absent using a stainless steel wire attached to a bone graft embedded between two layers of the fascial graft used to repair the tympanic membrane defect. He has done over 40 of these cases and in only one has the prosthesis been extruded. The operation is called malleomyringo–stapedioplasty and very accurate reconstruction can be obtained by this technique. (*Figure 11.14*)

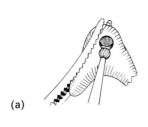

(a)

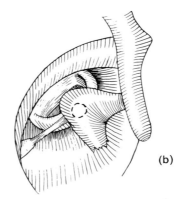

(b)

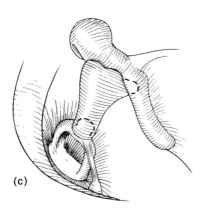

(c)

Figure 11.12 Incus transposition. (a) The new incus is refashioned with a fine polishing burr; it can be placed in position (b) as a 'horizontal' incus or (c) as a vertical incus. The 'horizontal' incus is the easier method but is less stable

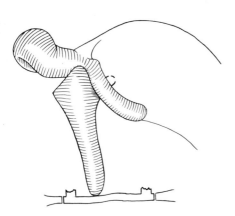

Figure 11.13 Missing incus and super-structure. A homograft malleus can be fashioned as shown and placed in contact with a mobile footplate. If the footplate is fixed it is removed and a vein or fascial graft placed over the oval window

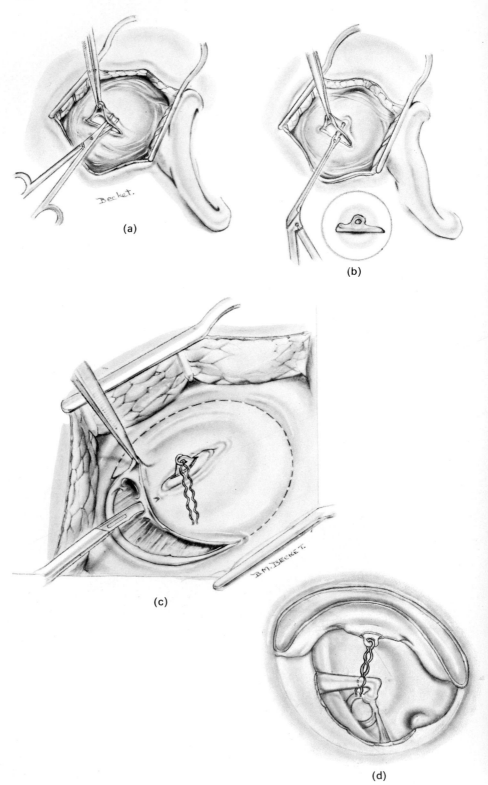

(a)

(b)

(c)

(d)

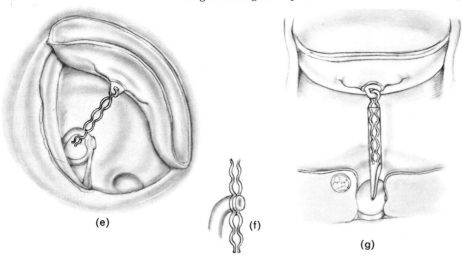

(e)

(f)

(g)

Figure 11.14   Schiller's operation of malleomyringoplasty and ossicular reconstruction.
(a) A tunnel is constructed between the loose areolar tissue layer and the underlying temporalis fascia after making a small incision through the areolar layer of the fascia. (b) The malleus replacement graft is inserted into the tunnel created until it is completely buried beneath the loose areolar layer and temporalis fascia tissue layers. The approximate shape of the bone graft is shown in the insert. (c) The requisite layer of composite graft is dissected from the underlying temporalis muscle. It is easier to attach and fix wire to the prosthesis before the composite graft is excised. (d) The composite graft reproduces the tympanic membrane and the handle of the 'malleus' positioned in the middle ear with its posterior section reflected forwards. The prosthesis connects the malleus replacement bone to the long process of the incus. (e) The prosthesis connects the graft to the stapedial crus. (f) The ossicle is embraced between the indentations of the corrugated limbs of the prosthesis. (g) If the crura are missing the wire clip prosthesis is inserted into a piece of polythene tubing which rests on the stapes footplate

Surgical management of active attico–antral disease

Introduction

The management of attico–antral disease is simplified if the particular case can be classified under one of the following headings:

(1) Reasonably safe: the disease appears inactive, limited and accessible.
(2) Potentially dangerous: the disease appears active, usually with otorrhoea, and is not clearly accessible for treatment from the meatus.
(3) Dangerous: active disease extends beyond the tympanum into the attic or mastoid segments so that it is not accessible; this group includes all cases with symptoms suggesting an early complication.
(4) Uncertain: there is temporary difficulty with the assessment, possibly on account of an acute pyogenic exacerbation or an otitis externa.

The potentially dangerous or uncertain cases can usually be re-assessed a reasonably safe or dangerous following further observation and with treatment by aural toilet or microscopic suction clearance. The use of ear drops is not recommended for chronic attico–antral disease unless required for treatment of an associated otitis externa; then, drops containing polymyxin B sulphate, neomycin and hydrocortisone may be indicated. The insufflation of boracic powder containing 1 per cent iodine following aural toilet may help to dry out the tympanic region. If granulations persist after suction they may be reduced with 10 per cent silver nitrate on a fine cotton tip or by trichloracetic acid applied very sparingly and precisely. An acute pyogenic exacerbation of chronic infection may require treatment with an appropriate antibiotic but such a case must be regarded as potentially dangerous.

The cooperation of the patient should be enlisted by an explanation of the nature of the disease and its prognosis with regard to both safety and influence on the hearing. In the reasonably safe group it is sufficient to stress the need for prolonged follow-up observation at 3-, 6- or 12-monthly intervals, as indicated for the particular case. At each visit the condition of the ear is re-assessed and any fresh accumulation of keratin removed. The patient is warned to keep water out of the ear and to report for earlier examination if there is a recurrence of otorrhoea, an increase of deafness or any vertigo, pain or headache.

In the dangerous group the patient is not ill, unless there is a threatening complication, and he may consider a mastoid type of operation an unnecessarily serious proposal. It is explained that it is relatively safe to operate while the disease is quiescent and that the object is to prevent those very dangers of intracranial complication associated in the public mind with mastoid disease. The social benefit of a dry ear and freedom from a foetid discharge is readily appreciated. The hearing position is also discussed and it is stressed that, while the elimination of disease must take priority, tympanoplastic procedures may enable the otologist to preserve or improve the hearing. If the patient has a reasonably safe ear and the main complaint is deafness, then the indications for tympanoplasty in one or more stages are fully assessed and explained.

In children and in some adults it may be advisable to concentrate on the control of active disease so that a hearing aid can be worn in comfort. The very deaf elderly patient, whose only hearing ear has poor cochlear function and dangerous disease, is a special problem. The risk to cochlear function is slight when excision of disease is confined to the mastoid and epitympanum. The mesotympanic disease may then be treated conservatively by aural toilet and the patient will still be able to use a hearing aid.

Microscopic suction clearance

Suction clearance is both a detailed microscopic examination of the ear with suction toilet and a surgical method of treatment. It is never a definitive procedure and the extent of the intervention varies according to the type and extent of disease and with the experience, enthusiasm and skill of the responsible otologist. For example, it may reasonably include an atticotomy or ossiculectomy where such bone removal is necessary to provide access to limited disease.

Although general anaesthesia may be advisable for children and nervous adults, especially for a first examination, suction clearance is usually an out-patient or 'office' procedure. It should be explained to the patient that there are distinct advantages in carrying out suction clearance with no anaesthesia or with limited local anasthesia. The patient's cooperation is of value since the disease may hide sensitive structures or landmarks which must be conserved. He is instructed to complain at once if there is any pain or vertigo, indications that the procedure is being unwisely extended. The otologist is thereby trained to exercise that delicacy of touch in instrumentation which is essential if any useful information or benefit is to be gained. There is therefore a common interest on the part of patient and otologist that suction clearance should be carried out with no pain and with only minimal and tolerable discomfort.

TECHNIQUE

The approach is permeatal, preferably through a blackened slotted speculum. The ear is cleaned with 1 per cent Cetavlon and, when necessary, local anaesthetic is injected into the outer posterosuperior meatal wall. The external meatus is cleared of wax and keratin. Any keratin over the surface of the drumhead, or possibly hidden in an attic or posterior tympanic recess, is engaged by fine suction cannulae and peeled off or extracted. It may be necessary to loosen adherent or impacted crusts or keratin with a fine-angled probe before they can be removed by suction. When using small cupped crocodile forceps or dissectors for the removal of granulations or impacted cholesteatoma, the view must be kept clear of blood with a fine angled suction cannula in the free hand. Full advantage is taken of the mobility, angulation of view and the selection of magnifications available when using the microscope by the permeatal approach.

OBJECTIVES AND LIMITATIONS

(1) To remove accessible disease including keratin, granulations and cholesteatoma matrix where possible from the tympanic region, attic and aditus. It is an odd feature that there is usually an excess of deep meatal keratin so long as active attico–antral disease persists and this should also be removed.

(2) To note where disease extends beyond reasonable access, for example in relation to attic, aditus and sinus tympani.

(3) To preserve what remains of the mucosal layer of the tympanic membrane, especially where this has survived in a healthy state underneath a mass of cholesteatoma. If the membrane is destroyed, the condition of the mucosa on the medial tympanic wall is assessed.

(4) To observe the state of the individual ossicles, the mobility of the ossicular chain and where possible the labyrinthine windows.

(5) To assess the extent to which spontaneous healing by the tympanic mucous membrane has established a closed, air-containing tympanic cavity, in continuity with the eustachian tube. The patient may be able to assist by performing Valsalva's manoeuvre.

(6) The tympanic physiology can now be determined by relating the sound pressure transformer mechanism of the tympanum, with provision of sound protection for the round window. Alternatively, a defective tympanic membrane may be persuaded to heal in a physiological manner, assisted by further suction clearance. Careful observation indicates that better hearing by type 3 and type 4 physiology

can occur by spontaneous healing than is ever achieved by a planned tympanoplasty.

(7) The limitations of suction clearance should be self-evident. Subjective and objective improvement is usually noted, so that patient and otologist are easily lulled into a state of false security. With the potentially dangerous case the otologist must accept the responsibility, after repeating microscopic suction clearance a few times, to advise operation where the disease has not become reasonably safe. Treatment for this limited period, however, reduces the activity of the disease and gives an understanding of potential tympanic physiology which will be of value at operation.

PREVENTION OF ATTIC CHOLESTEATOMA

Schiller has described a method of rectifying and strengthening specified abnormalities of the pars flaccida by means of a temporalis fascia graft and he gives the following indications for this operation.

(1) If a mass of epithelial debris accumulates in the pit of a retracted pars flaccida. Particularly so if it persists in reforming in spite of repeated suction clearance or, if the mass is encountered in the sound ear of a patient who has previously been subjected to mastoid surgery for cholesteatoma.

(2) If the surface epithelium of the pars flaccida is destroyed by desquamated hyperkeratotic plaques which persist in reforming after suction clearance.

(3) If conditions (1) or (2) are encountered in a patient who is unable to attend repeatedly for observation.

(4) If a clean attic perforation is detected and all evidence of attic disease has been excluded.

Spontaneous healing

It is significant that hearing by type 2, 3 or 4 mechanisms achieved through spontaneous healing is often better than that obtained by tympanoplasty. This observation applies to limited disease, possibly treated by microscopic suction clearance and also to more extensive attico–antral disease, suitably treated by modified radical mastoidectomy. This useful hearing usually depends upon a tympanum of very odd appearance, closed by a thin 'false' two-layer membrane; somehow the ossicles have remained freely mobile and where only the stapes footplate survives, it is covered by a thin epithelium without intervening fibrous tissue.

The less favourable hearing after tympanoplasty may be due to fibrosis limiting the mobility of the ossicles and drumhead; in type 4 conditions it commonly happens that the oval window niche fills in with a thick cushion of fibrous tissue. Despite these problems a reasonable measure of success should attend carefully-planned tympanoplasty operations. The surgeon has a difficult task. He must be radical about excision of disease, conservative with spontaneous healing responses, sensitive about cochlear function, assured that his reconstruction will achieve stable healing, and conscious always that the patient has little conception of these problems and expects to recover his hearing and to be cured of his ear discharge.

Wide access techniques

Wide access techniques for the treatment of active inaccessible chronic disease may be regarded as the complement of the narrow transcanal techniques already described for the treatment of healed chronic otitis media. Any form of surgery adopted for the treatment of active chronic suppurative otitis media must satisfy three important principles:

(1) Access to the disease must be adequate.
(2) Excision of all irreversible chronic disease must be complete.
(3) The technique must be compatible with long-term safety and security. In the final part of this chapter a detailed description of combined approach tympanoplasty is given. The preservation of an intact canal wall and the deliberate enclosure of the mastoid cavity are features of this technique which are at variance with the established wide access techniques which will now be described.

SURGICAL APPROACH

The principles governing the choice of soft-tissue approach and bone access have already been discussed. The wide access must not only be sufficient to give surgical exposure of the disease, but it must also create post-operative meatal access to a tympanomastoid cavity having a smoothly bevelled outline, so that healing by granulation and epithelialization may be easily accomplished. If part of the middle-ear cleft is conserved and enclosed, provision should be made, directly or indirectly, for its ventilation via the eustachian tube. An atticotomy may provide adequate access to deal with limited attic disease; some surgeons have become very skilled in the performance of this operation by a permeatal approach but for most an endaural approach gives more 'freedom of manoeuvre'. If the disease extends beyond the attic a decision must be taken either to remove more bone until the antrum is exposed (attico–antrostomy), or to explore the mastoid outline first and then to have a fresh look at the state of the tympanic segment (modified radical mastoidectomy).

DISSECTION OF DISEASE

In relation to the mastoid and attic, complete excision of the disease should be possible. The disease in question includes cholesteatoma, cholesterol granuloma, mucosal hyperplasia, granulation tissue and osteitis or sequestration of any part of the temporal bone or ossicles. Fortunately in these cases the mastoid is not usually well pneumatized but when it is, the cells must be thoroughly opened up until the healthy bone of the mastoid outline is reached. Limited exposure of healthy lateral sinus or dura is relatively harmless, provided the fact is immediately recognized so that they are not injured. Bleeding from the lateral sinus produced by minor trauma is characteristically very profuse; it is arrested by immediate direct pressure with a small pack followed by a muscle graft. When the lateral sinus or dura is exposed by disease, there is usually reactive fibrous thickening, with or without symptoms of a perisinus or extradural abscess. Further bone should be removed until a healthy margin of dura or lateral sinus is reached.

If mastoid tip development creates a cavity problem, the tip is removed and the soft tissue allowed to fall in. Fortunately this is seldom necessary since it causes a stiff neck and considerable post-operative pain. One clear indication for removal of the tip is when the disease has extended through its deep surface to form a Bezold's abscess beneath the sternomastoid muscle.

Accurate dissection of disease in the tympanum requires microscopic control. The simple principle to follow is that the disease is uncovered as completely as the surgical anatomical conditions permit. This may involve removal of the 'bridge', the outer attic wall and the deep posterior meatal wall, superficial and anterior to the descending part of the facial nerve. This latter exposure of the sinus tympani should be delayed until the horizontal part of the facial canal has been identified and the anaesthetist can watch the face in case there is a warning twitch.

Consider the common situation where attic cholesteatoma invades the tympanum. A fine-angled dissector is introduced at the level of the aditus and peels the matrix forwards and downwards while the field is kept clear with a small suction cannula. The surgeon must be constantly alert so that he will recognize and conserve any mucosal barrier shutting off the tympanum from disease. If cholesteatoma goes superficial to the malleus and incus, leaving the ossicular chain and tympanum intact, the operation is completed as a modified radical mastoidectomy with type 2 mechanism (*see Figure 11.4*). If undermined by cholesteatoma or if the long process is defective, the incus is removed and the head of the malleus is cut off at the neck. This gives excellent access to the epitympanum so that further dissection towards the mesotympanum is easier. The horizontal part of the facial canal, the handle of malleus and the stapes are useful landmarks, and if there is an intact mucosal barrier closing the tympanum at this level, the operation is completed as a modified radical mastoidectomy with type 3 mechanism. However, cholesteatoma may continue across the facial canal into the oval window niche and delicate dissection, with straight or angled needles, lifts the matrix to uncover the stapes. As soon as one edge of the footplate can be watched in case of any slight movement, the remainder of the stapes is cleaned without danger of dislocation. Commonly the head and one or both crura are destroyed but if the round window niche and the tympanum are closed off by a mucosal barrier, the operation is completed as a modified radical mastoidectomy with type 4 mechanism. Similarly more extensive disease may be removed and an air-containing hypotympanic tunnel survives to connect the round window niche to the eustachian tube.

When cholesteatoma infiltrates more extensively and is associated with secondary infection of the mesotympanum, the main problem is to assess the state of the tympanic contents. Any healthy remnant of the drumhead is conserved and as the fibrous annulus nearly always survives, together they provide a useful 'frame' for a new tympanic membrane. Slight mucosal swelling may recover, once disease in the tympanum and mastoid has been removed. Long-standing chronic infection causes the mucosa to become oedematous and polypoid and there is no real hope that it can revert to normal. When tympanoplasty is being considered it is wiser to remove all such doubtful mucosa and to rely on regeneration from any healthy mucosal remnants in the hypotympanum and eustachian tube. Fortunately, mucosa over the promontory and in the anterior part of the tympanum, being more remote from the main attico–antral disease, frequently survives in good condition.

With widespread disease and no hope of reconstruction, it is the duty of the otologist to carry out a complete *radical mastoidectomy*. Removal of the fibrous annulus and deep meatal wall provides access to the tympanic part of the eustachian tube, peritubal cells, hypotympanic cells and sinus tympani which are then meticulously cleared of disease with a fine curette or even a small cutting burr. The tensor tympani semicanal and muscle, the stapedius and pyramid are also removed. Finally, there remains only the stark outline of the anterior osseous labyrinth, with oval and round windows cleanly dissected, crossed by the facial nerve. Should the labyrinth be invaded, the disease is followed above and below the facial nerve which may be the only surviving structure.

CHOLESTEATOMA MATRIX

Majority opinion amongst otologists favours complete removal of the matrix, regarding it as having potential infiltrative or erosive qualities not possessed by ordinary meatal skin. The opposite view is strongly argued by Baron (1953) and supported by Plester (1961) and others. Baron recommends full exposure and marsupialization of the cholesteatoma sac as in a modified radical mastoidectomy. Matrix is retained to protect the middle-ear structures and to promote rapid healing of a sclerotic mastoid cavity. It may even be retained over exposed dura, lateral sinus, facial nerve or labyrinth fistula. Matrix is removed when necessary to provide access to a pneumatized mastoid, diseased perilabyrinthine, retrofacial or petrous tip cells, and also if there are infected granulations under the matrix or if an intracranial complication is suspected.

In a modified radical mastoidectomy with good access to the tympanum and mastoid, it appears reasonable to imitate spontaneous healing by preserving healthy matrix close to the tympanic membrane, especially when this helps in the creation of a successful type 2, 3 or 4 hearing mechanism. Matrix may also be safely used to supplement meatal skin flaps in the provision of epithelial cover for fascial tympanoplastic reconstructions. However, when in doubt, it is always safer to remove matrix since a well constructed temporal fascia tympanoplasty readily becomes epithelialized from adjacent meatal skin flaps.

Wide access tympanoplasty

Most of our early experience in tympanoplasty has developed within the limitations imposed by the concept that a wide access tympanomastoid cavity was inevitable. For details of techniques for the repair of the tympanic membrane and ossicular chain the reader is referred to transcanal tympanoplasty and combined approach tympanoplasty.

TYPE 2 RECONSTRUCTION

While some form of 'bridge' is an asset for the protection of the ossicular chain and for the support of a fascial graft, it is not an essential precondition for a type 2 conservation or reconstruction. After excision of disease there may be an intact ossicular chain with a small tympanic membrane defect on one side of the incus. Such a defect should be closed with a small plug of fascia or connective tissue or by the dissection and rotation of a flap of deep meatal skin. Under suitable conditions more ambitious type 2 reconstructions may be attempted with the use of fascia and homograft ossicles or cartilage.

TYPE 3 AND 4 RECONSTRUCTIONS

Since type 3 and 4 mechanisms have a small or flat middle ear they fit more easily into the concept of a nicely epithelialized, wide access, tympanomastoid cavity. This applies especially where the ear is known to have good hearing and it has been possible to conserve an established type 3 or 4 mechanism. A type 3 reconstruction is considered when at the completion of the dissection of disease the mesotympanum is exposed, with healthy mucosa over the promontory, and there is an intact mobile stapes. Sufficient epithelium is elevated from any remnant of the tympanic membrane and handle of malleus to make a bed for the fascial graft. It may be necessary to extend the dissection to the anterior meatal skin when the perforation reaches the anterior sulcus. Fascia is fitted on the plane of the drum remnant and the medial wall of the attic; the fascia should be tented slightly by the projecting head of the stapes. Should there be healthy mucosa over the medial tympanic wall no protection or support for the graft is necessary. However, if the mucosa is deficient so that the graft will easily adhere to it, then a piece of silicone sheet is fitted over the medial tympanic wall from the eustachian tube to the labyrinthine windows, a hole being cut in it for the stapes. Finally meatal skin is fitted marginally over the fascia and both are secured with gelfoam.

Type 3 tympanoplasty can give useful hearing improvement with a hearing level around 25 dB and the results are more certain in the hands of the surgeon with limited experience. This procedure is of value, is relatively easy to perform and is safe. It is possible when the ear is healed to contemplate further surgery with a view to restoration of the ossicular chain.

A type 4 reconstruction is considered when the only stapes remnant is a freely mobile footplate. The object is to exteriorize the footplate and provide sound protection for the window. This is the 'kleine Pauke' of the German writers. Any mucous membrane which remains over the lower aspect of the oval window niche and over the tensor tympani semicanal is dissected and everted to provide a mucosal lining for the upper part of the new tympanic cavity. The channel between eustachian tube and round window is outlined with silicone sheet and then covered with fascia. The fascia should extend for a few millimetres on to the meatal wall; above, it should cover the tensor tympani semicanal but not the oval window niche. A piece of thin meatal skin or matrix is placed over the stapes footplate extending on to the adjacent fascia. If rapid epithelialization of the oval window niche can be encouraged this will prevent it becoming filled in with fibrous tissue. The meatal skin flaps should overlap the fascia marginally and the reconstruction is supported with gel-foam.

Type 4 reconstruction seldom produces useful hearing gain and most surgeons today will carry out one of the methods of ossicular chain repair either as a primary, or second stage procedure.

TYPE 5 TYMPANOPLASTY

Where there is marked tympanosclerotic fixation of the drumhead and ossicular chain, especially where the stapes itself is much involved, restoration of a mobile and functioning tympanic membrane and ossicular chain may not be possible. Under these conditions, given good cochlear function, the simplest and safest method to restore hearing may be by fenestration of the lateral semicircular canal. Such a type 5 tympanoplasty can only be safely performed in two stages and this requires a wide access technique. A decision is reached at the first operation when chronic disease is eliminated; access is provided to the prominence of the lateral semicircular canal, the incus and the head of malleus are removed, and a type 3 reconstruction is completed ignoring the fixation of the stapes. Then some six months later, when the ear is securely healed, a small flap is raised and a fenestra is created in the lateral semicircular canal. It is an odd paradox that a fenestration operation is now seldom performed for deafness due to otosclerosis yet it may still be of value in chronic otitis media. Although type 5 tympanoplasty may be a safer procedure than stapedectomy in tympanosclerosis as regards preservation of cochlear function, it should be remembered that fenestration of the lateral semicircular canal produces certain disabilities. The patient may not swim or dive, the cavity requires meticulous after-care and the hearing level at the best will be around 25 dB.

STAPEDECTOMY

When a fixed stapes is recognized during an operation for repair of the tympanic membrane, a stapedectomy may be planned as a second stage operation provided that the malleus and incus are intact and mobile and there is good cochlear function.

The above account of tympanoplasty according to the principles of Wullstein and Zöllner written by the late Ian Thorburn is an excellent description of classic tympanoplasty.

Although the hearing results of these older methods are not as good as those obtained in the new techniques, which will be described later, useful hearing improvement is frequently obtained, particularly in type 3 tympanoplasty. These older methods have proved to be safe over a long period of time and are technically easier to perform. They still have a useful place in otology.

The fixed stapes may be the result of otosclerosis or tympanosclerosis and it is the author's experience that there is a considerable risk of delayed sensorineural deafness after stapedectomy when the stapes is fixed by tympanosclerotic deposits.

Hearing and mastoid cavity problems in tympanoplasty

HEARING

A main objective in the development of tympanoplasty has been the restoration of hearing. Success in this respect may be judged partly in relation to conservation of existing serviceable hearing and partly by the restoration of poor hearing to a serviceable level. Serviceable hearing may be defined as an average loss of 40 dB or better over the speech frequencies 500, 1000, and 2000 Hz (ISO).

An alternative yardstick is the closure of the air–bone gap. This could reasonably apply to type 1 or type 2 tympanoplasties but is more difficult to realize in type 3 or 4 because of the loss of lever advantage. Reliable statistics are not readily available but it will be generally agreed that the hearing reaches a serviceable level in about 80 per cent with type 1 and 2 reconstructions, 40 per cent with type 3 reconstructions and 15 per cent with type 4 reconstructions. Excellent restoration of hearing, comparable to that achieved in otosclerosis surgery, may follow two stage stapedectomy and fenestration operations, but there is an understandable reluctance to open the labyrinth where there has been previous chronic ear disease.

MASTOID CAVITY PROBLEM

Healing of an open mastoid cavity takes place by second intention. The large exposed bone surface is slowly covered by vascular granulation tissue, which fills in and smooths out any irregularities. The deep part of the granulation tissue is organized into a fibrous tissue matrix, while new formation on the surface ceases when epithelium grows in from the marginal meatal skin. Even a large radical cavity should heal readily in this way, provided there is no residual disease and no significant secondary infection. Any exuberant granulations are removed with forceps, caustic agents being avoided.

With a modified radical mastoidectomy local epithelialization of the tympanic segment readily occurs and the mastoid segment heals by granulation and epithelial growth. With an atticotomy or attico–antrostomy the cavity healing problem is much easier, especially when it has been partly lined by a deep meatal skin flap.

The mastoid cavity, healed by second intention, is much smaller than the original operation cavity. The published results of experienced otologists indicate that satisfactory healing occurs in about 70 per cent of cases. Any procedure which promotes rapid epithelialization, such as use of matrix, skin or vein grafting, will prevent granulation and maintain the cavity at its original size. This is important, since it is accepted that the 'satisfactory' cases will have a cavity problem for the rest of their lives. This means attendance every 6–12 months to have wax and keratin removed; otherwise saprophytic infection is apt to occur.

In recent years, much interest has been shown in 'the problem of the mastoid cavity'. It is, however, not often necessary to create a large cavity in the mastoid process and this problem of difficulty of healing of the mastoid cavity is one that the surgeon has produced himself. However, there are some cases, for example cholesteatoma in children with a pneumatized mastoid, when it is difficult to avoid making a large cavity if disease is to be adequately removed.

The methods of dealing with a large cavity to promote healing are:

(1) Obliterative methods.
(2) Lining of the cavity with a viable flap.

Muscle flaps

Some years ago, obliterative methods received much attention and techniques of using pedicled muscle flaps to line the cavity first described by Kisch (1932) were revived by Rambo (1958), Thorburn (1960) and Guilford (1961).

In 1969, the author collected the results of obliterative mastoid operations using pedicled muscle flaps from 162 surgeons in this country and presented a paper to the Third Workshop in Microsurgery of the Ear in Chicago. The complications were numerous and included recurrence of cholesteatoma in 24 cases and in one of the latter cases there was no cholesteatoma at the original operation (*Tables 11.1–11.4*).

Table 11.1   Noninfective complications

Haematoma	6
Necrosis flap	13
Meatal stenosis	6
Severe post-operative pain	6
Persistent pain	2
Peculiar sensation in ear	1
Vertigo on chewing	2

Table 11.2   Infective complications

Recurrence cholesteatoma	24
Continued discharge	12
Reformation cavity and discharge	8
Recurrent discharge from mastoid	8
Abscess beneath flap	2
Infection stripping up flap	3
Pedunculated granuloma in cavity	2
Infection donor site	1
Failure to epithelialize	1
Recurrent bone sepsis	1
Labyrinthine irritation and perisinus infection	1
Meningitis	1
Cerebral abscess	1

Table 11.3   Pathology of cases treated by myoplasty

Unhealed radical cavities	16
Unhealed fenestration cavities	4
Tympanoplasty with unhealed mastoid cavities	6
Mastoiditis with cholesteatoma	6
Tympanoplasty with primary myoplasty	8

Table 11.4   Complications after myoplasty in 198 cases (Thorburn: 198 cases, 86 primary and 113 secondary operations)

Donor site haematoma	very few		
Partial graft slough	3 cases	1.5%	
Meningitis	1 case	0.5%	3 months after operation
Ear not consistently dry	23 cases	12.0%	
Recurrence of cholesteatoma[1]	11 cases	5.5%	
6 cases tympanum only involved			
5 cases mastoid involved			

[1]In one of the latter cases, there was no cholesteatoma at original operation.

The long-term results of this procedure are obviously poor but muscle and fascia can be used as free grafts to line a large mastoid cavity. After a period of time, the tissue will shrink and produce a fibrous lining which acts as a support for the growth of squamous epithelium from the edges.

BONE GRAFTS

Schiller and Singer (1960) described the use of cancellous bone strips taken from the iliac crest to obliterate the cavity. Schiller (1977, personal communication) makes the following comments on bone grafts for obliteration of mastoid cavities.

'I have not done an obliterative procedure for many years, simply because I have not had the need to do one. I personally have never obliterated large cavities or any cavity which had been created to remove cholesteatoma. My obliterative attempts were confined to cases on whom I had done fenestration operations or on whom I had found the cellular system to be filled with cholesterol granulation tissue. I do not do the fenestration operation now and I have not seen cases with cholesterol granuloma for years.

Although it has its limitations, I have no doubt that cancellous bone is the best material to use to obliterate a large cavity.

The limitations of using autogenous cancellous bone are as follows:

(1) It necessitates taking a hip graft and this proves to be extremely painful for the patient for about ten days.

(2) After observation of a series of patients, it is found that shrinkage of or resorption of bone occurs in 75 per cent of cases. This left a moderately large cavity which, however, was epithelialized and the ears remained dry.'

Because of the disadvantage of having to take cancellous bone from the hip, Schiller did a series of cases using Kiel Calf bone. In almost all these cases, the bone became completely resorbed. In the other cases, partial revascularization of small pieces occurred, no solid blocks of bone were formed and the pieces had to be removed.

The mastoid cavity can be obliterated with autogenous bone paté. Bone dust is obtained from the mastoid cortex and squamous portion of the temporal bone and the dust is collected and mixed with the blood seeping from the bone and surrounding muscle (*Figure 11.15*). Within a few weeks, the graft becomes a solid bony external auditory canal and mastoid cortex. This technique should not be used in the presence of active purulent drainage or cholesteatoma.

RECONSTRUCTION WITH HOMOGRAFT EXTERNAL AUDITORY CANAL BONE
This method has been found to be useful in the management of large mastoid cavities which are free of infection. The posterior bony external auditory canal may be replaced with or without a homograft tympanic membrane and ossicular chain. All the homograft bone must be covered with autogenous fascia to promote the growth of skin.

Lining of mastoid cavity with a pedicled skin flap

The use of free skin grafts whether of full thickness or split skin to line a mastoid cavity is contraindicated as the skin will only survive in part and the presence of hair follicles and sweat glands gives rise to chronic infection necessitating removal of the parts of the graft that have taken at a later date. Pedicled skin flaps have been used by many workers to line the mastoid cavity. The author (1958, 1959) described a method using a skin flap consisting of the skin of the post-aural region. It was found that rapid healing occurred if the flap was large enough to line the cavity completely. However, if the cavity was too large for it to be fully lined by the flap, healing failed to occur in the uncovered areas. The use of extrameatal skin in this area has the other disadvantages previously described and methods such as this cannot be recommended.

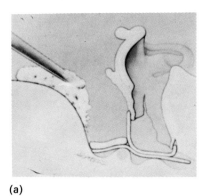

(a)

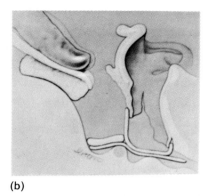

(b)

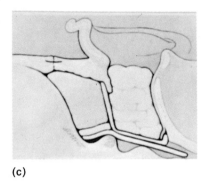

(c)

Figure 11.15 (a) Bone dust is collected and mixed with blood which seeps from the bone and surrounding muscle. (b) The pile of bloody bone pâté is blotted with a dry sponge to create a thick 'mortar'. (c) The bone pâté 'mortar' is packed into the cavity to reconstruct the external auditory canal and mastoid cortex

An obliterative mastoid tympanoplasty technique described by Smyth and Kerr (1969) has been recommended by them as an alternative to combined approach tympanoplasty.

Using a post-aural incision, a large periosteal flap pedicled anteriorly upon the auricle is elevated. The meatal skin cuff is preserved but the posterior bony meatal wall is taken down completely. After the disease has been excised a tympanoplasty is performed using a large piece of fascia (4 × 2 cm); this should extend from the tympanum to occupy the position of the removed posterior canal wall (*Figure 11.16*). The fascia is supported from behind by the pedicled periosteal flap which also fills the mastoid cavity. The meatal skin cuff is placed superficial to the fascia so that it is impossible for it to undermine the obliterative flap. Healing is usually secure in three weeks and hardly any post-operative care is required. Smyth reports the results of this technique in 119 ears with old unhealed radical or modified radical cavities: 12 cases gave some initial difficulty requiring minor revision operations in ten; with this proviso all ears healed securely, many with closure of the air–bone gap. With this technique, as with any other obliterative or closed technique, there is still an obligation upon the surgeon to be sure that he has cleared all disease, especially cholesteatoma, from the cavity which is to be obliterated. At least there is access which should give the surgeon, well trained in micro-surgery of the ear, every possible chance to clear disease and reach a healthy mastoid outline.

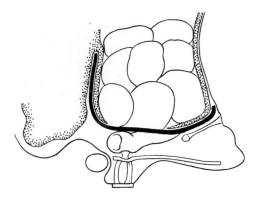

Figure 11.16 This shows the use of fascia to repair the tympanic membrane and to define the posterior canal wall, supported by the periosteal flap in the mastoid and so arranged that the meatal skin is superficial and cannot undermine the periosteal flap

Combined approach tympanoplasty (CAT)

Combined approach tympanoplasty has been developed and promoted by Jansen, Smyth, Corgill, House and Sheehy as an alternative to wide access techniques in the management of those cases of chronic suppurative otitis media which, because of their activity and extent, are unsuitable for transcanal tympanoplasty. The cochlear function should of course be good enough to justify functional reconstructive surgery.

The advantages claimed for combined approach tympanoplasty are:

(1) That since it retains a normal external auditory meatus with no access to the mastoid cavity, those after-care cavity problems inherent in classic radical or modified radical mastoid surgery are eliminated.

(2) That the reconstruction of a tympanic cavity of normal size and depth also makes possible the reconstruction of a sound transducer mechanism which should close the air–bone gap in a large proportion of cases.

If these claims for combined approach tympanoplasty can be substantiated and are shown to stand the test of time, they appear to present a revolutionary change in our attitude to the management of chronic otitis media. However, this may not be so much a revolution as the natural evolution from our experience with micro-surgical techniques in tympanoplasty over the past two decades. It must be emphasized that the successful employment of this technique requires considerable experience in the management of chronic suppurative otitis media and a high standard of technical competence. Indeed it may be difficult for some, because of their general commitments and limited experience with chronic ear disease, to acquire the necessary technical skill.

The main criticism levelled against combined approach tympanoplasty comes from certain senior otologists, for example Baron and Schuknecht in the USA and Beales in the UK, who consider that in chronic otitis media with an established cholesteatoma, it is not possible to be certain that all traces of this disease have been removed. It is, therefore, considered foolhardy and dangerous to reconstruct a closed tympanomastoid cavity which cannot be kept under observation, as has been the custom with conventional wide approach techniques.

In a recent paper, Smyth (1976) has followed up his results, over a period of 15 years, of 532 closed operations in cholesteatomatous ears. The operations were performed between 1961 and 1974 and over 80 per cent have been followed up regularly. The investigation has provided clear evidence to support the critics of combined approach tympanoplasty on the grounds of a high complication rate in both adults and children, and it is obvious that some of the optimism previously expressed by this author and others about the ability to eradicate cholesteatoma and restore function by combined approach tympanoplasty cannot be sustained. Smyth states that the use of combined approach tympanoplasty in non-cholesteatomatous ears remains unchallenged where it provides considerable advantages in regard to healing and functional improvement. He believes that two alternatives are available if cholesteatoma is present. (1) Either combined approach tympanoplasty can be carried out as a staged procedure until the ear is shown to be free from cholesteatoma. This has the disadvantage that some patients will require multiple operations. The other alternative (2) is to remove the canal wall in all cases of extramesotympanic cholesteatoma. Many surgeons will today adopt this approach. Smyth in his study found that the overall known incidence of residual cholesteatoma in children is much greater than in adults and is of the opinion that this operation should not be performed in children with cholesteatoma.

The essential technical features and principles of combined approach tympanoplasty, based on the work of Smyth, are described in some detail. Attention is also directed to the modified technique described by Schnee (1963) and Richards (1971) in which the bony posterior canal wall is sectioned superiorly and inferiorly; it is kept attached to the meatal skin so that it may be moved forwards to provide better access to the tympanum. Finally the canal wall is replaced in its normal position and the operation is completed as in ·combined approach tympanoplasty. The reader is reminded that these are not techniques for the occasional ear surgeon and is advised to remain critical and to keep himself informed of any new developments in this field.

Technical details

Combined approach really implies combined access, transmeatal and transmastoid, on either side of an intact posterosuperior bony canal wall (*Figure 11.17*). The soft tissue approach is by a generous post-aural skin incision. The periosteal tissues are separately incised and elevated as a substantial flap pedicled either above on the temporal muscle, or anteriorly on the auricle. The bone over the mastoid cortex and root of zygoma is exposed. The meatal skin is preserved as an intact cuff; this is elevated from the posterosuperior aspect of the meatus and then in continuity with the surface squamous epithelium of any tympanic membrane remnant until a pocket for the subsequent placement of a fascial graft is provided. If necessary this tympanic dissection goes from the notch of Rivinus downwards and forwards to the anterior annulus where the inner deep meatal skin may be elevated for a few millimetres. If the view of the anterior junction of drumhead with annulus is obscured by a canal overhang, this is uncovered by further elevation of the meatal skin cuff and the excess bone is removed until the annulus is clearly seen.

A cortical mastoid operation is completed and care is taken to provide room for subsequent instrumentation by removal of bone in the upper posterior part of the

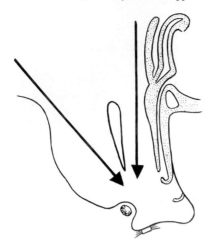

Figure 11.17   The arrows indicate the transmeatal and the posterior tympanotomy approach through the facial recess to the tympanum

mastoid. The bone dissection is expanded through the root of zygoma to the aditus and attic with exposure of the incus and head of the malleus. A posterior tympanotomy is now performed (*Figure 11.18*), providing access to the mesotympanum and hypotympanum by dissection of the facial recess. This is a space, triangular in outline (*Figure 11.19a*), created by the removal of bone between the descending portion of the facial nerve on the medial aspect, and the deep posterior canal wall with chorda tympani nerve on the lateral aspect (*Figure 11.19 b, c*); the fossa incudis superiorly forms the base of the triangle. Damage to the facial nerve is avoided by good visualization with the microscope, careful use of small cutting and diamond paste burrs on an angled handpiece, and familiarity with the normal anatomy of the facial nerve.

If there is an intact ossicular chain it is important that the cutting burr is not allowed to come into contact with the incus, since this may transmit acoustic energy sufficient to cause serious damage to cochlear function. If, therefore, an intact incus makes adequate dissection difficult, it should be removed.

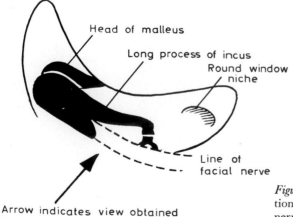

Head of malleus

Long process of incus

Round window niche

Line of facial nerve

Arrow indicates view obtained by posterior tympanotomy

Figure 11.18   Landmarks in the dissection of the facial recess—incus, facial nerve, the thinned deep bony posterior canal wall, stapes and round window niche

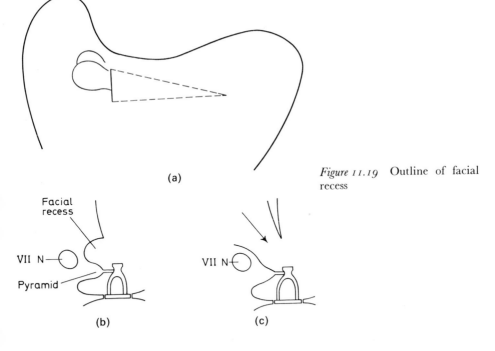

(a)

Figure 11.19   Outline of facial recess

Facial recess

VII N

Pyramid

(b)

VII N

(c)

Transcanal and transmastoid access must be such that cholesteatoma and diseased mucous membrane may be dissected more or less in continuity from any part of the middle-ear cleft. The removal of the incus and head of malleus may be necessary if these ossicles are involved in disease or to provide access to disease; this need not cause anxiety since techniques are available to reconstruct an alternative to the ossicular chain. It may be difficult to gain adequate access to the sinus tympani. This is a recess commonly infiltrated by disease, which lies posterior to the labyrinthine windows and medial to the descending portion of the facial nerve and pyramid (*Figure 11.3* and *11.18*). The facial nerve tends to interfere with access to the sinus tympani from the mastoid while the preserved deep posterior canal wall obstructs access from the meatus.

It is here that dissection of disease in continuity offers the best assurance that it is completely removed. The medial margin of the preserved canal wall may also hide cholesteatoma, hence the precaution is taken that it should be reduced to a knife edge with a diamond burr. Within the tympanum delicate dissection in continuity, under microscopic control, should ensure the complete removal of irreversible mucosal disease, cholesteatoma and granulation tissue; at the same time care is taken to conserve any healthy mucosa in the tympanum or mastoid, as well as useful remnants of the tympanic membrane or fibrous annulus.

In this respect the first objective is that the tympanomastoid cavity shall become lined with healthy mucous membrane which may have to grow from conserved mucosal remnants anywhere between the eustachian tube and the mastoid. The second objective is that the facial recess shall remain as a permanent opening between the tympanic cavity and the mastoid and so ensure free ventilation of the whole cavity from the eustachian tube.

The achievement of both these objectives is greatly enhanced by covering th
medial wall of the mastoid and tympanum with silicone sheet. This is specially
tailored so that it lies flat on the medial wall without any turned up edges which may
disturb the fit of the tympanic membrane graft. A notch is cut in the silicone sheet for
the tendon of the tensor tympani and a hole is provided for the oval window niche or
stapes. Present experience indicates that silicone sheet is well tolerated and may be left
in the ear indefinitely. Other advantages are that it prevents adhesion between the
medial tympanic wall and the newly fashioned tympanic membrane; also that in the
immediate post-operative period it promotes drainage of blood, serum and exudate
from the tympanomastoid cavity to the eustachian tube.

Any defect in the bony canal wall, caused either by instrumentation or disease
should be repaired with a thin sliver of homograft septal cartilage. Where previously
such a defect in the canal wall was not repaired, a retraction pocket was liable to
develop which went on to produce a recurrent cholesteatoma. Jansen (1963) states
that since care has been taken to repair any such defect in the canal wall, these
retraction pockets have not been observed.

In a one stage operation the repair of the tympanic membrane with fascia is carried
out following the ossicular reconstruction. For simplicity the technique is described
now as if this were the first part of a two stage operation. Dry temporal fascia is cut to
size so that it will cover the whole tympanic membrane area, extending well on to the
posterior canal wall. To prevent lifting of the fascia from the malleus a small incision
is made so that it goes underneath the handle. If the drum remnants and fibrous
annulus do not give adequate support anteriorly and inferiorly, the fascia should
extend for 1 or 2 mm on to the adjacent deep canal wall. At this level the canal skin
is now replaced over the margins of the fascia. It is important that the anterior angle
between drumhead and meatus be given firm support, for example with a piece of
silicone sponge. Attention to this point will prevent fibrous tissue thickening in the
angle—a condition called 'blunting' by Wright (1966); this may reduce the vibrating
surface of the drum and so contribute towards a poor hearing result.

The external auditory meatus is now examined through an aural speculum; the rest
of the meatal skin cuff is replaced over the posterior canal wall superficial to fascia and
to any cartilage repairing a defect in the canal wall. The deep meatal outline is
supported with gel-foam and in its outer part with cotton or ribbon gauze (*Figure
11.20*).

A meatoplasty incision for the purpose of enlarging the meatus should ordinarily be
avoided, since the ultimate outline will be determined by the shape of the bony
meatus. It is a notable advantage of this technique that the fit of the fascial graft, and
of any ossicular reconstruction, may now be precisely checked by examination
through the facial recess. Once this is seen to be satisfactory the periosteal flap is
sutured in position over the surface of the mastoid and the skin incision is closed with
superficial drainage.

The patient is given a five-day course of antibiotic. The dressing is renewed daily
under sterile conditions. The stitches are removed after five days when the patient
may be allowed home. He is instructed that clean cotton may be changed in the outer
meatus and when he reports three weeks after operation any dried gel-foam is
removed. The tympanic membrane and meatus should then appear healed.

While occasionally it is possible to retain an intact ossicular chain, defects are
common especially involving the incus. The majority fall into one of two categories:

(1) there is a malleus and an intact mobile stapes; (2) there is a malleus and only a footplate of stapes. Techniques for the repair of such ossicular defects have already been described.

ADVANTAGES OF COMBINED APPROACH TYMPANOPLASTY

The main advantage of this method (Beales, 1968) is the avoidance of a mastoid cavity and the possibility of the achievement of closure of the air–bone gap in tympanoplasty. This was not possible in the classic tympanoplasty of Wullstein and Zöllner. This method is the one of choice in the ear without cholesteatoma.

DISADVANTAGES OF COMBINED APPROACH TYMPANOPLASTY

If the operation is performed in the ear with cholesteatoma, the experience of 15 years has shown that there is a high incidence of recurrent cholesteatoma and this may be difficult to detect. There is evidence that a significantly smaller complication rate can be achieved through a combination of well-performed mastoidectomy and mesotympanic reconstruction.

This operation is contraindicated in cholesteatoma in children.

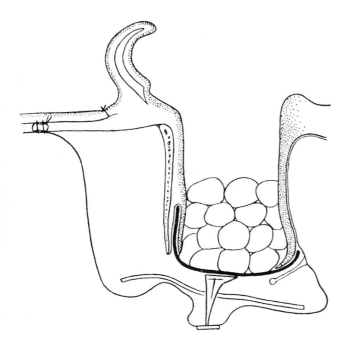

Figure 11.20 The graft which repairs the tympanic defect rests on the remnant of the tympanic membrane and on the posterior meatal wall, any defect in which has been repaired with cartilage. Silastic sheeting prevents adhesion between the fascial graft and the medial tympanic wall and encourages growth of tympanic mucosa. The meatal skin cuff is superficial to the fascia. Any defect in the ossicular chain is repaired either at the initial operation or at a later stage dependent upon the condition of the mucous membrane

Combined approach tympanoplasty is one of the most difficult techniques in aural surgery and must only be carried out by those with the necessary training and aptitude. Even if no cholesteatoma was present at the original operation, it is possible for retraction pockets to develop and give rise to cholesteatoma.

Careful long-term follow-up is essential and, if this is not possible, the method must not be used.

CAUSES OF FAILURE TO RESTORE HEARING IN TYMPANOPLASTY

Sensorineural deafness

Unfortunately with any surgical intervention for chronic ear disease, there is always some risk to cochlear function. This risk is present in all ages but is greater in older as compared to younger persons. The risk is minimized by taking extreme care with asepsis; by avoiding use of a cutting burr close to an intact ossicular chain; by respecting the hydrodynamics of the labyrinth in the care taken to be gentle in manipulation of the ossicles or in dissection and use of suction close to the stapes and the labyrinthine windows. Ototoxic antibiotics and sterilizing fluids should also be avoided both locally and systemically.

Conductive deafness

'Lifting' and 'blunting' have already been referred to as causes of conductive deafness. Failure of the ossicular mechanism to restore hearing may arise for a number of reasons:

(1) Dislocation of a part or the whole of the reconstruction.
(2) Cicatricial contraction may cause a loss of contact either with the tympanic membrane or with the head or footplate of the stapes.
(3) Fixation of the ossicular mechanism by fibrous tissue, hyaline or bone.
(4) Fixation of the footplate of the stapes by fibrous tissue, bone or otosclerosis.

The precise cause for a poor conductive hearing result may only be accurately determined by a revision tympanotomy operation. This should be carried out after a sufficient interval—approximately six months—so that the ear is soundly healed. Then it may be safe to open the labyrinth, should this be necessary to relieve a fixation of the stapes in the oval window.

Staging

Considering the nature and pathogenesis of chronic otitis media in the severely damaged ear, it is bound to be difficult to strike a balance between adequate excision of disease and reasonable functional conservation, especially if this is always attempted in one operation. Therefore, should the surgeon consider that there is any doubt about the adequacy of the excision of disease, or if there is a dangerous involvement of the stapes, it may be advisable to note this position carefully, and deliberately to leave the final dissection of disease and the repair of the ossicular chain to a second stage operation. The successful excision of extensive disease must often leave an ear with little or no mucous membrane. Surgery for such an ear should be staged so that measures are taken at the first operation to encourage regeneration of mucous membrane. Then, some months later, with an intact tympanic membrane and a mucosa-lined middle ear, it may be possible to rebuild a functioning ossicular mechanism. Alternatively, where the stapes is badly fixed by hyaline, staging may be oriented towards fenestration of the lateral semicircular canal. This does not fit with the philosophy of combined approach tympanoplasty since the posterior canal wall must be taken down at the first operation. With a severe conductive deafness due to tympanosclerosis, stapedectomy carries considerable risk that it may damage labyrinthine function since it is difficult to provide a secure seal for the oval window. It is safer, for the surgeon with experience in fenestration, to open the labyrinth over the prominence of the lateral semicircular canal where there can be no recessed or residual disease and to cover the fenestra with a healthy skin flap.

It must be appreciated and made clear to the patient that the fenestration operation has certain disadvantages and these have been mentioned previously. Many patients will prefer to have a tympanic membrane repaired by myringoplasty and to use a modern hearing aid.

References

Alberti, P. W. R. M. (1963). *Laryngoscope*, **73**, 605

Austin, D. F. (1965). *Archives of Otolaryngology*, **81**, 20

Austin and Smyth, G. D. L. (1964). *Journal of Laryngology*, **78**, 384

Baron, S. H. (1953). *Transactions of the American Academy of Ophthalmology and Otolaryngology*, Sept/Oct

Baron, S. H. (1967). *Archives of Otolaryingology*, **86**, 361

Baron, S. H. (1967). *Laryngoscope*, **77**, 905

Beales, P. H. (1968). *Journal of Laryngology*, **82**, 769

Beales, P. H. (1969). *Archives of Otolaryngology*, **89**, 195

Beales, P. H. (1969). *Archives of Otolaryngology*, **89**, 196

Beales, P. H. and Hynes, W. (1958). *Journal of Laryngology and Otology*, **72**, No. 11, 888

Beales, P. H. and Hynes, W. (1959). *Journal of Laryngology and Otology*, **72**, No. 8, 527

Corgill, D. A. and Storrs, L. A. (1967). *Transactions of the American Academy of Ophthalmology and Otolaryngology*, **71**, 53

Dawes, J. D. K. (1970). *Journal of Laryngology*, **84**, 583

Douek, E. (1976). *Operative Surgery—Ear*. London; Butterworth

Friedmann, I. (1956). *Journal of Clinical Pathology*, **9** 229

Friedmann, I. (1957). *Journal of Laryngology*, **71**, 313

Garcia-Ibanez, L. (1961). *Archives of Otolaryngology*, **73**, 268

Gibb, A. G. (1976). *Proceedings of the Royal Society of Medicine*, **69**, 155

Guilford, F. R. (1961). *Transaction of the American Academy of Ophthalmology and Otolaryngology*, **65**, 114

Harris, I., and Goodhill, V. (1967). *Laryngoscope*, **77**, 1191

Hough, J. V. D. (1970). *Laryngoscope*, **80**, 1385

House, W. L. (1960). *Archives of Otolaryngology*, **71**, 399

House, W. L., Glasscock, M. E. and Sheehy, J. L. (1969). *Transactions of the American Academy of Ophthalmology and Otolaryngology*, **73**, 836

House, W. L., and Sheehy, J. L. (1963). *Archives of Otolaryngology*, **78**, 96, 304

Jako, G. J. (1967). *Laryngoscope*, **77**, 306; **77**, 2022

Jansen, C. (1963). *Laryngoscope*, **73**, 1288

Jansen, C. (1968). *Journal of Laryngology*, **82**, 779

King, P. F. (1964). *Journal of Laryngology*, **78**, 849

Kisch, H. (1932). *Postgraduate medical Journal*, **8**, 270

Marquet, J. F. E. (1966). *Acta otolaryngologica*, **62**, 459

Marquet, J. F. E. (1968). *Laryngoscope*, **78**, 1329

Marquet, J. F. E. (1971). *Acta oto-rhino-laryngologica, Belgium*. In press

Plester, D. (1961). *Journal of Laryngology*, **75**, 881

Plester, D. (1963). *Archives of Otolaryngology*, **78**, 631

Pulec, J. L. (1976). *Operative Surgery—Ear*, pp. 117–122 London; Butterworth

Rambo, J. H. T. (1958). *Transactions of the American Academy of Ophthalmology and Otolaryngology*, Mar/Apl

Rambo, J. H. T. (1965). *Annals of Otology*, **74**, 535

Reijnen, C. and Kuipers, W. (1965). *Practical Otorhinolaryngology*, **27**, 306

Richards, S. (1971). *Acta oto-rhino-laryngologica, Belgium*

Sato, M. (1969). *Laryngoscope*, **79**, 295

Schiller, A. (1959). *Journal of Laryngology and Otology*, **72**, No. 7, 591

Schiller, A. (1970). *Archives of Otolaryngology*, **91**, 336

Schiller, A. (1977). Personal communication

Schiller, A. and Singer, M. (1960). *South African medical Journal*, **34**, 645

Schnee, I. M. (1963). *Journal of the Medical Society of New Jersey*, **60**, 1

Scott-Brown, W. G. (1971). *Diseases of the Ear, Nose and Throat*. London; Butterworth

Shea, J. J., Jnr. (1960). *Journal of Laryngology*, **74**, 358

Shea, J. J., Jnr. and Austin, D. F. (1961). *Laryngoscope*, **71**, 586

Sheehy, J. L. (1965). *Surgery of Chronic Otitis Media, Otolaryngology* Vol. 1, Chapter 10B. Ed. by G. M. Coates, H. P. Schenck and M. V. Miller, Hagerstown

Sheehy, J. L. and Patterson, M. E. (1967). *Laryngoscope*, **77**, 1502

Smyth, G. D. L. (1976). 'Post-operative Cholesteatoma.' In *Cholesteatoma* pp. 355–362. Ed. by B. F. McCabe, J. Sade, and M. Adamson. First International Conference, The University of Iowa, Iowa City, Iowa. June, 1976

Smyth, G. D. L. and Kerr, A. G. (1967). *Laryngoscope*, **77**, 330

Smyth, G. D. L. and Kerr, A. G. (1969). *Journal of Laryngology*, **83**, 1061

Smyth, G. D. L. and Kerr, A. G. (1970). *Journal of Laryngology*, **84**, 757

Smyth, G. D. L. and Kerr, A. G. and Jones, J. H. (1967). *Laryngoscope*, **77**, 1684

Smyth, G. D. L., Jones, J. H. and Kerr, A. G. (1967). *Journal of Laryngology*, **81**, 1325

Smyth, G. D. L., England, R. M., Gibson, R. and Kerr, A. G. (1967). *Journal of Laryngology*, **81**, 69, 75

Thorburn, I. B. (1960). *Journal of Laryngology*, **74**, 453

Thorburn, I. B. (1961). *Journal of Laryngology*, **75**, 885

Thorburn, I. B. (1963). *Journal of Laryngology*, **77**, 501

Thorburn, I. B. (1968). *Proceedings of the Royal Society of Medicine*, **61**, 395

Van den Broek, P. (1968). *The Fate of Incus Grafts in Rats*. (Thesis) University of Nijmegen, Holland

Wilson, D. F., Pulec, J. L. and van Vliet, P. D. (1966). *Archives of Otolaryngology*, **83**, 554

Wright, W. K. (1966). *Eye Ear Nose Throat Monthly*, **45**, 45

Wullstein, H. (1955). *Acta otolorayngologia*, **45**, 440

Wullstein, H. (1963). *Archives of Otolaryngology*, **78**, 296

12 Complications of infections of the middle ear

J D K Dawes

Pyogenic inflammation of the labyrinth

Pyogenic inflammatory lesions of the labyrinth have always been regarded as a serious complication of otitis media, because the perilymph communicates directly through the cochlear aqueduct with the subarachnoid space in the posterior fossa. The rare cases of meningitis following stapedectomy spread by this route. Spread from the labyrinth to the intracranial structures can occur by the perineural and perivascular channels to the internal auditory meatus, or occasionally along the aqueduct of the vestibule to produce a posterior fossa extradural abscess, or along the ductus endolymphaticus to produce a saccus empyema and a posterior fossa intradural abscess (*Figure 12.1*). Although all these routes have been implicated in various reports of intracranial suppuration, the labyrinth was found rarely at fault in the series studied by McGuckin (1935) and Dawes (1961).

Since the introduction of chemotherapeutic and antibiotic agents, acute otitis media arising in a normal middle-ear cleft must seldom cause acute suppurative labyrinthitis. In the past, severe acute otitis media which destroyed the labyrinth by uncontrolled

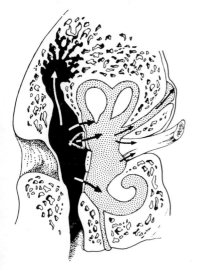

Figure 12.1

osteitis was uncommon. In all cases of acute labyrinthine disorder associated with acute inflammatory disease in the middle-ear cleft seen by the author, otitis media has in fact been but one manifestation of myringitis bullosa haemorrhagica, probably of virus origin (Dawes, 1951, 1953, 1963).

Acute otitis media may cause diffuse labyrinthitis if the stapes should be dislocated during an operation, or if post-operative infection should follow stapedectomy.

However, acute otitis media occurring in a previously damaged but healed middle-ear cleft may produce acute labyrinthitis by direct extension through a fistula previously produced by a spontaneously extruded cholesteatoma. Other fistulae may be the consequence of fracture through the labyrinth, or surgical fenestration, or injury to the stapedial footplate.

Even ear drops or water have been known to induce vertigo when a crack in the footplate or a surgical fenestra is exposed to the external auditory meatus.

Suppurative labyrinthine disorders usually follow chronic otitis media. Cholesteatoma may erode the labyrinthine capsule and so may invade any or all of its segments. The most common site of erosion is through the prominence of the lateral semicircular canal; less frequently erosions occur through the stapedial footplate, the promontory, or the superior and posterior semicircular canals (Dawes and Watson, 1978). As soon as an erosion has breached the bony labyrinth to reach the endosteum, it may be possible to elicit the 'fistula sign' by a sharp push on the tragus or the use of a Siegle's speculum. The resulting displacement of air may directly stimulate the labyrinth through the pathological fistula and cause a deviation of the eyes, or a short burst of nystagmus and a sensation of vertigo. This fistula sign cannot be always demonstrated even if exposure is extensive, because the opening may be protected against air displacement by a solid mass of cholesteatoma. Sterile cholesteatoma may insidiously erode and invade the whole labyrinth without the production of vertigo or discomfort, for the rate of erosion and invasion is so gradual that the labyrinthine system receives no stimulation. Similarly, slowly progressive destruction of the cochlea can occur with no more than a sense of progressive loss of hearing. The cholesteatoma after eroding through the endosteum at first may only be separated from the labyrinthine fluids by a serofibrinous exudate which later becomes a granulomatous membrane. The membranous labyrinth itself resists destruction and becomes thickened and, even though that part of the membranous labyrinth in direct contact with the cholesteatoma be destroyed, the adjacent parts become shut off and retain their function. An acute exacerbation of chronic otitis media may not at first completely break down the natural barriers of resistance but only produce a serofibrinous inflammatory reaction in the labyrinth (diffuse serous labyrinthitis). At this stage, the disease is reversible and the labyrinth and cochlea are capable of functional recovery. However, if the barriers are overwhelmed, a diffuse suppurative labyrinthitis will occur, leading to subtotal or total destruction of vestibule and cochlea. Occasionally the whole cochlea may sequestrate.

Spontaneous arrest of erosion may occur at any stage. The infection is overcome, osteoclasts invade the granulation tissue and the disease is shut off from the functioning remains of the labyrinthine system by new bone formation. This spontaneous arrest is unusual and may be incomplete, in that pus and cholesteatoma within the labyrinth and cochlea may become loculated by being separated from the main mass of disease in the middle-ear cleft. Such a loculated nidus within the labyrinth can be the cause of further extension of the disease.

Symptoms

As labyrinthitis affects both the vestibular and cochlear systems in different degrees the patient may have either disturbance of equilibrium or hearing loss as the dominant feature. Disturbance of equilibrium is the most striking feature both subjectively and objectively. The first evidence of labyrinthine upset may be no more than a momentary feeling of being off balance or stumbling. In more severe lesions the patient experiences a sensation of rotation or vertigo which may last minutes, hours or days. The more severe the vertigo, the greater the likelihood of observing horizontorotary nystagmus, with the quick phase usually towards the healthy side.

The patient tends to walk on a wide base and staggers to the side of the diseased labyrinth. The most severe forms of labyrinthitis, whether serous or suppurative, are heralded by an acute attack of vertigo and the patient may fall to the ground and vomit. He lies in bed curled up on the side of his sound ear, fearing to move in case he induces a more severe attack of vertigo. Vomiting may be persistent for a few days as also may horizontorotary nystagmus. Provided serious complications do not supervene, even in the worst attacks the patient after two weeks feels moderately comfortable, the vomiting having stopped, and although not yet stable he manages to walk around in daylight fairly well. In the dark he stumbles much more and with eyes closed and feet together he falls to the side of the lesion. Rapid movements of the head may induce short attacks of vertigo if any labyrinthine function has been retained. Full recovery of stability does occur within 4–6 weeks if the labyrinth has been totally destroyed, for the central neural mechanisms fully compensate for the loss of one labyrinth. When destruction is incomplete, the patient continues to suffer attacks of instability with each new flare up of infection.

In cases where semicircular canal system disease predominates the degree of loss of hearing depends on the extent of the labyrinthitis. When disequilibration is severe and long-lasting the increased deafness, which is of inner-ear type, may be severe or total and it remains so if destruction has been complete. When less severe, hearing may be retained or recover to its previous level. When vertigo is slight or of short duration the patient may not complain of any increase in hearing loss, and examination confirms that the loss of hearing is of middle-ear type, consistent with the degree of middle-ear damage.

Less commonly the cochlea is directly invaded and here inner-ear deafness may be severe whilst vertigo is only slight.

In cases of labyrinthine erosion, the patient may suffer momentary attacks of vertigo without significant deafness. For example, a ball of cholesteatoma destroying the stapes and projecting into the vestibule may remain in contact with the long process of the incus and transmit sound waves to the vestibule. Consequently it is of value in prognosis to determine the extent and type of hearing loss in a patient suffering from labyrinthine invasion by ear disease.

Investigations

Caloric and rotation tests are frequently recommended as a method of assessing the extent of labyrinthine damage. Both tests are superfluous since those cases which would be submitted to investigation clearly have symptoms suggestive of labyrinthine invasion. Mere clinical assessment decides whether or not surgery is indicated, and the extent of the surgical intervention is guided by the state of the hearing and the surgical findings. No value can be attached to caloric and rotation tests in the presence of potentially dangerous disease or in a patient who already has nystagmus. The syringing of water into the ear of a patient with labyrinthine symptoms complicating chronic ear disease may, in fact, break down the natural barriers limiting the invasion and may convert a circumscribed lesion into a diffuse suppurative labyrinthitis with its attendant risk of meningitis (Watson, 1952).

Clinical presentation

When vertigo occurs in a patient suffering from chronic middle-ear disease then the vertigo must be regarded as consequent on that disease until proved otherwise, even if an exploratory operation is necessary for proof. A cholesteatoma which has been infected throughout its progressive erosion into the labyrinth will produce vertigo as soon as the bony wall is breached, whereas a large fistula may have been insidiously produced by a sterile cholesteatoma before vertigo occurs, as a result of an acute exacerbation of the chronic otitis.

Fistulae of various sizes may be found quite unexpectedly at routine operation for chronic ear disease, and after careful questioning the patient may deny any pre-operative history of vertigo. Patients have even been known to walk into a consulting room to present the otologist with a sequestrated cochlea and to deny that there ever was any disturbance of equilibrium. Of course, loss of hearing is complete in these circumstances.

The first intimation that a patient has something wrong—apart from his discharging ear—may be that during washing or shaving he tends momentarily to lose his balance. The patient may himself discover that this was due to pressure on the tragus and may convincingly demonstrate the 'fistula sign' on request. At other times, during routine examination of the ear, mopping of cholesteatomatous debris and pus, or using Siegle's speculum, may elicit the 'fistula sign' and cause a sensation of vertigo or instability for the first time.

Microscopic inspection of the ear may demonstrate defects in the stapedial footplate, or erosions through the promontory. Aspiration of debris during microscopic assessment may immediately induce nystagmus and so convincingly demonstrate a fistula. If nystagmus occurs only after prolonged aspiration then it does not necessarily mean that a fistula is present, for prolonged aspiration has a cold caloric effect on the intact labyrinth. Where bone destruction is extensive, the actual fistula may be seen in the lateral semicircular canal.

Patients with spontaneously healed cavities produced by extensive cholesteatomatous erosion may notice vertigo or instability if a cold wind blows into the ear or if ear-drops are used. A healed fistula may occasionally be seen with the help of magnification.

More frequently, patients present complaining of intermittent attacks of vertigo of short and varied duration, often induced by rapid movements of the head; a fistula sign may be demonstrated. The hearing loss has not changed and is of the conductive type and of a degree in keeping with the findings of chronic middle-ear disease. The attacks of vertigo may last minutes, hours or days on each occasion but recovery to the previous level of function is usual between the attacks. Each attack of vertigo may be associated with an acute upper respiratory tract infection, swimming, taking a shower, or any factor which induces an acute exacerbation of the chronic otitis. Probably a mild serous labyrinthitis has occurred on each occasion.

In the presence of a fistula, severe labyrinthitis may arise at any time. It is not possible to distinguish diffuse serous from diffuse suppurative labyrinthitis at onset. Both show marked disturbances of equilibrium and severe hearing loss. Treatment should not be withheld merely because precise diagnosis must await future evidence. If hearing loss has not increased or if it has returned to its previous level, we can be sure that the labyrinthitis was serous, whereas if hearing loss is severe or total, the lesion has been destructive.

Post-operative vertigo may follow routine mastoid surgery even when there is no fistula. Presumably, drilling of perilabyrinthine cells or the surface of the bony semicircular canals has induced mild traumatic labyrinthitis. This post-operative vertigo, although occasionally associated with nystagmus, is of short duration. The duration of post-operative labyrinthine upset in the presence of a fistula is related to the size of the fistula, the degree of labyrinthine infection present or induced by surgery, the extent of the surgical interference and the normality of labyrinthine function prior to operation. Thus, a grossly diseased membranous labyrinth, although totally destroyed by surgery, produces only slight vertigo post-operatively, whereas an extensive purulent labyrinthitis surgically induced in an intact active labyrinth produces vertigo, vomiting and nystagmus which persist until either the infection is controlled or the labyrinth dies.

All cases of vertigo should be examined otologically, for occasionally both patient and attending physician are either unaware of the presence of insidious chronic ear disease or fail to relate the vertigo to the ear disease.

Differential diagnosis

The only suppurative complication of chronic ear disease likely to be confused with labyrinthitis is a cerebellar abscess, for not only may both lesions occur in the same

Table 12.1

	Labyrinthitis	*Cerebellar abscess*
Nystagmus	Fine horizontorotary towards the sound ear and increased on looking away. Gradually diminishes and disappears in 2–3 weeks	Coarse horizontorotary. Direction and type vary. Usually most marked towards the affected side. Is persistent while disease present
Vertigo	Experienced in plane of nystagmus and increased with higher degrees of nystagmus	At first associated with nystagmus but later is independent and persistent
Ataxia	Falling in direction of slow component. Disappears with cessation of nystagmus. Past-pointing with either hand in the direction of the slow component	Direction of falling usually constant and to side of lesion. No relation to nystagmus. Past-pointing usually present but only in hand on side of lesion
Dysdiadochokinesis	Absent	Present and marked
Joint sense	Normal	Usually lost or impaired

patient but vertigo, nystagmus and ataxia are common to both lesions. A surgical exploration of the ear is indicated in either instance; the operative findings and further progress of the case usually differentiate between them. It is worth noting that cerebellar abscess almost invariably follows a lateral sinus thrombophlebitis. The analysis of the symptoms and signs in *Table 12.1* may be helpful.

Labyrinthitis from acute ear disease is today very rare and when labyrinthine symptoms complicate an acute ear lesion it is usually found that the ear disease is myringitis bullosa haemorrhagica.

Management

An intensive course of antibiotics does not only control an infected labyrinth arising from *acute* otitis media but also the otitis media itself. Only if the otitic lesion cannot be controlled should the mastoid be explored.

The occurrence of labyrinthine disturbance in a patient with *chronic* ear disease indicates that the initial lesion has spread beyond the middle-ear cleft. This is an absolute indication for surgery in chronic otitis. Surgery should be directed to excision of the disease and, in particular, the whole cholesteatoma together with its matrix. Generally, this means a formal mastoid exposure by the endaural or post-aural routes. Occasionally the whole cholesteatoma can be removed by a permeatal route using aspiration, but this technique should only be used by the expert and even then with circumspection, and if any doubt exists as to the success of this procedure he should be prepared for formal exploration of the mastoid.

Antibiotics in themselves have no effect on chronic otitis media or the associated cholesteatoma but they may control an acute exacerbation or associated labyrinthitis; even more important they may localize the disease and protect other tissue planes such as the meninges from further spread. A broad spectrum antibiotic such as ampicillin, Septrin or Mysteclin, provides sufficient protection if a fistula is incidentally demonstrated, and given a high dosage will usually be adequate for the serous or suppurative lesions. A bacteriological swab taken at the time of operation is frequently of little help, for mainly saprophytic organisms dominate the culture and the active pyogenic organism is overlooked. However, the bacteriological findings may support a judgement that a change in drug is necessary and so offer a guide as to the most suitable antibiotic. The duration of therapy is determined by the patient's progress and not by any ideas about fixed duration of a course of treatment. Of course, it would be unwise to prolong the use of streptomycin or chloromycetin a day longer than necessary.

Before undertaking surgery the hearing level and condition of the other ear must be known, for if the affected ear is functionally the better, then within reasonable limits an attempt should be made to preserve the labyrinth and cochlea at operation, destroying them only when there is no possible alternative. The operative site can always be reviewed if there is any later doubt about the wisdom of the act of conservation.

If the hearing loss is of inner-ear type and severe or total, there is no point in attempting to preserve function.

By far the most common site of fistula is through the prominence of the lateral semicircular canal. Careful microscopically controlled dissection permits complete removal of the cholesteatoma matrix in many cases of small fistula without damage to the membranous labyrinth. If this is the whole extent of the erosion it may be hoped that, once the mild post-operative labyrinthine symptoms have settled and the mastoid cavity has healed, the patient may spontaneously develop a 'type 5 tympanoplastic mechanism' (*see* Chapter 11), a hope only rarely realized. A thickened membranous labyrinth may be preserved after cholesteatoma matrix has been carefully dissected away, even though the dome of the bony canal has been completely eroded, for once the chronic otitis has settled and healed the establishment of locally stable conditions may allow the labyrinth to resume its normal function undisturbed. Granulations in the neighbourhood of a fistula may be easily removed without incurring a penalty. In the majority of cases the labyrinth can be preserved and the hearing level maintained at its pre-operative level (Dawes and Watson, 1978).

As the fallopian canal is a close relation of the lateral semicircular canal a facial nerve exposure commonly accompanies a labyrinthine fistula and care must be exercised in cleaning the environment of the fistula so as to avoid damaging the nerve.

However, in all cases of graduated surgical interference it is worth remembering that the patient may develop more severe post-operative symptoms due to surgically induced spread of disease, and careful judgement must be exercised in each case to decide whether or not it is worth preserving the labyrinth. If post-operative vertigo is persistent, labyrinthine destruction can always be done later.

In more extensive cases not only is the membranous labyrinth locally destroyed but there may be extensive invasion of the canal system or vestibule by granulation tissue, cholesteatoma or pus, and the whole labyrinth may be completely invaded and destroyed with exposure of the internal auditory meatus and consequent cerebrospinal fluid leak. In any one case vestibule and cochlea may be invaded separately or together. In these more extensive invasions there is no hope of preservation of function; indeed, there is no function to preserve and the major concern is to be sure that all disease has been excised and that no loculus is left. Where a total loss of hearing is known to exist, even though there is no apparent extension beyond that seen even with a microscope, it is essential to open the whole labyrinth so that no loculus escapes attention.

It is extremely difficult to destroy the whole labyrinthine mechanism in the presence of granulation tissue and loculi and some patients, even after extensive labyrinthectomy, retain small functioning portions. They continue to have intermittent vertigo and even a fistula sign may clearly be demonstrated. More extensive surgery is indicated particularly if areas of infection persist, for complete excision of disease usually stops the vertigo. However, if the vertigo persists although the mastoid cavity is healed, the remaining parts of the labyrinth can be destroyed by an ultrasonic technique. Vestibular nerve section can be a more definitive procedure for control of vertigo in those rare occasions when the local disease has been satisfactorily eliminated.

For surgical destruction of the cochleolabyrinthine system in the presence of chronic ear disease, it is usually sufficient to open the dome of the lateral semicircular canal to expose the vestibule from above and then to remove the promontory between the oval and round windows to gain access to the vestibule from below. Through these superior and inferior vestibulotomies the membranous labyrinth can usually be destroyed and the bony labyrinth adequately drained. However, if there is extensive invasion with numerous granulations in the vestibule and cochlea the inferior vestibulotomy should be enlarged to include the cochlea, and the superior and posterior semicircular canals should also be widely opened to destroy the canals and provide drainage.

Otogenic intracranial complications

Extension of disease beyond the confines of the middle-ear cleft is so serious that the earliest possible diagnosis is essential to proper management. In the more advanced countries recognition of intracranial spread has been relatively easy for many years, although it is clear that therapy was seldom efficient before the advent of chemotherapeutic and antibiotic agents. In less advanced regions many patients still die undiagnosed and untreated.

In the past it was considered that 3 per cent of cases of acute otitis media, and 2 per cent of chronic lesions, were complicated by intracranial suppuration, but because chronic middle-ear disease was more common, it was held responsible for two-thirds of the total—always allowing that diagnosis of acute and chronic pathology was exact (*Table 12.2*).

Table 12.2   **Cases of aural suppuration and complications arising therefrom (Ear and Throat Department, Royal Infirmary, Edinburgh, 1907–26)** (after Turner and Reynolds)

Middle-ear suppuration	Intracranial complications	Percentage of complications
Total: 11 826	276	2.3
Acute suppuration: 3031	92	3.0
Chronic suppuration: 8795	184	2.0

Today, chronic ear disease still causes two-thirds of the intracranial complications (Dawes, 1961), although the overall frequency is greatly reduced; a figure of less than 0.15 per cent is given by Jeanes (1962). Most of the intracranial complications in childhood follow acute middle-ear infections.

Pathology of intracranial suppuration

Spread of infection from the middle-ear cleft to intracranial structures is usually direct and may be upward into the middle cranial fossa or backward into the posterior fossa. This direct form of spread passes through the tissue planes of dura mater, including blood sinuses, subdural space and pia-arachnoid mater finally to reach brain tissue. Infection may in passage involve one or several such tissue planes. As a rule, therefore, intracranial suppuration is adjacent to the temporal bone at the site of invasion. Rarely, otogenic intracranial suppuration lies remote from the invasion point; Pennybacker (1961) has seen this on only two occasions.

The pathogenesis of intracranial suppuration may be conveniently studied in three phases: (1) from the middle-ear cleft to the meninges; (2) across the meninges; (3) invasion of brain tissue.

MIDDLE-EAR CLEFT TO MENINGES
Fracture of the temporal bone may produce a preformed track, along which infection can readily spread to the meninges of the middle or posterior cranial fossa. Another

preformed path is the labyrinth itself and infection transmitted via this route produces lesions in the posterior fossa. More commonly it produces infection of the subarachnoid space, and only rarely has it been found to cause localized abscess in the internal auditory meatus or extradural abscess near the saccus endolymphaticus (*Figure 12.1*).

By far the most common method of extension of middle-ear disease is by osteitis or cholesteatomatous erosion. Acute disease in a well-pneumatized mastoid may destroy cell walls and so produce an abscess within bone which, in turn, may rupture through the mastoid cortex to form a post-aural abscess, a zygomatic abscess, or sometimes the digastric fossa is penetrated to produce what is known as Bezold's abscess. Variations in extent and distribution of cells in the mastoid determine the direction of spread. If the path of least resistance is through the tegmen, the osteitis will expose middle fossa dura which resists further spread and localizes the disease to form a middle fossa extradural abscess of varying size (*Figure 12.2*). The freedom of communication between an extradural abscess and mastoid abscess depends on the extent of necrosis of the tegmen. When the tegmen is inflamed but not destroyed the extradural abscess may be shut off from the mastoid disease. In like manner, osteitis extending backwards through Trautmann's triangle, or external to the lateral sinus, can produce either a freely communicating or a loculated posterior fossa extradural abscess. Destruction of the lateral sinus plate may expose the sinus to the mastoid abscess but if there is only osteitis in an intact plate an enclosed perisinus abscess may result.

In chronic ear disease the mastoid is relatively acellular but associated osteitis can produce extension of disease to the dura in a similar manner to acute otitis media. Cholesteatoma, a special factor in chronic disease, through insidious erosion of bone may expose the middle fossa dura or lateral sinus. If the erosion is caused by sterile cholesteatoma, the dura of either fossa may be lined by the cholesteatomatous matrix without inflammatory response; when the mass is infected the dura may respond by

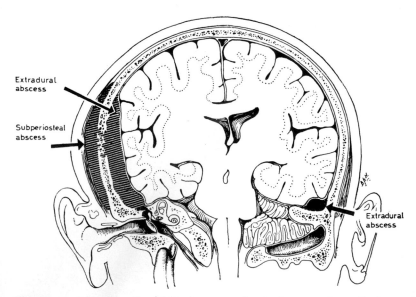

Extradural abscess

Subperiosteal abscess

Extradural abscess

Figure 12.2   Diagram of middle fossa extradural abscesses. A small abscess is demonstrated on one side. The opposite side shows the enlargement of the abscess and erosion through the vault of the skull to produce a subperiosteal abscess

producing granulation tissue at the point of contact. If an acute exacerbation of chronic disease should now occur, the intracranial structures are already exposed to the added infection. Cholesteatomatous erosion and osteitis may both contribute to passage of infection. Since suppurative intracranial disease, in particular thrombosis of dural veins including the lateral and superior petrosal sinuses, follows otitis media without obvious macroscopic osteitis of the interposing bone, arterial and venous routes of transmission must be considered. Arterial pathways are unlikely but the mastoid veins communicate with dural veins and with the lateral and superior petrosal sinuses. Thrombophlebitis of the mastoid emissary vein may lead to thrombophlebitis of the lateral sinus. Thrombophlebitis of the small venous channels in the Haversian canals is really an early stage of osteitis, necrosis of bone not yet having occurred, and therefore extension by thrombophlebitis of these channels from mastoid to dural vessels is really an osteitic extension.

ACROSS THE MENINGES

When disease reaches the dura, pachymeningitis results. Dura is very resistant and may become thickened and more adherent to bone in order to limit spread. Granulation tissue may form on the dura and the subdural space may react by obliteration to prevent spill. Because dura is so lightly attached to the calvarium, an extradural abscess in the middle fossa may become very large. On the petrous, however, dura is lightly attached laterally, but from the arcuate eminence medially it is firmly adherent. Hence, abscesses lateral to the arcuate eminence may increase in size by stripping of dura from the deep surface of squamous temporal and parietal bones. Abscesses medial to the arcuate eminence are small. Large abscesses may compress the temporal lobe or by osteitic erosion through the squamous temporal and parietal bones may produce a subperiosteal abscess (a typical Pott's puffy tumour) high up on the skull, well removed from the ear (*Figure 12.2*). In very young children, if the squamous temporal suture lines are not yet closed, a large extradural abscess with the squamous temporal bone lying within it, may be found.

Extradural abscesses in the posterior fossa are limited in size by firm attachment of dura in the subarcuate fossa and internal auditory meatus medially, and along the groove for the lateral sinus externally. Pachymeningitis may lead to thrombosis or thrombophlebitis of the dural vessels. In the posterior fossa an abscess in contact with the lateral sinus produces thickening of the wall with granulation tissue on the surface and mural thrombosis inside. These are nature's attempts to resist infection of the bloodstream. The thrombosis may fill the whole sinus and occlude it. The centre of the thrombus may break down and suppurate, and thrombosis may extend in both directions in an attempt to limit the spread of the disease within the lumen. The thrombosis may extend backwards into the sagittal sinus, forwards along the superior petrosal sinus to the cavernous sinus, or inferiorly down the jugular vein as far as the superior vena cava. During this progressive thrombosis, the clot may break down and throw off emboli to produce pyaemic abscesses. Such dissemination may be the cause of multiple pyaemic abscesses, peritonitis, empyema or suppurative arthritis.

If the dura fails to resist infection it necroses and infection of the subdural space may ensue. Before necrosis happens, the subdural space has usually been obliterated and the infection is transmitted directly across the space. Why the subdural space in some cases should become infected in preference to other tissue planes is unknown, but the explanation may be bacteriological in that the infecting organism is usually a streptococcus, the non-haemolytic forms being more common than the haemolytic forms. The subdural space can become infected without prior formation of an extradural abscess. A subdural empyema most commonly follows frontoethmoid sinusitis, the infection usually being carried by veins to the subdural space. Otogenic subdural empyema is often localized and frequently associated with other intracranial suppurations; by contrast, the rhinogenic lesion is often single and characterized by rapid diffusion throughout the space. The subdural space is co-extensive with the dura and initially a seropurulent effusion develops, rapidly spreading throughout the whole space and even passing beneath the falx cerebri to the opposite hemisphere (*Figure 12.3*). The effusion soon becomes purulent and, as the patient is usually recumbent, thick creamy pus collects near the falx and particularly at the junction of falx and tentorium cerebelli. Granulations may spread into the abscess to produce loculi. Sometimes the pus is absorbed and the subdural space obliterated by fibrous tissue. More commonly the abscess increases in size to become an intracranial space-occupying lesion, from which by venous extension an extensive cortical thrombophlebitis, and subsequently multiple small brain abscesses, may form.

Not all subdural empyemata are so extensive and in the gradual progress of infection across the meninges a localized abscess may arise at the portal of entry. In direct extension, infection may produce obliteration of the subdural and subarachnoid spaces and reach the brain, or it may spill into either space, most commonly into the subarachnoid space to cause leptomeningitis.

The preformed pathways to the subarachnoid space resulting from skull fracture have already been mentioned but more often the path of infection is directly across dura and subdural space of the middle or posterior fossa. The pia-arachnoid may develop adhesions to resist infection and, if successful, an encysted serous meningitis may occur in the posterior fossa. If such a cyst enlarges cerebellar symptoms may arise.

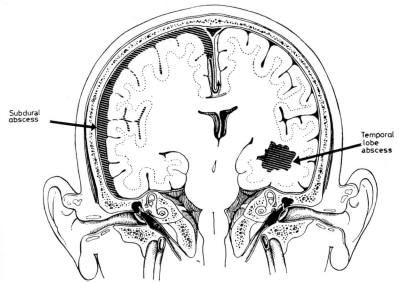

Subdural abscess

Temporal lobe abscess

Figure 12.3 Diagram to show a subdural abscess and a temporal lobe abscess. Note that a subdural abscess may spread throughout the subdural space and across to the opposite side, so producing diffuse cortical irritation and impairment of function, whereas a localized temporal lobe abscess usually only interferes with cortical function in the immediate neighbourhood

Adhesions in the subarachnoid space may localize leptomeningeal disease to form small abscess. Acute diffuse leptomeningitis may result from rupture of extradural or brain abscess.

Rupture of these various abscesses directly into the meninges produces severe, sometimes overwhelming, meningitis. Similar diffuse infections of the subarachnoid system occur with virulent organisms or where resistance is poor. The pia-arachnoid becomes inflamed, frank pus forms and collects mainly in the basal cisterns but also on the vertex of the brain, particularly in pneumococcal infections. The ventricular system may also become involved in diffuse purulent meningitis, and exudate may block the foramina of Munro, Magendie and Luschka and the aqueduct of Sylvius, and so obstruct free flow of cerebrospinal fluid. Exudate lying within brain sulci may affect the function of underlying grey matter and may be the cause of invasion of brain tissue. Paralysis, or loss of sensory function, may follow interference with cranial nerve roots by exudative collections. With full recovery of the patient these exudates may be absorbed, leaving minimal scarring.

Not all meningitis is purulent. In the early stages of invasion a serous effusion may occur which later goes on to suppuration if infection is not controlled. Serous meningitis may be a reactionary response to the presence of an abscess, for example, subdural abscess in contact with the pia-arachnoid. In a lesion of this kind bacteria may not be discoverable.

Localized leptomeningitis and loculation of generalized leptomeningitis were well recognized in the pre-antibiotic era. Cairns and Schiller (1949) held that there was confusion about the situation of subdural pus and concluded that some cases of purulent pachymeningitis had been described as leptomeningitis. Infected subdural effusions may complicate leptomeningitis (Hankinson and Amador, 1956; Jackson, 1962). These commonly occur in infants suffering from meningitis due to *H. influenzae*, pneumococcus and meningococcus (McKay, Ingraham and Matson, 1953).

Cholesteatoma may erode through the meninges without marked local reaction other than obliteration of subdural and subarachnoid spaces. Having reached brain tissue the cholesteatoma produces only superficial erosion. An acute exacerbation may now allow of primary invasion through any of the tissue planes with secondary spread to other planes. The author has seen a case where cholesteatoma actually invaded and filled the lateral sinus, tracked along it to the torcula, and eroded through the occipital bone to present as a suboccipital abscess.

INVASION OF BRAIN TISSUE

Invasion of the brain by progressive loss of tissue probably never causes more than superficial erosion of the cortex.

Thrombophlebitis of the lateral sinus may lead to retrograde extension along a cerebellar vessel and so produce cerebellar thrombophlebitis or abscess. This explains the common association of cerebellar abscess with lateral sinus thrombosis. A similar relationship exists between temporal lobe abscess and superior petrosal sinus thrombosis. Moreover, cerebral thrombophlebitis may produce single or multiple abscesses remote from the source of infection (*Figure 12.4*). Multiple brain abscesses complicating cerebral thrombophlebitis arising from subdural abscess have been described. Thrombophlebitis of a meningeal vessel at the portal of entry may be the cause of direct transmission to brain tissue. Eagleton considered that a high proportion of brain abscesses arose in this fashion.

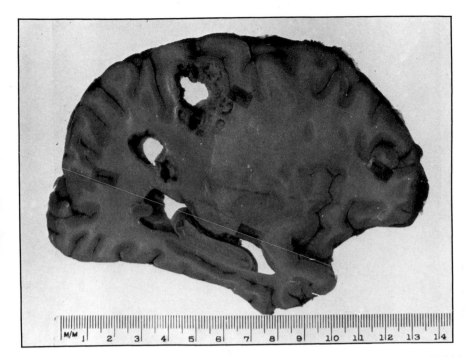

Figure 12.4   Multiple cerebral abscesses which arose from a lateral sinus thrombophlebitis

The perivascular route has been well described by Atkinson (1934), who considered that the majority of his abscess cases were transmitted by this route. A cortical artery on penetrating the grey matter carries with it a funnel-shaped cuff of pia-arachnoid to form the perivascular Virchow–Robin space in direct continuity with the subarachnoid space. Atkinson demonstrated that this space may be infected in the presence of local meningitis and form brain abscesses, although the cortical vessel itself

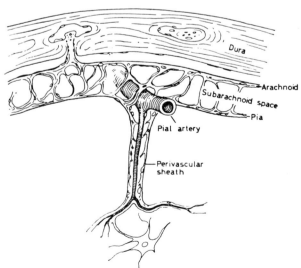

Figure 12.5 Diagram of a Virchow–Robin space (after Atkinson)

was microscopically normal. On this evidence he suggested that this perivascular space is a route of transmission of infection to the cerebral tissue (*Figure 12.5*).

Transmission from meninges to brain is either via the Virchow–Robin spaces or by thrombophlebitis. Arterial thrombosis is rare. If the vessel affected is the middle cerebral artery (*Figure 12.6*), infarction may occur; if an infected embolus is thrown off, a metastatic abscess may form.

The cerebrum and cerebellum receive their blood supply from two groups of end-arteries, a central perforating group of vessels and a cortical group. Because of their

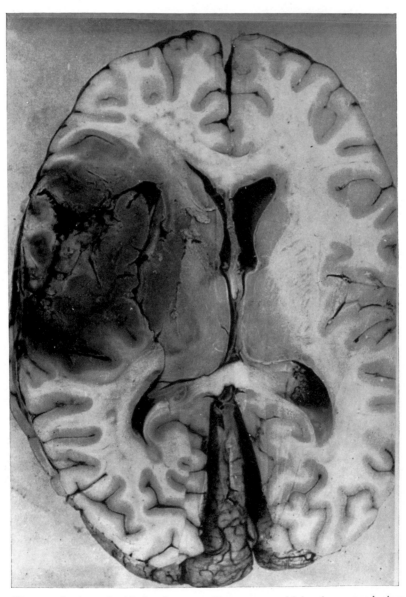

Figure 12.6   A cerebral infarction caused by a temporal lobe abscess producing arteritis of the middle cerebral artery

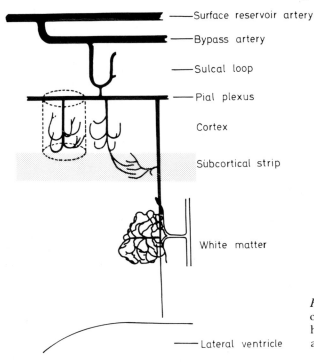

Surface reservoir artery

Bypass artery

Sulcal loop

Pial plexus

Cortex

Subcortical strip

White matter

Lateral ventricle

Figure 12.7 Diagram of the vascular pattern in the cerebral hemispheres (after Rowbotham and Hill)

distribution in the subcortical zone, a relatively vascular layer of white matter is found (*Figure 12.7*). It is in this vascular region that abscess formation begins. In the cerebellum this is usually in the centre of a lobule.

Before an abscess is formed, cerebral thrombophlebitis is present and if the infection is not controlled at this stage, focal necrosis and liquefaction proceed. In the most virulent form of the disease these changes spread along the line of vessels to cause phlegmonous encephalitis which, in turn, is accompanied by a massive swelling of the brain. Less severe forms produce localized non-suppurative encephalitis with brain oedema. Focal necrosis and liquefaction may be rapid enough to produce abscess formation (*see Figure 12.38*) and if reaction is good then microglial and vascular mesoblastic elements are mobilized to produce encapsulation. Once past the stage of acute abscess formation, the size of the abscess, the extent of brain oedema and the degree of encephalitis are indications of the continued battle between disease and resistance. An abscess expands by encroaching on white matter; a very large abscess may still have an intact compressed cortex of grey matter on its outer surface. A capsule can be detected within two weeks of onset of the abscess, and within five or six weeks the capsule may be well-formed and 2 mm thick. As the capsule forms, surrounding brain oedema subsides. When a chronic abscess has formed it may have a thick fibrous or calcified wall and act as a space-occupying benign tumour.

However, within the encapsuled abscess activity varies and the infection may break through the wall and form a new acute abscess, which may itself become encapsuled. By this process a multilocular abscess can form. In the cerebrum the abscess always tends to progress in the direction of the lateral ventricle, into which it may rupture to produce overwhelming infection in the ventricular system and subarachnoid space. If this rupture is valvular a periodic leak from the abscess may occur. This dramatic

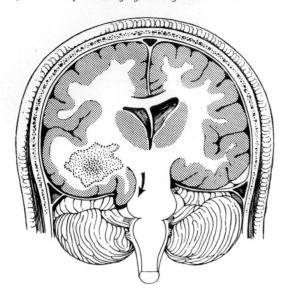

Figure 12.8 Diagram of a tentorial herniation due to a supratentorial hydrocephalus accompanying a temporal lobe abscess. The uncus has been displaced through the tentorium and is compressing the mid-brain

complication is no longer necessarily fatal (Dawes, Marshall and Robson, 1969). A cerebellar abscess may also be loculated and it may burst into the fourth ventricle.

As a brain abscess is adjacent to the temporal bone and has arisen by successive involvement of the tissue planes, the track from the mastoid to the abscess may be macroscopically easily recognized, the so-called 'abscess with a stalk'. Both cerebral and cerebellar abscesses may spontaneously discharge through the stalk into the mastoid but this external leak may be only periodic and inadequate.

As an abscess is a space-occupying and also space-consuming lesion associated with a massive cerebral oedema, a rise in intracranial pressure is not surprising. However, apart from this general external hydrocephalus the abscess and its surrounding oedema in the cerebrum may compress the lateral ventricle on the side of the lesion, and if this supratentorial hydrocephalus is great then the uncus may be displaced through the tentorium (*Figure 12.8*). Compression of the mid-brain at the tentorial level produces further obstruction to free flow of cerebrospinal fluid in the ventricles and a vicious circle leading to further increase of pressure in the ventricular system. If pressure is unrelieved, death must ensue from supratentorial hydrocephalus. Similarly, below the tentorium a cerebellar abscess may displace the flocculus into the foramen magnum to produce 'corking' with consequent failure of cardiovascular and respiratory centres.

Before supratentorial hydrocephalus becomes too severe the abscess and its associated oedema may have compressed the lateral ventricle so markedly at one point as to prevent free communication of a single part of the lateral ventricle (usually the anterior and inferior horns) with the remainder of the ventricular system. A local rise in ventricular pressure may occur, and on external drainage of the abscess the ventricle may itself rupture outwards through the abscess and cannula to the exterior. McGuckin (1936) reported three cases of spontaneous cure of brain abscess by this external ventricular rupture. Another more recent case has been recorded by Hanson and Dawes (1965).

From the description of the pathogenesis of intracranial suppuration, it is easy to see why at least one-third of all otogenic cases show multiple disease. Certain multiple combinations are readily understood, for example, perisinus abscess with lateral sinus thrombosis and cerebellar abscess, or middle fossa extradural abscess together with superior petrosal sinus thrombosis, subdural abscess and temporal lobe abscess. Either or both middle and posterior fossa abscesses may follow lateral sinus thrombosis if superior petrosal thrombophlebitis is present. During the course of the illness one feature may dominate the clinical picture and obscure the development of other lesions. Meningitis may be the sole otogenic complication or it may obscure the fact that a subdural abscess is developing, or indeed may be the presenting feature of a leaking brain abscess. In management, these factors must not be forgotten and the physician must watch for the development of new symptoms and signs indicative of other lesions. General symptoms and signs are considered apart from specific lesions, since the presenting picture in each may be similar.

Symptoms and signs

The invasion of intracranial structures, the establishment of disease within particular tissue planes, and the outcome, satisfactory or fatal, constitute a continued process, perhaps modified by treatment. This concept of continuity throughout the disease is essential to an appreciation of the whole natural history of infection in the individual patient. For descriptive convenience, the process may be considered in stages: (1) the stage of invasion; (2) the stage of established disease; and (3) the terminal phase. Early diagnosis and good management may reverse the disease process at any time during its natural history, but the earlier the diagnosis the more likely will be rapid recovery without morbidity. Ideally, therefore, the diagnosis should be suspected during the stage of invasion because countermeasures taken then may prevent invasion into any one of the tissue planes. Once the disease has become established, then more accurate diagnosis is possible but treatment tends to be less effective and more likely to demand surgical intervention. The rate of spread is variable. It may occur within 24–48 h or may be delayed for weeks. Once established the disease may be rapidly fatal, progress at variable speed, or may become so localized as to cause the patient little trouble for years, before resuming a rapid and possibly fatal progress. Even in these chronic cases, there is often an intermittent history. Although the pattern of events follows certain pathological rules, there is no such thing as the typical case. Therefore, a careful chronological history dating from the onset of the disease—taken from the patient or relatives—is essential and may indeed be so informative that the disease pattern is obvious. Some of the tissue planes crossed or infected produce more obvious symptoms and signs than others, but even in the cerebrum itself focal signs are obvious only if the dominant hemisphere is involved. It is not surprising that physical signs are found only in established disease; sometimes they may be late in the natural course of events and at other times they may be manifest within hours of onset.

STAGE OF INVASION

There is no one picture pathognomonic of the invasive stage, but certain features indicate that intracranial structures are under attack. A patient with uncomplicated acute middle-ear disease is not really ill, and with chronic ear disease he is not even unwell. The simple fact that the infected ear is producing symptoms or signs not strictly related to the ear itself, or even that the patient himself is ill, therefore implies that suppuration has extended beyond the confines of the middle-ear cleft. In chronic disease, earache indicates that something has gone wrong and if the pain is due to pus under pressure in the middle-ear cleft an intracranial lesion is impending. The development of headache is important and indicates that intracranial invasion has already occurred. The site and severity of the headache is variable. In adults it is a striking feature but children may complain little. Vomiting and nausea may accompany the headache and suggest a rise in intracranial pressure. Drowsiness occurs if the brain tissue is involved and the relationship should be accepted until proved otherwise. Changes in temperature and pulse rate must be carefully noted.

The symptoms of intracranial suppuration arise from infection and compression. Headache, vomiting and drowsiness in the early stages are evidence of invasion and change of intracranial pressure; temperature and pulse rate changes are indicative of infection. Headache alone may be due to rise in intracranial pressure, or be a symptom of meningeal irritation in the early phases of leptomeningitis or subdural abscess.

STAGE OF ESTABLISHED DISEASE

In the early stage of localization of disease the symptoms of the invasive phase are continued. Headache may increase in severity, the intensity being intermittent. The site of the headache, although commonly vertical, may be frontal, temporal or occipital but the site is of no focal significance.

Projectile vomiting without nausea has been considered to be typical of intracranial disease. However, this form of vomiting is uncommon, and indeed vomiting may not occur at all. Sometimes the patient may vomit before making any complaint of headache.

Drowsiness may progress to *coma* when compression increases. The drowsy patient is usually uncooperative, tending to fall asleep during questioning and to resent disturbance.

Frequent recording of pulse rate and temperature (at least four-hourly) is necessary if transient rises and falls are not to be missed. As rises in temperature and pulse rate accompany infection, and falls in both accompany cerebral compression, varied patterns are recorded (*Figure 12.9*). After the first few days the temperature in brain abscess tends to vary from 35.6°C (96°F) to 37°C (99°F), but if the temperature reading occasionally reaches more than 38.9°C (102°F) some other tissue plane is also involved. If the pulse rate is maintained at 80/min or less then cerebral compression must be suspected, but when intracranial tension is high the rate may fall into the 40s. McGuckin (1935) was inclined to believe that, with a pulse rate steadily over 80 and intracranial tension high, the lesion was more likely to be in the posterior fossa; in his series the pulse recordings tended to be lower in temporal lobe lesions. At the other extreme where infection predominates, as in lateral sinus thrombophlebitis, the patient has a 'swinging' temperature with high peaks and a pulse rate correspondingly high (usually above 100/min). It is worth noting that a rise in pulse usually accompanies a rise in temperature. Sudden rises in temperature may be accompanied by rigor and the ensuing rapid fall by intense sweating. When records are inadequate these sudden changes may be missed but careful history-taking may elicit descriptions of shivering bouts. The occurrence of rigors undoubtedly means that the patient has thrombophlebitis somewhere. In leptomeningitis, diffuse severe infection and increased

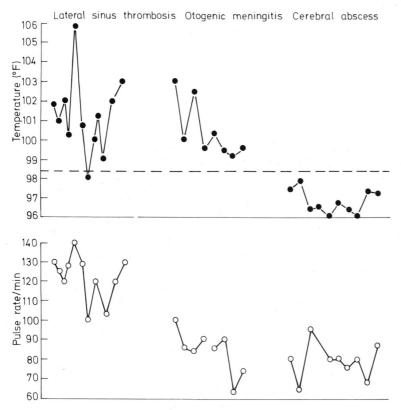

Figure 12.9 Temperature and pulse charts of typical cases. The upper chart shows temperature in degrees Fahrenheit, and the lower chart pulse rate/min

intracranial pressure co-exist, and the typical temperature chart shows a persistently raised temperature with small peaks and a relatively slow pulse.

The general appearance and condition of the patient may be helpful in reaching a diagnosis. In brain abscess the patient is drowsy and listless and never feels well, although at times he is rather better than at others; he has no appetite, progressively loses weight and may eventually be rather emaciated. The meningitic patient is obviously ill with severe headache, is very irritable and curls up facing away from the light. The patient with sinus thrombophlebitis between attacks of rigors may be sitting up in bed taking active notice of his surroundings and looking remarkably well. This temporary well-being may mislead the doctor.

Giddiness is a common complaint in a patient who has a cerebellar complication of ear disease even in the absence of labyrinthitis, and it presumably results from disturbance of cerebellar function. Occasionally, giddiness may accompany a temporal lobe lesion.

Epileptic fits—focal or generalized—are certain evidence of cortical irritation. Frequently the fit may start locally on the contralateral side and then spread to involve a whole limb or both limbs of that side. The starting points indicates the area of cortex involved. Fits occurring in the early phase of the illness suggest that cerebral thrombophlebitis is present. The fits may be so frequent as to suggest status epilepticus. After a bout of fits, the patient is drowsy and here the presence of hemianopia, haemianaesthesia and hemiplegia indicate cerebral damage. If the dominant hemisphere is involved, then aphasia may be present. The onset of fits is sometimes so rapid that there has been no time for abscess formation and thus far the patient may not look seriously ill. Signs of cerebral damage may disappear quite quickly. In the not too ill patient with rapid clearance of residual physical signs there has probably been no more than a cerebral thrombophlebitis. On the other hand, a subdural abscess may also produce cerebral thrombophlebitis. If, after the fits in an obviously ill patient, there is a persistence or progression of physical signs often associated with meningeal irritation, then the presence of subdural abscess must be presumed. In all such cases, further investigation by lumbar puncture, angiography or temporal burr-hole is urgently required for accurate diagnosis.

Neck rigidity results from irritation of basal meninges and is frequently found in leptomeningitis but may accompany subdural empyema or cerebellar abscess. When present it is a useful physical sign and, if associated with Kernig's sign, it is usually diagnostic of leptomeningitis. The length of time from onset of the illness to development of neck rigidity will suggest whether the patient has leptomeningitis alone, or a leaking brain abscess. Neck rigidity may be absent in the early stages of leptomeningitis for when a lesion exists near the vertex a few days may pass before the basal meninges are sufficiently irritated to produce rigidity. In cerebellar abscess the head may also be held in an unusual posture, to one side or forwards.

Nystagmus, a common finding in cerebellar abscesses, is frequently said to be slow and coarse on looking to the side of the lesion and rapid and fine on looking to the other side. However, there is no typical form of cerebellar nystagmus for, although it is horizontorotary, it may be coarse or fine in either direction. In cerebellar lesions the nystagmus may be accompanied by ipsilateral muscle weakness and incoordination of purposive movements of the limbs as demonstrated by testing for dysdiadochokinesia or the finger–nose test. If the patient can walk ataxia will be noted. Temporal lobe lesions occasionally produce horizontorotary nystagmus.

Aphasia is absolute evidence of involvement of the dominant hemisphere, either by cerebral thrombophlebitis or abscess formation. Aphasia may vary greatly from day to day, or hour to hour, presumably because of fluctuations in cerebral oedema around the abscess or thrombophlebitis area. The grossness of aphasia is no indication of the type of lesion. As a rule nominal aphasia is present but the patient may have to be tested with a large number of objects before the defect is observed. He may fail to name some objects but can describe their use. The observer is left with the feeling that the patient has the word on the 'tip of his tongue'. If he is told the name of an object he may easily repeat the name. Compound words provide the crucial tests—a bunch of keys may be called keys, a fountain-pen simply a pen, a box of matches just a match. Two-syllable spondee words such as penknife, armchair, inkwell, are often the first type of object to be misnamed, or the name cannot be recalled. Sometimes patients cannot recall the names of their children or the name of their street. One object may be named and then the same word repeated for all subsequent objects, perhaps ending with a new word having no obvious connotation. This phenomenon is called 'perseveration'.

Papilloedema is regarded as clear evidence of raised intracranial pressure. However, it does not develop until at least 2–3 weeks after the beginning of abscess formation.

It is a late sign. Occasionally, it is seen early in the natural history of intracranial infection, in which event it is a sign of otitic hydrocephalus, a common accompaniment of thrombosis of the larger lateral sinus or sagittal sinus or the only remaining functioning blood sinus.

Other physical signs appear late in the natural history of the disease, although only a few days may have elapsed in chronological history. A tender jugular vein surrounded by swollen lymph nodes may develop and as thrombosis extends so does the level of tenderness. Oedema around the jugular vein may migrate with extending thrombosis (*phlebitis migrans*). A case has been observed in which phlebitis crossed the middle line through the pre-tracheal space to the other side. Embolic abscesses in the lungs may be heralded by pain in the chest, dyspnoea, productive cough and signs of consolidation; an empyema may form and multiple joint swellings appear. An engorged orbit with a proptosed chemotic eye due to cavernous sinus thrombosis may also complicate spreading sinus thrombophlebitis (*Figure 12.10*). Persistent and

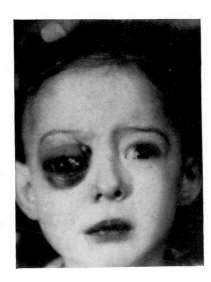

Figure 12.10 Child with cavernous thrombophlebitis complicating lateral sinus thrombophlebitis

progressively developing hemiplegia may follow the extension of a temporal lobe abscess, upwards to affect the motor cortex or inwards to invade the internal capsule (*Figure 12.11*). Rapidly developing diffuse physical signs which occur with cerebral or cerebellar thrombophlebitis or subdural abscess present a contrasting clinical picture to the slower progression of physical signs accompanying brain abscess.

The rate of progress and rapidity of change in the clinical picture are always factors worthy of note; when linked with a good understanding of pathology they provide clues for accurate diagnosis.

THE TERMINAL PHASE

This phase is regarded as ending in death. A leptomeningitis or pyaemia may have overwhelmed the defence mechanisms. A brain or subdural abscess may, by virtue of its size, produce a marked supratentorial hydrocephalus with the unci herniating one after the other through the tentorial opening to compress the midbrain and produce dilated fixed pupils, low temperature, slowing pulse and Cheyne-Stokes breathing in

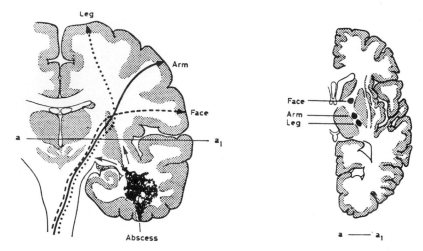

Figure 12.11 Diagram illustrating sequence of paralysis caused by an abscess in the temporosphenoidal lobe. When the abscess extends superficially the face is first affected, then the arm and the leg, but if the abscess spreads inwards towards the posterior part of the internal capsule the order of paralysis is reversed, the leg is first affected, then the arm and lastly the face

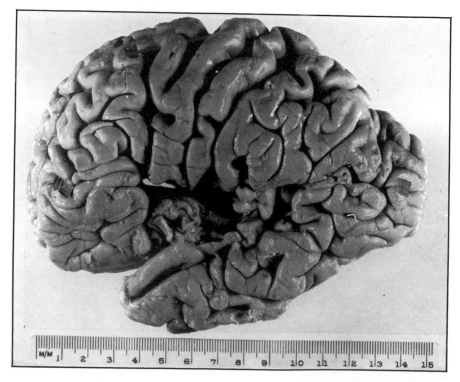

Figure 12.12 The left cerebral hemisphere shows a ragged abscess cavity situated at the lower end of the fissure of Rolando, involving the lower ends of the ascending and inferior frontal convolutions; the abscess has ruptured into the lateral part of the lateral ventricle

a deeply comatose patient. A similar picture may occur in cerebellar abscesses when tonsillar coning occurs. Shortly before death the temperature and pulse rate may suddenly rise and the latter may become uncountable.

Another commonly fatal end is when an overwhelming infection of the sub-arachnoid space follows rupture of an abscess into the ventricular system (*Figure 12.12*).

Management and investigations

It should be possible to suspect the presence of otogenic intracranial spread within 24–48 h of onset from the history alone; treatment should be immediate and investigations may run concurrently. To delay treatment until investigations are complete may allow the disease to progress so far that therapy must be less effective and diagnosis so obvious that investigation becomes unnecessary. In the case of quiescent chronic brain abscess diagnosis cannot be made accurately without careful enquiry, and provided that the risky investigations are carried out in a hospital where immediate neurosurgical treatment is available, little harm results. Between these early and late phases, a variety of problems presents and each requires individual management. The dominant clinical picture on presentation will demand its own specific treatment and if other associated lesions are uncovered these must also be treated as the need of the moment demands. Despite the differences, principles of treatment can be defined and followed.

In cases of intracranial suppuration following acute otitis media, treatment of the complication by antibiotics with or without surgery usually cures the otitis media. However, the ear lesion is important for it is the source of infection, and in uncontrolled acute and chronic ear disease surgical exploration of the middle-ear cleft is essential. In chronic disease, a persistent nidus of infection untouched by antibiotics exists, and until it is removed infection of intracranial tissue planes cannot be effectively controlled.

In acute otitis media, the intracranial infection is due to the organism producing the ear disease and, for this reason, antibiotics employed to cure the intracranial complication usually cure the acute otitis media. In chronic ear disease a multiplicity of saprophytic and potentially pyogenic organisms may infect a cholesteatoma; the intracranial infection may not be due to any of these, however, but rather to the pyococcus causing the acute exacerbation. The pyococcus may be readily grown from the intracranial tissue planes but not demonstrated amidst the variety of organisms in the ear. Frequently pus obtained from a brain abscess of subdural and subarachnoid infections is sterile.

All patients suspected of otogenic intracranial spread must be given antibiotics in high dosage. Penicillin remains the antibiotic of choice, for it is bactericidal to cocci, and if the pyococci are reputedly resistant they are often only relatively so. Therapy must not await full bacteriological studies although it may be varied when information becomes available. Bacteria are not always found in the intracranial tissue planes and the clinical response to antibiotic therapy may be the only guide. However, the blood–brain barrier reduces the effectiveness of systemic penicillin in subarachnoid or cerebral infections. As the blood–brain barrier has little effect on sulphadiazine or sulphamezathine, one of these drugs can usefully be given in combination with systemic penicillin. Streptomycin, a synergistic drug in respect to penicillin is effective against cocci and *H. influenzae* and can be combined with penicillin and sulphamezathine. Chloromycetin, a broad spectrum antibiotic, is extremely effective against *H. influenzae* and is particularly useful in the treatment of meningitis and can readily be combined with penicillin therapy. However, as cases of aplastic anaemia have been reported following its use, adequate blood studies should be done for protection if its use is prolonged or intermittent. The use of these drugs in suitable combinations provides an effective cover for destruction of the usual infecting organisms, namely, staphylococcus, streptococcus, pneumococcus and *H. influenzae*. Penicillin, in the adult, is given in doses of 1–2 megaunits six-hourly with 0.5 g streptomycin twice daily or sulphamezathine 500 mg six-hourly, or both, for the first few days and then 500 000 units six-hourly thereafter. For the child, dosage is scaled down. Sulphamezathine cannot easily be given to the vomiting patient and is therefore omitted. Vomiting may be induced by sulphonamides and, where the symptom is important in diagnosis, sulphonamides should be either withheld or withdrawn. Antibiotics need only be changed if the clinical response is unsatisfactory, or if there is definite laboratory evidence of insensitivity. Laboratory findings may indicate the choice of drug and perhaps suggest a change to tetracyclines. Chloromycetin can usefully be combined with penicillin but should not be continued for too long a period. Antibiotics should be continued until the disease is cured and not merely masked. Penicillin may be continued for long periods, but streptomycin or chloromycetin should not be continued beyond the tenth day unless absolutely necessary. Sulphonamides may replace streptomycin or chloromycetin if prolonged treatment is desirable.

During the first three days after the onset of intracranial disease, a brain abscess will not yet have developed, and the major problems are those of extradural infection, leptomeningitis and sinus thrombophlebitis. Cerebral or cerebellar signs will, in this early state, result from thrombophlebitis and, if adequate antibiotics are given, the thrombophlebitis will usually be controlled before focal necrosis and liquefaction produce an abscess. In this crucial phase antibiotics, supplemented by surgery to the ear, may rapidly control the intracranial extension. Medical treatment must start at once and the ear must be explored at the optimum moment in the ensuing 12–24 h, much depending on the patient's condition. Signs of gross cerebral compression are usually absent in the acute phase and lumbar puncture may be safe enough. For convenience the puncture may be done most safely immediately after mastoid surgery.

The mere fact that symptoms or signs suggestive of intracranial spread are present is, in itself, a definitive indication for exploration of the middle-ear cleft in chronic ear disease. At operation, it is essential to expose the middle fossa dura and the lateral sinus even if the bone is macroscopically intact for—as discussed in pathogenesis—extradural and perisinus abscesses may lie behind an intact tegmen or sinus plate. For adequate exposure the post-aural approach is often the best. All cholesteatoma is excised from the middle-ear cleft and just enough tegmen removed to expose dura for inspection. In the presence of a large middle fossa extradural abscess enough tegmen should be removed to give wide drainage, but in the case of a small abscess or dural granulations, the exposure may be limited to little more than the extent of the lesion. When dura is necrotic it may be incised crucially to see if a small subdural abscess needs drainage. When a perisinus abscess is present, sufficient of the lateral sinus plate should be removed to expose normal sinus wall beyond the abscess. A mural or solid thrombus of the sinus may be left, provided normal dura has been exposed. Necrotic sinus wall should be widely exposed and incised so that any necrotic or suppurating thrombus may be aspirated. It is not necessary to remove the whole clot since it is a protective mechanism. Control of the blood-stream infection will depend on the effectiveness of the antibiotics given.

Any tracks of disease are thoroughly investigated and excised. If the labyrinth is grossly invaded it is destroyed. Trautmann's triangle may need to be excavated to remove disease extending to the posterior fossa. The epitympanum must be carefully examined and tracks to the petrous apex opened, or if towards the middle fossa dura exposed. At the end of this operation the mastoid cavity is packed with BIPP gauze and the post-aural wound left open. While the patient is still under anaesthesia, lumbar puncture can be performed.

Lumbar puncture is a valuable investigation and often confirms the clinical diagnosis. If cerebrospinal fluid pressure is high or the fluid opalescent or turbid an intrathecal injection of 5000 units of penicillin in 5 ml of normal saline is given. A smear of centrifuged cerebrospinal fluid should be examined to determine whether cocci or bacilli are present. If cocci are found the antibiotics need not be changed unless the sensitivity reactions as determined after culture indicate that they should be. When bacilli are found chloromycetin should be given together with penicillin as the organism is likely to be *H. influenzae* and streptomycin only given if meningitis should prove to be tuberculous. If no organisms are found on culture there may be no need to continue intrathecal injections of penicillin. However, even in the absence of gross meningitis intrathecal penicillin can be a useful adjunct to systemic penicillin, for it is the only satisfactory method of increasing the penicillin level in the cerebrospinal fluid and thereby giving adequate protection against surgical dissemination of the infection. A rise in spinal pressure with only a slight increase in cell count and protein is consistent with a diagnosis of brain or subdural abscess. However, a normal spinal fluid may exist in the presence of a subdural or brain abscess.

If there is clinical evidence of marked cerebral compression, lumbar puncture may be dangerous. Tests of the Queckenstedt, Tobey–Ayer and Lillie–Crowe type are superfluous, for the mastoid operation has demonstrated the presence or absence of sinus thrombophlebitis. These tests are at best unreliable and should never influence a decision to operate. Patients with septicaemia due to thrombophlebitis may haemolyse their blood, and periodic blood transfusions are advisable when their haemoglobin falls.

Antibiotics supplemented by surgery control such lesions as extradural abscess, leptomeningitis and sinus thrombophlebitis. If these are the only problems then a satisfactory outcome can be expected. Post-operatively a constant watch should be kept for evidence of other lesions, such as cerebral, cerebellar or subdural abscesses. As a temporal lobe abscess may interfere with the lower fibres of the optic radiation an upper quadrant hemianopia may be detected by simple confrontation. When the patient is cooperative, visual field defect is best detected by perimetry (*Figure 12.42*). If the dominant hemisphere is likely to be involved frequent testing for nominal asphasia is advisable, for reasons already described. Cerebral thrombophlebitis or subdural abscess may be heralded by epileptiform fits and diffuse paralytic lesions. The rapidity of the appearance of this diffuse clinical picture probably excludes abscess formation within the temporal lobe but further investigations are necessary Nowadays the simplest and quickest method of detecting the presence of intracranial abscess is by the use of an EMI scanner. When this investigation is not readily available then other less satisfactory methods should be used. Ordinary x-rays of the skull occasionally show displacement of the pineal gland to the opposite side and an electroencephalogram, provided that the sphenoid electrode is included, usually demonstrates changes in the cerebral hemispheres which may be diagnostic of a brain abscess. Arteriography in skilled hands carries little risk and is the best technique for localizing supratentorial lesions such as brain or subdural abscess. Ventriculography and air encephalography are much riskier procedures, particularly if cerebral compression is evident, and should only be carried out where neurosurgical facilities are available. They are useful to exclude space-occupying lesions and occasionally may demonstrate lesions when other methods have failed (Pennybacker, 1961).

Not all cases present early, but provided the patient is fit enough and there is no evidence of marked cerebral compression, this method of approach is very safe. If there is clear evidence of a temporal lobe abscess, clinically or arteriographically, at the time of admission to hospital, the operation on the ear and tapping of the abscess may be done under the same anaesthetic. The temporal lobe abscess or large subdural abscess can be tapped through the clean field of a temporal burr-hole (*Figure 12.13*). A blunt brain cannula is used for tapping the brain abscess and one or two attempts may be necessary before successful entry. At the time of tapping, the consistency and thickness of the abscess wall should be assessed for information about the chronicity of the abscess. Pus is aspirated and 50 000 units of penicillin are injected into the abscess

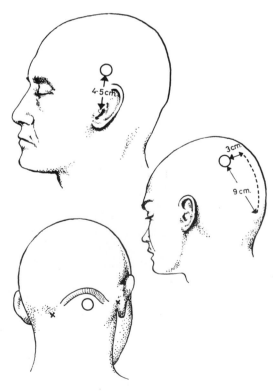

Figure 12.13   Common sites of burr-holes used in the management of otogenic brain abscesses

cavity and the progress of the abscess can be assessed by serial EMI scanning. If no scanner is available 2 ml of Steripaque is mixed with the penicillin and injected into the abscess cavity through the same cannula that was used for drainage. As the abscess wall takes up some of the radio-opaque material serial radiography can provide a visual assessment of progress. Aspiration of pus produces immediate improvement in headache, the patient becomes more awake and focal signs lessen or disappear. Repeated aspiration, using a pointed needle when the temporal wound is healed, leads to a general improvement, for the abscess shrivels up or becomes encapsulated and brain oedema becomes less. Serial scanning or radiographs after the use of Steripaque demonstrate any improvement. If, despite repeated aspiration, the abscess continues to increase in size, most neurosurgeons prefer to excise the lesion. When the abscess shrivels up and only a crenated scar can be seen radiologically, excision is probably unnecessary. Occasionally a crenated scar is seen but the patient's cerebral condition does not show the expected improvement; here loculation of the abscess or the presence of a subdural abscess should be suspected. Repeated investigation may demonstrate the cause. If a loculus is found, it must be aspirated or excised. Before a brain abscess is pronounced as cured the cerebrospinal fluid and air encephalogram must be normal.

Cerebellar abscess is similarly treated by repeated aspiration through a burr-hole made midway between the mastoid process and the external occipital protuberance (*Figure 12.13*). Many cerebellar abscesses complicate lateral sinus thrombosis and if thrombosis is found on exploration, a careful watch should be kept for the development of cerebellar signs. If cerebellar signs supervene then the patient probably has thrombophlebitis which may respond to adequate antibiotic therapy alone. If the response is poor or signs progress an abscess may be present. When intracranial pressure rises rapidly and pushes the cerebellar tonsils into the foramen magnum, urgent tapping of the abscess is required either through a suboccipital burr-hole or through the posterior fossa dura adjacent to Trautmann's triangle (*Figure 12.14*). When the transmastoid route is used, the abscess may be tapped through its stalk. Lumbar puncture should not be done in the presence of cerebellar abscess.

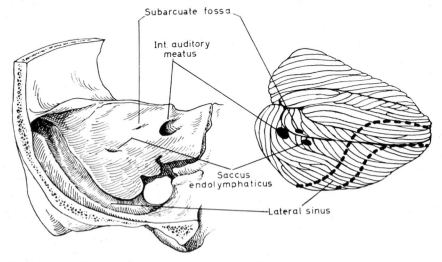

Subarcuate fossa

Int. auditory meatus

Saccus endolymphaticus

Lateral sinus

Figure 12.14   Diagram to illustrate the relations of the posterior surface of the temporal bone to the cerebellum

Occasionally, in a patient who develops a rapid increase in cerebellar signs and cerebral compression, a brain needle passed through the suboccipital burr-hole or Trautmann's triangle unexpectedly leads to a spurt of cerebrospinal fluid under pressure from a subarachnoid cyst. All signs of compression and cerebellar dysfunction may clear up immediately.

Once a subdural abscess is suspected arteriography should be done, but if this method is not available or there is evidence of rapidly increasing intracranial tension with diffuse signs, a temporal burr-hole should be made and the subdural space inspected. The earlier the subdural lesion is treated and drained the less it is likely that loculation will occur in the neighbourhood of the falx. As many as six burr-holes may be necessary on one side of the skull for adequate drainage and irrigation of a large subdural abscess. Small polythene tubes are inserted through the burr-holes to irrigate the subdural space with penicillin solution containing 500 units/ml. A drainage opening through the tegmen into the subdural space provides dependent drainage when the patient is sitting up. The infected effusion complicating meningitis, if recognized early, clears up rapidly with proper drainage and irrigation.

One of the great advantages of early mastoid surgery is that the focus of infection can be removed and lesions in adjacent planes drained, whereas the neurosurgical approach does not deal with the source, with small extradural abscesses or sinus thrombophlebitis.

The approach to management so far has considered either patients presenting with the acute picture of meningitis and sinus thrombophlebitis and subsequent development of brain and subdural abscesses, or patients with brain or subdural abscesses not showing gross evidence of cerebral compression in the early days. In either case a mastoid operation could be performed, and the acute lesions controlled by antibiotics, in which event cerebral lesions may never develop or may never demand urgent interference. However, brain abscess may be the dominant feature in the clinical picture and stupor, coma, slow pulse and even pupillary changes may be present, or meningitis may have followed a prolonged history of invasion and be already consequent on a leaking brain abscess. In such cases the brain abscess must be treated first and urgently, preferably through a temporal or suboccipital burr-hole. Neurosurgeons are generally opposed to draining cerebral or cerebellar abscesses by transmastoid routes. There is the fear of planting a brain abscess by exploring the brain through an infected field and the risk of the development of a brain fungus in the wound. The danger of planting a brain abscess, although real, is not a common occurrence. Brain fungus is of greater concern and is most likely to follow extensive removal of bone.

In the past, removal of the tegmen in continuity with the neighbouring part of the squamous temporal bone was used to gain access for drainage of a temporal lobe abscess. Drainage was by tube and consequently large herniations developed. However, even with much more limited removal of the tegmen and repeated aspiration small herniations into the mastoid develop. As a rule, these can be excised and the dura repaired by fascia but undoubtedly the surgical method is at fault, for brain fungus can easily be avoided if temporal lobe abscesses are always drained through a temporal burr-hole. For cerebellar abscesses, access was often obtained by extensive removal of bone external to the lateral sinus. Wide exposure of the cerebellum was achieved but a larger cerebellar fungus followed. However, a small incision in the dura of Trautmann's triangle with repeated aspiration does not produce cerebellar fungus; it is a useful approach for those otologists unskilled in neurosurgical techniques and gives a more direct approach to a cerebellar abscess. It is therefore recommended that abscesses should be drained through a clean field via temporal or suboccipital burr-holes, but an approach through Trautmann's triangle to a cerebellar abscess may be useful under unusual circumstances. Certain neurosurgical techniques should be learnt by all otologists, for there is no doubt that their use is occasionally required when a neurosurgeon is not available. Pennybacker (1961) points out that the treatment of brain abscess is a neurosurgical problem and that the patient should pass into neurosurgical hands as soon as possible. To transport a stuporose or comatose patient is inadvisable, but by giving 1 g of urea/kg of body weight in a solution of invert sugar intravenously, intracranial pressure may be reduced in 20 min. The reduction in pressure may last for several hours, usually long enough for the patient to be transferred safely. Alternatively a 25 per cent solution of mannitol, or a large dosage of dexamethasone may be used. If this intravenous injection does not improve the patient, then the abscess must be tapped immediately. The advantage of transmastoid drainage was that it was a lifesaving measure which could be easily performed by the relatively unskilled.

Throughout management it has been stressed that treatment should never be withheld merely because clinical diagnosis is as yet incomplete. Thus, to await a positive bacteriological culture from the cerebrospinal fluid or a positive blood culture in thrombophlebitis is to court disaster. Similarly to await the full development of a brain or subdural abscess before starting treatment means that the best time for prevention has been lost. The best way to manage otogenic intracranial complications is to recognize that invasion is occurring or impending and to institute treatment at once. Adequate therapy not only controls meningeal and bloodstream infection; it may also play a great part in controlling spreading encephalitis. When mastoid surgery is indicated, the operation should be performed at the earliest moment and if the post-aural wound is packed open, surgery may be completed at a later date when disease is controlled and time is unimportant.

Techniques of investigations

Lumbar puncture is the easiest method of obtaining cerebrospinal fluid for examination; it is not a routine measure to be undertaken lightly, since quite apart from mere discomfort, severe headache or root pain may follow and if adequate care is not taken meningitis may be induced. When intracranial pressure is marked lumbar puncture may precipitate herniation of the unci through the tentorium, coning of cerebellar tonsils into the foramen magnum, or rupture of an abscess into a ventricle. Any of these accidents may be fatal, and immediate surgery for relief of intracranial tension is the only hope of saving the patient. The dangers are greater in the presence of cerebellar abscess even when the clinical evidence of raised tension is slight. However, as changes in the cerebrospinal fluid may be of immense value to complete diagnosis and intrathecal injections of antibiotics are a useful adjunct in treatment, lumbar puncture is often necessary. Lumbar puncture done early in the course of invasion provides a satisfactory base-line for comparison with later diagnostic or therapeutic findings. Whenever lumbar puncture is undertaken, the reason for doing it and the risks entailed should be clearly understood.

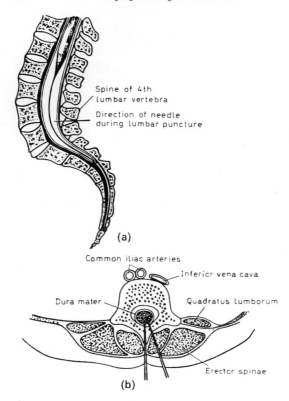

Spine of 4th
lumbar vertebra

Direction of needle
during lumbar puncture

(a)

Common iliac arteries

Inferior vena cava

Dura mater

Quadratus lumborum

Erector spinae

(b)

Figure 12.15 Lumbar puncture: (a) showing direction of needle: (b) horizontal section through fourth lumbar vertebra showing structures concerned. A needle is shown in each of the two positions described in the text

In the adult at the level of the lower border of the first lumbar vertebra the spinal cord ends and rapidly tapers as the conus medullaris, before continuing as the filum terminale to the second sacral vertebra (*Figure 12.15*). Between the second lumbar and second sacral vertebrae there is a large subarachnoid cavity which contains only the filum terminale, the spinal roots of the corda equina, and cerebrospinal fluid. It is this subarachnoid cavity which is tapped from behind in lumbar puncture. The two widest interlaminal spaces are between the third and fourth and the fourth and fifth lumbar vertebrae.

INSTRUMENTS (*Figure 12.16*)
A spinal needle and stilette should be about 8 cm long and 1.2–1.5 mm in diameter. The needle may be fitted with a three-way stopcock and a stilette which passes through the stopcock, for then the needle can be fitted to a manometer without loss of cerebrospinal fluid. The stilette should not be withdrawn until the lumbar theca is pierced. The test tubes for collection of fluid and a manometer graduated up to 300 cm must be at hand. Antibiotics given intrathecally must be prepared and checked beforehand. Instruments must be sterile and autoclaving is the best method of ensuring sterility.

POSITION OF PATIENT
Whether lumbar puncture is done in the sitting position or in the left lateral position, it is most important to obtain maximum flexion of the lumbar spine so that the

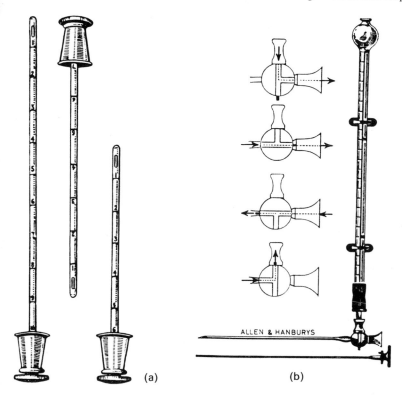

Figure 12.16   (a) Jefferson's brain cannulae with stilettes. (Reproduced by courtesy of H. K. Lewis); (b) Cerebrospinal manometer (Greenfield's), with three-way stopcock. (Reproduced by courtesy of Allen and Hanburys Ltd)

intervertebral spaces may be at their widest. The sitting position is the least useful for patients with intracranial suppurative disease and therefore, as the left lateral position has to be adopted most often, it is best to become accustomed to this technique. The patient lies on the left side, with the knees drawn well up to the chin, and near the edge of the bed or operating table; the spinal column should lie exactly in the horizontal plane. This position is difficult to maintain in a healthy patient, and support at the flexed knees and back of the neck may be needed to maintain flexion. In a meningitic, uncooperative, semicomatose or anaesthetized patient the flexed position must be firmly maintained by an assistant. A swab soaked in iodine is used to draw a line between the highest point of the iliac crests. This line crosses the interval between the third and fourth vertebrae. Another mark is placed at the fourth–fifth interspace. The skin is now sterilized, the patient towelled and an injection of local anaesthetic (procaine, lignocaine) given at the site of election, the third or fourth lumbar interspace. The needle, with stilette in position, is introduced midway between the spinous processes of the selected interspace, and thrust forwards and slightly upwards in the sagittal plane. Resistance is met from the supraspinous and interspinous ligaments and at about 4–5 cm there is further resistance from the ligamentum flavum; after a further advance of about 0.5 cm the theca is pierced. Some surgeons prefer to insert the needle about 1 cm from the midline to avoid the resistance of supraspinous and interspinous ligaments and, by inclination of the needle towards the midline, the theca is penetrated at the same site. When the needle is thought to have penetrated the theca the stilette is removed; if in the right position cerebrospinal fluid will flow, but if no flow is obtained the needle should be rotated through a quarter of a circle. If fluid still does not flow the stilette should be replaced, the needle withdrawn and another attempt made. Failure to obtain fluid usually means that the puncture has not been correctly performed. Particular difficulties are met in patients with scoliosis, arthritis, dorsal muscle spasm as in meningitis, or in obstreperous people. If blood flows from the needle it means that the venous plexus has been punctured. To obtain blood-free fluid it is best to use another needle, or at least to clear the old needle with sterile water. As soon as fluid flows, the stopcock is turned so that fluid enters the manometer to record the pressure. Any tests of pressure in response to jugular compression which are thought to be necessary are now performed and then up to 2–3 ml are run off into each test tube for examination. Finally the needle is withdrawn and a piece of collodion gauze placed over the site of entry.

Cisternal and ventricular puncture

Cisternal puncture rarely needs to be performed by the otologist, for the usual indications are related to the practice of neurosurgery. Puncture of the cisterna magna permits the cisternal fluid pressure to be compared with that in the lumbar theca, the introduction of opaque media or air into the subarachnoid space for neuroradiological studies, and intrathecal injection of antibiotics when it is the best route available. Cisternal puncture must not be done if the patient has a cerebellar abscess or if intracranial pressure is high.

Ventricular puncture is most commonly used for the injection of air for ventriculographic studies; occasionally it is used for the injection of antibiotics or as a surgical method of reducing supratentorial hydrocephalus prior to excision of a space-occupying lesion. Only rarely is it used to collect cerebrospinal fluid, and then usually to obtain specifically ventricular fluid.

TECHNIQUE OF CISTERNAL PUNCTURE

The occipital hair is shaved and the skin cleansed. The instruments used are similar to those used for lumbar puncture and should be sterile. The head is flexed and held by an assistant, either with the patient in a sitting or lying position and 1 per cent procaine or 1 per cent lignocaine injected in the midline between the occiput and the axis. The spine of the axis, which is the highest spinous process palpable, should be marked and the needle introduced in the midline about 1.25 cm above this and directed towards the glabella. At a depth of about 3 cm resistance from the posterior atlanto-occipital ligament is met and the needle is advanced by approximately a further 0.5–1 cm to enter the cisterna magna. The stilette is withdrawn and cerebrospinal fluid aspirated by gentle suction with a syringe, since a free flow occurs only if fluid pressure is raised. The posterior surface of the medulla lies about 6.5–7 cm from the skin surface in the adult and the needle must not be advanced beyond 6.5 cm.

TECHNIQUE OF VENTRICULAR PUNCTURE

Ventricular puncture is a neurosurgical procedure and full theatre technique should be maintained throughout. The scalp must be fully shaved and the skin prepared; two

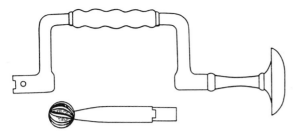

Figure 12.17 The Hudson brace and burr

points, 8–9 cm above the external occipital protruberance and 3 cm on each side of the midline, are marked (*see Figures 12.13* and *12.34*). Sufficient local anaesthetic is injected at each mark to permit a 3–4 cm incision. An incision carried right down to the bone is made between compression swabs and a self-retaining retractor inserted to control local bleeding. The burr-holes are made with a Hudson perforator and burr (*Figures 12.17* and *12.18*); the dura is inspected, the dural vessels coagulated by diathermy and a cruciate incision made. The brain cannula is introduced and aimed at the pupil on the same side; the ventricle is reached at a depth of about 5 cm and cerebrospinal fluid withdrawn. The normal ventricle is always tapped first.

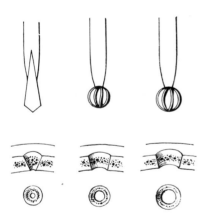

Figure 12.18 Method of producing a burr-hole by using first a perforator, after which the hole is enlarged by burrs of increasing size (after Rowbotham)

In the infant before closure of the anterior fontanelle, a short lumbar puncture needle introduced through the outer corner of the fontanelle (at least 1 cm from the midline to avoid the superior sagittal sinus) and directed downwards and slightly outwards, reaches the lateral ventricle at a depth of 3–5 cm.

Examination of the cerebrospinal fluid (*see Table 12.3*)

Changes in pressure recordings, cellular and biochemical elements of the cerebrospinal fluid must always be correlated with the clinical picture and not studied in isolation.

Pressure changes

The normal pressure range is 60–150 mm of fluid in the adult, and 45–90 mm of fluid in the child. The pressure is raised in the presence of an abscess, otitic hydrocephalus,

Table 12.3 The cerebrospinal fluid in certain intracranial complications of otitis media and mastoiditis

Disease	Appearance	Cells	Protein	Sugar	Chlorides	Organisms	Pressure
Leptomeningitis	Turbid or purulent, clots on standing	Greatly increased, mainly polymorphs	Increased, may be up to 200 mg/100 ml	Reduced or absent	Reduced to 650 or 600 mg/100 ml	Usually present	Raised
Tuberculous leptomeningitis	Clear, a fine coagulum on standing	10–400/ml; lymphocytes predominate	Increased, 200–300 mg/100 ml	May be diminished	Reduced, often below 600 mg/100 ml	Seldom present	Raised
Cerebral abscess	Clear	Up to 30/ml; lymphocytes predominate	Moderate increase	Normal	Normal	Absent	Raised
Cerebellar abscess	Clear	Up to 30/ml; lymphocytes predominate	Moderate increase	Normal	Normal	Absent	Usually raised
Purulent pachymeningitis	Clear	100–300; mainly polymorphs	Increased, 80–120 mg/100 ml		Normal	Absent	Raised
Otitic hydrocephalus	Normal	Normal	Normal	Normal	Normal	Absent	Raised

meningitis and encephalitis. Lateral sinus thrombosis produces a rise in cerebrospinal fluid pressure only if an associated lesion is present or the sinus obstruction is itself the cause of otitic hydrocephalus.

Cerebrospinal lumbar pressure is lowered if a spinal block has occurred following meningeal adhesions complicating meningitis, or in consequence of excessive dosage of intrathecal antibiotics. The block usually occurs in the spinal meninges or at the level of the foramen magnum.

QUECKENSTEDT'S TEST

Normally when both jugular veins in the neck are compressed the manometric reading rises quickly to 300–400 mm and on release of pressure, falls as quickly to normal. This can only occur if there is free circulation of fluid throughout the ventricles and subarachnoid cavity. No rise can occur if there is a complete block between the lumbar theca and the cranial subarachnoid space; or if the block is only partial, then the rise and fall in pressure readings are delayed.

TOBEY–AYER TEST

In unilateral sinus thrombosis pressure on the jugular vein of the normal side produces a quick rise of pressure equivalent to that of bilateral jugular pressure in the normal subject. Compression of the vein on the affected side produces little or no rise of pressure. Observation of the change in fluid pressure during alternate unilateral compression of the jugular vein is occasionally helpful in determining which sinus is thrombosed in bilateral ear disease.

Temporary reduction in fluid pressure may tide the patient over a crisis. One of the best methods is by intravenous injection of 1 g/kg body weight of urea. Other agents injected intravenously are 100 ml of 15–20 per cent hypertonic saline solution, dexamethazone, 25 per cent mannitol solution, or 50 per cent glucose in normal saline solution; 50–75 ml of 50 per cent solution of sodium chloride can be given per rectum and retained for 15 min.

The macroscopic appearance of the cerebrospinal fluid is of great value. Turbidity indicates the presence of large numbers of cells or organisms, or both. Clear fluid indicates that marked inflammatory involvement of the subarachnoid space has not yet occurred. The presence of coagulum indicates the development of a clot of fibrin and occurs when there is a cerebrospinal fluid block; it may also be noted in meningitis and polyneuritis. A yellow stained fluid suggests such lesions as subarachnoid haemorrhage, tumour adjacent to the ventricular system, or spinal block. Blood in the fluid may be due to needle-puncture of a venous plexus or to subarachnoid haemorrhage. In the former, the supernatant fluid is clear and the later specimens are even clearer, whereas in subarachnoid haemorrhage the fluid is equally stained in all specimens and the supernatant fluid is xanthochromic.

The normal cell content of the cerebrospinal fluid does not exceed 5 cells/mm³. Excess of cells (pleocytosis) in the cerebrospinal fluid suggests meningeal irritation but not necessarily frank meningitis. Meningitis characteristically produces increase of polymorphonuclear cells but in more chronic infections such as a brain abscess or subdural abscess, lymphocytosis predominates. The greater the number of polymorphonuclear cells present the more acute the lesion whereas predominance of lymphocytes may indicate a virus aetiology or a suppurative lesion close to the meninges. Polymorphonuclear cells may be seen in the presence of brain abscess or subdural abscess, in large numbers if ventricular rupture has occurred but in small numbers if such lesions are merely irritating ependyma or meninges by their proximity. However, in brain abscess, extradural and subdural abscess, and sinus thrombophlebitis the cerebrospinal fluid may be normal.

The protein content of cerebrospinal fluid is usually directly related to the cell content but a disproportionate relationship may be seen in virus meningo-encephalitides. A very high protein content in a case not frankly purulent may follow a spinal block, polyneuritis or Landry's paralysis. Although the chlorides fall in pyogenic meningitis, marked falls in chloride content are usually seen only in tuberculous meningitis. The sugar content of the fluid falls sharply in pyogenic meningitis and very slightly, if at all, in tuberculous meningitis.

One of the specimens collected in a test tube should be set aside for bacteriological study. After spinning down the turbid fluid in a centrifuge, a smear stained by Gram's method should be examined microscopically to determine whether or not intracellular or extracellular organisms are present and whether these are cocci or bacilli. This information is valuable when positive, as it may guide antibiotic therapy while awaiting culture studies. Today, however, positive bacteriological cultures are often unattainable despite the presence of frank meningitis. Immediate guides to therapy must be the pressure of cerebrospinal fluid and its cell content. Study of the clinical picture and the fluid findings together may, for example, establish a diagnosis of meningitis or may raise the question of another lesion, such as brain abscess or subdural abscess. A clinical picture of headache, marked neck rigidity and focal manifestations, with disproportionate changes in the cerebrospinal fluid, will suggest subdural abscess.

The electroencephalogram

The electroencephalogram has largely been superseded by EMI scanning in the diagnosis of intracranial abscesses. If encephalographic evidence is to be reliable it must be produced by those skilled in technique and experienced in interpretation. When a temporal lobe abscess is suspected, a sphenoid electrode should be used. A high proportion of brain lesions may be located by this method. In the very acute lesion a marked unilateral disturbance may be present but characteristically a well-defined focus of delta activity is found. A characteristic electroencephalogram of a posterior fossa lesion may indicate a cerebellar abscess but a normal electroencephalogram may be recorded in the presence of a cerebellar lesion.

Radiology

The radiology of otogenic intracranial disease has been completely revolutionized by the invention of computerized axial tomography by G. Hounsfield of EMI.

In centres possessing such a machine this is the investigation of choice not only for the initial diagnosis but also for follow-up examinations to ensure that treatment has been adequate.

On an EMI scan an abscess shows up as a low density area surrounded by 'finger-like' areas of oedema. The lesion and its surrounding oedema occupy a considerable amount of space and therefore the ventricles are shown to be markedly displaced. After the intravenous injection of Conray contrast medium the capsule enhances and shows as a dense rim. These appearances are illustrated in *Figure 12.19* and *Figure 12.20*. If there is no ring enhancement in the low density area after the injection of

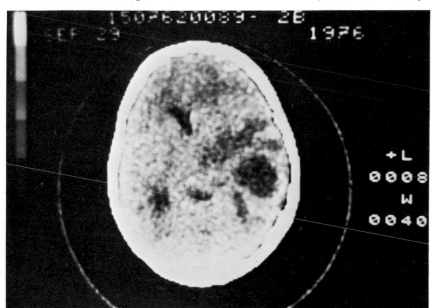

Figure 12.19   EMI scan of a patient with a left temporal lobe abscess. The abscess shows as a round low density area surrounded by 'finger-like' oedema. Note the gross displacement of the lateral ventricles

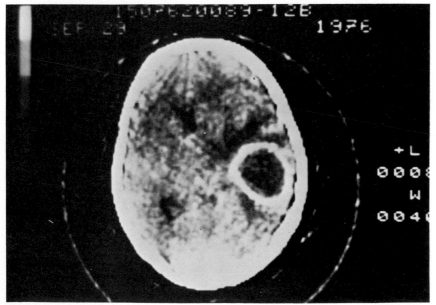

Figure 12.20   Same patient as in *Figure 12.19* after intravenous injection of contrast medium. The abscess capsule takes up the contrast medium and shows as a high density ring shadow

Conray this usually indicates an area of cerebritis which has not yet progressed to true abscess formation.

Abscesses in the posterior fossa on EMI scans usually show displacement of the fourth ventricle by the abscess itself, dilatation of the lateral ventricles and third ventricle due to obstruction of the CSF pathways and after contrast injection a similar enhancement to supratentorial abscesses. These appearances are illustrated in *Figures 12.21 (a–c)*.

Scans after adequate treatment show dissolution of the abscess capsule, diminution of the oedema and a return of the ventricular system to a more normal position. These appearances are shown in *Figure 12.22*.

Whether an EMI scanner is available or not, mastoid radiographs are of little value in otogenic intracranial disease since they seldom add anything useful to careful clinical assessment. Radiographs may delineate the tegmen and lateral sinus plate and so assist the search into assessing the distance between the posterior meatal wall and the sinus. However, in any planned operation due allowance must be made for the possibility of a forward lateral sinus or a low middle fossa dura. A cholesteatoma may or may not be demonstrated by plain radiographs even when it is known to be present. Even tomography of the skull may fail to show quite marked cholesteatomatous destruction.

Plain x-rays of the skull are similarly of little value; probably the only helpful sign is a displaced pineal confirming the presence of a space-occupying lesion on one or other side (*Figure 12.23*).

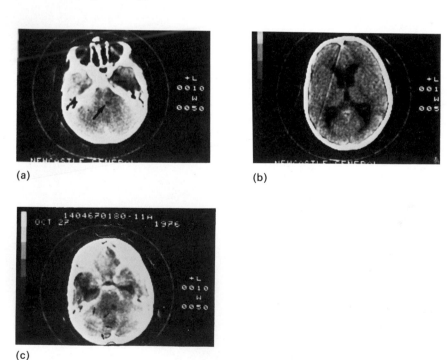

(a)

(b)

(c)

Figure 12.21   EMI scan of a patient with a cerebellar abscess. (a) The fourth ventricle is displaced to the right (arrow). (b) The lateral and third ventricles are dilated. (c) An abscess cavity is shown in the left cerebellar hemisphere

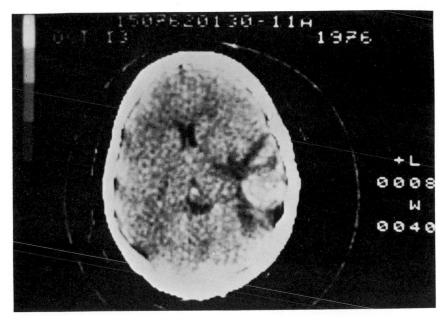

Figure 12.22　The same patient as in *Figures 12.19* and *12.20* after treatment. The scan is taken after an intravenous injection of contrast medium. The low density central area has disappeared and the capsule is dissolving. The lateral ventricles are now almost in normal position

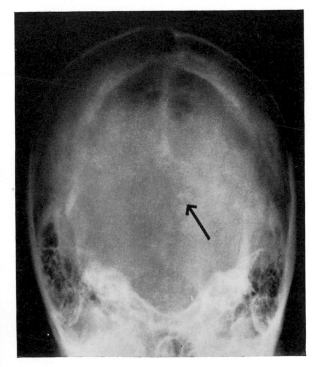

Figure 12.23　Half-axial projection: displacement of calcified pineal. (Reproduced by courtesy of Dr. G. L. Gryspeerdt)

Angiography

When computerized axial tomography is not available some form of angiography will be necessary to confirm the presence and the site of an abscess. If this is suspected to be supratentorial the angiography will be via the carotid artery. If it is suspected to be in the posterior fossa vertebral angiography will be necessary. In either case an injection of a water soluble contrast medium into the carotid or vertebral artery is performed and serial radiographs are taken. Abscesses appear as space-occupying lesions, commonly in the temporal lobe, without any evidence of pathological circulation (*Figures 12.24* and *12.25*).

Sinus thrombosis may be seen as defective filling of the sinus in the emptying phase (*Figure 12.26*).

Vertebral angiography is less reliable in the diagnosis of infratentorial mass lesions than is carotid angiography in the diagnosis of supratentorial mass lesions and in cases of doubt some form of ventriculography may have to be performed.

If a cerebellar abscess is present the radiological findings will consist of dilatation of the lateral ventricles and third ventricle and displacement of the fourth ventricle. These appearances are illustrated in *Figures 12.27* and *12.28*.

Pyography

When computerized tomography is not available follow-up of abscesses is best undertaken by pyography (*Figure 12.29*). At the time of aspirating the abscess a radio-opaque contrast medium is injected (the one in current use is sterile Micropaque) into the abscess cavity. The contrast medium is taken up by the wall of the abscess and

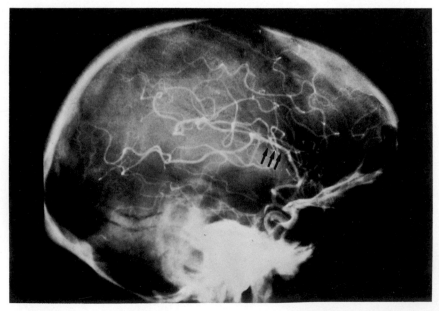

Figure 12.24 Upward displacement of the middle cerebral artery (arrow) by a temporal lobe abscess

radiographs taken at intervals permit the visualization of changes in size and shape. Thorotrast was used previously and behaved similarly and *Figures 12.30* and *12.31* demonstrate the outline of the ventricular system when the abscess leaked into the ventricle.

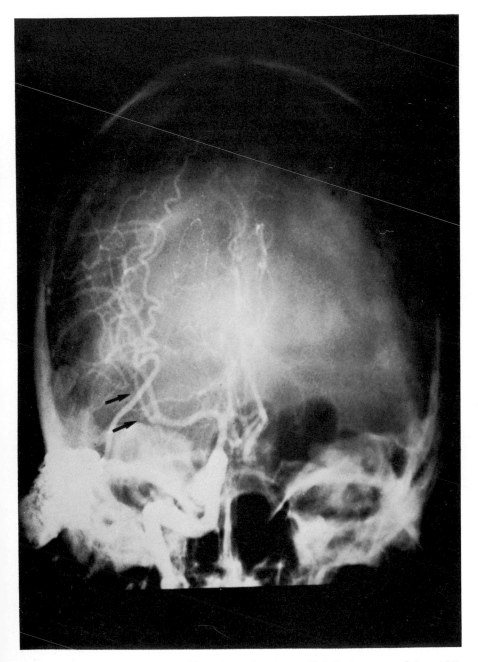

Figure 12.25 Same patient as in *Figure 12.24* showing medial displacement of the middle cerebral artery by the abscess

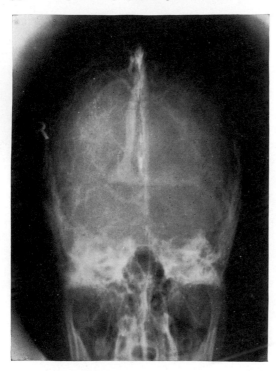

Figure 12.26 Right carotid angiogram: half-axial projection. Note the filling of the sagittal sinus and left lateral sinus; the right lateral sinus failed to fill because of a confirmed sinus thrombosis

Pneumoencephalography (*Figures 12.32* and *12.33*)

Cerebrospinal fluid can be partially replaced by air which acts as a negative contrast medium and is suitable for outlining the ventricles and subarachnoid space. The air shows as a shadow against solid cerebral tissue. Air or oxygen may be introduced through the ventricle, the cisterna magna or lumbar theca. High intracranial pressure or a posterior fossa abscess are contraindications but if pneumoencephalography is absolutely essential for localizing an abscess it must always be undertaken where neurosurgical facilities are available, in case an emergency is precipitated. When a brain abscess partly obliterates a ventricle, then the ventricle cannot be filled and information is inadequate. Arteriography should always precede pneumoencephalography. Pneumoencephalography as a diagnostic investigation of brain abscess has been superseded by more modern methods of investigation but occasionally may be useful to confirm that the disease has fully recovered.

Ventriculography (*Figures 12.34–12.36*)

The ventricle is punctured and replaced by air after 10 ml of fluid are withdrawn; air replacement proceeds until no more fluid can be aspirated. The other ventricle is then filled with air after a lapse of a short period to allow equalization of pressure. At all times the surgeon, having seen the result of the ventriculograms, should be prepared to proceed with surgery appropriate to the underlying disease.

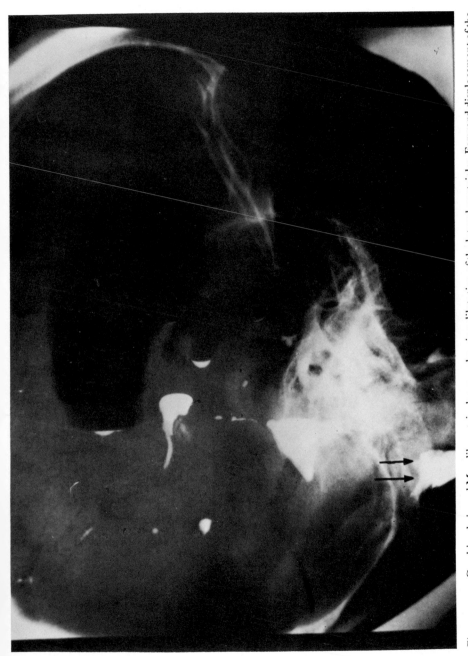

Figure 12.27   Combined air and Myodil ventriculogram showing dilatation of the lateral ventricles. Forward displacement of the fourth ventricle by a cerebellar abscess is demonstrated. Tonsillar herniation due to raised intracranial pressure is marked by the arrow

Encephalography (*Figures 12.32* and *12.33*)

This can be done either by the suboccipital or lumbar route. The cisternal route is less distressing to the patient, but it is easier and more convenient to use the lumbar route. Using the cisternal route, cerebrospinal fluid is replaced by air up to 30 ml, whereas

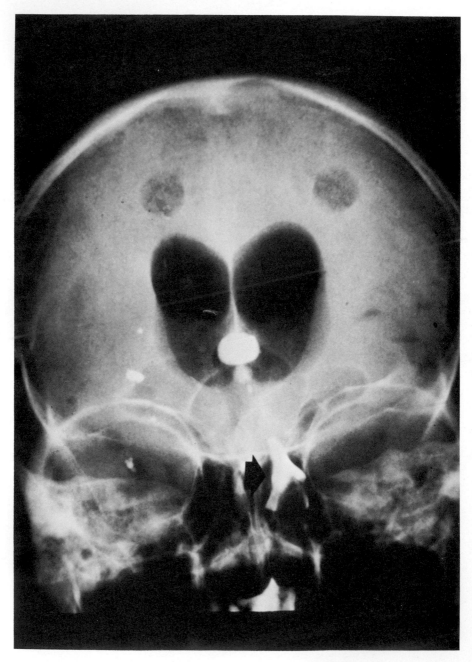

Figure 12.28   Same patient as *Figure 12.27* showing displacement of the fourth ventricle to the left (arrow)

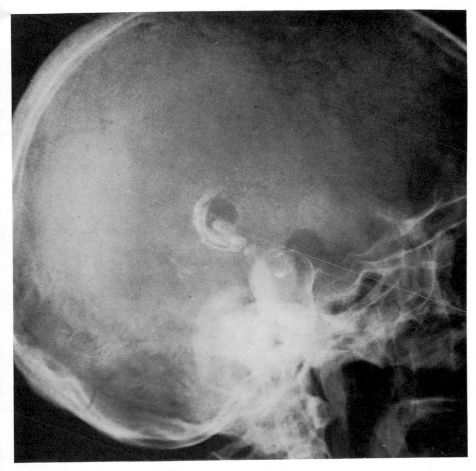

Figure 12.29   Steripaque in a multilocular temporal lobe abscess

using the lumbar route 45–50 ml of air are used in the replacement. Much larger quantities have been used but the amount used is usually determined at the time by the radiologist.

Radiological investigations should be clearly necessary before being undertaken; their greatest value is in localizing an abscess which is not adjacent to the mastoid. EMI scanning is the most useful method of investigation when available. Otherwise arteriography is the most informative, and, after aspiration of an abscess pyography is essential to check progress. Pneumoencephalography is nowadays virtually no longer required.

Extradural abscess

Extradural abscess, the most common otogenic intracranial complication, is a collection of pus between dura and bone (*see Figure 12.2*). It arises from acute or chronic otitis media and may develop in the middle or the posterior fossa. The lesion may be single or associated with other suppurations and it arises by direct extension

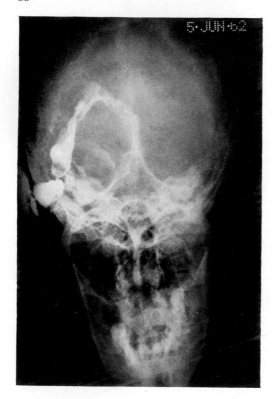

Figure 12.30 Pyogram. The abscess ruptured into the lateral ventricle. The patient survived

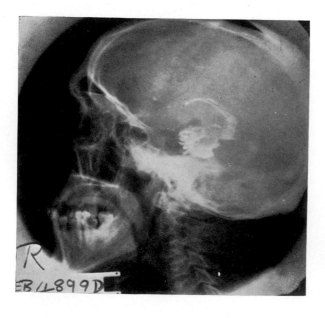

Figure 12.31 Pyogram. Lateral projection of abscess at same stage as *Figure 12.30*. The ventricle is outlined by Thorotrast

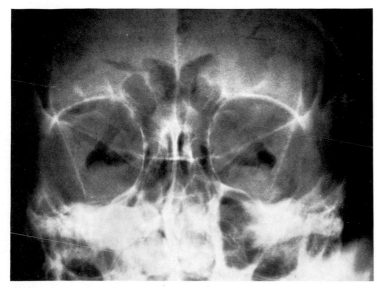

Figure 12.32 Air encephalogram. Antero-posterior brow up projection. Normal appearances. Both temporal horns have been deliberately filled with air. (Reproduced by courtesy of Dr. G. L. Gryspeerdt)

consequent on osteitic or cholesteatomatous erosion. The abscess may be separated from the mastoid by inflamed bone or it may freely communicate with the middle ear.

Symptoms and signs depend on speed of formation, situation, duration and extension of the abscess. Middle fossa collections are large only when lying lateral to the arcuate eminence, since here the dura may be readily stripped from the petrous and squamous bones. In most cases the disease is limited to the upper surface of the tegmen.

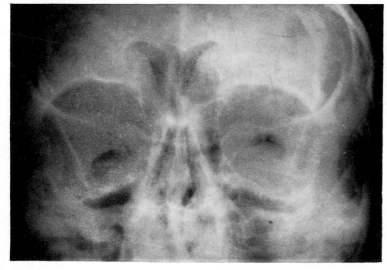

Figure 12.33 Air encephalogram. Antero-posterior brow up projection. Left temporal lobe lesion. Note typical displacement of the septum pellucidum to the opposite side and elevation of the ipsilateral temporal horn. (Reproduced by courtesy of Dr. G. L. Gryspeerdt)

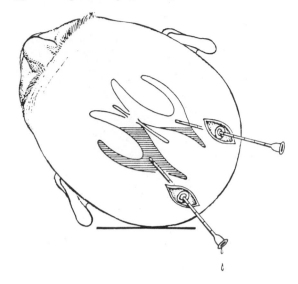

Figure 12.34 Technique of ventriculography. Ventricular puncture and replacement of fluid by air. Note the position of the head to ensure complete replacement (after Rowbotham)

There are no specific symptoms of middle fossa extradural abscess. Indeed, many cases are symptomless.

Headache in acute or chronic otitis media may be the only suggestive feature. A slight rise of temperature may also be noted. Almost all patients are ambulant, although they may feel unwell.

When a communicating abscess freely discharges into the external auditory meatus an intermittent history of headache and malaise, relieved by episodes of profuse otorrhoea, may be obtained.

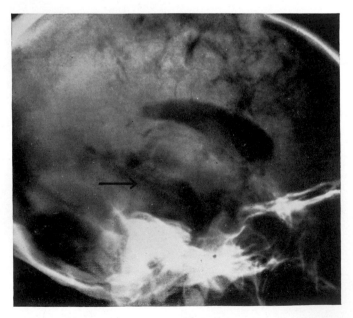

Figure 12.35 Ventriculogram. Lateral brow up projection. Normal appearances. The aqueduct is indicated by an arrow. (Reproduced by courtesy of Dr. G. L. Gryspeerdt)

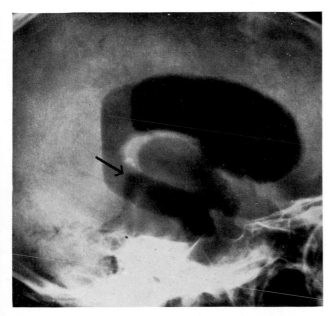

Figure 12.36 Ventriculogram. Later brow up projection. Left cerebellar abscess involving vermis. The supratentorial ventricular system is dilated. The lower part of the aqueduct is displaced forwards and kinked in the mid-part (see arrow). (Reproduced by courtesy of Dr. G. L. Gryspeerdt)

Very large middle fossa lesions may produce persistent headache and vomiting and, if prolonged, even papilloedema and more rarely focal signs. When focal signs and papilloedema are present, it is essential to exclude cerebral or subdural abscess before considering extradural abscess as the sole complication. A large abscess may erode the squamous temporal or parietal bone to form a subperiosteal abscess. In infants, when the suture lines have not closed, the extradural abscess may communicate freely with a large post-aural abscess.

Small collections overlying the petrous apex irritate and interfere with the function of the fifth and sixth cranial nerves causing trigeminal pain and diplopia (*Gradenigo's syndrome*) (*Figure 12.37*).

The posterior fossa dura is firmly attached to the petrous temporal bone at the internal auditory meatus, the subarcuate fossa and the edges of the bony grooves for the lateral sinus. Posterior fossa extradural abscesses are commonly perisinus in situation and most of them freely communicate with the mastoid disease. If localized to the sinus groove deep to bone the abscess may compress and obliterate the lateral sinus. A large abscess may expose dura both medial and lateral to the sinus. An abscess deep to Trautmann's triangle may be separate from or confluent with the perisinus abscess. Posterior fossa collections situated more medially between the internal auditory meatus and the subarcuate fossa are uncommon and usually arise from cholesteatomatous erosion with partial destruction of the labyrinth.

There are no symptoms typical of posterior fossa extradural abscess, although headache and rise of temperature may raise suspicion. Intermittent profuse otorrhoea with relief of headache and malaise may occur. No specific symptoms result from the deep medially located abscesses.

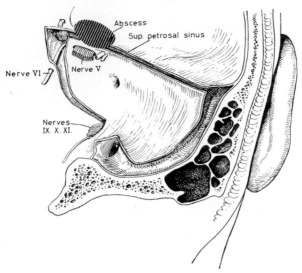

Figure 12.37   Diagram of the relations of the petrous apex.
Note the proximity of an apical extradural abscess and the
superior petrosal sinus to the fifth and sixth cranial nerves

Untreated abscesses may reach the surface behind the mastoid process (Cittelli's abscess) or reach the neck through the jugular foramen or even present in a retropharyngeal situation. These are very late events, more often seen in sinus thrombosis. Perisinus abscesses are frequently found on exploration for suspected sinus thrombosis or other intracranial extension.

As freedom of communication between an extradural abscess in either cranial fossa with mastoid disease is variable it is necessary, when exploring for suspected intracranial invasion, that parts of the tegmen and sinus plate be deliberately removed to exclude hidden abscess. More often a track leading to the lesion is found and mere removal of mastoid cortex may release a quantity of pus under pressure from a communicating extradural lesion. Once located, the abscess must be adequately drained into the mastoid and all surrounding necrotic bone removed. Dural or perisinus granulation tissue should be left untouched. Suitable antibiotic therapy should be given and further developments awaited. When an extradural abscess is the sole complication of otitis media, rapid recovery as in routine mastoidectomy may be expected.

In chronic ear disease the indication for surgery is obvious but in a patient with acute otitis media suffering from headache antibiotics alone may cure the lesion if it is communicating but, should symptoms persist, the mastoid should be explored.

Sinus thrombophlebitis

Sinus thrombophlebitis at one time carried a very high mortality and even today it may be fatal if uncontrolled. The lateral sinus is the most frequently infected of all the intracranial sinuses. Of 97 patients with proved thrombophlebitis, 89 were confined to the lateral sinus and the jugular bulb; in three of these thrombosis had extended to the superior petrosal sinus and in one it had reached the cavernous sinus. Seven of the patients had isolated superior petrosal thrombosis, one of which had extended into the cavernous sinus (Dawes, 1961). Lateral sinus thrombophlebitis arises by direct extension of disease from the mastoid and, in about half the cases, is preceded by perisinus abscess. In approximately 45 per cent there are associated lesions in the cerebrum, cerebellum, meninges or subdural space; 70 per cent of cases arise from chronic ear disease. Today, because of efficient antibiotic therapy, there is rarely need for surgery when thrombophlebitis complicates acute otitis media. Therefore, although lateral sinus thrombophlebitis may be suspected the diagnosis is not always confirmed.

Any of the pyococci may cause sinus thrombophlebitis, but generally *Streptococcus pyogenes* is found. The cocci are the cause of those cases complicating acute otitis media but in the chronic ear, although they may precipitate the acute exacerbation, other organisms, such as the *E. coli*, *B. proteus* or *Ps. pyocyaneus*, may be found. The organism grown from the chronic ear itself cannot be regarded as the causative agent with certainty and only when an organism is cultured from the thrombus or bloodstream can we be sure about the aetiological agent.

Thrombosis of a sinus is a response to infection of the vessel wall and is nature's attempt to exclude the disease from the bloodstream. Sometimes thrombosis may prevent invasion, but perhaps more often the process extends to occlude the whole lumen. The thrombus, in turn, may suppurate to form an intrasinus abscess which is excluded from the general circulation by an occlusive thrombus on either side of the abscess. As infection spreads both within the wall and the lumen, thrombosis extends into adjoining vessels to reach the confluence of the sinuses posteriorly, or the superior petrosal sinus and the cavernous sinus anteriorly, or the jugular bulb and the veins of the neck inferiorly. Septicaemia, pyaemia or invasion of other intracranial tissues may supervene at any stage. As the cerebellar veins drain into the lateral sinus, cerebellar thrombophlebitis or abscess may arise by retrograde extension. Similarly, a superior petrosal sinus lesion may be the precursor of cerebral thrombophlebitis or brain abscess. If cortical thrombophlebitis spreads far afield, then a brain abscess may be well-removed from the point of invasion (*see Figure 12.4*).

Clinical picture

The clinical picture as seen at any moment represents the extent of the thrombosis and the balance between the rate of progress of the disease and the patient's natural resistance, local and general. Consequently, a variety of clinical types can be recognized but as the disease is a continuous process, a rapid or gradual change from one type to another may occur.

A rigor is certain evidence that the bloodstream has been infected and indicates that natural resistance has failed. The temperature suddenly rises to 39–40°C (103–104°F) and falls again rapidly; these rapid changes are accompanied by fast pulse, severe shivering and profuse sweating and the patient feels and looks very ill. Even if a temperature record is not available, the history of a shivering bout (which may be so marked as to shake the bed) or profuse sweating, suggests that a rigor has occurred. In unchecked disease rigors recur and pyrexia is of remitting type with high peaks accompanied by corresponding rises in pulse rate (*see Figure 12.9*). Between these episodes the patient may seem well, alert or euphoric. In the absence of rigors, a high remitting temperature with corresponding pulse changes should be sufficient for diagnosis of sinus thrombophlebitis.

This striking evidence of septicaemia and pyaemia may be accompanied by embolic abscesses in the lungs, other viscera, subcutaneous tissues, or the pleuroperitoneal and joint cavities.

The picture of fulminating sinus thrombophlebitis can occur soon after the onset of virulent acute otitis media and indeed so quickly that no attempt to limit the spread of the disease is discernible. When surgery was commonly employed for control of the infection, sometimes no evidence of sinus thrombosis was found at operation.

More often, lateral sinus thrombophlebitis complicates uncontrolled acute otitis media or mastoiditis associated with perisinus abscess. In these cases recurrence of earache, development of headache, or rise in temperature and pulse rate, followed by remitting temperature, usually precede the appearance of rigors and pyaemia by a few days.

When disease is less virulent or natural resistance is high, symptoms may develop more gradually. When progressive thrombosis is effectively limiting the infection, oedema or even abscess over the site of exit of the mastoid emissary vein may form. This localized swelling is well back on the mastoid. Similarly there is time for peri-adenitis to develop round the jugular vein, and the level of tenderness along the jugular vein indicates the extent of the thrombophlebitis. An abscess developing post-aurally or around the jugular vein may be found to communicate directly with an intrasinus abscess or an abscess within the lumen of the jugular bulb or vein. As the thrombophlebitis extends down the jugular, the level of tenderness gets lower, and a localized oedema may follow the progressive thrombosis even to the root of the neck or across the middle line—a phlebitis migrans. A marked perivenous inflammatory reaction within the jugular foramen may cause paralysis of the ninth, tenth and eleventh cranial nerves. However, once the patient's resistance is overcome, rigors and embolic abscesses develop.

If the lesion extends forwards through the superior petrosal sinus, or from the jugular bulb via the inferior petrosal sinus, cavernous sinus thrombophlebitis may develop. The first evidence is a slight proptosis of one eye which becomes progressively worse with venous engorgement and chemosis and later extends to involve the other side through the circular sinus (*see Figure 12.10*).

Thrombosis of the larger of the lateral sinuses, or of the only remaining lateral sinus, or extension of the sinus thrombosis to the superior sagittal sinus via the confluence of the sinuses, produces marked alteration in the intracranial haemo-dynamics and consequently a high rise in fluid pressure. Thus a typical otitic hydrocephalus develops.

At any time during the course of lateral sinus thrombophlebitis, evidence of an acute cerebellar lesion may appear and so dominate the clinical picture that underlying symptoms and signs of thrombophlebitis may be overlooked.

Similarly, the presence of meningitis in the early stages of invasion of intracranial tissue planes may obscure the presence of lateral sinus thrombosis. A relatively inactive sinus lesion, when associated with marked focal signs of cerebral disease, may not be suspected until the mastoid is explored.

Although these clinical pictures have been described in relation to acute otitis media, any one of them may appear as a complication of chronic ear disease; the symptoms and signs of sinus involvement are the same.

Sinus thrombosis may be so insidiously formed in chronic ear disease that its presence may not give rise to symptoms or signs attracting the attention of patient or doctor. The complication may only be discovered during an operation performed solely for control of chronic ear disease. Occasionally, cholesteatoma itself may track along the lumen of the sinus to give rise to an abscess in the suboccipital region of the neck, and may present as such.

Although embolic abscesses occur late in the natural history of the disease they may be the presenting feature. Lung abscess or empyema may cause the patient to seek advice. Here the doctor may regard the prodromal septicaemic symptoms as part of the chest disease and the chronic ear lesion may have remained unmentioned by both patient and doctor. On occasion it is only on request for an otological opinion that the significance of the ear disease is appreciated. By the time the full diagnosis is made the patient may be moribund or dead. It is only awareness of the fact that embolic abscesses arise from sinus thrombophlebitis that permits correct interpretation of the history. Rarely, a patient presents with a lung abscess after the acute otitis has ceased to discharge on antibiotic therapy, and only an astute observer may recognize that chest pain, productive cough and radiological findings are otogenic.

Post-operative sinus thrombosis has frequently been reported in the literature but careful analysis of these histories indicates that clinical evidence of pre-operative thrombosis was frequently present and that operative exposure of the lateral sinus was inadequate. Occasionally, post-operative thrombosis may follow surgical injury to the sinus in the presence of infection but when injury is recognized antibiotic therapy should prevent serious consequences.

As a patient may present at any stage of the illness, a careful history of the events in chronological order is essential to proper understanding of the illness.

Laboratory investigations are of little help to diagnosis or surgical decision. The degree of leucocytosis is variable, lumbar puncture in the absence of otitic hydrocephalus is normal unless other tissue planes are involved, and the Tobey–Ayer test is only really useful in bilateral ear disease. Usually a carefully taken history will indicate which lateral sinus is thrombosed if the patient has bilateral ear disease; failing an adequate history, the Tobey–Ayer test may help but can only do so if the sinus itself is occluded by a thrombus. When the clinical history and cerebrospinal fluid pressure changes are in conflict, one should rely on the former. Very occasionally it may be necessary to explore both mastoids to find which lateral sinus is thrombosed. Repeated blood cultures can be done in an attempt to identify the infecting organism. To await results of blood culture (often negative in any case) before making a diagnosis or starting treatment is to court disaster.

The Lillie–Crowe test has been advocated as a method of deciding which lateral sinus is involved. When one lateral sinus is occluded by thrombosis, digital compression of the opposite jugular vein will produce dilatation of the retinal veins as seen at retinoscopy.

Ophthalmoscopic examination is essential in patients with suspected intracranial disease, since in extensive thrombosis with otitic hydrocephalus, papilloedema may be seen early.

The superior petrosal sinus may be primarily involved, or it may be invaded by extension from the lateral sinus. Superior petrosal lesions are frequently associated with middle fossa extradural abscesses and because of the close anatomical relationship of the sinus to the trigeminal nerve the patients may complain of pain in the lower jaw (*Figure 12.37*) (Bauer, 1951; Harpman, 1955).

Superior petrosal sinus thrombophlebitis may itself cause lateral sinus thrombosis and it may not be possible to distinguish between them. It is worth remembering that pain in the lower jaw in a patient with lateral sinus thrombophlebitis probably means that there is also a middle fossa extradural abscess or a superior petrosal lesion, or both. Temporal lobe cerebral thrombophlebitis or abscess may complicate a superior petrosal lesion.

Otogenic cavernous thrombophlebitis follows thrombophlebitis of the lateral sinus, the superior petrosal sinus or jugular bulb. At first, the eye on the affected side becomes proptosed, the retinal veins are engorged, the peri-orbital tissues become swollen, chemosis develops and later the other eye also becomes involved (*see Figure 12.10*).

Jugular bulb thrombophlebitis most commonly follows a lateral sinus lesion but may arise directly. No specific signs can be related to phlebitis beginning in the jugular bulb, but the presence of ninth, tenth and eleventh nerve paralysis and tenderness of the jugular vein in the neck indicates its involvement.

Sequelae

As a rule no sequelae directly follow sinus thrombosis. However, if the patient has survived one lateral sinus thrombosis and later develops sinus thrombosis of the other side, then he will have permanent papilloedema; he may retain little more than macular vision, and is liable to have epileptic fits, particularly when the head is lowered. Cavernous sinus thrombophlebitis, if not treated early enough, may cause blindness in the eye more severely afflicted—if the patient recovers. In general the prognosis of sinus thrombophlebitis is good, provided treatment is started early enough and antibiotics are given in adequate dosage. The majority of patients who die from sinus thrombophlebitis have a 'chronic ear', and death results from infection of other intracranial tissue planes or because the organisms causing the pyaemia do not respond to the antibiotics.

Management

The important points in management are to *suspect* the presence of sinus thrombophlebitis, treat the disease as such, and decide whether surgical exploration is indicated.

As the control of a bloodstream infection is dependent on adequate treatment, at least one to two million units of penicillin are given six-hourly, supplemented by 0.5 g of streptomycin twice daily or sulphamezathine 2 g six-hourly for the first two days and 1 g six-hourly thereafter. The treatment must be continued until full recovery has occurred even though this may be several weeks. Streptomycin should not be continued beyond the tenth day but penicillin and sulphamezathine can be continued longer with safety. This broad cover of antibiotics should control infection by any of the pyogenic cocci or the *H. influenzae*.

At the time the patient presents, a swab taken from the external auditory meatus can be cultured, or if surgery is contemplated a suitable bacteriological swab may be obtained at the time of operation. Frequently the patient has already shown a dramatic response to treatment before sensitivity tests are completed. Only if the response has been unsatisfactory or there is a definite indication from the bacteriological report, is it necessary to change the antibiotic. Chloromycetin is useful for treating coccal or influenzal infections but there is a risk of causing aplastic anaemia if treatment is too prolonged. The tetracycline group may be useful but in severe infections there must be a definite reason for preferring them to penicillin or streptomycin for, in effect, they are bacteriostatic and not bactericidal.

Antibiotics given in high dosage to control thrombophlebitis are likely to cure the acute otitis media. Today many patients have been given antibiotics before coming to hospital. Often the dosage has been inadequate. A disease unresponsive to oral penicillin may very well respond to heavy dosage of penicillin given intramuscularly, particularly when supplemented by the synergistic drugs streptomycin or sulphamezathine. Failure to respond to other drug groups may indicate change of antibiotics, preferably to those given in high dosage by intramuscular injection, namely penicillin and streptomycin.

Once the patient is admitted to hospital, the temperature and pulse rate must be recorded at least every 4 h, and any change carefully noted. The patient himself must be examined whenever there is a change in his condition, and the central nervous system should be assessed daily. Evidence of infection of tissue planes, other than the intracranial sinuses, may demand special techniques, such as lumbar puncture or exploratory burr-holes. Progressive development of local physical signs directly related to sinus thrombophlebitis, or evidence of extension to other sinuses, may suggest a review of medical management or the need to drain a perisinus or intrasinus abscess. When thrombophlebitis complicates otitis media of some standing, mastoid exploration is essential. It is probably safer to explore in all cases of acute otitis media when the intracranial complication is not showing rapid improvement on antibiotics alone. Once the mastoid is explored, the bacteriological findings may dictate a change in management, especially when progress is unsatisfactory.

In chronic middle-ear disease, the mastoid must be explored. Intensive medical treatment should first be started and the mastoid explored some hours later. A high blood concentration of antibiotics tends to limit any spread of infection consequent on surgery. Delaying surgery too long may permit the disease to spread, for antibiotics control only an acute exacerbation by pyococci or *H. influenzae*—not the destructive cholesteatomatous disease itself. Ideally, sinus thrombophlebitis should be suspected and the ear explored either before thrombosis has occurred or in the stage of mural thrombus. This view may not be realistic because the majority of cases already have an extensive thrombosis when first seen.

Although a preliminary x-ray of the mastoid may be useful to determine the situation of the lateral sinus, it is not essential. A post-aural incision is made and the whole mastoid process fully explored. A hammer and gouge or drill technique is used to excavate the mastoid, removing all mastoid air-cells. On perforating the cortex, pulsating pus under pressure may well up from a perisinus abscess. In the presence of such a communicating perisinus abscess the position of the sinus itself is readily seen. All necrotic bone and sufficient of the normal sinus plate are removed so that the whole extent of the perisinus abscess is uncovered to provide free drainage. If normal dura has not been exposed then more bone should be removed. As a rule bone removal need not extend beyond the superior genu at the sinodural angle or further than the jugular bulb itself. In the case of bulb thrombosis it is usually necessary only to drain the peribulbar abscess, for if too much bone is removed the facial nerve may be easily injured, particularly as venous bleeding in sinus thrombosis can be troublesome enough to obscure the nerve. The middle fossa dura is also deliberately exposed by removal of part of the tegmen antri, the sinodural bony angle being left intact.

Whenever the mastoid is explored for suspected intracranial disease the lateral sinus should be deliberately exposed even if it requires removal of an intact sinus plate. It is tempting to leave a thick sclerotic intact plate but there is no doubt that a perisinus abscess or a sinus thrombosis with an intrasinus abscess may exist deep to the apparently healthy bone. These are the cases which at one time were described as post-operative sinus thrombosis. The only case of post-operative otitic hydrocephalus due to sinus thrombosis which I have seen occurred in a patient where a definite pre-operative diagnosis of sinus thrombophlebitis was made but the sinus plate was not removed at operation as it appeared healthy and intact. When a diseased sinus deep to an intact sinus plate is overlooked then a second operation is needed to uncover it (Bauer, 1951). Having exposed the lateral sinus and middle fossa dura it is sometimes advisable to remove bone from Trautmann's triangle medial to the sinus in case this route is required to drain a cerebellar abscess or an encysted arachnoiditis.

Once part of the sinus plate has been removed the exposure can be easily enlarged by bone nibblers, provided that the sinus dura is first gently freed from the bone by a blunt-angled probe. The state of the sinus can then be assessed. A healthy sinus is blue in colour, uniform in texture and easily compressible. When only mural thrombus is present the sinus may appear normal or its surface may be covered by granulation tissue. The wall may be slightly discoloured and the sinus feel hard, in which case a palpable thrombus is present which may be occluding the whole vessel. In such cases the sinus need only be widely exposed, the mastoid cavity packed with BIPP gauze and the post-aural wound left open. When the wall is necrotic the sinus must be opened, the intrasinus abscess drained and all necrotic sloughs removed, but it is not necessary to suck out the limiting thrombus at either end for this acts as a protective mechanism. If the sinus wall is destroyed only the necrotic and loose clot should be removed by suction. Cholesteatoma, which has invaded the sinus, must be completely removed. If, during the removal of the diseased clot or cholesteatoma, profuse bleeding should occur the sinus must be obliterated by packing BIPP gauze between bone and sinus wall. The mastoid cavity and wound are also packed open with BIPP gauze.

Although occasionally an intrasinus abscess is very extensive, extending into the transverse sinus or jugular bulb, adequate drainage of the abscess into the mastoid suffices. Antibiotics should control the bloodstream infection.

Should the patient deteriorate despite surgery and adequate medical management, the lateral sinus must be re-explored and incised, and all clot removed so that free bleeding occurs from the upper end which is then packed off. The clot in the lower part should also be removed but free bleeding is frequently not seen. The superior petrosal sinus should also be exposed.

Adequate exposure of the lateral sinus may demand another incision extending posteriorly from the post-aural incision.

When necessary, the jugular vein may be ligated above the common facial vein. Ligation may not limit a thrombophlebitis, for the disease once in the jugular vein easily bypasses the point of division by using the venous collateral circulation. Furthermore, the vein is neither readily exposed nor ligated because it is surrounded by inflamed lymph nodes, and often thrombosis has already spread beyond the elective site.

To expose the internal jugular vein a 5–7.5 cm incision is made along the anterior border of the sternomastoid muscle downwards from the mastoid tip, the muscle retracted, and the vein dissected free and divided between ligatures. The upper end of the cut jugular vein may be opened to drain an intrasinus abscess which has tracked downwards. Ligation of the internal jugular was not required in any of the 89 cases of lateral sinus thrombosis reported by Dawes (1961).

Where sinus thrombosis has continued to progress, anticoagulant therapy has been recommended. Theoretically anticoagulants prevent the formation of further clotting—but only at the cost of inhibition of what is essentially a protective mechanism. In some cases the extent of thrombosis is so great that danger to life may arise from a downward extension to the superior vena cava or become a danger to the eyesight by spread to both cavernous sinuses. When extension is truly threatening, anticoagulants may have some place, but generally thrombosis is encouraged and infection controlled by a combination of antibiotics and surgery.

If a normal lateral sinus is injured surgically, the tear is usually small, and bleeding, although profuse, may immediately be controlled by a pack while a piece of temporalis muscle is cut and hammered to form a stamp graft. This graft is applied directly to the dural surface of the sinus and held in position by a pack which may be safely removed after a week. Bleeding from a large tear is controlled by packing between sinus plate and vessel wall to obliterate the sinus. The pack may usually be removed safely inside a week but the surgeon must be prepared to re-pack if bleeding recurs.

Whenever septicaemia or pyaemia is present, the patient's blood haemolyses and repeated blood transfusions may be required. This is a supportive measure but if it is ignored the patient's resistance to infection may be constantly reduced as haemolysis continues.

Otitic hydrocephalus

Otitic hydrocephalus occurs most frequently in children and adolescents as a complication of acute or chronic ear disease. In nearly all cases a sinus thrombosis which has upset the intracranial haemodynamics, is present.

The intracranial sinuses form the venous drainage system of the cerebral tissues and convey blood to the neck through bony foramina. By far the largest quantity of the intracranial venous blood leaves the skull through the jugular foramina and the largest contribution to the internal jugular vein is provided by the lateral sinus. In the extreme case of an occluding thrombus in both lateral sinuses or jugular bulbs a marked rise of intracranial venous pressure must occur, for the collateral venous drainage cannot expand rapidly to accommodate increased flow because the maximum size of exit depends on the size of the bony foramina. Much of the venous drainage is carried in the superior sagittal sinus which drains into the right or left transverse sinus. One transverse sinus is usually larger than the other and so transmits the greater amount of the venous flow. The right is more often the larger in a ratio of 6:4 or 7:3. Occasionally one side is very large and receives almost all the venous blood from the sagittal sinus; if this transverse or lateral sinus is thrombosed then a rise in intracranial venous pressure must follow, for the venous blood cannot drain adequately into the small sinus of the opposite side. Thrombosis may extend from the lateral sinus to the superior sagittal sinus with similar effects. Once the sagittal sinus has been involved, the efficiency of the arachnoid granulations is impaired and cerebrospinal fluid absorption is reduced. The rise in intracranial venous pressure and the reduced absorption of cerebrospinal fluid lead to an increase in cerebrospinal fluid pressure. This rise produces the clinical picture of otitic hydrocephalus.

Symptoms and signs

The patient complains of headache in varying degree, nausea and vomiting, blurred vision and occasionally diplopia.

The most striking physical sign is the presence of papilloedema seen after the onset of the intracranial complication. Papilloedema may be as much as 5–6 dioptres and patches of exudate or small haemorrhages may be seen. This clinical picture may occur during the acute phase of sinus thrombophlebitis or may be noticed later when the disease is under control. Between attacks of vomiting the patient looks well and pyrexia—noted early in the illness—may be short-lived. Indeed, the impression gained is that thrombosis has prevented spread of infection to the bloodstream but in so doing has produced a marked rise of intracranial tension. Apart from papilloedema, the only finding may be that of transient paralysis of the sixth nerve.

Cerebrospinal fluid obtained by lumbar puncture is under markedly increased pressure (over 300 mm of fluid) but is bacteriologically and biochemically normal. Skull radiography and angiography show no abnormality. The electroencephalogram is normal, and despite the name no hydrocephalus is demonstrated by pneumoradiography.

Differential diagnosis

Virus meningo-encephalitis is the only lesion likely to produce a similar picture. In both otitic hydrocephalus and virus encephalitis the cerebrospinal fluid may be normal but, in the former, pressure is markedly increased and focal neurological signs are absent. The mere presence of aural disease does not exclude meningo-encephalitis for the encephalitic picture may complicate myringitis bullosa haemorrhagica. Papilloedema in brain abscess does not appear in less than two weeks.

Management

Active medical and surgical treatment is directed against sinus thrombosis. The papilloedema tends to improve but, if persistent, optic atrophy and blindness may result. Therefore, lumbar puncture at intervals of 48 h may be used to reduce cerebrospinal fluid pressure but, if ineffective, subtemporal decompression may be necessary. When bilateral sinus thrombosis is present, the otitic hydrocephalus is permanent; optic atrophy results, perhaps leaving only macular vision, and if the patient stoops an epileptic fit may be induced. Little can be done to help these unfortunate patients.

Cerebral and cerebellar thrombophlebitis

Cerebral thrombophlebitis has frequently been called otogenic non-suppurative encephalitis and, under this title, the literature is extensive. Borries' (1949) clinical concept of this disease was that of a lesion showing the symptoms and signs of brain abscess without intracerebral suppuration. He regarded non-suppurative encephalitis as a pre-abscedal lesion passing through the stages of brain oedema, simple encephalitis, haemorrhagic encephalitis and phlegmonous encephalitis, to terminate in brain abscess. Although Borries thought that this was a pre-abscedal type of otogenic encephalitis 'this did not deny the existence of an autonomous non-suppurative encephalitis'. Dawes (1953), in a clinical study, distinguished two types of otogenic encephalitis: bacterial encephalitis—better known as cerebral thrombophlebitis— and virus encephalitis which complicated myringitis bullosa haemorrhagica and never progressed to suppuration. Viral and bacterial encephalitis often cannot be distinguished on a pathological basis. Here, we are concerned only with that cerebral thrombophlebitis which precedes abscess formation, wherein the patient's resistance and good therapy may prevent actual suppuration.

Cerebral thrombophlebitis may arise from lesions in dural veins, or from subdural abscess. Lateral sinus thrombosis is almost invariably the cause of cerebellar complications.

The onset of cerebral thrombophlebitis is heralded by the sudden appearance of focal epileptic fits in the course of intracranial invasion from suppurative ear disease. Fits begin focally, and spread to the whole of one side of the body or become generalized. Fits may occur at intervals of hours or days, or may be so frequent as to constitute a status epilepticus. After a fit headache may be increased, the patient may become drowsy, disorientated, possibly comatose, or restless, irritable and even temporarily violent. Focal signs, such as flaccid hemiplegia, hemianopia, hemianaes-thesia or aphasia (if the dominant hemisphere is involved), follow the fit and persist for a variable time. In cerebellar thrombophlebitis, giddiness, vomiting, nystagmus, incoordination and ataxia, suddenly appear and gradually clear away.

However, not all cases present so dramatically. Symptoms and signs may progress more slowly and, where improvement is not observed within two or three days, one must assume that focal liquefaction has moved on to abscess formation. Certain symptoms, for example aphasia, may be so transient as to be overlooked.

When focal signs have persisted after a bout of fits, arteriography may be necessary to exclude subdural or brain abscess. Exclusion of subdural abscess may require exploratory burr-holes. Electroencephalography is of doubtful significance since the electrical changes do not differentiate between the lesions and may only indicate the presence of a focal lesion.

Differential diagnosis

The presence of a subdural abscess must be excluded and this may readily be done by arteriography or exploratory burr-holes. However, the encephalitis of myringitis bullosa haemorrhagica is very similar in the dramatic onset of epileptic fits, the general condition of the patient and the appearance of focal neurological signs. Cerebral thrombophlebitis usually arises after intracranial extension is well advanced. A history of headache and drowsiness over several days may precede the explosive appearance of significant symptoms. In the first type of encephalitis complicating myringitis bullosa haemorrhagica the symptoms of the ear infection and brain involvement may present almost simultaneously; in the second type of 'post-infective 'encephalitis' it is almost impossible to make the distinction from cerebral thrombophlebitis but since treatment is much the same there is little cause for concern.

Slower progressive forms of cerebral thrombophlebitis may lead to brain abscess and careful investigation by arteriography or exploratory burr-holes may be necessary for distinction.

Management

Correct and adequate drug therapy should control cerebral thrombophlebitis but the ear lesion must be treated as the local condition demands.

Diseases of the meninges

Purulent pachymeningitis and subdural abscess (*see Figure 12.3*)

Purulent pachymeningitis, infected subdural effusions and subdural abscesses are different stages in invasion of the subdural space. Subdural infection may be the dominant intracranial lesion but often it is associated with invasion of other tissue planes, particularly in chronic otitic disease.

Subdural invasion may be localized at the portal of entry or infection may spread rapidly throughout the subdural space. At first the effusion may be serous or seropurulent but soon becomes purulent. Creamy pus tends to gravitate to the falx cerebri or to the junction of the falx with the tentorium cerebelli. Spontaneous healing may follow with subsequent formation of granulations and, finally, fibrous obliteration between dura and pia-arachnoid. More commonly the purulent exudate is split up into loculated abscesses by adhesions. These chronic abscesses can occur over the convex surface of the brain, between the hemispheres along the falx, or at the junction of the falx and tentorium. The subdural infection may cause thrombophlebitis of cortical vessels and, finally, multiple small abscesses in cerebral tissue adjacent to loculated subdural abscesses.

Pyococci usually cause these subdural infections but by far the most common organism found is a streptococcus, particularly of the non-haemolytic variety.

Clinical features

Subdural extension is usually preceded by the general clinical picture of otogenic intracranial invasion. Diffuse infection of the subdural space produces rapid deterioration in the patient. Headache suddenly becomes severe, drowsiness goes on to coma, a local paralysis of an arm or leg develops which, within hours, may spread to become a flaccid hemiplegia with an upper motor neurone facial paralysis. Aphasia and hemianaesthesia may be noted and, if the patient can cooperate, hemianopia may be detected. This rapid progression of signs indicative of functional impairment occurs over a period of hours, far too quickly for a brain abscess to have formed. The dramatic change in the patient's clinical picture may be heralded by epileptic fits starting locally and spreading rapidly to involve one side of the body. Fits may not occur early but once observed they may recur with increasing frequency when associated cortical thrombophlebitis produces marked cerebral irritation. In the fully developed picture, neck rigidity and Kernig's sign may prove less arresting than impairment of cerebral function and cerebral irritation. Papilloedema is rare but cranial nerve palsies, due to collections of exudate, may be present. The eyes frequently deviate to the unaffected side, conjugate deviation towards the affected side may be lost and ptosis may be present; the pupils are perhaps unequal but signs of oculomotor paralysis suggest that tentorial herniation has occurred.

The site of the major subdural empyema can usually be determined from analysis of Jacksonian fits and the extent of paralysis present. Fits starting in the face and arm, with aphasia or other major paralysis affecting the arm, suggest that the subdural empyema is on the convex surface of the brain. Similarly, fits starting in the leg, associated with major paralysis of the limb with homonymous hemianopia, suggest that the empyema has collected alongside the falx cerebri.

The clinical picture above should suggest the diagnosis, but lumbar puncture may be useful for confirmation. Cerebrospinal fluid pressure is raised and the fluid clear or turbid, depending on the degree of pleocytosis (usually less than 500 cells/ml). No organisms are found on culture and the sugar content is normal. The great value of these fluid findings may be to exclude purulent leptomeningitis. However, subdural effusion may complicate meningitis, particularly in children (Hankinson and Amador, 1956; Jackson, 1962). The change in the clinical picture establishes the diagnosis.

DIFFERENTIAL DIAGNOSIS

The striking feature of subdural empyema is one of rapid change in the clinical picture with marked evidence of cerebral irritation, as indicated by epileptic fits and impairment of cerebral functions, particularly paralyses. In leptomeningitis, signs of meningeal irritation are dominant and paralyses in the absence of subdural empyema are rare. Epileptic fits and evidence of impaired cerebral function may suggest cerebral thrombophlebitis. Angiography and exploratory burr-holes may be necessary for differentiation. Subdural empyema is an extremely serious lesion. If there is any doubt exploration through burr-holes is imperative.

MANAGEMENT

The indications for exploration of the mastoid are as in other otogenic intracranial infections. However, subdural empyema urgently demands surgical drainage. Therefore, if the patient shows evidence of diffuse subdural suppuration this must be drained first, and the mastoid explored later. Ideally, the patient's ear disease should be controlled before a subdural empyema has developed, by exploration of a chronic ear disease if there is the slightest suggestion of intracranial extension.

Intensive therapy, in various combinations of penicillin and streptomycin, sulphamezathine or sulphadiazine, should begin at once but if diffuse subdural infection is present drainage of the space must be undertaken immediately to prevent loculation. In a case described by Jackson (1962) the diagnosis was made early and an exploratory burr-hole released an infected subdural effusion. Usually the diagnosis is made at a later stage, by which time pus is creamy and much thicker. Pennybacker (1961) advocates that a number of holes, up to six on one side, be burred in the skull, and that small tubes should be inserted through these, partly to drain the subdural space but mainly to irrigate the space with a suitable antibiotic. It must be stressed that systemic penicillin seldom controls an infection of the subdural space. Wood (1952) insists that it is essential to explore both sides of the skull and that the burr-holes should be sited according to clinical localization of the empyema. He recommends that the burr-holes should be made in the following positions:

(1) Posterior parietal burr-holes 8 cm above the external occipital protuberance and 3 cm from the midline.
(2) Just within the frontal hair line 4 cm from the midline.
(3) Low in the temporal fossa.

Once the holes are made, the dura is opened through a cruciate incision and pus is aspirated. Saline is then washed from one burr-hole to another to clean the subdural space. Pools of pus alongside the falx are aspirated through soft rubber catheters from another burr-hole placed 1.5 cm from the midline just behind the coronal sutures. Finally, fine rubber or polythene catheters are placed in the subdural space and the scalp wounds sutured in layers.

The subdural space is irrigated twice daily using 10 ml of penicillin solution containing 500 units/ml; 5000–10 000 units of penicillin are also injected intrathecally, daily for the first few days, since systemic penicillin does not readily cross the blood–brain barrier.

Epileptic fits are controlled by sodium phenobarbitone, given intramuscularly at first and later orally in reduced dosage for six months.

Whenever possible, these cases should be managed by the neurosurgeon with the full cooperation of the otologist. However, the urgency of treatment may be such that the otologist has to initiate it.

Leptomeningitis

Dawes (1961) recorded a series of 98 cases of otogenic meningitis, of which three-fifths arose from chronic otitis media. In 60 per cent of the cases, otogenic meningitis was the only major intracranial complication. The meningitis resulted from acute or chronic ear disease in almost equal proportions. However, in the remainder, meningitis was associated with some other major intracranial lesion, and four-fifths of the multiple lesions arose from chronic ear disease. More recently Brydoy and Ellekjaer (1972) studied 136 cases of otogenic meningitis and found that 81 per cent of cases arose from acute otitis media.

Otogenic meningitis occurs at all ages. In the younger age group acute otitis media is the usual cause, whereas in the older age group chronic ear disease is more often responsible. Cawthorne (1939) found that 67 per cent of all cases of otogenic meningitis occurred under the age of 16.

In approximately 70 per cent of cases reported by McLay (1954) and Dawes (1961) and in over 60 per cent of those recorded by Jeanes (1962) and 59 per cent of Brydoy and Ellekjaer's cases no bacteria were cultured from the cerebrospinal fluid. This is in sharp contrast to the 114 cases reported by Stewart (1929) when positive cerebrospinal fluid cultures were obtained in 92 per cent. As a sterile cerebrospinal fluid in the presence of meningitis is found, whether the patient has or has not antibiotics prior to admission to hospital, McLay (1954) was forced to conclude that the infecting organisms today are of a relatively non-invasive type.

The organisms most frequently found are pyococci and *H. influenzae* and occasionally *B. proteus* and pseudomonas. Of the cocci *Streptococcus pyogenes* used to be the most common but today pneumococcus is more frequently found (Brydoy and Ellekjaer 1972). The streptococcus is least commonly found. Pneumococcus has the reputation of causing vertical meningitis.

Meningismus, serous meningitis and purulent meningitis are all different stages in infection of the meninges.

The pathology of meningeal infection has already been described but recapitulation of some features is advisable.

Although preformed pathways to the subarachnoid space of congenital or traumatic origin do occur, the majority of cases of otogenic meningitis arise by direct extension of ear disease through bone. The rate of extension of an infection to the leptomeninges will depend on the virulence of the organism, the natural resistance of the patient, the type of ear lesion and any already established exposure of the meninges. A virulent infection causing acute otitis media or an acute exacerbation of a chronic otitis media may rapidly invade the meninges whether a preformed pathway is present or not. An ear disease which has been present for some time may have prepared the way by osteitic erosion and indeed may have eroded through to the subarachnoid space itself to produce cerebrospinal fluid leakage. Leptomeningitis may arise at any time in the course of acute or chronic ear disease. In labyrinthogenic meningitis the labyrinthine walls have been first breached, surgically or by disease, and here the aqueduct of the cochlea, which communicates with the subarachnoid space in the posterior fossa, may act as a preformed pathway if local resistance is inadequate.

Once the meningitis has become purulent, exudate most commonly collects in the basal cisterns but occasionally on the vertex. The exudate may interfere with free flow of cerebrospinal fluid producing blockage at the ventricular foramina or at the junction of the cerebral and spinal subarachnoid spaces. The site of blockage determines the extent and type of hydrocephalus. A block in the ventricular system may cause local or generalized internal hydrocephalus and obstruction external to the ventricular system may produce varying degrees of external hydrocephalus. Local collections of exudate around the exit points of the cranial nerves may lead to impairment of their function. An exudative collection within a cerebral sulcus can, by infection of the Virchow–Robin space, lead to the formation of a brain abscess. Although exudates on the surface of the brain cause impairment of cerebral function, really massive exudates are difficult to distinguish pathologically from subdural collections and clinically must always be regarded as subdural empyemata.

CLINICAL FEATURES

The patient first complains of headache, generalized or localized, sometimes described as a 'bursting pain'; he is obviously unwell, anxious and fearful. The temperature is usually raised to 38.3°C (101°F) or 38.9°C (102°F). No other physical signs are found in the early stages. Within hours the patient becomes more ill, is restless and irritable, and may vomit; flexion of the neck on the body is resisted and he lies curled up facing away from the light which disturbs him. As the disease progresses headache and vomiting may increase, the patient may cry out in pain or be delirious. The neck becomes so stiff that head and shoulders may be raised from the bed like a rigid block.

The temperature remains high and the pulse rate is relatively slow. Kernig's and Brudzinski's signs are evident and abdominal reflexes may be lost. A child with severe meningitis may cry out in pain and have opisthotonic attacks. Drowsiness and coma supervene, the respiration becomes irregular and eventually of Cheyne–Stokes type, the pupils dilate and death follows.

This progressive picture of meningitis was all too common before chemotherapeutic agents and antibiotics became available. The preceding otological history is important for evidence of other intracranial infections may be recognized, and if the history has been prolonged the meningitis may well be due to a leaking brain abscess. Major ventricular rupture of a brain abscess produces a rapidly developing meningitic picture of overwhelming infection with quick onset of coma. A leaking abscess may produce an intermittent picture of relapsing meningeal irritation which, on each occasion, responds to treatment before finally ending in major rupture of the abscess if the real process has been overlooked.

Paralyses of limbs, or other focal signs, are not necessarily due to infection of the subarachnoid space and clinically these findings should always be regarded as evidence of subdural empyema or brain abscess. Epileptic fits do not occur in meningitis alone and when they are observed subdural abscess or overdosage of intrathecal penicillin should be considered.

In the early days of the meningeal infection the absence of neck rigidity is not significant for neck rigidity is only marked when the basal cisterns are involved and the cervical nerve roots irritated. Vertical meningitis may be present for two or three days before neck rigidity is noticed.

Papilloedema should not be regarded as a physical sign of otogenic meningitis. When papilloedema is present it probably indicates that the meningitis has followed an intraventricular leakage of a brain abscess.

Provided that there is no clinical contraindication, lumbar puncture provides essential information in diagnosis. The cerebrospinal fluid pressure is raised and the fluid is usually turbid but if an abscess has ruptured almost frank pus may be obtained by the lumbar tap. A cell count should be done immediately, and a direct film, prepared from centrifuged cerebrospinal fluid, should be stained by Gram's method. From this direct film useful bacteriological information may be obtained. Cocci or bacilli may be seen and, if cocci, their response to the Gram stain assessed. A large number of intracellular Gram-negative cocci is suggestive of meningococcal meningitis. An occasional Gram-negative coccus may be a degenerated Gram-positive coccus. However, the treatment of meningococcal and pyococcal meningitis is similar and a positive growth on culture may supply the final answer. Unfortunately, organisms are found only on direct film or on culture in about 30 per cent of cases of meningitis. The biochemical findings include raised protein and lowering of the sugar content and chlorides. Reduction of sugar content is definite evidence of bacterial activity. A normal sugar content in the presence of a turbid fluid suggests that an abscess may be leaking.

DIFFERENTIAL DIAGNOSIS

The differentiation of meningitis from subdural and brain abscess on clinical grounds and the evidence afforded by cerebrospinal fluid changes have been discussed. The importance of the clinical history and the progress of the illness must not be forgotten. As meningitis may obscure the presence of infections of other intracranial tissue planes, the slightest suspicion may call for other investigations. Electroencephalography is useful when findings are positive but a negative electroencephalograph does not exclude the presence of brain abscess or subdural abscess. An angiogram is most useful but if the patient is rapidly deteriorating or too ill to transport then exploratory burr-holes must be made.

PROGNOSIS

Before the era of modern medical therapy, very few cases of otogenic meningitis recovered. Nowadays, recovery rates of 74 per cent and 85 per cent have been recorded (McLay, 1954; Watson, 1948). McLay demonstrated the effectiveness of combining penicillin with sulphonamides, as opposed to the use of sulphonamides alone.

Table 12.4   Causes of death in otogenic meningitis

	Uncontrolled infection	Late diagnosis	Unexplained	Mismanagement
Acute suppurative otitis media 9 deaths	6 (all prior to 1949)	2 moribund	1	—
Chronic suppurative otitis media 26 deaths	6 (5 prior to 1947)	15 { 4 moribund / 8 temporal lobe abscesses / 2 cerebellar abscesses / 1 subdural abscess	3	2

Of the 98 cases of otogenic meningitis recorded by Dawes (1961), 35 died. When meningitis was the sole complication of acute or chronic ear disease, three-quarters of the patients recovered; there was a slightly more favourable outlook when it was a complication of acute otitis media. Much the highest death rate occurred in cases of multiple complications and these were seen in 38 of the 98 cases. Of the 38 multiple lesions 31 were caused by chronic ear disease. Otogenic meningitis associated with other major complications in chronic ear disease had a mortality rate of almost 50 per cent. These are difficult problems to manage. Dawes (1961) analysed his series further (*Table 12.4*) and, allowing for those cases which were admitted in the early days of antibiotic therapy and were possibly undertreated, the majority died as a result of late admission during the course of the illness or because a cerebral or cerebellar abscess remained obscure or had ruptured into the ventricle to cause the meningitis.

A high proportion of the deaths in McLay's series (1954) resulted from inadequate treatment or because a cerebral or cerebellar abscess was already present.

With the wide range of antibiotics available and known to be effective against the common organisms causing otogenic meningitis, meningitis should be controllable and the danger lies in failing to recognize and treat some additional lesion.

MANAGEMENT

As with all otogenic intracranial complications the most important factor is to make an early and complete diagnosis and institute treatment immediately on the slightest suspicion of intracranial extension. Throughout treatment a careful watch must be maintained for evidence suggestive of another intracranial lesion; the patient must not be discharged from hospital until the cerebrospinal fluid is normal and there is no suspicion of a residual intracranial lesion.

Acute otitis media usually responds to the treatment instituted for control of the complicating meningitis. However, the ear should be assessed carefully to be sure that the response is satisfactory and if doubt exists the mastoid should be explored. Chronic ear disease must be explored and, apart from excision of disease, deliberate exposure of the middle fossa dura and lateral sinus is necessary to exclude lesions at either site. The timing of the ear exploration in chronic ear disease is important. If there is merely suspicion of an intracranial lesion, antibiotic treatment is started, and within a few hours the ear is explored. Diagnostic lumbar puncture should be done immediately after operation whilst the patient is still under general anaesthetic.

If meningitis is manifest, medical treatment is started first and the ear explored approximately 24 h later. The antibiotics are used at once to control further infection which may be spread by surgical exploration, but to delay the operation beyond 24 h may allow the meningitis to gain a firmer foothold and prolong the morbidity.

Early excision of the otitic focus gives adequate control of the lesion which is continually spilling into the subarachnoid space; failure to control the ear lesion allows re-infection of the meninges and increases the problem of management. Dramatic improvement often follows exploration of the ear. Exploration of the ear permits control of a cerebrospinal fluid leak by plugging the hole with muscle (Alberti and Dawes, 1961), and also of any inner-ear infection when the labyrinthine walls are breached and the aquaductus cochleae may act as a preformed pathway.

ANTIBIOTIC THERAPY

Systemic antibiotics are given in high dosage. Penicillin one to two million units six-hourly by intramuscular injection is combined with sulphadiazine or sulphamezathine in dosage of 2 g four-hourly. Sulphadiazine and sulphamezathine readily cross the blood–brain barrier and are effective against pyococci and *H. influenzae*. However, sulphonamides given alone do not effectively control all cases of meningitis and are best combined with penicillin which is more effective against pyococci. As penicillin does not readily cross the blood–brain barrier the systemic dosage should be supplemented by daily intrathecal injections of 5000–10 000 units of penicillin in 5 ml of normal saline solution. Six-hourly penicillin may be effectively combined with 0.5 g streptomycin given twice daily. These are synergistic drugs and in combination are more effective against those pyococci which may be relatively insensitive to penicillin and sulphonamides alone. In severe cases, penicillin, sulphadiazine and streptomycin may be given together. Streptomycin is also effective against *H. influenzae* and intrathecal injections of 50 mg of the drug may help to control this type of disease. Wilson (1948) recommended combined use of penicillin, sulphonamides and streptomycin for the management of meningitis due to *H. influenzae*. Chloromycetin and the tetracyclines are more efficient in the management of influenzal meningitis.

When a case of otogenic meningitis is admitted to hospital the patient must immediately be started on penicillin, sulphonamides and streptomycin in combination.

Lumbar puncture is done and if the cerebrospinal fluid is turbid a prepared intrathecal injection of 5000 or 10 000 units of penicillin given. If no organisms are found in direct film or culture, the combined systemic antibiotic therapy known to be effective against all the common infective agents must be continued and daily intrathecal injections of penicillin given. Each specimen of cerebrospinal fluid obtained must be examined histologically, biochemically and bacteriologically. Changes in the fluid indicate response to treatment when the patient's general condition is so poor that it cannot be accurately assessed, and may first raise the suspicion that another major intracranial lesion is present when there is a difference betweeen the expected and the actual response. Demonstrable insensitivity is the only good reason for change of drugs. Organisms grown from a suppurating cholesteatoma may not be those actually causing the meningitis but may suggest that chloromycetin or tetracycline may be more effective. In practice, chloromycetin is indicated only if the meningitis is due to *H. influenzae* or resistant cocci. Failure in clinical response to surgical and medical treatment usually means the presence of another major intracranial disease or meningitis due to insensitive organisms; the latter is uncommon. Streptomycin should not be continued beyond the tenth day since permanent vestibular or cochlear damage may result. This rule must be abandoned if the organism is sensitive only to streptomycin and if control of infection by the drug must be continued beyond the desirable time limit because the saving of the patient's life is more important than the minor risk of labyrinthine disability. Intrathecal penicillin must be given daily at first. If clinical and cerebrospinal fluid changes indicate rapid improvement, intrathecal injections may be stopped before the fluid is quite normal. Systemic therapy must be continued in reduced dosage for at least 7–14 days after the patient is clinically normal. The cerebrospinal fluid should be normal and, ideally, an air encephalogram taken to exclude the presence of brain abscess before the patient is discharged from hospital.

Excessive dosage of intrathecal penicillin may cause epileptic fits and death. The dose should never exceed 10 000 units in 5 ml of normal saline at any one time. When doses of 50 000–100 000 units were commonly given in the early days of penicillin, adhesions developed in the subarachnoid system and cerebrospinal fluid blocks developed. A similar block may also follow exudative obstructions. In either case intrathecal penicillin given by the lumbar route no longer circulates, and intraventricular penicillin given via parietal burr-holes becomes necessary.

Occasionally the intraventricular route is needed in cases of pneumococcal meningitis if loculation arises from exudate.

The presence of a brain abscess or subdural abscess requires specific surgical measures.

Circumscribed serous meningitis

This is a rare otitic complication, usually of chronic ear disease. Dawes (1961) found only two cases in his series. Adhesions developing in the subarachnoid spaces in response to local irritation may produce local cyst formation. Although, theoretically, they may occur anywhere in the subarachnoid space, symptoms rarely arise from a supratentorial lesion. They are most frequently found in the lateral basal cisterns and are commonly adjacent to the bone of Trautmann's triangle.

The patient complains of headache which may fluctuate, but as the cyst becomes enlarged headache is more persistent and the patient may vomit. He looks remarkably well but gradually he develops symptoms and signs of a posterior fossa lesion. Giddiness, ataxia, spontaneous deviation of arms, poor performance in finger–nose tests, dysdiadochokinesia and nystagmus develop. Homolateral muscle weakness may be detected. Indeed, the clinical picture is that of a space-occupying lesion in the posterior fossa, and a false diagnosis of cerebellar abscess is usually made.

Treatment of the ear disease is as in other intracranial complications but, because a posterior fossa lesion is manifest, the dura in contact with Trautmann's triangle should be exposed. A small incision in the dura and insertion of a brain needle releases the cerebrospinal fluid under pressure. One tapping is usually enough. Similarly, if the suboccipital route is preferred a burr-hole is made as for drainage of a cerebellar abscess and the brain needle releases cerebrospinal fluid and not pus as expected.

Spontaneous cure of circumscribed serous meningitis may occur if the cyst bursts into the general subarachnoid space. Fluctuations in symptoms are probably due to recurrent leak of fluid into the subarachnoid system.

Otogenic brain abscess

Brain abscesses, cerebral or cerebellar, which arise by direct extension or by thrombophlebitis from middle-ear infection, most commonly complicate chronic ear disease. As the infection traverses intracranial tissues, several planes may be invaded and consequently the majority of brain abscesses are associated with other intracranial lesions (*see Figures 12.38–12.40*).

Otogenic brain abscess is nearly always situated adjacent to the temporal bone. Extension of infection to the middle fossa produces an abscess within the temporal lobe which may be adherent to the dura covering the tegmen tympani. Cerebellar abscesses formed by spread to the posterior fossa lie within the anterior part of the lateral lobe of the cerebellum (*Figures 12.39* and *12.40*) and are adherent to dura in the region of Trautmann's triangle or the lateral sinus (*see Figure 12.14*). If the abscess should communicate with the ear through a track, it is sometimes referred to as an abscess with a stalk.

Metastatic otogenic brain abscesses are situated at a distance from the portal of entry and have reached their location by thrombophlebitic extension or by an embolus from an infected arterial thrombus (*see Figure 12.4*). They are very uncommon.

Direct extension of cholesteatoma through the meninges may produce superficial cortical erosion which, although not truly a brain abscess, has sometimes been classified as such. Both adjacent and metastatic abscesses form within the subcortical strip of white matter and expand by further destruction of white matter towards the ventricles. Subsequent to the initial cerebral thrombophlebitis, cerebral oedema and encephalitis precede focal necrosis and liquefaction. Patients with little resistance may develop phlegmonous encephalitis, wherein massive cerebral oedema with spreading encephalitis and perivascular liquefactive necrosis occur. In response to abscess formation, microglial and mesodermal elements of the blood vessels are mobilized to limit spread by capsule formation. A capsule may be recognizable in two weeks and may be 2–3 mm thick within 5–6 weeks. Later, the capsule is formed of fibrous tissue

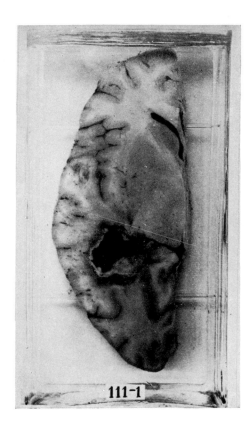

Figure 12.38 Acute temporal lobe abscess showing a poorly developed capsule and surrounded by marked hyperaemia

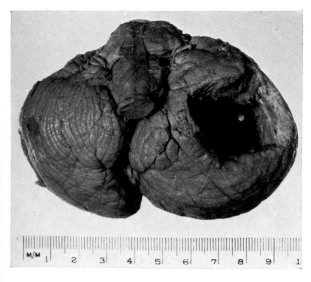

Figure 12.39 Large cerebellar abscess with marked thinning of the cerebellar cortex

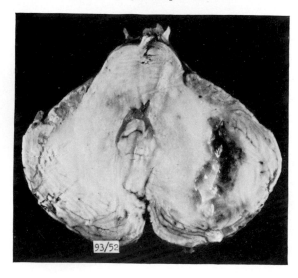

Figure 12.40 Acute cerebellar abscess. (Reproduced by courtesy of the Department of Pathology, Newcastle upon Tyne)

which may undergo hyaline degeneration and calcification. At any time, renewed activity in the abscess may produce an increase in size, or penetration of the wall to form daughter abscesses. Finally, an abscess may rupture into a ventricle or subarachnoid space (*see Figures 12.12, 12.30* and *12.31*). More rarely a ventricle distended by loculated hydrocephalus may rupture through the abscess to the exterior. An expanding abscess or a rapid increase in the surrounding cerebral oedema may cause a rapid rise in intracranial pressure and lead to tentorial herniation or impaction of the flocculus into the foramen magnum (*see Figure 12.8*). These in turn may cause fatal haemorrhages in the vital centres of the brain stem.

BACTERIOLOGY

The bacteria most commonly found in brain abscesses are the pyococci *Staphylococcus aureus* and *albus* and *Streptococcus pyogenes* and the pneumococcus. As diseases caused by these pyococci are highly susceptible to antibiotic therapy, Gram-negative bacilli, *E. coli*, *B. proteus* and *Ps. pyocyaneus* are being found more frequently. Sometimes a pyococcus is associated with a bacillus in the pus taken from the abscess, and these mixed infections are usually due to chronic ear disease. Foul-smelling or gas-containing pus is produced by the saprophytic *B. proteus* and *E. coli* and occasionally *Cl. welchii*. Frank pus may be sterile on culture and only degenerate organisms seen in a smear; yet the abscess may remain clinically active. Rarely have abscesses been reported as being caused by moulds such as actinomyces, or fungi such as aspergillus.

CLINICAL FEATURES

The natural history of brain abscess is that of a progressive process with periods of relative inactivity depending on the degree of local resistance. The initial invasion of brain tissue may be obscured by the more striking features of another intracranial lesion such as meningitis or sinus thrombophlebitis. The clinical picture depends on the rate of progress of the disease, the time after onset of presentation, the activity or quiescence of the abscess itself, the success or failure of capsule formation and the response to any treatment already given. The symptoms and signs produced by brain abscess are those of increased intracranial tension and certain focal symptoms and signs dependent on the part of the brain affected. The picture varies with the size of the abscess and the degree of surrounding oedema. Daily or hourly changes in physical signs are largely the result of variable cerebral oedema.

The initial symptoms and signs of invasion of cerebral tissue are headache and vomiting followed by drowsiness. These symptoms are not specific and are readily obscured by lesions of more dramatic onset. At this stage lumbar puncture may be helpful because an increase in pressure, protein and cell count support the diagnosis. Unfortunately the cerebrospinal fluid may show no change. Within 2–3 days of onset the symptoms arise from non-suppurative encephalitis which may respond to antibiotics alone. Persistence or recrudescence of the symptoms suggests the establishment of an abscess.

Virulent lesions progress rapidly, drowsiness and slow cerebration give place to stupor and coma, and finally death from either tentorial herniation or ventricular rupture. In marked supratentorial hydrocephalus with tentorial herniation, there is a progressive dilatation first of the ipsilateral pupil and later fixed dilatation of both pupils. In the absence of other intracranial lesions, the temperature is subnormal and the pulse increasingly slow, perhaps no more than 40/min. Just before death the temperature and pulse rate may suddenly rise. Therapy may slow down this rate of progress, and the more typical picture seen is that of gradual progression of symptoms and signs culminating in a final rapid deterioration.

The headache is persistent though of varying severity; its site is not of localizing value although it may be situated in the neighbourhood of the lesion. Vomiting may recur at intervals and be persistent during the more active phases of the abscess. The patient is apathetic, drowsy and often falls asleep during questioning and examination. The temperature is subnormal and the pulse rate slow. Although the patient may try to cooperate he lacks concentration and the history may be difficult to elicit. It is always advisable when possible to supplement the patient's history by another taken from the relatives.

After 2–3 weeks papilloedema may be found. The finding not only stresses the presence of raised intracranial pressure but indicates the abscess is of at least 2–3 weeks' duration.

In an abscess of long duration the patient may have become emaciated.

During this progressive picture focal signs, if carefully sought, may be elicited. These findings are of great importance, for the preceding symptoms and signs are common to abscesses in both the middle and posterior cranial fossae.

CEREBRAL FOCAL SIGNS

Visual fields
As a temporal lobe abscess may interfere with the fibres of the optic radiation, perimetry may demonstrate the presence of homonymous hemianopia (*Figure 12.41*). The defect is commonly in the upper quadrant but may be in the lower quadrant, and only when the abscess is enormous is a complete homonymous hemianopia found (*Figure 12.42*). Full cooperation is required for this test but unfortunately most patients seen by the otologist are in the acute stage of abscess development and rarely give the necessary cooperation. Testing of visual fields by confrontation requires less effort and it may readily demonstrate gross visual defects.

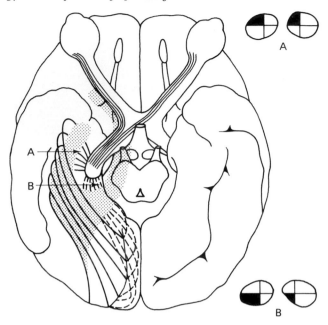

Figure 12.41 Diagram of optic radiations. Lesions at A or B produce the field defects shown in the insets

Aphasia
The speech centre is situated in the dominant temporal lobe and an abscess together with the surrounding cerebral oedema may interfere with the function of the associated fibres. Nominal aphasia and perseveration are the most common defects. Numerous objects should be used if partial aphasia is to be detected. Even if the correct

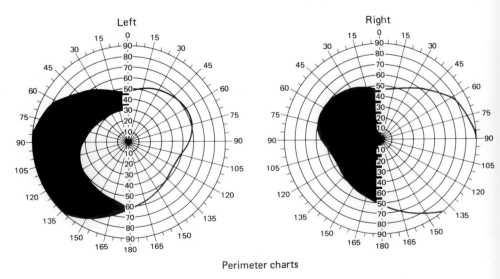

Perimeter charts

Figure 12.42 Visual field defect of patient whose abscess was illustrated in *Figures 12.30* and *12.31*

name of the object eludes the patient he may describe its use, recognize the name and may then repeat it if once mentioned by the observer. The degree of aphasia varies greatly even in the individual patient and frequent testing is essential.

INVOLVEMENT OF THE MOTOR TRACTS
As the abscess or surrounding encephalitis extends the motor tracts may be involved. Expansion upwards may involve cortical centres and contralateral upper motor facial paralysis may appear. As the lesion expands, the upper limb and finally the lower limb become paralysed.

Expansion inwards of an abscess produces progressive paralysis in reverse order, leg, arm and finally face, by direct interference with the pyramidal tracts in the internal capsule (*see Figure 12.11*).

Ocular paralyses are of special interest. Sixth nerve paralysis may accompany any intracranial lesion in which pressure is raised, or may follow a direct inflammatory lesion along the course of the nerve, for example, superior petrosal thrombophlebitis. Paralysis of oculomotor nerves is a late manifestation of brain abscess and is associated with supratentorial hydrocephalus producing tentorial herniation with mid-brain compression and displacement. Early dilatation of the ipsilateral pupil is followed by fixation and the opposite pupil may become involved.

CEREBELLAR SIGNS
Nystagmus, ipsilateral loss of muscle tone and muscular incoordination are typical. In addition, the patient may have complained of subjective vertigo or instability.

NYSTAGMUS
Nystagmus is commonly slow and coarse with the quicker phase towards the diseased side. This is far from constant and all types of horizontorotatory nystagmus are found.

ASYNERGIA
The ambulant patient staggers to the side of the lesion and may hold his head forwards or tilted to one side. The bed-fast patient frequently lies curled up on the side of the lesion with his eyes deviated towards the opposite side. Testing for muscle weakness soon demonstrates atonia, and tendon jerks on the side of the lesion are usually increased.

Muscle incoordination is best detected by purposive tests. A marked dissimilarity between the two sides is very evident, the ipsilateral side showing gross incoordination and the opposite side almost normal. Attempts to pick up a cup with the affected hand lead to overshooting of the mark and spilling of the contents. In the finger–nose test, particularly with closed eyes, the affected hand misses both the finger and nose, and waves from side to side. Dysdiadochokinesia is easily demonstrated by rapid pronation and supination of the forearms. On asking the patient to swing his fully extended arms alternately upwards and downwards from above his head to the level of the bed, an observer facing him will notice a spontaneous deviation of the ipsilateral limb in an outward direction.

Speech defects
Only if the abscess is of long duration is slurring of speech, and less often slight difficulty in swallowing, encountered.

The development of neck rigidity and marked signs of meningeal irritation in a comatose patient suggests that meningitis is due to leaking brain abscess. Unfortunately patients still present at this late meningitic stage, no significance having been attached to the preceding history.

At any stage in the slow progress of a manifest brain abscess, encapsulation may establish quiescence. The patient may have no more than persistent or intermittent headache, occasional vomiting and papilloedema. These provide evidence of raised intracranial pressure and localizing signs may be difficult to detect. The clinical picture may not be related to an aural lesion when chronic ear disease is present; if produced by acute ear disease the acute incident may have long been forgotten. Clinical examination may demonstrate a visual field defect or aphasia, but because of chronicity a diagnosis of brain tumour may be considered. Other investigations may only confirm the presence of a space-occupying lesion and the true diagnosis may only be reached at the time of excision of a well encapsuled chronic abscess.

After the more acute phases of meningitis or sinus thrombophlebitis have been treated and cured, an unsuspected brain abscess may be dormant for many years, producing no obvious changes other than those in personality or behaviour. Such an abscess is picked up later only by investigation of personality changes or recurrence of symptoms suggestive of the presence of a suppurative space-occupying lesion.

INVESTIGATIONS

Provided there is no evidence of a marked rise of intracranial pressure, lumbar puncture may be performed. An EMI scan is the most valuable investigation for demonstration of the presence of an abscess. Angiography is the second most valuable investigation. Occasionally plain radiographs of the skull may show a displaced pineal body or even gas within the abscess. Ventriculography is occasionally useful in the diagnosis of posterior fossa abscesses.

DIFFERENTIAL DIAGNOSIS

During the course of any otogenic intracranial suppurative disease a constant watch should be kept for symptoms or signs suggesting the presence of brain abscess, and particular note must be made of changes in the pulse and temperature, for a subnormal temperature and slow pulse may be the first signs.

A rapid development of wide focal signs is more characteristic of subdural empyema or cerebral thrombophlebitis and, depending on the urgency for surgical exploration, a cerebral angiogram or exploratory burr-holes will usually confirm the diagnosis.

Severe meningitis late in the history of the illness suggests that it is due to a leaking brain abscess.

Lateral sinus thrombophlebitis may produce a cerebellar abscess and the awareness of this association leads one to suspect that nystagmus or slight muscular inco-ordination is due to the cerebellar lesion. However, as lateral sinus thrombophlebitis by involvement of the superior petrosal sinus may cause a temporal lobe abscess, symptoms not directly related to the sinus lesion assume a new significance.

Otitic hydrocephalus may be confused with brain abscess, but the early onset of papilloedema, the characteristic cerebrospinal fluid picture and the absence of localizing signs, negative electroencephalogram and angiograms soon make the distinction clear.

Brain tumours occur occasionally in patients with ear disease and, apart from typical angiographic changes, the diagnosis may be accurately determined only on surgical exploration.

Cerebellar abscess may be confused with tuberculous meningitis in children but the typical cerebrospinal fluid changes and the finding of the tubercle bacillus in the fluid make the distinction.

PROGNOSIS

The patient's relatives should always be warned that the prognosis may be grave. In the series of 30 otogenic temporal lobe abscesses reported by Dawes (1961), 90 per cent of the cases followed chronic ear disease and more than 70 per cent of the abscesses were associated with another major intracranial disease. When the abscess was the sole otogenic complication seven out of the eight cases recovered but two-thirds of those with multiple lesions died. It is also interesting that the three patients with abscesses due to acute ear disease recovered. Of the ten cerebellar abscesses recorded all followed chronic ear disease, the three singular lesions recovered and three of the seven multiple lesions caused death. One may therefore conclude that multiple major intracranial lesions associated with abscess increase the gravity of the prognosis. Seeking to explain the high mortality Dawes (1961) analysed the cases further (*see Table 12.5*).

Table 12.5   Causes of death in otogenic temporal lobe abscess

	Uncontrolled infections		*Late or no diagnosis*	
1944–1948 8 deaths (62 per cent mortality)	3	2 pyaemias 1 meningitis	5	1 moribund 2 meningitis 1 subdural undiagnosed 1 undiagnosed
1949–1953	1		4	1 moribund 2 meningitis with late diagnosis 1 pyaemia
1954–1960 2 deaths (22 per cent mortality)			2—Both	meningitis with late diagnosis

A marked improvement in mortality rate has occurred in the later years. Many of the deaths from uncontrolled infections occurred in the early days of antibiotic therapy. Others who died were either sent to hospital very late in the course of the illness, or the presence of severe meningitis obscured the presence of a brain abscess, or the presenting meningitis was the direct result of ventricular leak or rupture. It seems probable that if intracranial invasions had been suspected and the patients referred for treatment at an earlier date, many more cases would have been saved.

Wood (1952) also stressed the multiplicity of intracranial lesions in his series of 33 abscesses, for 60 per cent of the cases were accompanied by another intracranial lesion. His mortality rate was 22.9 per cent and if the three cases which were moribund on admission were excluded from the series the mortality rate would have been reduced to 14.3 per cent.

Jeanes (1962) reported 15 brain abscesses with a mortality rate of 40 per cent. Seven of the 15 abscesses were complicated by meningitis.

Pennybacker's latest figures published in 1961 showed a remarkable improvement in mortality (*see Table 12.6*).

Table 12.6   Brain abscess due to mastoid infection

	1938–1950			1950–1960		
	No. of cases	*Deaths*	*%*	*No. of cases*	*Deaths*	*%*
Temporal lobe abscess	31	10	32	24	1	4
Cerebellar abscess	19	8	42	11	1	9
Total	50	18	36	35	2	5.7

In Pennybacker's series (1961) brain abscesses form the large majority of the cases reported, very few cases of meningitis and lateral sinus thrombosis being treated. When compared with Dawes' series it would seem that Pennybacker dealt with a selected group, which may well have been the surviving residue of a much larger group of multiple intracranial lesions. However, a mortality rate of less than 6 per cent is a remarkable achievement.

Provided a patient survives the acute phases of an intracranial invasion and a diagnosis of brain abscess is made early enough, then with proper management the chance of survival should be good.

Epilepsy and even status epilepticus may occur in those patients recovering from a temporal lobe abscess.

If a temporal lobe abscess was originally large enough to have destroyed the lower part of the optic radiation then a permanent quadrantic visual field defect may remain. All other neurological defects consequent upon the brain abscess disappear as recovery becomes complete.

After a cerebellar abscess the patient rarely remains ataxic.

TREATMENT

As a detailed outline of treatment of brain abscess has been considered earlier only a summary is included here.

The appropriate antibiotic should be given in large dosage at first to enable localization of the abscess. Throughout the whole length of treatment, antibiotics should be continued in reduced dosage adjusted to the degree of activity within the abscess.

Once the abscess has been diagnosed and localized it should be tapped by a brain cannula through an appropriate burr-hole. The contents should be aspirated and replaced by 50 000 units of penicillin in 1 ml, mixed with 2 ml of Thorotrast or Steripaque. Thorotrast permits the progress of the abscess to be assessed radiologically, even if an EMI scan is unavailable. The first aspiration usually relieves the headache, stupor and focal signs, and further aspirations are indicated if symptoms and signs re-appear, or the abscess has increased in size as seen in the radiograph. An increase in size may be seen radiologically before symptoms recur. After the first few days further aspirations must be carried out through the wound using a sharp needle. This sharp needle may puncture a vessel and so cause serious haemorrhage or it may implant infection outside the capsule; the abscess wall is not as readily assessed when using a sharp needle as compared with the blunt brain cannula. Repeated aspiration produces a shrinking down of the abscess to a crenated scar adherent to the dura at the portal of entry. This scar does not require excision.

If repeated aspiration does not produce cure, it may well control the lesion pending encapsulation. A persistent chronic abscess not responding to aspirations is best excised.

Occasionally an abscess is multilocular. An EMI scan or pyogram may indicate loculation; persistence or increase of brain symptoms and signs with reduction in the size of the treated abscess may also be suggestive. The new loculus may be treated by aspiration or the whole multilocular abscess excised. Because of the risk of loculation, no patient should be discharged home until the cerebrospinal fluid is normal and an air encephalogram has demonstrated that no further brain lesion exists.

The ear is always an important factor in otogenic brain abscess. Neither local extradural abscesses nor sinus thrombophlebitis can be treated by merely aspirating a brain abscess and it is wise to control the chronic ear disease and the associated intracranial lesions as early as possible, for once the ear is controlled further spillover into neighbouring tissue planes ceases. Control of the ear disease during the early stage of brain invasion, supported by adequate medical therapy, may prevent the establishment of an abscess. Even if the brain abscess demands priority in treatment the ear disease must also be controlled by surgery, either at the time of draining the abscess or as soon as the patient is fit enough to withstand further operation.

In all cases of established abscess it is worth while starting anticonvulsive therapy and continuing this for six months in an attempt to prevent the development of epilepsy.

As patients with brain abscesses are often very ill attention must be given to general care. Electrolyte balance must be carefully watched and an adequate fluid intake and output maintained. Intravenous therapy should, in general, be avoided for it may increase the cerebral oedema.

Intercurrent chest infections or hypostasis in a comatose patient must be treated by posturing the patient on his side, head down, so that the secretions drain from the mouth. Bronchoscopy may be necessary to aspirate the secretions on rare occasions. Frequent change of posture and physiotherapeutic measures may all help for a relative anoxia may increase cerebral oedema. Assisted respiration may be required.

Pneumocoele

A pneumocoele is rarely associated with otitis media. For air to enter and be retained in the intracranial tissue planes, a valvular communication must exist between the middle-ear cleft and involved plane. Such a communication may follow skull fracture or surgical injury (Horowitz, 1964). Although any intracranial tissue plane may be involved, it is probable that air most commonly percolates into the subarachnoid space and traumatized areas of cerebral tissue. Eventually the pneumocoele may communicate with the ventricles.

The patient may only complain of headache. Diagnosis is made by a skull x-ray demonstrating loculated air within the cranial cavity.

The mastoid should be explored and the valvular track plugged by muscle; the pneumocoele then gradually absorbs and the patient fully recovers.

Meningo-encephalitis of myringitis bullosa haemorrhagica

Myringitis bullosa haemorrhagica has a characteristic clinical appearance and although the aetiological agent has not been determined it is thought to be a virus. However, as myringitis bullosa haemorrhagica may be secondarily infected by the pyococci any of the suppurative complications of middle-ear disease may occur. Apart from these another distinct group of non-suppurative complications are associated with the bullous lesion and these may be regarded as of viral origin. The non-suppurative complications are meningo-encephalitis, and single or multiple cranial nerve lesions.

As in the case of mumps two types of meningo-encephalitis occur. The first type appears close to the onset of the bullous lesion and the second 'post-infectious' type 2–3 weeks later. This post-infectious encephalitis can rarely be differentiated from a pyogenic cerebral thrombophlebitis and each individual case should be treated as a suppurative intracranial lesion.

NEUROLOGICAL SYMPTOMS AND SIGNS

Headache is common and usually severe and may be relieved by lumbar puncture.

Drowsiness, stupor and coma may develop.

Mental disturbances, such as slow cerebration, confusion, disorientation, restlessness or even violence have occurred, and emotional disturbances may be present.

Focal signs

Aphasia, hemiplegia, hemianopia, and loss of extensor plantar response have all been found.

Epileptiform fits of motor or sensory type are of frequent occurrence.

Meningeal irritation, although frequently present, may be fleeting in character.

The cranial nerve lesions

Single or multiple cranial nerve lesions may accompany myringitis bullosa haemorrhagica. The lesions may be transient or permanent. Most commonly the facial and auditory nerves are affected. Typically, a lower motor neurone paralysis results from facial nerve involvement.

The cochlear or vestibular divisions of the auditory nerve may be affected individually or together. A cochlear division lesion causes an inner-ear deafness which is greatest at onset and, although the hearing loss frequently remains permanent, varying degrees of recovery occur within three months. The deafness is accompanied by tinnitus. The severity of the injury to the vestibular division is reflected in the severity and persistence of the vertigo accompanying the lesion. The vertigo is, as a rule, non-recurring and the patient, even after a totally destructive lesion, recovers fully within six weeks unless his neural compensatory mechanisms are deficient. When the whole auditory nerve is affected the patient suffers deafness, vertigo and tinnitus.

Nystagmus usually accompanies the vertigo of a lesion in the vestibular division, but it has been seen in cases where no injury to the auditory nerve could be detected. Nystagmus in these latter cases has usually been associated with a more diffuse meningo-encephalitis and may well have arisen from a lesion in the brain stem affecting the medial longitudinal bundle. Ptosis and ocular palsies of transient type have been noted during the course of the meningo-encephalitis.

Trigeminal pain, paraesthesia and loss of sensation in the trigeminal distribution have been recorded. The pain may persist for some weeks after the bullous lesion has disappeared.

Vagal paralyses have also been known to occur.

A lumbar puncture may be informative even in the absence of meningeal irritation. Pressure recordings are variable, but a protein-cell count disproportion, or lymphocytosis, support a diagnosis of virus meningo-encephalitis. Occasionally, the increased cellularity is a polymorphonuclear leucocytosis. No changes occur in the sugar or chlorides. However, a diffuse meningo-encephalitis may not be accompanied by changes in the cerebrospinal fluid.

CLINICAL PICTURE

The usual onset of severe encephalitis is sudden: headache, epileptic fits, coma or extreme irritability develop within a few hours of the appearance of the aural lesion. Diffuse cerebral involvement with focal signs and cranial nerve lesions of transient type follow. Recovery gradually occurs even in the most severe and diffuse lesions.

Headache and meningeal irritation may accompany severe vertigo, deafness, multiple or single cranial nerve lesions. The greater the number of cranial nerve lesions the more evident is the associated encephalitis.

Frequently singular nerve lesions accompany the bullae.

DIAGNOSIS

The sudden onset of meningo-encephalitis or cranial nerve lesions during the course of a non-suppurative disease of the ear usually makes diagnosis easy. The only difficulty likely to arise is when the encephalitis or cranial nerve lesions occur during the phase of a secondary infection of the myringitis bullosa haemorrhagica. In these late cases the complications should be regarded as of suppurative origin, unless the character and diffuseness of the complications are such that no suppurative lesion would be likely to cause them.

TREATMENT

There is no specific treatment for meningo-encephalitis.

PROGNOSIS

All known cases of meningo-encephalitis due to myringitis bullosa haemorrhagica have recovered without sequelae, other than hearing loss. By analogy it has been assumed that the meningo-encephalitis is similar to that of other virus diseases, and also that the accompanying cranial nerve lesions are due to damage at the nuclear level.

Facial paralysis

Facial paralysis occurs not infrequently as a complication of otitis media, whether acute or chronic. The pathology, diagnosis and treatment are described in Chapter 27.

References

Alberti, P. W. R. M. and Dawes, J. D. K. (1961) *Journal of Laryngology*, **75**, 123

Atkinson, E. M. (1934) *Abscess of the Brain.* London; Medical Publications

Ballance, C. A. (1919) *The Surgery of the Temporal Bone.* London: Macmillan

Bauer, F. (1951) *Journal of Laryngology*, **65**, 199

Borries, G. V. Th. (1949) *Acta Otolaryngologica, Stockholm*, **37**, 483

Brydoy, B. and Ellekjaer, E. F. (1972) *Journal of Laryngology*, **86**, 871

Cairns, H. (1949) *British Medical Journal*, **1**, 968

Cairns, H. and Schiller, F. J. (1948) *Proceedings of the Royal Society of Medicine*, **41**, 805

Cairns, H. and Schiller, F. J. (1949) *Journal of Laryngology*, **63**, 96

Cawthorne, T. E. (1939) *Journal of Laryngology*, **54**, 444

Davis, E. D. D. (1951) *Journal of Laryngology*, **65**, 646

Dawes, J. D. K. (1951) *Myringitis Bullosa Haemorrhagica; its Relationship to Cranial Nerve Paralyses.* M.D. Thesis; Durham.

Dawes, J. D. K. (1953) *Journal of Laryngology*, **67**, 313

Dawes, J. D. K. (1961) *Proceedings of the Royal Society of Medicine*, **54**, 314

Dawes, J. D. K. (1963) *Proceedings of the Royal Society of Medicine*, **56**, 777

Dawes, J. D. K., Marshall, H. F. and Robson, F. C. (1969) *Journal of Laryngology*, **83**, 981

Dawes, J. D. K. and Watson, R. T. (1978) *Journal of Laryngology*.

Eagleton, W. P. (1924) *Surgery, Gynecology and Obstetrics*, **39**, 653

Eagleton, W. P. (1926a) *Journal of the American Medical Association*, **87**, 1954

Eagleton, W. P. (1926b) *Cavernous Sinus Thrombo-Phlebitis.* New York; Macmillan

Fraser, J. S. (1924) *Journal of Laryngology*, **39**, 253

French, L. A. and Chou, S. N. (1974) *Advances in Neurology*, **6**, 257

Golding-Wood, P. H. (1952a) *Journal of Laryngology*, **66**, 71

Golding-Wood, P. H. (1952b) *Journal of Laryngology*, **66**, 496

Gucek, R. R. (1974) *Annals of Otology, Rhinology and Laryngology, Supplement*, **83**, **10**, 1

Hankinson, J. and Amador, L. V. (1956) *British Medical Journal*, **2**, 122

Hanson, H. G. de G. and Dawes, J. D. K. (1965) *Journal of Laryngology*, **79**, 912

Harper, A. R. (1951) *Journal of Laryngology*, **65**, 89

Harpman, J. A. (1950) *Journal of Laryngology*, **64**, 319

Harpman, J. A. (1955) *Journal of Laryngology*, **69**, 180

Horowitz, M. (1964) *Journal of Laryngology*, **78**, 128

Horowitz, S. (1949) *Journal of Laryngology*, **63**, 363

Jackson, J. McG. (1962) *Journal of Laryngology*, **76**, 641

Jeanes, A. (1962) *Journal of Laryngology*, **76**, 388

Kornblat, A. D. (1972) *Laryngoscope*, **82**, 1541

Macewen, W. (1893) *Pyogenic Infective Diseases of the Brain and Spinal Cord.* Glasgow; Maclehose

McGuckin, F. (1935) *Otogenic Brain Abscess.* M.D. Thesis; Durham

McGuckin, F. (1936) *Lancet*, **2**, 1387

McKay, R. J. Jnr., Ingraham, F. D. and Matson, D. D. (1953) *Journal of the American Medical Association*, **152**, 387

McLay, K. (1954) *Journal of Laryngology*, **68**, 140

Newland, W. J. (1965) *Journal of Laryngology*, **75**, 28, 120, 729

Northfield, D. W. C. and Cawthorne, T. E. (1942) *Proceedings of the Royal Society of Medicine*, **35**, 794

O'Connell, W. J. (1960) *Journal of Laryngology*, **74**, 121

Pennybacker, J. (1951) In *Modern Trends in Neurology.* London; Butterworths

Pennybacker, J. (1961) *Proceedings of the Royal Society of Medicine*, **54**, 309

Reid, J. L. and McGuckin, F. (1946) *Journal of Laryngology*, **61**, 273

Schiller, F., Cairns, H. and Russell, D. S. (1948) *Journal of Neurology, Neurosurgery and Psychiatry*, **11**, 143

Smith, A. B. (1950) *Journal of Laryngology*, **64**, 12

Smith, H. V., Schiller, F. and Cairns, H. (1946a) *Proceedings of the Royal Society of Medicine*, **39**, 613

Smith, H. V., Schiller, F. and Cairns, H. (1946b) *Journal of Laryngology*, **61**, 313

Stewart, J. P. (1929) *Journal of Laryngology*, **44**, 225

Symonds, C. P. (1927) *Journal of Laryngology*, **42**, 440

Symonds, C. P. (1931) *Brain*, **54**, 55

Symonds, C. P. (1937) *Brain*, **60**, 531

Turner, A. L. and Reynolds, F. E. (1931) *Intracranial Pyogenic Diseases.* Edinburgh; Oliver and Boyd

Tutton, G. K. and Shepherd, W. H. T. (1949) *British Journal of Surgery*, **36**, 240

Watson, D. (1948) *Proceedings of the Royal Society of Medicine*, **41**, 155

Watson, D. (1952) *Journal of Laryngology*, **66**, 247

Wilson, C. (1948) *Lancet*, **2**, 445

Wood, P. H. (1952) *Journal of Laryngology*, **66**, 71, 496

Yadar, Y. C. and Blatia, M. L. (1968) *Journal of Laryngology*, **82**, 1031

13 Tumours of the middle-ear cleft and temporal bone

John S Lewis

According to all published reports cancer of the ear is a very rare condition. An early excellent review of the literature was presented by Peale and Hauser in 1941. According to these authors, Wilde and Roudot, Schwartze, Lucae, Kidd, and others, in the period around 1775, were the first to discuss carcinoma of the middle-ear cleft. In 1883, Politzer gave a comprehensive description of cancer of the ear, as manifested in his patients. Kretschman, in 1886, gave an anecdotal description of reported cases, and included four of his own. Between 1804 and 1889, 121 otitic tumours were recorded, according to Zeroni (1924), and Newhart (1917) found 34 cases of the middle ear reported between 1899 and 1917. In 1921, Broders made a statistical analysis of 63 cases of epithelioma of the ear, which was the first comprehensive article published on the subject in the English language. Yates in 1936, published a report of 14 cases reported between 1917 and 1924, and 24 cases between 1924 and 1936. In 1943, Figi and Hempstead reported 48 malignant tumours of the middle ear and mastoid from 1922 to 1941. Grossman, Donally and Snitman, in 1947, reported six cases of squamous carcinoma of the middle ear and mastoid. Garnett Passe reported a case of primary carcinoma of the eustachian tube in 1948, and reviewed two other cases in the literature. Mattick and Mattick in 1951, discussed their experience with ten cases of cancer of the middle ear and mastoid. In 1954, Figi and Weisman describing a wide experience with the surgical management of ear cancer and chemodectoma at the Mayo Clinic, cited 124 cases of cancer of the middle ear and mastoid covering the period from January 1907 through December 1951. By way of contrast, more than 13 000 patients were treated for cancer of the stomach at that clinic in the same period. Among 212 000 cases of aural disease seen between 1905 and 1924, at the Manhattan Eye, Ear and Throat Hospital in New York, Robinson (1931) found a diagnosis of tumour in only 48, or a ratio of 1:4000. Schall (1934) found that in a 12-year period at the Massachusetts Eye and Ear Infirmary, only 15 patients out of 90 040 with pathological conditions of the ear, had neoplasms. Furstenberg (1924) found cancer of the middle ear in only two out of 40 000 patients in the Department of Otolaryngology at the University of Michigan Medical School. Tod (1907) quoting from the records of the London Hospital, where 20 000 cases are seen annually found only one case. Lodge (1955) and his co-workers found six cases of cancer of the temporal bone reported in a population of one million people, and estimated that

0.006 per thousand of living persons suffer from aural cancer at a given time. Towson and Shoftstall (1950) point out that the proportion of cancer of the middle ear and mastoid to all otologic pathological conditions is 1:5000 to 1:20000.

Pathology

Zizmor and Noyek (1969) have attempted to present a serviceable classification of tumours and other osseous disorders of the temporal bone. The author has added additional tumours to the classification.

(*1*) *Benign tumours*
    (a) Epithelial-primary cholesteatoma
    (b) Mesenchymal
        (1) Jugulo-tympanic paraganglioma (glomus tumour, chemodectoma)
        (2) Osteoma
        (3) Hemangioma
        (4) Neurogenic tumours
        (5) Xanthoma
        (6) Giant cell tumour
        (7) Benign osteoblastoma
(*2*) *Malignant tumours*
    (a) Primary
        Epithelial
        (1) Squamous cell carcinoma
        (2) Adenocarcinoma
        (3) Melanoma
        Mesenchymal
        (1) Sarcoma
        (2) Multiple myeloma
        (3) Hemangioendothelioma
        (4) Malignant xanthoma
    (b) Secondary
        Direct extension from:
        (1) Nasopharynx
        (2) External ear
        (3) Parotid
        (4) Temporo-mandibular joint
        (5) Meningioma
        Distant metastasis from:
        (1) Kidney
        (2) Lung
        (3) Prostate
        (4) Breast
        (5) Uterus

Each of these tumours will be discussed as to their pathology, natural history, treatment and prognosis.

Malignant epithelial and glandular tumours

Lodge (1955) and his associates consider that cancers of the middle-ear cleft and mastoid are comparable to Marjolin's ulcer, with its chronic sanious discharge producing cellular irritation that develops into cancer. Coachman (1951) has reported a patient with squamous carcinoma of the middle ear secondary to cholesteatoma. Indeed ten of the author's 150 cases had associated cholesteatoma.

Cancer of the middle ear and mastoid have approximately the same sex distribution, although cancer of the auditory canal is slightly more common in females. Broders (1921) found the median age for cancer of the ear to be 61 years. In the author's series the median age was 55 years. The age span was nine months to 76 years. In 1952, Aub *et al.* presented a case of epidermoid carcinoma of the middle ear in a radium dial painter which appeared 31 years following exposure. Beal *et al.* in 1965 described another case of epidermoid carcinoma of the middle ear and mastoid in a radium dial painter and mentioned that there have been eight other similar cases. Ruben *et al.* in 1977 reported a case of temporal bone carcinoma following radiation therapy to the head and neck area. He stated that the US Armed Forces Institute of Pathology has at least one temporal bone in which there is a malignant tumour which was probably radiation induced. As far back as 1917, it was recognized that up to 85 per cent of patients with cancer of the middle-ear cleft and mastoid had associated chronic otitis media, many of whom had been operated on for this condition previously. The author has treated three primary carcinomas of the mastoid bone, two epidermoid carcinomas, and one angiosarcoma. Clairmont and Conley (1977) reported only one case of primary carcinoma in the mastoid bone as compared to 61 cases of malignancy of the external auditory canal and 25 cases of cancer arising in the region of the middle ear.

Cancer of the middle-ear cleft and temporal bone is almost invariably squamous carcinoma. Lindahl (1955) reported that a search of the medical literature as far back as 1894 revealed a total of only eleven published cases of adenocarcinoma. Adenocarcinoma frequently arises from ceruminous gland tumours in the auditory canal, but primary adenocarcinoma arising in the middle-ear cleft is a rarity. Occasionally adenocarcinoma will extend directly into the temporal bone and middle ear from the deep lobe of the parotid gland.

DIAGNOSIS

The patient with the typical epidermoid carcinoma of the middle ear presents with a prolonged period of otorrhoea, which has a sanguinous tinge, becomes infected, and then begins to have ear pain. Aural polyps may grow along with the cancer and mask the true nature of the disease. Hearing loss progresses. Facial paralysis follows with erosion of the mastoid bone. Labyrinthine symptoms with vertigo and sensorineural hearing loss indicate advanced disease. Primary carcinoma of the mastoid presents with mastoid swelling, pain and occasionally facial paralysis. There may be additional external swelling due to invasion of the parotid and sternomastoid muscle. Approximately 10 per cent of cases have parotid node or cervical node metastases.

Routine mastoid films are diagnostic in 40 per cent of cases with demonstrable bone destruction (*Figure 13.1*). Tomograms demonstrate more clearly involvement of mastoid, petrous and erosion through the tegmen into the middle cranial fossa. Carotid angiography will demonstrate in its venous phase involvement of the lateral sinus. C.T. scan will also highlight the extent of tumour involvement.

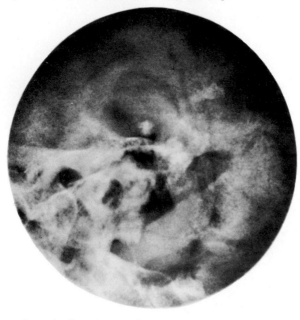

Figure 13.1 X-ray showing extensive destruction of the mastoid from cancer of middle-ear cleft

A typical case recently operated by the author was a 49 year old male first operated for chronic mastoiditis 29 years previously. The ear continued to drain and three months prior to admission he suddenly began to bleed from the ear and noticed a partial facial palsy. A large granuloma was removed from the auditory canal by his local otologist which was reported as benign. He was subjected to a radical mastoidectomy and the mastoid and middle ear were filled with friable granulation tissue, which on paraffin section was reported as epidermoid carcinoma. At the time of referral he still had the partial facial paralysis. Temporal bone resection revealed cancer extending through the tegmen tympani into the middle cranial fossa with extension along the facial ridge and into the petrous pyramid, attic and filling the mastoid cavity.

TREATMENT PLAN

After careful analysis of presenting symptoms, objective findings, biopsy and both routine and tomographic radiological evaluation, a treatment plan should be decided. Radical surgery and a curative dose of radiation therapy have in our experience given the best results.

RADICAL SURGERY

Anatomy

The temporal bone petrous process lies in a venous lake surrounded (1) posteriorly and inferiorly by the lateral sinus and its sigmoid portion which extends downward to the jugular bulb at the base of the skull (2) superiorly and inferiorly by the petrosal venous sinuses, and (3) medially by the cavernous sinus. The carotid artery courses through the anteromedial aspect of the petrous tip and is seldom encountered in the resection. The facial nerve is sectioned both in the temporal bone and in the parotid gland. Occasionally the vagus nerve is traumatized at the skull base. In transection of the petrous process the cochlea and semicircular canals are usually removed.

Surgical treatment—subtotal resection of the temporal bone

The operation consists of more than a petrosectomy. It is an *en bloc* resection of the involved portion of the auditory canal, middle ear, mastoid, petrosa along with temporo-mandibular joint, parotid and base of zygoma. Temporal bone resection is a combination of intracranial and extracranial surgical *en bloc* resection of cancer-ridden bone (*Figures 13.2, 13.3* and *13.4*). The initial exposure of dura and petrous pyramid is through a temporal craniotomy. The external ear and external auditory meatus are swung superiorly through a U-shaped incision, exposing the squamous portion of the temporal bone, the base of the zygoma and temporo-mandibular joint. The muscular attachments to the mastoid are transected, and a partial parotidectomy is performed to give clear definition to the styloid process and the temporo-mandibular joint. The facial nerve in the parotid may be tagged in its distal portion for facial-hypoglossal anastomosis either at the termination of the resection or at another sitting.

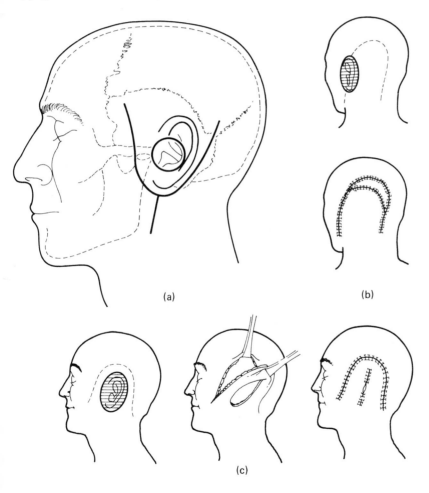

(a) (b) (c)

Figure 13.2 (a) U-shaped incision where the external ear may be saved. (b) Sacrifice of the external ear and coverage with a posterior-based scalp flap, from parietal–occipital region. (c) Sacrifice of the external ear and coverage by bipedicle flap. (Rob and Smith, *Operative Surgery—Ear*, Butterworths, 3rd edn, p. 134)

Petrous remnant

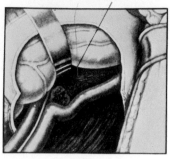

Figure 13.3 Combined intracranial–extracranial resection of the temporal bone. (Rob and Smith, *Operative Surgery—Ear*, Butterworths, 3rd edn, p. 134)

The styloid process is a key landmark, for deep to it lies the carotid artery. It is transected along with its muscular attachments. The base of zygoma is sectioned, and the neck of the mandible severed with a gigli saw. The temporal muscle is preserved for coverage of dura. A temporal craniectomy is carried out. A high-speed air-drill with a large cutting burr is utilized to expose the lateral sinus through the mastoid process and trace it to the jugular bulb level.

The path of least resistance for cancer extending from the middle ear is through the thin roof of the tegmen tympani into the middle cranial fossa. Cerebrospinal fluid, between 60 and 100 ml are withdrawn from previously placed malleable spinal needles to allow the dura and brain to be separated from underlying petrous bone. If dura is involved, it should be freed from the petrous roof with electro-cautery, dura

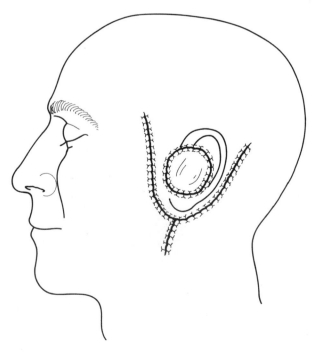

Figure 13.4 Closure of incision and skin graft creating new auditory canal. (Rob and Smith, *Operative Surgery—Ear*, Butterworths, 3rd edn, p. 134)

subsequently resected as a separate specimen, and the defect repaired with fascia. Occasionally the tumour has extended into brain or base of skull and is unresectable. This area should be marked with silver clips for post-operative radiotherapy. The Stryker saw is then utilized to cut through the petrosa lateral to the carotid canal and medial to the arcuate eminence. The transection is completed with a curved chisel. Bleeding is controlled, and the dura is carefully scrutinized for tears. Temporal muscle is mobilized and rotated over the dura. The defect is covered either with a split thickness skin graft or a posterior based scalp flap rotated into the defect. A lateral tarsorrhaphy is then carried out to protect the cornea.

If the patient has not been radiated, a post-operative course of supravoltage radiotherapy in the range of 6000 rad is administered approximately four to six weeks after surgery.

Complications of surgery

Haemorrhage   Hypotensive agents contribute greatly to the reduction of blood loss; the systolic blood pressure is kept at 80–90 mmHg throughout the procedure. Surgical procedures in this area result in considerable bleeding, with the median blood loss between 2500 and 3000 ml. Fortunately haemorrhage is chiefly of venous origin and can be controlled by local suture. The site of bleeding is usually the sigmoid sinus, and the use of vascular silk with a tampon of temporal muscle or Surgicel controls the bleeding. The smaller petrosal sinuses may be electrocoagulated. On rare occasions if the jugular bulb is transected in chiselling towards the skull base, a large pack may be inserted, left in place for five days and then removed. Secondary skin grafting may be then carried out.

Infection   The excision site is always covered by a skin graft. The graft is prone to infection, especially when patients have received pre-operative radiation. The most common organism is *Pseudomonas aeruginosa*. Adequate administration of carbenicillin and gentamicin is indicated. Occasionally portions of the skin graft are lost and must be replaced by secondary skin grafts. A permanent temporal decompression remains. When the entire pinna has been sacrificed a scalp flap is utilized to cover the defect.

Loss of facial nerve function   The facial nerve is severed both in the temporal bone and the parotid gland. The distal end of the nerve in the parotid substance may be utilized for facial hypoglossal anastomosis at the termination of the procedure or at a later date. A fascial sling procedure for support of the facial musculature is a useful procedure for late facial rehabilitation. The lateral tarsorrhaphy prevents corneal ulceration.

Deafness and vertigo   Hearing loss is complete following this procedure. Vertigo may last from 5 to 15 days, and there may be a period of unsteadiness for several months.

Carotid artery thrombosis occurred in one of our patients due to trauma to the carotid vessel during surgery. A unilateral hemiplegia resulted. Cerebral herniation may be prevented by the use of both temporal muscle flap and scalp flap rotated into the defect.

End results

With the use of hypotensive anaesthesia, high-speed air-drills in the dissection and antibiotic therapy the mortality rate has dropped in the last ten years from 10 per cent to under 5 per cent. With a total experience of over 100 cases the five-year cure rate is 28 per cent for all cases and 25 per cent for those with squamous carcinoma. Indeed Conley and Schuller (1977) have claimed a five-year cure rate of over 36.8 per cent utilizing temporal bone resection and supravoltage radiotherapy carried to 6000 rad in a group of 19 patients with middle-ear malignancy. Lederman (1965) reported a five-year survival rate of 30.7 per cent for petromastoid malignancies treated by radiation therapy alone. Our experience with 51 cases treated by radiation and mastoidectomy was 6 per cent five-year cure. However, Holmes (1965) and Figi and Weisman (1964) have reported five-year survivals of 30 per cent. Radical surgery combined with radiotherapy in our opinion gives the patient the best palliation and the best chance of cure.

Malignant melanoma

A series of 36 patients with melanoma of the external ear has been reported by Sylven and Hamberger (1944). The median age on admission (including two children, 10 and 12 years of age, respectively, and 34 adults) was 55 years. Of the 36 patients, 21 were male. Two additional cases of melanoma of the ear are reported in the literature: one by Friedmann and Radcliffe (1954) and the other by Cordes and Masing (1953). Our series includes two cases of melanoma arising from the posterior surface of the auricle, the lesions measuring less than 2 cm in diameter. One patient had proved positive neck nodes on admission. In a third patient the lesion arose in the auditory canal and metastasized to neck nodes. A fourth patient was a nine month old infant with melanoma of the middle ear. This undoubtedly represented transplacental implant from the mother, who subsequently died of widespread melanomatosis.

Except for the small lesions arising on the external ear, where wide local excision and neck dissection suffice, melanomas are best handled by combined temporal bone resection and radical dissection of the neck. The prognosis for melanomas arising from the ear is extremely poor.

Mesenchymal tumours

Primary sarcomas of the temporal bone are rare. A comprehensive review of the literature by Naufal (1973) revealed 211 reported cases. In 89 cases the histologic picture was that of undifferentiated sarcoma including spindle-cell, round-cell, atypical, and anaplastic types. Sixty-four cases were reported as rhabdomyosarcomas; all occurred in young children. There were 17 cases of fibrosarcoma, 7 of which originated in the nerve sheath. Tumours of the bone included 12 osteogenic sarcomas and seven Ewing sarcomas. There were eight tumours of vascular origin, six primary reticulum sarcomas, five myxosarcomas, one chondrosarcoma, one liposarcoma, and one meningeal sarcoma. The author reported an additional case of chondromyxosarcoma of the middle ear, osteogenic sarcoma of the temporal bone, and two cases of early aural rhabdomyosarcoma.

Embryonal rhabdomyosarcoma of the middle ear is a rare, highly malignant tumour found in patients in the pediatric age-group. In general, the overall prognosis and response to therapy as previously reported in the literature would appear to differ significantly from other embryonal rhabdomyosarcomas of the head and neck region, especially those arising in the orbit. Only 42 cases arising in the temporal bone have been documented in the world literature since the original description of this tumour in the middle ear by Soderberg (1932). The extremely morbid nature of embryonal rhabdomyosarcoma and its natural history have been discussed by many authors. The histologic patterns have been defined by Horne and Enterline (1966). Potter (1966) presents excellent hypocycloid body section radiography in evaluating the extent of involvement of bone in middle ear and of mastoid lesions. He thought that while radiotherapy might cause the visible aural tumour to regress, it did not significantly affect cases with demonstrated involvement of bone.

This tumour is lethal. When one reviews the reports, it appears that most of the cases were undertreated. Radiotherapy in curative doses at the 6000-rad tumour dose level plus concomitant chemotherapy offers the best chance for long-term survival. Cyclophosphamide, vincristine, and dactinomycin combined therapy plus radiotherapy is the treatment of choice. The tumour may rapidly invade the petrous apex, mastoid, middle ear, and bony and membranous labyrinth and may extend into the middle and posterior cranial fossae. Metastasis is early and is usually to lung and bones. Survival for five years is rare.

MULTIPLE MYELOMA

Multiple myeloma is a disease of the haemopoetic cells of the bone marrow and small translucent areas are frequently seen in the skull and mastoid on x-ray. Diagnosis is made on raised serum protein, raised globulin and the appearance of Bence-Jones protein in the urine. The bone marrow smear is diagnostic with the appearance of plasmacytes, myelocytes and erythroblasts. Chemotherapy and radiotherapy to discrete lesions is the modern treatment to the long bones.

MALIGNANT HEMANGIOENDOTHELIOMA

This rare bony tumour rarely affects the skull and mastoid. It usually involves the long bones and is treated by radiotherapy and chemotherapy. This diagnosis was given to malignant glomus tumours prior to their proper identification by Rosenwasser and Otani in 1945.

Secondary tumours of the mastoid and middle ear

Secondary tumours may reach the temporal bone either by direct extension or by distant metastases. Direct extension of cancer of the deep lobe of the parotid gland into the auditory canal and middle ear is not unusual. The patient may present with 'Bell's Palsy' which is not properly investigated. The deep lobe of the parotid is palpated, a mass felt, and needle biopsy will identify the tumour. Cancer of the nasopharynx may extend up the eustachian tube into the middle ear and present as a friable bleeding tumour which ruptures through the eardrum. Radiotherapy is the treatment of choice, but is usually only palliative at this late stage of the disease. Extensive cancer of the external ear frequently invades the mastoid, and offers a poor prognosis for cure by both surgery and radiotherapy. Rarely do malignant tumours of the temporo-mandibular joint invade the middle ear and mastoid. These are usually malignant synoviomas.

The most common cancer to metastasize by blood stream to the temporal bone is the hypernephroma. Other temporal bone metastases are from lung, breast, prostate, uterus and colon. Ear pain is a common first symptom and may present before the primary lesion is discovered. Neurologic symptoms rapidly follow with involvement of cranial nerves. Radiotherapy will relieve pain and give palliation to the patient.

MENINGIOMA

Involvement of the middle-ear cleft and mastoid by meningioma is due to invasion from an overlying meningeal tumour. Symptoms and signs derive from involvement of adjacent brain or impingement on structures within the temporal bone. Karam and Salman (1964) reported a case and stated that Cushing and Eisenhardt (1958) found no involvement of the middle ear in 313 histologically verified meningiomas. Punt (1965) reported a case of meningioma of the middle ear and quoted Nager (1964) as having cited seven previous cases. Fairman (1971) reported a case in a 16 year old male who presented with paralysis of the last four cranial nerves and was found to have meningioma involving the middle ear, petrosa and the occipital bone with obliteration of the anterior condylid foramen. No deformation of the brain was present on encephalogram. Treatment was by radiotherapy, and the disease was still arrested at the five year follow-up period.

Benign tumours

Epidermoids of the temporal bone

Epidermoids or congenital cholesteatomas are believed to result from aberrant epithelial rests during the closure of the neural groove and are distributed along the neuraxis. They occur most frequently in the intracranial cavity, the spinal canal, and the diploe of the skull. When they arise in the base of the skull, the temporal bone is the most common site. In the temporal bone the origin may be in the squamous, mastoid, or petrous portions, or in the middle-ear cleft. Onset of symptoms peaks at around age 15 but the majority are found somewhat later; males are affected more frequently than females.

Primary cholesteatomas are similar to secondary cholesteatomas in that they are lined with keratinizing squamous epithelium. This results in the pathological manifestations of the condition: accumulation of desquamated material causes the cyst to enlarge and erode the surrounding bone. The continuous desquamation also gives the cyst its characteristic concentric lamellar or 'onion skin' appearance on cross-section.

Symptoms may result from the slow growth and resultant obliteration of structures or from irritation and inflammation produced by rupture of the capsule. Thus the spectrum of symptoms may range from progressive hearing loss or vestibular dysfunction to sudden facial paralysis, trigeminal neuralgia or acute arachnoiditis.

Epidermoids of the temporal bone are radiographically characterized by regular bone destruction with sclerotic margins frequently in an otherwise normal, well-pneumatized temporal bone. As they may spread along clefts and canals and into less dense spaces the radiolucent lesions may be lobulated or with finger-like projections. Enlargement of the internal auditory canal is rare with epidermoids, but when they arise in the petrous apex, there may be a well-defined destruction of the entire apex.

Treatment of primary cholesteatoma, as for acquired cholesteatoma, should consist of complete surgical removal of the cyst. If there is good residual hearing and all evidence of tumour has been removed, radical exteriorization may not be necessary. Of course, disease must be completely removed and therefore pursued until this is certain, even should this entail exposure of areas of dura by removal of overlying bone.

Glomus tumours (jugulo-tympanic paragangliomas)

The glomus tumour was first accurately identified by Rosenwasser in 1945, following the definitive work of Stacey Guild (1941) in describing the glomus jugularis. Since then, many names have been suggested for this tumour: glomus jugulare tumour (Winship, Klopp and Jenkins, 1948), non-chromaffin paraganglioma (Lattes and Waltner, 1949), chemodectoma (Mulligan, 1950; Glenner and Grimley, 1974), the last two authors recommended the elimination of the term 'non-chromaffin' and designation of the term paraganglioma according to the site of origin. These tumours arise from widely distributed paraganglionic tissue which is presumed to originate from the neural crest (*Figure 13.5*). Carotid bodies and related paraganglia have been ascribed a homeostatic role by sensing fluctuations in blood pH and oxygen tension. The glomus tumour is the most common benign tumour of the ear, and is designated as a tympanic paraganglioma, arising from the tympanic branch of the glossopharyngeal nerve or from the dome of the jugular bulb. It may grow intraluminally into the jugular bulb. According to Lack *et al.* (1977), of over 600 000 cases examined in the Surgical Pathology Department of Memorial Sloan-Kettering Cancer Center from 1967 through 1975, there were only 69 cases of head and neck paragangliomas (incidence 0.012 per cent) of which eight cases were of the jugulo-tympanic type. According to Bickerstaff and Howell (1963) 10 per cent jugulo-tympanic tumours are multicentric. Rarely do patients with glomus tumours have signs and symptoms of a pheochromocytoma. Dellelis and Roth (1971) reported a case in which a functioning glomus tumour contained 9.4 mg of noradrenaline/g of tissue. Despite this concentration of catecholamine, the chromaffin reaction was negative.

According to Snyder and Mawr (1961) 70 per cent of cases occur in women. The median age is 45–50 years. In 1974, Busby and Hepp reported a glomus tympanicum tumour in a 12 month old infant.

The common presenting symptoms are hearing loss and pulsating tinnitus which seldom recedes. Seventh and twelfth cranial nerve palsies were seen in two of the authors' cases. A jugular foramen syndrome is present in the large tumours of the jugulo-tympanic type, with cranial nerve deficits of the last five cranial nerves and the facial nerve on occasion. Dizziness is unusual and should be investigated by angiography. A patient of the author with a jugulo-tympanic tumour discovered 18 years ago and untreated, recently developed vertigo. She showed tomographic and angiographic evidence of a contralateral carotid body paraganglioma. Arterial

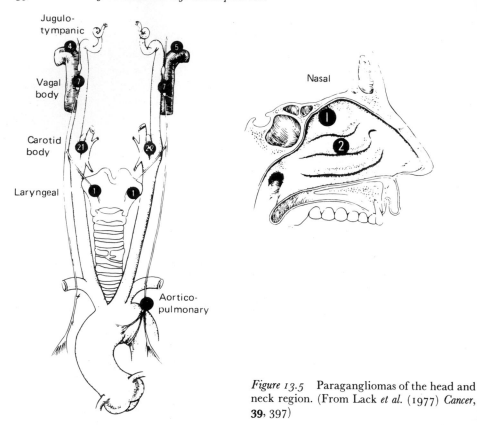

Figure 13.5   Paragangliomas of the head and neck region. (From Lack *et al.* (1977) *Cancer*, **39**, 397)

shunting from the vertebral basilar system to the highly vascular carotid body paraganglioma produced a steal-syndrome resulting in vertigo.

The small glomus tympanicus tumour confined to the middle ear appears as a mulberry coloured tumour in the inferior segment of the drum within the confines of the middle-ear cavity. Tumours arising from the jugular bulb erode the floor of the middle ear and auditory canal and present as vascular tumours in this area. They may also present with a jugular foramen syndrome, with facial paralysis, sensorineural hearing loss and perhaps an arterial bruit (*Figures 13.6* and *13.7*). Tomography and angiography outline the extent of the tumour. Open biopsy is associated with haemorrhage and is best performed in a hospital setting. Pain is a very uncommon presenting symptom, unless infection is also present. If the patient has severe primary hypertension, tests should be carried out to rule out a possible pheochromocytoma with noradrenaline secreting properties. The neck should be palpated to determine the presence of an associated carotid body tumour. A family history is sometimes significant. The author has two sisters as patients both of whom had glomus tumours associated with carotid body tumours.

The tumours are grey to mulberry colour when removed with areas of haemorrhage. Histologically, paragangliomas from all sites have epithelioid cells with finely granular eosinophilic cytoplasm and small round oval nuclei. Rarely does malignant change occur with mitotic figures. Irradiation of the glomus tumour produces swelling of the endothelial cells lining the blood vessels, with occasional focal disappearance of the

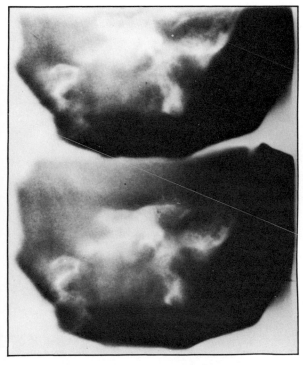

Figure 13.6 Tomogram of jugulo-tympanic paraganglioma (glomus jugulare tumour) with marked widening of the jugular foramen

cells and thrombi in the vessels (*Figure 13.8*). Fibrosis is present if the radiotherapy is given many months before removal. These findings correlate with the marked reduction in blood loss if the tumour is radiated pre-operatively. Treatment of Group 1 cases, the so-called glomus tympanicus tumours confined to the middle ear is by

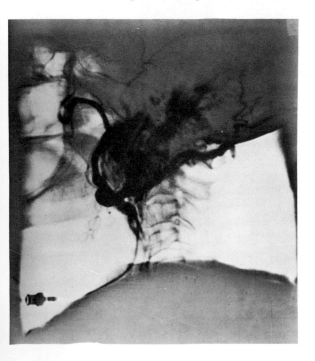

Figure 13.7 Angiogram showing venous phase of same tumour in the jugular bulb region

removal under magnification by the trans-tympanic route. The author has used cryosurgical probe to remove the tumour by this route without bleeding.

Group 2 cases arise from the region of the jugular bulb and extend into the middle ear and mastoid. Neurological deficits may be present with the associated jugular foramen syndrome. These patients are first given pre-operative radiotherapy between 5000 and 6000 rads supravoltage therapy. If the angiogram shows the principal blood supply to come from the ascending pharyngeal branch, the external carotid artery will be secured close to the bifurcation. The surgical approach depends on the pre-determined size of the tumour. If a medium sized tumour is present, a mastoidectomy with the extended facial recess approach may be utilized. However, if a large tumour is present, a combined extracranial and mastoidectomy approach first described by Shapiro and Neuss in 1963, and subsequently modified by Gardner *et al.* in 1977, is the best approach. The muscle attachments to the mastoid are severed, jugular bulb exposed extracranially, and then with a mastoid approach, the facial nerve is dissected out of its canal and rerouted. The sigmoid sinus is plicated with bleeding controlled with Fogarty catheters above and below the tumour. The tumour is removed with a segment of vein. The intraluminal segment of tumour if present is removed.

Group 3 cases have intracranial extension. A combined suboccipital and transtemporal approach, described by Hilding and Greenberg in 1971 is utilized. The seventh nerve is rerouted, and the tumour is removed piecemeal. It is necessary to ligate the sigmoid sinus to control bleeding. Results: It is imperative in the surgical management of large glomus tumours that a team approach with a neurosurgeon be the mainstay of treatment. The patient is left with permanent sensorineural hearing loss, although facial nerve function is usually preserved. The patient must be followed carefully because local recurrence is frequent.

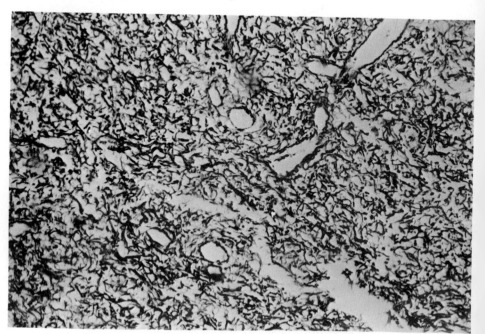

Figure 13.8 Glomus tumour, irradiated six weeks previously having received 6000 rad supravoltage radiotherapy

The author has several poor risk patients with large jugulo-tympanic paragangliomas, with cranial nerve deficits, who received 5000–6000 rad of supravoltage radiotherapy and who have been followed for more than 15 years without surgery and without further progress of disease symptoms. The biological behaviour of each case is variable. Approximately 4 per cent of cases become malignant according to Bersanyi (1962) and Winship, Klopp and Jenkins (1948). However, even the malignant tumours may be slow growing and be followed clinically beyond 15 years.

Osteoma

Osteoma usually arises in the bony portion of the external auditory canal in the region of the tympanomastoid suture line. It causes symptoms by encroaching on the external auditory meatus or middle-ear cleft, usually producing a conductive hearing loss. Marrocco (1948) described a case of multiple osteomas of the mastoid process and referred to 27 cases in the literature. In his cases the tumours grew from the inner table of the mastoid process. The tumour usually grows from the outer table of the mastoid forming an external swelling and can easily be removed. Cortical or hard osteoma presents as a dense, ivory-like oval or lobulated mass. It may block the external auditory canal and press through the tympanic membrane into the middle ear. Such obstruction may contribute to inflammatory processes in the middle ear.

Osteoma of the temporal bone is generally well defined, in contrast to the radiological appearance of more diffuse reactive hyperostosis associated with meningioma, and the osteoblastic changes associated with fibrous dysplasia and Paget's disease of bone.

In treatment osteoma should not be confused with exostoses. They should be removed surgically with a high-speed air-drill if they cause obstructive symptoms.

Hemangioma

Hemangioma of the temporal bone is indeed rare. It may involve the middle ear, mastoid or petrous pyramid, or by extension from adjacent structures. Hemangioma may produce pulsating tinnitus synchronous with the pulse and hearing loss. According to Zizmor and Noyek (1969) the following radiographic signs have been noted: (1) Osteolysis and decalcification of bone; (2) dilated vascular grooves in adjacent bone and a large mastoid emissary vein; (3) honeycombed or soap-bubble lucencies of bone; (4) spoke-like lines of increased density in the temporal squama; (5) spicules and striations of bone perpendicular to the periosteum of the temporal squama; (6) enlarged external or internal auditory canals.

Treatment is usually surgical or with cryotherapy.

Neurogenic tumours

These tumours arise from the nerve sheath of the eighth nerve, usually the vestibular nerve, or more rarely from the seventh nerve. According to Kettel (1963) in discussing neurinomas of the facial nerve, he described 25 per cent of tumours arising from the horizontal portion of the facial nerve and 75 per cent of tumours arising from the vertical portion. According to Fairman (1971), a tumour arising from the horizontal part of the facial nerve causes deafness due to early invasion of the middle ear. The labyrinth may be destroyed before a facial palsy occurs. A neuroma of the vertical portion of the facial nerve causes a facial palsy which may be the only symptom for many years. Treatment is excision of the tumour and nerve graft of the facial nerve.

Xanthomas

Xanthomatoses have been divided into two groups by most authors depending on the serum cholesterol concentration. Patients with high cholesterolaemia may have a deposition of cholesterol in skin, tendons, blood vessels and reticulo-endothelial system. Those seen in patients with normal cholesterol concentration include osseous xanthoma in which the temporal bone may be involved. Koch and Lewis (1956) have reported a case of xanthoma with hyperlipaemia and hypercholesterolaemia with deposition of cholesterol masses in the skin and tendon sheaths and a massive replacement of the mastoid by xanthoma.

Xanthoma of the external auditory canal may become malignant. The author had such a case in a 67-year-old male who underwent multiple local excisions for benign xanthoma of the auditory canal. The patient underwent temporal bone resection when the last local excision was reported as malignant. Within six months the patient had pulmonary metastases, and he died of disseminated disease.

Giant cell tumour

Primary giant cell tumour of the mastoid and middle ear has been reported by Rosenwasser (1969). These tumours most frequently involve long bones; the sites of predilection are the lower end of the femur, the upper end of the tibia, the radius, the mandible, the humerus, the small bones of the hands, the sacrum and rarely the patella. Invasion of soft tissue and the presence of old and recent haemorrhage are usual findings. The deposition of iron pigment in the haemorrhagic areas produces a brownish colour, hence the term 'brown tumour'. According to Rosenwasser (1969) these tumours are always benign and can be treated by curettage. However, Hutter, Worcester and Francis (1962) in a review of 76 cases reported a 62 per cent recurrence rate following conservative surgery and a 30 per cent incidence of cancer. Hutter indicates that giant cell tumours can only be diagnosed as such after a thorough appraisal of clinical, roentgenographic, operative, gross and microscopic pathologic data.

Benign osteoblastoma

A case of benign osteoblastoma of the temporal bone was reported by Ronis *et al.* (1974). It involved the auditory canal and middle ear, and was removed by curettage, thus preserving the facial nerve. These tumours were previously named 'osteogenic fibroma' by Lichtenstein (1956) and Golding and Sissons (1954) or 'giant osteoid osteoma' by Dahlin and Johnson (1954). Lichtenstein and Jaffe (1956) proposed the name 'benign osteoblastoma' to indicate the prominence of osteoblasts with no relation to a fibroma. The growth is primarily a tumour of children and adolescents. Byers (1968) reported only four other cases of benign osteoblastoma of the temporal bone in the medical literature.

Osseous disorders of the temporal bone

Fibrous dysplasia

This disease entity was first described by Lichtenstein and Jaffe to designate an ill-defined group of bony changes which were previously designated by such varying terms as osteogenic or ossifying fibroma, fibrous osteoma, or osteofibroma. Whether these growths really represent tumours or whether they are due to a failure of bone to heal in the ordinary way due to a mesenchymal deficiency is unclear. Fibrous dysplasia usually is considered to be either monostotic or polyostotic, referring to whether one or more than one bone is involved. Occasionally, the polyostotic type occurs as Albright's syndrome, which is characterized by multiple involvement of the long bones, pigmentation of the skin, and the early development of secondary sex characteristics in females. This type is very rare, and few of the cases reported have had involvement of the facial bones. The monostotic type of fibrous dysplasia may occur in the long bones and the facial bones or membranous bones, and this latter type usually involves the temporal bone.

Paget's disease

Paget's disease of the temporal bone is more common than fibrous dysplasia. It usually involves the vault of the skull, but involvement of the base of the skull and petrous bone is frequent. Paget's disease gives rise to symptoms by involving the cochlea and compressing the cranial nerves, especially the eighth nerve in the internal auditory meatus, with resulting profound sensorineural deafness. A predilection to sarcomatous change has been noted in Paget's disease.

Eosinophilic granuloma

Eosinophilic granuloma or histiocytosis X is a disease of unknown aetiology characterized pathologically by histiocytic proliferation. Clinically there are three variants: eosinophilic granuloma, Hand–Schüller–Christian disease, and Letterer–Siwe disease. These three variants have related manifestations but are symptomatically and prognostically different.

Eosinophilic granuloma is characterized by single or multiple osteolytic skeletal lesions. Histologically the lesions consist primarily of proliferation of histiocytes and eosinophils. The tumour occurs chiefly in children or young adults, although it may be found in patients of all ages. The lesions may occur in soft tissues (especially in the lungs and the gastrointestinal tract) as well as in bone. Involvement of the temporal bone may present as a polypoid mass in the posterior canal wall, with little or no pathology in the middle ear. Initially aural discharge is noticed, but as the disease progresses, pain and infection ensue with erosion of the posterior canal wall. Punched-out lesions in the mastoid or temporal bone are present on x-ray and are frequently interpreted as cholesteatoma. Therapy consists of conservative surgery, radiation therapy, steroids, and chemotherapy, usually with vinblastine sulphate (Velban).

Letterer–Siwe's disease is a rapid, fatal process occurring in children under three years of age. The main clinical findings are enlargement of the spleen, liver, and lymph nodes; a secondary anaemia; purpura; destructive skeletal lesions, especially of the skull; and a downhill febrile course.

Hand–Schüller–Christian disease was originally described as a triad manifested by destruction of the skull, exophthalmos, and diabetes insipidus. The latter two components are the result of destructive involvement of the sphenoid bone. Exophthalmos and diabetes insipidus are not mandatory in the description of the disease. Hand–Schüller–Christian is a chronic disease which ends fatally in 15 per cent to 20 per cent of cases. It usually occurs in childhood, but may occur later in life.

Giant cell reparative granuloma

Giant cell reparative granuloma of the temporal bone is a rare condition. According to Wolfowitz and Schmaman (1973) a history of trauma frequently precedes the onset of symptoms, and the reparative granuloma is a response to injury. It is not possible histologically to differentiate the giant cell reparative granuloma from a giant cell tumour with certainty. The process may involve the entire temporal bone. A combination of conservative surgery and post-operative radiotherapy appears to be the treatment of choice.

Osteopetrosis

Osteopetrosis, also known as Albers–Schönberg disease (marble bones), is a rare hereditary disease with congenital and familial abnormality in the development of bone. The bones are hard and brittle; they contain large amounts of calcium salts, and the long bones break like chalk. The mastoid air-cells may not develop, with resultant deafness and facial paralysis. Myers and Stool (1969) have reported a case in a two and a half year old child who became deaf and did not have facial paralysis.

Acknowledgment

The author acknowledges the assistance of James Grillo, MD, in the preparation of the section on Primary Cholesteatoma.

References

Aub, J. C., Evans, R. D., Hempleman, L. H. and Mortland, H. S. (1952) 'Late effects of internally deposited radioactive materials in man', *Medicine*, **31**, 221

Beal, D. C., Lindsay, J. R. and Ward, D. H. (1965) 'Radiation induced carcinoma of the mastoid', *Archives of Otolaryngology*, **8**, 9

Bersanyi, S. J. (1962) *Laryngoscope*, **72**, 1336

Bickerstaff, E. R. and Howell, J. S. (1963) *Brain*, **76**, 576

Broders, A. C. (1921) 'Epitheliomas of the ear: a study of 63 cases', *Surgical Clinics of North America*, **1**, 1401

Busby, D. R. and Hepp, V. E. (1974) 'Glomus tympanicum tumor in infancy', *Archives of Otolaryngology*, **99**, 377

Byers, P. D. (1968) 'Benign osteoblastic lesions of bone', *Cancer*, **22**, 43

Clairmont, C. and Conley, J. J. (1977) 'Primary carcinoma of the mastoid bone', *Annals of Otology*, **86**, 306

Coachman, E. H. (1951) 'Carcinoma secondary to cholesteatoma', *Archives of Otolaryngology*, **54**, 187

Conley, J. J. and Schuller, D. E. (1977) 'Reconstruction following temporal bone resection', *Archives of Otology*, **103**, 34

Cordes, C. and Masing, H. (1953) 'Primary melanoma of the middle ear', *Archiv für Ohren-, Nasen und Kehlkopfheilkunde*, **162**, 553

Cushing, W. M. and Eisenhardt, L. (1958) *Meningiomas*. Springfield, Ill.; Thomas

Dahlin, D. C. and Johnson, E. W. (1954) 'Giant osteoid osteoma', *Journal of Bone and Joint Surgery*, **36**-A, 559

Dellelis, R. A. and Roth, J. A. (1971) *Archives of Pathology*, **92**, 73

Fairman, H. D. (1971) In *Diseases of the Ear, Nose and Throat*, Scott-Brown, 3rd edn., p. 343. London; Butterworths

Figi, F. A. and Hempstead, B. E. (1943) 'Malignant tumors of the middle ear and mastoid process', *Archives of Otolaryngology*, **37**, 149

Figi, F. A. and Weisman, P. A. (1954) 'Cancer and chemodectoma of the middle ear and mastoid', *Journal of the American Medical Association*, **156**, 1157

Friedman, I. and Radcliffe, A. (1954) 'Otosclerosis associated with malignant melanoma', *Journal of Laryngology and Otology*, **68**, 114

Furstenberg, A. C. (1924) 'Primary adeno-carcinoma of the middle ear and mastoid', *Annals of Otology, Rhinology and Laryngology*, **33**, 677

Glenner, G. G. and Grimley, P. M. (1974) 'Tumors of the extra-adrenal paraganglion system (including chemoreceptors)'. *Second Series Atlas of Tumor Pathology*, Fasc. 9. Washington, D. C., A.F.I.P.

Golding, J. S. R. and Sissons, H. A. (1954) 'Osteogenic fibroma of bone, a report of two cases', *Journal of Bone and Joint Surgery*, **36**-B, 428

Grossman, A. A., Donally, W. A. and Snitman, F. (1947) 'Carcinoma of the middle ear and mastoid process', *Annals of Otology, Rhinology and Laryngology*, **56**, 709

Guild, S. R. (1941) 'Hitherto unrecognized structure, the glomus jugularis in man', *Anatomical Record Supplement*, **2**, 79

Holmes, K. S. (1965) 'Carcinoma of the middle ear', *Journal of Faculty of Radiologists*, **16**, 400

Horne, R. C. and Enterline, H. T. (1966) 'Rhabdomyosarcoma: clinical pathological study and classification of 30 cases', *Cancer*, **19**, 221

Hutter, R. V., Worcester, J. N. and Francis, K. G. (1962) 'Benign and malignant giant cell tumors of bone', *Cancer*, **15**, 653

Jaffe, H. L. (1956) 'Benign osteoblastoma', *Bulletin of Hospital for Joint Diseases*, **17**, 141

Karam, F. K. and Salman, S. D. (1964) 'Meningioma of the middle ear', *Archives of Otology*, **80**, 177

Kettle, K. (1946) 'Neurinoma of the facial nerve', *Archives of Otolaryngology*, **44**, 253

Kettle, K. (1950) 'Sarcoma of the facial nerve', *Archives of Otolaryngology*, **52**, 778

Kettle, K. (1963) 'Facial nerve surgery', *Archives of Otolaryngology*, **77**, 327

Koch, H. J. and Lewis, J. S. (1956) 'Hyperlipemic xanthomatosis with associated osseous granuloma', *New England Journal of Medicine*, **255**, 387

Kretschman, F. (1886) 'Uber Carcinoma das Schafenbeines' (1886), *Archiv für Ohrenheilkunde*, **24**, 231

Lack, E. E., Cubilla, A. L., Woodruff, J. M. and Farr, H. W. (1977) 'Paragangliomas of the head and neck region, a clinical study of 69 patients', *Cancer*, **39**, 397

Lattes, R. and Waltner, J. G. (1949) 'Non-chromaffin paraganglioma of the middle ear', *Cancer*, **2**, 447

Lederman, M. (1965) 'Malignant tumors of the ear', *Journal of Laryngology and Otology*, **79**, 85

Lichtenstein, L. and Jaffe, L. (1956) 'Osteoblastoma: a category of osteoid and bone forming tumors or osteogenic sarcoma', *Cancer*, **9**, 1044

Lichtenstein, L. (1972) *Bone Tumors*, 4th edn., p. 97. St. Louis; Mosby

Lindahl, J. W. S. (1955) 'Carcinoma of the middle ear and meatus', *Journal of Laryngology*, **69**, 457

Lodge, W. O., Jones, H. W. and Smith, M. N. (1955) 'Malignant tumors of the temporal bone', *Archives of Otolaryngology*, **61**, 535

Marrocco, W. A. (1948) 'Multiple osteoma of the mastoid cavity', *Archives of Otolaryngology*, **47**, 673

Mattick, W. and Mattick, J. (1951) 'Some experience in the management of cancer of the middle ear and mastoid', *Archives of Otolaryngology*, **53**, 610

Mulligan, R. M. (1950) *American Journal of Pathology*, **26**, 680

Myers, E. N. and Stool, S. (1969) 'The temporal bone in osteopetrosis', *Archives of Otolaryngology*, **89**, 460

Naufal, P. E. (1973) 'Primary sarcomas of the temporal bone', *Archives of Otology*, **98**, 44

Newhart, H. (1917) 'Primary carcinoma of the middle ear, report of a case', *Laryngoscope*, **227**, 543

Passe, Garnett (1948) 'Primary carcinoma of the eustachian tube', *Journal of Laryngology and Otology*, **62**, 314

Peale, J. C. and Hauser, C. H. (1941) 'Primary carcinoma of the external auditory canal and middle ear', *Archives of Otolaryngology*, **34**, 254

Politzer, A. (1883) *Textbook of Diseases of the Ear*, p. 729 Trans. and Ed. by Cassells, J. P. Philadelphia; Henry C. Lea's Son & Co.

Potter, G. D. (1966) 'Embryonal rhabdomyosarcoma of the middle ear in children', *Cancer*, **19**, 221

Punt (1965) quoted by Fairman, H. D. In *Diseases of the Ear, Nose and Throat*, Scott Brown, 3rd edn p. 343. London; Butterworths

Robinson, G. A. (1931) 'Malignant tumors of the ear', *Laryngoscope*, **41**, 407

Ronis, M., Oband, M. and Bucko, M. I. *et al.* (1974) 'Benign osteoblastoma of the temporal bone', *Laryngoscope*, **84**, 884

Rosenwasser, H. (1964) 'Carotid body tumor of the middle ear and mastoid', *Archives of Otolaryngology*, **41**, 64

Rosenwasser, H. (1969) 'Giant cell tumor involving the middle ear', *Archives of Otolaryngology*, **96**, 726

Ruben, R. J., Thaler, S. U. and Holzer, N. (1977) 'Radiation induced carcinoma of the temporal bone', *Laryngoscope*, **87**,

Schall, L. A. (1934) 'Neoplasms involving the middle ear', *Archives of Otolaryngology*, **32**, 548

Snyder, G. G. and Mawr, B. (1961) 'Paraganglioma of the middle ear and mastoid', *Archives of Otolaryngology*, **73**, 54

Soderberg, F. (1932) 'Rhabdomyome Epipharynge avant Envahi Procilis et les Meninges', *Acta Otolaryngologica*, **18**, 153

Sylven, B. and Hamberger, C. A. (1944) 'Malignant melanoma of the external ear, 36 cases treated between 1928–1944', *Annals of Otology, Rhinology and Laryngology*, **59**, 631

Tod, in discussion on Whitehead, A. L. (1907–8) 'A case of primary epithelioma of the tympanum following chronic suppurative otitis media', *Proceedings of the Royal Society of Medicine* (Sec. Otol.), **1**, 34

Towson, C. E. and Shoftstall, W. H. (1950) 'Carcinoma of the ear', *Archives of Otolaryngology*, **51**, 724

Winship, T., Klopp, C. T. and Jenkins, W. H. (1948) 'Glomus jugulare tumors', *Cancer*, **1**, 441

Wolfowitz, B. L. and Schmaman, A. (1973) 'Giant cell lesions of the temporal bone, with a case report', *South African Medicine*, **47**, 1397

Yates, E. C. (1936) 'Primary carcinoma of the middle ear', *Kentucky Medical Journal*, **34**, 501

Zeroni (1924) cited by Furstenberg, A. C. 'Primary adenocarcinoma of the middle ear and mastoid', *Annals of Otology, Rhinology and Laryngology*, **33**, 677

Zizmor, J. and Noyek, A. (1969) 'Tumors and other disorders of the temporal bone', *Seminars in Roentgenology*, **4**, 2

14 Diseases of the otic capsule— I. Otosclerosis

Andrew W Morrison

Introduction

Many different diseases of diverse aetiology can affect the bone of the otic or labyrinthine capsule. Most of them are generalized diseases which involve the temporal bones as part of the skeletal system; a few of them, otosclerosis in particular, are confined to the otic capsule. Irrespective of the pathogenesis they have one thing in common, their ability to cause deafness and vestibular symptoms. This chapter will be devoted to otosclerosis, the next to some of the others.

Definition

Otosclerosis is a common hereditary localized disease of the bone derived from the otic capsule. Mature lamellar bone is removed by osteoclasis and replaced by unorganized woven bone of greater thickness, cellularity and vascularity. An otosclerotic focus may cause no symptoms, its presence being detected by post-mortem histological section; it may replace the footplate of the stapes causing progressive osseous ankylosis and conductive deafness; it may involve other parts of the labyrinthine capsule giving rise to sensorineural changes, both cochlear and vestibular; and it may produce a combination of these effects, which are sometimes referred to as 'histological', 'stapedial', 'cochlear' and 'combined' otosclerosis.

History

As early as 1704, Valsalva associated deafness with stapedial fixation, and Toynbee (1861), from his extensive temporal bone dissections, noted the common occurrence of stapedial ankylosis in the fenestra ovalis causing deafness. Magnus (1876) gave an early description of both the macroscopic pathology and the familial pattern. It was Politzer (1894) who introduced the term 'otosclerosis' and gave the first revolutionary account of the histological findings. Later these were confirmed by Siebenmann (1912) who proposed the more accurate pathological term 'otospongiosis', still preferred and used by many European otologists.

It is quite remarkable that, before the end of the nineteeth century the stapes had been approached surgically by Kessel (1878), Boucheron (1888), Miot (1890) and Faraci (1899) with varying manoeuvres to attempt mobilization, and by Blake (1892) and Jack (1893) who both described stapedectomy without stapes replacement. These were voices in the wilderness, but it is not perhaps so surprising that their work was forgotten for 50 years, since the 'best' otological opinion at that time either advised against surgery or failed to recognize the disease. This, after all, was still the era of 'dry catarrh' or 'chronic adhesive catarrh' and the reign of that remarkable instrument, the eustachian catheter.

Although opening of the lateral semicircular canal for otosclerosis was described by Jenkins (1914), Holmgren (1923), Bárány (1924) and Sourdille (1932), the prejudice against surgery was not overcome until Lempert (1938) popularized the one stage fenestration operation, designed to bypass the footplate obstruction by creating a new window in the lateral canal allowing sound waves to enter the cochlea via the canal and vestibule. The operating microscope, first used by Holmgren in 1923, was re-introduced and Lempert's pioneering work was taken up by Shambaugh (1940), Hall (1945), Shambaugh and Juers (1946), House (1948), Passe (1949), Cawthorne (1951) and others, and fenestration techniques were still evolving as late as 1957 (Lempert). During this half century asepsis, chemotherapy and antibiotics had been added to the otologist's armaments.

The second phase in the development of otosclerotic surgery was the revival of permeatal mobilization of the fixed stapes by Rosen (1952, 1953). The operation was seldom effective in restoring hearing for any length of time though, like the fenestration operation, it still has a minor place in otology. Its merits were threefold—it emphasized the concept of respecting normal anatomy and physiology; it introduced the approach, first described by Lempert (1946) which, with minor modifications, forms the basis of today's lateral (permeatal) tympanotomy; and it acted as a stimulus for the development of the modern operating microscope.

With improved vision surgeons became more adventuresome. Footplate surgery was conceived by the anterior crurotomy of Basek and Fowler (1956) and by the partial stapedectomy (with polythene tube from incus to fractured footplate) of House (1959) and Hall (1958) and was finally born when the whole stapes was removed by Shea (1958) and replaced by an oval window graft and polythene strut. Prosthetics had entered the field of reconstructive ear surgery. The eustachian catheter was forgotten.

Pathology

Sites of development

The otic capsule which becomes incorporated in the petrous part of the temporal bone, ossifies in cartilage from 14 or more centres which fuse to form a protective shell for the labyrinth and the maximum size is reached by the fifth month of fetal life

(Anson and Donaldson, 1967). The bone is considered as the hardest in the body and consists of three layers: (a) an *outer periosteal layer* of dense lamellar bone which continues to thicken until adult life; (b) a *middle endochondral layer* which hardly changes from birth to old age, which shows almost no new bone formation unless it be pathological, and which contains a number of fibro-cartilaginous rests; (c) a thin *inner endosteal layer* of lamellar bone which likewise shows little developmental change, and lines the cavities of the labyrinth.

The areas of residual cartilage, described by Bast and Anson (1949), are the acknowledged sites of origin of otosclerotic foci and the most important of these is the very constant fissula ante fenestram, a slit of fibro-cartilage, found only in man, passing through the whole thickness of the otic capsule from the vestibule to the middle ear, anterior to the oval window and posterior to the processus cochleariformis. The other sites of residual cartilage are much less constant though nevertheless

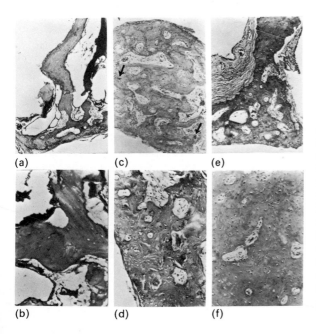

(a)   (c)   (e)

(b)   (d)   (f)

Figure 14.1 Histopathology of otosclerosis: (a) early otosclerosis affecting lamina stapedialis; (b) normal footplate; (c) active otosclerosis—arrows indicate osteoclasts; (d) higher power showing large vascular spaces and increased cellularity; (e) active footplate focus demonstrating classic features, including the thickening; (f) late 'healed' otosclerosis. Mature lamellar bone still very thick and cellular. All footplate biopsies

important in relation to otosclerosis. The fossula post fenestram, structurally similar to the fissula ante fenestram, is situated posterior to the oval window and is present in 67 per cent of ears though it seldom extends through the thickness of the otic capsule to the tympanic cavity. The posterior margin of the cochlear or round window in the region of the cochlear aqueduct is another; also the infracochlear region below the internal auditory meatus; and rarely areas of otic capsule surrounding the semicircular canals.

Otosclerosis can also arise, however, in the footplate of the stapes itself. Strickland, Hanson and Anson (1962) and Hanson, Anson and Strickland (1962) have given an account of ossicular development. The footplate has a dual origin, the lateral or middle-ear aspect together with the head, neck and crura developing from the mesenchyme and cartilage of the dorsal end of the second arch; and the medial or vestibular aspect developing from the cartilage of the otic capsule. This otic capsular area of the footplate is called the lamina stapedialis, and most adult bones have residual cartilage on the vestibular surface. Normally the periphery of this aspect of the footplate differentiates to produce the annular ligament, and failure to do so causes congenital stapedial fixation sometimes encountered alone, sometimes in association with other ossicular abnormalities or with congenital meatal atresia and microtia. In cases of partial differentiation it is usually the posterior part of the footplate which remains ankylosed and this anomaly should not be confused with otosclerosis. *Figure 14.1a* shows a footplate with early otosclerosis still confined to the lamina stapedialis and for comparison a normal footplate (*Figure 14.1b*).

The distribution and relative frequency of foci can be assessed from the temporal bone sections studied by Guild (1944) and Nylén (1949). The following percentages are approximations from both series. By far the commonest site was in relation to the fissula ante fenestram (85 per cent) and about half of these were causing stapedial ankylosis. The next commonest sites were the round window (35 per cent) and the cochlear capsule (35 per cent) followed by the promontory continuous with the oval window (17 per cent), the internal auditory meatus (15 per cent), the footplate of the stapes—primary focus—(7 per cent), and the semicircular canals (7 per cent). Operative experience suggests that primary footplate pathology is more frequent than this, and that round window otosclerosis is much rarer.

Histopathology

Otosclerosis is a pathological enigma, the enigma being the occurrence of apparently normal healthy new bone in a localized area commonly causing conductive and, not infrequently, sensorineural deafness.

The actual light microscopic findings are fairly straightforward, the appearances being those of new bone formation such as might be seen following fractures or in response to infection or other trauma. The mature lamellar bone is removed by histiocytes, in what is sometimes called the active phase of otosclerosis (*Figure 14.1c*) and replaced by immature woven bone of increased thickness, vascularity and cellularity (*Figure 14.1d*). The really prominent features are the large vascular spaces surrounded by more basophilic staining bone and the remarkable cellularity. It used to be thought that osteoclasts were extensively involved in the active resorptive phase.

Histological and electron microscopy studies of the early microfoci by Causse and his colleagues (Bretlau *et al.*, 1971; Chevance *et al.*, 1972) have shown that the histiocytes involved in the early lytic process are rarely osteoclasts. The osteoclasts are abundant in the pseudo-Haversian rebuilding phase.

Frost (1962) has estimated that otosclerotic bone has five times as many osteocytes as lamellar bone. The increased thickness even in the early stages of footplate pathology (*Figure 14.1c*) can be compared with the normal (*Figure 14.1b*). In the histologically quiescent phase there is an attempt at organization into Haversian systems but the bone remains greatly thickened and cellular (*Figure 14.1f*). When involving the stapes the 'healing process' probably increases the ankylosis.

This account gives the impression of an orderly sequence of events, but some otosclerotic foci show all stages of activity in differing areas.

Otosclerotic bone has been grown *in vitro* in tissue culture by Rundle and Lawrence (1961) who found the osteoblasts smaller with nuclei containing denser chromatin, compared with cultured osteoblasts of normal otic capsule. Later, however, Lawrence and Arbor (1965) found no difference in appearance in tissue culture between otosclerotic and normal osteoblasts, though it is interesting to note that their sections of the otosclerotic tissue culture bone still showed all the classic features of the temporal bone pathology including continued osteoclasis. Presumably an abnormal enzyme system persisted in the tissue culture.

Electron microscopy has added little to our knowledge of otosclerosis. Reydon and Smith (1968) thought the dense band in the collagen period was wider than normal, but no alteration in periodicity was found by Young (1966), by Clarke (1969), or by Frank, Klotz and Höhling (1968). The latter workers showed by electron diffraction that crystals in otosclerotic bone were large and atypical and consisted of hydroxyapatite. Clarke (1969) using scanning electron microscopy demonstrated microscopic osteophytes and crystal-like projections on the vestibular surface of the otosclerotic footplates. Chevance *et. al.* (1970) have provided a comprehensive account of the ultrastructure and Schuknecht (1974) a detailed description of the histopathology of otosclerosis.

Since the turn of the century well over 50 theories have been advanced regarding pathogenesis, the most recent being a re-statement of the claim for microscopic areas of avascular necrosis (Wright, 1977). Numerous histochemical and biochemical studies of otosclerotic bone and of various physiological body fluids from otosclerotic patients have been carried out by many investigators, until recently with unrewarding results. Causse *et al.* (1977) have summarized their work on the analysis of some 2000 perilymph specimens, the samples being taken during stapedectomy. They have found higher concentration of the proteolytic enzyme trypsin (derived from the lysosomes) and lower concentrations of alpha-1-antitrypsin. Their results indicate that when the balance of these two enzymes is upset, the disease process is triggered. Their arguments are convincing and will be referred to further below.

Macroscopic pathology

The causation of the conductive deafness is easily understood and accepted. Stapedial ankylosis arises from any focus involving the footplate, annular ligament and adjoining otic capsule. With the passage of time the focus spreads to the crura and gradually obliterates the oval window. At operation otosclerotic 'exostoses' are frequently seen anterior to this area in relation to the fissula ante fenestram occasionally posterior to the oval window but only rarely involving the round window (perhaps 1–2 per cent of cases). Four degrees of stapedial otosclerosis are recognized macroscopically—type 1 is an early lesion, at least half the footplate being thin; in type 2 there is involvement of the whole footplate but it can still be scored, fractured and removed; type 3 shows marked thickening though the diseased footplate can still be visually differentiated from the margins of the oval window niche; type 4 is obliterative, the bone being continuous with the otic capsule and the crura grossly involved.

Table 14.1 shows the footplate pathology encountered in a consecutive sample of 510 personal stapedectomies. The same criteria were used to classify the macroscopic pathology, which is compared with the severity of air conduction deafness in the operated ear. It will be seen that, although all degrees of ankylosis are encountered in the three categories of hearing loss (moderate, severe and subtotal), there is a definite

Table 14.1   Footplate pathology (510 cases)

Type of pathology	Loss < 75 dB Mean 250–4000 Hz (ISO) 320 cases (per cent)	Loss > 75 dB Mean 250–4000 Hz (ISO) 160 cases (per cent)	Subtotal deafness 30 cases (per cent)
1	34	16	7
2	49	38	10
3	15	26	33
4	2	20	50
Total	100	100	100

tendency for a thicker footplate to be associated with greater hearing loss. This association does not necessarily imply a causal relationship as we shall see when describing cochlear otosclerosis.

Table 14.2 compares the types of footplate otosclerosis with the duration of deafness in decades, and, though the correlation is not as obvious as in *Table 14.1* there is a tendency to encounter grosser pathology with longer duration. The rapidity of spread of an otosclerotic focus must influence this and it can vary greatly from patient to patient. It usually follows a slow relentless course which can best be recorded in decades rather than years. The great majority of footplates fall into types 1 and 2, and the inference from *Table 14.2* is that during the first 30 years of deafness only a

Table 14.2   Footplate pathology (510 cases)

Type of pathology	Duration of deafness			
	< 10 years 178 cases (per cent)	11–20 years 148 cases (per cent)	21–30 years 112 cases (per cent)	> 30 years 72 cases (per cent)
1	47	23	21	3
2	46	49	39	26
3	7	18	24	45
4	0	10	16	26
Total	100	100	100	100

minority of patients (23 per cent) develop advanced disease. Gristwood and Venebles (1975) consider that there is a high incidence of obliterative footplate disease in patients from South Australia. Their figures for this stage are 11.9 per cent. The frequency from the figures in *Table 14.1* is 10.4 per cent, not a significant difference. Donaldson (1976), reporting on the experience from St. Thomas's Hospital, classified 6.2 per cent as type 4 footplates, though they classified a relatively higher percentage as type 3. Sometimes progress can be remarkably rapid, and such otosclerotic bone is likely to be more vascular; and if the bone of the promontory is involved, it gives rise to the classic Schwartze sign, a pink tinge of the tympanic membrane on otoscopic examination. At the other pathological extreme 'healing' may occur and the progression halt.

Pathology of cochlear otosclerosis

It has long been recognized that the conductive deafness of otosclerosis can be complicated by a sensorineural loss, sometimes moderate, sometimes severe, occasionally total. The clinical aspects will be described later, but it should be noted now that this is a common phenomenon. Total or subtotal deafness is not a rarity and accounted for 6 per cent of the 510 cases in *Tables 14.1* and *14.2*. It has been considered that this loss was due to obliteration of both round and oval windows and, indeed, this is a very logical explanation which may still appply in some cases. Generalized otosclerosis of the otic capsule might also involve the spiral ganglia or compress the contents of the internal auditory meatus.

Rüedi (1962, 1963) was the first to draw attention to the cochlear pathology in otosclerosis. His observations have now been confirmed by many investigators who have been able to correlate the clinical and subsequent histopathological findings. They include Altmann, Kornfeld and Shea (1966), Schuknecht and Gross (1966), Linthicum (1966), Nager (1966), Lindsay and Beal (1966) Holleman and Harrill (1967), Sando *et al.* (1968) Myers and Myers (1968), Keleman and Linthicum (1969) and Schuknecht (1971, 1974). Sensorineural loss occurs when the otosclerotic focus spreads to involve the inner endosteal layer of the otic capsule adjacent to the spiral ligament. Degenerative changes occur in the spiral ligament, stria vascularis and hair-cells. The process may be localized or spread from the basal towards the apical coil. Loss of spiral ganglion cells supervenes. The changes are usually more marked with increasing age and appear to be unaffected by previous stapes surgery. Secondary labyrinthine hydrops is sometimes observed and even rupture of the saccule or cochlear duct.

There seems to be no doubt that if the lamellar endosteal bone supporting the spiral ligament is replaced by active otosclerotic bone then sensorineural loss supervenes. The explanation of these changes is still uncertain. Anastomotic shunts have been described between the vessels of the spiral ligament and those of the pathological bone. Normally the two circulations are quite separate. These shunts could lead to vascular stasis or abnormal metabolites in the inner-ear fluids or they might alter the electrical potentials. It has also been suggested that the involvement of the spiral ligament has mechanical effects on the cochlear duct. The enzymatic concept proposed by Causse *et al.* (1977) envisages an upset to the normal equilibrium of trypsin/antitrypsin in the inner-ear fluids, disturbing the relative metabolic isolation of the cochlea. The higher ratio of trypsin causes the hair-cell loss and other changes. Certainly their analytical studies show a definite relationship between this enzymatic ratio and the clinical evidence of sensorineural loss in stapedial otosclerosis.

When we consider sensorineural deafness due to cochlear otosclerosis, without stapedial involvement, there is less agreement among the authorities. The strongest advocate for the frequent existence of this entity is Shambaugh (1969), and against it Schuknecht (1971, 1974). Gross (1969), analysing the temporal bones of patients with unexplained sensorineural deafness, has not been convinced that the histological otosclerotic foci seen were of significant incidence or size to explain the inner-ear changes. Schuknecht and Kirchner (1974) came to the same conclusion. However, on the basis of Causse's enzymatic concept, proteolytic enzymes could spread from a focus through the canaliculi to the inner-ear fluids. Given the present state of histopatho-logical and pathogenic knowledge on this subject, uncertainty must exist. Statistical evidence in favour of pure cochlear otosclerosis is presented under 'Genetic Factors and Natural History' below.

Interest in the pathological inner-ear changes has centred on the cochlea, virtually to the exclusion of the vestibular labyrinth. In the fenestration era it was recognized that otosclerotic foci could spread to involve the fenestration site. Wolff and Lempert (1965) reviewed bone biopsies taken from the lateral canal and found definite otosclerosis in 17 per cent and 'incipient' otosclerosis in a further 10 per cent. This is not surprising considering the proximity of the oval window. The occasional finding of labyrinthine hydrops and of degenerative changes in the supporting structure and neuroepithelium of the vestibular labyrinth (Altmann and Kornfeld, 1965; Bretlau and Jørgensen, 1968; Johnsson and Hawkins, 1973) helps to explain the relative frequency and diversity of vestibular symptoms in patients with otosclerosis, whether 'stapedial', 'combined' or 'pure cochlear'. In the latter, of course, the clinical picture would be indistinguishable from idiopathic hydrops or Menière's disease.

Genetic factors and natural history

The natural history will be considered with relevant genetic factors since these are frequently interrelated. The progress of the disease tends to be similar within a sibship, while wide variations occur from one family to another. Larsson (1960), Morrison (1967), Morrison and Bundey (1970) and Gapany-Gapanavičus (1975) have examined these factors in some detail.

Racial distribution and prevalence

Otosclerosis has only been demonstrated in *Homo sapiens* and is predominantly a disease of Caucasoid man, being a very common cause of deafness throughout Europe, the Balkans, the Middle East and the subcontinent of India, together with the Caucasian peoples of North and South America, Australia, New Zealand, South Africa and elsewhere. It also occurs, though less frequently in the negrito peoples of Malaya, New Guinea and the Philippines and in the Japanese, a mixed race of mongol, ainu and negrito blood.

It is relatively rarely found in mongoloid and negroid man, though it is encountered in the Negro population of America and the West Indies, presumably due to hybridization. In this latter group the disease is ten times less frequent than among Caucasians. Causse *et al.* (1977) have suggested that the racial distribution of otosclerosis may be related to inherited deficiency of alpha-1-antitrypsin (AA), a deficiency which is rarely found in mongoloid man. In a sample of their otosclerotic patients they found 27 per cent with serum deficiency of AA. Enzymatic polymorphism, however, is much more complex than this. There are many different phenotypes of AA polymorphism, though it is true that a similarity has been found in black Africans, Asians, Finns, Lapps, Greenland Eskimos and Eastern Island Natives (Fagerhol, 1975), who all have relatively few non-M alleles. Caucasians, on the other hand, have high frequencies of the Pi[s] allele.

Elucidation of the incidence is befogged by the differentiation into 'histological', 'stapedial' and 'cochlear' otosclerosis. In Caucasians, Guild (1944) found post-mortem 'histological' otosclerosis in 38 out of 585 temporal bones (6.5 per cent) and 'stapedial' otosclerosis in 6 out of 585 (1 per cent). 'Cochlear' otosclerosis was not recognized. Schuknecht and Kirchner (1974) found 'histological' otosclerosis in 4.4 per cent of 734 ears from whites, excluding subjects under five years and persons with 'stapedial' otosclerosis.

The prevalence of the 'stapedial' condition has been estimated at about 0.5 per cent by Shambaugh (1949) and by Cawthorne (1955), at 0.3 per cent by Morrison (1967) and by Hall (1974) and at 0.24 per cent by Pearson, Kurland and Cody (1974). It should be emphasized that this means that between 3 and 5 per 1000 of the adult Caucasian population have clinical conductive deafness due to stapedial otosclerosis.

Estimation of the frequency of 'cochlear' otosclerosis is more difficult. Shambaugh (1969) considers that pure sensorineural impairment will prove to be as frequent as stapedial otosclerosis. At first acquaintance this figure seems staggering, but increasing awareness of the entity and of its clinical and radiological manifestations makes the idea more acceptable. If 'histological' otosclerosis occurs in 4.4 per cent to 6.5 per cent (say 5.4 per cent) of adult temporal bones and 'stapedial' otosclerosis in a further 0.24 per cent to 0.5 per cent (say 3.5 per cent), then the 'histological' condition is 15 times more frequent than the 'stapedial' disease. Only 1 in 15 with 'histological' foci would require to develop secondary sensorineural deafness to make the 'cochlear' variant as frequent as the 'stapedial'.

A combination of conductive and senorineural loss in otosclerosis is very common. This has been mentioned in the section on pathology (p. 411). Of the 510 patients shown in *Table 14.2*, 37 per cent had some degree of sensorineural loss and 6 per cent had subtotal deafness. Furthermore the commonest single cause of severe adult deafness (air conduction loss greater than 75 dB for the speech frequencies) is a combined stapedial and cochlear otosclerosis (Morrison, 1969a).

Age of onset

Whether conductive, sensorineural, or combined, the deafness of otosclerosis is essentially a disease of adults. The hearing loss is first noted in 91 per cent of cases between the ages of 15 and 45 years, with the peak in the third decade. In 2 per cent the onset is under 10 years, in 3 per cent between 10 and 15 years, and in 4 per cent over 45 years. The age of onset is the same for males and females.

Sex distribution

It is common clinical knowledge to otologists that otosclerosis is encountered more frequently in females than in males and a sex ratio of about 2 to 1 has been noted by most authorities. These observations, however, relate to out-patients or surgical experience and do not reflect the true sex ratio of the deafness. There are several reasons for this apparent contradiction.

When a large number of otosclerotic families is investigated and all the brothers and sisters of deaf patients, or propositi, are examined it is found that the ratio nears equality (32 per cent of all males and 40 per cent of all females in the sibships). When the propositi are excluded the ratio becomes exactly 1 to 1. Furthermore 'sporadic' cases, with no otosclerosis in other family members, have an equal sex ratio.

It seems that females with otosclerotic deafness are more likely to seek medical advice. Firstly, there are more females in the population under enquiry, especially with increasing age; secondly unilateral otosclerosis or definite asymmetry of deafness is much commoner in males (20 per cent of male cases) than in females (9 per cent of female cases); thirdly, the male working and living in a noisier environment and because of the phenomenon of paracusis is less likely to be aware of his disability; and fourthly, hormonal influences can operate during pregnancy to initiate or increase the hearing loss.

Pregnancy and otosclerosis

In 12 per cent of otosclerotic females who have had one or more pregnancies the hearing loss is first noticed during one pregnancy, and in a further 42 per cent deafness increases during at least one pregnancy. From the prognostic viewpoint, it can be indicated that there is only a 50:50 chance of hearing deteriorating during any given pregnancy, and multiple pregnancies do not appear to increase the risk to hearing.

The initiation of, or increase in deafness is usually noted about term or in the puerperium. In this context it is noteworthy that during pregnancy the raised oestrogens, which cause fragility of the lysosomal membranes with release of enzymes, might initiate or activate the otosclerotic foci. The deafness of otosclerosis can also increase in patients with thyrotoxicosis.

Mode of inheritance

The familial pattern of this common disease has been recognized for about a century, yet the simple mode of inheritance has almost escaped recognition amid the bewildering variety of postulated theories, all striving to adhere to strict mendelian ratios. In the majority of families the evidence in favour of an autosomal dominant inheritance is conclusive. The subject is simplified by considering separately the families with other affected members and the truly sporadic cases.

In two-thirds of patients, upon adequate enquiry, there are secondary cases in the family and the disease can be traced directly or indirectly through two, three or even four generations. If the abnormal gene were always manifest one would expect half the parents, siblings and children to be affected, a quarter of the grandparents, grandchildren, aunts, uncles, nephews and nieces to be deaf and an eighth of the first cousins to be involved. In fact about half their members have clinical otosclerosis as demonstrated in *Table 14.3*; but the other half will carry the abnormal allele and may pass the disease to the next generation. For simple genetic counselling it can be stated that if two otosclerotic parents have issue about half of their children will develop the clinical condition; and if an otosclerotic marries a non-otosclerotic about a quarter of their offspring will become deaf (*Figure 14.2*).

The degree of manifestation varies from family to family, and even this appears to be genetically determined. Some families are encountered with 100 per cent manifestation, the full penetrance giving strict mendelian dominant ratios, while other families show degrees of manifestation of as little as 10 per cent. It is tempting

Table 14.3   Manifestation in otosclerosis

Relationship to propositi	Number affected	Number normal	Total	Expected ratio	Expected affected	Degree of manifestation (per cent)
Parents	64	228	292	1:2	146	43.8
Grandparents	44	361	405	1:4	101.25	43.4
Aunts, uncles, nephews, nieces	100	864	964	1:4	241	41.5
Children	7	19	26	1:2	13	53.8
Cousins	18	355	373	1:8	46.6	38.6
Siblings excluding propositi and sporadic families	75	250	325	1:2	162.5	46.1
Total	308				710.35	43.3

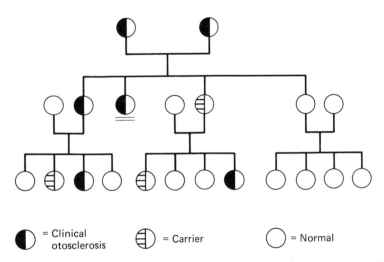

= Clinical otosclerosis   ⊕ = Carrier   ◯ = Normal

Figure 14.2   Inheritance of otosclerosis. Diagrammatic representation of a typical family tree. Dominant inheritance with manifestation of clinical otosclerosis in half the expected ratio. 'Carriers' can transmit the disease

to postulate that 'sporadic' cases are simply a continuation of this process. In any given case a detailed family history is the best guide to prognosis for other family members, and this applies to the natural history as well.

Variable expressivity

Clinical severity must not be confused with manifestation which follows the all-or-none law. Once the gene for otosclerosis is manifest any degree of clinical severity may be encountered. As would be expected with an hereditary disease, the variable expressivity is mainly between and not within families. There is a striking similarity in the age of onset of deafness and rapidity of its progress in any given family—this is especially noted within the sibship, but is less obvious from one generation to the next. Concordance in monozygotic twins has been described by many authors. Familial ipsilateral otosclerosis and familial asymmetry of deafness are other examples of this expressivity.

Cochlear otosclerosis, either without stapedial involvement or with minimal fixation also follows a dominant hereditary pattern. Families are not infrequently encountered having the expected ratio of members with pure sensorineural loss and the rapidity of progress, audiometric pattern and arrest of deafness are often similar in the sibships. Pure cochlear otosclerosis is rarely encountered in families whose other members all have clinical stapedial otosclerosis, yet it does occur in 2 per cent of families investigated. Combined stapedial and cochlear otosclerosis, on the other hand, is a common familial phenomenon.

Progression of deafness

The macroscopic footplate pathology has been compared with the degree of deafness (*Table 14.1*) and with the duration of deafness (*Table 14.2*). There is also a positive correlation between the duration of deafness and the hearing loss (*Figure 14.3*) which provides a clue to the general prognosis of stapedial and combined otosclerosis. There is a slow but relentless progression of hearing loss over the decades, and this applies to both familial and sporadic cases for males and females. The disease may progress more rapidly in females in the first 20 years (Morrison, 1967).

Shambaugh (1963), from his extensive experience, considers that both stapedial and cochlear otosclerosis do not progress inexorably in all cases and this observation

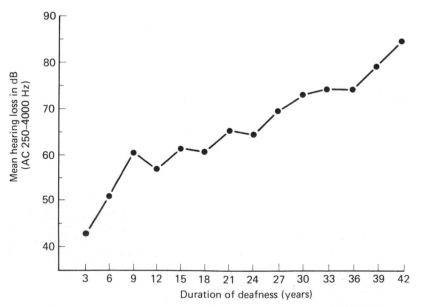

Figure 14.3   Progression of deafness. Graph showing the mean hearing loss in both ears for the speech frequencies against the duration of deafness in years. Data from 510 stapedectomies in 466 patients. Demonstrates relentless progression, best measured in decades

cannot be denied. Of his patients with untreated stapedial disease 96 per cent showed no increase in conductive deafness over 10–23 years, and 27 per cent showed no progression of sensorineural loss but three-quarters did show a progressive sensory deafness.

In many families the progression of deafness is so slow that even two decades is not enough to measure progress. *Figure 14.4* shows the spread of cases presented, in simpler form, in *Figure 14.3*. There can be no doubt that in the great majority of patients the hearing loss increases with the passage of time, and that eventually varying degrees of sensorineural loss supervene. A small percentage (less than 5 per cent) are fortunate

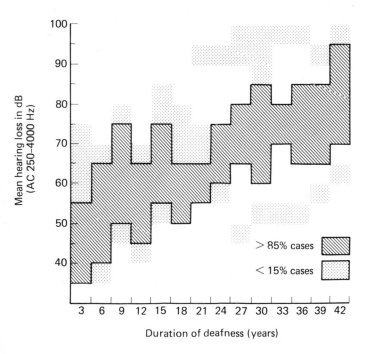

Figure 14.4 Progression of deafness. Mean hearing loss in both ears for the speech frequencies charted against the duration of deafness in years. Data from 510 stapedectomies in 466 patients—85 per cent of cases show steady deterioration over many decades. In 15 per cent progression is either more rapid or halts

in not progressing beyond the 50–60 dB level after four decades, but an equal or greater percentage show what is sometimes referred to as *malignant otosclerosis*. In these cases the onset is usually in adolescence, the progression rapid, the Schwartze sign positive, the sensorineural involvement severe within a few years, and the family history similar. Gristwood (1966) found obliterative footplate disease in the majority of these patients.

Total or subtotal deafness occurs in a fair proportion of patients (*see Table 14.1*), sometimes after many decades, sometimes more rapidly as in malignant otosclerosis and very occasionally quite suddenly. The sudden losses are encountered in cochlear and combined otosclerosis and are presumably due to spontaneous membranous labyrinthine rupture.

Isolated or sporadic otosclerosis

Sporadic cases account for about one-third of patients seen and, without the family history as a guide, the prognosis is more elusive. They show all the features already described. Only after detailed enquiry can otosclerosis be classified as isolated. Not infrequently the existence of other deaf relatives is denied at the first consultation but is subsequently forthcoming, and actual examination of other relatives often reveals unsuspected otosclerosis.

There are a number of explanations for these sporadic cases. The most obvious is a misdiagnosis. Many conditions simulate otosclerosis and this will be discussed under differential diagnosis. A very small number (1 out of 25 sporadic cases) will represent new mutations. The majority of sporadic cases would appear to be isolated because their relatives have only histological otosclerosis. This can be expressed in another way—otosclerosis is not manifest in other family members because of the modifying influence of other genes. Morrison and Bundey (1970) have presented theoretic statistics which explain this relationship to the incidence of histological otosclerosis.

Other genetic factors

There is no evidence of either association or genetic linkage between otosclerosis and the common blood groups, the hair or iris colour, or the common genetic markers. Detailed studies of the relationship with a variety of recently recognized enzymatic polymorphisms are required. Chromosome studies show normal karyotypes. The special relationship with osteogenesis imperfecta will be described later.

Because otosclerosis is a very common condition it is found at times in patients with either common hereditary disorders such as diabetes mellitus and colour blindness and sometimes with rarer alleles such as retinitis pigmentosa or albinism. These associations are quite coincidental.

Clinical features

Some aspects of the clinical features have been described under Pathology (p. 406) and Natural History (p. 412). This basic knowledge of otosclerosis is essential for proper management.

History

A detailed history is the first step in examination, and this should include enquiry into the age of onset of deafness, its rate of progression, the degree of social and occupational handicap, if relevant the influence of pregnancy, the presence or absence of tinnitus or vertigo, and the presence of paracusis. *Paracusis* is the phenomenon of hearing better in the presence of background noise. In this circumstance the conversational voice is raised above the noise level and above the threshold of the patient with conductive deafness. Another indication of conductive loss is frequently obtained during preliminary history taking. The patient often has a quiet voice of good tone which, being transmitted by bone conduction, is subjectively loud enough. If sensorineural loss supervenes, paracusis usually disappears but the relatively quiet voice may persist even in patients with marked combined otosclerosis. Indeed when patients present with subtotal deafness this characteristic speech, if present, can be a most helpful diagnostic feature.

Past history of ear disease, of head or blast injury, of exposure to noise, of ototoxic drugs administered, of bone or joint disease and of previous illnesses may be relevant to the differential diagnosis and for management.

A detailed family history is desirable and invaluable in assessing the prognosis when relatives are affected.

Clinical assessment of deafness

Unless there is concomitant disease, the upper respiratory tract is healthy and the tympanic membranes normal in appearance. The presence of minor atrophic or tympanosclerotic changes, though raising the possibility of alternative diagnoses, does not exclude otosclerosis. The *Schwartze sign*, a pink flush on otoscopic examination, is due to reflection from vascular bone on the promontory. It is seen in about 2 per cent of new cases, usually young adults with widespread active disease, and it carries a poor prognosis.

A quick assessment of hearing loss using conversational and whispered voice, or amplified speech, together with the traditional tuning fork tests give helpful preliminary information on the degree of handicap. In pure stapedial otosclerosis the Rinne test is negative and in unilateral or asymmetrical deafness the Weber is lateralized to the deafer side. The absolute bone conduction test (ABC) is normal. In pure cochlear otosclerosis the Rinne test is positive and the ABC reduced, the Weber being lateralized to the better hearing ear. In combined otosclerosis the Rinne test is negative and the ABC reduced.

Because sophisticated methods of investigation are available, these simpler tests should not be ignored. There are certainly two instances when they are of assistance. The first is the example of predominantly unilateral stapedial otosclerosis with poor bone conduction, simulating sensorineural deafness, when the Weber is referred to the deaf side. The clinician is alerted and further investigation confirms the true nature of the lesion (*Figure 14.5*).

The second example, shown in *Figure 14.6*, is encountered in subtotal combined deafness. Most clinical audiometers in routine use record bone conduction to the 50 or 60 dB level (only a few record up to 80 dD). If the patient's voice has reasonable quality and the Rinne test is negative with the 256 fork, then stapedectomy may be indicated and surprising results can be achieved.

A good case history and clinical examination followed by pure-tone and possibly speech audiometry are normally adequate for diagnostic purposes. Tympanometry is very helpful especially prior to surgery and occasionally the middle-ear muscle reflexes are invaluable. Polytomography is not required in the routine assessment of stapedial otosclerosis though it is sometimes necessary in unilateral disease or in the differential diagnosis, while it is essential in the evaluation of pure cochlear otosclerosis.

Pure-tone audiometry and speech audiometry

One of the classic clinical features of otosclerosis is the symmetry of the hearing loss which is readily demonstrated by pure-tone air and bone conduction audiometry. In

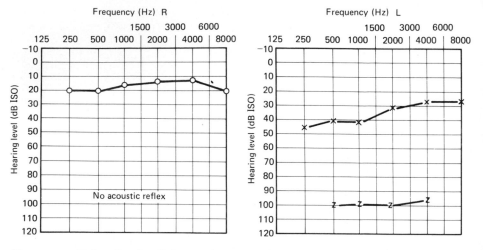

Figure 14.5   Value of tuning-fork tests. A woman of 56 who presented with a five-year history of left tinnitus and hearing loss. Despite the absence of an air–bone gap on either side the Weber was consistently referred to the left. Speech discrimination was 100 per cent on both sides. On the right side the compliance value was 0.36 cm³, on the left 0.25 cm³. The acoustic reflex (Z–Z) could not be elicited by supraliminal stimulation of the right with the probe tone in the left. Polytomography confirmed the diagnosis and showed early promontory irregularity and radiolucency on both sides. She was treated for four months with sodium fluoride 20 mg daily. The hearing has remained unchanged but tinnitus has improved

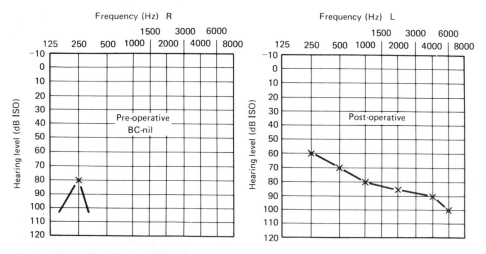

Figure 14.6   Value of tuning-fork tests. Subtotal bilateral deafness due to combined stapedial and cochlear otosclerosis. No recordable BC on audiometry, but definite Rinne negative with 256 and 512 forks. The compliance value in this ear was 0.20 cm³. Polytomography confirmed the diagnosis. Result of stapedectomy indicates the surprising cochlear reserve

early stapes fixation the air conduction graph is flat or gently rising, and in uncomplicated stapedial fixation this pattern persists with increasing ankylosis (*Figure 14.7*). The difference between the air- and bone-conduction levels is called the *air–bone gap*. Speech discrimination remains good.

With the passage of time some sensorineural loss usually supervenes and a wide

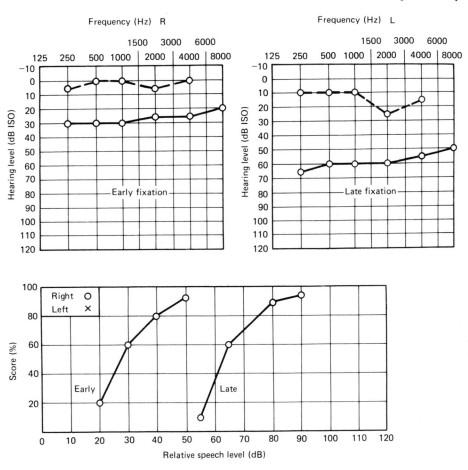

Figure 14.7 Pure stapedial otosclerosis. Pure-tone audiograms giving examples of early and later stapedial fixation. Note the Carhart notch at 2000 Hz on bone conduction. The speech audiogram shows a shift to the right from lowering of the threshold but maintained good discrimination

variety of patterns can result. These are perhaps best seen by considering the types of bone conduction curve encountered, bearing in mind that the air pattern tends to parallel at a lower level.

In a series of 510 cases, the bone conduction was normal in 15 per cent. In 33 per cent there was a Carhart notch at 2000 Hz (Carhart, 1950). A further 6 per cent showed notches at 1000 Hz, at 500 and 2000 Hz or at 1000 and 2000 Hz. In 20 per cent there was a general reduction and about half of these demonstrated notches. A further 20 per cent had loss of bone conduction over 1000 Hz and in patients followed for some years, this could be seen as a progression from a Carhart notch. Finally, in 6 per cent there was either no recordable bone conduction or a reading at only one or two frequencies.

When the mechanisms of bone conduction are not fully understood it is difficult to dogmatize on the aetiology of the Carhart notch. The accepted theory has postulated that some bone conducted sound reaches the cochlea by vibration of the skull, the middle-ear air, the drum and the ossicles. This middle-ear contribution to bone conduction is reduced by the mass of otosclerotic footplate bone giving rise not only to notches but to an overall reduction which simulates sensorineural loss.

This has a practical bearing on otosclerotic surgery for after successful stapedectomy small notches can disappear and there can be a general rise in bone conduction threshold, giving post-operative overclosure of the air–bone gap of the order of 10 dB. Shambaugh (1951), in the fenestration era, described a formula for estimating the cochlear reserve from the corrected bone conduction threshold which can equally be applied today in cases of pure stapedial otosclerosis.

It is evident, however, that the majority of cases with reduced bone conduction have combined otosclerosis. Of the patients in this series, who had good stapedectomy results, only one-third showed a post-operative improvement in bone conduction. The other two-thirds had no change and notches, general reductions or other patterns persisted despite closure of the gap. This is in agreement with Sataloff (1966) who considers that the Carhart notch can arise from a cochlear rather than a mechanical defect.

Associated with the reduction in bone conduction (BC) there is usually a falling off in speech discrimination though it remains fairly good until the BC is very poor. Examples are shown in *Figure 14.8*. Owens, Sooy and Egger (1972) have analysed speech discrimination and bone-conduction thresholds in otosclerosis and related them, in different age groups, to the results of stapedectomy. The falling BC graph carried a poor prognosis for post-operative discrimination even if the air–bone gap was closed by surgery. The question of age will be considered below.

Tympanometry and acoustic reflexes

Any ossicular fixation will reduce tympanic membrane mobility. Visualized through a Siegle's speculum, drum movement in response to positive and negative pressure can be judged by some, but the method is crude and of little scientific or clinical value. The impedance presented by the middle ear to a sound wave of low frequency is determined mainly by the stiffness of the middle-ear system, and the compliance is greatest when the drum is relaxed by equal pressure on its two surfaces. The electro-acoustic bridges are designed to estimate this compliance in cubic centimetres and to give information on middle-ear pressure and acoustic reflexes. The subject is covered more fully in Chapter 1.

Brooks (1969) has defined the normal limits of compliance as from 0.3 to 1.5 cm^3; values below 0.28 cm^3 or above 1.72 cm^3 are considered abnormal. It must be emphasized that the most important single factor in determining compliance is the condition of the tympanic membrane itself. Excessive laxity without ossicular discontinuity or loss can give readings in excess of 1.72 cm^3, while fixation, for example due to tympanosclerosis, can record compliances of less than 0.28 cm^3 even in the presence of ossicular loss.

In otosclerosis the drum is usually normal though minor abnormalities may be detected on otoscopic microscope examination. The middle-ear pressure is normally zero or atmospheric. It will be seen from *Table 14.4* that in otosclerosis a fairly wide range of compliance values is encountered. Despite this spread of data, there is merit in carrying out a tympanogram for two reasons. Firstly if the compliance is greater than 0.6 cm^3 it is highly probable that the footplate of the stapes will be relatively thin

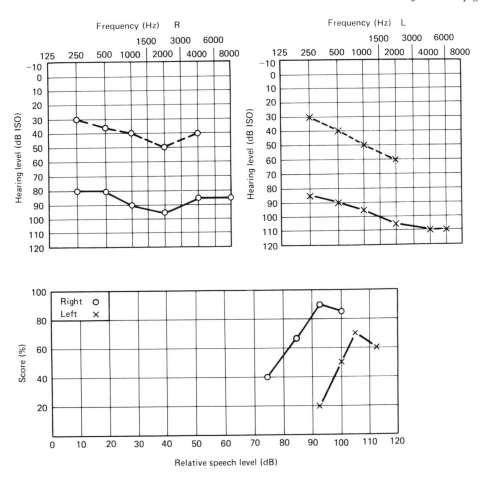

Figure 14.8   Pure-tone and speech audiograms in combined otosclerosis. With the elevation of BC threshold there is some reduction in speech discrimination. The falling BC graph carries a poorer prognosis. When BC becomes worse than shown in this left ear, discrimination deteriorates rapidly

Table 14.4   **Footplate thickness at operation related to pre-operative compliance**

Compliance	Footplate thickness			
(cm³)	*1*	*2*	*3*	*4*
Over 1.0	15	7	1	0
0.8–1.0	9	12	0	0
0.6–0.8	14	9	2	0
0.4–0.6	10	20	5	4
0.2–0.4	9	24	14	10
Below 0.2	2	5	12	8

(Data from 192 Stapedectomies)
Figures are the number of ears in each group

and that surgery will be less complicated, while if the compliance is less than 0.2 cm³ there is a reasonable likelihood of encountering a fairly thick or even obliterated footplate. If hearing loss is symmetrical this information may help select the side for surgery. Furthermore trainee otologists can gain their earlier experience with the less difficult operations.

Secondly the tympanogram is a very useful aid in differentiating some middle-ear problems which can mimic otosclerosis, such as tympanosclerosis, the fixed malleus/incus syndrome, secretory or adhesive otitis or ossicular discontinuity. (Morrison, 1975). In many of these reduced mobility states the middle-ear pressure is on the negative side and the tympanogram may even appear flat.

In stapedial otosclerosis one would normally expect to find absent stapedial or acoustic reflexes in response to supraliminal stimulation. This is indeed so, for as little as 15–25 dB of conductive deafness due to stapedial fixation will result in failure to elicit the reflex. This fact is of inestimable value in detecting the earliest stages of conductive deafness due to the disease (*see Figures 14.5* and *14.9*). There is another merit in attempting to elicit the acoustic reflexes especially in a unilateral lesion; a false Rinne negative is uncovered in seconds.

Polytomography

The radiographic changes of otosclerosis are best demonstrated by hypocycloidal polytomography. Linear tomography is adequate for many purposes but it does not show as much detail of the otic capsule.

The radiological evidence of fenestral otosclerosis has been described by Jensen, Rovsing and Brunner (1966) and by Valvassori (1969). There may be apparent enlargement of the window due to the osteolytic process (*Figure 14.9*) or a nodule of bone in the footplate area (*Figure 14.10*) or varying degrees of narrowing or obliteration of the fenestra (*Figures 14.11, 14.12* and *14.13*). Three variants of capsular otosclerosis are normally recognized: changes limited to the basal coil (*Figures 14.9* and *14.10*), diffuse involvement of the cochlear capsule (*Figure 14.12*) and more widespread changes in the whole labyrinthine capsule (*Figure 14.13*). The first of these is by far the most common. Demineralization of acute otosclerotic bone results in areas of radiolucency while sclerotic changes are seen in areas of thickened lamellar bone. As would be expected from the histopathology, the two are frequently combined in the same ear.

Shambaugh (1971) considers that recalcification of a focus may result in normal radiographic appearances. This, though it may well be so, confuses the diagnostic criteria for pure cochlear otosclerosis, but explains the not infrequent finding of normal x-rays in patients with obvious combined stapedial and cochlear otosclerosis. Naunton and Valvassori (1969), in patients with stapedial or combined otosclerosis, have been able to correlate the bone conduction levels and the evidence of capsular otosclerosis in 74.3 per cent. Gunkovich and Rosenfeld (1974) have been able to make similar correlations in 69.6 per cent.

In summary, positive polytomographic evidence of cochlear otosclerosis, with or without stapedial involvement, can be a helpful diagnostic tool; negative radiological evidence does not exclude the possibility.

Cochlear otosclerosis

Pure cochlear otosclerosis, without stapedial involvement, is a difficult condition to identify. Whereas it has been argued under 'Pathology' that there is statistical evidence to suggest that cochlear otosclerosis should be encountered as frequently as the stapedial variant, clinical experience refutes this. Morrison (1975) presented the clinical features in 50 patients in whom the diagnosis of cochlear otosclerosis had been made; this compared with a personal clinical experience of some 1600 patients with stapedial disease. Three diagnoses of sensorineural cochlear otosclerosis have been' made for every 100 with stapedial involvement. It has also been noted above in the

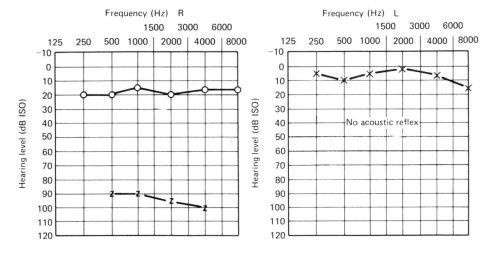

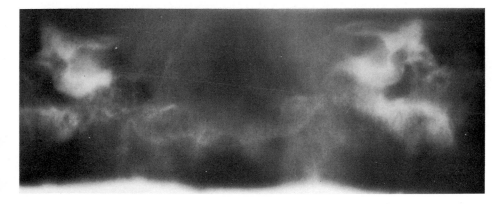

Figure 14.9   A man of 25 who complained only of right tinnitus of 18 months' duration. He had visited many hospitals and had undergone psychiatric treatment to no avail. His hearing was near normal and discrimination 100 per cent. The absent acoustic reflex pointed to the diagnosis which was confirmed by postero–anterior hypocycloidal polytomography. On the left side the oval window margins are sharp and normal and the promontory bone of the basal coil normal; on the right the oval window margin is larger and hazy and there is loss of definition of the basal coil due to the radiolucency. His symptom improved with prolonged fluoride therapy. His main help came from the explanation of his symptom which he learned to tolerate

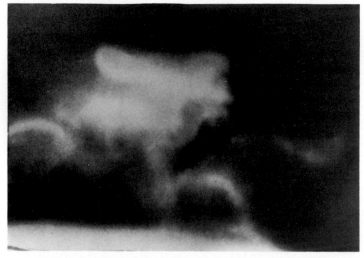

Figure 14.10 Fenestral otosclerosis. Hypocycloidal polytomography, demonstrating the basal coil of the cochlea and the oval window area. The centre of the footplate is occupied by a visible 'nodule' of otosclerotic bone. There is some irregularity and radiolucency of the basal coil. From a woman of 26 with bilateral combined otosclerosis. The poor air–bone gap precluded stapedectomy. She was treated with repeated courses of sodium fluoride. The hearing level has remained stable for the past five years at about the 45-dB level

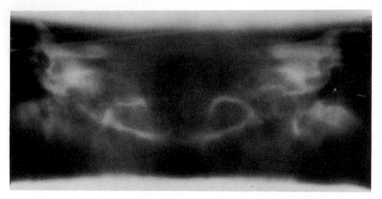

Figure 14.11 Fenestral otosclerosis in a man of 32. Hypocycloidal polytomography demonstrating the basal coil of the cochlea and the oval window area. The margins of the window can be clearly seen in the right ear which had normal hearing though the promontory is suspect. On the left the oval window could not be seen on any of the tomographic cuts, being obliterated by otosclerotic bone, confirmed surgically. Unilateral stapedial otosclerosis is commoner in males

section on Genetic Factors and Natural History that sensorineural deafness presumed due to cochlear otosclerosis was found in only 2 per cent of families with stapedial disease. Daniel (1969), examining the prevalence of stapedial otosclerosis in some areas of the USA with a high fluoride content in the drinking water (1.9 parts/million) and comparing it with the prevalence in low fluoride areas (0.6 parts/million or less), found the incidence of stapedial otosclerosis to be significantly greater (four times) in

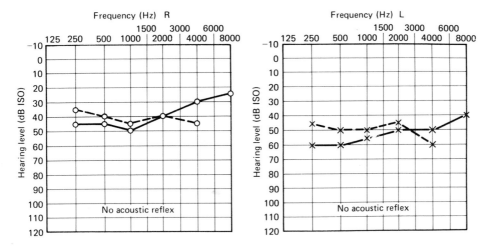

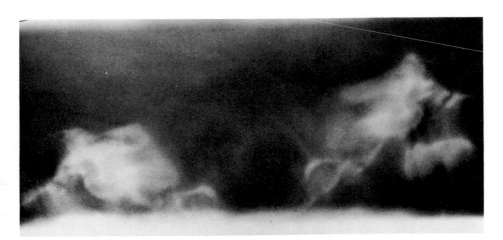

Figure 14.12 Diffuse capsular otosclerosis with stapedial involvement. A woman of 32 with a two-year history of left deafness, tinnitus and transient episodes of positional vertigo. Her father had had a stapedectomy. Note the low-tone deafness with almost no air–bone gap and the absent acoustic reflexes confirming the diagnosis. Compliance was 0.35 cm^3 on each side. Polytomography showed narrowing of the oval window on the right with an adjacent nodular focus of otosclerosis and some irregularity and thickening of the basal coil. On the left the oval window was apparently widened and there was thinning and radiolucency of the basal coil due to active otosclerosis. The hearing loss has stabilized over the past six years with three courses of sodium fluoride 20 mg daily

low fluoride areas, whereas there was no difference in the overall prevalence of hearing loss. This is further statistical evidence to suggest that pure cochlear otosclerosis cannot be a sizeable problem.

Cochlear otosclerosis is characterized by progressive sensory loss, usually bilateral and symmetrical. Progression is normally slow and, as in stapedial disease, may remain stationary for quite long periods of time. The distribution of age onset is similar to stapedial otosclerosis and there is a slight preponderance of females. Some

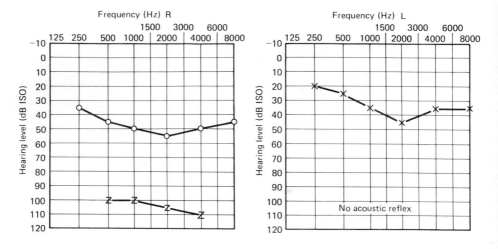

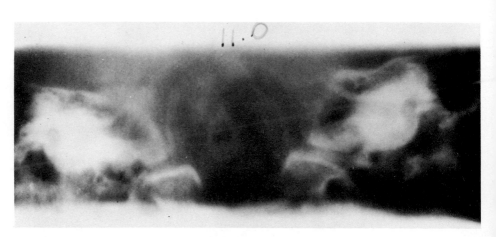

Figure 14.13   Widespread labyrinthine otosclerosis. A woman of 41 with a 25-year history of progressive bilateral deafness and right tinnitus. She had experienced attacks of right positional vertigo for four years. Her father had stapedial otosclerosis. There was a positive Schwartze sign on the right. Note the trough-shaped audiograms, the absent acoustic reflex indicating some stapedial involvement on the right and the present reflex showing no stapedial involvement on the left. There was no air–bone gap. Polytomography confirmed the widespread labryinthine otosclerosis on the right including the stapedial changes. On the left the oval window is clearly defined but the bone of the cochlear capsule is thick and mottled. She was treated with sodium fluoride 20 mg twice daily for six months and the course repeated a year later. Hearing loss has stabilized for the past seven years

aspects of the history and physical findings help to suggest the diagnosis. For example there is usually a dominant family history (70 per cent) and relatives may have proven stapedial disease (12 per cent); the deafness may have started or increased during pregnancy or following the use of oral contraceptives (29 per cent); or there may be a Schwartze sign (8 per cent). The commonest pattern of pure-tone audiogram is a high-tone one, notches and troughs being encountered almost as frequently, flat- or low-tone losses being less frequent. Carhart's (1966) findings are in agreement. Tinnitus and vertiginous symptoms are common (*see below*).

In some cases there is little doubt about the diagnosis, especially when reinforced by the typical polytomographic changes; in others the appearance of the basal coil may be considered within the limits of normal variation (Lloyd, 1973). The clinician is then obliged to base the diagnosis on anamnestic and clinical data, an unsatisfactory state of affairs. While admitting that lack of diagnostic acumen and facilities may be responsible for the difficulty in identifying pure cochlear otosclerosis with greater frequency, one is inclined towards the Schuknecht view that it is a relatively rare otological entity.

Specialized hearing tests

In stapedial otosclerosis the picture is one of conductive deafness. The Békésy is type 1; tone decay is absent or minimal; the speech discrimination score is high (90–100 per cent); the SISI score is low (0–10 per cent); loudness discomfort levels cannot be obtained; and in unilateral deafness there is no recruitment on binaural loudness balance. The stapedial reflex is not elicited.

In pure cochlear otosclerosis the patterns are those of end-organ disease. The Békésy is usually type 2; there is moderate tone decay of up to 20 dB at the frequencies involved; speech discrimination scores of 80–90 per cent are encountered with moderate deafness, of 50–80 per cent with more severe changes and of 0–30 per cent with subtotal loss; the SISI score is high (60–100 per cent); loudness discomfort may be present at 100–110 dB with affected frequencies; and in unilateral cases full recruitment is present. The stapedial reflex is present.

In combined stapedial and cochlear otosclerosis there is, as expected, a combined effect and the results of specialized tests vary with the degree of conductive and sensorineural loss at any given frequency.

Tinnitus

Tinnitus is almost a universal phenomenon and the majority of patients with otosclerosis, on questioning, will admit to occasional subjective tinnitus. It becomes a definite and sometimes very disturbing complaint in about 25 per cent of patients with stapedial otosclerosis and about 50 per cent of those with combined or cochlear disease.

It is encountered especially in the older age group with combined otosclerosis and in those with an early age of onset and cochlear involvement. In pure cochlear otosclerosis and in stapedial otosclerosis arising in pregnancy it can be the presenting symptom. It would appear to be associated with sensorineural loss, though some patients with this complication and quite severe deafness have no complaint of tinnitus. Donaldson (1976) found pre-operative tinnitus in 23 per cent of patients with a type 1 footplate, in 27 per cent of type 2 and in over 40 per cent of types 3 and 4. This confirms the relationship of tinnitus to the extent of fenestral and cochlear involvement.

A good stapedectomy result or the use of a hearing aid, by presenting background masking, usually makes the patient less aware of head noises, but there is no guarantee of this outcome. Failed surgical cases and those with a 'dead ear' usually develop severe tinnitus and depression is not infrequent.

Vertigo

Like subjective tinnitus, transient giddiness is a common experience and it is difficult to know how much significance to place on this symptom in otosclerosis. Cawthorne (1955) found that 25 per cent of cases had momentary dizziness induced by postural change or head movement, though their caloric responses were normal. Fisch (1965) using ENG techniques, demonstrated spontaneous or positional nystagmus in 28.8 per cent of 66 patients pre-operatively, and these cases had poorer cochlear function than the remainder. Shambaugh (1967a) in his text book states 'Endolymphatic hydrops is not uncommon as a complication of advanced cochlear otosclerosis', but he does not indicate its prevalence. Paparella and Chasin (1966) describe a variety of vestibular symptoms in otosclerosis and they rightly argue in favour of a common pathology. Donaldson (1976) found vertigo in 3.9 per cent of their patients.

Excluding vague transient symptoms, definite subjective vertigo was encountered in 6 per cent of the patients with stapedial or combined otosclerosis discussed under 'Pathology', p. 406.

By far the commonest clinical picture was a true benign paroxysmal positional vertigo on lying on one side in bed or on upward gaze and head tilting to one side. This occurred in 4.5 per cent of all cases and, if the symptom was present at the time of examination, objective positional nystagmus showing fatigue could be elicited from one side, usually the side with the poorer hearing and more sensorineural loss. This group tended to have either large notches or loss of bone conduction over 2000 Hz.

The second group of 1.5 per cent had more prolonged symptoms which, on history, could not be differentiated from Menière's disease. A few had episodes of vestibular failure lasting longer than one would expect with labyrinthine hydrops. In this small group the hearing losses were more variable, though they tended to be severe. The therapeutic implications are discussed below.

Transient episodes of vertigo, often positional, occur in 20 per cent of patients with pure cochlear otosclerosis, while the symptoms of hydrops are found in 6 per cent. Disease of the otic capsule should be kept in mind when the patient has sensory or sensorineural deafness and symptoms of Menière's disease. This subject is more fully covered in the next chapter.

Sudden and fluctuant hearing loss

In stapedial otosclerosis the hearing loss is normally slowly progressive. Fluctuant deafness, though rare, can occur when there is cochlear involvement and especially so in those patients with secondary endolymphatic hydrops. An example is shown in *Figure 14.14*.

Sudden total or subtotal deafness is an even rarer natural phenomenon in otosclerosis. It is due to rupture of the saccule or cochlear duct adjacent to an area of endosteal disease. Schuknecht (1971) shows a perfect example of this.

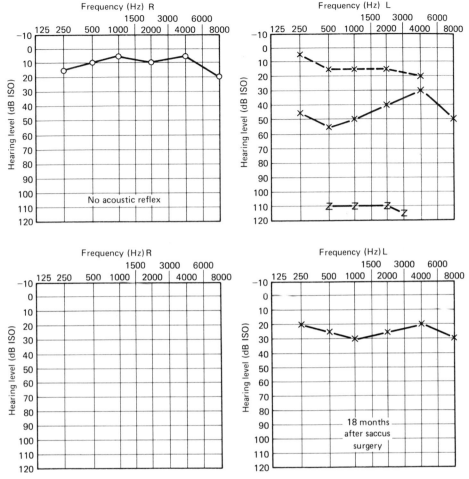

Figure 14.14 Combined otosclerosis with secondary hydrops. A woman of 58 who presented with a five-year history of left deafness and tinnitus and attacks of paroxysmal vertigo. She had been thought to have classic Menière's disease. The audiogram and acoustic reflexes were typical of unilateral otosclerosis (above). Left fenestral and capsular otosclerosis was confirmed on polytomography. There was directional preponderance of caloric induced nystagmus to the right. She was treated with sodium fluoride for three months. Hearing improved by 10 dB in the low frequencies and vertigo settled. A few months later there was a relapse which responded for a few hours to glycerol dehydration. A left saccus drainage operation was then performed. The patient has remained well for 18 months and the hearing loss has improved (lower audiogram)

Differential diagnosis

Otosclerosis, with its varied clinical and pathological manifestations, can mimic a remarkable number of diseases causing both conductive and sensorineural deafness. It is important to make the correct diagnosis pre-operatively since the surgical management of these conditions is frequently different; indeed there are circumstances when stapedectomy is strongly contraindicated. The subject is best considered under four groupings—other causes of ossicular immobility, ossicular discontinuity, some bone disorders, and the differential diagnosis of cochlear and severe combined otosclerosis. Reference should be made to the appropriate chapters for fuller descriptions of these conditions.

OSSICULAR IMMOBILITY

In isolated congenital ossicular fixations, without meatal atresia, the deafness dates from birth, bilateral cases having retarded speech. Unilateral cases are usually diagnosed in later childhood or even adolescence. Unlike adolescent otosclerosis they are non-progressive but the pure-tone audiogram can be identical, including the Carhart notch. By far the commonest is congenital footplate fixation mentioned under 'Pathology of Otosclerosis'. An example is shown in *Figure 14.15*. It is important to recognize the entity as stapedectomy should be avoided if possible due to the high risk of sensorineural loss and perilymph flooding (Morrison, 1971). Footplate mobilization is the treatment of choice and even fenestration may be preferred to stapedectomy. Congenital fixation of the malleus–incus complex is much less frequent.

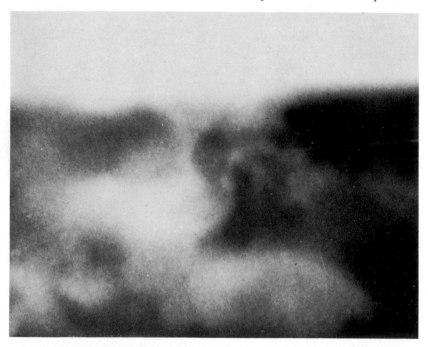

Figure 14.15   Congenital stapes fixation. Hypocycloidal polytomography showing the basal coil and footplate area. The oval window is filled with bone thick enough to be seen on tomography. The stapes arch (never normally seen) is abnormal and readily visualized. The patient was an adolescent male with a conductive deafness of 65 dB, recently noticed. Surgery was not advised.

Ossicular fixations due to past disease can take several forms. The fixed malleus head can usually be diagnosed before surgery from a history of past disease, asymmetry of deafness, and visible attic scarring or a small retraction pocket in this site. Out-patient examination with the operating microscope is invaluable in demonstrating some of these minor changes. At times the drum appears quite normal but there may be evidence of past disease on the other side. Goodhill (1966) described the *fixed malleus syndrome* and Morrison (1969b) found it in 2 per cent of tympanotomies. The stapes should not be damaged since treatment consists of removal of the incus and malleus head followed by incus transposition.

Resulting from past otitis media there can be fibrous or *fibro-osseous footplate fixation*. In these cases, which usually show obvious tympanic membrane changes, footplate mobilization is sometimes feasible for there is less likelihood of re-ankylosis than in otosclerosis. If necessary stapedectomy will give good results provided the malleus–incus complex is fully mobile or can be made so. *Tympanosclerosis* is usually fairly obvious. On otoscopic examination the drum is opaque and white plaques are visible. The tympanosclerotic tissue can affect not only the medial surface of the drum and the promontory but surround and immobilize any or all of the ossicles. This abnormal tissue can be dissected out but it may involve intact canal wall techniques and the stapes should be preserved with great care. Another variant resulting from past suppuration is *chronic adhesive otitis*. The drum can look surprisingly normal. There is not only tympanosclerosis but dense fibrous adhesions which make identification of landmarks impossible. Some of these ears defy surgical correction, and the less experienced should hesitate before embarking on a possible stapedectomy in patients with a past history of suppuration and visible tympanic membrane abnormalities. In all these other forms of ossicular fixation, the tympanogram is abnormal.

Before leaving the sequelae of suppuration, another warning note is necessary. Patients are often seen with bilateral conductive deafness, one tympanic membrane looking normal or nearly so, the other showing a dry central perforation. A diagnosis of otosclerosis plus chronic perforation is made. The statistical chances of this dual pathology are about 5/million of the adult population. The stapes can indeed be fixed as can other parts of the chain but it is better to assume that the ankylosis is not due to otosclerosis. Myringoplasty is permissible. A staged stapedectomy carries a 50 per cent risk to the inner ear (Morrison, 1975).

Chronic secretory otitis media may look very like otosclerosis and upper tone loss of air and bone conduction is often present in long-standing cases. Microscope examination can reveal minor changes in drum translucency and radiology will demonstrate cloudiness of the mastoid cells and the middle-ear cleft. The tympanogram is typical.

OSSICULAR DISCONTINUITY

A history of deafness, usually unilateral, following head injury or previous cortical mastoidectomy, should indicate the possibility of *ossicular dislocation*. A variety of lesions can result but dislocation of the incus is the most frequent. If the stapes has been involved there may be perilymph leak and progressive sensorineural loss superimposed on the conductive loss. It is important to recognize this rare trauma because surgery is urgent.

In *congenital ossicular absence* there are also a variety of lesions. Absence of the stapes superstructure with or without the long process of the incus is the commonest. Polytomography may demonstrate ossicular absence or dislocation or reveal fracture lines, but radiology is often disappointing. An incus need only be dislocated 1–2 mm to cause marked deafness. An intact scarred drum is quite frequently found with *post-inflammatory loss of the long process of the incus*. Other sequelae of old suppuration can co-exist.

Higher than normal compliance values are obtained on acoustic impedance measurements in all these ossicular discontinuities, provided the drum is not sclerotic.

BONE DISEASES SIMULATING OTOSCLEROSIS

Some of the bone diseases which involve the otic capsule can be confused with otosclerosis. They are described in the next chapter.

The deafness, blue sclerotics and brittle bones triad of van der Hoeve and de Kleyn (osteogenesis imperfecta), has some similarities. Stapedectomy does have a place in the management but should be delayed until a long time has elapsed from the active stage. Paget's disease of bone, or osteitis deformans, can produce deafness and vestibular symptoms very like otosclerosis. It should be suspected in patients when the age of onset is over 50 years. Surgery is sometimes indicated but not stapedectomy. In both conditions the hearing loss may be conductive, sensorineural or more often a mixture of the two.

The other diseases of the labyrinthine capsule cause sensorineural deafness and vestibular lesions (*see* Chapter 15).

SENSORINEURAL DEAFNESS

The differentiation of pure cochlear otosclerosis from the dominant hereditary deafnesses which present in adult life can be difficult. In the absence of a Schwartze sign, or a family history of stapedial otosclerosis, or definite polytomographic evidence of capsular otosclerosis, it must be assumed that a progressive sensorineural hearing loss is due to one of the dominant inner-ear diseases. Some of these are very rare such as Alport's syndrome, the Flynn–Aird syndrome or Norrie's disease. In a few families the deafness of retinitis pigmentosa presents in adolescence or early adult life. These classified variants should present little diagnostic difficulty. Nor should there be problems about excluding those patients with either osteitis deformans or osteogenesis imperfecta who have sensorineural rather than conductive deafness.

Most of the unclassified (i.e. no described syndrome, with deafness the only manifestation) sensorineural hearing losses have a dominant inheritance. As with the majority of non-fatal dominant diseases, the degree of manifestation varies from family to family. In some pedigrees the full 50 per cent of individuals are affected, while in others the figure may be as low as 10–20 per cent. There is, however, a striking similarity in the clinical features within any given family. This applies to the age of onset, the pattern of pure-tone hearing loss, the rapidity of progression, the ultimate severity and the age at which the progress halts. Occasionally the lesion is right or left sided in the family.

Middle frequency losses occur in about 50 per cent of these dominant cases, flat audiograms are seen in about 20 per cent, and low frequency or high-tone notches are encountered in about 10 per cent. These variants carry a relatively good prognosis in so far as the loss seldom exceeds 70 dB, remains sensory and discrimination continues to be fairly good. Tinnitus and vertigo are not a problem. In approximately 20 per cent of these families the prognosis is not so good; the hearing loss is high tone with evidence of secondary neural degeneration after a period of some years. In this latter group tinnitus is often troublesome and a few develop vestibular changes on one or both sides. Konigsmark (1969) has drawn attention to the importance and prevalence of these hereditary forms of adult deafness which are much more likely to be encountered than pure cochlear otosclerosis.

Severe combined otosclerosis resulting in total or subtotal hearing loss has to be differentiated from a number of diseases which start in adult life and which have a similar end-result for hearing. These include late syphilis of the temporal bone, unrecognized ototoxicity, Menière's disease if there are infrequent vertiginous episodes, neurofibromatosis, a few of the progressive hereditary diseases, and a number of rarities.

Treatment

Fortunately the great majority of patients with otosclerotic deafness can be assisted by either surgical or non-surgical methods, and even those with total or subtotal deafness can be given some support and guidance, and a little hope for the future.

Medical treatment

FLUORIDES IN TREATMENT

Any treatment which can arrest the progression of deafness in cochlear or combined otosclerosis must be given serious consideration. Even those who deny the existence of the pure cochlear disease admit to the frequency and severity of the combined variety. It is one of the common causes of profound adult deafness (Morrison, 1969a).

The rational basis for fluoride therapy is threefold. We have already noted Daniel's (1969) finding of a fourfold frequency of stapedial otosclerosis in low-fluoride drinking water areas compared with high-fluoride areas. The second basis comes from the experimental work of Shambaugh and his associates (Shambaugh and Petrovic, 1967; Shambaugh, 1971). Their work on the remodelling cycle in young rat bones showed that sodium fluoride in optimum dosage promoted new bone formation and had an inhibiting effect on bone resorption.

The third rationale follows the reports of change in the clinical and radiological state in patients with cochlear or combined otosclerosis following fluoride therapy. These include Shambaugh and Scott, 1964; Shambaugh, 1966, 1967a, 1971; Linthicum, House and Althus, 1973; Kovács and Gömböri, 1973; Shambaugh and Causse, 1974; and Morrison, 1975.

The Chicago experience now spans over 12 years of fluoride treatment to over 2000 patients, and Causse in France has treated a similar number of patients. Despite the long natural history of this disease some meaningful figures are beginning to emerge.

At first Shambaugh's philosophy was to use sodium fluoride 40–60 mg daily in patients with stapedial otosclerosis and a Schwartze sign. Following the development of polytomography with visualization of the otic capsule, evidence of capsular disease whether alone or combined was taken as an indication for therapy. Progression of the cochlear component of the hearing loss was also used as a criterion especially by the French group. Efforts were made to achieve radiological improvement in mineralization of the otic capsule and to this end 40–60 mg sodium fluoride (sometimes higher doses) were administered daily for 1–2 years. X-ray improvements were reported in 23.5 per cent, no change was noted in 71 per cent and deterioration seen in 5.5 per cent.

Of over 4000 patients treated between Chicago and Beziers, only a handful have experienced some recovery of the sensorineural component of the hearing loss, but it has stabilized in 80 per cent. In about 20 per cent the sensory loss has progressed. In a much smaller control group, however, progression of sensorineural deafness was noted in a much higher percentage. Among those who stabilized on fluorides were some who relapsed 2–7 years later. Daily maintenance therapy of 20 mg is now advised in these patients.

Shambaugh's current practice is to prescribe calcium gluconate 0.5 g and vitamin D 400 units thrice daily before meals, together with enteric-coated sodium fluoride 20 mg twice or thrice daily after meals. Therapy is continued for two years and four years if necessary. A skeletal survey for evidence of fluorosis is conducted every two years.

The Los Angeles group advises 25 mg of sodium fluoride daily and claim arrest of hearing loss in a small number of patients with cochlear otosclerosis followed for a few years. Morrison (1975), using 20–60 mg sodium fluoride daily, reported the results of a double-blind trial in 40 patients with cochlear otosclerosis followed from 2–5 years. The treated group were statistically better than the control group with a probability of 0.02. The hearing gains, however, were only of the order of 15 dB at three or more frequencies. The present practice is to prescribe 20 mg once daily after meals for three months and to repeat the course of therapy as indicated at yearly intervals; this is used for cochlear and combined otosclerosis and for stapedial disease when surgery is not indicated.

In the present state of our knowledge it seems that sodium fluoride therapy has a place in the management of otosclerosis. The indications might be summarized as follows.

(1) Pure cochlear otosclerosis when confirmed by clinical, anamnestic *and* polyto-mographic evidence.
(2) Stapedial otosclerosis, without sensorineural loss, when surgery is not indicated or is refused.
(3) Combined otosclerosis, whether evidenced as a poor or falling bone conduction level, as a positive Schwartze sign or as secondary hydrops, with or without radiological evidence. These situations can be encountered both before and after surgery.

OTHER NON-SURGICAL MEASURES

The use of a transistorized hearing aid with an insert air conduction receiver gives excellent results in most patients with deafness, whether stapedial, cochlear or combined. Speech discrimination scores are often high and even patients with moderate sensorineural loss obtain considerable benefit. Rarely in conductive deafness due to otosclerosis better discrimination is achieved with a bone conductor aid, and such aids are sometimes required in the presence of bilateral fenestration cavities. Hearing aids should be advised when surgery is awaited, refused or contraindicated (*see below*). Insert hearing aids are indicated post-operatively in a group of patients with combined otosclerosis when stapedectomy can produce only a moderate threshold improvement. Three aspects of prescribing or advising a hearing aid should not be forgotten—their use does not prevent the natural progression of the deafness; in more severe deafness the amplification required can cause discomfort and, perhaps the main reason for surgery—the deaf prefer 'natural' hearing to the use of an aid.

When hearing aids are used, auditory training and rehabilitation are very helpful. Patients with severe to total deafness and those with a poor prognosis should be advised to have lip-reading instruction. Binaural aids can improve discrimination.

High-powered bone conductors or vibrotactile devices, with appropriate training, may assist the profoundly deaf by providing additional cues to lip-reading.

Advanced cases often have troublesome tinnitus and depression. They all require sympathy and understanding, many need antidepressive therapy and some the guidance of a social worker.

Surgical treatment

In the past few years attitudes to stapedectomy have (or should have) changed in several ways. It is now recognized that violation of the oval window carries a definite risk to the inner ear and that opening the vestibule should not be undertaken lightly.

In the early stapedectomy area—the 1960s—thousands of patients presented themselves as potential candidates for this new and highly rewarding surgery. Problems, of course, were encountered from the earliest days; with the passage of time the frequency and sometimes severity of these iatrogenic disorders began to appear in otological clinics and later in the literature. At least to most otologists the days of the 96–98 per cent success rate are long since gone and many never claimed such results.

An examination of failure rates and of the causes of failure is a healthy sign for the future, and a constant reminder that a realistic prognosis should be presented to each patient who, on medical and otological grounds is a suitable subject for such surgery. The patient must make the final decision.

The diminished number of patients now seeking or referred for stapedial surgery has resulted in less opportunity for the trainee to become familiar with this form of micro-surgery. Medico–legal consequences can flow from complications which, at one time, were more readily defensible.

In recent years, at least in Great Britain, a fair percentage of the patients now seeking advice belong to a younger age group and have less severe hearing losses than their counterparts of the 1960s. There are now more opportunities to observe the progress of the disease, to evaluate the results of fluoride therapy, to assess the response to hearing-aid rehabilitation and, in carefully selected patients, to attempt the less invasive mobilization techniques. With few exceptions the first stapedectomy should also be the last; the individual patient's disability should be bad enough to warrant the risks of surgery.

CONTRAINDICATIONS TO STAPEDECTOMY

The following list of contraindications may be helpful by including guidelines on the preferred lines of management.

(1) Stapedectomy is contraindicated by *general medical diseases* when the patient is unfit for surgery or where expectations of life is limited. Local anaesthesia may widen the scope for surgery in the former situation.

(2) At one time *old age*, in itself, was not considered a definite contraindication. Common sense dictated that the elderly were best advised to rely on hearing aids, even though excellent stapedectomy results had been reported in octogenarians.

In a significant contribution from Owens, Sooy and Egger (1972), the authors have compared pre- and post-operative speech discrimination in different age groups. It should be emphasized that these calculations were all made on 'good' stapedectomy results with 'closure' within 20 dB or better of the air–bone gap. Under the age of 60, 3.5 per cent of patients showed some reduction in discrimination, while over the age of 60, 22.4 per cent had a poorer post-operative discrimination. Their figures show that over the age of 70 there is a 40 per cent chance of discrimination becoming worse, and between 60–70 age groups a 20 per cent chance of deterioration.

The problem of perilymph fistula will be examined later. Morrison (1975) found the mean age of 14 patients with early fistula, dating from the time of surgery, to be 56 years (range 30–81 years), while the mean age of 24 patients with late developing fistula was 38 years (range 25–62 years). It seems likely that the risk of primary fistula formation from failure of the oval window to seal off properly is greater over the age of 55 years.

In the light of these two sets of statistical data, one can argue strongly against stapedectomy over the age of 55–60 years.

(3) Stapedectomy should never be performed in *children*; even if the fixation is thought to be due to otosclerosis. The diagnosis is likely to be congenital fixation. Bilateral cases should be fitted with hearing aids at least until adolescence. Polytomography can assist in assessing the severity of the problem. If there is total undifferentiation of the oval window, lateral canal fenestration may be considered. An x-ray showing abnormal development of the vestibule, cochlear duct or internal auditory canal is a contraindication to any surgery. If the stapes footplate looks thin on tomography and if compliance values are not too low on tympanometry, then stapes mobilization may be effective. In congenital fixation the risk of post-stapedectomy sensorineural loss is high especially if pre-operative bone conduction levels are lowered.

These remarks apply to isolated congenital lesions of the stapes. The broader topic of congenital malformations of the ear is covered in Chapter 6.

(4) The stapes should never be damaged if the conductive loss is due to *other ossicular lesions*, such as the fixed malleus or incus, incus dislocation or erosion. The place of stapedectomy in the management of post-inflammatory and tympanosclerotic stapes fixation is more difficult to define. It is sometimes permissible to mobilize the stapes or its footplate during tympanoplastic surgery, but even this carries a risk to the inner ear. Staged stapedectomy for 'chronic ear disease' or its sequelae is sometimes employed. While emphasizing that this should not be undertaken lightly, Paparella and Jurgens (1972) report acceptable results, though Morrison (1975), with poor late results argues in favour of fitting a hearing aid even if the primary surgery has resulted in an intact ear.

Patients are occasionally encountered with bilateral stapedial otosclerosis and *poor eustachian tube function* in one ear. This malfunction is detected only by tympanometry which reveals a persistent negative middle-ear pressure on one side. In this situation it is advisable to operate on the ear with the atmospheric middle-ear pressure rather than the poorer hearing ear, assuming hearing loss to be nearly symmetrical.

(5) Stapedectomy has little or no place in treating the deafness of *Paget's disease of bone*—ossicular mobilization or reconstruction is preferred. In osteogenesis imperfecta stapedectomy is indicated only after a considerable interval from the last fracture.

(6) *Other local pathologies* may exclude stapedectomy. It should not be carried out in the presence of external otitis, and the vestibule should never be opened or the footplate damaged during myringoplasty. Concomitant external canal exostoses may require a first stage operation, though if the exostoses are small it is possible to proceed to stapedectomy.

(7) Stapedectomy is not necessary in *early fixation* when the hearing loss is, say, less than 40 dB and the handicap is minimal. The position can be reviewed from time to time. Some otologists would advise mobilization in such cases arguing that this degree of pathology is likely to be amenable to the conservative operation. Re-ankylosis will occur with the passage of time, possibly making the subsequent stapedectomy more difficult; and if the arch is fractured during mobilization, premature stapedectomy becomes necessary. Each case must be judged separately, but there is a place for mobilization in such circumstances. (*Figure 14.16*)

(8) On the same basis, i.e. minimal handicap, it can be argued that there is little place for surgery in unilateral or predominantly *unilateral otoscleroris*. Many patients find unilateral deafness a great social or even occupational handicap and binaural hearing has the advantages of better speech discrimination and sound localization. If the patient complains of the hearing loss then surgery should not necessarily be refused, provided there is good speech discrimination pre-operatively.

(9) Stapedectomy should never be carried out on the patient's *only hearing ear*, for no technique, even mobilization, is free from the small but definite risk of immediate or delayed sensorineural loss or 'dead ear'. In severe combined otosclerosis of longstanding one ear may be 'dead' from gradual or sudden spontaneous loss, or as a result of previous surgery; for years the patient has been helped by an aid on the other side. The time can come when the only hearing ear is of no value with the best available aid and, ironically, in this circumstance stapedectomy is sometimes worth considering.

(10) In *combined stapedial and cochlear otosclerosis* when there is a poor air–bone gap (taking into account the possible 10 dB of cochlear reserve) stapedectomy is contraindicated. Such patients should be treated with fluorides.

  If the hearing loss is moderate (say less than 50 dB), if compliance is over 0.8 cm^3 (*see Table 14.4*), and if polytomography shows a good oval window then mobilization may have a place. In patients with subtotal deafness due to severe combined otosclerosis the sort of result shown in *Figure 14.6* is exceptional. Nevertheless, for those involved in experimental cochlear implantation in such patients, it raises the issue of a preliminary trial stapedectomy. Morrison (1969a) reported four such results from 21 operations for subtotal deafness and more recently Sellers (1972) has achieved similar results in two out of ten cases. If stapedectomy is considered in these patients, they must be given a realistic prognosis.

(11) When there is *vertigo* and clinical evidence of *labyrinthine hydrops* as part of the picture of combined otosclerosis, stapedectomy should not be carried out for fear of a 'dead ear'. Since the saccule may be distended and impinging on the footplate, it is likely to be damaged during dissection. The correct management is fluoride therapy and endolymphatic sac surgery. If vertigo remains controlled, stapedectomy can be performed as a second stage procedure. Gristwood (1972)

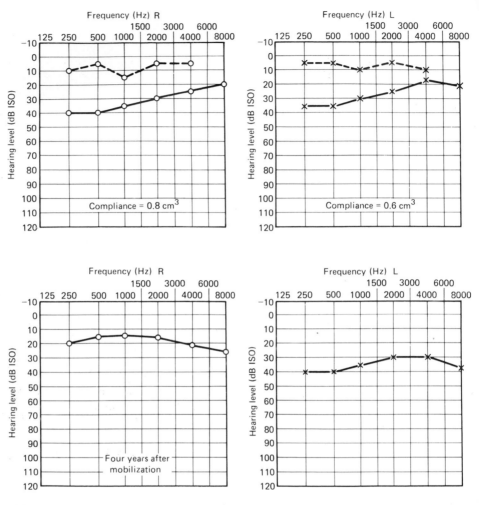

Figure 14.16   Mobilization for stapedial otosclerosis. The patient was a young cardiologist who could not adjust to an amplified stethoscope. Stapedectomy was not indicated with this degree of hearing loss. Fluorides did not alter the thresholds. For otosclerosis, compliance was high especially on the right and on polytomography the oval window looked normal. Mobilization was easily effected and so far there is no evidence of refixation.

reports successful stapedectomy following preliminary saccus decompression. The author now has experience of five such cases without injury to the inner ear.

These remarks do not apply to the commoner picture of benign positional vertigo in otosclerosis. Then it is usually better to perform stapedectomy on the affected side and at least half the cases have post-operative freedom from vertigo.

(12) *Revision stapedectomies* will be considered later, but it is very inadvisable to reopen the vestibule for the same reason. Fine adhesions often exist, following the original operation, between the footplate area and the saccule or cochlear duct. Reclosure of the oval window by otosclerosis is best treated by considering fenestration, or stapedectomy on the other ear after an appropriate interval, and provided the original side has adequate speech discrimination.

(13) Many arguments can be put for and against *operation on the second ear*. Sensorineural losses are encountered as late as five to ten years after stapedectomy and, as a general guide, a five-year interval seems reasonable. The 510 operations described under 'Pathology of Otosclerosis' have been followed for a minimum of three years and a maximum of 18 years. In the early years 15 per cent had bilateral operations and in the later phase less than 5 per cent. In the past seven years the author has rarely operated on a second ear (less than 1 per cent of cases). Though stapedectomy techniques are becoming standardized, some evolution is still taking place and there is no urgency about operating on the second ear.

(14) Several references have already been made to the young adult with rapidly spreading stapedial and cochlear otosclerosis, a *positive Schwartze sign*, and a poor prognosis. Stapedectomy is often difficult due to spongy vascular bone, and refixation is more likely to occur. There is much to be said for delaying surgery until the footplate focus matures (polytomography can help in the assessment), with the aid of fluoride therapy.

(15) There is no indication for stapedectomy *during pregnancy*. In some pregnant women who have increased deafness and tinnitus, there is a Schwartze sign and notches suggesting early cochlear otosclerosis. It is advisable to wait 6–12 months after parturition. Fluorides should not be given during pregnancy.

(16) It may be inadvisable to perform stapedectomy on professional sportsmen or women or on those whose occupations involve considerable physical strain. Flyers may be included in this category. The risks of perilymph fistula are almost certainly higher in these groups. Surgery can be postponed.

INDICATIONS FOR SURGERY

Despite this formidable list of contraindications the great majority of patients with conductive deafness due to *stapedial otosclerosis* are suitable for stapes surgery and normally the poorer hearing ear is selected. *Stapedectomy* is the treatment of choice. There should be an adequate air–bone gap and a good cochlear reserve. One of the main indications for stapedectomy as opposed to the use of a hearing aid (which gives excellent results in otosclerosis) is the patient's desire for 'normal' rather than artificially amplified hearing. The otological surgeon however, must not be talked into surgery, if there are contraindications, even if the patient is 'willing to take a risk'.

The commonest traumatic ossicular lesion is dislocation of the incus, but *fracture of the stapes* is not uncommon (*see* Chapter 7). If the fracture involves the arch, replacement may be effected by a wire or piston prosthesis to the mobile footplate. If the fracture involves the footplate or if the footplate is dislocated with perilymph leakage, *stapedectomy* may be the most effective way of sealing the leak and achieving some hearing gain.

There is a limited but definite place for *stapes mobilization* in the surgical management of stapedial or combined otosclerosis. This has been discussed above.

The indications for *primary saccus surgery* in otosclerosis with secondary endolymphatic hydrops have also been mentioned.

Fenestration of the lateral semicircular canal is so rarely performed today that an account of the operative technique will not be included. The reader is referred to the very full description by Shambaugh (1967a). Regrowth of footplate otosclerosis with fixation of a stapedectomy prosthesis would be one indication. Morrison (1975) encountered this problem in only nine out of 177 stapedectomy failures and in all of these cases there was a mixed conductive and sensorineural loss; the poor cochlear reserve precluded fenestration. In some well prescribed congenital deformities of the ear fenestration is indicated.

For the total or subtotal deafness encountered in some patients with severe combined otosclerosis, House (1976) has reported the results of *cochlear implantation* mainly with a single channel unipolar scala tympani electrode. This form of artificial electrical auditory stimulation, despite its use in a few highly specialized units for a number of years, must still be regarded as in the developmental and assessment stage. Nevertheless the limited transfer of information does hold some prospect of help for these unfortunate patients.

STAPEDECTOMY

When stapedectomy is advised the operation and convalescence should be explained briefly to the patient and the prognosis given for that particular case. In general terms about 85 per cent can expect closure of the air–bone gap, about 4 per cent can expect sensorineural problems and the remainder are likely to be unchanged or somewhat better. At worst patients with subtotal deafness and little or no recordable bone conduction can be given almost a 20 per cent chance of being able to hear fairly well with a hearing aid post-operatively.

Some otologists use prophylactics antibiotics, usually ampicillin or tetracycline, others use none. Leonard (1967) found all the inflammatory complications in patients on prophylactic treatment and no such infections in the control group. It would almost appear that prophylactic antibiotics are contraindicated.

No pre-operative local preparation is necessary. Wax or debris is removed in theatre under magnification with less trauma. The skin of the pinna and canal may be cleaned with an antiseptic solution: 0.1 per cent tincture of thiomersal is suitable. Many otologists prefer to avoid introducing chemicals into the ear canal.

Anaesthesia depends upon the preference of the otologist, and the general health of the patient. General anaesthesia with some hypotensive technique gives a beautiful dry field and there is virtually no risk if the patient is fit, if pre-operative investigations have excluded anaemia and cardiovascular abnormality and if the patient is kept supine. It must be emphasized that some hypotensive anaesthetic methods are safer than others and that problems may arise unless the anaesthetist has complete control of the situation. A more simple general anaesthetic can be combined with local, or the operation can be performed with sedation and local anaesthesia.

Under local anaesthesia, 1 per cent lignocaine with 1 in 200 000 adrenaline is injected to balloon the meatal cuff of skin and periosteum down to the annulus. The tympano–mastoid and tympanosquamous suture lines will limit this effect and at least two injection sites are necessary, the posterosuperior being the more important. Once the middle ear has been opened, topical anaesthetic must be applied; though 4 per cent lignocaine with adrenaline is adequate, better middle-ear anaesthesia is obtained with a specially prepared 10 per cent solution.

Routine operative technique

Most footplates are relatively thin (types 1 and 2 macroscopic pathology) and the normal operative procedure is shown in *Figure 14.17*. Lateral (permeatal) tympano-tomy is now fairly standardized. Through a speculum a widening skin flap is elevated

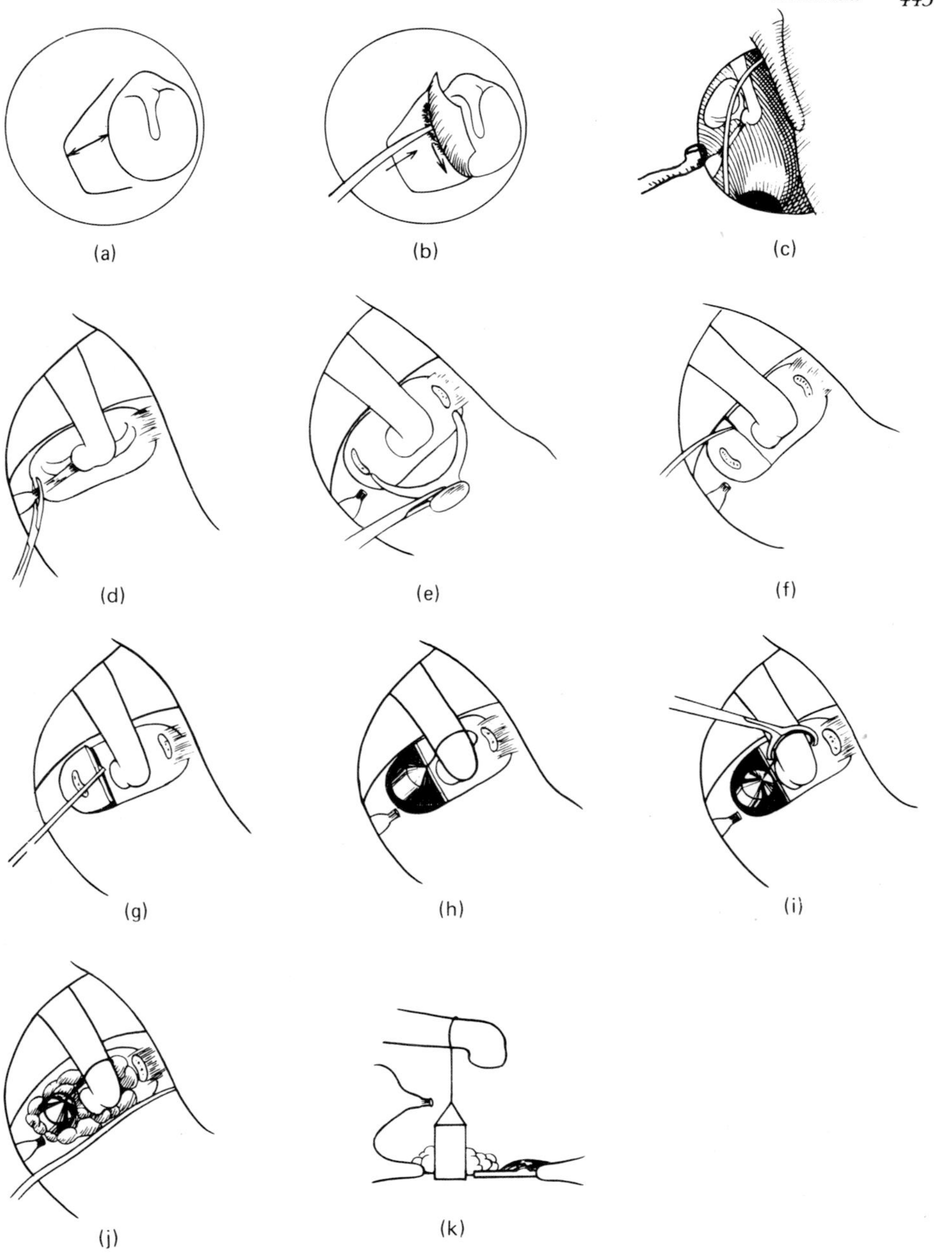

Figure 14.17   Stapedectomy technique: (a) the incision; (b) elevation of tympanomeatal flap; (c) exposure of middle ear; (d) division of incudostapedial joint and stapedius tendon; (e) removal of stapes superstructure; (f) splitting the footplate; (g) removal of posterior third of footplate; (h) placement of McGee piston; (i) crimping of wire loop; (j) testing mobility and applying gel-foam; (k) demonstrating correct piston length. For detailed description see text

towards the drum (*a*). Lateral to the annulus the bony meatus often dips medially away from the operator (*b*). This minor anatomical feature is important in avoiding tears of the flap or drum. The middle ear is entered posterosuperiorly by incising the mucosa. Care is taken to avoid the long process of the incus. A blunt dissector is swept inferiorly, in the middle ear, lifting the annulus from its sulcus attachment; the superior part of the flap is elevated from the outer attic wall towards the neck of the malleus. Occasionally the chorda tympani is swept forward with the tympanomeatal flap though more often it is seen crossing the long process of the incus. Bone is removed with curette, microdrill or nibbling forceps to give the desired exposure of the incus, stapes, stapedius tendon and facial nerve (*c*). The chorda tympani can frequently be left undisturbed but if it is traumatized or interferes with access it should be divided without hesitation. The extent of bone removal depends upon the disposition of the incus and stapes; in 10 per cent of ears no removal is required, in 70 per cent some bone and in 20 per cent several millimetres. It is for this reason that the upper edge of the skin flap should be 3–4 mm above Shrapnell's membrane.

The next important step is examination of the footplate and gentle palpation of the ossicles to note mobility. The fixed malleus syndrome or other ossicular abnormality being excluded, the incudostapedial joint is disarticulated and the stapedius tendon divided near the pyramid (*d*). The head, neck and crura of the stapes are then displaced on to the promontory, the stress fracturing the crura near the footplate (*e*).

Mucous membrane is not removed; the footplate is divided with a sharp pick (*f*), and its posterior third removed (*g*). The chain is reconstructed with a McGee stainless steel piston 0.6 mm in diameter and usually 4.5 mm long. The piston almost fills the vestibular opening (*h*). The wire hook is firmly crimped on the long process of the incus, care being taken to avoid crushing or dislocation (*i*). Finally satisfactory movement transmitted from the malleus handle is checked and the lateral displacement of the handle confirms that the piston is not too short (*j*). Formalin-free gel-foam or fat is applied to the oval window area. The piston should just enter the vestibule (*k*). The tympanomeatal flap is replaced and blood clot removed from the meatus. It is customary to insert a narrow ribbon gauze meatal pack impregnated with suitable dressing for 48 h.

The patient is out of bed the following day and may be discharged on the third or fourth day. Sudden head movements may cause transient dizziness and should be discouraged for a few days. In the uncomplicated case convalescence is quick and uneventful.

Special operative situations and problems

Fortunately the majority of stapedectomies present little technical difficulty. Many anatomical, physiological and pathological variations can be encountered. When a number are combined in the same case they may present such obstacles that it is wiser to stop rather than proceed. Such decisions require experience and judgement.

Anatomical variations of the facial nerve are not uncommon. Dehiscences of the fallopian canal are frequent. In about 0.5 per cent of middle ears there is a sizeable dehiscence so that the nerve bulges down and obscures the arch and footplate. In lesser degrees of this abnormality (*Figure 14.18*) it is possible to displace the nerve gently upwards and complete the operation. If footplate surgery is likely to be blind it is wiser to abandon the operation. Another situation arises when the fallopian canal is intact but bulging down. By altering the direction of vision it is usually possible to gain accesss to the footplate.

Very rarely the facial nerve takes an anomalous course, either splitting to surround

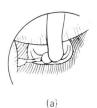

(a)

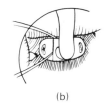

(b)

Figure 14.18 Abnormal facial nerve: (a) nerve protruding through large dehiscence resting on crura and obscuring the footplate; (b) nerve displaced to allow footplate surgery

the stapes or coursing inferior to the oval window. Nine such cases have been reported in the world literature (Hoogland, 1977).

A persistent stapedial artery of sufficient size to prevent completion of the operation is very rare. It is likely to be encountered two or three times/1000 stapedectomies. A small vestigial vessel is not infrequently seen. It should be recognized since damage may cause troublesome bleeding. Davies (1967) has described the developmental anatomy.

Perilymph flooding is also a rare problem. Most authorities suggest that it might happen once in 500 stapedectomies; Schuknecht (1971) indicates a frequency of 1 in 300. The author has not yet encountered this problem during surgery for otosclerosis but has met it on opening the vestibule in congenital fixation (Morrison, 1971). Many authors since Sooy (1960) have reported this congenital anomaly. The usual explanation is an abnormally patent cochlear aqueduct which allows CSF to flow through the cochlea into the vestibule. Another possibility is a direct communication between the internal meatus and vestibule. Polytomographic evidence of an abnormally shaped vestibule should warn against stapedectomy.

If perilymph flooding should be encountered, the use of a spinal drain, the intravenous administration of mannitol and the raising of the patient's head should control the flow enough to allow sealing of the window and placement of a prosthesis. There is likely to be post-operative vertigo and severe sensorineural loss. Persistent CSF otorrhoea will require further surgery to stem the flood though it may stop spontaneously after a few days.

In children the cochlear aqueduct is more patent and minor degrees of abnormal patency may persist into adult life. During stapedectomy in some adults there is a pulsatile escape of perilymph into the middle ear rather than flooding. This phenomenon is not so rare. To avoid a perilymph fistula the whole or most of the footplate should be removed and a vein or other tissue sheet applied before placement of the prosthesis.

Bleeding during stapedectomy can cause problems. The benefits of a dry field cannot be overemphasized. Surgery is quicker, the footplate can be visualized without interruption, the vestibule is open for the shortest possible time, blood does not enter the vestibule and the avoidance of repeated suction helps prevent mucosal trauma and later adhesions. Each surgeon cooperating with the anaesthetist must decide upon the safest and most reliable method of achieving a dry field. Pre-operative fluoride therapy is probably of help in reducing the vascularity of active otosclerotic bone.

The floating footplate can cause great technical difficulty and result in damage to the inner ear. It is most likely to occur during attempts to needle a hole in the centre of a uniformly thick type 2 footplate. Some authors advise puncturing the plate prior to arch removal. When presented with this problem it may be possible to tilt the footplate by applying pressure to one of the crural attachments, so that a hook may extract or fracture the plate. Alternatively a fine hook may be insinuated through an inferiorly placed marginal burr-hole.

If the technical difficulty of removing a floating or hinged footplate is not resolved fairly quickly, it is wisest to abandon the attempt rather than run the considerable risk of severe sensorineural loss and vertigo from inner-ear damage. An acceptable result can follow reconstruction with a prosthesis from the incus to the floating footplate. A remarkable result can follow reconstruction while part or all of the footplate remains slightly hinged inwards. The alternative management is the application of fat without any attempt to reconstruct.

Obliterative otosclerosis is a fairly common finding, likely to be encountered in about 10 per cent of operations. Besides type 4, some type 3 footplates require to be drilled. Employing the method of slowly drilling a hole just large enough to accommodate a piston of 0.6 mm diameter, the results of this surgery are among the best obtained. The final opening into the vestibule should be done with fine needles and hooks (*Figure 14.19*). For the less experienced, drilling is an added anxiety. Some pre-operative indication of footplate pathology may be supplied by the compliance value (*Table 14.4*). Valvassori (1973) favours pre-operative multidirectional polytomography in all patients, and claims a high degree of accuracy for radiographic assessment of oval window pathology.

Obliteration of the round window by otosclerotic bone is a very rare operative finding. No attempt should be made to remove this bone.

Removal of the stapes 'in toto' should be avoided, since there is a risk of the sudden

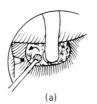 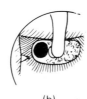 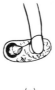

(a)   (b)   (c)

Figure 14.19 Obliterative otosclerosis: (a) slow controlled drilling without pressure; (b) vestibule opened posteriorly; (c) reconstruction with a slim piston

inner-ear pressure change disrupting the membranous labyrinth. If the stapes should mobilize during the preliminary testing and there is a likelihood of its being removed '*in toto*', then the footplate should be divided or pierced before the arch is removed.

Tympanic membrane tear

On completion of the operation a small tear in the drum is occasionally encountered though it is rare if the wedge flap is used. A slit need only be covered with gel-foam. A larger tear can be closed by rotating the flap and covering with gel-foam (*Figure 14.20*). Healing is almost invariable and minute deficiencies do not interfere with function. Chronic perforations are more likely to result from inadequate flaps together with bone removal. If such a deficiency is seen at the end of the operation temporal fascia should be placed medial to the drum and on to the adjoining bony meatus.

Revision operations will be discussed more fully under 'Complications of Stapedectomy', p. 453. When reopening, a larger flap should be raised. The drum is usually adherent to the long process of the incus and must be carefully dissected off. Adhesions must be cut and not torn. As a general rule the vestibule should never be reopened at revision operations.

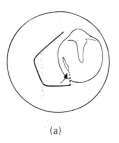

(a)

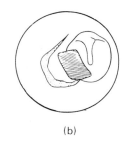

(b)

Figure 14.20 Repair of tympanic tear: (a) inferior incision into the tear; (b) flap rotated and area covered with gel-foam

Incus replacement

The need for an incus replacement prosthesis arises in otosclerosis when stapedectomy is indicated in the previously fenestrated ear. It can also arise during stapedectomy if the incus is dislocated, if its long process is fractured or, in revision operations if it has undergone partial necrosis.

In the fenestrated ear (*Figure 14.21*) the meatal incision is carried over the facial ridge and lateral semicircular canal (*a*). The incus and head of malleus have been removed at the original operation. When the middle ear is entered and bone removed the stapes is found at a higher level than the appearance of the tympanic membrane suggests—the outer attic wall is missing and the pars flaccida rotated 90 degrees. An incision is made through the periosteum of the malleus handle (*b*). The drum and periosteum are elevated to provide a tunnel. A House malleus wire or similar fabricated prosthesis usually 5.25 mm long is tightened on the handle (*c*). The stapes and its whole footplate are removed, the oval window covered with vein graft (intima

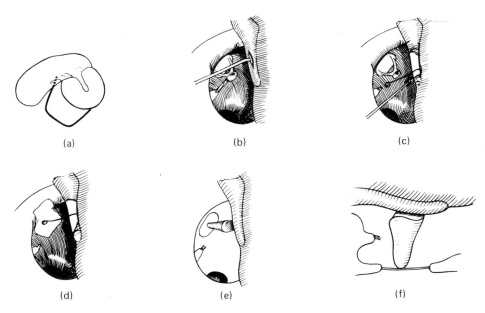

(a)   (b)   (c)

(d)   (e)   (f)

Figure 14.21 Incus replacement: (a) incision and flap in the fenestrated ear; (b) elevating periosteum from handle of malleus; (c) fitting of House malleus wire; (d) stapes removed. House wire resting on oval window vein graft; (e) homograft incus type 2 as alternative to wire prosthesis; (f) homograft incus type 2 between malleus handle and vestibular membrane. For fuller description see text

facing vestibule) and the stainless steel or tantalum prosthesis rotated into position (*d*). The flap is replaced. This can be a very difficult operation as the malleus handle may be very short and, having little support, is very mobile during manipulation. Furthermore a proportion of the wires slowly become dislodged and protrude through the drum. A similar type of prosthesis can be used in stapedectomy if the incus is damaged; technically easier than in the fenestrated ear and giving somewhat better results.

Unilateral stapedectomy may be considered in patients with bilateral fenestrations, no fistula sign, a large air–bone gap, a dry cavity with intact drum and dislike for or intolerance of a hearing aid. The results are not comparable with primary stapedectomy largely due to technical difficulties. In ten patients followed for four years or longer only four have closure of the air–bone gap, three are improved, two are slightly worse and one has a 'dead ear'. These numbers are small but the results are very comparable to those quoted to Guilford (1969) and Sheehy (1969). Willis (1975) advises the additional technique of using tragal cartilage blocks to increase the depth of the middle ear. Most otologists, however, have abandoned this form of surgery.

A much simpler reconstruction employs a homograft incus, the long process being removed, the short process resting on the vein graft and the articular facet wedged behind the malleus handle (*e*). This type 2 incus transposition can also be used in primary stapedectomy when the patient's own incus is damaged, and in some revision operations when it is rested on a mobile vestibular membrane (*f*). Care must be taken to avoid damaging the membrane. A cartilage strut may be used in the same way. The results of this surgery are likewise disappointing and it is seldom employed.

MODIFICATIONS IN STAPEDECTOMY TECHNIQUE

A number of variations in stapedectomy technique are used by different authorities. Some of them are shown diagrammatically in *Figure 14.22*. In competent hands each gives a high percentage of good results. Minor modifications are still taking place. Factors to be considered are the stability of sound conduction and the risk of sensorineural deafness.

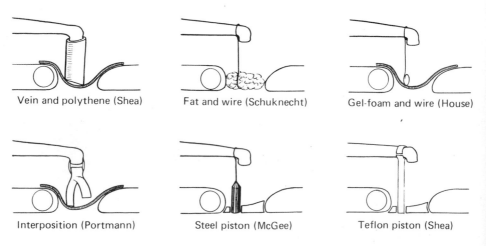

Vein and polythene (Shea)   Fat and wire (Schuknecht)   Gel-foam and wire (House)

Interposition (Portmann)   Steel piston (McGee)   Teflon piston (Shea)

Figure 14.22 Diagrammatic representation of some of the many types of stapedectomy. See text for full account

Mechanical stability

Shea's original vein and polythene strut operation (Shea, 1958), though representing a major otological advance, has now been abandoned because of its inherent mechanical instability. Disarticulation of the incudopolythene arthroplasty either from slipping or pressure necrosis of the lentiform process occurred in 8 per cent of cases, and a further 14 per cent gave improved but indifferent long-term results (6–15 years). These figures come from a personal series of over 200 such operations. Walsh (1967) had a similar experience.

The Portmann (1961) interposition operation and the somewhat similar anterior crurotomy have the disadvantage of being technically more difficult and of being applicable to only a proportion of cases with limited disease. Hough (1976), however can remove the anterior crus, seal the window with perichondrium and replace the posterior crus in between 80–90 per cent of cases. Long-term results reported by Fisch and Rüedi (1968) showed recurrence of conductive loss in 9 per cent. Nevertheless the risk of sensorineural deafness must be small with this method and there is no foreign body to slip or cause incus necrosis. The technique is still used by many otologists in suitable cases.

The fat and wire reconstruction described by Schuknecht, McGee and Colman (1960) and the House (1962) gel-foam and wire method have the same mechanical advantage as the McGee or tef-wire pistons. When the wire loop is crimped on the incus it rarely becomes dislodged but it can cause pressure necrosis. For good sound transmission crimping has to be firm. Care must be taken to avoid damaging or dislocating the incus.

The Shea (1963) Teflon piston has the great advantage of simplicity in application. If the incus long process is slender the Teflon ring is rather loose and can fall off. Though Shea (1969a) had never encountered incus necrosis or displacement with this piston, Morrison (1975), reviewing the results of different prostheses found this to be its mechanical weakness. Furthermore Shea (1971) has changed to a Teflon-cup piston for better mechanical linkage.

A prosthesis, and in particular a piston, which is too long is mechanically unsound. It must become attached to and not pass through a vibratable membrane (*Figure 14.23*). A piston which is too short is equally unsuitable. For this reason some surgeons use special instruments to measure the distance from the footplate to the lentiform process of the incus and modify the prosthesis length according to the results. It must not be forgotten that measurements *before* opening the vestibule must take the footplate thickness into account, and this can be very variable.

Another mechanically unstable situation arises when, usually following complete footplate removal, a 'submucosal fistula' forms. The prosthesis may be the correct length, and nature effects a seal in the oval window niche lateral to the anatomical footplate site. This produces the same mechanical inaptitude as the overlong piston. Small footplate openings which do not disturb the middle-ear mucosa prevent this development.

Sensorineural problems

Factors which might result in sensorineural deafness must now be considered.

Techniques which call for the removal of all or most of the footplate must carry increased risk of surgical trauma to the inner ear. This applies particularly to type 3 and 4 footplates. It was largely for this reason that the drilled hole and piston

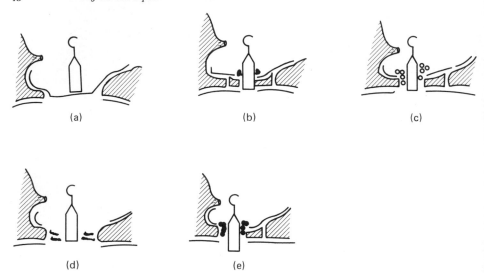

Figure 14.23 Prevention of perilymph fistula. (a) the whole footplate has been removed and the oval window is covered by a vein graft prior to placement of the prosthesis; (b) a small hole has been made in the plate; the piston fills the hole and is surrounded by gel-foam; (c) the posterior half of the plate has been removed; to avoid the risk of fistula the piston is surrounded by a tissue graft such as fat; (d) the whole footplate has been removed and the prosthesis surrounded by absorbable gel-foam—the risk of fistula formation is high in this situation; (e) the piston is too long—this is mechanically unsound and there is every prospect of either early or late fistulas

prosthesis was devised. McGee (1965) foresaw this when describing his early results for obliterative otosclerosis.

The first vein and polythene procedure had one excellent principle which has returned to stapedectomy surgery. That principle was the tissue sealing of the oval window. Hearing gains were frequently immediate and there was little risk of early fistula formation. Struts were easily fabricated at the time of surgery to provide a good fit and flat base. Late fistula problems were very rarely seen with these 'home-made' prostheses. Some of the pre-fabricated polythene struts were sharp pointed. They could and did pierce the oval window membrane up to many years later causing sudden sensorineural deafness, tinnitus and vertigo. Such late problems are still presenting. The Interposition operation also seals the oval window. The fat and wire technique is similarly designed though small fistulas are occasionally encountered.

Stapedectomy methods which employ a piston or wire either with no attempt to graft the oval window or with the use of gel-foam only, carry the greatest risk of early fistula formation. By way of confirmation, Shea (1969a), analysing his results for obliterative otosclerosis, found that the incidence of sensorineural problems was two and a half times greater (6.7 per cent) with large openings into the vestibule than with small fenestrae (2.5 per cent); the percentage with closure of the air–bone gap was higher in the latter group. For some time now Shea (1969b, 1971) has returned to vein grafting and Teflon or Teflon-cup pistons and the early fistula problem has largely disappeared.

From time to time in the history of stapedectomy, attempts have been made to return to mobilization in carefully selected cases in order to avoid inner-ear complications. House (1967), with the same objective, described the results of reconstruction with a wire or similar prosthesis on to a fragmented footplate in selected cases. House (1977) now favours the use of vein or other suitable tissue to seal off the vestibule.

When pistons are used to reconstruct the ossicular chain, it is advisable to employ one of the modifications shown in *Figure 14.23*. As an alternative to fat, if the chorda tympani has been sacrificed during surgery, an excised length of this nerve is an excellent tissue to encircle the base of a piston and effect a seal. The dangers of a large unsealed opening into the vestibule are shown to very good effect in *Figure 14.24*.

No single stapedectomy or partial stapedectomy technique is free from potential mechanical or iatrogenic inner-ear complications. Whereas there is considerable choice and scope for modification according to the circumstances in any given case, the principles of the surgery are now fairly established.

STAPEDECTOMY RESULTS AND COMPLICATIONS

Results

It is important to put this subject into perspective. Results should not be glorified nor is there any need to be a prophet of gloom.

One difficulty which arises in attempting to estimate or compare results is the definition of 'closure' of the air–bone gap. Overclosure and complete closure are easily understood. Most authors include within 10 dB of the pre-operative bone conduction level as 'closure', though some include within 15 dB or even 20 dB. On the last of these definitions a patient with, say, a 30 dB gap who had a 10 dB gain, would be classified as a success.

Reference has been made to a comparison of pre- and post-stapedectomy speech discrimination. Closure of the air–bone gap, especially in older patients and in those with a pre-operative high-tone sensorineural component, can be associated with poorer post-operative discrimination or distortion of sound. It would seem logical to use both pure-tone and speech tests to assess results. However, many different forms of speech material can be used and extensive tests are costly and time consuming. It is suggested that, with the smaller number of patients now presenting for stapedial surgery, more comprehensive testing and analysis is indicated.

The success criterion of 'within 10 dB of closure or better' presents another difficulty in assessing results. Many patients have poor (or even no) recordable bone conduction pre-operatively yet, if the air–bone gap is wide enough they can achieve considerable gain from surgery. Closure of the gap will leave many of these patients still handicapped by deafness.

With these reservations in mind, most of the published British stapedectomy series of results fall within the success range 80-90 per cent. For example Holden, Hood and Taylor (1967), 88 per cent; Ludman (1968), 92 per cent; Dawes and Curry (1969), 90 per cent; Morrison (1969a), 70 per cent for vein and polythene, 88 per cent for piston reconstruction; and more recently Donaldson (1976), 82 per cent.

Hammond (1976) has drawn attention to the poor long-term follow-up rates after stapedectomy especially in the USA. The figures available show a falling percentage of good results with the passage of time. For example House and Greenfield (1969) reported 91 per cent closure at four months reduced to 75 per cent at five years;

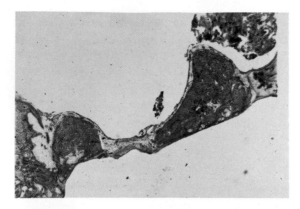

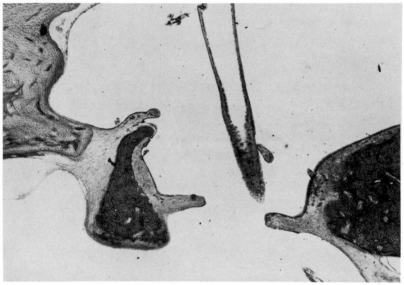

Figure 14.24   Good footplate healing and fistula formation. Autopsy specimens of both temporal bones from the same patient on whom bilateral stapedectomies, with Teflon pistons, had been performed during life. In the upper section a small hole had been made in the footplate and there is a strong membrane. She had an excellent and lasting hearing result on this side. In the other ear (lower section) there is a much larger footplate hole and a posterior fragment of footplate has been depressed into the vestibule; on this side there is a large fistula. After the second stapedectomy the patient had experienced no hearing gain and had developed progressive sensorineural deafness and intermittent vertigo. The ear had not been re-explored (Sections by kind permission of Professor L. Michaels, Institute of Laryngology and Otology, London)

McGee (1969) had 89.5 per cent good results at one year reducing to 83.8 per cent at six years; and Hough (1969) reported 95 per cent closure at six months reduced to 85 per cent at five to seven years. Cody (1967) noted a similar trend.

In the third edition of this book the author wrote 'This era of otosclerotic surgery spans a decade. We have seen from the natural history that this interval of time can be insignificant. Whether or not stapedectomy will prevent the natural progression of deafness common to most patients with this disease, the next decade may reveal'. That decade is now over without a definite answer. The majority of patients with a good initial result continue to hear well though perhaps 10–20 per cent of them have poorer thresholds of hearing. A small percentage have been unfortunate in developing late conductive or sensorineural problems.

Complications

The advances in middle-ear micro-surgery during the past two decades have brought relief to many thousands of deaf patients. When considering the complications and problems which may follow stapedectomy, this important fact must not be forgotten.

Post-operative *otitis media* is a very rare complication, having a frequency of something like 2 or 3/1000 operations. The use of a prophylactic broad-spectrum antibiotic is reassuring. Labyrinthitis and meningitis are even rarer complications though they have been reported (Leonard, 1967).

Post-operative *granuloma* is a difficult problem since its aetiology remains speculative. It may be bacterial in origin. Most of the reports on this condition have come from Schuknecht's unit (Kaufman and Schuknecht, 1967; Schuknecht, 1971; Schuknecht, 1974; Burtner and Goodman, 1974). He considers it to be one of the common early complications of stapedectomy and to have a frequency approaching 2 per cent. This has not been the experience of others (Shea, Hough and House, 1969). It may result from the use of gel-foam containing variable amounts of formalin, yet it is recorded following techniques which use no gel-foam. It may be due to foreign-body reaction (glove powder, Teflon dust or unidentified particles) as suggested by Dawes and Curry (1974) and by Burtner and Goodman (1974). It may have an autoimmune basis as described by Gromer *et al.* (1974). In two of the only four cases seen by the author, Gram-negative organisms were cultured from the granuloma.

The complication is suspected between the third and tenth post-operative days when the patient complains of some local discomfort, increasing deafness and vertigo. The drum and meatal flap look red and bulky. Urgent re-exploration is indicated to excise the granulation tissue for culture and to remove the prosthesis and seal off the oval window (if this has not already been done). In cases where there has been no effective seal, the granulation tissue invades and destroys the inner ear. Schuknecht (1971, 1974) considers that prompt action may save the inner ear.

Haemotympanum is a not uncommon post-operative finding. No treatment is necessary. It can be readily diagnosed on inspection of the drum. The patient can be reassured that there will be only some delay in hearing improvement.

A transient, partial, delayed-onset *facial paralysis* may be encountered once or twice in every 1000 operations performed under general anaesthesia. The incidence might be higher when local anaesthesia is employed, bearing in mind the frequency of fallopian canal dehiscence. Reassurance is the only treatment necessary. If there is immediate complete post-operative facial paralysis then it is likely that the nerve has been damaged. The management of facial paralysis is fully covered in Chapter 27.

It is surprising how seldom patients complain of *loss or alteration of taste* when the chorda tympani has been divided. They are as likely or more likely to notice this when the chorda has been bruised or stretched unduly. Bull (1965) found that 93 per cent of patients were symptom-free within a year.

Delays in hearing recovery are not uncommon. The normal convalescence following stapedectomy should be examined before looking into the early sensorineural complications.

Following almost every stapedectomy, even when a tissue graft has been employed, there is probably a leak of perilymph into the middle ear. As soon as nature has produced an intact footplate membrane the hearing discrimination returns. During this early interval, which may be a matter of one to several weeks, sounds are heard loudly in the ear but there is some distortion and indifferent discrimination. Fluctuation is not uncommon. Pure-tone audiograms performed within the first ten days usually show incomplete closure of the air–bone gap and a high-tone loss. There is normally rapid improvement of these audiological signs over the next few weeks and high-tone loss and discrimination continue to improve over several months.

Many patients after stapedectomy have transient *vertigo* on sudden head movement, the symptom disappearing in a few days or, at most, a week or two. At rest there is no clinical nystagmus or subjective vertigo. During these first few days nystagmus may be elicited to the same or the opposite side when fixation is abolished by the use of Frenzel glasses. Operations on the stapes, even mobilization, can affect the vestibular labyrinth over the longer term. Fussing and Peitersen (1965) found evidence of vestibular damage in 5 per cent of patients after mobilization and in 23 per cent after stapedectomy; there were still minor caloric test abnormalities in 3 and 13 per cent of these patients respectively a year later.

The picture just described for the very early recovery after stapedectomy— fluctuant hearing loss, indifferent discrimination, a persisting air–bone gap, high-tone loss and transient vertigo on movement—has all the classic features of a perilymph fistula. Provided there is a quick and continuing improvement in all these signs and symptoms no action is necessary. Indeed, provided the surgical principles have been followed during the operation, it would be most unwise to reopen the middle ear. During this healing period the patient should be advised to avoid strain or exertion. Balancing and labyrinthine exercises are the worst possible thing. Flying is inadvisable within the first two weeks.

Sensorineural hearing loss

The tragic case of severe hearing loss after stapedectomy is one which otologists most fear. Despite every care and precaution and even in the most experienced hands such iatrogenic problems are bound to occur.

Immediate losses

Direct surgical trauma to the structures of the inner ear is less likely to occur with increasing operative experience. The microanatomy of the footplate area must be fully understood and no attempt made to pass instruments more than 1 mm into the vestibule. In 1959 and 1960 micro-surgical instruments were still crude and microdrills were developing. Even today one sometimes sees instruments more suited to tympanoplastic than to footplate surgery. Attention to such detail is essential. Before commencing on the vital footplate dissection, the field should be dry, the exposure adequate and binocular vision available.

To give some indication of the frequency of direct surgical trauma, Morrison (1962) reported two cases from the first 50 stapedectomies (4 per cent), both in patients with obliterative disease following attempts to remove large bone chips from the vestibule with instruments which were crude by today's standards. In the next 50 operations there was one similar case (2 per cent). In the next 500 operations there were no immediate losses from direct surgical trauma (0 per cent); in the subsequent 400 stapedectomies one inner ear was damaged attempting to deal with an inwardly hinged plate (0.25 per cent).

Indirect surgical trauma should be avoidable if the causes are kept in mind. They have already been mentioned. There is a risk of disruption of the membraneous labyrinth if the stapes is removed '*in toto*'. The result is likely to be a severe high-tone loss and poor discrimination, even if the air–bone gap is closed in the lower frequencies. In the presence of *secondary labyrinthine hydrops* the distended saccule is at risk. Stapedectomy without prior management of the hydrops, will almost certainly destroy the ear. *Reopening the vestibule* in revision surgery carries a very high risk. This will be discussed below. The *noise or vibration trauma* from drilling is less readily defined. It is well recognized that a fast rotating cutting burr applied to any part of the intact ossicular chain can cause sensorineural loss. The very slowly rotating burr which should be used on the obliterated footplate seems unlikely to have this consequence. The rare case of *perilymph flooding* has been discussed.

Early perilymph fistula　This was undoubtedly one of the common causes of early post-stapedectomy hearing loss. Some of the factors predisposing to early fistula have already been examined (*Figures 14.23* and *14.24*). To summarize they are inadequate closure of the fenestration in the footplate, a prosthesis which is too long, increased perilymph pressure and possibly surgery in older patients. A fragment of footplate which is displaced or hinged into the vestibule could act in the same manner as a lengthy prosthesis and prevent healing. Now that these factors are understood it is hoped that the frequency of this problem will diminish.

The symptoms and signs of fistula vary according to the size of the hole. Large untreated fistulas result in sudden or rapid hearing loss, tinnitus and vertigo. Fluctuation is not likely to be a feature. The hearing loss in the early stages will appear to be conductive though it soon becomes sensorineural and finally subtotal or even total. Early surgical repair can be effective (*Figure 14.25*). Morrison (1975) reviewing 14 large fistulas dating from the time of stapedectomy found that referral was regrettably late, that the hearing losses were profound when first seen and that repair had little effect apart from curing vertigo. Where records were available it was noted that the surgeon had experienced one or more technical difficulties during the operation. The management of troublesome tinnitus in these patients is covered below.

A small fistula dating from the primary surgery is more likely to be encountered and managed at a later stage. The correct management depends on the clinical course. Some patients probably have a minute fistula following stapedectomy and the only evidence of this is a failure of good closure of the air–bone gap, some fluctuation in hearing and good though poorer discrimination than might be expected. Some distortion may be a feature. Provided the result is acceptable and there is no progressive deterioration, these patients should simply be kept under observation. Needless to say the other ear should not be operated on.

Late losses
Perilymph fistula　Most authorities would now agree that the main cause of late sensorineural deafness, after stapedectomy, is perilymph fistula. An examination of

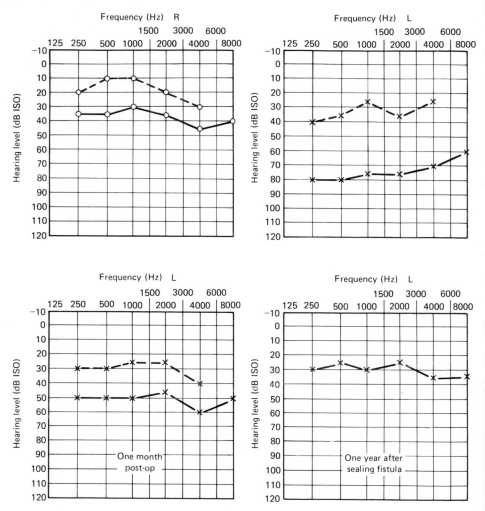

Figure 14.25   Early perilymph fistula. Pre-operative audiograms (above) from a man of 37 with a 15-year history of progressive left deafness and a two-year history of right deafness. Several difficulties were encountered during the left stapedectomy. Bleeding was troublesome throughout. The oval window niche was deep and narrow. On removing the posterior part of the footplate perilymph pulsated into the middle ear. Blood and perilymph continued to obscure vision. The chain was reconstructed with a McGee piston and surrounded with gel-foam. There was failure of closure of the air–bone gap, intermittent vertigo and tinnitus. The ear was reopened one month later. Hypotensive anaesthesia was used. Perilymph was escaping freely around the piston. The remainder of the footplate was removed, the window sealed with a vein graft and a new piston applied. This satisfactory outcome (bottom right) is unusual and can be achieved only with early repair

some of the documented cases of fistula (Hemenway *et al.*, 1968; House and Greenfield, 1969; Moon, 1970; Harrison *et al.*, 1970; Shea, 1971) indicates that no technique is devoid of this complication.

Harrison and his colleagues in Chicago have found that the longer the period of follow-up in a series of stapedectomy patients, the greater becomes the percentage who develop a fistula. In 1967, Harrison *et al.* quoted about 1 per cent with fistulas while in 1970 this had risen to 3 per cent. Fully 50 per cent of their fistulas were encountered more than two years after surgery. In 1969a, Shea put the frequency at 0.9 per cent, while in 1971 he quoted a figure of 2.4 per cent. In 1971, Morrison, in the third edition of this volume quoted 0.7 per cent of fistulas, while in 1975, the percentage had risen to 2.82.

Hemenway, Hildyard and Black (1968) analysing the predisposing factors found no cause in about 50 per cent. In the remainder the same stresses which can result in spontaneous labyrinthine fistula were operative. These included pressure changes from flying, mountaineering, lifting heavy objects, coughing and sneezing, and head injury. An analysis of the operative findings in 24 cases of late perilymph fistula is presented diagrammatically in *Figure 14.26*. Sometimes a mechanical fault causes the

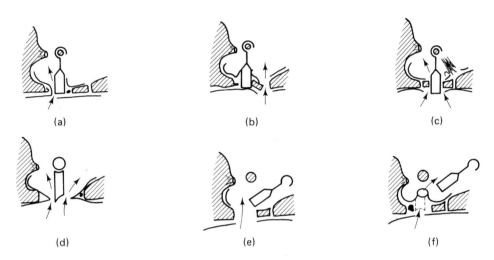

(a)   (b)   (c)

(d)   (e)   (f)

Figure 14.26 Types of late perilymph fistula–findings in 24 revised cases. Small fistulas are most commonly seen in situations (a) (6 cases) and (b) (2 cases); there is no obvious cause for the development of late fistula apart from lack of adequate strength in the membrane, a depressed fragment of footplate or a piston which may be too long. These patients have lesser degrees of hearing loss and the classic fluctuating features. The other situations tend to result in large obvious fistulas; these patients have sudden more severe deterioration without fluctuation. In (c) (4 cases) adhesions cause the membrane to rupture. In (d) (3 cases) a sharp polythene tube pierces the membrane. In (e) (7 cases) the prosthesis becomes dislodged from the incus and tears a large hole in the footplate membrane. In (f) (2 cases) there is a similar event but the perilymph escapes through a mucosal tube. For simplicity McGee pistons or polythene struts (d) have been shown in the diagrams though these problems have been encountered with all types of prosthesis

fistula. The oval window membrane can be pierced by a sharp-pointed prosthesis or by medial retraction of a piston from adhesions. Displacement of the prosthesis can also result in a fistula.

As with early fistulas, the symptomatology and management depend upon the size of the fistula, the degree of hearing loss and the rapidity of onset. The classic features of a small fistula have been described. In addition some patients with a late-developing small fistula complain intermittently of clicking or dripping noises in the ear. The fluctuant deafness may be worse on awakening and improve during the day. Nystagmus may be demonstrable with Frenzel glasses. If a negative pressure of

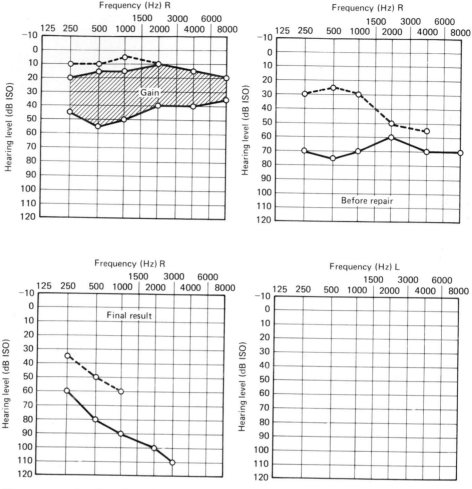

Figure 14.27   Small perilymph fistula. A man of 44 who had a good stapedectomy result (top left). Four years later he developed sudden fluctuant hearing loss and slight vertigo and tinnitus (top right). Tympanotomy one month after the deterioration showed perilymph leaking from the lower margin of the oval window adjacent to the piston. The piston was removed, the fistula sealed with vein and a 4-mm Teflon piston replaced. He had post-operative vertigo for several days and progressive sensorineural deafness. The final result (lower left) is unchanged four years later.

— 200–300 mm water is applied to the drum with an impedance bridge there may be subjective unsteadiness. Fluctuations in speech discrimination are another feature of a small fistula.

The management of small fistulas may be conservative or surgical. There is much to be said for a wait-and-see attitude in the supervision of suspected small fistulas which date from surgery. The risks of more severe disturbance to the inner ear are considerable with revision surgery (*Figure 14.27*). At operation the footplate area must be examined under high magnification in a dry field. A small fistula is confirmed when moisture reappears after aspiration. The prognosis for hearing after this sort of fistula repair are not good. Harrison *et al.* (1967) reported only 24 per cent improved, with

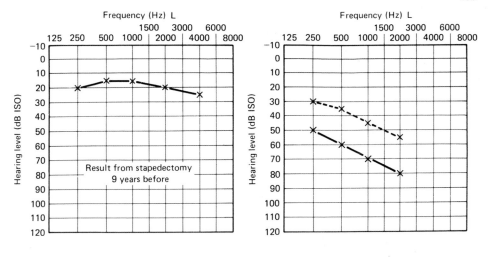

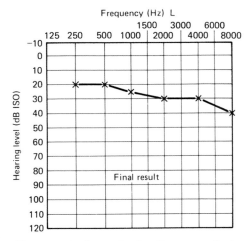

Figure 14.28   Large fistula of late onset. Early repair. A vein and polythene-tube stapedectomy had been performed nine years before with a good lasting result (top left). The patient suddenly developed deafness, tinnitus and vertigo while gardening (top right). Compliance in this ear was 4.10 cm³. The ear was reopened within a week. The tip of the incus was necrosed. The tube was free in the middle ear. There was an obvious perilymph flow through the mucosal cuff (*see Figure 14.26 f*). The cuff was excised, the fistula closed with fat and a McGee piston applied. Four months later the hearing deteriorated again but there was no vertigo. The ear was opened again. The wire had come off the incus but there was a well healed window membrane. A homograft bone strut was placed between the membrane and the drum (*see Figure 14.21*). The result is very acceptable and has been maintained for four years

further sensorineural loss in 30 per cent. In the author's experience there is a 60 per cent chance of further deterioration if the prosthesis is removed. This is unacceptable. Such cases are now managed by gently scarifying the edges of the fistula and surrounding the area with a small fat or fibrous tissue graft and gel-foam *without* disturbing the assembly. No deterioration has occurred with this management, though from six such repairs the symptoms suggest residual fistula in four.

Late large fistulas present the clinical picture of sudden or rapidly progressive severe deafness not always associated with vertigo. These are not 'vascular' or 'viral' in origin. Delay in reoperating on these cases is a mistake for early repair can be effective (*Figure 14.28*). The sort of findings encountered are shown in *Figure 14.26*. With early surgery—say within a month—there is a 40 per cent chance of salvaging the hearing. With late repair the only advantage is to settle vertigo. Many otologists, especially in North America, argue that these repairs and other types of revision surgery should be performed under local anaesthesia. Any indication of vertigo would be a warning not to proceed with piston removal.

Many of these unfortunate patients have *severe and persistent tinnitus*. Provided there is no useful function in the inner ear and already marked hypofunction of the vestibular end-organ, eighth nerve section should be seriously considered. Eight such translabyrinthine operations have been performed. The cochlear nerve section has abolished tinnitus in two, resulted in an acceptable tinnitus level in five, while only one is unchanged. In this last patient the cochlear and facial nerves were impossible to separate and the cochlear section was incomplete. There is obviously some risk to the facial nerve with this operation and pros and cons of surgery must be carefully weighed and discussed with each patient.

Cochlear otosclerosis   Late sensorineural loss, usually slowly progressive, but occasionally quite marked over a period of several months, may be due to the natural history of the disease. Rapid progression during pregnancy, the development of a Schwartze sign, similar changes in the unoperated ear and polytomographic evidence of diffuse capsular otosclerosis would all suggest this diagnosis. In such cases flouride therapy is indicated.

The rare occurrence of sudden *rupture of the cochlear duct* in combined otosclerosis has been described. Clinically it can only be suspected, after stapedectomy, when there is x-ray evidence of capsular involvement and when re-exploration has revealed a 'normal' middle ear. Armstrong (1967) reported three such sudden total losses in the unoperated ear.

Summary

The experience of the past two decades indicates that, considering all the causes of iatrogenic sensorineural deafness after stapedectomy, the overall risk of such loss both early and late must be of the order of 4 or even 5 per cent in reasonably competent hands. It could well be higher with the less experienced surgeon. When advising stapedectomy to the patient this 1 to 20 risk must be explained. It is to be hoped that recent modifications in the surgery will improve on this position.

POST-OPERATIVE CONDUCTION FAILURES AND REVISION OPERATIONS

Conductive deafness, occasionally persisting after stapedectomy, though usually developing subsequently occurs with about the same or somewhat greater frequency than sensorineural deafness. The incidence from failure to mobilize or from refixation was high (75 per cent) after attempted mobilization operations; with the vein and polythene stapedectomy it occurred in about 17 per cent; while after the piston or wire or other methods currently used, it is of the order of 5 to 6 per cent. As with sensorineural complications the longer the period of follow-up the higher is this figure likely to become.

Before proceeding it should be noted again that a perilymph fistula with a developing air–bone gap can simulate a conductive loss. *Post-operative adhesions* also give rise to a mixed conductive and sensorineural hearing loss.

Incus dislocation or fracture during stapedectomy will produce an indifferent result. The management of this problem is discussed under 'Incus Replacement'.

In the early days of stapedectomy it used to be thought that division of the stapedial tendon and removal of the stapes might result in avascular *necrosis of the tip of the long process of the incus*. Morgenstein and Manace (1968) suggested that medial fixation from regrowth of otosclerosis would have mechanical effects on the incus tip. Such regrowth is relatively rarely seen. Although loss of the incus tip can follow any of the techniques used it was commonest with the polythene strut and is more frequent with crimped wire than with Teflon piston or interposition operations. Pressure necrosis seems the likely pathogenesis.

A *slipped prosthesis* is the most frequent cause of recurrent conductive deafness, sometimes of sudden onset. The hearing loss is usually entirely conductive and of the order of 50–60 dB. Compliance values are high. Polythene struts disarticulated in 6 per cent of cases. Teflon pistons fall off the incus occasionally. Crimped wire is less likely to disarticulate. On the other hand a persisting air–bone gap of 20–30 dB can be due to failure to crimp a wire prosthesis sufficiently well.

Occasionally a *short piston* fails to reach the oval window membrane. Willis (1976) reviewing a large number of stapedectomy operations found that if a 4-mm prosthesis was used there was a 10 per cent frequency of mechanical failure (and a 1 per cent fistula rate), while if a 4.5-mm prosthesis was employed there was a 2 per cent mechanical failure (and a 5 per cent fistula rate). There would appear to be a need for a 4.25-mm piston.

Schuknecht and Feldman (1970) described a series of 154 revision operation findings. The commonest problem was a slipped piston (50 cases). If 35 cases are excluded where the footplate had not been removed, the next commonest assembly fault was incus necrosis (15 cases). Adhesions were found in 13, a fixed malleus in seven, and secondary closure of the oval window by otosclerosis in only four instances. The other problems were mainly sensorineural.

Morrison (1975) reviewing 177 stapedectomy failures of which 100 were revised found four cases of *regrowth of fenestral otosclerosis*. The other causes of conductive failure were similar to those quoted by Schuknecht and Feldman, though there were five tympanic membrane perforations. Especially with the failures of late onset there was frequently more than one problem in the same ear, for example slipped piston with perilymph fistula or adhesions plus unexplained sensorineural deafness.

Revision operations

The results of revision surgery for late failures are disappointing. Donaldson (1976) reporting on the experience from St. Thomas's Hospital indicates that about half these patients were helped; Schuknecht and Feldman (1970) achieved improvements in only 40 per cent of all their revisions; and Morrison (1975) in only 50 per cent of the revision operations for simple conductive loss.

The surgical procedure adopted depends on the findings and on the surgical ingenuity of the operator. There are, however, certain principles to be kept in mind. Reopening of the vestibule carries a 50 per cent risk of inner-ear damage, whether the footplate is redrilled for new otosclerotic growth or if the membrane is simply pierced to insert a new prosthesis. Shambaugh (1967a) advises fenestration in the former situation. If a new prosthesis of bone or cartilage strut is being placed on a good window membrane, the fitting must be exact without pressure on that membrane. Myringoplasty after stapedectomy carries a 20 per cent risk to the inner ear; if surgery is indicated great care must be taken to avoid ossicular movement during the repair.

Provided these risks are avoided, it is certainly worth attempting to reconstruct the sound conducting apparatus after an assembly failure. With care there should be little risk of sensorineural deafness and at least a 50 per cent chance of gain. The division of adhesions, even if quite extensive, rarely results in much improvement.

The indications for revision operation must be carefully weighed for each patient. As much pre-decision information as possible should be obtained from previous records, from audiological and tympanometric assessment and from polytomography. If primary stapedial surgery can, on occasions, be difficult, revision operations can be even more taxing.

References

Altmann, F. and Kornfeld, M. (1965) *Annals of Otology, Rhinology and Laryngology*, **74**, 915

Altmann, F., Kornfeld, M. and Shea, J. J. (1966) *Annals of Otology, Rhinology and Laryngology*, St. Louis, **75**, 5

Anson, B. J. and Donaldson, J. A. (1967) *The Surgical Anatomy of the Temporal Bone and Ear*. Philadelphia; Saunders

Armstrong, B. W. (1967) *Archives of Otolaryngology*, **86**, 156

Bárány, R. (1924). *Acta otolaryngologica Stockholm*, **6**, 260

Basek, M. and Fowler, E. P. Jnr. (1956) *Archives of Otolaryngology*, **63**, 589

Bast, T. H. and Anson, B. J. (1949) *The Temporal Bone and the Ear*, Springfield, Illinois.; Thomas

Blake, C. J. (1892) *Transactions of the American Otology Society*, **5**, 306

Boucheron, E. (1888) *Union Medical, Paris*, **46**, 412

Bretlau, P., Causse, J., Jørgensen, M. B. and Chevance, L. G. (1971) *Archiv fur Klinische u. experimentalle Ohren-, Nasen- u. kehlkopfheilkunde*, **198**, 301

Bretlau, P. and Jorgensen, M. G. (1968) *Journal of Laryngology*, **82**, 65

Brooks, D. N. (1969) *International Audiology*, **8**, 563

Bull, T. R. (1965) *Journal of Laryngology*, **79**, 479

Burtner, D. and Goodman, M. L. (1974) *Archives of Otolaryngology*, **100**, 171

Carhart, R. (1950) *Archives of Otolaryngology*, **51**, 798

Carhart, R. (1966) *Annals of Otology, Rhinology and Laryngology*, St. Louis, **75**, 559

Causse, J., Chevance, L. G., Bretlau, P., Jørgensen, M. B., Uriel, J. and Berges, J. (1977) *Clinical Otolaryngology*, **2**, 23

Cawthorne, T. E. (1951) *Journal of Laryngology*, **65**, 53

Cawthorne, T. E. (1955) *Journal of Laryngology*, **69**, 437

Chevance, L. G., Bretlau, P., Causse, J. and Jørgensen, M. B. (1970) *Acta Otolaryngologica*, Suppl. 272

Chevance, L. G., Causse, J., Bretlau, P., Jørgensen, M. B. and Berges, J. (1972) *Acta Otolaryngologica*, **74**, 23

Clarke, J. A. (1969) *Journal of Laryngology*, **83**, 1045

Cody, T. (1967) *Archives of Otolaryngology*, **85**, 184

Daniel, H. J. (1969) *Archives of Otolaryngology*, **90**, 585

Davies, D. G. (1967) *Journal of Laryngology*, **81**, 649

Dawes. J. D. K. and Curry, A. R. (1969) *Journal of Laryngology*, **83**, 641

Dawes. J. D. K. and Curry, A. R. (1974) *Journal of Laryngology*, **88**, 213

Donaldson, I. (1976) *Journal of Laryngology*, **90**, 915

Fagerhol, M. K. (1975) 'The genetics of alpha-1-antitrypsin and its implications'. In *Aspects of Genetics in Paediatrics'*. Ed. by D. Barltrop, London; Fellowship of Postgraduate Medicine

Faraci, G. (1899) *Archivos italiano Otologica*, **9**, 209

Fisch, U. (1965) *Acta Otolaryngologica*, **60**, 515

Fisch, U. and Rüedi, L. (1968) *Practical Oto-rhino-laryngology*, **30**, 325

Frank, R. Klotz, G. and Höhling, H-J., (1968) *Annals of Otolaryngology*, **85**, 159

Frost, H. M. (1962) In *Otosclerosis*. Ed. by H. F. Schuknecht. London; Churchill

Fussing, T. and Peitersen, E. (1965) *Acta Otolaryngologica Stockholm*, **60**, 265

Gapany-Gapanavičus, B. (1975). *Otosclerosis: Genetics and Surgical Rehabilitation.* New York, Toronto; John Wiley and Sons

Goodhill, V. (1966) *Transactions of the American Academy of Ophthalmology and Oto-Laryngology*, **70**, 370

Gristwood, R. E. (1966) *Journal of Laryngology*, **80**, 1115

Gristwood, R. E. (1972) *Journal of the Oto-laryngology Society of Australia*, **3**, 396

Gristwood, R. E. and Venables, W. N. (1975) *Journal of Laryngology*, **89**, 1185

Gromer, R., Kietzer, G., Oda, M. and Paparella, M. (1974) *Archives of Otolaryngology*, **100**, 168

Gross, C. W. (1969) *Laryngoscope*, **79**, 104

Guild, S. R. (1944) *Annals of Otology, Rhinology and Laryngology*, **53**, 246

Guilford, F. R. (1969) 'Incus Replacement in Stapes Surgery'. In *Otolaryngologic Clinics of North America*. Philadelphia; Saunders

Gunkovich, V. A. and Rosenfeld, L. G. (1974) *Archives of Otolaryngology*, **99**, 281

Hall, I. S. (1945) *Journal of Laryngology*, **60**, 200

Hall, I. S. (1958) Personal communication

Hall, J. G., (1974) *Acta Otolaryngologica*, Suppl. 324

Hammond, V. (1976) *Journal of Laryngology*, **90**, 23

Hanson, J. R., Anson, B. J. and Strickland, E. M. (1962) *Archives of Otolaryngology*, **76**, 200

Harrison, W. H., Shambaugh, G. E. Jnr., Derlacki, E. L. and Clemis, J. D. (1967) *Laryngoscope*, **77**, 836

Harrison, W. H., Shambaugh, G. E. Jr., Derlacki, E. L. and Clemis, J. D. (1970) *Laryngoscope*, **80**, 1000

Hemenway, W. G., Hildyard, V. H. and Black, F. O. (1968) *Laryngoscope*, **78**, 1687

Holden, H. B., Hood, W. G. and Taylor, L. R. S. (1967) *Journal of Laryngology*, **81**, 593

Holleman, I. L. Jnr. and Harrill, J. A. (1967) *Laryngoscope*, **77**, 493

Holmgren, G. (1923) *Acta otolaryngologica, Stockholm*, **5**, 460

Hoogland, G. A. (1977) *ORL*, **39**, 148

Hough, J. V. D. (1969) *Archives of Otolaryngology*, **89**, 414

Hough, J. V. D. (1976) *Journal of Laryngology*, **90**, 15

House, H. P. (1948) *Annals of Otology, Rhinology and Laryngology, St. Louis*, **57**, 41

House, H. P. (1959) *Laryngoscope*, **69**, 1085

House, H. P. (1962) *Archives of Otolaryngology*, **76**, 298

House, H. P. (1967) *Laryngoscope*, **77**, 1410

House, H. P. (1977) Personal communication

House, H. P. and Greenfield, E. C. (1969) *Archives of Otolaryngology*, **89**, 420

House, W. F. (1976) *Annals of Otology, Rhinology and Laryngology*, **85**, Suppl. 27

Jack, F. L. (1893) *Transactions of the American Otological Society*, **5**, 474

Jenkins, G. J. (1914) *Journal of Laryngology*, **29**, 520

Jensen, J., Rovsing, H. and Brunner, S. (1966) *British Journal of Radiology*, **39**, 669

Johnsson, L-G. and Hawkins, J. E. Jr. (1973) *Excerpta medica*, **276**, 177

Kaufman, R. S. and Schuknecht, H. F. (1967) *Annals of Otology, Rhinology and Laryngology, St. Louis*, **76**, 1008

Keleman, G. and Linthicum, F. H. Jr. (1969) *Acta Otolaryngology*, Suppl. 253

Kessel, J. (1878) *Arch. Ohrenheilk.*, **13**, 69

Konigsmark, B. W. (1969) *New England Journal of Medicine*, **281**, 713

Kovács, I. and Gömböri, B. (1973) *Excerpta medica*, **276**, 192

Lawrence, M. and Arbor, A. (1965) *Archives of Otolaryngology*, **82**, 136

Larsson, A. (1960) *Acta otolaryngologica Stockholm*, Suppl., 154

Lempert, J. (1938) *Archives of Otolaryngology*, **28**, 42

Lempert, J. (1946) *Archives of Otolaryngology*, **43**, 199

Lempert, J. (1957) *Archives of Otolaryngology*, **66**, 35

Leonard, J. R. (1967) *Laryngoscope*, **77**, 663

Lindsay, J. R. and Beal, D. D. (1966) *Annals of Otology, Rhinology and Laryngology, St. Louis*, **75**, 436

Linthicum, F. H. Jnr. (1966) *Annals of Otology, Rhinology and Laryngology, St. Louis*, **75**, 512

Linthicum, F. H. Jr., House, H. P. and Althus, S. R. (1973) *Journal of American Medical Association*, **244**, 1482

Lloyd, G. A. S. (1973) 'Polytomography of the Temporal Bone'. In *Recent Advances in Otolaryngology* 4th ed. Edinburgh and London; Churchill Livingstone

Ludman, H. (1968) *Journal of Laryngology*, **82**, 313

Magnus, A. (1876) *Archiv fur Ohrenheilkunde*, **11**, 244

McGee, T. M. (1965) *Archives of Otolaryngology*, **81**, 34

McGee, T. M. (1969) *Archives of Otolaryngology*, **89**, 423

Miot, C. (1890) *Review of Laryngology*, **10**, 49, 83, 145, 200

Moon, C. N. Jr (1970) *Laryngoscope*, **80**, 515

Morgenstein, K. M. and Manace, E. D. (1968) *Laryngoscope*, **78**, 600

Morrison, A. W. (1962) *British Medical Journal*, **1**, 1804

Morrison, A. W. (1967) *Annals of the Royal College of Surgeons of England*, **41**, 202

Morrison, A. W. (1969a) *Proceedings of the Royal Society of Medicine*, **62**, 959

Morrison, A. W. (1969b)) *British Journal of Hospital Medicine*, **2**, 1395

Morrison, A. W. (1971) *Acta oto-rhino-laryngology, Belgium*, **25**, 898

Morrison, A. W. (1975) *Management of Sensorineural Deafness*, London and Boston; Butterworths

Morrison, A. W. and Bundey, Sarah, E. (1970) *Journal of Laryngology*, **84**, 557

Nager, G. T. (1966) *Annals of Otology, Rhinology and Laryngology, St. Louis*, **75**, 481

Naunton, R. F. and Valvassori, G. E. (1969) *Archives of Otolaryngology*, **89**, 372

Nylen, B. (1949) *Journal of Laryngology*, **63**, 321

Owens, E., Sooy, F. A. and Egger, D. T. (1972) *Annals of Otology, Rhinology and Laryngology*, **81**, 157

Paparella, M. M. and Chasin, W. D. (1966) *Journal of Laryngology*, **80**, 511

Paparella, M. M. and Jurgens, G. L. (1972) *Transactions of the American Academy of Otolaryngology and Ophthalmology*, **76**, 147

Passe, E. G. (1949) *Journal of Laryngology*, **63**, 495

Pearson, D., Kurland, L. T. and Cody, D. T. R. (1974) *Archives of Otolaryngology*, **99**, 288

Politzer, A. (1894) *Zeitschrift Ohrenheilkunde*, **25**, 309

Portmann, M. (1961) *Archives of Otolaryngology*, **74**, 11

Reydon, J-L. and Smith, Catherine A. (1968) *Laryngoscope*, **78**, 95

Rosen, S. (1952) *Archives of Otolaryngology*, **56**, 610

Rosen, S. (1953) *New York State Journal of Medicine*, **53**, 2650

Rüedi, L. (1962) In *Otosclerosis* Ed. by H. F. Schuknecht. London; Churchill

Rüedi, L. (1963) *Archives of Otolaryngology*, **78**, 499

Rundle, F. W. and Lawrence, Merle (1961) *University of Michigan Medical Journal*, **27**, 96

Sando, I., Hemenway, W. G., Hildyard, V. H. and English, G. M. (1968) *Annals of Otology, Rhinology and Laryngology, St. Louis*, **77**, 23

Sataloff, J. (1966) *Hearing Loss*. Philadelphia; Lippincott

Schuknecht, H. F. (1971) *Stapedectomy* Boston; Little, Brown

Schuknecht, H. F. (1974) *Pathology of the Ear*. Harvard; Harvard University Press

Schuknecht, H and Feldman, M. (1970) *Laryngoscope*, **80**, 1251

Schuknecht, H. F. and Gross, C. W. (1966) *Annals of Otology, Rhinology and Laryngology, St. Louis*, **75**, 423

Schuknecht, H. F. and Kirchner, J. C. (1974) *Laryngoscope*, **84**, 766

Schuknecht, H. F., McGee, T. M. and Colman, B. H. (1960) *Annals of Otology, Rhinology and Laryngology, St. Louis*, **69**, 597

Sellers, S. L. (1972) *South African Medical Journal*, **46**, 434

Shambaugh, G. E. Jr. (1940) *Illinois Medical Journal*, **81**, 104

Shambaugh, G. E. Jr. (1949) *Archives of Otolaryngology, Stockholm*, Suppl., 79

Shambaugh, G. E. Jr. (1951) *Archives of Otolaryngology*, **54**, 699

Shambaugh, G. E. Jr. (1963) *Archives of Otolaryngology*, **78**, 509

Shambaugh, G. E. Jr. (1966) *Annals of Otology, Rhinology and Laryngology, St. Louis*, **75**, 579

Shambaugh, G. E. (1967a) *Surgery of the Ear*. 2nd edn. Philadelphia; Saunders

Shambaugh, G. E. (1967b) *Annals of Otology, Rhinology and Laryngology, St. Louis*, **76**, 599

Shambaugh, G. E. Jr. (1969) In *Otolaryngologic Clinics of North America*, p. 27. Philadelphia; Saunders

Shambaugh, G. E. Jr. (1971) *Journal of Laryngology*, **85**, 301

Shambaugh, G. E. Jr. and Causse, J. (1974) *Annals of Otology, Rhinology and Laryngology*, **83**, 635

Shambaugh, G. E. Jr. and Juers, A. L. (1946) *Archives of Otolaryngology*, **43**, 549

Shambaugh, G. E. Jr. and Petrovic, A. (1967) *Acta Otolaryngologica*, **63**, 331

Shambaugh, G. E. Jr. and Scott, A. (1964) *Archives of Otolaryngology*, **80**, 263

Shea, J. J. Jr. (1958) *Annals of Otology, Rhinology and Laryngology, St. Louis*, **67**, 932

Shea, J. J. Jr. (1963) *Laryngoscope*, **73**, 508

Shea, J. J. Jr. (1969a) 'A Technique for Stapes Surgery in Obliterative Otosclerosis'. In *Otolaryngologic Clinics of North America*. Philadelphia; Saunders

Shea, J. J. Jr. (1969b) 'Stapes Surgery Symposium'. In *Proceedings of the Centennial Symposium Manhattan Eye, Ear and Throat Hospital*. Vol. 2. *Otolaryngology*. Ed. W. F. Robbett. St. Louis; Mosby

Shea, J. J. (1971) *Transactions of the American Academy of Ophthalmology and Oto-laryngology*, **75**, 31

Shea, J. J. Jr., Hough, J. V. D. and House, P. H. (1969) 'Stapes Surgery Symposium'. In *Proceedings of the Centennial Symposium Manhattan Eye, Ear and Throat Hospital*. Vol. 2. *Otolaryngology*. Ed. W. F. Robbett. St. Louis; Mosby

Sheehy, J. L. (1969) 'Stapes Surgery When the Incus is Missing'. In *Otolaryngologic Clinics of North America*. Philadelphia; Saunders

Siebenmann, F. (1912) *Papers of the International Otology Congress*, **9**, 207

Sooy, F. A. (1960) *Annals of Otology, Rhinology and Laryngology*, **69**, 540

Sourdille, M. (1932) *Revue d'Laryngologie, Paris*, Suppl.

Strickland, E. M., Hanson, J. R. and Anson, B. J. (1962) *Archives of Otolaryngology*, **76**, 100

Toynbee, J. (1861) *Med-Chirurgerie Transactions*, **24**, 190

Valsalva, A. M. (1704) *De aure humana tractatus*. Utrecht

Valvassori, G. E. (1969) *Radiology*, **92**, 449

Valvassori, G. E. (1973) 'Otosclerosis'. In *Otolaryngologic Clinics, North America*, Philadelphia; Saunders

Walsh, T. E. (1967) *Pacific Medical Surgery*, **75**, 188

Willis, R. (1975) *Archives of Otolaryngology*, **101**, 320

Willis, R. (1976) *Journal of Laryngology*, **90**, 31

Wolff, Dorothy and Lempert, J. (1965) *Journal of Laryngology*, **79**, 613

Wright, I. (1977) *Journal of Pathology*, **123**, 5

Young, B. A. (1966) Personal communication

15 Diseases of the otic capsule— II. Other diseases

Andrew W Morrison

Introduction

In this chapter the diseases to be described are of a generalized nature, the temporal-bone involvement forming only a part of the clinical picture. Attention is directed towards the otological manifestations and management of these conditions. Therefore care must be taken not to leave the impression that the non-otological features are of lesser significance. Indeed in some instances, for example syphilis, the generalized disease frequently dictates the management of the patient; while in others, for example osteitis deformans, disability from otological involvement is relatively infrequent.

The majority of these diseases, if they do affect the otic capsule and its contents, result in inner-ear problems. In a few there is a middle-ear component and superficially there is a resemblance to otosclerosis. The latter group will be described first.

Osteogenesis imperfecta

Osteogenesis imperfecta, fragilitas osseum or the syndrome of van der Hoeve and de Kleyn (1918) is a relatively rare disease having a frequency of 2–4/100 000 of the population (Morrison, 1967; Smårs, 1961). It belongs to a group of hereditary disorders of collagen, with a dominant mode of inheritance, incomplete manifestation and varying degrees of expressivity from family to family.

One of the largest recent studies of osteogenesis imperfecta was that of Smårs (1961) from Sweden, containing findings from 190 surviving cases (106 males and 84 females). The clinical features from his data can be summarized as follows. There was a tendency to fractures in 95.8 per cent (the other 4.2 per cent had blue sclerae); blue sclerotics were found in 84.2 per cent; hyperlaxibility was noted in 44.7 per cent; deafness was encountered in 22.6 per cent; a tendency to bruising was observed in 31.1 per cent; and 15.3 per cent had the characteristic dental changes. Rather surprisingly the combination of blue sclerae and deafness without fractures was not observed.

Although only a few of Smårs' 43 deaf subjects were examined by otologists, several important figures about the hearing defect in osteogenesis were elicited. The percentage with deafness increased from 6.8 per cent under 20 years of age to 50 per cent over 50 years of age. Pregnancy increased the hearing loss in three patients. There was no relationship between hearing loss and the severity of the osteogenesis imperfecta as indicated by physical handicap. Deafness was equally common among sporadic and familial cases.

The author has now examined eight families and six sporadic cases, providing a total of 61 affected individuals. Some of these cases have previously been reported (Morrison, 1967 and 1975). The findings are summarized in *Table 15.1*. Almost half the cases of osteogenesis imperfecta had deafness. The hearing loss bore no relationship to the presence, frequency or severity of fractures. Deafness started as early as six years and as late as 51 years of age, with a peak in the third decade. Deafness alone, or deafness and blue sclerae together, *without* fractures were the only manifestations of the disease in 16 of the family members. Stoller's (1962) analysis of 58 cases is similar.

Table 15.1   Association of osteogenesis, blue sclerae and deafness

	Multiple fractures	Blue sclerae	Deafness	Total cases
Sporadic cases	6	3	1	6
Affected individuals in 8 families	30	45	27	55
Totals	36	48	28	61

Because of the superficial resemblance of the deafness in osteogenesis to the deafness of otosclerosis there has been a natural tendency for otologists to consider them as different manifestations of the same disease. Hlavácek and Chtádek (1963), for example, claimed that of 292 patients with otosclerosis no fewer than 22 per cent had blue sclerae, 12 per cent had a tendency to fractures and 1.7 per cent had the full van der Hoeve syndrome. A similar argument based on the temporal bone pathology has been advanced by Wullstein, Ogilvie and Hall (1960) and by Ogilvie and Hall (1962). The temporal bone changes are more widespread, however (*Figure 15.1*), and the deafness, though nearly always having a conductive component, tends to be more severe than in otosclerosis and to have a greater sensorineural element.

It must be remembered that blue sclerae, though classically associated with fragilitas osseum, occur as an isolated family disorder and also in association with Marfan's syndrome (McKusick, 1955), as well as with otosclerosis. Morrison and Bundey (1970), however, examining 240 families with otosclerosis found only one of these families with blue sclerae affecting some of its members. Furthermore, osteogenesis imperfecta frequently manifests itself as a widespread collagen disease involving bone, joints, sclerae, teeth, blood vessels and skin. There is no evidence of skeletal abnormalities, of the characteristic amelogenesis nor of any haemorrhagic diathesis in patients with otosclerosis. Sporadic cases are frequent in otosclerosis (perhaps 1 in 3) but rare in osteogenesis imperfecta. Otosclerosis is known only to occur in man, whereas osteogenesis imperfecta is found also in other animals including dogs and pigs.

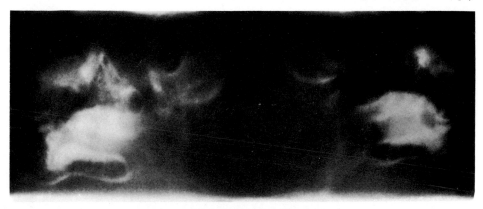

Figure 15.1   Osteogenesis imperfecta. Postero–anterior hypocycloidal polytomogram showing diffuse involvement of the whole labyrinthine and otic capsule by the disease. There are mottled areas of sclerosis and lysis. On the left side the oval window area is better defined though still involved

The superficial similarity in temporal bone histology between the two conditions could be extended to include osteitis deformans and osteitis fibrosa cystica—two very different diseases. Studies by Clerc and Chevance (1965) involving several staining techniques, have shown significant differences in the microscopic pathology of the stapes footplate in otosclerosis and in osteogenesis imperfecta. They conclude that microscopic fractures of the footplate and subsequent healing are the important causes of the stapedo–vestibular fixation in osteogenesis imperfecta. Altmann and Kornfeld (1967), from histological and histochemical evidence, also consider them to be different diseases.

Clinical features and treatment

As noted, the hearing loss in the van der Hoeve syndrome may start in childhood or be delayed well into adult life. It usually progresses from the third decade. Of the deaf patients in *Table 15.1*, some 40 per cent had quite severe sensorineural involvement when first seen, apart from any element of conductive hearing loss. Healed fractures of the handle of the malleus were seen in two of the 29 patients. Only four were considered to have an air–bone gap which justified stapedial surgery. Despite the widespread changes in the otic capsule (*Figure 15.1*), a Schwartze sign has not been seen in any of these patients, nor, surprisingly, have any of them had vertiginous symptoms.

A typical example of one of the patients is shown in *Figure 15.2*. As in otosclerosis the acoustic reflexes cannot be elicited. Compare this with the state of affairs in Paget's disease of bone (p. 468). Note the very high compliance values, outside normal range, despite the ossicular fixation. This is assumed to result from the abnormal collagen causing excessive laxity of the drum. It might account for a few decibels of high-tone conductive deafness. On closer examination, therefore, the hearing loss in osteogenesis imperfecta may be distinguished from otosclerosis.

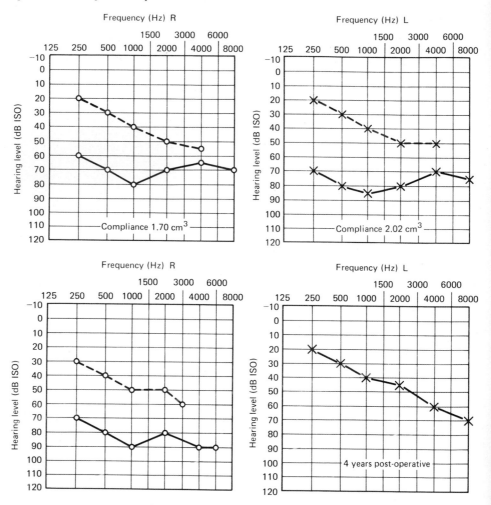

Figure 15.2   Osteogenesis imperfecta. Pure-tone audiograms (above) from a woman of 52 with a 14-year history of progressive bilateral deafness which started during her first pregnancy and became worse during her second pregnancy. She has blue sclerotics and in childhood had suffered from several fractures after trivial trauma. Her mother had osteogenesis imperfecta and deafness. Her first child was normal. Her son, aged seven, had blue sclerotics and had already suffered three fractures. Note the high compliance values compared with otosclerosis. Polytomography showed all the classic features (*see Figure 15.1*). A left total stapedectomy was performed after removing a floating footplate. Reconstruction with a McGee piston and fat graft. The hearing result is maintained four years later (below) though the other side has deteriorated

There is no known medical treatment for the condition. Very severe cases die '*in utero*'; severe cases are badly crippled in childhood; in the average case fractures, which heal normally, cease to occur in adolesence, though the skull involvement continues into adult life causing the typical 'soldier's helmet skull' and deafness; and in mild cases there are only two or three childhood fractures, or possibly blue sclerae and deafness as the only manifestations.

There is conflicting evidence in the literature on the surgical findings. In the author's limited experience, the footplate of the stapes resembles otosclerosis, but thick vascular bone had not been encountered. The footplate fixation, has in all cases, been classed as type 1 or 2 and, as in the case in *Figure 15.2*, there has been a 50 per cent incidence of 'floating footplate'. This observation has also been made by Kosoy and Maddox (1971) who had generally satisfactory results from stapedectomy in four out of five patients.

Generally good results have been recorded by Stoller (1962), Hoogland (1962, 1963), Shea, Smyth and Altmann (1963), and Patterson and Stone (1970) for example. The continuing disease process, however, and the likelihood of some sensorineural loss should be explained to the patient before surgery.

It is axiomatic that surgery be delayed until many years after all 'spontaneous' fractures have stopped. Even so, at surgery the long process of the incus looks thin and weak and must be managed with great care.

Opheim (1968) seems to have been the first to observe degeneration of the stapedial crura. Similar changes have been noted by others including Patterson and Stone (1970). These changes might have resulted from spontaneous fractures of the arch which, even in healthy subjects, do not produce osseous healing. This possibility should be borne in mind if surgery is contemplated.

Amelogenesis imperfecta is found in about 15 per cent of patients with osteogenesis imperfecta. There is an irregular formation of dentine which results in cracking of the overlying enamel. The teeth are yellow, opaque and irregular. To the inexperienced eye the changes resemble tetracycline staining. Amelogenesis imperfecta can occur as the only manifestation of the disease. Two patients have been encountered with amelogenesis imperfecta and associated inner-ear problems. Both demonstrated abnormal sclerosis of the otic capsule on polytomography, both complained of tinnitus and paroxysmal vertigo attacks and one had moderately severe sensorineural deafness. Clinically they resembled 'idiopathic' Menière's disease.

The *other inherited disorders of collagen*, Marfan's syndrome, the Ehlers–Danlos syndrome and pseudoanthoma elasticum do not appear to involve the otic capsule though rare cases of otosclerosis associated with the Ehlers-Danlos syndrome have been reported (Mair, Schrøder and Johannessen, 1974), and Schuknecht (1974) notes that both conductive and sensorineural deafness have been recorded in Marfan's syndrome.

Osteitis deformans

Paget's disease of bone, of unknown aetiology, is characterized by spreading osteolytic and osteoblastic changes affecting mainly the pelvis, lumbosacral spine, skull and femoral and tibial bones. Although the condition may be widespread in the skeleton, it tends to affect localized areas.

Woodhouse (1973) estimated that perhaps three quarters of a million people have the disease in Britain. Collins (1956) found evidence of it in 3.7 per cent of 650 post-mortem examinations of people over 40 years of age. Symptoms, however, seem to occur in only 5 per cent of those affected. It is mainly a disease of Caucasians and there is a familial pattern (Barry, 1969), most probably a simple autosomal Mendelian dominant inheritance (McKusick, 1966). Hereditary factors are difficult to estimate because of incomplete genetic manifestation and the late age of onset. The disease is rarely seen before the age of 40 years and is more commonly encountered after the age of 55 years.

The pathological changes are explained by the excessive osteoclastic and osteoblastic activity resulting in a greatly increased rate of bone resorption and deposition. Thus adjacent areas of osteolytic and sclerotic bone with increased vascularity replace the normal Haversian systems. This gives rise to bone softening, a tendency to fractures and deformity, bone pain, typical biochemical changes and the classic radiological picture of thickened cortex, mottled appearance and the loss of normal architecture. The temporal bone is involved, sooner or later, in perhaps 50 per cent of those with clinical manifestations.

When one considers these general features it is not surprising that otosclerosis has been considered as a very localized and less severe variant of Paget's disease.

The histopathological changes in the temporal bone also have a resemblance to otosclerosis. They have been described by, among others, Kornfeld (1967), Rüedi (1968), Davies (1968), Lindsay and Lehman (1969) and by Schuknecht (1974). Apart from the general loss of bone architecture, when the endosteal layer of the otic capsule is involved by osteitis, degenerative changes occur in the stria vascularis with atrophy of the structures of the cochlear duct and vestibular labyrinth. Both secondary endolymphatic hydrops of the cochlear duct and saccule, and atrophy of the membranous semicircular canals have been described. Schuknecht (1974) reviews the 24 recorded cases of temporal bone histology in Paget's disease. Only two showed osteitis in the stapes footplate and only one of these two involved the annular ligament of the stapes. The footplate seems to be relatively immune from involvement in Paget's disease, though the remainder of the ossicular chain is affected.

Clinical features

Considering the frequency of the disease it is surprising how seldom the deafness of Paget's disease is encountered in otological practice. Morrison (1975) found it to be the cause of deafness in about one out of every 200 deaf patients. Three to four cases of Paget's deafness are seen for every 100 with otosclerosis.

When there are obvious skeletal changes (bowing of the legs, kyphosis, short stature and enlarged skull), bone pain and sometimes enlargement of the temporal arteries, the diagnosis is straightforward. However, osteitis deformans can be symptomless apart from the otological features. In these circumstances the diagnosis could readily be missed, and patients with a large element of conductive deafness could be considered to have otosclerosis. The deafness of Paget's disease normally starts after the age of 45 years, a less usual age for the development of otosclerosis.

In patients with Paget's deafness there are usually obvious signs in the plain skull radiographs. These, however, are not inevitable. Davies (1968) reviewing 236 patients with the disease, found skull involvement in 165 and deafness in 97. Of the 97 with deafness there was no plain x-ray evidence of Paget's in 14; vertigo was a complaint in 35 and tinnitus, often pulsatile, in 31.

It is also customary, when there is deafness in Paget's disease to find elevation of the serum alkaline phosphatase from the osteoblastic activity, and an increase in the total urinary hydroxyproline from osteoclastic activity. The serum calcium level is usually normal even though the rate of turnover of bone calcium is enormously increased and calcium is lost from the skeleton.

There is normally a mixture of conductive and sensorineural deafness, though one may predominate. In the earlier stages of its development the disease causes a conductive deafness in some 70 per cent of affected ears, though there is always a high-tone sensory loss (*Figure 15.3*). The hearing loss is usually fairly symmetrical. In the earlier stages when the deafness is not so severe as to make it impossible to initiate the stapedial reflex, this reflex is always present. This does not occur in otosclerosis, nor in osteogenesis imperfecta when as little as 15–20 dB of deafness due to stapedial fixation abolishes the reflex. Another example of persistence of the acoustic stapedial reflex is shown in *Figure 15.4*, despite up to 40 dB of conductive loss.

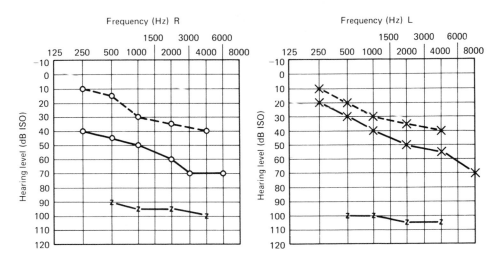

Figure 15.3 Paget's disease. Pure-tone audiograms and acoustic reflexes (Z–Z) from a woman of 74 with a two-year history of progressive bilateral deafness, intermittent tinnitus and, during the first year, attacks of transient paroxysmal vertigo. Compliance on the right side was 0.80 cm^3, and on the left 0.55 cm^3. She had no other symptoms. The diagnosis, suspected on the history and classic audiological findings, was confirmed by plain x-rays of the skull and by the finding of a significantly raised serum alkaline phosphatase. In view of her age and the absence of other symptoms she was given a hearing aid

The causation of the conductive component of the deafness seems to be involvement of the ossicles, mainly the malleus head by osteitis deformans (*Figure 15.5*). Fixation of the malleus/incus in the attic seems possible but unlikely, since even in cases with a marked middle-ear deafness, though the compliance values are low, the tympanogram still shows a peak at atmospheric pressure. With malleus/incus fixation the tympanogram is usually flat or peaked on the negative side of the graph. Davies (1968) noted that the air–bone gap averaged 30 dB in females and 20 dB in males. His finding that the gap tends to be greatest at 500 Hz is confirmed by the author's experience.

In about 20 per cent of patients the otological manifestation is a progressive sensory hearing loss. Even in this group of patients, however, there may be a conductive element (*Figure 15.6*). A Schwartze sign may be present. Specialized tests, at least in the earlier stages, show that the inner-ear loss is mainly sensory. With long-standing

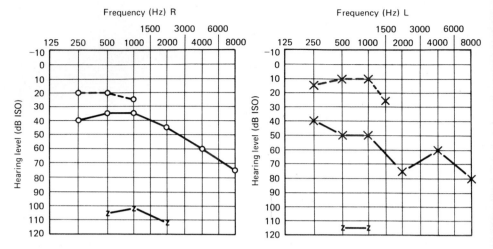

Figure 15.4   Paget's disease. Pure-tone audiograms and acoustic reflexes (Z–Z) from a woman of 57 with a 15-month history of progressive bilateral deafness. Note the presence of the acoustic reflexes despite the severity of the conductive loss. Also note the typical high-tone sensorineural deafness. On the right side compliance was 0.35 cm^3, and on the left 0.16 cm^3. She had long established Paget's disease affecting the skull, maxillae, pelvis and long bones. Bone pain was not a significant feature. Surgery to the left ear was declined and a hearing aid was supplied

skull disease the hearing loss can become subtotal (*Figure 15.7*). Secondary neuronal degeneration seems likely in the later stages of the disease, and if there is sufficient softening and deformity of the skull base the nerves may even be involved in the internal auditory meatus.

The vertigo in patients with osteitis deformans is seldom a very prominent feature. It can mimic Menière's disease when it is presumably due to secondary hydrops. More often, however, it consists of transient episodes of vertigo or unsteadiness. Davies (1968) considered it more likely to arise from vertebro–basilar insufficiency secondary to bone disease of the cervical spine. If this were so, one would expect this symptom to progress and continue, whereas in Paget's disease the vertiginous episodes have a reasonably good prognosis and tend to settle after a number of years.

Treatment

There are several factors which argue against *stapedectomy* in the treatment of the conductive deafness of Paget's disease. Firstly there is the lack of post-mortem histological evidence of stapedial fixation; secondly there is the almost inevitable sensorineural deafness which is present and which progresses; thirdly there is the age group of these patients to be considered; and fourthly there is the experience gained from surgical treatment.

Sellars and Fine (1975) who argue in favour of stapedectomy reported three operations. There was failure of closure of the air–bone gap in all three and in one an 18-month improvement after surgery was followed by total bilateral deafness. The other two were still moderately better 2–3 years after surgery. From an earlier report

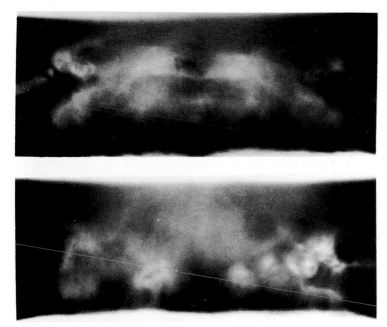

Figure 15.5 Paget's disease of the otic capsule. Hypocycloidal macrograms from two different patients with osteitis deformans. Note the extensive demineralization and osteoporosis in both, making it difficult to identify specific features. In the upper film the enlarged head of malleus is visible on both sides. In the lower film, on the left, the basal coil, vestibule and oval window are just discernible. In Paget's disease the conductive element of the hearing loss is due to ossicular involvement rather than stapedial ankylosis. Otic capsular disease causes a variable sensorineural component in all cases

Waltner (1965) recorded some improvement in only three out of five stapedectomies and none had closure of the air–bone gap. Follow-up was not longer than one year. Sparrow and Duval (1967) reported one stapedectomy for Paget's disease—the footplate was histologically normal and the patient had some hearing gain for a few months only. Davies (1968) reports two stapedectomies for this disease; in one there was a very temporary 15-dB gain and in the other there was failure to close the air–bone gap. Morrison (1975) reported two stapedectomies on patients with 40–50 dB air–bone gaps. In each case the stapes was found to be normal. Both had a very temporary hearing gain followed by progressive conductive and sensorineural loss.

Stapes or rather *ossicular mobilization* may have a place in the temporary management of a few of these younger patients with a good air–bone gap. Goodhill (1960) achieved a moderate hearing gain after mobilization. Sparrow and Duval (1967) also reported a mobilization improvement which was still present six years later. Morrison (1975), on the other hand, mentioned two good hearing results after mobilization which reverted slowly to the pre-operative levels within a few months and which, with the passage of years, developed increasing sensory loss on both sides.

If any surgery is indicated for the conductive deafness of osteitis deformans, one would imagine it to be removal of the incus and malleus head with appropriate incus replacement.

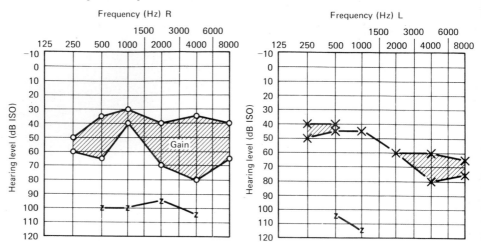

Figure 15.6   Sensory deafness in Paget's disease and the hearing gain with calcitonin therapy. A woman of 69 with a one-year history of headaches and progressive bilateral deafness, and a six-month history of episodic vertigo. Skull radiographs confirmed the diagnosis (not previously made). Her alkaline phosphatase was 66.5 units per cent. Caloric responses were normal. When first seen there was an air–bone gap of 10–15 dB on both sides. The acoustic reflexes were present (Z–Z). Compliance on the right was 0.1 cm³ and on the left 0.15 cm³, confirming a middle-ear component. Apart from these complaints she was found to have a high output heart failure.

She was treated with porcine calcitonin 80 units i.m. daily for a period of four months. Hearing gain on the right (shaded area) was obvious at one month and reached the level shown at four months. Her alkaline phosphatase fell during treatment to 34.5 units per cent, but there was no obvious radiographic change. Her heart failure was not significantly improved. Over the next year there was some loss of the hearing gain though she remained better than the pre-treatment level

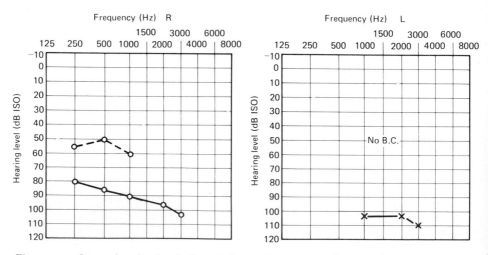

Figure 15.7   Severe hearing loss in Paget's disease. Pure-tone audiograms from a woman of 77 with a 30-year history of headaches; progressive bilateral deafness and, during the first ten years, episodes of vertigo. She had all the typical deformities and the classic radiographic and biochemical changes. She derived some benefit from the use of a body-worn aid on the right. On account of the severity of the hearing loss and the persisting headaches, daily calcitonin injections were started. She found outpatient travelling difficult and therapy was stopped after two weeks without benefit

Medical therapy with calcitonin holds some promise for the future. At present a major limiting factor is the need for daily or twice daily injections continuing for many months, given to patients who are mainly elderly and often infirm. Permanent replacement or maintenance treatment would be most costly. In the case of calcitonin of porcine or salmon origin, there is also the risk that antibody formation may interfere with treatment.

The subject is reviewed by Woodhouse (1974) who considers that, in Paget's disease, uncontrolled bone pain and hypercalcaemia are the indications for calcitonin therapy. Deafness is not mentioned. There are, however, reports of hearing improvement with this treatment (Shai, Baker and Wallach, 1971; Moffatt, Morrow and Simpson, 1974; Morrison, 1975). To be effective in preventing the development of widespread skeletal disease and severe hearing loss it seems likely that younger adults with evidence of rapidly progressing Paget's disease would be the best candidates for long-term therapy. When other patients are first seen with extensive disease, temporary amelioration of symptoms with shorter-term therapy seems logical. The otologist should cooperate with the metabolic physician in the management of these patients.

Woodhouse (1973) indicates that calcitonin may be important in the differentiation of bone cells and in the process of remodelling of bone. In the treatment of Paget's disease, calcitonin produces an immediate fall in the urinary hydroxyproline from a rapid slowing of osteoclastic activity. The raised serum alkaline phosphatase starts to fall after one to two weeks from reduced osteoblastic activity. With continued therapy there is a reduction in the rapid turnover of calcium and a gradual remineralization of bone. Longer-term responses vary from patient to patient and according to the severity of the disease. As Woodhouse (1974) points out, dosage schemes are not fully worked out yet and this form of treatment should still be considered experimental. It is encouraging that, so far, no serious side effects or toxic reactions have been reported.

Other diseases affecting the temporal bones

Osteitis fibrosa cystica or von Recklinghausen's disease of bone

This is very rarely seen in otological practice. Primary hyperparathyroidism, usually due to adenoma, causing hypercalcaemia normally presents as renal colic or with gastrointestinal symptoms. Bone pain from osteitis fibrosa cystica is less usual and sometimes the condition is found by accident. There are few if any physical signs and the diagnosis can on occasion be difficult even for the physician. The plasma calcium levels are high and, when there is osteitis fibrosa cystica, the alkaline phosphatase is raised. A minority of patients show radiological change, the skull and phalanges being mainly involved. The loss of bone calcium produces a mottled appearance not unlike Paget's disease. The usual treatment is to locate and remove the parathyroid adenoma, though some symptomless cases are kept under observation.

Secondary hyperparathyroidism can occur in chronic renal failure or in osteomalacia with the administration of vitamin D or calciferol.

Rüedi (1968) has described the temporal bone changes in four ears from two patients with osteitis fibrosa cystica. The pathological features were similar to those

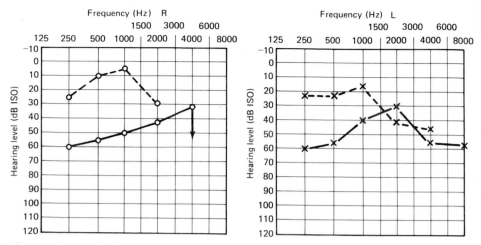

Figure 15.8   Osteitis fibrosa cystica. Pure-tone audiograms from a man of 46, with no previous history of ear disease, who presented with one month's history of rapidly progressive bilateral hearing loss. Both drums looked dull and had white patches which, in retrospect, must have been calcium deposits. The patient had no other complaints. He was seen in the mid 1960s before the impedance bridge was in regular use. Diagnostic myringotomy, as an outpatient, revealed no fluid in either middle ear. He defaulted from follow up. Some months later it was learned that he had been admitted to another hospital with terminal hypercalcinosis

found in the temporal bone in Paget's disease. Otological presentation must be exceptionally rare and, as in the case in *Figure 15.8*, the diagnosis could readily be missed.

Idiopathic osteoporosis

Henkin, Lifschitz and Larson (1972) recently described the otological findings in seven patients with idiopathic osteoporosis. All had sensorineural deafness greater than would be expected for their ages. All had low normal compliance values. On tomographic study the otic capsule showed relative sclerosis in five of these patients and the degree of sclerosis bore a relationship to the severity of hearing loss. These findings raise the question of the relationship of senile osteoporosis to that variant of presbyacusis described by Schuknecht (1974) in which there is spiral ligament atrophy similar to that seen adjacent to areas of otosclerosis, Paget's disease, or inflammatory osteitis.

Osteopetrosis

Abnormalities of bone causing increase of hard tissue at the expense of soft tissue are classified as osteopetrosis or 'marble bones'. The disease is uncommon. It is seen chiefly in infants as a recessive hereditary disease which is usually fatal in consequence of profound anaemia. A less severe form, probably due to a dominant inheritance (Johnson *et al.*, 1968) is also seen. It was described first by Albers-Schönberg (1904) whose name is frequently given to the disease.

There is marked thickening of the calvarium and skull base with narrowing of the foraminae. This results in cranial nerve lesions with the optic, trigeminal and facio-acoustic being mainly involved. The temporal bone pathology is described by Schuknecht (1974) and the clinical features by Hamersma (1973), who has encountered a remarkable number of cases in South Africa.

In the more benign form, the head is usually enlarged by adolescence and there may be recurrent facial palsies. In this variant there is rarely anaemia and the lifespan may be normal. Headaches are a feature. Conductive deafness, due to ossicular immobility and stapes fixation (Jones and Mulcahy, 1968) occur at an early age and there is usually a progressive sensorineural loss possibly due to compression of the acoustic nerves. The diagnosis is readily made on radiological examination, which shows the increased skull dimensions, the extreme sclerosis with loss of diploeic spaces and the absence of pneumatization. There is no known treatment though decompression surgery for the seventh and eight nerve lesions may have to be considered.

Another rare cause of 'osteopetrosis' described by Weir (1977) is recessive hypophosphataemic vitamin D-resistant rickets. Sensorineural deafness is described in some of the cases due to extreme narrowing of the internal auditory meatus.

Fibrous dysplasia of the temporal bone

This is also rare. It is more frequently seen by otolaryngologists affecting the upper jaw.

It is a chronic disease, of unknown aetiology, which usually manifests itself in childhood, adolesence or early adult life, which develops and progresses very slowly and which often reaches a static phase in middle age. Females are more often affected. The term *fibrous dysplasia* was first used by Lichtenstein and Jaffe (1942). It used to be considered as a variant of hyperparathyroidism though as early as 1931, Hunter and Turnbull, naming it osteitis fibrosa, recognized it as a separate entity characterized by localized fibrous 'tumours' of bone with no generalized skeletal involvement and without the biochemical changes seen in osteitis fibrosa cystica. Nevertheless if several bones are involved, hyperparathyroidism must be carefully excluded.

The characteristic histological appearance is of bone replaced by fibrous tissue with variable osteoclastic and osteoblastic activity. Radiologically the picture varies with the histology from lytic areas to sclerosis. The swellings are seen as moderately dense soft tissue masses.

The rarity of temporal bone involvement is pointed out by Williams and Thomas (1975). Probably less than 20 cases are recorded. They are reviewed by Schuknecht (1974). The author has seen only one such monosteal case. There is usually slowly progressive painless swelling in the mastoid or temporal fossa with obliteration or stenosis of the external auditory meatus. Initially the hearing loss is conductive. The otic capsule, however, is not immune and eventually the inner ear may be involved. Biopsy confirms the diagnosis. Mastoid surgery is usually necessary for cosmetic reasons and to re-establish the external meatus. Multiple operations frequently ensue.

Tumour or tumour-like lesions can affect the otic capsule and the structures of the inner ear. *Carcinoma* may arise in the middle ear (*Figure 15.9*) or present as a secondary deposit in the temporal bone. *Embryonic sarcoma* or primary bone tumour (*chondrosarcoma* or *osteogenic sarcoma*) arising in this area is very rare. Tumours of the jugular bulb

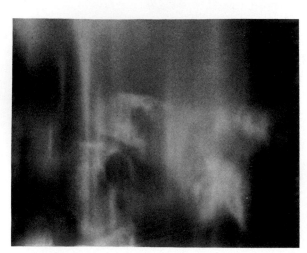

Figure 15.9   Primary squamous carcinoma of the middle ear. Left temporal bone tomogram from a man of 67 who presented with a one-month history of progressive left deafness, earache, unsteadiness and partial facial weakness. There was no past history of ear disease and the tympanic membrane was normal. There was total hearing loss on this side. The extensive destruction of the otic and labyrinthine capsule is shown. Transmastoid biopsy confirmed the diagnosis. No other primary was found or subsequently revealed itself. Initial response to radiotherapy was good

(*chemodectoma* or *neurinoma*) may enlarge upwards and erode the cochlear capsule. *Developmental cholesteatoma* of the petrous apex, growing insidiously from birth, usually presents in the third decade when erosion of the cochlea causes sensorineural hearing loss, often of sudden onset, tinnitus, dull pain and vertiginous symptoms. Similar destruction is sometimes seen from *trigeminal neurinoma* or *meningioma* of the cerebello–pontine angle. In the case of meningioma the tumour can invade the temporal bone. Diseases of the reticulo–endothelial system such as *eosinophil granuloma or plasmocytoma* are occasionally seen invading the temporal bone and inner ear. They cause extensive osteolytic destruction. *Wegener's granuloma*, though rare in this site, has a similar destructive effect.

Osteoradionecrosis of the temporal bone can occur months to many years after therapy which includes one or both temporal bones in the irradiated field. This disease with illustrative case histories has recently been reviewed by Ramsden, Bulman and Lorigan. (1975). Apart from irradiation atrophy of the membranous inner ear, sequestration and suppuration may involve the otic capsule.

Late syphilis

Late syphilitic osteitis involving the otic capsule, whether congenital or acquired, is not infrequently encountered in otological practice. Untreated it carries a poor prognosis. To be treated it must be diagnosed. To be diagnosed it must be suspected. To be suspected it must be in the forefront of the clinician's mind when presented with any patient who complains of deafness, tinnitus or vertigo.

Pathology

There are now many comprehensive descriptions of the temporal bone histopathology in late syphilis, mostly from congenital cases (Mayer and Fraser, 1936; Goodhill,

1939; Perlman and Leek, 1952; Karmody and Schuknecht, 1966; Mack *et al.*, 1969; Schuknecht, 1974). All three layers of the otic capsule are involved by osteitis with patchy resorption of bone and inflammatory infiltration. As in all gummatous lesions there is endarteritis and infiltration with lymphocytes, plasma cells and giant cells. The spiral ligament and modiolus are commonly involved. The striking feature is usually the hydrops of the cochlear duct, saccule and utricle. Atrophic changes occur in the spiral ligament, the organ of Corti, the cristae of all the semicircular canals and in the cochlear and vestibular nerves. Cellular damage in the organ of Corti is frequently complete, though the structures in the middle coil may survive longer. Connective tissue is frequently seen in the perilymphatic spaces especially the basal end of the scala tympani. There may be ruptures of the basilar membrane or of Reissner's membrane. The extent of neuronal degeneration varies from moderate to total (*Figures 15.10* and *15.11*). The pathogenesis of the hydrops is probably the obliteration of the endolymphatic duct in the region of its sinus. Mayer and Fraser (1936) emphasized that gummatous infiltration in this site is common.

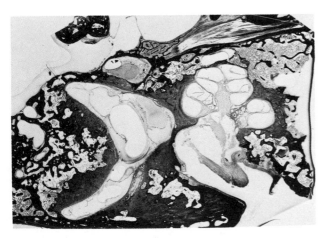

Figure 15.10   Horizontal section of the left temporal bone showing the features of late syphilis in a woman aged 70 with congenital syphilis and long-standing bilateral sensorineural deafness. There is patchy destruction of all three layers of the otic capsule, and a gumma adjacent to the posterior canal; also hydrops of the cochlear and vestibular labyrinths. In the basal coil of the cochlea there is degeneration of the organ of Corti, atrophy of the stria vascularis and loss of the spiral ganglion. (Photomicrograph by kind permission of Professor H. F. Schuknecht, Boston, USA)

The persistence of *Treponema pallidum* has been demonstrated in several sites in late-treated human syphilis. (Collart, Borel and Durel, 1962a, b, c; Smith and Israel, 1967 a, b; Smith, Israel and Harmer, 1967; Goldman and Girard, 1967; Rice, Jones and Wilkinson, 1968; Dunlop, King and Wilkinson, 1968). These sites include lymph nodes, the liver, the temporal artery, the anterior chamber of the eye and the cerebrospinal fluid. It seems likely that the spirochaetes demonstrated in the temporal bone by Mack *et al.* (1969) were also persistent *T. pallidum*. This has significant therapeutic implications.

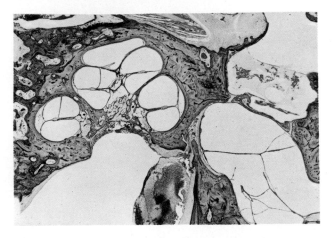

Figure 15.11   Horizontal section of right temporal bone in late syphilis in a man aged 48 with a 30-year history of progressive bilateral deafness which had been total on this side for ten years before death. There is marked hydrops and the saccule is distended to the footplate of the stapes; also advanced degeneration of the organ of Corti and near-total loss of cochlear neurons. Similar changes affect the sensory epithelium and neural elements of the vestibular system. (Photomicrograph by kind permission of Professor H. F. Schuknecht, Boston, USA)

Prevalence

The numbers of *new* cases of congenital syphilis presenting for treatment each year in England and Wales are to be found in the Annual Reports of the Chief Medical Officer. In 1931 there were 2439 new congenital cases, in 1950 there were 1223, in 1968 there were 254, in 1972 (England only) there were 159 notifications and in 1976 (England and Wales) there were 137 cases (provisional figure).

The figures have declined dramatically in the past 50 years and appear to be stabilizing at about 150 new cases each year. The majority of these patients are diagnosed in their first, second or third decades. Let us assume that they have a life expectancy of as little as 40 years. From the notification figures of the last 40 years or thereabouts it can be calculated that, in England and Wales with a population of about 49 million (Census, 1971), there are currently about 50 000 cases of diagnosed congenital syphilis. This is a figure of 1 in 980 or 0.1 per cent. Karmody and Schuknecht (1966) estimate that about one in three patients with congenital syphilis develop otological manifestations, often many years after the initial diagnosis. This proportion could well be higher. In addition there must be a number of undiagnosed cases in the population and some must have escaped the notification network.

Compared with congenital syphilis, temporal bone involvement in late acquired disease is less common. Three cases of the former are likely to be seen for one of the latter. Newly notified cases of *late* acquired syphilis, however, are more frequent than new congenital ones. In 1972, for example, there were 2.50/100 000 of the population in England compared with 0.34/100 000 congenital cases. The diagnosis of late acquired syphilitic ear disease is probably missed quite often, especially in elderly male patients.

In a consecutive series of 1550 adults and children with hearing loss, Morrison (1975) found evidence of syphilitic ear disease in 21 (1.4 per cent); and in those with sensorineural deafness the percentage was as high as 2.5 per cent. If the notification trends continue, however, it is likely that fewer congenital cases will be seen, at least in the UK, in the next 20 years.

Natural history

With a few exceptions the clinical picture and prognosis are the same in congential syphilitic and late acquired ear disease. The temporal bone is affected 10–60 years after the primary infection. Congenital cases present with otological manifestations from childhood to old age, though the great majority are seen before the age of 50 years. Acquired cases are mainly seen over the age of 40 years.

Congenital syphilitic deafness is commoner in females (Hahn, Rodin and Haskins, 1962; Karmody and Schuknecht, 1966; Morrison, 1975). Acquired syphilis affecting the ear is twice as common in males.

For a long time it has been recognized that the natural history is one of slow relentless progression to profound bilateral deafness; there are occasional fluctuations and sometimes sudden deafness. The great majority of patients with late syphilis of the temporal bones have had previous antitreponemal therapy which does not appear to affect this prognosis. The rapidity of progression of deafness is quite variable. Within the first five years of otological manifestations , the hearing loss may be as little as 40 dB or as great as 120 dB. After 15 years these patients would be fortunate to have a hearing level of 70–80 dB on either side. An example of this progression is shown in *Figure 15.12*.

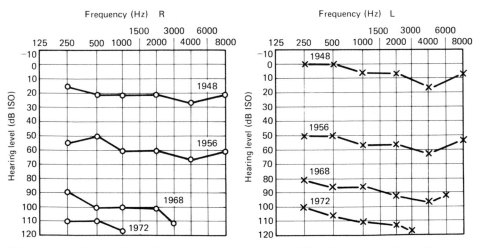

Figure 15.12 Progression of deafness in late acquired syphilis of the temporal bone. Pure-tone audiograms from an elderly male patient whose primary infection was in 1928 when he was treated with bismuth and arsenicals. Between 1948 and 1956 when he was experiencing attacks of vertigo and progressive deafness, he was retreated many times with penicillin. He was treated again in 1968. Steroids were not used

Fluctuations in hearing and in speech discrimination (Hahn, Rodin and Haskins, 1962; Dawkins, Sharp and Morrison, 1968) are a definite feature of late acquired and congenital syphilitic deafness and occur in about a third of cases. Sudden total or severe loss—presumably due to cochlear duct rupture or acute hydrops—is seen in 20 per cent of affected ears. Some patients are unfortunate enough to experience this sudden loss on both sides. Acute auditory failure due to late syphilis is seldom seen in an ear with previously normal hearing; it is more likely to occur when the otological symptoms have been present for a few years. Tinnitus, a common symptom in those patients, is a more prominent feature after sudden loss.

In most congenital cases the onset of deafness is bilateral and the progression symmetrical. This sort of symmetry is seen in only 50 per cent of acquired cases. In the latter, symptoms frequently remain unilateral for a number of years. Eventually both sides become involved.

Vestibular disturbances can be the presenting feature and an important part of the natural history. At some stage of the disease vestibular symptoms or signs are seen in the majority of patients, usually accompanying the onset of deafness in one or other ear. The vestibular manifestations fall into two roughly equal groups. In the first there are paroxysmal attacks of rotary vertigo lasting from 15 min to several days. On the history these episodes can be indistinguishable from Menière's disease. The acute attacks of longer duration are frequently misdiagnosed as 'vascular accidents' or 'viral infections'. In the second group slowly progressive bilateral destruction of the vestibular end-organs results in progressive imbalance and unsteadiness of gait, especially in the dark. The ataxia can vary in severity. In congenital cases with bilateral blindness it can be a great problem. In younger patients when vestibular destruction is gradual and compensation is good the evidence of vestibular loss may come only from testing.

Otological and vestibular features

In both congenital and acquired late syphilis of the ear, the commonest pattern of pure-tone hearing loss is high tone accounting for 35 per cent of affected ears (*Figure 15.13*). Flat audiograms are seen in 25 per cent, total or subtotal deafness in 20 per cent and low-tone loss or a peaked audiogram in 20 per cent.

Considering the pathological tendency to hydrops and the greater likelihood of hair-cell preservation in the middle coil, it seems surprising that there is not a higher frequency of flat, low-tone or peaked hearing losses. When the data from earlier cases is examined (deafness of less then two years' duration), it is found that the frequency of these audiogram types rises to about 60 per cent (*Figure 15.14*). Schuknecht (1974) has noted this similarity in type and progression of hearing loss compared with Menière's disease.

Specialized tests of hearing indicate that, for a surprisingly long time, the deafness remains predominantly sensory. There is little or no tone decay in the lower frequencies and decay of 10–20 dB in the higher; the Békésy tracing is usually type 2; loudness discomfort levels and the acoustic stapedial thresholds remain within the normal limits of approximately 80–100 dB ISO; and speech discrimination patterns are in keeping with an end-organ lesion. Subjective fluctuation of hearing level may be reflected only in a change in discrimination with variable distortion of sound.

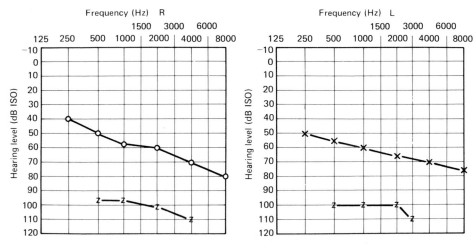

Figure 15.13   Late congenital syphilis. Pure-tone audiograms and stapedius reflex threshold (Z–Z) from a man of 55 with a four-year history of progressive bilateral deafness and episodic vertigo. He had evidence of old interstitial keratitis. Note the symmetry of the hearing loss and its sensory nature. High-tone deafness is the commonest pattern when hearing loss has been present for several years

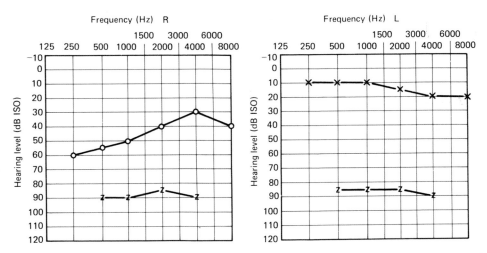

Figure 15.14   Late acquired syphilis. Pure-tone audiograms and stapedius reflex threshold (Z–Z) from a woman of 56 who complained of right deafness and tinnitus of three months' duration and sudden onset. The lesion is sensory. Low-tone deafness is found in many early cases. Acquired syphilis is more likely to affect one ear before the other

When there is asymmetry of hearing loss recruitment can be demonstrated by alternate binaural loudness balance testing; in this situation tonal inequality between the ears can often be demonstrated for the lower frequencies.

Transtympanic electrocochleography (EcochG) has now been carried out on many patients with hearing loss due to late congenital or acquired syphilitic ear disease. The reader is referred to Chapter 1 for details of technique. Ramsden, Moffat and Gibson (1978) have described the findings in the first 27 ears studied in this way. Most of these patients had flat, peaked or high-tone losses. As might be expected the hearing thresholds were confirmed and the cochlear microphonics (CM) were of small amplitude, mostly less than 3μV. The greater the hearing loss, the smaller was the CM. In 80 per cent of the ears tested there was a large negative summating potential (SP) mainly affecting the descending limb of the compound action potential (AP). In idiopathic Menière's disease the negative SP mainly affects the ascending limb of the AP (Gibson, Moffat and Ramsden, 1977). However, these findings must *not* be taken as pathognomonic since both patterns of negative SP are encountered in hydrops whatever the underlying pathology. Nevertheless they can raise suspicions.

As the hearing loss becomes more severe, there is increasing evidence of secondary neuronal degeneration (*Figure 15.15*). Speech discrimination becomes worse, tone decay increases, decay of the acoustic reflexes finally progresses to inability to elicit the reflex and no AP or CM can be demonstrated on transtympanic EcochG. Even in the presence of total hearing loss, however, some neurones survive in at least some of these patients as evidenced by their response to promontory electrical stimulation or cochlear implantation (House, 1976).

Almost all the patients with vestibular symptoms have objective vestibular signs. During the earlier, more acute phase latent nystagmus may be elicited with Frenzel glasses or on electronystagmography. The commonest finding, however, is progressive diminution in the sensitivity of both labyrinthins to caloric stimulation. Bilateral absent Hallpike responses in a patient with only moderate hearing loss is a very suspicious sign.

Hennebert's sign—a fistula sign with an intact drum and no evidence of middle-ear disease—has been commented on by a number of writers (Asherson, 1931; Perlman and Leek, 1952; Kerr, 1969; Schuknecht, 1974; Morrison, 1975), since Hennebert's original description in 1911. Like the Tullio phenomenon—transient vertigo and nystagmus on sudden noise stimulation—which is sometimes seen in late syphilis of the ear, it may be due to energy transmission through the footplate of the stapes directly on to the distended saccule. These signs are certainly worthy of search but they are not diagnostic and, in the author's experience, only occasionally found in late syphilis.

Other signs of congenital syphilis

The great majority of patients who subsequently develop late congenital syphilitic ear disease have previously had ocular manifestations, usually interstitial keratitis (IK), sometimes choroidoretinitis. The first attack of acute IK is usually experienced between the ages of 5 and 25 years. The diagnosis is usually made then and treatment given. The symptoms of the inner-ear disease usually commence 10–40 years later. Infrequently the ophthalmic and the otological symptoms start together or are separated by a few years. More than one attack of IK is common (*Figure 15.16*).

Understandably these patients wish to forget their earlier ophthalmic problems and the causation. When they present many years later with deafness, tinnitus or vertigo they do not relate to the previous experience and will not volunteer the information even if directly or indirectly asked. Indeed many patients with corneal opacities will ascribe them to 'old eye injury'. Sometimes the evidence of previous IK is obvious in one or both eyes, though frequently slit-lamp examination is necessary to reveal the

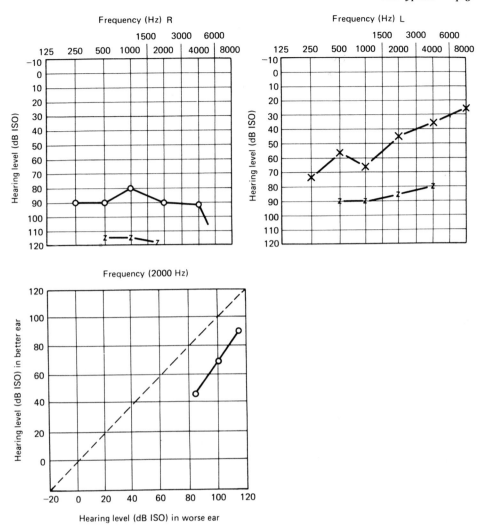

Figure 15.15 Secondary neuronal degeneration in late syphilis. Pure-tone audiograms, stapedius reflex threshold (Z–Z) and loudness balance tests in a man of 51 with acquired syphilis. There was a 20-year history of right deafness and a ten-year history of left deafness. The asymmetry of the stapedius reflex, the incomplete recruitment on loudness balance and tone decay of 30 dB(+) on the right indicated the neuronal element. Speech discrimination was 65 per cent on the left and 20 per cent on the right

tell-tale vessels. The opinion of an ophthalmologist is essential, for on occasion, this will be the only other evidence of congenital syphilis (very rarely all the serological tests are negative).

By comparison the other stigmata of congenital syphilis are less frequently encountered. Hutchinson (1863) whose name has been given to the dental formation which is characteristic of congenital disease (*Figure 15.17*), did, in fact, give one of the early descriptions of the ocular and otological signs and symptoms. The saddle nose and frontal bossing which constitute the 'typical facies' of congenital syphilis are even

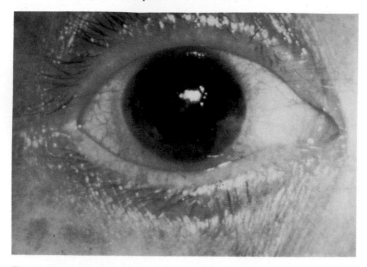

Figure 15.16 Acutely inflamed eye due to relapse of IK with old kerato-iritis; classic of congenital syphilis. First attack of IK is usually in adolescence and deafness starts 10–30 years later. Of patients with congenital syphilitic deafness 90 per cent have previously had IK

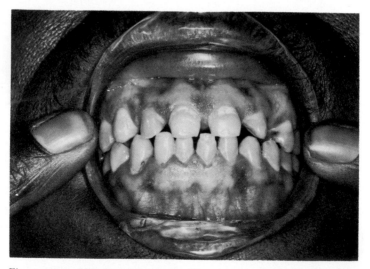

Figure 15.17 Hutchinsonian teeth. The permanent incisors are thickened antero-posteriorly and are wedge or screw-driver shaped. They are sometimes notched. Hutchinsonian teeth are found in 19 per cent of patients with congenital syphilitic deafness

less frequently seen (*Figure 15.18*), while Dubois' sign, Clutton's joints or sabre shins are rarely encountered.

Late neurosyphilis

Florid tabes dorsalis and general paralysis of the insane are rarely seen today, largely due to the earlier and more adequate treatment of primary and secondary syphilis.

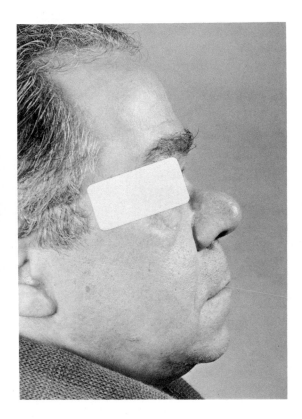

Figure 15.18 Saddle nose and frontal bossing. Sometimes described as facies typical of congenital syphilis, but only found in 10 per cent of those with deafness

Neurosyphilis has always been regarded as a rare consequence of congenital infection. Less florid evidence of neurosyphilis, especially in acquired disease, can often be found in patients presenting with deafness or vertigo. A full neurological history and examination are likely to bring these to light. There may be a history of 'lightning pains', bladder disturbances, ataxia, paraesthesiae, visual loss, headaches, personality change or depression. Examination may reveal Argyll–Robertson pupils, absent ankle jerks, loss of vibration sense, loss of pain sensibility in the tendo Achilles, early optic atrophy, or tremors of the lips and tongue.

In patients presenting to otologists with late-onset deafness these neurological signs and symptoms have been attenuated by previous treatment(s) and a careful search is necessary to find even one or two of them. It should be emphasized that if there is evidence of neurosyphilis it is almost always a coincidental finding and has nothing to do with the causation of the hearing loss. The pathology is in the temporal bones. A better perspective of the relationship can be obtained by examining the subject from the venereologist's or neurologist's viewpoint. Catterall (1977), reviewing the subject, found hearing loss to be very rare in patients with late neurosyphilis.

Polytomography in syphilitic ear disease

Attempts to demonstrate syphilitic osteitis in the temporal bones, even with polytomography, have been unrewarding. Patients with short and long histories of hearing loss have been examined radiologically. There is, perhaps, a tendency for sclerotic changes to be seen though most of the studies have been considered as normal.

Laboratory tests

SEROLOGICAL TESTS

There are now many *'screening' tests* for syphilis including the Cardiolipin Wasserman Reaction (CWR), the Venereal Disease Research Laboratory Slide test (VDRL), the Reiter Protein Complement Fixation Test (RPCFT), the Automated Reagin Test (ART) and the Rapid Plasma Reagin test (RPR). Although they are useful, in late previously-treated syphilis they are frequently negative, and false-positive results can be obtained. Late syphilitic ear disease should never be diagnosed on the basis of these tests alone and it is unwise to discuss this diagnosis with the patient on the basis of screening test results.

Relying on say one or two of these tests only, it is likely that about 40–50 per cent of cases of congenital disease will be missed and that about 20–30 per cent of late acquired infection will escape recognition.

Acute false-positive results are a temporary phenomenon, for example following vaccination or infection. Chronic false-positive results may indicate the presence of autoimmune disease.

Despite these limitations the tests have some value and the VDRL test in particular, being performed in graduated dilutions, can give some indication of the activity of the disease and of the immune responses.

The more *specific tests* for syphilis are the Treponema Pallidum Haemagglutination test (TPHA), the Treponema Pallidum Immobilization test (TPI) and the Fluorescent Treponemal Antibody test (FTA). At one time the FTA test was used by diluting the patient's serum 200 times. This FTA-200 test is seldom used now. The FTA absorbed test has become the most sensitive test for syphilis (Dunlop, King and Wilkinson, 1968); the patient's serum is diluted five times after absorption of non-specific group antibodies.

Of these tests the FTA-ABS is the one which should be requested in patients suspected of having late previously-treated syphilis of the temporal bones. The TPHA appears to be almost as effective.

TESTS ON THE CEREBROSPINAL FLUID

It is normally advisable, though perhaps not essential, to hospitalize patients with a diagnosis of late syphilitic ear disease. A number of tests on the CSF are indicated to search for evidence of late neurosyphilis. There may be a rise in the lymphocyte count or protein level, or elevation of the IgM or IgA. The non-specific or specific tests for syphilis may be positive in the CSF, or the Lange curve may be abnormal. A search may be made for treponemes.

In late congenital syphilitic ear disease the CSF is usually normal (since there is usually no neurosyphilis). Morrison (1975) reported the specific tests for syphilis as negative in 95 per cent of cases, though minor protein abnormalities were found in 10 per cent and treponemes in 8 per cent. In late acquired syphilitic ear disease higher percentages of abnormality are likely to be encountered since there is a greater likelihood of associated neurosyphilis.

Yaws

Yaws, due to *Treponema perpenue* (indistinguishable from *T. pallidum*) is transmitted by direct contact usually in childhood. In geographical distribution it is found in parts of Africa, Central America, the West Indies and SE Asia. There is a history of infection in childhood with weeping skin lesions which are slow to heal. They leave paper thin scars distributed particularly on the lower legs. With increasing immigration into the UK, yaws is no longer such a rare disease.

The late manifestations of yaws are so similar to those of syphilis that it would be surprising if the temporal bones were not similarly affected. The serological tests give the same results. As yet there are no confirmatory temporal bone histology reports.

A similar endemic non-venereal type of syphilis, probably transmitted by the use of communal drinking utensils, is found in parts of Arabia.

Clinically there is no doubt that some patients are seen, especially from the West Indies, with all the otological features of late syphilitic ear disease and positive serological tests. They have none of the stigmata of congenital syphilis, no history of primary infections but the typical cutaneous scarring of yaws. Equally, patients are seen from these areas with both congenital and acquired syphilis. Treatment is the same for all groups.

Transmission of disease

It is always advisable to investigate and treat these patients in cooperation with a venereologist. It is surprising how often he can elicit a history of previous infection and details of past treatment, information which may have eluded the otologist.

There is also the important aspect of managing family members and contacts. In congenital disease siblings should be examined and also the parents, if alive. Patients with congenital syphilis can be reassured that there is no risk of their spreading the disease; though the incidence of miscarriage in congenital syphilitic mothers may be high, the infection is not passed to a third generation.

In the case of acquired syphilis, spouses, contacts and possibly children may have to be examined; the risk to the fetus must be explained to women of childbearing age.

Early syphilis

One variant of early syphilis of the ear is virtually unknown today. It is an otolabyrinthitis of congenital origin (Rodger, 1940), presenting at or soon after birth. The infection involves the middle ear and labyrinth as part of a generalized severe infection. A fatal outcome is usual.

The other variant which is still encountered and which will probably become more common is meningoneurolabyrinthitis or *acute meningovascular syphilis* as it is more commonly named today. It is a relatively early manifestation of the disease occurring during or shortly after the secondary stage. If there has been no recognized primary sore or secondary rash it would present as an early latent case. It usually occurs within the first two years of infection and is found predominantly in males.

The vessels of the meninges and brain are affected by endarteritis with perivascular infiltration of plasma cells and lymphocytes. As part of the basal meningitis the infection may involve the eighth nerve and spread from the spiral ganglion into the cochlear duct. The membranous labyrinth can be infiltrated with inflammatory cells.

The clinical picture is one of acute syphilitic meningitis with headaches and fever. Ocular palsies, facial paralysis or deafness, tinnitus or vertigo of sudden onset may occur as the presenting symptoms. If very acute the infection may simulate a bacterial leptomeningitis, though cases seen by the author have had no photophobia or vomiting and no significant fever or neck stiffness. They have sought advice because of headaches and acute auditory failure, either unilateral or bilateral. One had an associated third nerve palsy. An example is shown in *Figure 15.19*. Catterall (1977) indicates that, even untreated, the acute infection runs a benign course though deafness may be a permanent sequel. He emphasizes that diagnosis may be difficult on account of the multiplicity of possible presenting features. For the otologist, however, it is enough to suspect early (or late) syphilis in every case of sudden onset eighth nerve symptoms.

Being early, the serological tests for syphilis in the blood are strongly positive. In the CSF there is usually a moderate lymphocytosis, some elevation of the protein level, an abnormal Lange curve and positive serological tests (even the non-specific ones).

It seems likely that more cases of acute syphilitic meningitis will be seen in the future. The prevalence of acute acquired syphilis remains a problem and an increasing

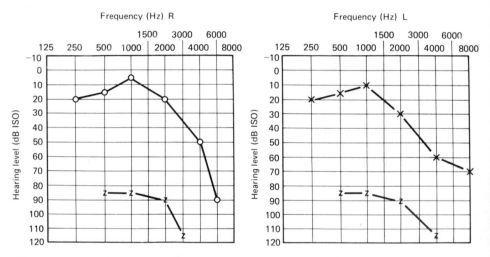

Figure 15.19 Acute meningovascular syphilis. Pure-tone audiograms and stapes reflex (Z–Z) thresholds from a heterosexual male patient, aged 33, with a two-week history of headaches, bilateral hearing loss and tinnitus and acute vertigo on sudden movement. After abolishing fixation there was nystagmus to right and left. Caloric responses were absent at 20 °C. The high-tone loss was partly sensory and mainly neural. Tests for syphilis were strongly positive in the serum and the CSF. The CSF contained 13 cells/mm³, protein of 80 mg per cent, a positive Pandy test and a meningitic Lange curve (5443211 0). He was treated with i.m. cephaloridine 500 mg four times daily for 17 days and steroids for three months. On withdrawing the steroids he had two weeks of erythromycin 500 mg four times daily. There was a moderate improvement in the pure-tone audiogram on both sides and speech discrimination on the right improved from 65–90 per cent. The acoustic reflex threshold at 4 kHz also improved.

A year later the tests for syphilis were still positive in the CSF which was otherwise normal. He was re-treated with penicillin and probenecid

one. In England, in 1971, there were 2.5 new cases/100000 of the population, in Canada there were 2.6 and in the USA, 11.5. In 1974 the Annual Report drew attention to the worldwide increase in the prevalence of early syphilis, especially in homosexual males. Provisional figures for England and Wales show that there were 2543 new early cases in 1976; in a population of approximately 49 million (Census, 1971), this is about 5.2/100000 of population; 84.5 per cent of these new cases were found in males.

Treatment of late syphilis of the ear

STEROIDS

There is now ample clinical evidence that steroids alone sometimes improve the hearing in late syphilitic deafness. In 1952, Perlman and Leek reported some success with ACTH; in 1962, Hahn, Rodin and Haskins reported 50 per cent of their cases improved with prednisone therapy; in 1966, Karmody and Schuknecht found temporary benefit following systemic steroids; in 1968, Dawkins, Sharp and Morrison found it difficult to assess the results due to the frequency of fluctuation; in 1969, Morrison reported that 50 per cent of the patients treated with steroids had definite hearing gains, but that relapses were being encountered; in 1973, Kerr, Smyth and Cinnamond reported early favourable results in a small number of patients treated with ACTH; and in 1975, Morrison reported the longer-term results in over 100 patients, analysing the different regime results.

From the earlier reports it appeared that the deafness of late syphilis was to some extent reversible by steroids alone and that there might be an immunological basis to part of the hearing loss. The finding of treponemes in the eye, the CSF and possibly in the temporal bone in late syphilis alters the immunopathological concept, especially when it is realized that experimental animals have been infected by treponemes from such sources. This work has been reviewed by Dunlop (1972), though Catterall (1977) questions the pathogenicity of these organisms. In their excellent monograph as long ago as 1936, Mayer and Fraser suggested that the deafness was resistant to antitreponemal drugs because the spirochaetes were protected by the chronic inflammatory reaction. It seems logical to deduce that late syphilitic ear disease is due to persistent low-grade temporal bone infection and that steroids are of temporary benefit only by virtue of their local anti-inflammatory properties.

There is now both clinical and experimental evidence that systemic steroids, presumably by diminishing the immune responses of the body, can precipitate or reactivate the lesions of late syphilis. Steroids are given to experimental animals to increase the yield of treponemes for use in specific serological tests. Collart, Borel and Durel (1962 a, b, c) found that the lesions of syphilis were precipitated in penicillin-treated rabbits by the subsequent administration of steroids. Dunlop, King and Wilkinson (1968) found that all patients with late ocular disease, from whom treponemes were recovered from the aqueous humour, had been treated with local and/or systemic steroids, which they considered may have reactivated the disease. In the otological field, Morrison (1969, 1975) has reported relapses or even increased hearing losses after the withdrawal of steroids in many patients.

Studies on bacteria *in vitro* indicate that penicillin has its greatest bactericidal effect upon organisms when they are dividing rapidly. Dunlop *et al.* (1968) suggests that in late syphilis the spirochaete, dividing less rapidly than it does in early infections, is less susceptible to antitreponemal therapy. He points out that steroids given in late syphilis might render the treponeme more sensitive to antibiotics, presumably because, being reactivated, it will be dividing more rapidly.

These observations and arguments form the rationale of the currently advised treatment. Whatever treatment(s) have been given in the past, the patient is admitted to hospital for parenteral antitreponemal antibiotic therapy together with steroids for 17 days. Antibiotic/steriod therapy, by reducing the immune responses of the body both systemically and in the local lesion, allows the treponemes to multiply and be more effectively destroyed. The possibility of a Herxheimer reaction is minimized. Steroids are continued on an out-patient basis with regular monitoring of pure-tone and speech thresholds. If there is no evidence of improvement in auditory or vestibular symptoms and signs within 4–6 weeks, the steroids are withdrawn, with a 10-day course of antibiotic cover. Should there be a good response to initial treatment, normally seen within the first four weeks, steroids are continued for many months in small dosage, and sometimes indefinitely. Patients receiving long-term steroids are re-treated annually with antibiotics. Termination of steroids is always accompanied by a further course of antitreponemal drugs.

Therapy normally consists of prednisone, 10 mg thrice daily for the first week and 25 mg daily for the next three weeks. No advantage has been found with higher dosage. For long-term therapy 2.5–7.5 mg daily seems to be acceptable. Most patients learn to modify the dose according to fluctuations in their hearing (*Figure 15.20*).

Steroids are sometimes contraindicated or not tolerated. Morrison (1975) was unable to use steroids in 17 per cent of cases for reasons of hypertension, gastric ulceration, diabetes, pulmonary tuberculosis, anxiety depression, pregnancy or glaucoma. In addition, in the earlier stages of these enquiries, a number of patients were treated with antitreponemal antibiotics only, to form a small control group.

ANTITREPONEMAL ANTIBIOTICS

In the pre-penicillin era Moore (1933) found that arsenicals had no effect in preventing advancing deafness in late congenital or acquired syphilis, though he did report temporary success in treating the sudden deafness due to early meningovascular disease. By 1947, Moore considered that penicillin was the treatment of choice for all the stages of syphilis, and, by and large, this view is held by most venereologists today. Other antibiotics such as erythromycin, the tetracyclines, chloramphenicol, cephaloridine, ampicillin, and carbomycin are antitreponemal but as Catterall (1977) points out no long-term controlled trials have been carried out and none of these antibiotics is considered to be as effective as penicillin. The route of administration is important. Intramuscular therapy, in adequate dosage, is known to be effective. Any form of oral therapy carries the risk of inadequate blood levels either from failure to take the prescribed course or from variable absorption.

Benzylpenicillin G, 500 000 units intramuscularly six-hourly, or procaine penicillin, 600 000 units twice daily for at least 17 days is the treatment of choice for late syphilis. The addition of probenecid, 0.5 g four times daily helps to raise the blood and CSF levels by blocking the excretion of penicillin.

Although erythromycin is considered by some to be the most effective alternative it has the disadvantage of oral administration. Morrison (1975), found a 10 per cent incidence of penicillin allergy in patients with late syphilitic ear disease. This is not

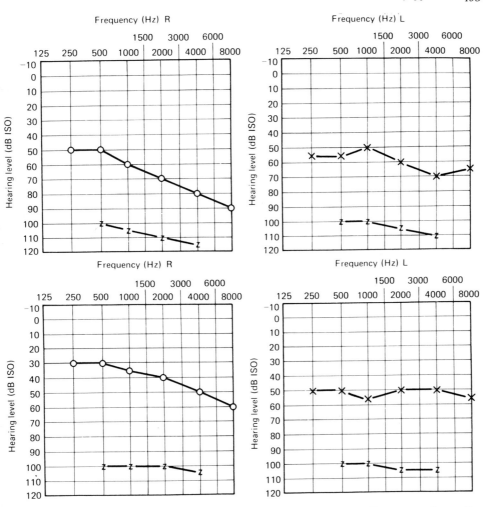

Figure 15.20 Congenital syphilis: response to treatment. Pure-tone audiograms and stapedius reflex thresholds (Z–Z) before treatment (above) and nine years after treatment (below). The patient, when first seen, was a woman of 58 with a history of progressive bilateral deafness from the age of 11 years and she had a seven-year history of increasing unsteadiness. IK had been treated with arsenicals when she was 17. She had been treated with penicillin for her hearing loss when she was 47, but it continued to deteriorate. When seen the caloric responses were absent. Old IK was confirmed on slit lamp examination and treponemes were found in the anterior chamber of the eye. Her CSF was normal. In the blood the VDRL, TPI and FTA were positive. She was treated for 17 days with benzylpenicillin G 0.5 mega-units and probenecid 0.5 g six-hourly together with steroids. Within a month the pure-tone levels had improved and discrimination was significantly better on the right. She was able to discard her hearing aid. Steroids have been continued for nine years at 2.5–5 mg prednisone daily. She is retreated with oral antibiotics annually

surprising considering that so many of them had previously been treated with penicillin, sometimes many times. The advantages of cephaloridine, as an alternative to penicillin, are the intramuscular route of administration and possibly the high levels of this antibiotic in bone. The dosage is 500 mg four times daily for a minimum of 17 days.

Antibiotic administration to cover the withdrawal of steroids or for annual therapy in patients on long-term steroids, is acceptable by the oral route. Erythromycin 2 g, cephalexin 2 g, or ampicillin 2 g daily for 10 days is acceptable though intramuscular therapy is used for withdrawal cover after long-term steroids.

It is always advisable for the patient to be kept under observation and this is especially important if evidence of neurosyphilis has been detected. Venereologists normally make annual checks on the blood and CSF in these cases for many years. Re-treatment is dictated by the findings.

RESULTS OF TREATMENT

Although the deafness and vestibular damage resulting from late syphilis of the ear still carries a poor or guarded prognosis, the current regime holds out some prospect of halting the relentless progression of symptoms and signs. It should be emphasized that the spectacular recovery shown in *Figure 15.21* is very rarely achieved.

In the past 13 years over 200 patients with late syphilis of the ear have been treated by the author, some with penicillin (or other antibiotics) alone, some with steroids alone, some with a combination of antitreponemal antibiotics and steroids for relatively short periods and some with the combined therapy followed by long-term steroids. The following results and principles of management seem to have emerged.

(1) The hearing gains which can be expected with modern treatment are of the order of 20–30 dB, mainly in the frequencies below 3 kHz. There is a coincidental improvement in discrimination. Speech discrimination may improve without a pure-tone threshold change.

(2) Penicillin or cephaloridine alone is valueless in terms of obtaining an improved hearing result, and there is no definite evidence that they prevent the progression of the otological manifestations. Nevertheless antitreponemal therapy must be given even if steroids are contraindicated.

(3) Steroids alone undoubtedly influence the course of the temporal bone disease. Hearing gains are achieved in about a third of treated cases though 50 per cent of ears showing improvement subsequently deteriorate some time after withdrawal of the drug.

(4) Steroids together with intramuscular penicillin or cephaloridine offer the best prospect of altering the prognosis. Over 50 per cent of ears show an initial gain. Even with this regime there is a significant relapse rate—of the order of 30 per cent of those responding.

(5) The relapse rate following withdrawal of steroids is twice as high (50 per cent) if terminal antitreponemal drugs are not given (20 per cent, if they are used).

(6) Retreatment following relapse is rarely effective in achieving a gain though further deterioration may be prevented.

(7) After initial therapy, long-term steroids with annual antibiotics offer the prospect of maintained hearing levels. Even in this group of patients 25 per cent of ears show some deterioration after intervals of 2–13 years.

(8) Sudden hearing loss carries a poorer prognosis for treatment. Fluctuant hearing loss (as would be expected from the potential reversibility) carries a better prognosis.

(9) Following treatment the prognosis is better when the otological history is

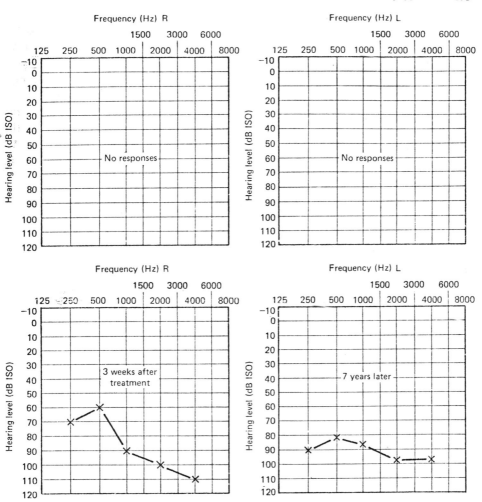

Figure 15.21 Congenital syphilis. Response to treatment. Pure-tone audiograms from a woman of 44 who had been totally deaf in both ears for one year. Prior to this there was an 11-year history of fluctuant and progressive hearing loss and severe attacks of vertigo. She had evidence of old IK. The CWR, VDRL and FTA were positive in the blood. CSF was normal. The total deafness was confirmed by repeated tests. She was allergic to penicillin and was treated with cephaloridine and steroids. There was a spectacular recovery within three weeks on the left side only. She continues to take 5 mg prednisone daily. Speech discrimination on the left varies from 30–40 per cent. She is retreated with i.m. cephaloridine or oral cephalexin each year

relatively short (less than two years) compared with when it is long (more than ten years).

(10) Vestibular symptoms are dramatically controlled in 50 per cent of those treated with antitreponemal drugs and steroids, in 25 per cent of those treated with steroids only but in almost none of the patients treated with penicillin alone.

As yet there is no unequivocal evidence about the changes which occur in the inner ear when there has been a good response to antitreponemal/steroid therapy. Transtympanic EcochG offers the opportunity of gaining information. A number of tracings have now been carried out (in the same ears) before and following 17 days of treatment (Ramsden, Moffat and Gibson, 1978). Ears showing a good hearing response have demonstrated a considerable increase in the amplitude of the CM. Larger CM voltages have been recorded without objective or subjective hearing gain. Abolition of the typical negative SP has also been recorded without hearing change. Ears which have shown no EcochG change have not improved with treatment.

Further work is required along these lines. The initial observations suggest the possibility that treatment may be having a beneficial effect on the inner ear (and the longer-term prognosis) even when there is no demonstrable audiological (pure-tone, stapes reflex or speech threshold) change. It would also appear that improvement in hearing is not necessarily related to diminution of the hydrops.

Cogan's disease

The disease first described by Cogan (1945 and 1949) and now bearing his name is considered a non-syphilitic interstitial keratitis (IK) with fluctuant and progressive cochleovestibular damage. It is extremely rare. Young adults are usually affected, and the ocular and otological manifestations frequently start together. The onset is usually sudden. The corneal changes are relatively mild, whereas the progression of deafness may result in total bilateral hearing loss. Tinnitus is troublesome and paroxysmal attacks of vertigo can be severe.

The pathological changes have been described by Crawford (1957), Fisher and Hellstrom (1961) and by Wolff *et al.* (1965). Generalized arteritis, similar to periarteritis nodosa, is described. In the temporal bones there is hydrops, degeneration of the organ of Corti and severe neuronal loss, with new bone formation in the scala tympani and other areas of the perilymphatic space. Osteogenesis is not specific to Cogan's disease; it is sometimes encountered in otosclerosis, and secondary to infections, trauma and tumours involving the otic capsule.

In recent years cases have also been described by Cody and Williams (1960), Serrins, Harrison and Chandler (1963) and by Smith (1970). It is mostly agreed that the disease, though of unknown aetiology, probably has an autoimmune basis and that the best prospects for saving some hearing are obtained by large doses of steroids.

The clinical picture has so many similarities to congenital syphilis that one wonders if some of the earlier described cases—before the advent of the FTA tests—were, in fact, instances of this disease.

References

Albers-Schönberg, G. (1904). *Münchener medizinische Wochenschrift*, **51**, 365

Altmann, F. and Kornfeld, M. (1967). *Annals of Otology, Rhinology and Laryngology*, **76**, 89

Annual Report, Chief Medical Officer for the year 1968. (1969). 'On the State of the Public Health'. Appendix C. London; HMSO

Annual Report, Chief Medical Officer for the year 1972. (1973). 'On the State of the Public Health'. London; HMSO

Annual Report, Chief Medical Officer 1974. (1975). 'On the State of the Public Health'. London; HMSO

Asherson, N. (1931). *Journal of Laryngology*, **40**, 326

Barry, H. C. (1969). *Paget's disease of Bone*. London; Livingstone

Catterall, R. D. (1977). *British Journal of Hospital Medicine*, **17**, 585

Census (1971). London; HMSO

Clerc, P. and Chevance, L. (1965). *Annales d'oto-laryngologie* **82**, 413

Cody, D. and Williams, N. (1960). *Laryngoscope* **70**, 447

Cogan, S. G. (1945). *Archives of Ophthalmology*, **33**, 144

Cogan, S. G. (1949). *Archives of Ophthalmology*, **42**, 42

Collart, P., Borel, L.-J. and Durel, P. (1962a). *Annales d'Institut Pasteur, Paris*, **102**, 596

Collart, P., Borel, L.-J. and Durel, P. (1962b). *Annales d'Institut Pasteur, Paris*, **102**, 693

Collart, P., Borel, L.-J. and Durel, P. (1962c). *Annales d'Institut Pasteur, Paris*, **102**, 953

Collins, D. H. (1956). *Lancet*, **2**, 51

Crawford, W. (1957). *Pennsylvania Medical Journal*, **60**, 835

Davies, D. G. (1968). *Acta otolaryngologica*, Suppl. 242

Dawkins, R. S., Sharp, M. and Morrison, A. W. (1968). *Journal of Laryngology*, **82**, 1095

Dunlop, E. M. C. (1972). *British medical Journal*, **2**, 577

Dunlop, E. M. C., King, A. J. and Wilkinson, A. E. (1968). *Transactions of the Ophthalmological Society, UK*, **88**, 275

Fisher, E. and Hellstrom, H. (1961). *Archives of Pathology*, **72**, 572

Gibson, W. P. R., Moffat, D. A. and Ramsden, R. T. (1977). *Audiology*, **16**, 389

Goldman, J. N. and Girard, K. F. (1967). *Archives of Ophthalmology*, **78**, 47

Goodhill, V. (1939). *Archives of Otology, Rhinology and Laryngology*, **48**, 676

Goodhill, V. (1960). *Laryngoscope*, **70**, 722

Hahn, R. D., Rodin, P. and Haskins, H. L. (1962). *Journal of chronic Diseases*, **15**, 395

Hamersma, H. (1973). *ORL*, **36**, 21

Hennebert, C. (1911). *Clinique Bruxelles*, **25**, 545

Henkin, R. I., Lifschitz, M. D. and Larson, A. L. (1972). *American Journal of medical Science*, **263**, 383

Illaváček, V. and Chtádek, V. (1963). *Acta. otolaryngologica (Stockholm)*, **56**, 75

Hoeve, J. van der, and Kleyn, A. de (1918). *Archives of Ophthalmology*, **95**, 81

Hoogland, G. A. (1962). *Nederlands tijdschrift voor geneeskunde*, **106**, 34

Hoogland, G. A. (1963). *Nederlands tijdschrift voor geneeskunde*, **107**, 11

House, W. F. (1976). *Annals of Otology, Rhinology and Laryngology*, **85**, Suppl. 27

Hunter, D. and Turnbull, H. M. (1931). *British Journal of Surgery*, **19**, 203

Hutchinson, J. (1863). *A Clinical Memoir on Certain Diseases of the Eye and Ear Consequent on Inherited Syphilis*. London; Churchill.

Johnson, C., Lavy, D., Lord, T., Vellias. F., Merritt, A. and Deiss, W. (1968). *Medicine*, **47**, 149

Jones, M. and Mulcahy, N. (1968). *Archives of Otolaryngology*, **87**, 116

Karmody, C. S. and Schuknecht, H. F. (1966). *Archives of Otolaryngology*, **83**, 18

Kerr, A. G. (1969). *Journal of Laryngology*, **83**, 435

Kerr, A. G., Smyth, G. D. L. and Cinnamond, M. J. (1973). *Journal of Laryngology*, **87**, 1

Kornfeld, M. (1967). *Practica oto-rhino-laryngologica*, **29**, 406

Kosoy, J. and Maddox, H. E. (1971). *Archives of Otolaryngology*, **93**, 115

Lichenstein, L. and Jaffe, H. L. (1942). *Archives of Pathology*, **33**, 777

Lindsay, J. and Lehman, R. (1969). *Laryngoscope*, **79**, 213

Mack, L. W. Jr., Smith, J. L., Walter, E. K., Montenegro, E. N. R. and Nicol, W. G. (1969). *Archives of Otolaryngology*, **90**, 37

McKusick, V. A. (1955). *Journal of chronic Diseases*, **2**, 491 and 500

McKusick, V. A. (1966). *Hereditable Disorders of Connective Tissue*, 3rd Ed. St. Louis; C. V. Mosby

Mair, I. W. S., Schrøder, K. E. and Johannessen T. A. (1974). *Journal of Laryngology*, **88**, 1061

Mayer, O. and Fraser, J. S. (1936). *Journal of Laryngology*, **51**, 168

Moffatt, W. H., Morrow, J. D. and Simpson, N. (1974). *British medical Journal*, **2**, 203

Moore, J. E. (1933). *The Modern Treatment of Syphilis*. London; Bailliére

Moore, J. E. (1947). *Penicillin in Syphilis*, Springfield, Illinois; Thomas

Morrison, A. W. (1967). *Annals of the Royal College of Surgeons*, **41**, 202

Morrison, A. W. (1969). *Proceedings of the Royal Society of Medicine*, **62**, 959

Morrison, A. W. (1975). *Management of Sensorineural Deafness*. London and Boston; Butterworths

Morrison, A. W. and Bundey, S. E. (1970). *Journal of Laryngology*, **84**, 921

Ogilvie, R. F. and Hall, I. S. (1962). *Journal of Laryngology*, **76**, 841

Opheim, O. (1968). *Acta Oto-laryngologica*, **65**, 337

Patterson, C. and Stone, H. (1970). *Laryngoscope*,
  80, 544
Perlman, H. B. and Leek, J. H. (1952).
  Laryngoscope, **62**, 1175
Ramsden, R. T., Bulman, C. H. and Lorigan, B. P.
  (1975). *Journal of Laryngology*, **89**, 941
Ramsden, R. T., Moffat, D. A. and Gibson, W. P.
  R. (1978). *Annals of Otology, Rhinology and
  Laryngology* (in press)
Rice, N. S. C., Jones, B. R. and Wilkinson, A. E.
  (1968). *Transactions of the Ophthalmological Society,
  UK*, **88**, 257
Rodger, T. R. (1940). *Journal of Laryngology*, **55**,
  168
Rüedi, L. (1968). *Acta otolaryngologica*, **65**, 13
Schuknecht, H. F. (1974). *Pathology of the Ear.*
  Harvard; Harvard University Press
  medical Journal, **49**, 1256
Serrins, A. J., Harrison, R. S. and Chandler, J. R.
  (1963). *Archives of Otolaryngology*, **78**, 785
Shai, F., Baker, R. K. and Wallach, S. (1971).
  Journal of Clinical Investigation, **50**, 1927
Shea, J. J., Smyth, G. D. L. and Altmann, F.
  (1963). *Journal of Laryngology*, **77**, 679
Smårs, G. (1961). *Osteogenesis imperfecta in Sweden.*
  Stockholm; Scandinavian University Press

Smith, J. (1970). *Laryngoscope*, **80**, 121
Smith, J. L. and Israel, C. W. (1967a). *Journal of the
  American medical Association*, **199**, 980
Smith, J. L. and Israel, C. W. (1967b). *Archives of
  Ophthalmology*, **77**, 474
Smith, J. L., Israel, C. W. and Harmer, R. E.
  (1967). *Archives of Ophthalmology*, **78**, 284
Sparrow, N. J. and Duval, A. J. (1967). *Journal of
  Laryngology*, **81**, 601
Stoller, F. (1962). *Laryngoscope*, **72**, 855
Waltner, J. G. (1965). *Archives of Otolaryngology*, **82**,
  355
Weir, N. (1977). *Journal of Laryngology*, **91**, 717
Williams, D. M. L. and Thomas, R. S. A. (1975).
  Journal of Laryngology, **89**, 359
Wolff, D., Bernhard, W. G., Tsutsumi, S., Ross, I.
  S. and Nussbaum, H. E. (1965). *Annals of Otology,
  Rhinology and Laryngology*, **74**, 507
Woodhouse, N. J. Y. (1973). 'Paget's Disease and
  Calcitonin Therapy', *Ninth Symposium on Advanced
  Medicine.* Ed by G. Walker. London; Pitman
  Medical
Woodhouse, N. J. Y. (1974). *Journal of Hospital
  Medicine*, **11**, 677
Wullstein, H., Ogilvie, R. F. and Hall, I. S. (1960).
  Journal of Laryngology, **74**, 67

16 The deaf child

Ian G Taylor

Consideration of the deaf child embraces first identification of a hearing impairment, then assessment of its nature and degree. Appropriate medical and surgical treatment must never be isolated from the basic need that the deaf child must be helped to live in the world around him.

It must be understood that development of a normal baby is highly dependent upon hearing, and that social, emotional and intellectual development is bound up with the functioning of the normal auditory system. Ewing and Ewing (1950) have described in detail the effect of a hearing disability on a developing child, even to the importance of hearing on physical attributes of breathing, a sense of rhythm, walking, eating and drinking and personal habits. Hearing deprivation has its greatest effect on linguistic development. Being able to understand speech and speaking is *the* one function of human behaviour which sets man apart from all other living creatures. Lack of this ability must make an early diagnosis of deafness a necessity, to ensure that medical or surgical management and the appropriate rehabilitation and education are made available.

Speech acts as a vital factor in the formation of personal–social relationships. The child's growing awareness and growth of speech secures for him a system of communication with others. It is a sobering thought, when considering deaf children, that normal children will have a basic functional use and understanding of spoken language by the age of three years.

In the hearing child of three years the vocabulary is necessarily limited but there is a use of grammar and syntactics, as well as a working understanding of the semantic structure of the language.

The development of speech is thought by Lenneberg (1964) to be due to biological capacities which are specific to the human species. Lenneberg shows how difficult it is to suppress the acquisition of speech in children even in unfavourable environments and in the presence of severe handicaps.

All languages have principles of syntax and semantics which are learned through social transmission. It must be assumed that man is well-structured for acoustic signals. This is an important concept which must influence our views about the development of communication skills with deaf children. Further consideration will be given to this aspect later when reference is made to the educational management of deafness. As hearing impairment affects linguistic development the medical profession must be vitally interested in securing an early diagnosis to determine (1) the nature and (2) the degree of hearing loss.

It is important to distinguish between a conductive and a sensorineural deafness. In the first instance medical and surgical treatment can remove or reduce the degree of loss.

In sensorineural cases, the degree of hearing loss is most important in the subsequent management of the child and the family, particularly in the choice of an appropriate hearing aid. Another question vital to the parents concerns the cause of the hearing loss. Accurate diagnosis must include identification of the causative factor wherever possible so that advice can be given as to whether or not there is a genetic factor present, with a high probability of other children being born deaf.

The early identification of deafness

Screening tests

If deafness could be identified in the newborn it would have two clear advantages. Firstly, early help could be given to the baby and the family. Secondly, as many babies are now born in hospital, a test of hearing at that time would ensure a high rate of early identification. To this end methods of screening hearing in the newborn have been developed, but the procedures are still controversial. The result of mass screening programmes are inconsistent and may be misleading. Barr *et al.* (1978) refer to the recommendation of the Joint Committee for Infant Hearing Screening which recommends that, instead of such mass programmes, infants at high risk for hearing impairment should be identified by means of history and physical examination.

Test procedures for the newborn involve stimulation of the awake or lightly sleeping baby with short bursts of sound in the region of 70–100 dB sound pressure level (SPL) and the assessment of the reaction by noting a startle or auropalpebral response.

Bench and Boscak (1970) point out that 10–20 per cent of normal full-term neonates emit a spontaneous startle response and also that there is a high rate of false negatives. Bench and Boscak investigated these problems by application of the signal detection theory which allows for a calculation of the optimum performance of the ideal detector. They investigated the effects of stimulus intensity and the effect of the pre-stimulus-aroused state. The results of these observations indicated that the signal detection was affected by both the sound pressure level of the stimulus and the state of the baby before stimulation.

Fisch (1971) in a similar context, discussing the complexity of the nature of reaction to sound stimuli, pointed out that a child reacts to a test stimulus only when he is ready to respond. To quote '. . . environmental influences and internal determinants interact and create the condition of readiness to respond, a condition which can vary greatly according to these influences.'

In a further study of the neonates' responses to auditory stimuli judged in relation to stimulus onset and offset, Collyer and Bench (1974) concluded that it is difficult to judge responses to the onset of an auditory stimulus and even more difficult to judge the offset response. Lewis (1971), working with infants from 12 weeks to 12 months, found a deceleration of heart-rate responses for both onset and offset auditory stimuli on first presentation. With repeated presentations, onset responses were habituated, but not those to offset.

Collyer, Bench and Wilson (1974), in a group of six month old babies, studied the responses to a range of stimuli including a 2 kHz pure tone at 40 and 70 dB SPL and a female voice at 65 dB SPL. They reported that the female voice elicited the most responses and this is in line with most clinical observations. An earlier paper by Robson (1970) had demonstrated that normal babies at nine months respond very poorly to pure tones whatever their intensity. Any screening test of hearing must aim at determining the child's capacity to hear speech, and therefore should encompass both frequency and loudness measurement.

In practice it is now well established that babies respond to very quiet sounds by locating the source of the sound from about the age of 7–9 months. This is the developmental age when the child is sitting unsupported. The characteristics of the response have been well described. The baby responds by turning towards the source of the sound. The best responses are evoked when the sound is made at 2–3 ft from the head on the imaginary plane which runs through the two ears. If sounds are made on other planes the baby tends first to look along the horizontal plane and then up or down, depending on the actual sound point. This developmental phenomenon appears to be associated with the gaining of the upright posture—the baby having a reference plane in order to establish the complete image of space perception (Taylor, 1958). At the age of nine months sounds behind the head or above the head often do not evoke a response from a baby. A non-response will often be experienced to loud sounds or sounds which do not appear to have 'significance'.

A screening test must ensure that the sounds to which a baby responds must be made very quietly indeed so that the loudness of the sound approximates to the zero of the pure-tone audiogram. It is advisable to monitor the sound levels with a sound-level meter.

The frequency-specificity of the sound source must be carefully regarded. Low-frequency sounds can be produced by the laryngeal voice without whisper, and to a certain extent by the sound of a spoon on a cup.

High-frequency sounds can be produced by using the unvoiced and unforced consonant 's' and by the rattle specially made for this purpose. This rattle contains a number of glass beads which strike against each other when the rattle is very gently shaken. The noise output of the rattle may be calibrated in terms of frequency and sound pressure level. The frequency spectrum of the noise has been analysed, using third-octave filter equipment, over the range 125 Hz–40 kHz. The noise output of the rattle reaches a maximum at approximately 10 kHz when a sound pressure level of 35 dB is obtained from a distance of 1 m. At frequencies below 5 kHz the sound pressure level is less than 5 dB SPL at a distance of 1 m. Consequently, a person with a binaural flat hearing loss of 30 dB HTL (Hearing Threshold Level) or greater, would not detect the rattle noise when the rattle is correctly shaken in very quiet surroundings at a distance of 1 m.

The middle-frequency range can be covered by using a chime bar which has a specific response in the middle range for 2–4 kHz.

Although this type of test has now been established with some variations in the British Isles since the 1930s using two people, there have been tests described involving the use of one person only. Such a test has been described recently by Stensland Junker *et al.* (1978). If carried out with care and efficiency in good acoustic conditions it can be expected that 1–2 per cent of babies will fail the test due to hearing impairments either of a conductive or sensorineural type.

Barr *et al* (1978) reported that, of 30 000 infants, 1.5 per cent did not pass the test. Of these, 20 were found to have a severe bilateral hearing impairment and in only five cases had the parents observed or suspected a lack of sound reaction. The rest were thought to have not responded on account of upper respiratory tract infections and secretory otitis media, or because of conditions which would explain lack of response to the sound stimuli other than a hearing impairment.

'At risk' factors

Children known to have a family history of deafness, children whose mothers gave a history of a virus infection in pregnancy, particularly rubella, children in whom there was a perinatal problem such as jaundice or anoxia or prematurity, children with cerebral palsy or meningitis, or who were late to talk or had defective speech may be regarded as potentially deaf—'at risk'.

Howarth (1958) was able to demonstrate in Lancashire a significant difference between 'at risk' babies and others. The difference was of the order of 14 times greater incidence of deafness in the 'at risk' group as compared with the other babies. While this statistic is a striking one it must be remembered that the primary objective in a screening test of hearing must be to identify the babies with impaired hearing *in the first year of life*. To include in the tests children who are not talking does admit those who are considerably older than nine months.

There are further reasons for not confining the tests to children who fall into the above special categories. Results depend on the responsiveness of the baby to environmental sound, and whilst the primary function of the test is to find babies with hearing impairments, the screening test may also reveal those children who do not respond on account of abnormal mental states.

It should also be remembered that mild and moderate degrees of conductive deafness are found frequently in babies. If the screening test is performed efficiently, it will also find those babies with conductive deafness.

In the very young the screening procedure is directed at three attributes of normal hearing; that the baby responds to very quiet sounds, that the responses are to sounds where the frequency corresponds to the frequency range of the pure-tone audiogram, and that there is an accurate localization of the sound source.

At a later stage in development when normal children are showing development of understanding of the spoken word it is necessary to modify the procedure whilst maintaining the principles. At the age of 18 months to two and a half years the criteria for passing a screening test satisfactorily are to have shown that the child can understand very quiet speech when the instructions are given at a distance of 3 ft from the ear; that there is a clear response to high-frequency sounds; and that the ability to localize is present.

When the child is three years of age, and in normal circumstances has grasped the rules of the mother tongue, he is deemed to have passed the test if he is able to show understanding of very quiet speech at 3 ft: to respond to low- and high-frequency sounds by such an action as placing a brick in a box when a sound is heard; and also to locate the sound source.

Screening procedures for hearing should be undertaken ideally at the ages of 7–9 months, at two and a half to three years and at, or just before, school entry at five years.

At the age of five years it is usual to screen the hearing of children using pure-tone audiometry. According to Leith (1973) the pure-tone levels should be

250 Hz	500 Hz	1000 Hz	2000 Hz	4000 Hz
20	20	15	15	15

These levels indicate a rather strict interpretation of screening for hearing in the ordinary school environment, in view of the ambient sound levels usually encountered.

Harrison (1971) suggested that testing at 250 Hz should be discontinued on account of the ambient sound levels, and that signal presentation levels should be maintained at 20 dB re BS Audiometer Zero. Increasing the signal level reduced the efficiency of the test as a screening device.

It is assumed that screening tests are designed primarily to identify those children who will have difficulty in hearing speech. For this reason both pre-school and school-age screening test procedures are based on our knowledge concerning the clinical threshold levels and the frequency range of the sounds of speech.

It has been recognized that children with pathological conditions of the middle ear may have normal auditory acuity (Eagles, 1961). The use of pure-tone sweep frequency testing will measure auditory acuity but will not necessarily identify those children with some degree of middle-ear disease unless the otological condition is sufficient to interfere with the transmission of sound through the middle-ear mechanism. Screening tests should therefore be carried out in conjunction with an otological examination of the ears, and each should be considered as complementary to the other.

Eagles (1973) expressed the view that in primary-school years, yearly examinations are desirable. In older children the interval between examinations can be greater. He records that approximately one half of the children who had abnormal otoscopic findings evinced no recorded change in their hearing sensitivity. On the basis of otoscopy approximately 39 per cent of the children studied needed medical attention because of ear conditions.

Brooks (1977) has investigated the value of middle-ear impedance measurement in screening. He has reported (1976) on the examination of 80 children. Of these, 41 maintained very stable patterns of middle-ear function. About one sixth exhibited persistent or recurrent episodes of middle-ear effusion. The results of a larger study by Ferrer are awaiting completion.

Leith (1973) commenting on the use of electro-acoustic impedance as a screening test concludes, from her comparative study of this method and a sweep frequency pure-tone screening test, that both tests were equally acceptable to children. She found that the sweep test was less time-consuming than the acoustic impedance test. She concludes that each method estimates different capacities of aural function which are possibly complementary.

Diagnostic tests (*See also* Chapters 1 and 2)

PURE-TONE AUDIOMETRY

This is the most extensively used measurement of auditory function. The value of determining the air and bone conduction levels for each ear separately has been greatly helped by the establishment of satisfactory masking techniques using narrow band masking. Hood (1962) described the method of masking now commonly used in clinical practice, based on the criteria of masking efficiency as expressed by Denes and Naunton (1952), and Fletcher's so-called critical frequency bands. Hood's method is logical, scientific, and simple to apply even with young children.

From the age of three, mentally normal children can be tested with pure tones. Sometimes it is necessary to modify the techniques which would be appropriate for adults. It is time-saving if pure tones can be introduced to children under five years of age by demonstrating the idea of responding to a signal, by teaching the child to respond to a signal by some suitable activity, such as placing a brick in a box. A free field audiometer can be used as the sound source for this purpose. As soon as a consistent response is secured then pure-tone audiometric testing can proceed. It can be advantageous in young children to help the child's attention by holding one ear-piece to the ear in order to focus the child's attention on the ear under test. It is usual to be able to proceed from this to complete headphone placement and to complete the thresholds for air conduction and bone conduction.

It is usual to measure air-conduction responses followed by bone-conduction testing. However, in very young children when their attention factors are relatively short, it is advisable to proceed to bone-conduction testing first in order to secure at the first examination a vital measurement which will differentiate between a conductive and a sensorineural deafness when raised levels have been demonstrated in a free field test. If it is possible to establish bone-conduction thresholds, pure-tone narrow band masking can then be introduced through an insert receiver. In this case when testing young children it is best to place the insert in the non-test ear with little or no verbal explanation to the child. The masking noise can be successfully raised whilst attention is drawn by the tester to those pure tones presented to the test ear. The basis for success with young children is to limit verbal explanation to a minimum until the child is of an age when verbal facility is well established.

ELECTRO-ACOUSTIC IMPEDANCE BRIDGE MEASUREMENT

This should now be regarded as a normal procedure in clinical practice. The principles of the measurement of middle-ear function by measurement of the acoustic impedance properties of the middle ear are comprehensively described by Feldman and Wilber (1976). Details are given in Chapter 1.

The common conditions of childhood affecting middle-ear function are those which cause blockage of the eustachian tube such as serous otitis media.

With a blocked eustachian tube it is usual to find a negative pressure with normal or decreased compliance. In the early stages of this condition it is possible to demonstrate the return to normal pressure by using the Valsalva manoeuvre.

When the eustachian blockage has become established and when fluid accumulates in the middle ear, the pressure is found to be increasingly negative and the compliance markedly decreased. In the extreme the actual negative pressure is greater than the instrument can register and the curve is flat.

Whilst in the early stages of eustachian malfunction little is to be observed otoscopically, clear otoscopic features are usually evident in the established condition.

In the event of a perforation of the tympanic membrane no seal is possible and no pressure gradient is obtained.

In children other abnormalities of the middle ear occur less often. They are:

(1) Ossicular fixation, either congenital or acquired. The pressure is normal, and the compliance may be normal or decreased.
(2) Ossicular discontinuity due to trauma or disease. The pressure is normal but the compliance will be increased.
(3) Eardrum abnormalities. Where the drum has lost the middle elastic coat the compliance will be increased although the pressure will be within normal range.

The stapedial reflex

The stapedius muscle is innervated by the facial nerve. The afferent arc is the auditory nerve.

The pathway of the acoustic reflex arc in rabbits has been described by Borg (1973) but the pathways in man are less clear although it is clear that the physiological function of the stapedial reflex is activated concurrently with the speech musculature. Anderson (1976) refers to Borg's (1974) view that its perceptive role, helping to distinguish external sounds when a person is talking, has the greatest significance for man. It has been shown, when the stapedius reflex is paralysed on one side, as in Bell's palsy, that the speech discrimination score diminishes. This is due to the masking of the lower frequency sounds over the high.

However, in clinical practice, the ability to elicit the stapedial reflex has proved to be of use in certain limited conditions.

Chiveralls and Fitzsimons (1973) investigated the stapedius reflex action in normal subjects. Their study of 47 normal young adults showed a mean stapedial reflex threshold over the frequency range 500 Hz–4 kHz to be 88 dB hearing level. This was a broad agreement with Lidén (1970) and Jepsen (1955) although some 5–10 dB higher. Chiveralls and Fitzsimons considered that because of the wide range of reflex threshold in the normal population a raised or absent threshold cannot be considered pathological. These findings and observations are important in the interpretation of data in the clinical situation of measured hearing loss.

In the presence of a sensorinerual loss it is sometimes assumed that the identification of the stapedius muscle contraction using an electro-acoustic impedance bridge at a stimulus level within the normal range is an indication of abnormal loudness function. Lidén (1970), in a study of the stapedial reflex in patients with either cochlear or retrocochlear lesions, claims that 'it could be inferred that loudness recruitment established by means of the stapedial reflex is equivalent to the presence of a lesion in the cochlea'.

Despite this claim further evidence would be valuable before we can equate the phenomenon known as loudness recruitment in the adult with an acquired lesion in a child who has a congenital sensorineural deafness. Taylor *et al.* (1973) were unable to demonstrate uncomfortable listening levels in children born deaf, although this phenomenon is well documented in adults with acquired cochlear lesions.

The stapedial reflex as a significant measure in paedoaudiology is limited to two areas. *Firstly,* demonstration of this reflex in the presence of a sensorineural deafness would suggest the presence of an abnormal loudness function. In most children this observation is not found to be associated with any of the well-recognized experiences found with adult abnormal loudness recruitment. *Secondly,* in the rare event of congenital stapedial fixation or in otosclerosis in childhood, suspicion of the presence of a stapedial fixation can be aroused by the absence of a change in the impedance reading when the contralateral ear is stimulated, especially when the pressure and the compliance are found to be normal and where it has been determined from pure-tone audiometry that a conductive deafness exists.

One interesting use of the stapedial reflex has been proposed by Niemeyer and Sesterhenn (1974). They used stimuli of pure tones in octave intensities from 125–8000 Hz, and white noise and a 24-tone mix to produce the stapedial reflex in a group of 50 normally hearing adults and ten normally hearing children.

They found that the reflex threshold for pure tone was 70–85 dB above normal hearing threshold, while for white noise and for the 24-tone mix the thresholds were between 40 and 50 dB above the threshold of audibility. Their work was extended to the investigation of 125 subjects with sensorineural hearing loss. From this work they calculated the mean hearing threshold by the formula—

$$\text{Hearing threshold} = \text{stapedius reflex (pure-tone) (SRT)} - 2.5 \text{ dlz}$$

dlz = the difference level between the mean SRT for pure tones from 0.5–4 kHz and the SRT for white noise.

They claimed that this was an accurate method of determining the threshold except in cases of falling pure-tone audiograms.

Shaw (1977) reported a study of 35 normally hearing subjects and of 29 hearing-impaired subjects. Shaw showed that within the normally hearing group prediction was accurate for 86.6 per cent and within the hearing-impaired group 61.5 per cent. Shaw concludes that the error in prediction when using this method prevents it being used by itself for definitive diagnosis.

SPEECH AUDIOMETRY

It has been known for many years that standardized tests of speech discrimination have a distinctive role in diagnostic procedures. Care must be taken to define the exact nature of the word lists or sentence material used in any test of speech discrimination. The American literature refers to the use of spondee word lists which are not appropriate for use in the English-speaking population.

In some word lists the standardization is based on the whole word being identified correctly. In others the scoring of each word is determined by the correct number of phonemes recognized correctly.

Watson (1957) has published word lists which are to be scored right or wrong whether or not the whole word is identified correctly. Boothroyd's (1968) lists are standardized to score each word as being three separate parts, each part identified correctly scoring one, and the highest score for a word being three marks. Whatever method is used it is most important to adhere rigidly to the author's original method of standardization.

It should be realized that in the scoring of a phonemic basis it is theoretically possible to score 66.6 per cent correctly without recognizing one word correctly. If the same list was scored on whole word recognition only, the score in this case would be 0 per cent. (*See* Chapter 1 for details of hearing tests.)

In disorders of the nerve fibres the speech discrimination capacity is very much poorer than would have been expected. This type of disorder is not found commonly in childhood. In children it is often noticed that the speech discrimination curve is normal when the results of pure-tone testing would suggest a sensorineural loss. This finding is commonest in children between the ages of nine and 12 years of age and is usually an indication of a non-organic hearing loss. This finding should alert the doctor to an underlying psychological disturbance which often has roots in problems at school or is a symptom of an anxiety state. These children are often reported as having an unusual facility for lip-reading.

The true nature of the problem can be resolved by testing the lip-reading capacity in controlled conditions where the subject is placed in a position where he is able to see the spoken word but the sound of the voice is not heard. In these conditions it quickly becomes apparent that there is no lip-reading capacity and indeed the patient is dependent on his hearing for speech discrimination.

ELECTRIC RESPONSE AUDIOMETRY

Although clinical interest in electric response audiometry (ERA) mushroomed with the advent of the averaging computer, the early work on the electrical activity of the auditory system laid the foundation for this great step forward (Davis, 1976).

Characteristics of the three major auditory-evoked responses

Each of the three major auditory-evoked responses may be recovered optimally by the use of certain band-width constraints associated with respective amplifier gain figures in the signal recovery system.

The curve illustrates the continuity of the three major responses in the time domain when the stimulus is in the form of a 60 μs click at 80 dB SPL. The curve is a composite, based on the three responses originally studied in isolation. For clarity both amplitude and time axes are non-linear. Amplitude calibrations are included in the delineated time zones.

A typical brain-stem evoked response (BSER) six-wave complex is elicited in a recording band-width of 550 Hz–3.3 kHz. The overall system gain in use is 105 dB.

The sixth wave of the BSER merges into a post-auricular response recorded in a 22–80 Hz bandwidth, this requiring a system gain of 60 dB.

Finally at 50 ms after the stimulus the post-auricular myogenic response (PAM) gives way to the cortical slow-vertex response recorded in a band-width of 3–30 Hz and a typical system gain of 88 dB.

The middle-latency intracranial responses (fast-vertex response) would appear at the same time location as the PAM. However, their recovery is dependent upon only small myogenic potentials being present and in general they demand low intensities of stimulation to avoid the masking effect of the PAM.

The 60 μs click stimuli used to elicit the BSER and PAM responses are non-frequency specific, i.e. a wide range of frequencies are produced by the click covering the range from below 200 Hz to above 8 kHz. The slow-vertex response is however produced as a result of stimulation by pure-tone bursts, which in this case are of 300-ms duration with controlled rise and fall times. Such stimuli are, of course, highly frequency specific.

The cortical slow vertex response can be elicited by the use of pure tones. Because of this, examination of the auditory signal is more frequency specific than it is when using the other responses where the sounds used to evoke responses lack the frequency specificity to the same extent.

Beagley (1976) has provided a very comprehensive account of the present state of the use of electric response audiometry (ERA) as practised in this country. He has found, using ketamine anaesthesia, that the electrocochleogram is valuable if used selectively with those children who cannot be tested by conventional methods and who need sedation. He advocates the electrocochleogram rather than attempting an evoked cortical response in children with epilepsy and athetoid cerebral palsy where the clarity of the ERA tracing is impaired. Indeed, he goes so far as to question whether or not ERA has a place in the assessment of hearing loss in children.

The possibilities of the brain-stem evoked response remain to be explored and further work is necessary before its value in clinical practice is established.

In an attempt to bring into perspective the place of the various test procedures it should be stressed that the well-tried conventional triad of pure tones, speech discrimination tests, and impedance measurement remain the first line in our diagnostic procedures. The place of the electric response procedures remains in a secondary role when the more conventional test procedures cannot be applied, and where it is essential to estimate the state of the auditory system. In the writer's experience these occasions are few in number. The degree of dependence on electric response audiometry is in some respects a failure of the tester's expertise in conventional test procedures.

ACOUSTIC CONDITIONS FOR TESTS OF HEARING

Since screening procedures depend on the response of children to sounds of minimal intensities, it is most important that they should be done in suitable surroundings. The clinics in which pre-school children are given screening tests should be sited in quiet localities whilst the internal noise in the building must be kept to a minimum whilst testing is in progress. Preferably the room in which tests are made should have some acoustic treatment to avoid reverberation (John, 1957). All these matters are even more important in clinics where diagnostic tests are being made. The test room, as well as being acoustically treated, should be insulated from noise sources in the building. Sweep-frequency testing of school-age children is normally undertaken in the schools, where good acoustic conditions are difficult to find. More failures in these tests result from the noisy background than through hearing impairment in the children. The only guidance that can be offered is that strenuous efforts must be made to insist on the optimum conditions that are available. Special noise-attenuating headphones may help to reduce the masking effect of the low-frequency ambient noise.

Guidance to parents of young deaf children

The methods of diagnosis outlined above are all designed to secure the identification of deafness at the earliest age possible. In practice the results are disappointing. Taylor (1977) reported in one clinical centre over the period 1968–74 the age at which a positive diagnosis of deafness was made as shown in the *Table 16.1*. This experience is not unique and is unacceptable. A diagnosis of deafness late in childhood has serious consequences for the deaf child and his family, the most significant being the time and opportunities lost when language should have been developing.

Table 16.1   **Ages at the date of referral for hearing tests of children who were enrolled under the parent guidance scheme of the Department of Audiology**

	Years										
Years of referral	6/12– 9/12	9/12– 1	1– 1½	1½– 2	2– 2½	2½– 3	3– 3½	3½– 4	4– 4½	4½– 5	5 and above
1968–1974	23	27	59	68	65	78	41	33	30	13	19

During the first four years of life, before school entry, a great deal of help can be made available to parents to help them understand the nature of their child's problem, to overcome their first reactions and to come to terms with the problem.

A guidance programme does not only take account of the educational needs of the child but must also accommodate the needs of the parents. The guide develops a close relationship with the parents as well as with the child.

Broomfield (1976) suggests that the 'reaction of families during the first months and year after a diagnosis of deafness in a child makes it clear that a guidance worker should be primarily concerned with the psychology of the handicap and only secondarily with the educational treatment of deafness'.

Luterman (1973) suggests that for the parents to deal positively with their child's needs they must be allowed the luxury of working through their own feelings of guilt, fear and confusion.

When the diagnosis of deafness is made some parents suffer a period of shock and immobility, while others who have themselves been convinced that their child is deaf, feel a sense of relief that at last their suspicions have been confirmed. At this initial stage the parents need emotional support. To have someone there who can share their feelings is a great help. If that same person is also knowledgeable about the educational management then a strong bond can be developed on which the pre-school years can be based. It must be the major goal that language-competence is achieved by the time the child is five years of age. To achieve this depends on a number of critical factors. The proper fitting of a satisfactory hearing aid is obviously vital. The parents must be helped to understand the goal of language acquisition and how they can furnish the optimum conditions for its realization.

It is a necessary part of the parents' task to talk to their children as often as possible in order to give the child the experience of auditory clues which we know are vital to the recognition of what we call our mother-tongue. Spoken language is a continuous flow which has important acoustic features which are vital for the understanding of what is said.

Speech is our basic mode of communication. It is a system in which a stream of sound signals radiated from the lips of one person is detected by the ears and interpreted by the brain of another person. The sound stream is a sequence of phonemes which are the separate speech sounds in a language. In English there are some 40 phonemes, each of which has its own sound pattern. A change of phoneme changes a word, e.g. man, ban, fan, are three different words because of the different sounds of the initial phonemes. Similarly in mean, moan, moon the change of meaning is due to the different sounds of the vowel phonemes. Our recognition and understanding of speech is partly a matter of our hearing the different sound patterns of the different phonemes. It is also a matter of our brains interpreting relationships between phonemes in sequence.

In learning to understand speech and to talk our brains acquire an enormous store of information about the ways in which the sound of one phoneme is joined to the sound of another phoneme. We learn that the linking sound is characteristic of a pair of phonemes and that there is a distinct relationship between phonemes in sequence. In the word *mat* we consciously hear only the three sounds represented by the letters m, a and t. Our ears can also detect the linking sounds, called transitions, and if listening conditions prevent us from hearing the whole sound pattern in each phoneme our brains will use information contained in the transitions.

In understanding speech we do not have to hear every sound—if we did listening and conversation would be an intolerable exercise. Fortunately speech contains far more information than is necessary to understand a message. We say that speech is highly redundant. The information contained in the transitions linking phonemes is an example of redundancy. Other examples are the time relationships between phonemes, syllables and words in sequence and the ways in which word sequences are ordered according to the syntax of a language.

Deafness may make some speech sounds inaudible or only partly audible to a child even when using powerful hearing aids. However, even severely deaf children usually have some residual hearing and hearing aids can amplify speech so that the child can hear that part of the sound stream which his residual hearing will allow. Much of the redundancy in speech will be contained in the limited range of frequencies audible to the child. Deaf children must be helped to exploit this 'redundant' information and to learn to interpret it.

The residual hearing of severely deaf children is usually better for lower frequencies than for higher frequencies. Such children may not be able to hear even the amplified sounds of some consonants. However, if they can hear the relatively low frequency vowel sounds they can also hear the transitions of those vowels and learn to interpret them. Again, more information is contained in the time-patterning of speech and if a child can be enabled to hear any sound he can perceive rhythmic patterns and learn to interpret them.

An important word in the last paragraph is *learn*. Learning to interpret the information contained in speech is not something which is done consciously, either by hearing or by deaf children. It is done unconsciously in the process of listening to speech. For the hearing child the learning is easy because he receives the whole of the sound patterns of speech during most of his waking life. In the deaf child it is much more difficult because he receives only a part of the sound pattern and that, unless special efforts are made, for only short periods of time. Nevertheless, when special efforts are made to talk to deaf children to enable them to hear speech as much as possible, the vast majority of them can learn to talk and to communicate through speech. (One recognizes that this may not be true in the case of some deaf children with additional, complicating handicaps such as an inability of the brain to process acoustic information.)

With the deaf child fitted with a suitable hearing aid there will necessarily be a limitation to the acoustic and visual clues he will receive. Understanding of the spoken language will develop if the parents are encouraged to use normal patterns of speech. The development is not dependent on exceptional intelligence of the child or the parent but on the consistent application from the earliest age of the maximum use of any residual hearing, watching for speech and consistently speaking to children using normal sentences as we would when speaking to hearing children.

When speaking to deaf children it is tempting to modify the speaking patterns, often subconsciously, in a way which may truncate sentences, or to speak in a way which is grammatically correct, corresponding to a written form of language, or in the worst situation to use single word utterances. Another possibility is that the speech patterns used might be distorted by slowing down the rate of utterance, thus interfering with the time features of speech.

It is important to remember that in parent guidance it is not the total amount of talk which is important but the amount of talk which makes clear to the child the correspondence between linguistic and non-linguistic events.

Tizard *et al.* (1972) showed that it was the amount of informative talk by adults, their willingness to answer children's questions and the amount of active play they initiated which resulted in the better comprehensive and expressive language scores by the children. It was not the total amount of talk to children that made the difference.

Howarth (1977) summarized the essential work for parents with a deaf child as follows:

(1) To use consistently the best possible hearing aids.
(2) To make time for conversations which are meaningful as outlined above.
(3) To ensure that conversations are real exchanges of meaning which are necessary to parent and child. The child has to see that something happens as a result of speaking.
(4) To understand the child's mind in order to anticipate and respond to his incomplete and often unintelligible part in the conversation.
(5) To say back in well-formed English what he tried to say himself.
(6) To recognize that the form of their spoken language will be appropriate to the language level of their children if they do not think about it and do not consciously modify it because the child is very young or very deaf.

The fitting of hearing aids in children

Hearing aids have been available through the National Health Service since 1948. Although this provision was made, studies indicated that the use of hearing aids by children in school was unsatisfactory. Martin and Lodge (1969) reported in their survey that the number of non-working hearing aids was high. They advised that a competent hearing-aid technician should be assigned to a school or a group of schools to carry out continuous 100 per cent checks on all hearing aids and other acoustic equipment.

Another survey investigating the use of hearing aids in schools for the deaf and partially hearing in Great Britain showed that as many as 50 per cent of aids issued were inadequate for the needs of the children.

At the outset it should be remembered that the Medresco range of aids were designed primarily for use with adults. The Medical Research Council Report (1947) was based on experimental work with adults, who, in the main, suffered from acquired deafness.

It is likely that the degree of hearing loss found amongst congenitally deaf patients suffering from sensorineural hearing loss in special schools will be greater than many of the adult deaf population with acquired losses.

A survey by Hine (1973) of 5016 children in 55 special schools for the hearing-impaired in England, Wales, Scotland, Northern Ireland and Eire indicates the nature of the distribution of hearing losses in that population.

Although more powerful hearing aids were being made available an important development was the availability of commercial aids on the National Health Call-Off Contract in 1974. This was a significant step forward in making available aids which would be more suited to the hearing losses of children with congenital sensorineural deafness.

In the case of older hearing-impaired children who are capable of indicating differences amongst hearing-aid test procedures, the selection of a suitable aid can be made on the basis of differences using speech discrimination tests.

With babies and young children where such techniques are not applicable other methods for hearing-aid selection have to be adopted.

Boothroyd (1968) in his investigation had determined a method of analysis of speech which would allow an area to be plotted on the pure-tone audiogram form which would give an indication of the approximate spectral content of the speech signal.

Huntington (1975) indicated the application of this knowledge in hearing-aid fitting. He suggested that the aim when fitting a hearing aid is to lower or amplify this speech area so that the hearing-impaired child's pure-tone audiogram lies on or about the top of the area. This method will ensure that the aid chosen will reach the residual hearing capacity of the child.

Nolan (1977) has made available information on a wide range of commercial and National Health Service hearing aids so that the essential data are now available to the practising otologist in the prescription of hearing aids for children. Two major factors in the consideration of hearing aid selection are the maximum output and the frequency response. The earlier work on which the Medresco aids were designed suggests a maximum output of 120 dB (SPL). However, the majority of deaf children require a maximum output of 130 dB SPL.

Serious difficulties have been presented in achieving a satisfactory output with very deaf children on account of the difficulty with the production of moulds which should be accurately fitted so as to obviate acoustic feedback. Nolan and Tucker (1977) have suggested a method whereby the seal can be improved. It still remains true that the most important factor in the making of satisfactory ear moulds is the personal care which is expended in the preparation.

Nolan (1978) has drawn attention to the availability of sub-miniature receivers available through the National Health Service with three commercial high-power bodyworn aids. It is recommended that these receivers should be used routinely with children. These receivers have been shown to improve the ear-mould receiver system in terms of output available before feedback, wearability of ear moulds and the cosmetic aspects of the amplification system.

Markides (1974), considering the benefits of binaural aids, concludes that subjects with symmetrical conductive or symmetrical sensorineural hearing impairments and with average hearing levels of 50–90 dB benefited from binaural aids in terms of speech discrimination and localizing ability. In those subjects with a flat loss in one ear and a steeply sloping loss in the other, there was no advantage as far as speech discrimination was concerned but binaural hearing aids did help localization.

Markides (1974) reports that in patients with severe or total unilateral loss there were advantages with CROS (Contralateral Routing of Signals) hearing-aid systems.

The conventional bodyworn aids and the behind-the-ear aids present considerable problems to the user where the environmental noise is not controlled. John (1957) has indicated the effects of such environments on hearing-aid use and suggested ways of modifying these effects.

It was hoped that the introduction of the loop system in classrooms would help significantly with the noise problems. However, the loop field varies in strength from one part of the classroom to another and the teacher's signal is not contained within the classroom ratio. There remain considerable technical difficulties with this system which have largely been overcome in the radio-microphone system. The teacher, wearing a light microphone–transmitter transmits speech via radio waves to children equipped with wearable radio receivers and amplifiers. Mobility is maintained, constant strength signals are transmitted and there is no overspill since the transmission frequency is particular to the room where the teacher works. Since each child wears the same kind of receiver the characteristics of the system are known quantities. The problem of balancing teachers' voices and child's voice has been solved.

An additional feature of the high quality radio aid is the incorporation of linear dynamic compression circuiting which ensures undistorted output, even at high-intensity levels, but with an adjustable maximum output that protects sensitive listeners against uncomfortable or painful peak intensities. The radio aid is playing a major role in the situation where a hearing-impaired child integrates for lessons among normally hearing children.

Concern has been expressed about the possible damage to the residual hearing. Markides (1971) made a comprehensive survey of the literature and concluded that there was no conclusive evidence that hearing aids do or do not have any adverse effect on the users' residual hearing.

Hine and Furness (1975) made an examination of the annual pure-tone audiograms of 21 children aged 5–9 years in a school for the partially hearing where the natural means of communication is oral and where great emphasis is laid on the use of hearing aids. There were no cases of a statistically significant deterioration in measured threshold and it was concluded that the regular use of hearing aids had not damaged the residual hearing of any of these children. In fact, over one third of the children showed statistically significant improvement in measured threshold. They concluded that this improvement reflected an enhanced ability to attend to auditory signals.

Education of hearing-impaired children

Statistical data help us to appreciate the size of the population of children within the different educational provisions (*see Table 16.2*).

Table 16.2   Hearing impaired children in special schools and units in 1976

	Deaf	*Partially Hearing*	*Totals*
In special schools			
Day	1829	1302	
Residential	1678	942	
	3507	2244	5751
Attending 'designated special classes' (Partially Hearing Units)	278	3249	3527
In independent school by arrangements with Local Education Authorities	304	98	402
Home tuition, or in small groups	55	75	130
Awaiting admission to special school	93	200	293
	4237	5866	10103

N.B.   These figures do not include hearing-impaired children specifically placed in ordinary schools, or pre-school parent-guidance cases supervised by peripatetic teachers. This latter group could approximate to 20 per cent of those in the special schools and units, i.e. about 2000.

The growth of educational provision is evident from the following statistics. (Provisions vary between different educational authorities.)

Units:

England and Wales	1966	162 classes	
	1967	191 classes	
	1968	173 units	
	1971	212	
	1973–4	299	
	1975–6	369	
	1976–7	419	

Peripatetic teachers:

Her Majesty's Stationery Office Survey	1951	2	
England and Wales—New appointments	1955	1	
	1956	0	
	1957	1	
	1958	3	
	1959	3	
	1960	11	
	1961	9	
	1962	11	
	1963	21	
	1964	26	
	1965	31	
	1966	41	
	1967	177	
	1973–4	262 NDCS	283 NCTD
	1975–6	369 NDCS	363 NCTD
	1976–7	414	

(NDCS = National Deaf Children's Society; NCTD = National College of Teachers of the Deaf)

Special schools may be day or residential. A few of the special schools are specially designated as schools for the partially hearing. Generally speaking, they are all-age schools providing for deaf children from the age of 3–16, although there are a few separate primary schools and some separate secondary schools. There is a special grammar school for deaf and partially-hearing pupils. A report of the academic results from this grammar school has been published by Askew (1971). There is also a selective secondary school with a technical bias for boys. Many special schools are able to present successfully some of their pupils for the Certificate of Secondary Education and the General Certificate of Education.

There are a small number of schools catering specifically for deaf or partially-hearing pupils with additional handicaps.

About one third of children in special educational provision attend special classes attached to ordinary schools. These classes are in charge of qualified teachers of the deaf and the aim is to help the children to develop linguistically and academically so that they may integrate to as great a degree as possible into the regular classes in the school. If the integration is to be successful the pupils need to be socially as well as academically prepared for it. Some children may have reached this point by the end of the infant stage; others require a great deal of special help throughout the junior stage. For children who have been unable to achieve complete integration by the end (11 years) of the primary stage, some secondary units have been established. Here there is usually a somewhat different approach to the problem. The pupils are enrolled in ordinary forms and come to the special teacher for varying periods of extra tuition according to their needs. Most unit classrooms are acoustically treated and generally provided with various types of hearing-aid equipment, so that the pupils are enabled to make the best possible use of their hearing.

There are as many hearing-impaired children attending ordinary schools as there are in special schools and units. The function of the peripatetic teachers who supervise them is to advise the class teachers on their problems and how to deal with them, to give some auditory training, help with speech and lip-reading where this is required and to give some remedial help when possible. One of the major difficulties these children face is that of discriminating speech through an aid in ordinary classroom conditions. As has been mentioned previously, background noise, distance of teacher from the microphone of the child's aid and the reverberant qualities of untreated rooms all militate against the effectiveness of wearable hearing aids. One way to overcome these difficulties is the use of radio aids. A useful description of the problems of children in ordinary schools is given by Johnson (1962) and by Fisher (1971).

A review of educational treatment of deafness must consider the special place of *method of communication.* Much controversy surrounds this area of discussion which must be confusing to those not primarily involved in the educational profession. John and Howarth (1973) in a paper putting forward an argument for oral communication indicate the theoretical and practical reasons for supporting the general consensus view in this country for an oral approach to the teaching of hearing-impaired children. They indicate many of the weaknesses of a manual method.

Owrid (1971) has made clear that much confusion abounds in what comparative research studies are deemed to have demonstrated. He has pointed out the main weaknesses of the studies by Stuckless and Birch (1966), Hester (1964) and Quigley (1969) in putting forward the advantages of manual communication.

Markides (1976) has shown from his study of 30 deaf pupils from a manual school for the deaf, 30 deaf pupils from an oral school for the deaf and 30 hearing pupils from an ordinary middle school that the linguistic proficiencies of the deaf pupils from the oral school for the deaf were of equal standard and on certain occasions significantly better than the performance of the hearing pupils. He found that the pupils from the oral school for the deaf were better prepared, with regard to attitude, to live and work with the hearing society than the pupils from the manual school for the deaf. Markides (1976) like Owrid (1971) concluded that no evidence exists to show that manual and/or combined methods of educating deaf children are superior to the oral approach.

Manual communication

There is a great variety of manually-formed visual symbols for use in communication by and with hearing-impaired people. Some of these forms, such as the signs traditionally used in many residential schools for deaf children and in social clubs for deaf people, were developed many years ago; others are of very recent invention. Broadly they can be categorized in three groups: those which are transformations of spoken language as in finger-spelling; those which have developed from principally pictorial gestures and from mime as in signing; and those which attempt to provide, in addition to traditional signs, indications of the grammatical features of spoken language, for example, indicators of tense changes in verbs.

Finger-spelling

Forms of finger-spelling have been known for centuries. In the simplest form hand shapes represent letters of the alphabet. In the UK the two-handed alphabet is the more common. In the USA the one-handed alphabet predominates. Its advantage in freeing one hand may be gained at the expense of some loss of clarity. Finger-spelling does not of course match exactly the printed word since a page of text allows the eye to scan back and forth. Still less does finger-spelling match the spoken word with all its nuances of intonation, stress and rhythm. A great deal of practice is required to become a fluent finger-speller and more especially to be able to follow the rapid finger-spelling of another person.

Cued speech

Some sounds of speech, especially consonants, are not easy for a lip-reader to discern. A method of producing hand cues to sounds which are not clearly visible was invented by Forchhamer, a Dane, in the nineteenth century. Recently Cornett (1967) working at Gallaudet College in the USA has produced a system which aims by the use of hand cues to identify visually and completely the sounds of speech. It is a feature of the system, called Cued Speech, that the hand cues alone do not provide the full identification of a particular sound.

The hand cue must be interpreted in conjunction with the lip movements of speech. To this end the hand cues are formed close to the speaker's face. A problem of all combinations of hand symbols with speech is that the hand symbols are not produced as rapidly as speech sounds. It is claimed that in Cued Speech a cueing speed can be achieved which does not reduce the speech flow to levels which would be slower than a normal measured delivery. Cornett does not disguise the fact that to become fluent persistent practice is required.

Traditional signing and systematic signs

When residential schools for deaf children were established during the nineteenth century it was common for communication between teachers and supervisory staff and the children to be carried on by means of signs. Most of these originated in pictorial gestures. For example, a key might be signified by a turning motion of the hand. Some of the signs doubtless originated from gestures used by the children but many of them were provided by adults, hearing or deaf, who had knowledge of the native verbal language.

Consequently, the signs are usually readily translatable into words although the converse is not true. There are many words for which no exact counterpart in signing exists. Traditional signing provides a repertory of symbols which is limited when compared with the vocabularies of verbal languages. A more obvious difference between verbal language and signing is the absence in signing of grammar as the term is usually understood. There are principles governing the use of signs but those components of grammar, such as rules of word order and of inflection which are common to verbal languages, have little, if any, analogue in signing. In the translation of signs into verbal language considerable additional interpretive work is often needed if incomprehensible strings of words are to be avoided. In the translation of verbal language into signs the problem of words which have no sign counterpart arises whilst the difficulty of showing the inflections of words is even more acute. This difference between the grammatical constructions of verbal languages and patterns of signing has given rise to the invention of systems of signing which attempt to follow the grammatical patterns of verbal language. Such a system was foreshadowed in the work of the great eighteenth century educator of the deaf, the Abbe de l'Epée. Since his time several forms have been provided. In the UK Lady Paget, widow of Sir Richard Paget, developed her husband's ideas and together with Pierre Gorman (1969) produced the Systematic Sign Language. The aim of this system is to provide a repertory of signs which in addition to representing the root meanings of words will also provide indications of the inflections so that English may be represented grammatically by signs. Similar systems have been developed recently in the USA.

On superficial consideration, manual means of communication appear to have very clear advantages for people who have extremely restricted hearing. The evidence of experience, by contrast, points to their very severe limitations as substitutes for spoken language or the printed word.

As far as adults who have become deaf in later life are concerned, there is reluctance to turn to manual communication. Two obvious reasons could account for such reluctance. The difficulty which older people have in learning new skills compounds the inherent difficulty in achieving fluency in manual communication. In addition there may be unwillingness to adopt forms of communication which the deaf person may feel will separate him further from the society of hearing people which he is used to and with which he is likely to wish to remain in contact.

In the case of children who are very deaf the problem of communication remains the problem of learning a language. Very deaf children acquire gestures and traditional signs easily if they are in contact with these means of communication. They do not however readily acquire the grammatical features of systematic signing which are intended to provide the children with access to the grammar of verbal language. Similarly it is true of finger-spelling that it is extremely difficult to learn verbal language by this means. Briefly it may be said that those means which are easy for the very deaf child to learn, such as gestures, signs and pantomime, do not in themselves lead to knowledge of or skill in verbal language. Moreover, those means, which because they are forms of verbal language might lead to knowledge of the printed and spoken word, are no easier for the children to acquire than the direct form of the spoken or printed word.

Because of the difficulties of the systematic forms of manual communication some people have advocated mixtures which involve the use of virtually any form of communication. These mixtures are termed Total Communication in the USA. They have much in common with the Combined Methods which have been used widely in the past in residential schools in this country. Such methods have not solved the communication and educational problems of deaf children. Workers who have much experience of signing or finger-spelling emphasize the necessity for long and continued practice to achieve and retain fluency in manual communication. It is unusual for normally hearing people, including the parents of most deaf children, to have access to situations in which long practice in manual communication is available. Hence arguments which are based on the performance of children of deaf parents lose much of their force when extended to quite different linguistic and communicational situations.

A powerful and compelling argument for oral education has been argued by Furness (1972) in a cogent assessment of the reasons for wide variations in linguistic development and capabilities of deaf children. Furness points out that in many schools oral methods were introduced into older special schools and superimposed on a well-established manual system. He asserts that children will not develop through an oral method if the practice ground provides the facilities for active participation in the manual medium. Furness sees the special school as a centre where deaf children will go to be specially helped to do naturally what largely comes naturally to a hearing child.

Furness makes a fundamentally important distinction between the traditional methods of teaching language to deaf children and the concept of the incidental way of learning to talk as experienced by normal children. In essence a deaf child must learn to talk and not be taught to speak. This view of the need to talk is emphasized in the earlier section on parent guidance. With parents of deaf children we ask them to speak normally to their children. It is an extension of this practice that Furness argues so forcibly and it is the deviation from what we know of language development in the normal child that produces the problems in the education of deaf children.

Causes of childhood deafness

The clinician has considerable interest in the causes of congenital and acquired sensorineural deafness on two main counts. Firstly it is important to be able to give as accurate a statement as possible to parents, who have presented with one deaf child, what the possibility is of another child being born with the same disability. Secondly, the research of sensorineural deafness should be given active consideration.

Harrison, K. (1971) has presented a comprehensive classification based on pre-natal, perinatal, post-natal, and unknown causes. In early investigations of the causes of deafness, many cases were classified as congenital when, in actual fact, they were acquired. As early as 1894, Mygind recognized this error in classification. Many causes of deafness in children are now known and a suitable classification can be made in relation to the time at which the hearing mechanism is affected, that is pre-natal, perinatal and post-natal (*see Table 16.3*).

Table 16.3   Classification of causes

I. PRE-NATAL
  A. *Genetic*
      Scheibe   Michel
      Bing–Siebenmann   Usher's syndrome
      Waardenburg's syndrome   Endemic cretinism
      Pendred's syndrome   Klippel–Feil syndrome
      Mondini–Alexander
  B. *Non-genetic*
      Diseases occurring during pregnancy
          German measles and other virus illnesses
          Toxaemia
          Diabetes
          Nephritis
      Drugs taken during pregnancy
          Streptomycin
          Quinine
          Salicylates
          Thalidomide
II. PERINATAL
  Prematurity
  Haemolytic disease—kernicterus
  Birth trauma—anoxia
III. POST-NATAL
  A. *Genetic*
      Familial perceptive deafness (heredodegenerative
          deafness)
      Otosclerosis
      Alport's syndrome
  B. *Non-genetic*
      Infectious diseases
          measles
          mumps
          meningococcal or pneumococcal meningitis
          tuberculous meningitis
          trauma
      Otitis media—suppurative and non-suppurative
          (exudative)
      Ototoxic antibiotics—streptomycin, neomycin,
          kanamycin

It is often thought that genetic deafness is only congenital, meaning that the hearing mechanism has only been affected pre-natally. It is now known that genetic deafness may only become manifest post-natally, in childhood or even in adult life, e.g. familial perceptive deafness, otosclerosis and Alport's syndrome. The deafness that results from the above causes is usually perceptive (sensorineural). Amongst the post-natal causes there are some cases of conductive deafness resulting from otosclerosis, otitis media and trauma, and these can usually be treated surgically.

In all reported series there are considerable numbers which have to be placed in the 'unknown' group. Harrison (1959) and Livingstone (1962) both reported around 30 per cent of cases in which no cause could be determined. Fraser (1964) reported 38 per cent in a large group of 2355 severely-deaf children. Maran (1966) reported 28 per cent of unknown aetiology in 464 children with sensorineural deafness. He considered that the shape of an audiogram was of no value in relation to the cause but thought that it may aid further questioning in the unknown group. With better identification and understanding of genetic causes, more accurate diagnosis will be made in this unknown group.

Developmental abnormalities of the outer and middle ear are described in Chapters 4 and 6.

Paparella and Winter (1968) have suggested a classification of sensorineural deafness in childhood based only on the clinical considerations of aetiology. They have taken a broad perspective and have not attempted a detailed breakdown of types beneath the subheading classifications (*Table 16.4*).

In the differential diagnosis of sensorineural deafness in children the otologist should first determine whether the hearing disorder was present at the time of birth (congenital) or whether it developed subsequent to birth (acquired). A secondary diagnostic consideration is whether the deafness is of genetic or non-genetic origin and thus these subheadings should appear in the classification. Paparella and Winter state that at the moment there are many reports of sensorineural deafness in children which are not well established and these must necessarily fall into category III (unclassified) to await further clarification.

1. Prenatal

A. GENETIC

Ormerod (1960), in describing the pathology of congenital deafness, states that the following causes may be responsible:

Failure in the development of
(1) the bony cochlea,
(2) the membranous cochlea,
(3) the organ of Corti and the tectorial membrane,
(4) the middle ear, ossicular chain and external auditory meatus.

Interruption of development of
(1) organ of Corti and the tectorial membrane,
(2) the ossicles of the middle ear, and
(3) the external ear.

Degeneration of parts of the auditory apparatus which have already developed in some degree or reached maturity

Table 16.4   Proposed classification of sensorineural deafness in childhood

---

I. CONGENITAL
  Genetic
  Non-genetic
    inflammatory, toxic,
    metabolic, neoplastic
II. ACQUIRED
  Genetic
  Non-genetic
    inflammatory, toxic,
    metabolic, neoplastic, traumatic
III. UNCLASSIFIED

---

(1) the canal of the cochlea or scala media,
(2) the sensory end-organ including the tectorial membrane, and
(3) the nerve elements including the spiral ganglia over the basal nuclei.

Ormerod believed that amongst the causes of inherited deafness, those of the Scheibe (sacculo–cochlear) type appear to be the most common. The whole bony labyrinth and the membranous utricle and canals are fully formed and the latter are functioning. The cochlea and saccule show an early fetal type of sensory epithelium and the organ of Corti and saccular macula are represented by a mound of undifferentiated cells. The tectorial membrane is formed, but is distorted and flattened down over the organ of Corti and the stria vascularis is degenerate. The Scheibe type of deafness is not usually associated with other developmental abnormalities. In the Mondini–Alexander type, the cochlea is flattened, with development of the basal coil only and with a comparable underdevelopment of the vestibular structures. In the Bing–Siebenmann type, the bony cochlea and vestibule are fully formed, but the membranous internal ear is either malformed or is degenerate in both halves. It may be associated with abnormalities of the central nervous system.

In the Michel type, there is a total lack of development of the internal ear and this is the most severe deformity. This change may be associated with other abnormalities and with mental retardation.

Waardenburg's syndrome
The histopathology has shown the absence of the organ of Corti and atrophy of the spiral ganglion with a paucity of nerve fibres.

Pendred's syndrome
In one case described by Huidberg-Hansen and Jørgenson (1965) and reported by Lindsay (1973), histopathology showed pronounced hydrops of the cochlear duct. There were no hair-cells, total atrophy of the tectorial membrane, no nerve fibres and only a trace of ganglion cells. The Mondini type of deficiency was reported.

Usher's disease
Lindsay reports that the pathological change is restricted mainly to the cochlea and its nerve and vascular supply. The stria vascularis shows irregular areas of degeneration throughout. The organ of Corti is atrophied together with the epithelium

of the inner and outer sulci in the lower basal turn and degeneration decreasing in the upper turns. In the spiral ganglion peripheral and central fibres show severe atrophy. There are darkly stained occlusions in the stria vascularis.

Endemic cretinism

Lindeman (1965) reported that histological examination showed a nearly-normal organ of Corti and tectorial membrane, but that Reissner's membrane was depressed and the number of ganglion cells in the basal turn was decreased. The stria vascularis appeared abnormal.

Klippel–Feil

Abnormalities may involve the bony as well as the membranous labyrinth and the auditory nerves.

B. NON-GENETIC

German measles

Carruthers first reported the pathological changes in the ear. Lindsay and his colleagues (1953) examined both inner ears from four cases and found degenerative changes within the cochlear duct and saccule. The stria vascularis, the tectorial membrane and the organ of Corti showed different degrees of degenerative changes, whilst the wall of the saccule showed collapse and adhesions to the macula.

Lindsay (1965) considers that the virus invades the endolymphatic system without involving the perilymphatic spaces. He considers that the histopathological changes result from a haematogenous invasion during the course of a viraemia, and describes it as 'haematogenous endolymphatic labyrinthitis'. The changes are similar to those described in the Scheibe type.

Diabetes

Kelemen (1957) describes a primipara with severe diabetes who was rapidly becoming blind and whose pregnancy was terminated at four months. Examination of the internal ear of the fetus showed haemorrhages into the cochlea and vestibule. There was normal development of the end-organ and other parts but haemorrhage was certainly causing absorption of the cupula and presumably would in time have affected other parts, including the tectorial membrane.

Nephritis

Kelemen (1957) described the termination of pregnancy, at its fourth month, of a woman with severe nephritis and advanced coma. Examination of the internal ear showed changes similar to those in the diabetic case.

Drugs taken during pregnancy

Kern (1962) reported a case in which an ototoxic antibiotic, dihydrostreptomycin, administered in early pregnancy resulted in profound deafness in the fetus. It is considered that certain drugs can cross the placenta and damage the inner ear in the fetus.

II. Perinatal

PREMATURITY

In an important study Davies and Stewart (1975) identify two groups of low-birth-weight (LBW) babies. This term is normally taken to refer to babies of $\leqslant$ 2500 g and very low birth weight $\leqslant$ 500 g. 'Pre-term birth' as defined by Davies and Stewart indicates delivery before the 37th complete week of gestation. Infants are referred to as 'small-for-dates' (SFD) if their birth weight falls below the tenth percentile for gestational age on accepted standards of birth weight in relation to gestation, and are considered 'Appropriate-for-dates' (AFD) if weight lies between the tenth and 90th percentile. In the consideration of the pathology of deafness in premature babies there are often other factors co-existing which make the identification of one causative factor difficult. Such drugs as streptomycin and dihydrostreptomycin were used frequently in the earlier years at dosages which would now be considered high.

Lindsay (1973) when discussing the place of anoxia and hypoxia records that severe deafness has been known to occur in cases of breech presentation with the cord round the neck and producing anoxia or severe hypoxia.

Changes in the primary nuclei due to asphyxia have been reported. Lindsay (1973) concludes that the evidence that premature birth of a normal infant predisposes to deafness has not been clearly established, although the incidence of deafness among premature babies otherwise apparently normal, has been higher than in full-term births.

Fraser (1976) in a consideration of this problem concludes that the representation of premature babies in a series of deaf children has in fact become increasingly prominent. The deafness is thought to be due to haemorrhage into the inner ear following injury or stress during birth. Buch (1966) studied the temporal bones of 73 newborn infants and suggested that traumatic procedures played an important role in the aetiology of these haemorrhages. It is also possible that there may be damage to the cochlear nuclei.

In animal experiments Myers (1972) has described two forms of asphyxia in term monkeys. One form called acute total asphyxia implies sudden complete cessation of oxygen supply to the fetus. This results in damage predominantly to structures in the brain stem. The cerebral cortex and basal ganglia are either unaffected or damaged rather late. In the clinical situation a similar form of asphyxia may be associated with cardiac arrest. In partial prolonged asphyxia there is a gradual fall in the partial pressure of oxygen in the fetal blood. This type of asphyxia prolongs the clinical situation. In monkeys partial prolonged asphyxia causes brain swelling and damage to the cerebral cortex and basal ganglia.

The well documented experimental work of Ranck and Windle (1959) showed marked damage to the cochlear nuclei and the nuclei in the mid-brain in the monkey. The nature of these experiments would be classified under the heading of 'acute total asphyxia'.

HAEMOLYTIC DISEASE OF THE NEWBORN

Haemolytic disease of the newborn (HDNB) may result from either rhesus incompatibility or prematurity. Levine, Katzin and Burnham (1941) stated that rhesus incompatibility was responsible for haemolytic anaemia and jaundice in the newborn. Some of the cases of jaundice develop neurological complications resulting from yellow staining of the basal nuclei. This staining of the basal nuclei was first described by Orth (1875) and called 'nuclear jaundice'. Later, in 1904, Schmörl coined the term 'kernicterus'.

Crosse, Wallis and Walsh (1958) stated that there are about 500 cases of kernicterus due to prematurity in England and Wales each year. The cause is thought to be an hepatic immaturity. In these infants, the serum bilirubin is considerably raised. Normally, the bilirubin is conjugated with glycuronic acid, but if the liver is immature this cannot occur.

Claireaux (1950) put forward the hypothesis that in the kernicterus of rhesus incompatibility, cells of the nuclear masses are markedly affected by anoxia resulting from severe anaemia. This increases the cell permeability to bilirubin, to give rise to the typical yellow staining.

Gerrard (1952) carried out post-mortem examinations in two cases of kernicterus. The cochlear nuclei showed degeneration of the nerve cells, but the cochleas themselves appeared to be within normal limits.

Dublin (1951) examined the brains of seven newborn babies who had died as a result of kernicterus and he found damage in both the dorsal and ventral cochlear nuclei. There was also damage in the medial geniculate body and the auditory cortex and radiations. There was no damage to the hair-cells.

III. Post-natal

MEASLES

Lindsay and Hemenway (1954) reported the pathological findings in the inner ears of an infant who died from cardiac complications of measles. Histopathological changes were confined to the structures within the endolymphatic system. The organ of Corti and stria vascularis showed degenerative changes that progressed in extent from the apex (where the changes were confined to the stria, the hair-cells and the tectorial membrane) to the base (where the organ of Corti had been totally destroyed and only remnants of the tectorial membrane and stria remained). They describe the findings as an 'endolymphatic labyrinthitis' due to haematogenous invasion in the course of a viraemia.

MUMPS

Lindsay, Proctor and Work (1960) reported the histological findings in the ears of a child with profound deafness in both ears that had occurred during mumps. The findings represent the destructive effects of the mumps virus on the structures within the cochlear duct and saccule—the results of an inflammatory process that can be described as 'endolymphatic labyrinthitis'. There is still no satisfactory explanation as to why the deafness in mumps is usually unilateral.   Lindsay (1965) states that the histopathological changes found in cases of deafness due to maternal rubella, measles and mumps have indicated the hazard to the receptor organs in the ear from virus disease, either in the course of pregnancy or in early childhood. They also suggest a possible explanation for the Scheibe type of cochlear dysplasia on the basis of acquired degeneration *in utero* or early infancy as contrasted to a genetically-related defect.

It is evident from the histopathological findings in viral labyrinthitis that two basic types occur. In one, the infection extends primarily into the perilymphatic spaces and in the other the virus invades the endolymphatic system in the course of a viraemia without involving the perilymphatic spaces.

MENINGITIS

The cause of deafness in bacterial meningitis still remains obscure. In these cases the meningitis may be cured, but function of the labyrinth may be destroyed.

In tuberculous meningitis, Whetnall and Lucas (1952) demonstrated that there is extensive tuberculous infiltration in the sheath of the auditory nerve; and the basilar membrane, organ of Corti, Reissner's membrane and stria vascularis show marked infiltration with lymphocytes. It must also be remembered that when streptomycin and dihydrostreptomycin are used in the treatment of tuberculosis meningitis, the ototoxic effect is greatly increased if the antibiotics are given by the intrathecal route. Direct access to the inner ear by way of the cerebrospinal fluid and perilymph is indicated, and this could be one route of entry even after intramuscular administration. Other possibilities include secretion into the perilymph from the vessels of the spiral ligament, or into the endolymph from the stria vascularis or spiral prominence. Still another possible route is that from the vessels of the basilar membrane (the so-called vas spirale) into the cortilymph (Hawkins, Beger and Aran, 1965).

Trauma and *otitis media*, including suppurative and non-suppurative (exudative) are described in Chapters 9 and 10.

OTOTOXIC ANTIBIOTICS

Many drugs are known to cause sensorineural deafness in both children and adults. The most important group of drugs as far as deafness in childhood is concerned are those drugs in the aminoglycoside group of antibiotics. The nine aminoglycosides named by Leach (1962) which are known to be toxic to the labyrinth are dihydrostreptomycin, framycetin, kanamycin, neomycin, polymyxin B, nitocitin, streptomycin, vancomycin, and viomycin. Ballantyne (1973, 1976) indicates the need to add gentamicin to this list.

Szekely and Draskovitch (1965) examined 84 children between the ages of six and eight years who had received streptomycin in infancy; 43 had measurable high frequency losses, although only 14 showed evidence of residual vestibular damage.

Both streptomycin and dihydrostreptomycin are reported to cross the placenta and damage the fetal ear.

Ballantyne (1973) has stressed that the topical application of the aminoglycoside drugs may also be ototoxic. For further details see Chapter 21.

Discussion

Fraser (1976) has published an important study *Causes of Profound Deafness in Childhood*, which is the analysis of a study of 3533 individuals with severe hearing loss present at birth or of childhood onset. An early publication by Fraser (1970) presented a shorter form of this study. He reported on 2355 children in the British Isles (*see Table 16.5*).

Table 16.5   Causes of deafness in the 2355 children of the school study in the British Isles

Cause	Males	Females	Total
Not deaf	16	10	26
Genetically-determined deafness			
Autosomal recessive syndromes			
with goitre	65	68	133
with retinitis pigmentosa	16	12	28
with ECG abnormalities	7	9	16
others	3	4	7
Autosomal dominant syndromes			
with pigmentary anomalies	40	31	71
others	3	0	3
Clinical undifferentiated deafness			
where family history suggests			
single-gene inheritance			
autosomal recessive	145	164	309
autosomal dominant	66	61	127
sex-linked recessive	22	0	22
Malformation of complex causation			
Wildevanck's syndrome	2	18	20
other	9	3	12
Primarily acquired deafness			
pre-natally acquired (mainly rubella)	69	69	138
perinatally acquired	76	51	127
acquired after the end of the			
perinatal period	287	176	463
Total with tentative diagnosis of aetiology	826	676	1502
Residual groups of unknown cause	465	388	853
Total	1291	1064	2355

From Sensori-Neural Hearing Loss (1970). Reproduced by permission of the Ciba Foundation

Fisch (1976) reported on the relative proportion of causes of congenital deafness in 600 cases (*see Table 16.6*).

Table 16.6

Causes	No. of cases	%
Genetic	157	26.1
Unknown	151	25.1
Maternal rubella	144	24
Anoxia	82	13.6
HDNB	59	9.8
Other*	7	1.16

* This includes drug-induced deafness (thalidomide etc.)
HDNB = Haemolytic Deafness of the Newborn

Taylor *et al.* (1973) reported on a much smaller sample in a study of one school for the deaf in a specific investigation into a study of the so-called 'cause unknown' group (*see Table 16.7*)

Table 16.7

Cause	No. of cases
1. Familial	21 (4 with family history)
2. HDNB	16
Rubella	7
Anoxia or prematurity	13
3. Unknown	24
4. Meningitic	5
	86

It will be noted that there are considerable differences amongst these studies which can be understood in terms of the nature of each of the studies.

In the genetic group there is a higher percentage in the study by Fraser.

In the pre-natal group Fisch's study includes a much greater proportion than in either Fraser's or Taylor's. Both Taylor and Fraser undertook retrospective studies, when serological data would not be valid (if they had not been undertaken in the first four years of life). The method of recognizing rubella as a cause of congenital deafness apart from serological examination would be the finding of other stigmata known to be associated with this condition. It is likely that in Fisch's group the children were younger than in the other two studies and that more accurate records were available regarding the mother's recollection of a definite rash identified as caused by the rubella virus or a positive serological test.

Conversely, Fraser's study indicates a much lower incidence of perinatal causes of deafness compared with Taylor's and Fisch's. The probable explanation is the different availability of hospital records at the time of the studies.

Fraser has a much greater percentage of those children in the post-natal grouping compared with Fisch or Taylor.

In all three studies there is reported a significant proportion of 'cause unknown'. This is a particularly interesting group calling for greater consideration and study in that, on the grounds of logic, some children in this group are 'simplex cases' (i.e. only a single child or a sibling is affected). The basis for classifying children as having an autosomal genetic cause for their deafness is the identification of other affected members of the family.

Taylor *et al.* (1975) in a further investigation of the families of the 'cause unknown' group (from the original study) reported that the audiometric data and the statistical method of segregation analysis taken together tend to support the view that many, if not all, cases of deafness of undetermined cause are cases of autosomal recessive inheritance. In a more recent unpublished series of pre-school deaf chlidren it is evident that the rubella virus remains a most important causal agent in congenital sensorineural deafness. In this series of 70 children some one third have positive serology indicating congenital rubella infection. This finding is more in line with Fisch's figures of 24 per cent reported in his series. It is probably true that in one quarter of the children born with a congenital sensorineural deafness the rubella virus can be implicated.

The incidence of deafness arising from rhesus incompatibility is dropping rapidly since the introduction of immunization with anti-D vaccine and the improvement in antenatal management and exchange transfusions. It is now a rare clinical experience to see a child with athetoid cerebral palsy and deafness resulting from rhesus incompatability.

The relationship of low-birth-weight (LBW) infants and deafness is well summarized by Davies and Stewart (1970). Lubchenco *et al.* (1963) noted that 10.5 per cent of 63 survivors of very LBW children born 20–25 years ago were deaf. Drillien (1964) reported a similar incidence. More recently Stewart and Reynolds (1974) and Davies and Tizard (1975) reported deafness in 1–1.8 per cent LBW babies. Davies and Stewart point out the difficulties of evaluating the aetiological factors when ototoxic drugs were used. They conclude that since 1960 there has been an improvement in the prognosis for life and normal development of LBW infants. If this trend is continued we can expect to see a reduction in the incidence of deafness in this group of infants.

The prevention of rubella infection in pregnancy must hold out the other main hope for a reduction in the incidence of congenital sensorineural deafness. The most definitive statement concerning the policy of rubella immunization has been made by Dudgeon (1978), stating the present policy in this country. This policy of containment is different from that adopted in parts of the USA, which can best be described as an eradication policy. The effect of this approach is described by Krugman (1977).

The importance of the rubella virus has been highlighted in the publication of the National Congenital Rubella Surveillance 1971–1975 (Health Trends, 1977). It is estimated that 67 children with congenital rubella were born in each of the years 1970–1973. Of the 367 cases referred to the Surveillance Programme a sensorineural deafness was diagnosed in 217 (59 per cent), and in 127 no other defect was reported. This survey concludes that rubella infection relatively late in pregnancy causes isolated deafness and moderate intrauterine growth retardation, whilst earlier infection leads to multiple defects and more severe growth inhibition. In those babies with the single defect of sensorineural deafness about half have retinal pigmentation (Taylor, personal communication).

If the fetus is infected *in utero* it manufactures its own IgG and IgM antibodies, probably from about the 20th week of gestation onwards. These antibodies are present at birth together with maternal IgG. IgM antibodies continue to be found for about six months and their presence is instantly diagnostic of intrauterine infection. Maternal IgG disappears during the first six months but the infant continues to produce its own IgG, certainly for several years and probably for life. The antibody can usually be detected by the HAI (Haemagglutination-inhibition) test, and a positive HAI between the ages of six months and four years is therefore evidence of congenital infection in about 95 per cent of cases. However, in a proportion of children the titre of IgG antibodies declines after the first year or two and may fall below the level detectable by the HAI test. In such cases IgG antibody can still be detected by the more sensitive aminoflourescent techniques.

Cytomegalovirus is another agent which is thought to be a causal factor in congenital deafness. Tobin, Marshall and Peckham (1977) reported that in a series of 59 symptomatic congenital CMV (Cytomegalovirus) children, five had sensorineural deafness. These figures appear higher than those to be found in a similar series of congenital sensorineural deafness as yet unpublished when only one child in 70 has a positive urine test.

Incubator noise as a cause of deafness has been studied by Falk and Farmer (1973) who analysed the noise spectrum as found in incubation. They found noise in a 57.7 dB

A-weighting and 74.5 dB lower weighting with a peak at 500 Hz. They suggested that damage-risks criteria need to be established in infants, and incubators should be designed in accordance with these criteria. Douek *et al.* (1976) concluded that there is definite circumstantial evidence of the damaging effect of many incubators on the hearing of premature infants. This is one more of the several imponderables which surround the possible noxious factors in the perinatal period.

The clinical approach to diagnosis

Once the diagnosis of a sensorineural deafness is established a full clinical examination of the child is required, including serological examination for rubella antibodies and a urinary examination for the cytomegalovirus. First-hand study of the obstetric notes is most important. The clinical examination should include an examination of the retina by an ophthalmologist. Whilst the pigmentation from maternal rubella is characteristic, in older children suffering from Usher's disease the early identification of this retinal involvement is most important because of the poor prognosis and the need to alert teachers to the fact that the child will lose the sight and therefore lip-reading ability.

Fraser has drawn attention to the importance of examining of the head and neck in the identification of the many syndromes of which deafness is part. Valuable descriptions of these syndromes are available in the proceedings of the Second Conference on Clinical Delineation of Birth Defects, in which Konigsmark (1971) describes some 70 types of hereditary deafness. An additional valuable reference paper is given by Konigsmark (1969), and detailed clinical descriptions of the various clinical conditions associated with congenital and acquired deafness can be found in the publication by Fraser (1976).

References

Anderson, S.D. (1976). 'The Intratympanic muscles'. In *Scientific Foundations of Otolaryngology*. London; William Heinemann Medical Books Ltd.

Askew, R. (1971). 'Opportunities for continued education of the deaf in the United Kingdom', *The Teacher of the Deaf*, **69**, 175

Ballantyne, J. (1973). 'Ototoxicity. A Clinical Review', *Audiology*, **12**, 325

Ballantyne, J. (1976). 'Ototoxic drugs'. In *Scientific Foundations of Otolaryngology*. London; William Heinemann Medical Books Ltd.

Barr, B., Stensland Junker, K. and Svärd, M. (1978). 'Early discovery of hearing impairment: a critical evaluation of the BOEL test', *Audiology*, **17**, 62

Beagley, H. (1976). 'Application of Auditory Electroneurophysiological Tests'. In *Scientific Foundations of Otolaryngology*. London; William Heinemann Medical Books Ltd.

Bench, R.J. and Boscak, N. (1970). 'Some applications of signal detection theory to Paedo-audiology', *Sound*, **4**, No. 3

Boothroyd, A. (1968). *The selection of hearing aids for children* Ph.D. Thesis. University of Manchester

Borg, E. (1973). *Brain Research*, **49**, 101

Borg, E. (1974). 'The sound reception in mammals'. In *Symposium of the Zoological Society, London*, No. 37, London; Academic Press

Brooks, D.N. (1969). 'The use of the electro-acoustic impedance bridge in the assessment of middle-ear function', *International Audiology*, **8**, 563

Brooks, D.N. (1976). 'School screening for middle ear effusion'. *Annals of Otology, Rhinology and Laryngology*, Suppl. **25**, 223

Brooks, D.N. (1977). 'Middle ear impedance measurement in screening'. *Audiology*, **16**, No. 4, 288

Broomfield, A.M. (1967). 'Guidance to parents of deaf children—a perspective', *British Journal of Disorders of Communication*, **11** (2), 111

Buch, N.H. (1966). 'The inner ear of newborn infants (a histo-pathological study)', *Journal of Laryngology*, **80**, 765

Carhart, R. (1946). 'Monitored live voice as a test of auditory acuity', *Journal of the Acoustical Society of America*, **17**, No. 4, 339

Carruthers, D.G. (1945). 'Deaf-mutism as a sequala of a rubella-like maternal infection during pregnancy,' *Medical Journal of Australia*, **1**, 315

Chiveralls, K. and Fitzsimons, R. (1973). 'Stapedial Reflex Action in Normal Subjects', *British Journal of Audiology*, **7**, 105

Claireaux, A. (1950). *Archives of Disease in Childhood*, **25**, 61

Collyer, Y. and Bench, J. (1974). 'Newborn responses to auditory stimuli judged in relation to stimuli onset and offset', *British Journal of Audiology*, **8**, No. 1

Collyer, Y., Bench, J. and Wilson, I. (1974). 'A comparison of predicted and observed auditory responses in six month old infants', *British Journal of Audiology*, **8**, 37

Cornett, R.O. (1967). 'Cued Speech', *American Annals of the Deaf*, **112**, 3

Crosse, V.M., Wallis, P.G. and Walsh, A.M. (1958). *Archives of Disease in Childhood*, **33**, 403

Davis, H. (1976). 'Principles of Electric Response Audiometry', *Annals of Otology, Rhinology and Laryngology* Suppl. 28

Davis, P.A. and Tizard, J.P.M. (1975). 'Very low birth weight and subsequent neurological defect', *Developmental Medicine and Child Neurology*

Davies, P.A. and Stewart, A.L. (1975). 'Low birth-weight infants: neurological sequalae', *British medical Bulletin*, **31** (No. 1), 85

Denes, P. and Naunton, R.F. (1952). *Proceedings of the Royal Society of Medicine*, **45**, 790

Douek, E., Dodson, H.C., Bannister, L.H., Ashcroft, P. and Humphries, K.N. (1976). 'Effects of incubator noise on the cochlea of the newborn', *Lancet* Nov. 20, 110

Drillien, C.M. (1964). *The growth and development of the premature born infant.* Livingstone, Edinburgh

Dublin, W.B. (1951). *American Journal of Clinical Pathology*, **21**, 935

Dudgeon, J.A. (1978). 'Measles and rubella vaccine', *Archives of Disease in Childhood*, **52**, No. 12

Eagles, E.L. (1961). 'Hearing levels in children and implications for identification audiometry', *Journal of Speech and Hearing Disorders*, Suppl. **9**, 52

Eagles, E.L. (1973). 'A longitudinal study of ear disease and hearing sensitivity in children', *Audiology*, **12**, No. 5–6

Engström, H. (1951). *Acta oto-laryngologica*, **40**, 5

Ewing, I. R. and Ewing, A.W.G. (1950). *Opportunity and the Deaf Child.* London; University of London Press Ltd.

Falk, S.A. and Farmer, J.C. (1973). 'Incubation Noise and Possible Deafness'. *Archives of Otolaryngology*, **97**, 385

Feldman, A.S. and Wilber, L.A. (1976). *Acoustic Impedance and Admittance. The measurements of Middle Ear Function.* Baltimore; Williams and Wilkins

Fisch, L. (1971). 'The probability of response to test sounds in young children', *Sound*, **5**, 7

Fisch, L. (1976). 'Sex ratio and congenital deafness', In *Disorder of Auditory Function II.* London; Academic Press

Fisher, B. (1971). 'Hearing impaired children in ordinary schools', *The Teacher of the Deaf*, **69**, No. 407, 161

Fletcher, H. (1950). 'A method of calculating hearing loss for speech from an audiogram', *Acta Oto-laryngologica*, Suppl. **90**, 26

Fraser, G.R. (1964). *Research in Deafness in Children.* Oxford; Blackwell

Fraser, G.R. (1970). 'The causes of profound deafness in childhood'. In *Sensori neural hearing loss.* London; Ciba Foundation

Fraser, G.R. (1976). *The causes of Profound Deafness in Childhood.* London; Ballière Tindall

Fuller, A. (1960). 'Ototoxicity of neomycin aerosol; *Lancet*, **1**, 1026

Furness, H.J.S. (1972a). 'The Linguistic Potential of Deaf Children', *The Teacher of the Deaf*, **70**, No. 412, 107

Furness, H.J.S. (1972b). 'The Linguistic Potential of Deaf Children', *The Teacher of the Deaf*, **70**, No. 413, 186

Gerrard, J. (1952). *Brain*, **75**, 526

Gonzalez, G., Miller, N. and Wasilewski, V. (1972). *Annals of Otology, Rhinology and Laryngology*, **81**, 127

Gorman, P. and Paget, Lady G. (1969). *A systematic sign language.* 4th Ed. London

Harrison, D.R. (1971). 'An investigation into the effects of ambient noise in pure tone screening tests of hearing in schools', *Sound*, **5**, 94

Harrison, K. (1971). 'Deafness in Children'. *Scott-Brown's Diseases of the Ear, Nose and Throat.* Ed. by J. Ballantyne and J. Groves. London; Butterworth

Hawkins, J.E., Beger, V. and Aran, J.M. (1965). *Sensorineural Hearing Processes and Disorders*, p. 415. London; Churchill

Hester, M.S., (1964). 'Manual Communication', *Proceedings of the International Congress on the Education of the Deaf.* Washington D.C.; US Government Printing Office

Hine, W.D. (1973). 'How deaf are deaf children', *British Journal of Audiology*, **7**, No. 2, 41

Hine, W.D. and Furness, H.J.S. (1975). 'Does wearing a hearing aid damage residual hearing', *The Teacher of the Deaf*, **73**, No. 433, 261

Hood, J.D. (1962). 'Narrow band masking in bone conduction audiometry', *The technics of Audiological Tests.* Boerhaave; Kwartier-Leiden

Howarth, I.E. (1958). *Medical Officer*, **100**, 307

Howarth, J. (1977). 'The Development of Spoken Language', *Conference of National Deaf Children's Society.* Manchester; University of Manchester

Huidberg–Hansen, J. and Jørgenson, M.B. (1968). 'The inner ear in Pendred's syndrome', *Acta Otolaryngology,* **66**, 129

Huntington, A. (1975). 'Selecting Hearing aids for young children', *British Journal of Audiology,* **9**, 75

Jepsen, O. (1955). *Studies on the acoustic stapedial reflex in man.* (Thesis.) Denmark; University of Aarhus.

John, J.E.J. (1957). 'Design and Construction of Schools for the Deaf'. In *Educational Guidance and the Deaf Child.* Ed. by A.W.G. Ewing. Manchester; Manchester University Press

John, J.E.J. and Howarth, J.N. (1973). 'An argument for oral communication', *The Teacher of the Deaf,* **71**, No. 418, 102

Johnson, J.C. (1962). *Educating hearing impaired children in ordinary schools.* Manchester; Manchester University Press

Kern, G. (1962). *Schweizerische medizinishe Wochen-schrift,* **92**, 70

Kelemun, G. (1957). *Monatsschrift für Ohren-heilkunde u. Laryngo-Rhinologie,* **91**, 16

Kingman, S. (1977). 'Present status of measles and rubella immunization in the United States', *Journal of Paediatrics,* **90**, 1

Konigsmark, B.W. (1969). 'Medical progress: Hereditary deafness in man', *New England Journal of Medicine,* **281**, 713

Konigsmark, B.W., (1971). 'Syndromal Approach to the Nosology of Hereditary Deafness. Birth Defects.' *The National Foundation.* Baltimore; March of Dimes

Leach, W. (1962). *Journal of Laryngology,* **76**, 774

Leith, C. (1973). 'Screening tests of hearing for school age children', *British Journal of Audiology,* **7**, 1

Lenneberg, E.H. (1964). 'A Biological perspective of language'. *New Directions in the Study of Language.* Massachusetts; M.I.T. Press

Lewis, M. (1971). 'A developmental study of the cardiac response to stimulus onset and offset during the first year of life', *Psychophysiology,* **8**, 689

Levine, P., Katzin, E.M. and Burnham, L. (1941). *Journal of the American medical Association,* **116**, 825

Lidén, G. (1970). 'The stapedial muscle reflex used as an objective recruitment test; a clinical and experimental study'. In *Sensorineural hearing loss.* Ciba Foundation

Lindeman, R.C. (1965). *Sensorineural Hearing Processes and Disorders.* p. 451. London; Churchill

Lindsay, J.R., Carruthers, D.G., Hemenway, W.G. and Harrison, M.S. (1953). *Annals of Otology, Rhinology and Laryngology,* **62**, 1201

Lindsay, J.R. and Hemenway, W.G. (1954). *Annals of Otology, Rhinology and Laryngology,* **63**, 754

Lindsay, J.R., Davey, P.R. and Ward, P.A. (1960). *Annals of Otology, Rhinology and Laryngology,* **69**, 918

Lindsay, J.R., Proctor, L.R. and Work, W.P. (1960). *Laryngoscope* **70**, 382

Lindsay, J.R. (1965). *Sensorineural Hearing Processes and Disorders,* p. 445. London; Churchill

Lindsay, J.R. (1973). 'Profound Childhood Deafness', *Annals of Otology, Rhinology and Laryngology,* **82**, Suppl. No. 5

Livingstone, G. (1962). *Journal of Laryngology,* **76**, 469

Lubchenco, L.O., Horner, F.A., Reed, L.H., Hix, I.E. Jr., Metcalfe, D., Cohig, R., Elliot, H.C. and Bourg, M. (1963). *American Journal of Disease in Childhood,* **106**, 101, 115

Luterman, D. (1973). 'On parent education', *Volta Review,* **75**, No. 8, 504

Maran, A.G.D. (1966). *Journal of Laryngology,* **80**, 495

Markides, A. (1971). 'Do hearing aids damage the user's residual hearing?' *Sound,* **5**, 22

Markides, A. (1974). *The possibility of restoring binaural hearing advantage by means of wearable hearing aids,* (Ph.D. thesis.) University of Southampton

Markides, A. (1976). 'Comparative linguistic proficiencies of deaf children taught by two different methods of instruction—manual versus oral', *The Teacher of the Deaf,* **74**, 307

Martin, M.C. and Lodge, J.J. (1969). 'A survey of hearing aids in schools for the deaf and partially hearing units', *Sound,* **3**, No. 1, 2

Myers, R.E. (1972). 'Two patterns of perinatal brain damage and their conditions of occurrence', *American Journal of Obstetrics and Gynecology,* **112**, 246

Niemeyer, W. and Sesterhenn, G. (1974). 'Calculating the hearing threshold for different sound stimuli', *Audiology,* **13**, 421

Nolan, M. (1977). 'The performance of a wide range of hearing aids', *The Teacher of the Deaf,* **1**, No. 3, 108

Nolan, M. (1978). 'Sub miniature receivers for use with DHSS call-off contact bodyworn aids?' *The Teacher of the Deaf,* **2**, 3, 98

Nolan, M., Elzemety, S., Tucker, I. G. and McDonough, D. F. (1978). 'An investigation into the problems involved in producing efficient ear moulds for children', *Scandinavian Audiology,* **7**, 213

Nolan, M. and Tucker, I.G. (1977). 'A simple method of improving the acoustic seal of an earmould', *The Teacher of the Deaf,* **1**, No. 2, 72

Ormerod, F.C. (1960). *Journal of Laryngology,* **74**, 919

Orth, J. (1875). *Virchows Archiv für Pathologische Anatomie und Physiologie und für klinische Medizin,* **63**, 477

Owrid, H.L. (1971). 'Studies in manual communication with hearing impaired children', *The Teacher of the Deaf,* **69**, 407, 151

Parparella, M.M. and Winter, L.E. (1968). *Transactions of the American Academy of Otolaryngology,* **72**, 782

Quigley, S.P. (1969). The influence of finger spelling on the development of language, communication and educational achievement in deaf children'. *Institute of Research on Exceptional Children.* University of Illinois

Ranck, J.B. and Windle, W.F. (1959). 'Brain damage in the monkey macaca Mulatta by asphyxia neonatorum', *Experimental Neurology,* **1**, 130

Robson, J. (1970). 'Screening techinques in babies', *Sound,* **4**, No. 4, 91

Schmörl, G. (1904). *Verhandlungen der Deutschen pharmakologischen Gesellschaft,* **6**, 109

Shaw, S.D. (1977). *Predicting hearing loss from stapedial reflex measurements.* (Unpublished dissertation) Manchester; University of Manchester

Sheppard, S., Smithells, R.M., Peckham, C.S., Dudgeon, J.A. and Marshall, W.C. (1977). 'National Congenital Rubella Surveillance', *Health Trends,* **9**, 38

Stewart, A.L. and Reynolds, E.O.R. (1974). *Paediatrics, (Springfield),* **54**, 724

Strensland Junker, K., Barr, B., Maliniemi, S. and Wasy-Hocken-O (1978). 'BOEL Screening: a Program for the early detection of communication disorders', *Audiology,* **17**, 51

Stuckless, E.R. and Birch, J.W. (1966). 'The influence of early manual communication on the linguistic development of deaf children', *American Annals of the Deaf,* **3**, 452, 499

Szekely, T. and Draskovitch, E. (1965). *Zeitschrift für Laryngologie, Rhinologie, Otologie, u. ihre Grenzgebiete,* **44**, 15

Taylor, I.G. (1958). 'Localization of sound stimuli', *Speech Pathology and Therapy* **66**

Taylor, I.G., Brasier, V.J., Hine, W.D., Morris, T. and Powell, C.A. (1973). 'Some aspects of the Audiology of Familial Hearing Loss'. Disorders of Auditory Function. London; Academic Press

Taylor, I.G., Brasier, V.J., Hine, W.D., Chiveralls, K. and Morris, T. (1975). 'A study of the causes of hearing loss in a population of deaf children with special reference to genetic factors', *Journal of Laryngology and Otology,* **89**, No. 9

Taylor, I.G. (1977). 'How should Services for Hearing Impaired Children be Organised'. *Conference of National Deaf Children's Society.* Manchester; University of Manchester

Tizard, B., Cooperman, O., Joseph, P. and Tizard, J. (1972). 'Environmental effects on language development: a study of young children in long stay residential nurseries', *Child Development,* **43**, 339

Tobin, J.O'H., Marshall, W.C. and Peckham, C. (1977). 'Virus infection', *Clinics in Obstetrics and Gynaecology,* **4**, No. 2.

Tucker, I. G., Nolan, M. and Colclough, R. O. (1978). 'A new high-efficiency earmould', *Scandinavian Audiology,* **7**, 225

Watson, T.J. (1957). 'Speech Audiometry for Children'. In *Educational Guidance and the Deaf Child.* Ed. by A.W.G. Ewing. Manchester; Manchester University Press

Whetnall, E.M. and Lucas, H.A. (1952). *Proceedings of the Royal Society of Medicine,* **45**, 779

17 Traumatic lesions of the inner ear

H Ludman

Man has discovered many ways to damage himself and others. Most are accidental, a few murderously deliberate, and some an inevitable consequence of his exploration of alien environments. Although the inner ear is embedded in the densest bone in the body, the peculiar delicacy of its structure, and the fragile separation of its fluid-containing spaces from air in the middle-ear cleft, render it susceptible to injury from which it cannot be protected by its enclosure. Furthermore, it is tethered to a massive brain, which floats freely mobile relative to the skull base in which the labyrinth is rigidly incarcerated. This entails the risk of tearing neurovascular connections under the inertial strains of acceleration.

The head may be buffeted; the skull may be fractured through the labyrinth; the ear may be penetrated by projectiles: the inner ear may suffer unique injury from the effects of rapid pressure changes in the air of the middle ear, or in the cerebrospinal fluid within the head communicating through anatomical channels with the perilymph. The pathophysiology of some of these lesions may be studied in Volume 1.

From a purist point of view it would be agreeable if the effects of these injuries could be discussed fully under headings within a complete and consistent system of classification—according, for example, to the nature or environment of the injuring agent, or to the site or functional effects of the structural damage. Unfortunately no single consistent classification can offer such a basis for satisfactory treatment of this subject. Any single one would be artificial, and would impose rigidity and unnecessary repetition on the discussion, without allowing the selective emphasis of topics important to the otologist. Furthermore, practical requirements demand an interest in the particular *environmental hazards* causing injury. Full treatment of the subject can best be achieved under a 'hybrid' system of categorization, with some topics classified by site of lesion, and others according to the environmental circumstances of the injury, as follows:

(1) Labyrinthine membrane ruptures.
(2) Temporal bone fractures.
(3) Closed head and neck injuries—without fracture.
(4) Diving injuries.
(5) Blast injuries.
(6) Surgical trauma.

Labyrinthine membrane rupture

During the past ten years otologists have learned that sensorineural hearing loss and vestibular symptoms, following many different forms of trauma, may be asssociated with the operative finding of perilymph leaking into the middle ear through a fistula in the stapediovestibular ligament of the oval window, or in the round window membrane. It is generally accepted that this finding of perilymph fistula is evidence of damage to membranous structures within the labyrinth, in addition to the tear in the partition of separation between the inner and middle ear.

Perilymph fistula was first recognized as a complication of stapedectomy operations (House, 1967), but in 1968 Simmons suggested that this sort of lesion might explain two instances of sensorineural deafness after diving, and in the same year Fee described the finding of three oval window fistulae, two following head injury and one with no definite preceding trauma. Reports of oval window fistulae by Stroud and Calcaterra in 1970 were followed by three more accounts of surgically confirmed fistulae by Goodhill in 1971. Goodhill's experience of these lesions grew so that he was able, with colleagues, to write in 1973 of 15 fistulae, and to describe 47 examples in 1976.

The preceding trauma includes closed head injury, which accounted for two of the first cases described by Fee, and for about half of the cases Healy described with his colleagues in 1974. This cause has figured in many other descriptions. Gunshot wound is a fairly obvious possible cause, and an instance can be found in the account by Emmett, Staab and Fischer in 1977. Barotrauma, particularly associated with diving, is a very important cause which will be discussed in more detail later. Five cases were described by Freeman and Edmonds in 1972, and an instance with round window rupture was offered by Schuknecht and Gacek in 1973, while a full account of the problems of diving barotrauma can be found in Farmer's 1977 monograph. It is of great interest and importance that membrane rupture may apparently be caused by slight physical exertion—or even appear to be spontaneous, as in one of the first cases described by Fee in 1968. Some of Stroud's 1970 patients developed symptoms while laughing or singing; and Goodhill's 1976 account of 47 fistulae, found during the exploration of 59 ears in 76 patients with sudden sensorineural hearing loss, recognized antecedent activities that included lifting, coughing, sneezing, straining at stool or during micturition, and sexual intercourse. Common to all these forms of exertion, of course, is raised intracranial pressure. Blast and severe acoustic trauma have also been implicated.

Mechanism of membrane rupture

Goodhill, in his publications, has given us a clear account of the ways in which membrane ruptures may arise following pressure changes across the middle/inner ear partitions (*Figure 17.1*). By what he calls an 'explosive route' a rise in CSF pressure, from whatever cause, may be transmitted to the perilymph, with bulging and finally rupture of the oval or round window membranes. The route of transfer of fluid pressure from the CSF to the perilymph is most probably through the aqueduct of the cochlea to the scala tympani. Goodhill also suggests a route through the internal acoustic meatus and lamina cribrosa, but this is less likely. Certainly Harker's 1974 experiments, in which CSF pressure in cats was raised until bulging of the round

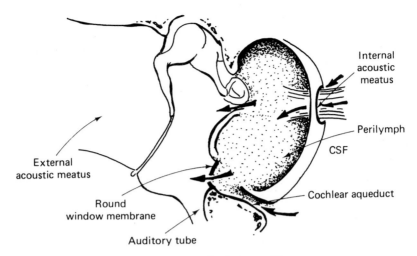

Internal
acoustic
meatus

Perilymph

CSF

External
acoustic meatus

Cochlear aqueduct

Round
window membrane

Auditory tube

Explosive routes

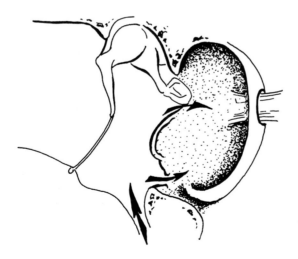

Implosive routes

Figure 17.1 Diagram of explosive and implosive routes for labyrinthine membrane ruptures. (Adapted from Goodhill, 1976)

window membrane was followed by rupture, showed that the transfer of dye in the CSF was through the cochlear aqueduct. Pressure operating in the opposite direction, from the middle ear to the labyrinth, is described by Goodhill as the 'implosive route'. This may arise when the middle-ear cleft is forcefully inflated by a successful Valsalva's manoeuvre. In contrast, attempts to inflate the middle ear that are unsuccessful, because of auditory tube blockage, raise the CSF pressure relative to the middle-ear air pressure, and may cause membrane damage through the 'explosive route'. CSF pressure also rises during straining, and with sudden compression and deformity of the skull in head injury.

Whichever the route of pressure transfer, the perilymph fistula must not be considered the cause of the inner-ear disturbance. Simmons, in his 1968 suggestion, implied that the labyrinthine damage would probably be complex, with ruptures of intralabyrinthine membranes—including the basilar membrane and Reissner's membrane—causing damage to intracochlear structures. As Goodhill has stressed, the finding of a fistula must be considered as evidence, at its lateral boundary, of more serious damage to the labyrinth. The fistula is not the sole or even the main cause of the auditory or vestibular disturbance. This important fact explains the poor hearing results that usually follow effective sealing of a perilymph leak.

Since the majority of preceding traumatic events are common and slight, we must consider why these ruptures appear to be relatively rare. It may be that they occur more commonly than believed, as Healy suggested in 1974, and that spontaneous healing is the rule. Alternatively a number of anatomical factors might be found in rare combinations, placing a few ears at greater risk than the majority. Congenital weakness of the window membranes, as Althaus suggested in 1977, might occasionally be associated with unusually large cochlear aqueducts. As Goodhill pointed out in 1971, the presence of a large cochlear aqueduct in the adult is the retention of an immature development feature, and this would allow an abnormally and undesirably rapid equalization of pressure between the CSF and the perilymph. Pullen, in 1972, noticed the absence of a well-formed round window niche in two cases, and Healy, in 1974, when he observed the same abnormality, suggested that perhaps the lack of a deep niche to protect the round window membrane might expose it to greater risk of pressure damage by the 'implosive route'. He also suggested that absence of the stapedius tendon could render the footplate more liable to rupture.

Site of fistula

Studies of the growing literature on this subject show that the oval window is more frequently the site of fistula than the round window: indeed in Goodhill's 1976 series only four of 47 fistulae were of the round window alone—19 involved both, but 24 affected only the oval window. Misconceptions that the round window is the more frequently damaged might perhaps stem from the title of Goodhill's 1971 paper: 'Sudden deafness and round window rupture'. As recently as 1977 Farmer reported that, following diving barotrauma, only round window fistulae have been described. However, Caruso and his colleagues have published an account in 1977 of oval window fistula from diving. Lateralization is interesting, particularly the finding by Goodhill of predominant involvement of the left ear. This could be explained by a larger aqueduct on that side, but Healy, in 1974, found the sides to be equally frequently affected.

Clinical features

There are no auditory or vestibular features that are pathognomonic of labyrinthine membrane rupture. The possibility should be suspected when certain forms of sensorineural deafness or of vestibular disturbance arise in circumstances that make the occurrence possible—after trauma or diving.

Auditory symptoms are, either the onset of sudden sensorineural hearing loss— often severe—or the development of a fluctuating hearing loss in no way different from that of endolymphatic hydrops. Vestibular symptoms do not necessarily accompany the hearing loss. Positional vertigo of the benign paroxysmal variety, episodic attacks of vertigo of a Menière-like kind, and instability of gait have all been described. Inner-ear barotrauma is always accompanied by pain from concomitant middle-ear barotrauma, and as Edmonds, Freeman and Tonkin recorded in 1974, the deafness and vestibular disturbances may not develop for hours, or even days after the diving exposure.

Audiological findings are of a sensorineural hearing loss, which may be severe. The initial loss (Fee, 1968) is often for low tones, eventually becoming more uniformly distributed, and indeed, as Althaus observed in 1977, it is often indistinguishable from that of hydrops. The Békésy pattern is most usually type II (Goodhill, 1976; Healy, Strong and Sampogna, 1974). Often there is disproportionately poor speech discrimination (Fee, 1968; Pullen, 1972; Healy, Strong and Sampogna, 1974).

Vestibular findings include a positive fistula sign, but this seems to be a fickle diagnostic indicator. Although Healy showed a positive fistula sign in over half his 1974 patients, Stroud and Calcaterra never found one, and it was a feature of one only of Althaus's six cases in his 1977 report. Positional testing often provokes nystagmus, of the benign peripheral variety, beating towards the underlying ear after a latent period, fatiguing after maintenance of the provoking position for a short while, and accompanied by severe vertigo. This finding may be present in more than 50 per cent of patients. Indeed, Healy elicited positional nystagmus in 13 out of his 19 cases, and he also described a positive Romberg sign of ataxia in 50 per cent of the series. On caloric testing canal paresis or directional preponderance is occasionally found.

Diagnosis

The ultimate diagnosis of labyrinthine membrane rupture, and its associated perilymph fistula, can be made only by the demonstration of perilymph leakage during a tympanotomy operation. The condition should be suspected under a number of different circumstances. The accounts already mentioned, particularly those of Healy in 1974, Goodhill in 1976 and Althaus in 1977, indicate that the possibility must be considered:

(1) In patients with sudden sensorineural hearing loss associated with or preceded by head injury, barotrauma, or unusual physical exertion. When the fistula test is positive the diagnosis is almost certain.
(2) In patients with vertigo after concussion.

Healy's 1974 paper emphasized the significance of vertigo and ataxia in this syndrome as presenting symptoms, and suggested that strong suspicion should also fall on:

(1) Patients with 'Menière's disorder' which is atypical in that there is persisting ataxia between the episodes of vertigo.
(2) All patients with ataxia without evidence of central nervous system disease.
(3) All patients seen with a diagnosis of 'benign positional vertigo'.

Although the diagnosis is conclusively made only by finding a perilymph fistula during tympanotomy, this is not as simple and clear-cut as might be thought, and there is still scope for uncertainty even during operation. This is because an actual membrane hole is rarely seen—its presence is inferred from the seepage of fluid. That leak may be extremely slow, so that tissue fluid exudation, or moistening by local anaesthetic injected into the meatal wall, may easily be misinterpreted as perilymph. Furthermore, mucosal strands in the round window niche sometimes create the illusion of a torn window membrane, and manoeuvres to see the window more clearly may actually cause damage with perilymph leakage. For all these reasons, diagnosis, except in the most florid instances, must be subject to scepticism.

Management

The management of patients suspected of membrane rupture, on grounds discussed above, must be governed by the following considerations:

(1) That operation is the only definitive way to make the diagnosis, but that, for the reasons indicated, presence or absence of a fistula cannot always be reliably identified.
(2) That some, perhaps many, fistulae heal spontaneously.
(3) That the results from surgical repair of fistulae are excellent for the relief of vestibular symptoms, but are poor for the restoration of hearing, and indeed involve a risk of further cochlear damage.

If the symptoms have developed slowly, or are not of recent onset, the management involves planning exploration of the middle ear to search for a fistula. The decision to explore must depend on the degree of suspicion, and the considerations listed above.

The sudden onset of symptoms, particularly sensorineural hearing loss, in circumstances suggesting membrane rupture, requires first of all a period of conservative management in bed. This should involve complete rest with the head raised. Rises in CSF pressure must be prevented by avoiding straining, coughing, nose blowing, or Valsalva's manoeuvre. The period of conservative management allows time for full assessment of the patient with investigations for other otological or possible general medical causes. It also provides time during which a fistula might heal spontaneously, or a disorder other than fistula might recover—either spontaneously, or under the influence of medication appropriate for the treatment of any cause revealed by investigation. In accordance with Goodhill's 1976 recommendations, systemic steroids should be administered, in the absence of medical contraindications, during this waiting period.

The middle ear should be explored if there is no improvement, or indeed if there is deterioration in hearing during the period of medical care. The ideal time for exploration is not certain, but Goodhill suggests waiting for 10–12 days following the stress or trauma. The results of operation seem to be poorer if delayed beyond two weeks. Auditory or vestibular symptoms arising from dives in which decompression sickness is unlikely should all be assumed to be due to membrane rupture, and Farmer in 1977 recommended that operative exploration should be performed if there is no improvement during 48 h of conservative management.

TECHNIQUE OF EXPLORATION

Exploration is through a standard tympanotomy approach. Each window requires careful inspection, and, as indicated earlier, it may be difficult to identify a fistula even at this stage. Careful observation under high power magnification is required, and observation for 5–10 min may be needed (Healy, 1974). Viewing with the patient in the head down position, and Valsalva's manoeuvre by the patient, if under local anaesthesia, may help to reveal the leak. Gel-foam pledgets make useful blotters, and gentle fine suction can be used to remove the fluid so that its reaccumulation can be observed (Goodhill, 1976). Emmet (1977) has described the use of an intrathecal radioactive tracer, picked up 24 h later on Ivalon sponges in the windows. Large fistulae are rarely seen, and Goodhill notes that, not only is there usually no visible hole in the round window membrane, but the round window reflex is usually present. The difficulties of identifying the actual fistula site are so great that, out of 18 oval window fistulae, Healy in 1974 could identify the exact location in four only. For the remainder he recommended total stapedectomy with reconstruction by closure of the oval window with fat or perichondrium, and a Teflon prosthesis. When a site can be identified, it should be sealed with mesenchymal tissue after elevation of the surrounding mucosa. Fat from the lobule of the ear, temporalis fascia, or tragal perichondrium are all suitable materials.

RESULTS

The incidence of finding fistulae in suspected cases has varied. Goodhill's 1976 account of 47 fistulae in 59 explorations may be taken as representative of the expectations of diligent suspicion.

Vestibular symptoms are usually completely relieved by closure of a fistula. Healy was successful in 100 per cent of cases in his 1974 series, and Althaus described vestibular relief in 83 per cent.

Tinnitus, as might be expected, is variably and unpredictably affected.

Hearing benefit is much less likely. Generally less than 50 per cent can expect improvement, and marked gain was found by Goodhill in only 25 per cent. Not surprisingly cochlear function may be damaged—this was Healy's experience in four of his cases—nearly 25 per cent.

As has already been stressed, the diagnosis is fraught with difficulty even at operation, so the extent to which radical measures are justified must partly be governed by the quality of the hearing that operation would place at risk. This exemplifies the dilemma facing the surgeon treating this disorder. The better the hearing the more important it is to close the defect; but the greater the hazard being chanced.

Temporal bone fractures

Eighty per cent of skull base fractures involving the petrous temporal bone run longitudinally through the roof of the middle-ear cleft towards the petrous apex. The accompanying aural damage is principally of the middle-ear structures, with conductive hearing loss. However, inner-ear damage with attendant sensorineural loss may occur, often with some recovery during the first few weeks after the injury, as described in 1956 by Schuknecht and Davison. The pattern of the sensorineural loss accompanying a longitudinal fracture, which does not transgress the otic capsule, has been attributed to 'cochlear concussion', and takes the form of localized hearing deficit at 4000 Hz, or of more widespread damage affecting many higher frequencies. Barber in 1964 found benign positional vertigo in 47 per cent of patients with longitudinal fractures. The labyrinthine damage from this variety of fracture produces symptoms in no way different from those of closed head injuries without fracture—as might be expected.

Labyrinthine damage is a much more frequent sequel to the less common transverse fractures of the temporal bone—those that run through the otic capsule and labyrinths at right angles to the long axis of the petrous pyramid. These fractures frequently follow blows to the occipital region of the skull, and are accompanied by facial paralysis in 50 per cent of instances. The attendant labyrinthine disruption usually destroys cochlear and vestibular function—totally and permanently.

The effects of the total hearing loss require no special discussion here. The vestibular destruction produces the clinical picture of sudden vestibular failure. The symptoms, when not modified by other effects of the head injury and intracranial damage, are violent vertigo accompanied by nausea, vomiting, and total prostration. At first the maintenance of erect posture is impossible, and the intense vertigo is exacerbated by any head movement. Slowly, balance is regained, so that after a few days the victim may be able to walk, but insecurely, holding on to nearby furniture. After ten days or so, walking may be stable, provided sudden movements are avoided. Some instability will persist and be exacerbated by attempts to walk in the dark, or when intellectual effort is impaired by fatigue, drugs, or intercurrent illness. Recovery is slower in the elderly; and indeed certain balancing skills may never be regained. Of course the vestibular function of the destroyed labyrinth does not recover: the restitution of equilibrium derives from a process of compensation. This depends partly on a reduction in the tonic activity of the undamaged labyrinth, under the influence of efferent stimuli from the brain; and partly on readjustment of the central integrating activity within the brain, so that the abnormal vestibular sensory information, available only from the intact labyrinth, may more accurately be interpreted. This compensation may suffer impairment, temporarily or permanently at any later period in life—with a return of vertigo and disequilibrium. Such breakdown in the compensating process may develop if other sources of sensory information about spatial orientation—such as vision—develop defects; or if the central computer integrating activity of the brain is degraded by fatigue, illness, drugs, or central nervous system degeneration. Combined defects of this kind explain the occurrence of vertigo or persisting imbalance in older age if one labyrinth has been destroyed in earlier life. The acquisition of compensation can be expedited by the application of the vestibular head exercises described in 1946 by Cawthorne and Cooksey for rehabilitation of patients after fenestration operations.

Traumatic loss of labyrinthine function is immediately followed by the appearance of a large amplitude third degree nystagmus, beating towards the undamaged ear. Compensation, as the symptoms subside, is associated with abatement of the nystagmus, which passes through second and then first degree stages of magnitude before disappearing during the first three weeks or so after the injury. For a long time afterwards, although the nystagmus is no longer visible when the eyes are examined in the light, it will reappear for inspection if the eyes are examined in the absence of optic fixation—in darkness, with Frenzel's spectacles or an infrared viewer, or by electronystagmography.

Head and neck injuries—without fracture

Closed head injuries are often followed by deafness, tinnitus and vestibular symptoms; especially when the injury has caused concussion. Auditory symptoms were found in as many as 50 per cent of patients by Toglia *et al.* in 1970. The commonest form of hearing loss is a bilateral high tone deficit, most profound around 4000 Hz, similar to that of acoustic trauma. Some recovery may occur over the first few weeks, especially at 8000 Hz, but it is rarely complete. Occasionally a severe unilateral hearing loss is found.

Vestibular symptoms include ataxia, but the commonest is positional vertigo of the benign paroxysmal variety—found by Barber in 1964 in more than 10 per cent of the victims of severe head injury without skull fracture. This may persist for some months.

Whiplash injuries of the neck produce auditory and vestibular symptoms similar to those following head injury, and as frequently, according to Toglia *et al.* (1970).

Mechanism

As earlier discussion has shown, closed head injuries may cause labyrinthine membrane rupture—as a result of the raised intracranial pressure, but at the time of writing it is not possible to say how commonly this is an important mechanism. Injuries may damage the vestibulo-cochlear system either in the peripheral labyrinth—so called 'labyrinthine concussion'—or in more central structures. The contribution of each to the overall pattern of damage probably depends on the mobility of the head at the time of injury—labyrinthine concussion following blows to the fixed head, and central damage being more common when the mobile head is violently accelerated (or decelerated). Striking the fixed immobile head causes a pressure wave through the base of the skull, and excessive movement of the stapes footplate due to ossicular inertia. The cochlear changes produced by this mechanism, described by Igarashi, Schuknecht and Myers in 1964, are injuries to the organ of Corti, similar to those caused by noise damage. Schuknecht *et al.* (1951) found that striking the fixed immobile heads of cats caused high-tone hearing losses, particularly around 4000 Hz, associated with histological damage in the appropriate site on the basilar membrane.

Rapid acceleration or deceleration of the head allows the brain to move relative to the skull, because of its inertia, often with a rotatory or swirling motion. Impact against irregularities in the base of the skull may bruise the frontal and temporal lobes; twisting of the brain stem may cause damage; and the eighth nerve may be stretched or torn. Makishima's experiments in 1975 and 1976, in which guinea-pigs were injured by violent head shaking—to be contrasted with hitting the fixed head with a mallet—produced haemorrhage and laceration of the eighth nerve, and haemorrhage within and around the brain. There were degenerative changes in the cochlear and vestibular neurones, and extravasation of blood into the scala tympani. Changes within the labyrinth, however, were conspicuously slight, and physiological tests indicated retention of intact peripheral cochlear function.

Whiplash injuries expose the head to the same sort of inertial acceleration damage, and additional harm, as Toglia suggested in 1970, might stem from injury to the sympathetic nervous system, and to vascular structures in the neck causing ischaemia of the labyrinths and their central nervous system connections.

Post-traumatic positional vertigo has been attributed by Schuknecht in 1962 and 1969 to 'cupulolithiasis'. Detached otoconia, following disruption of the otolith membrane, are said to settle into the ampulla of the posterior semicircular canal and displace its cupula when the head is in the provoking dependent position. As already noted, positional vertigo may be a feature of labyrinthine membrane rupture with perilymph fistula. Although Healy, in 1974, considered this an alternative mechanism to that of cupulolithiasis, and was unable to find displaced otoconia in post-mortem studies, there seems no reason for a conflict of opinion here, and the perilymph fistula may be taken as evidence of intralabyrinthine damage of which otolith membrane disruption may be one feature.

Clinical findings

Audiometric testing usually shows a bilateral high-tone hearing loss, most marked around 4000 Hz. This is in no way distinguishable from that produced by noise stimulation damage, and all audiological tests produce findings typical of a hair-cell lesion within the cochlea. Nystagmus of the peripheral benign type may be elicited by positional testing—a nystagmus associated with vertigo, preceded by a latent period, beating towards the underlying ear, and becoming fatigued after a short period of time. As Toglia has emphasized in 1970, ENG examination may, in a high number of instances, reveal a 'latent' nystagmus provoked particularly by neck rotation, but also by removal of optic fixation and positional testing. In nearly two-thirds of his patients caloric testing showed a unilateral canal paresis.

Diving injuries

Since 1873 when Smith first described 'Caisson disease', the unphysiological exposure of the body to large and rapid changes in pressure has been known to cause deafness and vestibular symptoms. This damage has been attributed to numerous different mechanisms (*see* Volume 1). They include nitrogen bubbling into the labyrinthine fluids and inner-ear blood supply during decompression; labyrinthine haemorrhage; pressure disruption of the inner-ear membranes; air embolism; unequal caloric stimulation; and excessive noise exposure. To these must be added general disturbances of equilibrium caused by hypoxia, hypercarbia, nitrogen narcosis, sensory deprivation, and alcoholic hangovers.

In 1973 Edmonds classified the pathophysiological causes of vertigo during diving into two main groups: those in which there is unequal vestibular stimulation, and those in which the vestibular responses are unequal. Farmer, in his 1977 monograph, has provided us with a practical division of the effects of diving trauma into those of:

(1) Transient vestibular dysfunction.
(2) Persistent inner-ear injury.

Transient vestibular dysfunction

This may arise from the following.

UNEQUAL CALORIC STIMULATION

This is as described by Edmonds and others in 1973. It occurs when equal entry of cold water into each ear is prevented by obstruction of one external acoustic meatus, or if the middle ear is irrigated by cold water after traumatic rupture of the tympanic membrane.

UNEQUAL MIDDLE-EAR PRESSURE EQUILIBRATION

Vertigo was described, from this cause during ascent by Lundgren in 1965 under the name of 'alternobaric vertigo'. Edmonds *et al.* in 1973, gave an account of the same symptom experienced during descent. It is a common disturbance, as was shown by Lundgren's report in 1974 that it affected nearly 17 per cent of divers in a large series. The vertigo can be relieved by returning to the previous depth, and probably never causes permanent damage. Some divers, prone to the disorder, can induce vertigo on the surface by performing Valsalva's manoeuvre.

HIGH PRESSURE NERVOUS SYNDROME

This is the name given to a syndrome, described by Brauer in 1968 and Bennett and Towse in 1971, of transient disequilibrium associated with deep helium–oxygen diving. It is characterized by vertigo, intention tremor and decrement of psychomotor skill, and it follows rapid compression in a helium–oxygen environment to depths in excess of 150 m. The symptoms recover within a few hours of decompression. Apparently the disorder is not related to excess or insufficient oxygen, or to raised blood carbon dioxide levels in the body. Farmer (1977) attributes it to a decrease in the cerebellar inhibition of the vestibular nuclei.

Persistent inner-ear injury

Following Farmer's suggestions, these injuries may conveniently be discussed according to whether they occur:

(1) During descent or ascent in relatively shallow diving with little likelihood of decompression sickness—or during compression in deeper diving (*inner-ear barotrauma*).
(2) At stable deep depths—a syndrome of sudden *unilateral vestibular* failure.
(3) During or after ascent or decompression from dives in which decompression sickness is possible (*otologic decompression sickness*).
(4) In relation to high levels of background noise.

Inner-ear barotrauma

This, with rupture of labyrinthine membranes, is the mechanism by which persisting damage may be suffered during relatively shallow ascent or descent (to depths as little as 2–3 m) or decompression from deeper diving. The subject of labyrinthine membrane rupture has already been discussed in this chapter. During diving the pressure differences that may be imposed on the inner-ear membranes are much greater and change more rapidly than can be expected on land or in air travel, so it is not surprising that membrane disruption should occur. During descent (or compression) the body fluid and CSF pressure rises along with that of the environment (*Figure 17.2*). The air pressure in the middle ear, however, does not rise unless clearance of air through the auditory tube is achieved. As Freeman and Edmonds observed in 1972, inner-ear barotrauma occurs only in association with the pain of middle-ear barotrauma. The tympanic membrane bulges inwards, and the round window membrane and stapes footplate outwards, towards the middle-ear air cavity. If the tube remains blocked it becomes locked by valvular collapse of its walls. Now, a forced Valsalva's manoeuvre will raise the CSF and perilymph pressure above that of the surrounding sea water, and increase still further the differential between the pressures in perilymph and air in the middle ear. This may cause rupture of the bulging round window membrane or the stapediovestibular ligament. Even without the added harmful effect of forced Valsalva's manoeuvre, continued descent with a locked auditory tube will raise the perilymph pressure level until eventually a window membrane ruptures into the middle ear—through the 'explosive route'. The critical pressure difference for this occurrence in man is unknown. Harker's 1974 experiments in cats, to which allusion was made earlier, showed a tendency for window membrane rupture at a pressure difference of about 120 mmHg, which would be met in diving to a depth of 1.58 m in sea water. During ascent the middle-ear air pressure rises relative to the body fluid pressure, and the membranes may be forced inward towards the labyrinth with possible rupture by the 'implosive route'.

Any diver who develops persisting giddiness or sensorineural deafness during or after a dive under these conditions, in which decompression sickness is unlikely, has almost certainly suffered labyrinthine membrane rupture, and must be treated appropriately. This hazard should be prevented by forbidding diving if there is any difficulty in clearing the auditory tube.

Treatment of labyrinthine membrane rupture has already been discussed. Farmer stresses that there is danger of further damage if, because of misunderstanding about the nature of the disorder, the diver is treated with hyperbaric oxygen. The conservative period of nursing in the raised head position should be followed by exploratory operation as early as 48 h after the dive if there is no spontaneous improvement, in accordance with Goodhill's recommendations in 1973.

Unilateral labyrinthine failure

This was described at stable deep depths by Sundmaker in 1973 in a few patients. The symptoms arise shortly after a change in breathing gases from a helium–oxygen mixture to a three gas mixture, at the same overall pressure, with nitrogen or neon added. Farmer suggests two possible mechanisms. First, the rapid rise in concentration

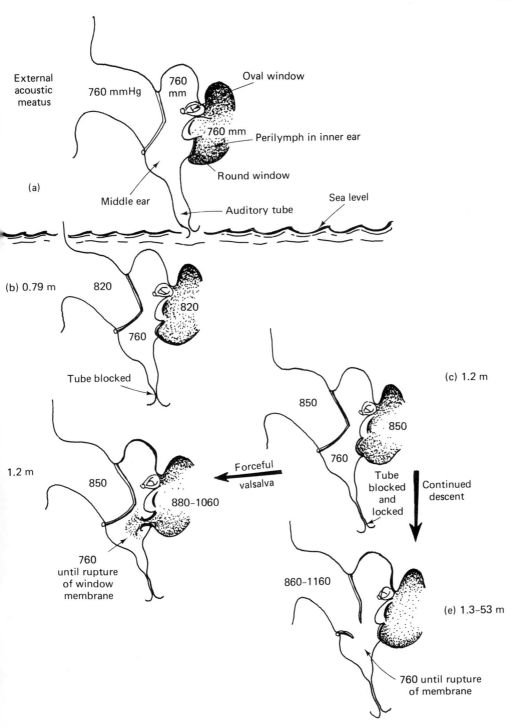

Figure 17.2 Effects of barotrauma during descent. (Adapted from Farmer, 1977)

of the added gas in the endolymph might produce an osmotic hydrops. Secondly, the new inert gas, diffusing in one direction across tissue barriers, may meet the inert gas already present, diffusing in the opposite direction and cause damage by bubble formation at tissue interfaces such as labyrinthine membranes.

Otologic decompression sickness

Inner-ear damage from inert gas bubbling during decompression was thought to be rare, but this cause is now well recognized. Farmer (1977) studied 23 vestibular and cochlear injuries shortly after decompression. He excluded patients whose injuries might fall into the previous categories, those who had made such rapid ascents that air emboli were possible, and those who had features suggesting central nervous system decompression sickness. His findings indicate that prompt recompression favours full recovery, and this implies that the injury is due to gas bubbling within the inner-ear fluid spaces or the internal auditory artery—rather than to haemorrhage into the labyrinth, structural disruption of the labyrinth, or ischaemia from vascular spasm. Sometimes symptoms arise, during decompression, after a switch from a helium–oxygen mixture to air. These may be due to counter-diffusion of inert gas, with bubbling at the partitions within the labyrinth, to which vestibular failure at stable depths has been attributed.

The treatment of otologic decompression sickness involves recompression. The ideal depth is not known, but empirically a pressure 3 atmospheres above that at which the symptoms arose is suggested by Farmer. If the symptoms appeared after a change of breathing mixture, recompression should take place in the atmosphere used before the change. It is doubtful whether any medication can be helpful, and drugs such as heparin, which have been advocated, might do harm. There is some reason for believing that parenteral diazepam may have a useful symptomatic effect, and that oxygen-enriched treatment gases should be used.

Injuries from noise exposure

These are outside the scope of this chapter, but it should be noted that noise levels within diving helmets can exceed 100 dBA, and, within compression chambers, breathing gases and ventilation equipment may produce sound levels above 120 dBA. Even at stable depths, ventilation equipment causes potentially damaging noise levels.

Blast injuries

Blast offers one example of so-called stimulation damage. It is characterized by a relatively prolonged duration—more than 1 ms (Ruedi and Furrer, 1947). Usually resulting from exposure to bomb explosion, similar effects are produced less dramatically by flat hand blows to the closed external ear. The physical character of blast is of an initial positive pressure wave lasting about 5 ms and reaching pressure levels up to thousands of pounds per square inch, followed by a much longer lasting negative phase, below atmospheric pressure, for up to 30 ms. The time scale of these pressure changes is demonstrated by the so-called Friedlander curve (*Figure 17.3*). The

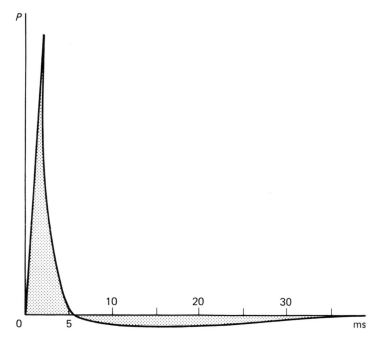

Figure 17.3 Blast wave-diagram of pressure–time relationships. (Adapted from Kerr and Byrne, 1975)

energy, represented by the area under the curve, is approximately equal in each phase.

Kerr and Byrne (1975) in Belfast have had the unfortunate opportunity to study the effects of blast, and have concluded that damage to the drum head occurs during the positive phase, and that its likelihood depends on the rate of rise, the peak value, and the duration of that phase.

Cochlear damage, causing a severe hearing loss and tinnitus is universal, but usually recovers within a short while; although after one explosion one third of Kerr's patients suffered a long-lasting high-tone loss. Since these were patients who all suffered perforation of the tympanic membrane, the traditional belief that rupture of the drum protects the inner ear from damage is no longer tenable. Teter, Newell and Aspinall (1970) also recorded high-tone hearing losses as the commonest auditory defect after blast exposure. As after closed head injuries, some recovery of auditory function may be expected during periods of a few months.

Vestibular symptoms were uncommon after blast injury in Kerr's experience, unless the head had been struck—when benign positional vertigo was frequently observed. Positional vertigo has however afflicted patients who suffered pure blast damage without any blow to the head. Perilymph fistula from the oval window might reasonably be expected as an associated finding in patients complaining of this symptom, and Strong described such an instance in 1973. The present writer has found positional vertigo of the benign paroxysmal type, recovering after several months, in a patient from one of the London restaurant explosions in 1975. No fistula could be found when the ear was explored during repair of an accompanying unhealed perforation of the tympanic membrane. That patient acquired, and still suffers from, a high-tone sensorineural hearing loss in the damaged ear.

Surgical trauma

The labyrinth may suffer accidental injury from mechanical, acoustic or thermal energy. During mastoid surgery severe injury will result from opening a fistula into the lateral semicircular canal, which, because of its position, is the most vulnerable part of the otic capsule. The risk is highest when the bone has previously been eroded by cholesteatoma. Provided the matrix is removed without opening the perilymph space, the labyrinth will probably not suffer, but transgression of the endosteum is often—and tearing of the membranous canal is invariably—followed by severe cochlear and vestibular damage. The oval window may be accidentally breached by displacement of the incus and stapes. Singleton and Schuknecht, in 1959, demonstrated that inward subluxation of the stapes footplate, in cats, caused injuries to the basal coil of the cochlea similar to those produced by blast or head blows.

Stapedectomy entails risk to the membranous structures within the vestibule, particularly during attempts to extricate inwardly displaced fragments of footplate. Severe functional loss can be expected to follow tears of the utricular wall, and contact injuries may produce 'cupulolithiasis', causing positional vertigo. After stapedectomy the ear is more vulnerable to damage by barotrauma, and there have been numerous instances of sudden sensorineural hearing loss following accidental cabin decompression during air travel. The causes of perilymph leakage from the oval window, already discussed, are more likely to operate on a surgically modified oval window covering. An ear whose hearing mechanism has been reconstructed by a direct columella from the malleus handle to the oval window niche is probably more vulnerable to drum movement caused by barotrauma. A report in 1975, by Sleekx and Shea, of oval window fistula due to pressure trauma in an air pocket two years after stapedectomy, was later followed by the post-mortem finding, in the same patient, of rupture of the wall of the saccule and loss of macular structures. This again stresses that window rupture, with perilymph leak, is evidence of intralabyrinthine membrane disorganization.

Acoustic trauma may be transmitted by contact between a rotating burr and an intact incus to the inner ear, as Paparella showed in 1962. This should be avoided, although the smaller the burr the less the risk.

Intentional injury to the labyrinth, for the relief of vertigo from episodic vestibular activity, may be accomplished by mechanical extirpation of membranous labyrinth material—either the utricle from the vestibule or the membranous lateral canal (Cawthorne, 1960)—or by ultrasonic destruction. Traditional teaching holds that the labyrinth is more easily destroyed in Menière's disorder than when it has been involved by chronic infection, but this may not be so. As the present writer has suggested (Ludman, 1971) the susceptibility to surgical destruction may be the same in the two groups of disorders; and persisting vertigo after chronic infection may stem from mechanisms other than survival of parts of the vestibular epithelium.

Symptoms

The auditory effect of surgical damage to the inner ear is sensorineural deafness. This may be severe or affect only high tones. Fluctuating hearing loss is the hallmark of leakage of perilymph.

Vestibular symptoms arising immediately after operation are those of sudden vestibular destruction (which has already been discussed) or the syndrome of benign positional vertigo. In addition, disequilibrium and attacks of vertigo after temporal bone surgery may be due to:

(1) Persistence of random labyrinthine activity from surviving epithelial structures.

(2) Failure of adequate compensation for loss of vestibular function.

(3) Direct neural stimulation of vestibular nerve endings in the medial wall of the vestibule (Ludman, 1971).

(4) The presence of a fistula into an intact vestibular system, causing vertigo by the Tullio phenomenon when the stapes remains mobile—labelled 'perilabyrinthitis' by Cawthorne in 1957. The stimulating effect of adjacent mucosal inflammation on a persistent fistula may produce similar symptoms.

(5) Secondary hydrops—causing episodic Menière-like vertigo in a patient whose ear has suffered severe previous cochlear damage. In the author's experience, the vertigo of this syndrome may not develop until many years after the original cochlear injury.

The elucidation of the particular cause requires careful consideration of the history of the events preceding and following the operation, together with evaluation of evidence for a persisting fistula, of signs of activity in the damaged labyrinth, and of the pattern of the vestibular disturbance.

References

Althaus, S. R. (1977) 'Spontaneous and traumatic perilymph fistulas', *Laryngoscope*, **87**, 364

Barber, H. (1964) 'Positional nystagmus especially after head injury', *Laryngoscope*, **74**, 891

Bennett, P. B. and Towse, E. J. (1971) 'The high pressure nervous syndrome during a simulated oxygen–helium dive to 1500 feet', *Electroencephalography and Clinical Neurophysiology*, **31**, 383

Brauer, R. W. (1968) 'Seeking man's depth level', *Ocean Industry*, **3**, 28

Caruso, V. G., Winkelmann, P. E., Correia, M. J., Miltenberger, G. E. and Love, J. T. (1977) 'Otologic and otoneurologic injuries in divers', *Laryngoscope*, **87**, 508

Cawthorne, T. E. (1957) 'Perilabyrinthitis', *Laryngoscope*, **67**, 1233

Cawthorne, T. E. (1960) 'Labyrinthectomy', *Annals of Otology Rhinology and Laryngology*, **69**, 1170

Cawthorne, T. E. and Cooksey, F. S. (1946) 'Vestibular injuries', *Proceedings of the Royal Society of Medicine*, **39**, 270

Edmonds, C. 'Vertigo in Diving'. In *The Use of Nystagmography in Aviation Medicine*. Ed. by Guedry, F. E. Jr. AGARD Conference proc. No. 128 (NASA) A24–1

Edmonds, C., Freeman, P.. Thomas, R. *et al.* (1973) *Otological Aspects of Diving*, p. 55. Sydney; Australian Medical Publishing Co.

Edmonds, C., Freeman, P. and Tonkin, J. (1974) 'Fistula of the round window in diving', *Transactions of the American Academy of Ophthalmology and Otolaryngology*, **78**, 444

Emmet, J. R., Staab, E. V. and Fischer, N. D. (1977) 'Perilymph fistulas secondary to gunshot wound', *Archives of Otolaryngology*, **103**, 98

Farmer, J. C. (1977) 'Diving injuries to the inner ear', *Annals of Otology, Rhinology and Laryngology*, Supplement 36, Vol. 86

Fee, G. A. (1968) 'Traumatic perilymph fistulas', *Archives of Otolaryngology*, **88**, 477

Freeman, P. and Edmonds, C. (1972) 'Inner ear barotrauma', *Archives of Otolaryngology*, **95**, 556

Goodhill, V. (1971) 'Sudden deafness and round window rupture', *Laryngoscope*, **81**, 1462

Goodhill, V. (1973) 'Inner ear barotrauma', *Archives of Otolaryngology*, **95**, 588

Goodhill, V. (1976) 'Sudden sensorineural deafness', *Proceedings of the Royal Society of Medicine*, **69**, 565

Goodhill, V., Harris, I. and Brockman, S. (1973) 'Sudden deafness and labyrinthine window ruptures', *Annals of Otology, Rhinology and Laryngology*, **82**, 2

Harker, L., Norante, J. and Rzu, J. (1974) 'Experimental rupture of the round window membrane', *Transactions of the American Academy of Ophthalmology and Otolaryngology*, **78**, 448

Healy, G. B., Strong, M. S. and Sampogna, D.

(1974) 'Ataxia, vertigo and hearing loss—a result of rupture of inner ear window', *Archives of Otolaryngology*, **100**, 130

House, H. P. (1967) 'The fistula problem in otosclerosis', *Laryngoscope*, **77**, 1410

Igarashi, M., Schuknecht, H. and Myers, E. (1964) 'Cochlear pathology in humans with stimulation deafness', *Journal of Laryngology and Otology*, **78**, 115

Kerr, A. G. and Byrne, J. E. T. (1975) 'Concussion effects of bomb blast on the ear', *Journal of Laryngology and Otology*, **89**, 131

Ludman, H. (1971) 'Destruction of the labyrinth and perilabyrinthitis', *Proceedings of the Royal Society of Medicine*, **64**, 849

Lundgren, C. E. G. (1965) 'Alternobaric vertigo—a diver's hazard', *British Medical Journal*, **2**, 511

Lundgren, C. E. G., Tjernstrom, O. and Ornhagen, H. (1974) 'Alternobaric vertigo and hearing disturbance in connection with diving: an epidemiological study', *Undersea Biomedical Research*, **1**, 251

Makishima, K. and Snow, J. B. (1975) 'Pathogenesis of hearing loss in head injury', *Archives of Otolaryngology*, **101**, 426

Makishima, K., Sobel, S. F. and Snow, J. B. (1976) 'Histopathologic correlates of otoneurologic manifestations following head trauma', *Laryngoscope*, **86**, 1303

Paparella, M. (1962) 'Acoustic trauma from the bone cutting burr', *Laryngoscope*, **72**, 116

Pullen, F. W. (1972) 'Round window rupture: a cause of sudden deafness', *Transactions of the American Academy of Ophthalmology and Otolaryngology*, **76**, 1444

Ruedi, L. and Furrer, W. (1947) *Das Akutishe Trauma*. Basle; S. Karger

Schuknecht, H., Neff, W. and Perlman, H. (1951) 'An experimental study of auditory damage following blows to the head', *Annals of Otology, Rhinology and Laryngology*, **60**, 273

Schuknecht, H. (1962) 'Positional vertigo: clinical and experimental observations', *Transactions of the American Academy of Ophthalmology and Otolaryngology* **66**, 319

Schuknecht, H. (1969) 'Cupulolithiasis', *Archives of Otolaryngology*, **90**, 765

Schuknecht, H. and Davison, R. C. (1956) 'Deafness and vertigo from head injury', *Archives of Otology, Rhinology and Laryngology*, **63**, 513

Schuknecht, H. and Gacek, R. R. (1973) 'Surgery on only hearing ears', *Transactions of the American Academy of Ophthalmology and Otolaryngology*, **77**, ORL 257

Simmons, F. B. (1968) 'Theory of membrane breaks in sudden hearing loss', *Archives of Otolaryngology*, **88**, 41

Singleton, G. and Schuknecht, H. (1959) 'Experimental fracture of the stapes in cats', *Annals of Otology, Rhinology and Laryngology*, **68**, 1069

Sleeckx, J. P. and Shea, J. J. (1975) 'Barotraumatic rupture of the saccule following stapedectomy', *Acta Otorhinolaryngologica Belgica*, **29**, 1046

Smith, A. H. (1873) *The Effects of High Atmospheric Pressure, Including Caisson Disease*, 1. Brooklyn, N.Y.; Eagle Print

Stroud, M. H. and Calcaterra, T. C. (1970) 'Spontaneous perilymph fistulas', *Laryngoscope*, **80**, 479

Sundmaker, W. (1973) *Vestibular Function*. Ed. by Lambertsen, C. Special Summary Program, Predictive Studies III Philadelphia, University of Pennsylvania

Teter, D. L., Newell, R. C. and Aspinall, K. B. (1970) 'Audiometric configurations associated with blast trauma', *Laryngoscope*, **80**, 1122

Toglia, J. U., Rosenberg, P. E. and Ronis, M. L. (1970) 'Post traumatic dizziness', *Annals of Otology, Rhinology and Laryngology*, **92**, 485

18 Noise and the ear
Peter W Alberti

Introduction

Noise

Noise is any undesired sound, and by extension noise is any unwanted disturbance within a useful frequency band, for example undesired electrical waves in a transmission or device. Noise is an erratic intermittent or statistically random oscillation. Since these definitions of noise are not mutually exclusive it is usually necessary to depend upon context for the distinction (NIOSH, 1973).

Noise thus has physical, physiological and psychological connotations, all of which differ. Physically it is complex sound having little or no periodicity. However, it can be measured and its characteristics analysed. Physiologically, acoustically and electronically noise is defined as a signal that bears no information and whose intensity varies randomly in time. Psychologically noise is any sound, irrespective of its wave form, which is unpleasant or unwanted.

Noise, like any sound, is defined in terms of its duration, frequency spectrum measured in Hz, and intensity measured in sound pressure level (SPL) and expressed in decibels (dB). It may be continuous, intermittent, impulsive or explosive. It may be steady-state or fluctuant. Two standard noises require definition.

White noise is a random sound with a spectrum containing a mixture of all frequencies, and a spectral density such that all frequencies are equally represented, i.e. there is constant power/cycle.

Pink noise is fabricated to contain a constant power/octave.

White noise has more power/octave in the higher than in the lower frequencies because there are an increasing number of cycles/octave as frequency is increased. It rises by 3 dB/octave. Conversely pink noise has relatively more energy in the lower frequencies than at high levels. This has practical application because the energy spectrum of pink noise closely resembles that of speech, which it therefore masks more effectively for a given total energy level than does white noise.

This chapter deals with the effect of sound—particularly excessive sound—on hearing, and the word noise will be used in all of the above ways, but is more often used to mean unwanted sound, by virtue of it being unpleasant, interfering or harmful.

In this sense noise need not fit any preconceived physical parameters; the sweetest music if played sufficiently loudly may become just a noise.

Unwanted sounds are of increasing importance in twentieth century society. The sound levels in urban communities are apparently rising at an exponential rate, and the nuisance value of unwanted sound is high. Excessive sound is one of the most common causes of hearing loss in the world—both from military and industrial sources.

Historical

'Civilization is noise.' So said Dan McKenzie (1916), and man's progress through the ages has been accompanied by activities involving ever-increasing noise intensity.

It has been suggested that occupational hearing loss due to noise dates at least from the Bronze Age (Hinchcliffe, 1967). Certainly man's discovery of the use of metals, first bronze, later iron, with the attendant noises of heating, hammering and forging these materials to fashion useful implements and weapons, occasioned perhaps the first situation in which human hearing was 'at risk' from occupational noise.

About A.D. 1300 appeared the second danger, gunpowder. The next threat was associated with the Industrial Revolution and the mechanization of factories, followed closely by the development of railways, the internal combustion engine, power-driven ships and aircraft. It is little recognized that after the Second World War there was a further Industrial Revolution when the results of technological and scientific discovery of the 1930s and 1940s were put into effect. Economies in size were made at the price of quantum increases in sound levels. Refineries, chemical plants, papermaking machinery, mining equipment, construction machinery, transportation, all became larger, more efficient and much, much louder. The machinery of war also became more devastating and more deafening. The Lee Enfield rifle of the Second World War is now known as the 'quiet rifle' compared with the modern carbines! Twenty-five years later we are reaping the rewards of the unwanted increase in noise in an epidemic of deafness.

The enormous power of sound was recognized in ancient times—witness the trumpet blasts that shattered the walls of Jericho, and the great horn of Alexander, so loud that it could summon soldiers at a distance of ten miles.

Recognition that deafness could be caused by noise was slow, although some of its effects on the ear were obvious. The book of Ecclesiasticus describes the 'smith sitting by the anvil, the noise of the hammer and the anvil is ever in his ears—without these cannot a city be inhabited'.

Martial, in the first century A.D., commented in his epigrams on the noise of ancient Rome and that 'blacksmiths with their hammer notes, keep up their din the whole day long'.

Physicians of the medieval medical school of Salerno noted:

'Our hearing is a choice and dainty sense,
And hard to mend, yet soon it may be marred,
Blows, falls, and noise . . . all these . . .
Breed tingling in the ears, and hurt our hearing.'

The first mention of deafness from cannonading is attributed to Alberti in 1591.

In his *De Morbis Artificium* Ramazzini (1713), reported that those who hammered copper for a living had their ears so injured by the perpetual din that workers of this class became hard of hearing. If they grew old at this work, they became completely deaf (Bell, 1966). He recommended the use of hearing protectors to prevent deafness occurring.

Nils Skragge, over 200 years ago, wrote a thesis on occupational deafness in coppersmiths and blacksmiths (Kylin, 1960), and Fosbroke in 1831 gave an accurate description of noise-induced deafness in blacksmiths coining the expression 'black-smith's deafness'. A good example of percussive noise injury was Admiral Lord Rodney who apparently became deaf for 14 days following the firing of 80 broadsides from his ship HMS *Formidable* in the year 1882. However, occupational hearing loss, and particularly noise-induced hearing loss, is basically a direct consequence of the first and second Industrial Revolutions. It was necessary to fabricate machinery before man-made noise reached large-scale deafening proportions. It soon became evident that heavy engineering, ship-building, boilermaking and the like were traumatic to hearing, and the general term 'boilermaker's deafness' was introduced. Indeed occupational hearing loss reached epidemic proportions in such ship-building areas as the Clyde and Tyne in Great Britain, so that in 1886 Thomas Barr of Glasgow, wrote 'it is familiarly known that boilermakers and others who work in very noisy surroundings are extremely liable to dullness of hearing. In Glasgow, we would have little difficulty in finding hundreds whose sense of hearing has thus been damaged, by the noisy character of their work. We have therefore in our city ample materials at hand for investigation of this subject'. Boilermaker's deafness is particularly interesting in that it did not exist until the invention of riveting, but has virtually disappeared again with the technological change which has introduced welding as a preferred method of joining sheets of steel.

The site and nature of the lesion were first described by Habermann (1890), in a man of 75 who had worked as a blacksmith for 20 years and whose occupation had exposed him to high intensity noise during his working life. Partial disappearance of the organ of Corti was found with destruction of the hair-cells, the most extensive damage being in the lower basal coil. There was a resultant atrophy of the auditory nerve, with complete degeneration of the spiral ganglion and the nerves in the osseous spiral lamina.

Soon after the introduction of audiometry, Fowler (1939) observed dips at 4 kHz and Bunch (1937) published probably the first audiometric data demonstrating the typical high-frequency loss acquired by those exposed to noise. Dickson, Ewing and Littler (1939) described the 'aviator's notch' at 4 kHz in pilots of piston-engined aircraft. Subsequently, efforts to correlate industrial noise levels and frequency spectra with the hearing levels of employees have been the subject of numerous reports.

Scope

The size of this problem is difficult to estimate, for there are no valid epidemiological data covering total populations. However, it is established that in the UK there are probably 100 000 individuals with noise-induced hearing loss—approximately 0.2 per cent of the total population. The US Department of Labour estimates that 26 per cent of 14.3 million production workers in the USA in 1973 were exposed to noise levels in excess of a 90-dB 8-h exposure/working day, and this excludes workers in mining, transportation, construction and the military. In the Province of Ontario, Canada, with a population of 8 million there were 2500 new claims for industrially induced hearing loss in 1976, and in Sweden there were a similar number of claims in the same year. The US army is paying more in pensions for hearing loss following the wars in S.E. Asia than for any other disability. Thus, a century after Thomas Barr, hearing loss from noise remains a disorder of epidemic proportion.

Definition of terms

Previous descriptions indicating the varying effects of noise on the ear have not always been clearly defined. Thus some authors have considered 'acoustic trauma' as a generic term covering all aspects of noise damage, whilst others have employed it in a strictly limited context. Here it will be reserved for permanent hearing loss produced by very brief exposure to very loud sound (Davis *et al.*, 1954, 1957).

A partial impairment of the sense of hearing is nowadays described by the term 'hearing loss' with the expression 'deafness' reserved for patients with profound or complete hearing loss.

Effects of sound stimulation

Stimulation of the ear with sound causes:

(1) Adaptation (transitory residual masking)
(2) Temporary threshold shift (TTS)   (a) fatigue
                                        (b) long-lasting TTS
(3) Persistent threshold shift
(4) Permanent threshold shift (PTS)

The subject of adaptation and TTS is well reviewed by Ward (1973) and by Burns *et al.* (1973).

Adaptation

Adaptation or pre-stimulatory fatigue, also known as transitory residual masking, is an immediate phenomenon which occurs when a sound is presented to the ear somewhat elevating the threshold. For fatiguing sounds of up to 90 dB sound pressure level (SPL) the greatest adaptation is produced for an identical test tone of identical frequency. The spread to either side of the fatigue tone is asymmetric with a greater effect being shown at frequencies above the fatigue frequency than below it. The amount of residual masking that remains after the fatigue tone ceases is proportional to the SPL of the fatiguer, but independent of its duration. The recovery is exponential in nature, and for fatigue sounds of up to 70 dB SPL occurs fully within 0.5 s. There are electrophysiological correlates of this adaptation which can be measured in animals as reductions in action potential; there appears to be a significant individual variation in the amount and length of adaptation which occurs (Kärjä, 1968).

Temporary threshold shift (TTS)

This is post-stimulatory fatigue. Like adaptation, it has in the past been referred to as auditory fatigue.

Some authors divide TTS into two distinct entities: fatigue, and temporary stimulation deafness.

FATIGUE

Transition from adaptation to fatigue has been considered to result from stronger or more extended exposures. A metamorphosis from the purely physiological process of adaptation to a state bordering on the pathological in fatigue has been envisaged, no clear distinction being drawn between the two. Another view, however, is that adaptation and fatigue can co-exist and should clearly be distinguished from each other. Fatigue denotes a decline in activity resulting from previous activity of the organ, according to Larsen (1953). If follows intensive sound stimulation, the maximum changes appearing 0.5–1 octave above the frequency of the pure-tone stimulus (*Figure 18.1*). The degree of fatigue increases progressively with stimulus duration and intensity, a balance not being achieved until abnormal sound intensities are applied. Recovery is slow and related to the degree of fatigue. If the stimulus is strong enough, irreversible changes may occur (Kärjä). There has been considerable controversy about the maximum point of TTS and whether the effect really is half an octave above the exposure tone. However, on balance this seems to be currently accepted (Burns *et al.*, 1973). Physiological fatigue shifts that last for more than 2 min can be considered as true fatigue. Much work has been done to attempt to relate these longer temporary threshold shifts to long-term permanent shifts. For the purpose of

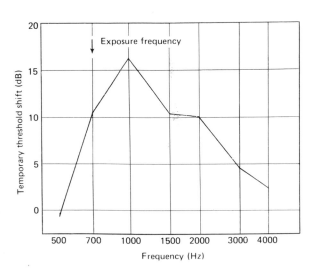

Figure 18.1   Temporary threshold shift at different frequencies, 5 min after the end of exposure to a tone of 700 Hz, for 5 min. Note the displacement upwards in frequency relative to the frequency of the exposure tone (From Ward, 1962). (Reproduced by courtesy of the Editor of *Journal of the Acoustical Society of America*)

this discussion physiological fatigue will be limited to TTS that lasts for more than 2 min, but that has completely recovered in less than 16 h, for this covers the situation of complete recovery after one day's work before beginning the next.

The amount of physiological fatigue is rarely above 30 dB. The recovery after physiological fatigue is exponential, rapid at first and then slowing down. The amount of TTS that occurs is more or less linearly related to the sound pressure level once the critical point is exceeded where it starts. This point seems to be between 70 and 75 dB for a 2-h exposure centred on 1000 Hz, although at frequencies below 1000 Hz the critical level may be higher. Ward (1973) gives a good discussion of this phenomenon and the exceptions to the rule. In general the higher the exposure frequency up to 4–6 kHz, the greater the TTS produced. The corollary to this statement is that damage risk criteria (DRC) generally suggest higher safe exposure levels at lower frequencies than at high frequencies. Greater temporary threshold shifts are produced by pure tones than by noise bands at frequencies below 2 kHz, because noise is a better stimulus for sustained middle-ear muscle contraction which protects the cochlea. The relationship between the sound pressure levels of noise band and pure tone to the amount of TTS produced is thus complex and no criteria developed for pure tones covers noise bands or vice versa. Impulse noise also produces TTS, which is similar to that for noise with the exception that TTSs for impulse noise grow linearly with time instead of exponentially, as do the TTSs for steady noise. Intermittent exposure, which is much more common than prolonged steady-state exposure, produces fairly complex results. For high-frequency sounds the amount of TTS produced is proportional to the total length of time of exposure. For example, exposure to 30 min of sound/h for 4 h at a high frequency produces TTS roughly equivalent to that produced by half the decibel level of a 4-h continuous exposure. For intermittent low frequency sounds, particularly those of considerable intermittency, the amount of TTS produced is less because the auditory muscle reflex provides additional protection and recovers between bursts of sound. It is possible to compute the amount of TTS produced by intermittent sounds, for it is additive to the amount of recovery which has taken place at the end of each exposure. The procedure is tedious and unnecessary except in experimental situations. If the intermittent sound exposure includes quanta of sound below the critical level necessary to produce a TTS, then those periods are treated as if in silence. Ward deals with the subject in considerable detail.

LONG-LASTING TTS—PATHOLOGICAL FATIGUE

If the amount of noise exposure is sufficient, then a more prolonged temporary threshold shift occurs which does not recover in 16 h, and does not have the decay characteristics of the short TTS. The cut-off point between short- and long-term TTS seems to be a TTS of approximately 40 dB. Above this level recovery does not occur within 16 h nor is it completely linear. This slope is initially much less steep than for short-term threshold shifts but after a variable period of time suddenly becomes steeper. This type of shift blends imperceptibly with permanent threshold shift. This type of loss is well discussed by Burns.

TTS PRODUCED BY PROLONGED EXPOSURE TO NOISE

A related topic is to ascertain how much hearing loss is produced by noise exposures greater than 8 h. How much threshold shift is produced by an infinitely extended exposure to noise? Is there for a given noise an asymptotic point where no further temporary threshold shift occurs irrespective of the continuation of sound? If such a point is found then at least one relationship has been established between TTS and PTS, i.e. at a fixed level after exposure to a given sound the permanent threshold shift cannot exceed the asymptotic point of the temporary threshold shift. Mills (1976a) undertook a detailed series of animal experiments to define such an asymptote in chinchillas exposed to an 80-dB sound for 90 days. The noise notch produced almost reached its final shape within five days, but grew a small but apparently significant amount in the remaining 85 days. Mills and his colleagues also studied the recovery of hearing following this exposure in their animals and found that most of the recovery had taken place by seven days, and indeed between seven and 60 days after cessation of noise exposure there was little change. However, from the 60th to 150th day there was a further slight but significant improvement in hearing. This suggests that some biological repair process was at work in the ear. If these results are transferable in man then they would have significance in the timing of audiometry for pension awards.

Melnick (1976) discusses human asymptotic threshold shifts (ATS) and concludes that they do occur in man from moderate levels of exposure to continuous noise, after 8–12 h of noise exposure. He believes however that recovery from levels of ATS of 30 dB or less is prolonged when compared to the recovery from similar magnitudes of threshold shift produced by short-term high-level exposure, and frequently is not complete within 24 h of cessation. He also points out that most experimenters suggest that, after some threshold noise level has been exceeded, TTS will grow at a greater rate/dB than the noise level is increased. He comments that the magnitude of threshold shift and the frequencies affected by a given noise depend upon the noise spectrum— the lower the frequency of the exposure noise, the broader the frequency band affected by TTS. There is considerable inter- and intra-subject variability in these experiments.

The practical implications of temporary threshold shifts mainly affect audiometry. How much temporary threshold shift is acceptable for screening audiometry in an industrial plant? How long should a worker be out of noise before a pension is awarded? How accurate is audiometry undertaken shortly after a 4-h jet airplane flight or motor bus trip? These are practical problems in North America and the less densely populated parts of Europe to which answers are not fully available.

ANIMAL CORRELATES

There is experimental evidence of morphological changes to match these psycho-acoustic findings. They will be described below.

Permanent threshold shift (PTS)

This is an irreversible elevation of the auditory threshold associated with permanent pathological changes in the cochlea. It is seen particularly in permanent noise-induced hearing loss, under which heading its specific characteristics are described.

Noise-induced hearing loss

There are many causes of hearing loss produced by noise and occupation, and the following classification covers most:

(1) Noise-induced temporary threshold shift (NITTS)
(2) Noise-induced permanent threshold shift (NIPTS)

Both of the above imply prolonged exposure to noise, which may be steady-state, impact or a mixture of the two.

In addition there is hearing loss caused by single intense sound sources classified as acoustic trauma, as for example a rifle shot, or in worse form blast trauma from an explosion. These produce variable hearing loss, some of which may recover. In blast injury there may be damage to the tympanic membrane and ossicles with a variable degree of injury to the cochlea.

Noise-induced temporary threshold shift (NITTS)

When a person is first exposed to hazardous noise, the initial change usually observed is an elevation of the threshold of hearing in the higher frequency range. Classically this appears as a steep isolated audiometric dip, the 'acoustic notch', at about 4 kHz (*Figure 18.2*).

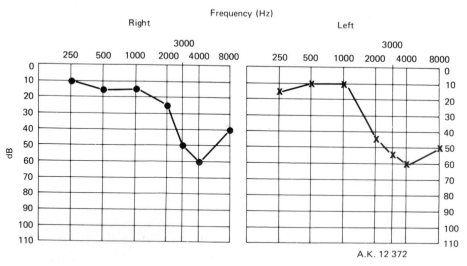

Figure 18.2   A typical 4-kHz notch found after exposure to noise

In the early stages of exposure this occurs as a temporary threshold shift, referred to also as noise-induced temporary threshold shift. After a rest period away from the noise the hearing usually returns to its former level.

Glorig (1958) has noted that individuals with normal hearing whose ears have never previously undergone prolonged noise exposure (green ears) demonstrate greater TTS than those whose ears have been exposed for long periods of time (ripe ears).

The recovery of hearing from a pathological temporary threshold shift was discussed in the previous section. There is a small but definite improvement for many days after removal from noise, but for practical purposes this is usually ignored because the amount of improvement found after the first day or two is less than the confidence limits of the audiometry used in testing. It should be emphasized that this is not true of massive threshold shifts produced by explosions, for here significant recovery continues for some weeks (*Figure 18.3*).

That recovery can continue for long periods after noise exposure was found by Miller, Watson and Cavell (1963) who observed additional recovery of 8–13 dB during the third and fourth months following exposure; Sokolovski (1969) found in cats recovery, usually not greater than 10 dB, up to about the 56th post-exposure day; and Ward (1969) found slight additional recovery in chinchillas between 20 and 40 days but did not consider this change statistically significant. It should be noted that these are animal studies and their relevance to man is debatable.

A relationship between TTS and PTS has been sought for years—both for scientific and empiric reasons, for if they are related, the former might be used to predict the risk of the latter. Unfortunately, no easy relationship has been delineated—the problems are well discussed by Ward (1976a). The lack of such a test bedevils hearing conservation programmes in industry, particularly in heavily unionized plants. At present the only way of determining whether a worker is unduly susceptible to the effects of a particular industrial noise is to test his hearing at regular intervals and note whether it deteriorates at a significantly greater rate than the norm. This may take six months to discover, at which time it may be very difficult to dismiss the worker, the only alternative if the plant has no quieter jobs.

Noise-induced permanent threshold shift (NIPTS)

For practical purposes this is the most commonly encountered hearing loss due to noise, one for which there are many synonyms: occupational hearing loss, industrial noise-induced deafness, chronic acoustic trauma, noise-induced hearing loss, permanent noise-induced hearing loss, stimulation deafness, occupational deafness, boiler-maker's deafness, etc.

Although it is often stated that continous employment in a potentially noise-hazardous environment for 10–15 years is necessary for an initial TTS to be established as a NIPTS (*Figure 18.4*) the actual data are of course entirely dependent upon (1) the noise levels, and (2) individual susceptibility. A point of practical importance is the quite uneven noise levels in industry, both within a single work period of 8 h and over a period of months or years as machinery and process varies. It is no accident that so few studies have been undertaken in which hearing loss has been quantified against prolonged constant industrial exposure, because there are singularly few industries where the noise level has remained constant over two or three decades. A notable exception is the extremely well-studied group of jute workers in Dundee (Taylor *et al.*, 1965).

A major study by Burns *et al.* (1970) has laid the basis for the *equal energy concept* which suggests that equal amounts of acoustic energy between a level which is totally

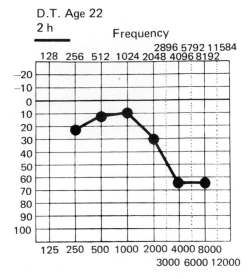

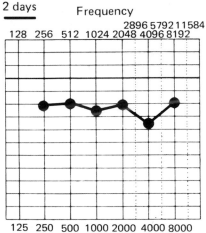

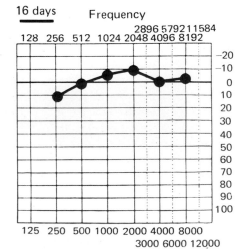

Figure 18.3 Serial audiograms of 22 year old laboratory technician exposed to an exploding retort showing recovery over a 16-day period

safe and one which is totally injurious produce equal amounts of hearing loss. If one can compute the amount of noise exposure, one can predict the risk to hearing. As a doubling of energy represents an increase in noise levels of 3 dB, it follows that for equivalent risk, the exposure time must be halved for each 3-dB increase. Burns *et al.* (1970) coined the term 'noise imission level' which is an index of the total noise energy

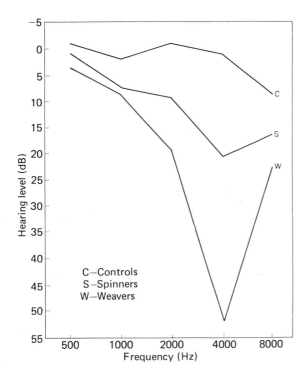

Figure 18.4 Median hearing levels of small groups of subjects employed at the same textile mill. Controls had not been exposed to noise; spinners and weavers had both spent ten years, on average, in their respective occupations. (From Burns, Hinchcliffe and Littler (1964), reproduced by courtesy of the Editor of *Annals of Occupational Hygiene*)

incident on the ear over a period of time. This has also given rise to the expression 'equivalent continuous noise level' expressed as L eq. It is suggested that all noise exposure to steady-state noise, and indeed to much impulse noise (Martin, 1976a) be related to a baseline 90 dBA weighting/40-h working week which allows for a good risk prediction. These findings are embodied in an International Standard ISO 1999, which gives the technique for adding various noise exposures experienced over minutes or hours to produce a L eq, to a steady-state 40-h noise exposure measured in dBA. It does this by computing a *partial noise exposure index:* (an index determined by a sound level and its duration within a working week, 40 h); and adding to produce a *composite noise exposure index:* (the sum of partial noise exposure indices for relevant sound levels over a working week, 40 h). These are then entered into a table to convert them to *equivalent continuous sound level* (L eq): (that sound level in dBA which if present for 40 h in one week, produces the same composite noise exposure index at the various measured sound levels over one week). It goes further and quantifies the risk to the exposed population of the given noise level and takes into account the amount of hearing loss which would be expected in a similar non-noise-exposed population.

Robinson and Shipton (1973) have further simplified matters by producing detailed tables for the estimation of noise-induced hearing loss, based on noise imission levels and ISO 1999 which they emphasize gives population data, but because of individual variations cannot be applied to individuals.

Impact noise

So far most discussion has concerned steady-state noise. Impact noise is as dangerous and just as frequent in the military and industrial complexes of the world; early examples were rifle shots and riveting. Steady-state and impact noise merge because if the time between impacts is sufficiently short the noise becomes, for practical purposes, steady-state. A good example of this is the diesel engine; the old single cylinder diesel engines which used to power fishing boats had a characteristic 'put-put' sound where each explosion in the cylinder produces a discrete sound, which should be contrasted with the modern 2-stroke supercharged diesel motor used in motor buses where there are still individual sounds, but they occur so close to each other that it sounds as one. The characteristic of impact sounds varies enormously, rise and decay times range from abrupt to gently sloped, all of which may alter the effect on the ear; contrast for example the crack of a high velocity rifle with the ring of a hammer hitting a metal tank.

One of the problems which has bedevilled work with impact noise is difficulty in the exact measurement of the sound itself. It may be so transient that although there is a high peak SPL it does not persist long enough to be fully registerable even on a modern impulse-measuring sound level meter.

This question of measurement is crucial to establishing appropriate damage risk criteria (DRC). Theoretically this question is extremely complicated for it depends upon the physical nature of the impact and its repetition rate. In practice Martin has shown that at least some impulse noises follow the equal energy concept which pertains for steady-state noise. A more basic question is the level of impulse noise which is safe, or alternatively the DRC at various levels of impulse noise. The work of Coles (1968) on hazardous exposure to impulse noise, particularly to gunfire noise, led to recommendations by the US National Academy of Sciences who proposed DRC for impulse noise which have been tentatively accepted, albeit with reservations. Henderson, *et al.* (1977) have recently questioned these findings and believe that the reverberation of the impulse is important—if the impulsive noise is short enough it is less damaging than if it rings, as for example by reflection from nearby hard surfaces.

It should also be noted that Ward (1976b, 1977) has been a most eloquent and persuasive antagonist of the equal energy concepts applied to steady-state and impact noise, and also the proposed DRC applied to impulse noise. He makes the point that most experimental work with equal energy concepts has been concerned with temporary threshold shifts and the relationship between these and the permanent threshold shifts are not known. However, notwithstanding these criticisms, at present DRC for steady-state and impact noise now seem to rest fairly firmly on the belief that the magnitude of permanent threshold shift is directly related to the square of any weighted sound pressure integrated over time (Burns *et al.*, 1970; Burns, *et al.*, 1977). The latter report also reconciles the major previous differences between the large American study by Baughn (1966), which was the basis for the International Standard ISO 1999.

Natural history of NIPTS

The relationship between NIPTS and NITTS is by no means clear and has been discussed above. Within the broad range of noise levels described as hazardous the average initial change is a temporary threshold shift which imperceptibly blends into permanent threshold shift. There is no arbitrary period of exposure beneath which no NIPTS may occur, nor any maximum exposure beyond which no further NIPTS will occur.

NIPTS usually commences around 4 kHz and gradually progresses at that frequency and spreads into neighbouring frequencies. At first it may be asymptomatic but if it spreads into the lower frequencies, 3 and 2 kHz, complaints appear. Initially subjects experience difficulty in discriminating speech in social gatherings or crowded places, but as the loss spreads into the lower frequencies they may have difficulty with sounds being too quiet. The notch may start anywhere between 3 and 6 kHz, and after a time the better hearing above the apex of the notch disappears so that the audiogram becomes flattened out in the higher frequencies. It must be emphasized that whilst a notch is often present in the hearing loss produced by NIPTS it is not a prerequisite for the diagnosis.

The mean hearing loss experienced is a function of the noise levels and length of exposure. 'Typical' audiograms are frequently shown in texts, but they are typical only of the group to which they apply. The typical audiogram shown in *Figure 18.4* is applicable only to the noise levels experienced by that particular group of weavers and the quite different audiogram shown in *Figure 18.5* is typical of the hearing of male hard-rock miners after 20 years of underground drilling with pneumatic tools. The two are quite dissimilar but each is characteristic of its group.

It has been said that a hearing loss after ten years of exposure to sound has progressed as far as it will—this statement is almost certainly not true. The hearing loss at 4 kHz appears to progress at a steady rate for about ten years, and then the rate of progression slows greatly (*Figure 18.6*). However, as the years progress the loss spreads into other frequencies and it takes up to 30 years to involve frequencies of 1 kHz and below to any great extent. The natural progression of an occupational hearing loss is thus: to increase fairly rapidly at 4 kHz and areas around it, then as the years pass to spread into other frequencies so that gradually what was a notched sensorineural hearing loss centred at about 4 kHz becomes a steeply sloping loss starting at about 500 Hz. Our own findings based on over 2000 heavy industrial workers, miners, papermakers and steel workers, show a 7.5-dB/octave drop from 500 Hz to 4 kHz after about 20 years of exposure (Alberti and Morgan, 1974).

Individual susceptibility varies enormously, and unfortunately there is no good way of predicting this. Damage risk criteria predict what will be safe for a certain percentage of the population, but they do not help with protection of total populations. The much mentioned 90 dBA/40 h exposure, which is described as 'safe' is safe for about 85 per cent of the population; conversely 15 per cent of workers exposed to this level for a prolonged period will develop a demonstrably handicapping hearing loss. In order to protect 95 per cent of the population an 85-dBA safe level must be adopted. It should be emphasized that all of these figures are on ears unprotected by hearing protectors. The individual differences in noise-induced hearing loss have recently been summarized by Mills (1976b).

The rate of progression depends upon the type of noise and individual susceptibility.

The type of progression for a particular noise is shown in *Figure 18.6* and the range covered by these curves in *Figures 18.7* and *18.8. Figure 18.6* shows quite clearly that

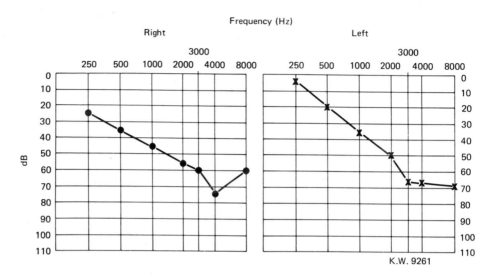

Figure 18.5   Audiogram of a 56 year old nickel miner exposed to about 20 years of hard rock drilling. This audiogram is typical of rock miners after this exposure

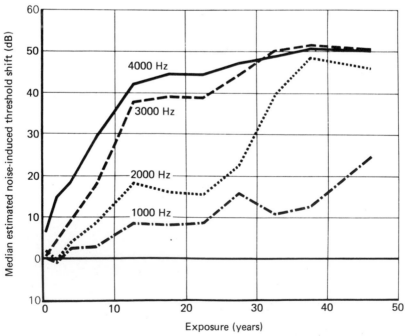

Figure 18.6   Estimated noise-induced threshold shift as a function of duration of exposure. (From Taylor, Pearson, Mair and Burns, 1965. In *Noise and Man* by W. Burns *et al.*, John Murray; London, 1968. p. 174). (Reproduced by permission of the publishers)

for that noise the hearing loss at 3 and 4 kHz increases linearly at one rate for a dozen years and then slowly tapers off, whilst the hearing loss at 2 kHz behaves in an almost opposite way—slowly increasing for 25 years and then relatively more rapidly to reach the same level at the higher frequencies after 38 years of exposure. At the end of a working lifetime the loss for 1 kHz is only just making itself manifest. However, there is tremendous individual variation, e.g. at 2 kHz the loss after 30 years of exposure shows a 30-dB difference in permanent threshold shift between 25th and 75th percentile (*Figures 18.7* and *18.8*). These graphs might be very different with different noise exposures. One of the difficulties of making predictions of this nature is the changing nature of industrial noise—machinery may be changed or malfunction, a silencer may blow, a bearing break, etc. There are a number of well-documented

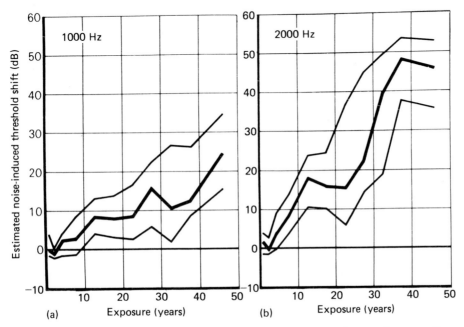

Figure 18.7   Estimated noise-induced threshold shift for particular frequencies, as median and quartile values, for different exposure durations (a) for 1000 Hz; (b) for 2000 Hz. (From Taylor, Pearson, Mair and Burns, 1965. In *Noise and Man* by W. Burns *et al.*, John Murray; London, 1968. p. 174). (Reproduced by permission of the publishers)

incidents of workmen dating a sudden change in their hearing levels to such temporary changes in work noise. In the resource industries, hard rock drillers will often attribute a noticeable worsening of their hearing to a particular period of drilling in which the noise levels were higher than usual. There seems to be an intensity level above which noise produces dramatic changes which may not recover. These are more usually associated with acoustic trauma, i.e. a single explosion or blast, but may be due to exposure of an ear to too intense a steady-state noise.

There are some people with 'tough' ears who seem to be able to withstand higher levels of exposure better than average, and others with relatively tender ears which are easily damaged. Audiograms of two such individuals are shown as *Figures 18.9a* and *b*. Both men had been hard rock drillers in a nickel mine undertaking work which so far as could be ascertained was identical, for a similar number of years. In addition the patient from *Figure 18.9a* had been a tank driver during the Second World War and yet he shows minimal hearing loss, which led to considerable difficulty as he was a strong trades unionist who felt that irrespective of his hearing loss he should be compensated for long exposure.

A fairly constant concomitant of industrial hearing loss is tinnitus, which is frequently present for some hours after noise exposure, but fortunately usually disappears. However, after many years of exposure or after intense exposure it may become permanent. This is a distressing symptom which is difficult to quantify and thus difficult to study. The recent introduction of tinnitus clinics, both in the USA and the UK, will hopefully bring some order to the problem. There seems to be no uniform characteristic of tinnitus produced by prolonged exposure to noise, descriptions running the full gamut of adjectives are used to describe the symptom.

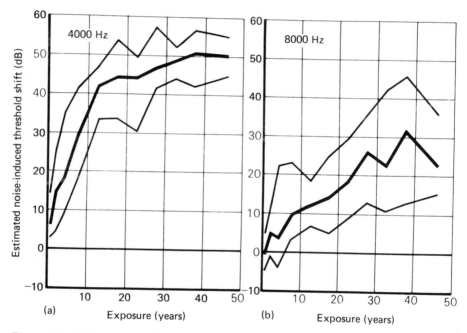

Figure 18.8   Estimated noise-induced threshold shift for particular frequencies, as median and quartile values, for different exposure durations. (a) for 4000 Hz; (b) for 8000 Hz. (From Taylor, Pearson, Mair and Burns, 1968. In *Noise and Man*, by W. Burns *et al.*, John Murray; London, 1968, p. 174). (Reproduced by permission of the publishers)

WORSENING OF HEARING AFTER CESSATION OF NOISE EXPOSURE

It is generally accepted that when noise exposure ceases the hearing will not worsen, and indeed may even improve. A disturbing report by Pfander (1975) indicates that there are individual cases of both acute and long-term progression of hearing loss following the cessation of acoustic trauma.

EXPLANATION OF THE 'ACOUSTIC DIP'

Several theories have been advanced to account for the occurrence of the characteristic high-tone notch.

Anatomical

The 4-kHz area of the basilar membrane which is that usually affected by noise lies in the basal turn of the cochlea. This bears the initial impact of sound waves stimulating the inner ear, particularly those of higher frequency which travel directly across the middle-ear space by para-ossicular conduction. At this point the basilar membrane is more firmly fixed, thus subjected to more torsion and so more liable to undergo degenerative changes. A weakness of the bony capsule corresponding with the critical 4-kHz dip has been demonstrated (Kelemen, 1962).

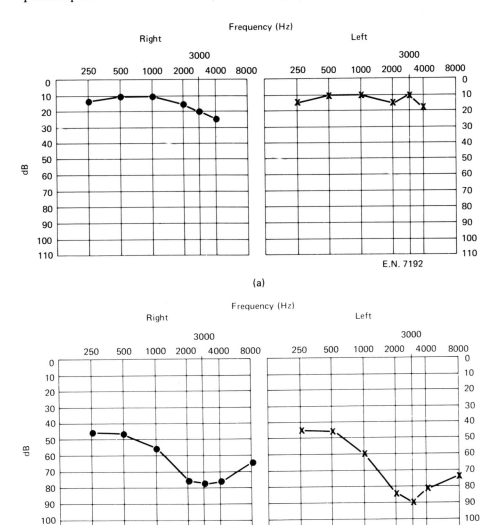

Figure 18.9 (a) Audiogram of 50 year old miner who had been a hard rock miner for 20 years and served as a tank driver during the war: he shows little hearing loss and is an example of 'tough' ears; (b) Audiogram of 54 year old miner with identical noise exposure to the man in (a) above. He has a profound loss and is an example of 'tender' ears. Both should be contrasted with *Figure 18.5*

Physiological

Summation of TTS curves resulting from several pure tones recorded in the same diagram, is found to occur at or above 4 kHz.

The sensitivity of the ear, however, decreases steeply above this frequency. The maximum effect, therefore, occurs exactly in the area around 4 kHz. If the stimulating sound is extremely loud, the dip takes place at 6 kHz (Lehnhardt, 1965). This accords with the observations of Nakamura (1964) that the greater the intensity, the higher are the frequencies reached by maximal TTS.

The acoustic reflex and the influence of the middle ear on dip production have been studied by Lehnhardt (1960). Fixation of the ossicles is caused by contraction of the intratympanic muscles when activated by sound stimulation. When noises in excess of 80 dB SPL are applied this results in a shift in the natural frequency of the middle ear towards the higher frequencies. If temporary inhibition of the middle-ear muscle reflex is produced by curarization, the sensitivity curve of the ear takes the same form as the threshold curve.

White noise exposure in such cases resulted in dips at 3 kHz instead of 4 kHz. It was therefore considered that in some instances the cause of dips below 4 kHz is hypofunction of the middle-ear musculature.

Physical

Resonance in the external auditory meatus increases the amplitude of sound waves between 2 kHz and 3500 kHz by about 20 dB compared with waves at other frequencies (Onchi, 1951). Such intensification may therefore be a factor.

Hydrodynamic causes were demonstrated by von Békésy (1953) to be responsible for the maximal sensitivity of the ear between 1 and 4 kHz. Stimulation in any specific frequency range activates regions of the basilar membrane responsive to higher frequencies as well, but not areas of the lower frequency specificity (Davis *et al.*, 1953; Hood, 1950; Littler, 1966)

SYNERGISTIC EFFECT OF OTOTRAUMATIC AGENTS

Various noxious agents may damage the ear. They include steady-state and impact noise, a variety of drugs, head trauma, ageing, various ear diseases including the premature degeneration of the cochlea found in many familial hearing losses, and infective degenerations of the ear. The question of how these various agents interact is complex and important. Is an ear which has already been damaged by noise more or less susceptible to further damage by an ototoxic antibiotic, or is the effect purely additive? Many of the answers are not known, but it is strongly suggested that for several of these ototoxic agents the effect of interaction is synergistic, i.e. the agents potentiate the effect of each other so that the cumulative result is greater than the mere addition of one to the other. Henderson *et al.* (1974) explored the interrelationship of continuous and impulse noise in carefully controlled animal experiments, which showed that simultaneous exposure to 'safe' impulse noise superimposed upon a 'safe' level of continuous noise had a devastating effect on the cochlea. The practical implication of this for factory workers working in a steady-state background of noise-utilizing impact instruments such as pneumatic chisels or drop forges is clear. Further examples include the use of rock drills in mines against a steady-state background noise from high-level ventilation noise. Similar interactions between ototoxic antiobiotics and noise exposure seem to exist. The effects of kanamycin have been particularly well studied and dosages of kanamycin, which in guinea-pigs produce minimal damage to the cochlea, are potentiated by noise levels which in the same animal produce barely perceptible damage, so that when given together the effect is profound. Interestingly and perhaps fortunately, salicylates and noise do not appear to potentiate each other. Much of the extensive literature on these subjects is reviewed by Hamernik and Henderson (1976). The practical implications of this type of experiment are far-reaching. The patient receiving ototoxic antibiotics should perhaps be advised not to work in noise whilst receiving them, and conversely an injured worker will be more susceptible to the ototoxic effects of antibiotics if the drugs are given immediately after noise exposure, as may occur following an industrial or military accident. Noise levels in newborn nursery incubators should reflect the possibility that neonates may receive ototoxic drugs (*see below*).

The damage risk criteria which have been discussed in some detail above, may also not be entirely valid if the noise is a mixture of steady-state and impulse noise. This may account for the demonstrated differences in growth of PTS at 4 kHz over time found in different surveys (Hamernik and Henderson, 1976).

REST INTERVALS

The intermittency of noise exposure and the length of time between exposure seems to be of importance. It has already been shown that the amount of recovery from temporary threshold shift between noise exposures is of importance and it may well be that 16 h is not long enough for complete recovery to occur. Thus, workers exposed to only 4 h of noise with 20 h rest may fare better in the long term than others exposed to 8 h of an equal amount of sound energy but with only 16 h in which to recover. Short exposures occur in many cyclical manufacturing processes and in some jobs where the total work time is less than 8 h (for example some musicians).

THE ACOUSTIC REFLEX

The acoustic reflex is specifically a reflex contraction of the stapedius muscle in response to loud sound. Its dynamic characteristics have been admirably reviewed by Borg (1976), and will not be further discussed here, except where they relate to noise exposure. The muscle when contracted attenuates the passage of sound through the middle ear by up to 30 dB. The contracted muscle however fatigues readily, particularly in response to high-frequency stimulation. Nevertheless, recovery is rapid and if the stimulus is repetitive then the muscle is said to contract repetitively. It is suggested that the middle-ear muscle reflexes may protect the ear against some of the harmful effects of noise, although the evidence in favour of such a statement is very contradictory and confusing. It has been suggested that conditioning of the reflexes prior to the impact noise may have a protective action; unfortunately the middle-ear muscle reflexes seem remarkably resistant to attempts to condition them.

SEX

There is no evidence of a sexual preponderance in sensitivity to NIPTS.

PRESBYACUSIS

The interrelationship between presbyacusis and noise-induced threshold shifts is not fully understood, controversial and of considerable practical importance in compensation planning. At the present time it is not known whether the effect of age and noise are additive, or synergistic.

In retrospective studies of noise-induced deafness, it is customary to apply presbyacusis correction curves such as those of Hinchcliffe (1958), on the basis that hearing losses due to noise and age are additive (*Figure 18.10*).

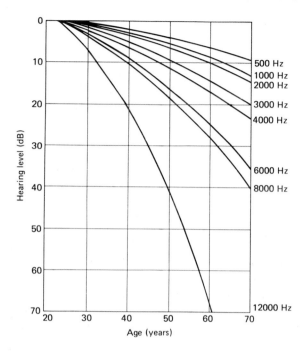

Figure 18.10 The relation between age and hearing level. The values apply equally to men and women up to age 54 years, and for frequencies up to 2000 Hz inclusive. At greater ages and higher frequencies the curves apply to women, but in the absence of noise-induced hearing loss it is probable that they would also apply to men. (From Hinchcliffe, 1958, reproduced by courtesy of the Editor of *Gerontologica*)

The current state of thought concerning presbyacusis is well reviewed by Corso (1976). He compares many studies of presbyacusis and discusses how it interrelates with NIPTS, suggesting that, as the latter usually reaches an asymptote in the late 50s or early 60s, all further hearing loss should be attributed to presbyacusis (unless other ear disease supervenes). He then debates the controversial question of what appropriate correction factor to apply in pension assessments. The orthodox view is to subtract from the total hearing loss the presbyacusis factor before evaluating a pension for hearing loss. In the writer's view this is only valid as long as the whole hearing loss is compensated—if a low fence is applied the technique is more debatable, for the hearing loss at age 60 from presbyacusis is less sensitive than the low fence; from presbyacusis alone the claimant would have no compensatable loss. In other words the low fence has already acted as a presbyacusis correction. The writer has seen many elderly claimants with severely handicapping hearing loss (> 45 dB average for 0.5, 1, 2 kHz), in whom a presbyacusis correction factor was applied of 0.5 dB/year for every year above 50, whose hearing loss was corrected below the compensatable level! Clearly, without noise exposure they would have had much less handicap. There is no one rule that can be applied to all formulae for compensating NIPTS—it should be evaluated separately with each compensation scheme.

ACOUSTIC TRAUMA

Acoustic trauma is irreversible. It may arise from short-term intense exposure or from one single exposure. Small arms, gunfire and major explosions, all associated with explosive pressure rises, may be responsible causing sudden aural damage (Burns *et al.*, 1968). Single loud sounds unassociated with explosion can cause perceptive deafness of this type. The piercing note of 'atmospheric' disturbances in a telephone receiver, or 'acoustic shocks' have been reported (Bunch, 1929; Fowler, 1939).

The effect of a single episode to acoustic trauma depends on its intensity and temporal characteristics. Many of the firework exposures recover, but certainly if the blast is intense enough a profound and permanent hearing loss may occur. The recovery takes place over many weeks and the clinician is cautioned not to make prognostic statements about the amount of recovery too early.

OTITIC BLAST INJURY

In this form of trauma, external-, middle-, and inner-ear structures can all be damaged. Blast is the sudden explosive force generated by bursing shells, detonating minefields, exploding bombs and mortars, and roaring guns. There is a qualitative similarity between a bomb explosion and a gun report (Rüedi and Furrer, 1947). However, the shock waves from an explosion are three times longer than those from the report of a 2-cm gun. Kerr and Byrne (1975) state that explosive material is changed suddenly from solid to gas resulting in a rapid positive pressure blast wave and a longer negative phase, the former lasting typically 5 ms and the latter 30 ms. Blast trauma to ears, they state, usually occurs only when the duration of the stimulation is greater than 1.5 ms and when this occurs middle-ear damage is relatively common. The important features are rise time, the absolute intensity of the peak pressure and the duration of the positive wave.

They give a graphic and remarkably well-documented account of the effect of a bomb blast in a restaurant in Belfast in which two people were killed, four lost both legs, and in which there were multiple ear injuries. Eighty people were subsequently identified, present in the restaurant at the time, who agreed to later examination. In general the closer the person to the bomb, the more likelihood of ear perforation, and in people with unilateral perforations the membrane perforated was usually the one facing the bomb. Most victims complained of severe temporary deafness which verged on the total for those most badly affected, which was usually short-lived. Virtually all complained of severe tinnitus following the blast. At least 60 tympanic membrane perforations were identified from this one explosion, which had protean characteristics. It used to be taught that traumatic perforations always had everted edges. However, in Kerr's series they were linear or cleanly punched or ragged, large or small and occasionally double, and the edges were both inverted and everted. These findings agree with stories related from the Vietnam war. Kerr advocates conservative management, with surgical repair reserved for those which did not clear spontaneously; 80 per cent healed spontaneously and the remaining ears were successfully closed by surgery. This once again points out the fallacy of the classic teaching that all traumatic perforations heal spontaneously—they do not. They also comment on the development of inclusion epidermoid cysts following this type of trauma, an experience which is also mirrored in S.E. Asia.

The inner-ear damage was also variable. Initially most had some degree of sensorineural loss which usually cleared quickly and completely. Many of the subjects who had a residual high frequency hearing loss were unaware of its presence. Kerr feels that tympanic membrane rupture did not protect the inner ear from sensorineural hearing loss but was impressed by the degree of recovery which occurred. The writer has similar experience with an unfortunately large number of miners exposed to accidental dynamite blasts underground who almost uniformly complain of an immediate profound hearing loss accompanied by tinnitus which usually but not always recovers. Several patients have now been seen in whom one ear became permanently deaf after a blast whilst the other recovered. It should be remembered that the deafness may be 'functional' (*see below*).

The Tullio phenomenon

This term is applied to vertigo induced by noise. As early as 1899 Deetjen discovered that the vibration from a Klein's whistle caused movement of perilymph in the semicircular canals. The classic experiments of Tullio culminated in his discovery (1929) that sound can stimulate the cristae direct. The literature on vestibular reactions provoked by intense noise was reviewed by Camis (1930). Tullio's original work was confirmed and extended by Huizinga in a long series of investigations (1934–1952). He found that in pigeons the Tullio phenomenon (vertigo provoked by intense sound stimulation) could be elicited after destruction of the cochlea, provided the conducting mechanism remained intact. Benjamins (1938) described a patient exhibiting the Tullio reflex, likewise stressing the fact that an intact middle-ear mechanism was necessary for its occurrence. Lindsay (1947) described two patients with labyrinthine fistulae who complained of unsteadiness in the presence of loud noises, and the occasional occurrence of the Tullio phenomenon was reported by Cawthorne (1949) when a two-stage operation for labyrinthine vertigo was performed. It was observed following construction of a lateral canal fistula provided the stapes was mobile and was abolished by subsequent avulsion of the membranous labyrinth.

Cases of dizziness on stimulation by the whistle of a train have been reported (Moulonguet and Poncet, 1947; Chadwick, 1966). The writer has recently seen a further case. It has been suggested that intense noise may cause sudden contraction of the intratympanic muscles causing massive jolting of the stapes which sets up violent motion in the perilymph which is transmitted to the semicircular canals provoking a sensation of sudden giddiness.

Patients with Menière's syndrome sometimes complain that they are afraid to go out because the roar of traffic makes them dizzy, or the noise from heavy lorries makes them feel unsteady. Although such statements are not uncommonly volunteered spontaneously by patients with Menière's disorder, the significance of such remarks is placed in proper perspective by Kacker and Hinchcliffe (1970) who remark that it is surprising that the occurrence of the Tullio phenomenon in this condition has not previously been reported. Under the heading 'Unusual Tullio Phenomena' they report three cases of the Tullio reaction occurring where only one mobile window opened into the inner ear on the vestibular side of the vestibular membrane and quote a case reported by Land (1957) in which a falling reaction could be induced in a patient by an acoustic stimulus when he lay on his side. The experiments of Bleeker and de Vries (1949) are noted, showing that a cristal microphonic, which parallels the frequency response curve for the Tullio phenomenon can be recorded from the cristae of the fenestrated semicircular canal in the pigeon.

The hypothesis suggested by Kacker and Hinchcliffe to explain the Tullio phenomenon sometimes observed in association with Menière's syndrome is that endolymphatic hydrops distends the saccule to such an extent that it lies in direct contact with the stapedial footplate without being cushioned by the perilymph, as has been described by Cody, Simonton and Hallberg (1967). There is thus direct continguity of the ossicular chain with the membranous labyrinth. Support for this hypothesis was given by the operative findings in a case of middle-ear trauma. The patient had noted a feeling of imbalance with loud sounds, particularly noticeable in a noisy bazaar and was found to have a subluxation of the stapes which had been driven into the vestibule, almost certainly in contact with the saccule.

Histological changes

Haberman followed up his original description in 1890 of degenerative changes in the organ of Corti in a blacksmith, by the publication of five further cases in 1906. In these, atrophy of the organ of Corti (*Figure 18.12*) and the nerves in the osseous spiral lamina of the lower basal coil were considered to be the result of noise damage. Since that time there have been many attempts to correlate hearing loss from noise with histological changes in the organ of Corti. In spite of considerable work, the picture remains disappointingly opaque. Bredberg and Hunter-Duvar (1975) provide a remarkably comprehensive survey of previous work. The reasons for the relative lack of information and conflicting reports are quite clear. There is considerable difficulty in obtaining and processing human temporal bones after noise exposure, uncontami-nated by other changes such as presbyacusis and post-mortem artifacts. Attempts to replicate industrial noise exposure damage in animals are complicated by the difficulty and considerable expense of conditioning them so that a behavioural hearing response may be obtained. There is considerable expense involved in training more than a few animals, and long-term experiments are difficult to perform. There is considerable interspecies variation in susceptibility to noise and the choice of experimental animals is therefore difficult; those which are cheap and readily conditioned do not necessarily react as human ears would to the same stimulus. In addition there is still considerable controversy about the normal functioning of the cochlea and without an adequate concept of its operation it is difficult to interpret the changes that are found.

In spite of these difficulties much work has been done. Recent technical advances allow examination not only by routine light microscopy, but also by phase contrast, transmission and scanning electron microscopic techniques. The latter in particular has produced dramatic illustrations of damage caused by noise. New methods of fixation of tissue allow material to be prepared both for phase contrast and electron-microscopic examination, so that the results of these techniques can be correlated in one experiment. It is important to realize that not only are hair-cells damaged by noise, but to a varying degree virtually all other cochlear structures have been implicated, including pillar cells, supporting cells, blood vessels, the stria vascularis, and nerve fibres related to the hair-cells. Damage to the organ of Corti by noise is a mixture of biochemical change and mechanical disruption, the proportions varying according to the intensity of the noise.

Békésy (1953) described some of the mechanical properties of the organ of Corti, and Tonndorf (1960) a shearing motion in the scala media. Beagley (1965b) has

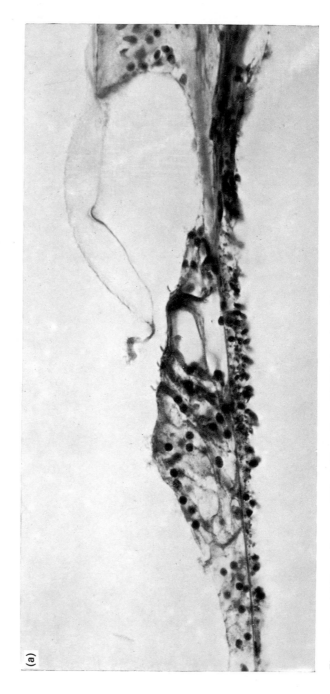

Figure 18.11 (a) Normal organ of Corti (From Igarashi, Schuknecht and Myers, 1964, reproduced by courtesy of the Editor of *Journal of Laryngology and Otology*)

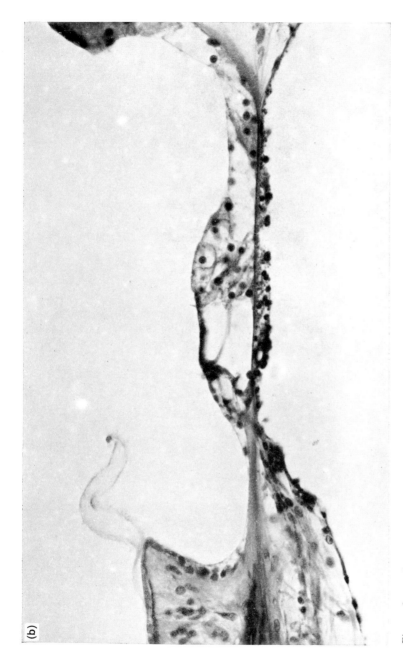

Figure 18.11 (b) Pathological organ of Corti. The outer hair-cells of the first and second rows are missing. (From Igarashi, Schuknecht and Myers, 1964, reproduced by courtesy of the Editor of *Journal of Laryngology and Otology*)

correlated these hydrodynamic observations with the type of damage found in different cellular structures following noise exposure. When a travelling wave passes along it, a radially-directed shear stress develops in the cochlear partition. The basilar membrane is fixed along each side of the spiral lamina and the spiral ligament, while the middle is not supported. This part is mobilized by the travelling wave with its maximal excursion somewhere near the middle. As the inner pillar cell is closely related to the fixed spiral lamina, with the outer pillar cell based on the more central part of the basilar membrane, the place of greatest movement, the whole triangle composed of both pillar cells and the structures attached to them will undergo a radially directed rocking movement, with the fulcrum near the base of the inner pillar cell. Beagley considers this may well explain why the supporting cells around the inner hair-cells are so often damaged and it is probably the reason why the outer hair-cells in the first row whose heads are attached to the phalangeal processes of both inner and outer pillar cells, are the ones most often injured.

Localized degeneration in the basal coil following noise exposure in a case documented with an audiogram showing a characteristic hearing loss most marked at 4 kHz was described by Igarashi, Schuknecht and Myers (1964). An area of partially degenerated hair-cells 5–12 mm wide was seen, the maximum injury taking place at a distance of 10–12 mm from the proximal end of the cochlea (*Figure 18.11*).

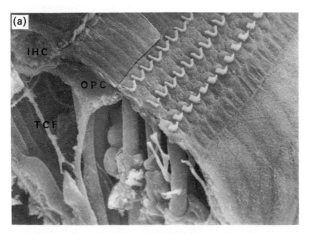

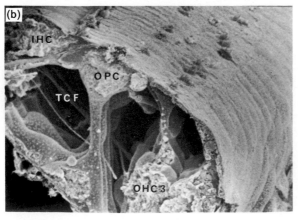

Figure 18.12 Chinchilla—scanning micrographs demonstrate (a) a normal and (b) an acoustically damaged organ of Corti from right and left ears of an animal ten weeks after exposure to a 120-dB tone. The right ear was protected from the exposure. Only a few deteriorated outer hair-cells (OHC3) remain in the damaged area of the left ear. IHC = inner hair-cell, OPC = outer pillar cell, TCF = tunnel crossing fibre. (Courtesy Dr. I. Hunter-Duvar, Hospital for Sick Children, University of Toronto.) Previously published in *Fundamentals of Hearing*, Ed. by Yost and Neilsen, 1977, New York; Holt, Reinhart & Winston. (Reproduced by permission of the publishers)

The spiral ganglion cells and the nerves in the osseous spiral lamina in corresponding regions appeared undamaged.

Progressively more severe damage with increases in the stimulating SPL were found in the cochlea by Miller, Watson and Cavell (1963). With low intensities there occurred swelling of vacuoles in Deiter's supporting cells and the internal phalangeal cells. Increased stimulation progressively affected the inner hair-cells, tunnel rods and external hair-cells, leading to collapse of the tunnel of Corti. Reisner's membrane sometimes ruptured. Finally, Deiter's cells and the external hair-cells were lifted from the basilar membrane and there was almost complete destruction and loss of the organ of Corti. Subsequent degeneration of spiral ganglion cells and peripheral nerve fibres appeared. It was observed by Bredberg (1968) that sensory cells could degenerate within an exceedingly short period of time following damage, probably less than 24 h. Complete disappearance of nerve fibres takes considerably longer.

Hunter-Duvar (1978) exposed conditioned chinchillas to 1 kHz pure-tone stimuli sufficient to result in temporary or permanent hearing losses ranging from 12 min at 120 dB to 3 h at 90 dB. Temporal bones were removed at post-exposure times ranging from immediately to nine months (*Figure 18.12*). He emphasized that animals, like humans, show a considerable range of susceptibility to acoustic trauma, some having tough ears and some having tender ears. He described permanent damage after 12–15 min exposure at 120 dB; within 1 h of exposure the cilia of inner hair-cells were in a state of disarray, the headplates of the inner hair-cells were sometimes ruptured, and the cilia of the first and second rows of outer hair-cells were agglutinated and in some cases were already undergoing autolysis (*Figure 18.13*). The reticular lamina of the phalangeal processes of the Deiter's cells bubbled up and collapsed, but no perforation was seen from the scala media into the tunnel of Corti. The hair-cell bodies and their supporting structures were so severely damaged that they were unrecognizable. After 24 h those inner hair-cells which had not fused had returned to an upright position, but the articular plates of the outer hair-cells had been ejected onto the surface of the organ of Corti (*Figure 18.14*). After these acute changes a certain degree of reorganization and repair takes place, so that between ten weeks and nine months after exposure in the missing areas of the organ of Corti the supporting cells had closed off completely the ends of the tunnel of Corti and the tunnel-crossing nerve fibres remained, even in the absence of outer hair-cells. Of considerable interest is the temporary damage which was noted in lesser degrees of exposure such as 90-dB stimuli, where patches of cilia on the outer hair-cells collapsed or bent over in the expected lesion area (*Figure 18.15*). Examination of animals with a similar noise exposure several weeks later showed predominantly normal cilia, and thus the inference may be drawn that intense noise exposure produces a temporary collapse of the cilia, which may recover. There were always a few missing cilia, so some clearly failed to return to their pre-exposure state. It took from 3–6 days for recovery of the cilia to occur. Hunter-Duvar comments on the rapidity of deterioration of the stereo-cilia on the first row of outer hair-cells which 'appear to agglutinate and then to be consumed during stimulation, leaving the cuticular plate and the tectorial membrane intact'.

Spoendlin (1976) reviewed an extensive series of personal experiments in which he attempted to correlate the anatomical changes produced by intense sound stimulation in the ears of guinea-pigs and cats. He has developed an ingenious technique which allows simultaneous interference contrast microscopy and electron microscopy and

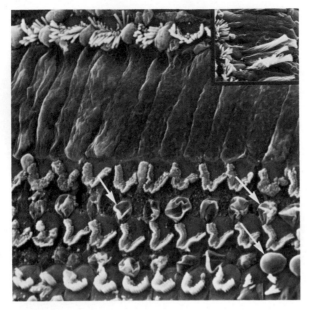

Figure 18.13 Chinchilla—scanning micrograph of a lesion area immediately after acoustic over-stimulation. Cilia on outer hair-cells are fused and undergoing autolysis. Phalangeal processes of Deiter's cells are seen to balloon and then collapse (arrows). Cilia of inner hair-cells are in disarray. Inset demonstrates how the heads of some pillar cells may burst and extrude fibres. (Courtesy Dr. I. Hunter-Duvar, Hospital for Sick Children, University of Toronto.) (From Hunter-Duvar, 1978, reproduced by courtesy of the Editor and publishers of *Acta Otolaryngologica* Suppl. 351)

which gives an accurate identification of the section of the cochlea which is being studied. His experiments were extensive and involved no less than 240 guinea-pigs and five cats, which had been exposed to different types of wide and narrow band stimuli for periods of 30 s to one week, and which were sacrificed for examination at time intervals ranging from immediately after the cessation of exposure to one year after its end. He described immediate damage including mechnical disruption of the organ of Corti with complete disintegration and multiple ruptures of the reticular lamina associated with disconnection from the basilar membrane. Weak points seem to exist particularly along the lateral attachment of the reticular membrane of the Hensen's cells as previously described by Beagley (1965), at the pillar heads and medial to the inner hair-cell cuticle. Frequently the whole organ of Corti was swept away from the basilar membrane and at exposure intensities of above 140 dB ruptures of Reissner's membrane occurred. Irrespective of the stimulation intensity he never found significant structural changes in the stria vascularis unless Reissner's membrane

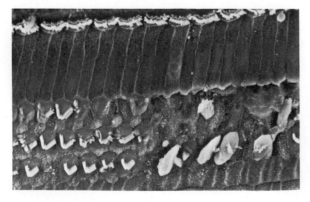

Figure 18.14 Chinchilla — lesion area 24 h after acoustic overstimulation showing cuticular plates of third row outer hair-cells which have been ejected onto the surface of the organ of Corti. Note the erect position of cilia of inner hair-cells in the lesion area. (Courtesy Dr. I. Hunter-Duvar, Hospital for Sick Children, University of Toronto.) (From Hunter-Duvar, 1977, *Morphology of the normal and the acoustically damaged cochlea. Scanning Electron Microscopy.* Vol.II/IITRI. Reproduced by courtesy of the Editor)

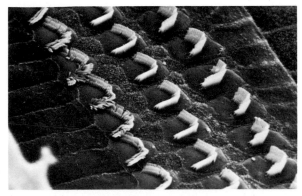

Figure 18.15 Chinchilla — cilia of the first row of outer hair-cells are shown to be bent over in the 1-kHz area when examined immediately after exposure to a 1-kHz tone at an intensity of 90 dB for 3 h. (Picture by courtesy of Dr. I. Hunter-Duvar, Hospital for Sick Children, University of Toronto)

was ruptured. This had been suggested by Duvall *et al.* (1974) that one of the mechanisms of damage in acoustic trauma was strial damage with disruption of the vessel transport mechanism; this however remains to be confirmed. Nevertheless their arguments are convincing and perhaps the discrepancy exists because of a difference in experimental animals, or because of differences in timing of the examination. Spoendlin also described different changes which occur after long exposure to sounds of below 120 dB SPL. Here he found signs of cellular damage with swollen outer hair-cell nuclei, particularly in the first row, followed after a delay by a degeneration of the individual hair-cells amongst normal neighbours scattered over quite large areas. He stressed that the primary changes were always confined to the sensory cells with nerve fibres remaining initially intact. A complicating factor is that scattered degeneration of this nature is found to a lesser degree as a spontaneous happening in normal animals.

Spoendlin emphasized the presence of two mechanisms, direct mechanical damage as a result of acoustic overstimulation with high intensity stimuli, and metabolic stress or exhaustion following lower intensity stimuli. He commented further that bending and fusion of sensory hairs is not necessarily a mechanical problem because it is also found after drug intoxication. In his experiments even slight distortion of the outer hair-cells did not necessarily recover completely, for distorted outer hair-cells were found as long as three months after cessation of noise exposure. He described the distortion of the inner hair-cells as being permanent without any recovery, for they were found as long as one year after noise exposure. However, the swollen afferent dendrites and the changes in the cell nuclei all recovered within a week. Spoendlin also commented upon the retrograde degeneration of cochlear neurones which he believed to be a secondary phenomenon induced by loss of inner hair-cells. Retrograde degeneration is important but never total, even if the whole organ of Corti disappears. He found at least 10 per cent of the neurone population in an apparently healthy state. He believed that loss of outer hair-cells had little effect on afferent cochlear neurone degeneration.

Spoendlin reviewed the tonotopic localization of damage in his animals and described well-defined localization found after even 30 s of exposure, which he believed demonstrated that the determining factors for localization were the mechanical properties of the cochlea, the most likely of which was the maximum volume displacement in the particular region. He found that narrow band exposures of the centre frequencies from 250–8000 Hz gave accurate tonotopical localization, but that the greatest damage was produced with bands in the lower and mid-frequency range. He also commented on intra- and interspecies variability in susceptibility to noise. The damage due to impulse noise showed greater variation, but the most significant feature was the length of rise time of impulse—the shorter the rise time, the less the damage.

Bohne (1976) has made extensive studies of the mechanism of noise damage in the inner ear and bases many of her findings on the wealth of data accumulated at the US Central Institute of the Deaf over a quarter of a century. Utilizing guinea-pigs and chinchillas she categorizes the damage according to three groups of exposure—very intense, intense and moderate. She reviews hypothesized mechanisms of injury under the headings of metabolic exhaustion, vascular change and ionic change. Cytoplasmic changes due to metabolic exhaustion have already been described. The theory of vascular changes has been raised on several occasions. The strial changes have already been discussed. Other suggested changes include diminution or the lack of red blood cells in the vessels below the basilar membrane in noise-exposed ears. However, there are significant species variations in the existence of this vessel and the findings are not consistent. Bohne makes a persuasive argument to support the hypothesis that ionic changes are responsible for some of the damage in occupational hearing loss. She suggests that noise exposure may interrupt the continuity of the reticular lamina, thus allowing endolymph and perilymph to intermingle so that cell membranes not normally exposed to high levels of potassium may be damaged by it. She suggests that in areas surrounding maximally damaged portions of the organ of Corti scattered outer pillar cells were damaged, and that they had grossly swollen or ruptured outer hair-cells adjacent to them. It is hypothesized that endolymph enters the fluid spaces of the organ of Corti through the resulting holes in the reticular lamina, thus coming into contact with the hair-cells and damaging them. Similar damage has been produced experimentally by Duvall, Sutherland and Rhodes (1969), by mechanically damaging the endolymphatic surface of the organ of Corti and allowing fluid to intermingle.

Lim (1976) noted occasional holes in the reticular lamina but did not find the cell changes described by Bohne, nor did he find the holes as regularly as required for this theory to be a major factor. Hunter-Duvar (1978) was unable to confirm the presence of the holes using the scanning electron microscope. Clearly, further work is required.

One of the major problems in attempting to correlate the effect of noise on the ultrastructure of the ear with the behavioural changes that occur is the considerable confusion that exists concerning the role of the afferent nerves. Contrary to previous belief it is now assumed that up to 95 per cent of the afferent nerve fibres in the cat connect with the inner hair-cells (Spoendlin, 1972), and in the guinea-pig between 80 and 85 per cent of the afferent fibres originate on the inner hair-cell (Morrison, Schindler and Wersall, 1975). The inner hair-cells are amongst the most resistant structures of the cochlea to change from noise, and yet hearing loss unquestionably occurs. The innervation patterns of the organ of Corti have recently been reviewed by Bredberg (1977) using the scanning electron microscope. Until a better relationship is hypothesized between structure and function in the normal, the pathological changes produced by noise will clearly not be elucidated.

Bredberg (1967) illustrates his results by plotting cochleograms (Engström, Ades and Andersson, 1966) which number the damaged hair-cell populations in the first, second, third and fourth rows and indicate their exact position in the cochlea. These are shown side by side with cochleas for a variety of workers in noise, shipyard employees, workshop mechanics, diesel engineers, etc. (*Figure 18.16*).

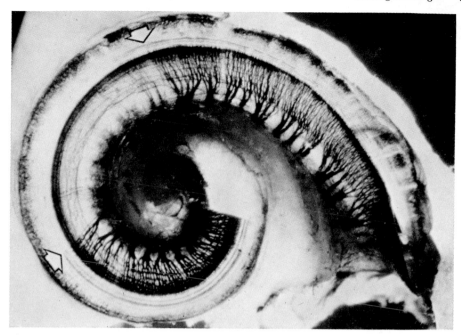

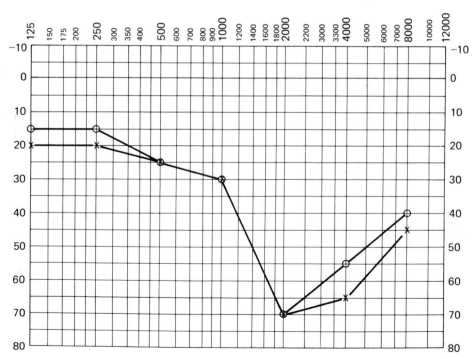

Figure 18.16 Cochlea and audiogram from a man aged 71 exposed to high intensity noise in a sawmill for several years. Note the dip in the audiogram from 2–4 kHz. The cochlea shows a complete degeneration of the nerves in the osseous spiral lamina as well as a corresponding degeneration of the organ of Corti 10.5–14.5 mm from the basal end (between arrows) (× 13). (From Bredberg, 1967, reproduced by courtesy of the Editor of *Journal of Laryngology and Otology* and Dr. Göran Bredberg)

How do these findings apply to humans? Johnsson and Hawkins (1976) have described some degenerative patterns in human ears exposed to noise. They found that the commonest anatomical correlative of 4-kHz dip was a relatively diffuse degeneration of the second quadrant of the basal turn, which if advanced showed a wide gap of more or less complete sensorineural degeneration affecting the second quadrant and displaying various degrees of extension towards the apex and base. The pattern they found associated with an abrupt high-tone loss showed more or less complete hair-cell and nerve degeneration in both the first and second quadrants; this was however rare. They felt they were able to differentiate the degenerative pattern from the diffuse losses found in presbyacusis and suggested that patterns with knife-sharp transitions between normal and damaged cochleas were characteristic of noise-induced losses. They emphasized the difficulty in making the correlations, and indeed of working with human material. They did not find any increase in strial damage. Other human correlations were reviewed by Bredberg and Hunter-Duvar (1975), who described much greater outer hair-cell loss than inner hair-cell loss. However, they also commented that there was no simple relationship between noise exposure and/or changes in threshold with the loss of sensory cells.

The current state of knowledge thus tells us something about the morphological changes due to noise exposure in chinchillas, guinea-pigs, and to a lesser extent cats. Because of significant species differences, primate material is urgently required, and is gradually being accumulated (Hawkins, Johnsson and Stebbins, 1976). A relative lack of hard data after so much intense work reflects the difficulty in working in such a small and inaccessible organ.

Biochemical changes

The biochemical mechanisms underlying the mechanism of hearing are ill understood, and their changes with pathological processes including intense noise exposure are unclear. The tissues are extremely difficult to isolate and analyse. The observer marvels at the audacity of the investigator in undertaking biochemical investigation in the ear, and applauds any degree of success because of the technical mastery that is involved, without really expecting to receive knowledge of the subtle changes produced by minor variations in stimuli to the ear. In spite of these strictures a certain amount of work has been done on the biochemical changes associated with noise exposure.

Loud sound produces changes in the basic energy-producing system by which the terminal pathways of metabolism are maintained. Oxygen acts as a limiting factor in preserving a metabolic balance within the ear. Sound stimulation results in a decrease in oxygen tension in the cochlea and an increase in the glucose content of the perilymph (Koide *et al.*, 1960).

Dreschner (1976) gives a general review of biochemical mechanisms in the ear, which includes an up-to-date review of membrane chemistry and oxidative energy exchanges as they apply to the ear. He attributes to Konishi, Butler and Fernandez, (1961) the discovery that cochlear potentials decrease with anoxia, and suggests that loud sounds may limit oxygen availability by decreasing cochlear blood flow. The effect of sound on blood flow has been described above and there is no uniform opinion about this. It is suggested that during loud noise glycogen is broken down to provide energy and that it is synthesized in periods of quiet. Unfortunately glycogen granules are not present in the ears of all species.

Schneider (1974) exposed 190 guinea-pigs to various amounts of white noise and then measured the concentration of lactate in the perilymph, which he found increased significantly after noise exposure whilst blood levels remained constant. He believes this supports the hypothesis that exposure to sound reduces cochlear blood flow, and thus the oxygen supplies to sensory cells which may cause metabolic breakdown and degeneration of sensory cells.

A most ingenious quantitive biochemical technique has been applied to the study of ears including normals and those damaged by noise, which is well described by Thalmann (1976). Much work has been done to demonstrate that the metabolic processes, aerobic and anaerobic, that exist elsewhere in the body also occur in the ear. This is an essential prelude to the investigation of pathological changes. He studied changes in guinea-pigs using their other ear as a control for the unilateral noise exposure and found no significant changes in the *in vitro* activity of lactic dehydrogenase or of glucose-6-phosphate dehydrogenase. ATP in the outer layer of the outer hair-cells was not significantly different in level from normal, and exposed ears for the steady-state levels of ATP, glutinate and aspartate overlap experimental and control ears. The work continues.

Changes in electrical potentials

Electrical potentials are produced by the cochlea and eighth nerve in response to sound. Intensive study of these phenomena, initially of the cochlear microphonics and more recently of action potentials of individual fibres of the eighth nerve, have been undertaken in an attempt to establish the mechanism of neural encoding and message transmission for the transducer in the cochlea to the brain. Attempts have also been made to establish electrical correlates of changes found after exposure to high levels of sound. These include older and more recent experiments.

Marked variation in the loss of sensitivity of the cochlear microphonic was found by Eldredge and Covell (1958) with moderate exposures of 500 Hz at 128 dB SPL for 20 min from the third turn of the cochlea in the guinea-pig, the area most affected by this frequency. The cochlear microphonic represents very closely the electrical equivalent of sound energy up to a given intensity (Davis *et al.*, 1958); thereafter it follows a decrease due to fatigue. For guinea-pigs the transitional limit at 500 Hz–2 kHz was 95 dB human threshold; for cats 75–90 dB at 250 Hz–3 kHz, and 100 dB at 5 kHz, corresponding well with the fatigue limits of the human ear (Kärjä, 1968).

That the recovery of sensitivity after giving the same exposure to guinea-pigs as Eldredge and Covell used is greater than the capacity to generate cochlear microphonic voltages was demonstrated by Beagley (1965a). He noted that the travelling wave resulting from a 500-Hz tone begins at the stapes, has its maximal amplitude in the third turn of the cochlea and falls away abruptly beyond. An inverse relationship exists between the cochlear microphonic threshold shift and the extent of separation of the Hensen's cells and Deiter's cells which tends to protect the inner ear.

More recent work has been summarized by Durant (1976). The cochlear microphonic is reduced by intense stimulation of the cochlea and this seems to be directly related to the sound pressure level and the common logarithm of the duration exposure. However, the relationship has not been clearly demonstrated over a wide range of exposure conditions. There appears to be a linear relationship between the change in cochlear microphonic and the intensity and duration of exposure when plotted in log coordinates; however when sound level input is increased significantly above that at which the maximum cochlear microphonic output is observed, a dramatic increase in loss of CM sensitivity is produced which deviates from the straight line relationship established at lower levels. Thus no simple function relating loss of CM sensitivity to intensity of the exposure exists which holds good for all intensities, and in all probability for all durations. Attempts have been made to establish DRC based on cochlear microphonic to determine what parameters lead to permanent versus temporary depression of the microphonics. No generally acceptable relationships have yet been established, although the point at which increasing stimulus intensity fails to produce an increase in the microphonic may represent the level of sound that can overload the cochlea. Studies to determine the rate of recovery of microphonic sensitivity suggest that this takes place in an exponential manner with a rapid partial recovery and more gradual later changes.

The endocochlear potential appears to be potentiated following exposure to intense sound unless Reissner's membrane is ruptured, when it is suggested it may become depressed. In truth the endocochlear potentials have been little studied following exposure to noise. No consistent picture is available of the changes in whole nerve action potential following exposure to noise.

Evans *et al.* have undertaken an elegant series of experiments along similar lines. The relevant material related to noise exposure was well summarized at a Benchmark Conference on the Effect of Noise on Hearing held in 1976 in Syracuse (Evans, 1976). In normal hearing, frequency selectivity has already been determined in large part at least, at the level of the cochlear nerve as the result of a postulated two-stage frequency filtering process in the cochlea. They are particularly interested in the second stage which seems extremely vulnerable to a wide range of potentially harmful agents including noise. They suggest that the first filter is the mechanical tuning curve of the basilar membrane itself, whilst the second filter is a cochlear neural tuning. The arguments in its favour are persuasive although circumstantial, for its method of action and its situation remain obscure. They have found the second filter, i.e. the tuning curves of individual cochlear neurones from which electrical measurements have been made, to be reduced in sharpness as a result of a wide range of noxious agents, including chronic administration of ototoxic antibiotics, hypoxia, a number of chemical poisons, alpha-adrenergic receptor blocking agents, and local damage to the cochlear partition. The cochlear action potential threshold is simultaneously raised but the cochlear microphonic does not necessarily follow. The fibres lose their sensitivity for their low threshold sharply-tuned segment leaving behind a high threshold, more broadly-tuned, segment. Evans speculates on the relationship between the loss of nerve tuning and the susceptibility to damage of the outer hair-cells by the same agents which disturb the second filter characteristics of the eighth nerve potential. The relative paucity of nerve fibres originating from outer hair-cells is a real problem, for most of the nerve recordings must come from fibres originating from inner hair-cells. This raises the speculation of an interaction between outer and inner hair-cells or between their innervations, although the anatomical basis of such an interaction remains unexplained. Evans suggests that the breakdown of the second filter may be the common denominator by which a wide range of different toxic agents interact to produce their effect in the ear; agents such as metabolic disorders, drugs, mechanical disturbances from noise, presbyacusis, disease, etc. He also believes it may account for the synergistic effects of noise and antibiotics.

The pioneering and continuing work of Kiang on the electrical changes in single cochlear nerve fibres has been extremely productive. Kiang, Liberman and Levine (1976) found that the response characteristics of auditory nerve fibres in cats exposed to intense sound were characterized by an elevation of the tuning curve tips occasionally associated with a hypersensitivity of their tails, i.e. sensitivity is reduced with a relative decrease in frequency specificity. They found that significant shifts of unit threshold could exist without significant loss of hair-cells, but conversely significant hair-cell loss was always accompanied by highly abnormal unit thresholds.

Specific non-industrial noise hazards

Small arms

Although Neely (1959) considered that the tympanic membrane could rupture at 160 dB, much higher sound pressure levels have been measured from firearms and gunfire. Their duration, however, is often extremely short.

Coles (1963) found an intensity of 174 dB at the firer's head with an automatic gun; Glorig and Wheeler (1955) that noise from firearms might attain 180 dB; Yarington (1968) recorded impulse noise attaining 190 dB from 105 mm howitzers; and Salmivalli (1967) 188 dB from field cannons and 185.6 dB from antitank guns.

The maximum permissible level which the ear can tolerate without sustaining permanent damage is dependent on the exposure time. Pfander (1965) considers 165 dB permissible for 0.003 s/day, but for 0.3 s only 145 dB can be tolerated.

Permanent damage may be caused on initial exposure. Stewart and Barrow (1946) found that over 20 per cent of gunners sustained acoustic trauma with their first round of firing.

Impulse noise, such as gunfire, produces TTS. Ward (1963) found that it grew linearly with exposure time, provided the interval between two impulses was sufficiently long. When due to continuous noise, the response was logarithmic. Murray and Reid (1946) found that sudden deafness after short exposure to gunfire, even if causing a 60 dB loss, usually recovered in 48 h, although it might take 60 h, and occasionally 20 days.

An asymmetrical hearing loss is characteristic of rifle and shotgun fire with differences of up to 20 dB noted between the two ears. This is due to the 'head shadow effect', the head diffracting sound waves when the sound source is to one side. The ear closer to the muzzle is deafened, the other one protected. In pistol firing, or carbine firing from the hip, where both ears are equally exposed, they are also equally affected.

Acoustic trauma has become much more prevalent in the modern army as weapons have become noisier. The standard use of semi-automatic carbines has made the old Lee Enfield seem by comparison an almost silent rifle. The addition of high background noise from armoured personnel carriers and troop transporting helicopters have given rise to noise levels which would not be tolerated in civilian life. Transportation to the battlefield in a helicopter transport, rapid skirmishes with the use of carbines, covering fire from 'Puff the Magic Dragon'—the helicopter gunship with its Gatlinberg machine guns firing 2000 rounds/min, all combine to make deafness from noise one of the more distressing long-term sequelae of the recent war in South Vietnam.

The notably severe hazards of 12-bore shotguns have been emphasized by Knight and Coles (1960). They produce peak SPLs of 155 dB at the firer's forward ear and together with 0.38 calibre pistols, peak SPL 157 dB, were considered capable of causing significant hearing loss bordering on auditory handicap, in about 10 per cent of individuals (Coles and Rice, 1966).

The writer attempted to obtain normal hearing subjects for a psychoacoustic experiment from a freshman medical student class of 80, in the southern USA, and found only 20 with hearing better than 30 dB at 4 kHz. None of the students were aged above 26. Those who had not been in the armed forces were ardent sports shooters.

Sociacusis

The increased diversity of modern leisure-time pursuits makes it necessary to distinguish not only occupational hearing loss incurred in employment, but also recreational hearing loss acquired in the enjoyment of noisy pastimes, and noise exposure experienced in modern communities as part of everyday life.

Individuals who work under comparatively quiet conditions during the day may spend their free time indulging in a variety of noisy spare-time activities, or live close to noisy highways.

The staid bank manager may be an enthusiastic shot on the grouse moor, and the anaemic salesman a tearaway in highpowered motorcycle scrambles. Sports cars can be particularly offensive noise weapons, SPLs inside vehicles and traffic noise in towns having been recorded as high as 115 dB (Lehnhardt, 1965). Hearing loss from the cumulative effect of social noise exposure has been termed sociacusis, and in evaluating the cause of hearing loss it should be taken into account, along with industrial and military exposure to noise, and presbyacusis.

Recreational noise exposure

Hazardous sound levels are an accompaniment of many enjoyable playthings of young and old alike; fire-crackers, model aeroplanes, engines, motorcycles, snowmobiles, racing cars, sport cars, all share high levels of noise, and indeed the noise may be half the fun. What entertainment would a silent fire-cracker be? Who would watch Grand Prix motor car racing if the motors were silenced? Who would go to a quiet disco? However, the otologist should be aware of the potentially hazardous nature of some of these pursuits.

(A) FIREWORKS

Chinese crackers are frightening from afar and deafening close at hand. Gjaevens, Moseng and Nordahl, (1975) examined the hearing of 791 Norwegian schoolchildren aged 12–14 before and after the Constitutional Day holiday, at which time fire-crackers are exploded with abandon. Follow-up examination showed that 0.7 per cent of the boys had a considerable permanent hearing loss. They make the point that the audiometric dips were very narrow and might have been missed in conventional screening audiometry. This is one of the reasons why fireworks are outlawed in North America, where other reports testify to their harmful aural effects (Glorig and Ward, 1961; Sataloff, 1952; Chadwick, 1966).

(B) MODEL AEROPLANES

Model aeroplane engines came under the scrutiny of Bess and Powell (1972), who undertook an acoustic analysis of the engine noise and found that the dBA levels exceeded DRC for a short exposure. They went on to examine model aeroplane operators and found that three subjects had considerable temporary threshold shift following a brief exposure to the noise. They strongly urge the wearing of earplugs during this type of recreation.

(C) SNOWMOBILES

A particularly noxious device has invaded the North American countryside in the winter—the snowmobile. These are single track vehicles powered by small and usually inadequately silenced motorcycle engines. A representative off-the-shelf machine was reported by Bess and Poyner (1974) as having a sound level at the driver's head of 86 dBA when idling, and 113 dBA at full throttle. The greatest energy was found within the speech frequency range. The sound levels exceeded DRC for a 2-h exposure. Careful analysis of sound levels during a ride showed that on one stock snowmobile the sound pressure level was 108 dB average with peaks in excess of 120 dB SPL. These matters are compounded in racing snowmobiles, which had idling SPLs of 112 dB and two-thirds throttle SPLs at the driver's head of 135 dB! At the place where most spectators were clustered around a racetrack, 6 m from the machines, the intensity levels averaged 106 dBA. Not surprisingly the mean hearing threshold of racing snowmobile drivers included quite a significant 6-kHz dip, and they once again demonstrated hearing levels in teenagers reduced to half for their age, which they attributed to wholehearted enthusiasm for this new sport.

TTS of varying degree was detected in 87 per cent of snowmobile operators after half an hour of use and typical machines were said to exceed federal safe levels for more than two and a half hours of riding (Chayney, McClain and Housen, 1973).

The Eskimo of northern Canada has adopted and replaced dog teams with snowmobiles. A study by Baxter and Ling (1974) found that up to 85 per cent of the adult male population had a sensorineural hearing loss which they attributed to repeated 12-h snowmobile safaris at full throttle on unsilenced machines, accompanied by firing of high powered rifles from the shoulder. Whilst manufacturers are steadily quietening snowmobiles, many still exceed reasonable noise levels.

(D) SPORTS

Motorcycle riding, drag racing, sport shooting and boxing amongst students came under scrutiny by Fletcher and Gross (1977). They used high-frequency audiometry to screen out hearing loss from those exposed to these sports when compared with a matched control group. Motorcycling produced most damage and sports shooting least. The latter surprising finding was attributed to the fairly routine use of ear defenders amongst sport shooters in the USA. They comment that there is no point in examining the hearing of boxers immediately after a bout because of the masking effect of the post-traumatic tinnitus which most of them experience but if tested some time later the boxer too showed some degree of high frequency hearing loss which was greatest in those who had been most traumatized.

Community noise exposure

The levels of noise experienced in the community are orders of magnitude less than those in industry, but they affect many more people. Full discussion of community noise levels, their effect, their measurement and their control, is beyond the scope of this chapter, although certain areas will be highlighted.

The problem of noise in our cities is not new. In the days of horse-drawn carriages with steel shoes and iron wheels on granite cobblestones the sound was deafening. Individuals sprinkled straw to deaden the noise in cases of illness, and communities replaced the granite with wooden blocks, only to have them removed as they became skid-traps for rubber shod automobiles.

A paper by Shaw and Thiessen, (1975) gives a balanced review of current problems and their solutions. They point out that there is a linear relationship between increasing power of machinery and the sound which it produces; thus a food blender produces the same amount of sound for its power as does a tractor-trailer or a quietened aeroplane. For example current mechanical power ranges from 200 W for a typical dishwasher to 5000 kW for a typical wide-bodied aeroplane—a factor of more than 10^5, but the acoustic power ranges from 30 μW for the dishwasher to 30 000 W for the larger aircraft—a factor of 10^9. Implicit in this suggestion is the belief that for a given power output sound can be reduced and the manufacturers of dishwashers have done a better job than the manufacturers of some aeroplanes. Shaw points out that the fraction of mechanical power which is lost as acoustic energy is extremely low even in the noisiest machinery, where it rarely exceeds 1000 parts/million.

The psychology of noise is important. Would the average housewife believe that a quiet vacuum cleaner worked as efficiently as her current noisy one? Not only have machines become more powerful and noisier, there are more machines in existence. The number of automobiles in the USA more than doubled in the 20-year period 1950–1970, as did the number of large trucks and lorries. Commercial jet aeroplanes increased from 200 in 1960 to 2000 in 1970. These are but examples of a widespread phenomenon; the spread of recreational vehicles, labour-saving devices, air conditioners, etc. has produced a quantum increase in the number of sound-producing sources in society at large. Sound levels in North America have increased greatly, particularly in the cities. Median daytime noise levels in the USA range from 20 dBA at the north rim of the Grand Canyon to 80 dBA outside the window of apartments near a freeway. The most ubiquitous source of high median noise levels is the motor vehicle. Shaw stresses that human welfare is dependent upon the ability to speak easily, and that for this to occur without tension a background level of no greater than 55 dB is required. Relaxed conversation at 3 m requires a background level of 45 dB or less, something which is rarely found. It is the writer's belief that air conditioning of buildings in North America with sealed windows, is as much an effort to sound-proof interiors from street noise as it is to provide a well-tempered climate. But even here the background noise of most air-conditioning systems in larger buildings is sufficiently high to require voices to be elevated and tensions raised.

There are excellent measures of noise nuisance value to which references are made. Shaw discusses at length the art of the possible—that which can be done with the existing technology without bankrupting a community. Heavy vehicles represent only 10 per cent of the traffic stream but produce almost 70 per cent of the sound. Thus, efforts aimed at heavy vehicle noise control, such as the quiet truck programmes of the USA and the EEC standards for vehicles which are being introduced will have this effect. Research has shown that tyre noise is of paramount importance, and different tread patterns are being developed. Urban transportation systems are taking care to control the noise—buses are becoming quieter again as communities react to the tyranny of a relatively unsilenced supercharged diesel motor in buses, and urban railways, both elevated and underground, are subjected to a wide variety of sound reduction techniques. The reduction in aircraft noise gives dramatic proof of what can be done, with the new generation of wide-bodied aircraft generating absolute amounts of noise below that of the less powerful 707s and DC8s. Perhaps the most important feature in implementing noise control is public awareness that noise is harmful and can be controlled. The books *Noise and Man* by Burns *et al.* (1973) and *Effects of Noise on Man* by Kryter (1970) provide adequate background reading, to which can be added innumerable government publications in all western countries. These are reviewed in pamphlet form on a two weekly basis by the *Noise Regulation Reporter*, published in the USA.

TRANSPORTATION NOISE

The noise levels in aircraft, buses, and subways are harsh. Many commuters spend considerable periods daily on subways where the sound levels are very close to 90dBA or even higher, particularly if the track is bad or on curves. Some representative levels are shown in *Table 18.1*. Modern engineering techniques are hardpressed to reduce the levels in the carriages and this may add substantially to the total daily noise exposure, for example 2 h of travelling with average noise levels of 90 dB added on to an 8-h work exposure will produce a hazardous situation.

HOBBIES

Home hobbies may be harmful: the 'do-it-yourselfer' with his power tools is well advised to wear ear defenders because the noise levels, particularly in the confined space of a workshop, are frequently well in excess of safe levels. This is particularly important in those who experience noise at work, because the social noise exposure is in addition to the daily aliquot during the period of employment. The man who has a 'safe' exposure of perhaps 88 dBA for an 8-h working day puts his ears at risk when he adds 2 h of 94 dBA noise from power tools in his home workshop, or 6 h of snowmobiling at 92 dBA. The writer was incensed to find a claimant for compensation for noise-induced hearing loss state he obtained it during working hours teaching the use of power tools to high-school students without wearing ear defenders, ultimately to reveal that his major noise exposure was the do-it-yourself project of building his own home—again without using ear defenders!

'POP' MUSIC AND ITS EFFECTS

Whether music gives pleasure or not is a subjective question. That it is a source of sound, and sometimes extemely high intensity sound, is however, beyond debate. Depending on one's attitude, music can give pleasure, can be intensely stirring or extremely irritating. The emotive comments both for and against the sounds of bagpipes, Bartok and 'beat' music are all familiar. However, the addition of electronic amplifiers to music, usually of the pop variety, has led to much greater SPLs than had previously been possible. Now the smallest group with its 200-watt amplifiers can make a more intense sound than a 100-piece symphony orchestra. It is indeed remarkable that all in a concert hall audience of 2000 can hear the solo violinist without any form of amplification, whilst in a room one tenth of the size a pop-music group requires amplification of an intensity that may be painful. The purpose of high intensity sound is to produce vegetative effects of a general kind quite apart from imposing the sound on the listener. In order to have a musical 'trip' it seems necessary to have the sounds of a sufficiently high intensity to be above 'safe' levels.

There has been considerable discussion in the literature about the potentially harmful effect of amplified music on the ears of both the musician and the audience. In the case of the musician the question is no different from any other form of occupational noise exposure—a sufficiently intense sound for a sufficiently long period of time will produce damage in an appropriately susceptible individual. The question of the audience is a more vexed one, and controversy exists about the potentially hazardous effect of listening to professionally amplified music. It is difficult to obtain an accurate measure of the total amount of noise exposure in discos; the sound contains many transients and is well distributed throughout the frequency range, with the maximum intensity below 2 kHz. This was shown by Lebo and Oliphant (1968), by Fearn (1973), and more recently by Bohne, Ward and Fernandez (1978). The sound spectra measurements are all very similar, being about 110 dB in the octave bands centred between 100 and 500 Hz, and gradually dropping to about 100 dB at

Table 18.1   Some transit car interior noise levels

Transit system	Conditions	Speed (mph)	Average noise levels (dBA)
San Francisco (BART)	Concrete aerial structure	60	76
	Subway—concrete track bed	60	80–82
Chicago Transit Authority			
New cars	Ballast and tie, welded rail	60	72
Old cars	Ballast and tie, welded rail	50	83
	Jointed rail		89
	Subway—concrete track bed	50	97
	Ballast and tie		87
Paris Metro			
New steel wheel	Subway—ballast and tie track bed	37	82
Rubber tyre cars	Subway—ballast and tie track bed	37	82

Adapted from: *Noise Regulation Reporter* **90**; Oct. 24 1977
From report by Paul Remington, to Noise-Con 77

2 kHz, and nearer 90 dB at 8 kHz. These sound levels are far in excess of those found in an average symphony orchestra hall, which is usually well below 95 dB, even in peaks (Lebo and Oliphant, 1968). The strategic positioning of loudspeakers in discotheques and rock concert arenas ensures much higher sound pressure levels in the far recesses of the hall. Rice (1969) summarized the findings of a pilot study on the effects of pop-group music on hearing by stating:

(1) The mean noise level was about 110 dBA; 5 dB less within the audience. Transient levels reached 122 dBA.
(2) Higher levels found close to loudspeakers were a more likely hazard to hearing.
(3) An exposure of one and a half hours is likely to produce a TTS close to the proposed ISO acceptable limit—equivalent to continuous noise exposure of 95 dBA.
(4) Habitual exposure may result in permanent loss of hearing.
(5) Little permanent loss was present in the groups tested, and the hazard to hearing of loud pop-group music was not considered a serious problem for the occasional, as opposed to full-time, professional habitual listener providing:
  (a) the exposures were not habitual or excessive,
  (b) TTS from one exposure had recovered completely before the next exposure,
  (c) tinnitus and difficulty in hearing conversation were not observed.

Some controversy exists concerning the relative hazards of continuous exposure to rock music and intermittent exposure, i.e. with pauses between musical pieces. Rintelmann *et al.* (1971) measured temporary threshold shift in 20 normal-hearing females following exposure to identical rock-and-roll music presented continuously for an hour, or presented in 3-min bursts with 1-min breaks in which only discotheque ambient noise was heard. Statistically the TTS was less after the intermittent noise exposure, but the recovery times were similar.

That temporary threshold shifts occur after exposure to pop music is well documented. In quite an elegant series of experiments Ulrich and Pinheiro (1974) tested teenagers before and after each of a series of rock concerts, and again some weeks later. TTS was discovered in all, but permanent hearing loss was found in only one ear of one teenager some weeks later. Whether this was related to noise or not is unclear. They review other similar work which seems to have similar conclusions, but point out that the absence of demonstrable threshold shift does not preclude permanent damage to the cochlear sensory structures.

Further inferential evidence that significant hearing loss is produced by pop-music attendance is reported by Hansen and Fern (1975) who undertook ENT examinations, hearing tests and a questionnaire survey of approximately 500 students, and found a statistically significant hearing loss in the group that admitted frequent attendance at pop-music entertainment. They also identified hearing loss from occasional employment in noise, and from gunfire, and emphasized that all the losses they discovered were unrecognized prior to the investigation.

There is an occupational hazard for disc jockeys (Chueden and Strauss, 1974) in discotheques and for pop musicians. Many of the latter use hearing protectors, but there are few good long-term studies either of the risk or of the effect on hearing.

Although the concert hall audience of a full symphony orchestra is not assaulted by damaging levels of sound, the musicians within the orchestra may well be. Those in the percussion section are subject to particularly high levels of impact noise and those unfortunate enough to be close to the more powerful brass instruments are subjected to transient peaks of well over 100 dB. However, both here and in military marching bands the noise levels are not considered much of a hazard. In a study of a Canadian military band it was discovered to the surprise of the investigator that many of the players had a hearing loss which looked suspiciously like noise-induced loss even though the band played for only 1 h/day. Close questioning showed that those involved were supplementing their incomes by playing an additional several hours/day with amplification in rock bands! (Novotny, 1976, personal communication).

Several animal studies have been undertaken to attempt to correlate histopatholog-ical changes with hearing loss produced by noise. Lipscomb (1969) exposed a guinea-pig to 88 h of disco noise in 58 days and described hair-cell destruction and irreversible permanent damage to 19 per cent of the cell population in one third of the second turn and 25 per cent of the third turn. More recently Bohne, Ward and Fernandez (1976) reported a series of experiments in which six chinchillas placed in a cage 1 m in front of a large loudspeaker and rotated at regular intervals, were exposed to live rock music for 2.5 h. Their ears were examined histologically and compared with chinchillas exposed to more standard laboratory sounds. Some animals were sacrificed acutely and others allowed to recover for some weeks before preparation. They conclude that the qualitative histological changes after exposure to rock music were identical to those found following exposure to 1 h of an octave band of noise centred at 4 kHz at 108 dB SPL. They found extensive damage in some cochleas including outer hair-cell loss, and in the specimens which were allowed to recover there was some strial atrophy.

However, the relationship between these findings and the findings in man are not clear. A New York disco operator on hearing of the damage produced in a guinea-pig's ear by disco noise was reported as stating that he would put up warning notices as soon as he had a regular clientele of guinea-pigs. Facetious as this comment may be it emphasizes the need for caution in interspecies comparisons, and in particular between chinchillas and man, for the ears of chinchillas are notoriously sensitive to the damaging effect of sound, much more so than primate and human ears.

The pervasive nature of popular music makes it an easy target for concern about its potential effect on hearing, and a significant amount of study has been made of the subject—both in human subjects and in animals. Whittle and Robinson (1974) give a very balanced assessment of the problems involved. They conclude that as with industrial noise, 'The determination of maximum permissible exposure rests on a judgment of the amount of hearing loss at various frequencies that should be accepted in certain percentages of the population, after a given number of years of exposure, and whether the effects of other noise exposure (e.g. occupational) should be taken into account.' They, in common with other authors are concerned that the usually employed criteria for the onset of hearing impairment are too lax for a voluntary occupation, and indeed quite significant degrees of subclinical hearing loss may occur before 'measurable' loss is found. They also point out that the mean age of those attending discotheques is low, so that significant noise exposure may occur some years before the commencement of employment. That this may indeed be a cause of hearing loss is suggested by Taylor (1976). He questioned new apprentices about their noise exposure and as a result divided them into two groups, one with significant noise exposure and the other without. Audiometry was performed and it was found that the exposed group had a significant loss at 6 kHz. Whilst minor degrees of hearing loss of this sort may by themselves not appear great, they are of significance when looked at in the total context of a lifetime of noise exposure and a lifetime of other ototraumatic assaults on the ear.

Weber, McGovern and Zink (1967) analysed 1000 school-age children with hearing loss. High-frequency hearing impairment among older children was considerably more prevalent than among younger ones. In an attempt to relate incidence of high-frequency hearing impairment to environmental noise exposure, Lipscomb discovered a marked increase in its incidence in the frequency region of 2 kHz and above as a function of age (Lipscomb, 1969).

Before the commencement of rifle training, Neiger and Fisch (1967) found a noise trauma curve (defined as a dip of at least 30 dB) in 19 per cent of young new infantry recruits before exposure. They noted a very close comparison between this figure and that for noise trauma found in schoolchildren, which they gave as 20 per cent. They believe that these figures are indicative of the increased noise levels in modern society and that these levels are responsible for a higher incidence of auditory noise trauma in the world today.

Medical noise

NOISE FROM DENTAL ENGINES AND SUCTION UNITS

The introduction of turbine-driven high-speed dental drills led to the suggestion that the sound levels generated might be harmful to the ear. One of the most recent studies by Welleschik (1976) suggests that the noise levels are well below those considered hazardous. However, the study of the drills used in temporal bone surgery has led to suggestions that sound levels to which the patient's cochlea may be exposed are potentially hazardous. Paulsen and Vietor (1975a, 1975b) measured airborne sound levels in close proximity to current high-speed temporal bone drills and also by means of strain gauges measured the bone conducted noise. They found that air conducted noise was higher than bone conducted noise, and that it was relatively independent of the type of drilling machine and handpiece. While free running most drills had levels of 85 dBA at 35 cm but when drilling bone large cutters had sound levels of up to 110 dBA at 15 cm. Kylen and Arlinger (1976) and Kylen *et al.* (1977) concluded that noise levels were primarily influenced by the size of the burr—the bigger the burr, the higher the noise. They found that a 6-mm cutting burr gave noise levels of 88–108 dB whilst these levels were reduced by 5–16 dB when the cutting burr size was reduced to 2 mm. The mean noise levels of diamond burrs were 5–11 dB lower than the mean levels of similar sized cutting burrs. They also point out that the noise levels around the cochlea were only slightly influenced by the localization of the drill within the ear, and also suggest that drill-induced noise levels in ear surgery cannot be reduced to any great extent. They suggest that the only way to minimize drill-produced noise trauma to the inner ear is to reduce the time which the drill is used. Certain suction units used during ear toilet and ear surgery also produce high sound pressure levels.

It is therefore possible that some of the sensorineural hearing loss which is routinely found in chronic ear disease after surgery may be due to the surgical therapy itself rather than to the disease process. However, Paparella *et al.* (1972) point out that diminished bone conduction with a slowly progressive sensorineural hearing loss is a common feature of chronic otitis media even if not operated on. Smyth (1977) reports on the changes in bone conduction hearing in 3000 consecutive tympanoplasties and believes that excessive manipulation of the ossicles rather than noise is the principle cause of a further hearing loss.

HAZARD FROM HEARING AIDS?

One possible cause of noise-induced hearing loss is a hearing aid, for it is suggested that high levels of amplification, and SPL, provided to alleviate hearing loss may be the cause of a further deterioration of hearing. Some hearing aids have enormous power output—above 140 dB—and maximum acoustic gains of up to 80 dB, particularly if the aids are produced for patients with conductive hearing loss. The evidence to prove that hearing aids do in fact damage hearing is inconclusive and has been well reviewed by Markides (1971).

Typical pros and cons are presented in papers by Jerger and Lewis (1975), who report a fairly well-substantiated case of a child suffering permanent damage to residual hearing due to the use of a powerful hearing aid. On the other hand Darbyshire (1976) in a study of 100 children with profound hearing loss tested their hearing before and after they wore one or two high-gain and high-output hearing aids over a period of three years, and was unable to detect clinically any statistically significant deterioration worse than occurred in the unaided ear. Titche, Windrem and Starmer (1977) review the current literature, concluding that in their own series no changes were found, but that there was a risk of further hearing loss occurring. The conclusion to be drawn is to provide an aid which is adequate for the job without being unnecessarily powerful.

COMPRESSION CHAMBERS

Compression chambers may also be an otological hazard, both from the standpoint of pressure equalization and, more insidiously, from noises close to the air entry valves. One well substantiated report (Hughes, 1976) of a military compression chamber tells of a soldier with his right ear close to the entry valve of a compression chamber who developed profound hearing loss.

HOSPITAL NOISE

The otologist should be aware that hospitals themselves can be extremely noisy and the source both of inconvenience and of hearing loss. From a nuisance standpoint Fife and Rappaport (1976) report that the length of hospital stay for simple cataract surgery during a period of construction noise, was compared retrospectively with two similar periods without construction noise. The hospital stay was significantly longer during the period of construction. This was equated with lack of rest and sleep disturbance. Ducel, Suter and Dupont (1976) comment upon high noise levels in intensive care units (ICUs). With the widespread use of open-plan ICUs noise levels certainly should be watched—the sound from monitoring equipment, respirators, suction pumps, and a variety of life-support systems are certainly sufficient to be sleep-disturbing and may be frankly injurious to staff employed for long periods of time. It should also not be forgotten that hospitals have quite extensive engineering facilities, including automatic dishwashing equipment, noisy central sterilizing plants, and in the more modern buildings large air-conditioning plants, all of which may exceed sound levels for 40 h of 90 dBA DRC (Maguire and Van Wagoner, 1977).

A more important cause of noise has been incubator and oxygen tents. League *et al.* (1972) give accounts of the acoustical conditions in incubators prevalent at that time, and in infant oxygen tents. They suggest that levels are high. This was particularly so in incubators used in premature nurseries where the sound levels were close to or exceeding those considered safe for an eight-hour exposure. What effect this has on the immature ears of the neonate is difficult to tell, and it is certainly feared that minor degrees of damage at that time, whilst not producing a detectable hearing loss, would initiate the destruction of some hair-cells at an earlier than normal age and ultimately lead to a premature hearing loss. The question is compounded by the synergistic effect of noise and ototoxic drugs which have frequently been given, particularly in the form of kanamycin, to premature infants. This was studied in animal experiments by Dayal, Kokshanian and Mitchell (1971). They demonstrated that guinea-pigs exposed to a combination of low frequency, low intensity noise (68–72 dB at 125 Hz) and low dosages of kanamycin (15–50 mg/kg body weight) had hair-cell damage, whereas with either agent acting alone those dosages did not produce damage. No follow-up studies in humans so exposed have yet been reported, but there is certainly need for caution.

Effects of infrasound, vibration and ultrasound

There are still wide gaps in our knowledge of the effects of frequency stimuli above and below the normal range of human auditory perception, usually regarded as ranging from about 20 Hz–20 kHz. Tones between 200 Hz and 10 kHz are perceived at very low threshold levels, but at either extreme of the low frequency range, SPLs must be comparatively high before sounds can be detected. It is difficult to determine at what level infrasound becomes inaudible; although it is stated that the human ear is incapable of hearing below 16 Hz there are those who claim to experience a sensation similar to sound at frequencies as low as 7–8 Hz. Whether this is genuine auditory sensation produced by the primary wave or whether it is caused by hearing harmonics is unknown. Certainly the ear is highly insensitive to low frequency vibrations, which is in part at least an evolutionary protective mechanism to prevent being deafened by the low frequency vibrations produced by blood coursing through the carotid arteries.

von Gierke (1965) commented that although work on the acceptability of infrasonic noise and of sonic boom associated with supersonic flight was in progress, all proposed schemes were based not on objective indications for various levels of risk of physiological damage but on subjective judgment of comfort or tolerability. Acceptable criteria for rating vibration exposure were not available and although criteria for ultrasound exposure were desirable, data were limited.

Technically, sound is a specialized form of vibration which stimulates the auditory sense. Normally noise is heard and vibration is felt, but physically they are similar (Westin, 1975). It is sometimes quite difficult to differentiate between infrasound and vibration.

Sources of infrasound

The ear is extremely insensitive to low frequency vibrations and is a poor detector of ubiquitous infrasound and vibrations which originate both from natural and man-made sources. By definition they are normally not heard and therefore man is usually unaware of their presence. Geophysical phenomena are a major source of infrasound, which include thunder, high winds and ocean waves. Natural phenomena such as earthquakes or volcanic eruptions and auroral discharges are also implicated. This and many other of the properties and problems of infrasound are well reviewed by Westin. The majority of geophysical phenomena seem to produce infrasound at extremely low frequencies—often below 4 or 5 Hz. The infrasound waves travel great distances without attenuation—the vibrations produced by thunder over the state of Oklahoma were detected in the Caribbean, and in water the propagation of long wavelength waves is equally distant. Man-made infrasound is common but infrequently detected, for most sound-measuring surveys do not extend the range of investigation into frequencies below 60 Hz, and even when they do, almost never test below 20 Hz because FM tape-recorders are required to record infrasound. Even the best normal tape-recorder is technically incapable of reproducing such low frequency vibrations, irrespective of their intensity. The automobile is one of the most common sources of infrasound, which is responsible for some of the unpleasant sensations experienced when driving at speed with windows open. Much heavy industrial machinery produces infrasound, including air-conditioning plants, fans, and many forms of transportation including jet aircraft, piston engines, rockets, etc.

The effects of infrasonic airborne sound are dependent upon its SPL according to Burns *et al.* (1968). They quote Gavreau, Condat and Saul (1966) who experienced nausea and vertigo, attributable to excitation of the semicircular canals. Sounds of 7, 16 and 250 Hz produced resonance of internal organs, intense irritation, interference with intellectual activity and visual disturbances. The effects are similar to those caused by low frequency mechanical vibration. An extensive list of alarming non-auditory effects were observed by Mohr and his colleagues (1965) but as far as the ear itself was concerned, apart from noting giddiness and nausea, they found no shifts in TTS_2 (hearing thresholds measured 2 min after exposure) in noise-experienced subjects wearing earmuff and earplug combinations. They considered that for short duration exposures of 150 dB SPL were well within the limits of human tolerance. Broad band and discrete frequency noise in the 1–100 Hz range was tested for short durations as high as 150 dB and, with the subjects wearing ear protectors, was well tolerated. Sound at 3–5 Hz was perceptible but not audible.

Burns has commented that the relevance of the observed effects of infrasound lies in whether they are found to occur in real situations in industry or near machines. In this respect Mohr *et al.* (1965) observe that with space rocket boosters the maximum energy occurs in the 1–100 Hz frequency range. The level of noise increases as the booster increases in size and thrust. They predict that very large boosters in the future will produce their maximum energy in the infrasonic range, below 20 Hz, and knowledge of its effect on the astronauts and space scientists is urgently needed, as well as effects on those on the ground nearby.

Exposure of subjects to intense sound below 22 Hz ranging from 119–114 dB SPL for 3 min was studied by Alford and his colleagues (1966). They concluded that auditory effects might be produced at a lower SPL as the frequency of the stimulus increased, and that the susceptibility to the auditory effects from intense tones in the low frequency range may be increased by the presence of a pre-existing hearing loss. Most of their subjects had a feeling of pressure in the ears and nystagmus occurred in the majority. Only one subject experienced brief tinnitus. With exposures exceeding 137 dB, a TTS of more than 10 dB was found in over half the subjects. These threshold shifts occurred at 2, 10, 12 and 22 Hz. It was demonstrated by Kylin (1960) that to produce a significant TTS in the lower frequency band 75–150 Hz, the SPL of the stimulating sound needed to be 20 dB more intense than that required to produce a similar TTS at frequencies above 2 kHz.

An account of nystagmus induced by stimuli in the 2–20 Hz frequency range has been given by Evans (1969). She considered the occurrence of the Tullio phenomenon as a response of the semicircular canals to low frequency sound. On existing biophysical considerations she considered the nystagmus to be a response of the otolith system to a slow alternating displacement.

Unfortunately, lack of information is one of the major conclusions to be drawn from any review of the effect of infrasound on man. The studies which have been undertaken are few, and confusing. It is extremely difficult to evaluate the effects of infrasound without including vibration and/or broad band noise, and what experiments there are—most of which have been reviewed above— are of a short-term nature. Inversely related to the hard data is the mythology which surrounds the effect of infrasound, ranging from making it the whipping boy for mood changes and ill health in periods of thunder storms, to fanciful tales of deathrays from high intensity, low frequency sounds, the proponents of which evoke the walls of Jericho being blown down by trumpets. Some of this mythology evolves around the possibility of infrasound establishing cavity resonances within the body. There is some evidence that in the range between 2 and 10 Hz it may be possible to excite various body cavities into resonance (Westin, 1975), which may be responsible for some of the reported unpleasant effects.

Vibration

The effects of vibration on man have been comprehensively reviewed by Goldman and von Gierke (1961). Fatigue and structural damage can be produced, as can nausea and disorientation. They are probably caused by transmission of vibration by the endolymph to the semicircular canals resulting in abnormal stimulation of the balance organ (Burns *et al.*, 1968). Vibration levels that are structurally safe for vehicles may be uncomfortable, annoying, or even dangerous for their occupants (Peterson and Gross, 1963). A modern review of vibration in transportation is given by Lyon (1973).

Many modern forms of transportation produce significant levels of vibration, not least the helicopter. Helicopters may vibrate in such a way that the eyes of the pilot shake, preventing him from seeing the instruments properly, and one type of military helicopter is reported as establishing resonances of the nasal vibrissae of its pilots, leading to constant nose-scratching and picking and resultant dermatitis from the pilot's oilstained glove!

A recently recognized hazard of intense vibration, particularly as seen amongst pneumatic drill operators, is the white hand syndrome which is now recognized as a fairly significant problem.

Ultrasound

Mention has been made elsewhere of the effects of ultrasound on disturbances of equilibrium. With regard to the effects of ultrasonic frequencies on hearing levels, Parrack (1966) considered that frequencies from 20–37 Hz should be harmless to human ears until approaching the 140 dB SPL. Around this intensity level, ultrasonic single frequency sounds gave no hearing sensation. Some TTS however occurred at half the frequency, and below, of the fundamental. Amongst non-auditory effects were sensations from vibration of the hairs in the external auditory canals and nostrils.

Sources of ultrasound are fairly widespread, both from jet aircraft, and amongst other industrial sources, sonic cleaners and dental drills. There is no hard evidence that any of these are harmful.

Non-auditory effects of noise

That noise can have an effect in systems far removed from the ear is well known and has been applied to hearing testing. Brain waves as generated in response to sound are currently much being studied, and in the past changes in respiratory rate, cardiac rate, and conditioning of the subject to the sound producing a change in skin resistance, have all had their day as methods of hearing testing. Sound has an alerting value which produces reflex responses, and these reflexes may be unconditioned or conditioned. The startle response in the infant to a loud sound is an example of the former, the downing of tools as the lunchtime buzzer goes in a plant is an example of the latter. There have been many suggestions that community and industrial noise have a deleterious effect on health, although it is extremely difficult to differentiate the effect of sound *per se* from other stressful stimuli. Kryter (1976) has written extensively on the subject, and has recently reviewed his and other findings. He suggests that there are two major schools of thought concerning the systemic effects of noise; (1) in which noise is treated as a reinforcer of innate reflexive responses, and (2) that noise directly stimulates or causes activation of the autonomic nervous system to such an extent that it endangers the health. The reflexive school suggests that there are two types of response to sound; (1) the orienting response in which the autonomic nervous system treats sound as an alerting signal and responds accordingly, and (2) the defensive response which becomes stronger as sound is increased. Knowledge of or meaning attributed to the sound is a potentiating factor. The experimental work reviewed suggests that these reflexes habituate so rapidly that they are unlikely to be unduly stressful. The second school suggests that the autonomic responses do not habituate and are a direct result of sound and become harmful. This is in keeping with stress-producing theories of Selye. Kryter is sceptical of the second group. There is however a certain amount of evidence which at least gives food for thought. Cohen (1973) studied the injury rate and the illness rate in a noisy and relatively quiet plant, and found that both were higher in the noisy plant. However, whether these were the direct result of noise or other factors in the plant remains totally open.

The effect of noise on sleep has been studied in some detail, although this is extremely difficult to do without having the experimental conditions interfere with the study because of the need for continuous EEG monitoring. The results are well summarized by Thiessen (1976). He suggests that for moderate intermittent levels of noise repeated through several nights, the probability of awakening as a result of the noise diminishes as the nights pass, i.e. there is a subconscious adaptation to the noise which becomes less disturbing, although even if the subject does not wake the alpha rhythm is disturbed by noise. Certainly the higher the background noise the more the likelihood of shifting in sleep level. It has been argued that disturbed or altered sleep is responsible for some of the deleterious effects of noise rather than the noise itself.

Cantrell (1975a) studied the effect on sleep and showed that noise louder than 35 dB can cause arousal in adults. He also points out that many factors other than noise influence arousal from sleep, including motivation, age, sex, time of sleep cycle, and stimulus meaning, for example baby crying or the telephone ringing.

He reviews the psychological and sociological effects of noise exposure, the results of which are again contradictory and confusing. Some authorities suggest that noise affects non-auditory work performance at much lower levels than others, but this seems to be tempered by the psychological type of the subject, the task involved and the motivation.

Cantrell (1975b) reviews the general adaptation theory which when applied to noise suggests that 'noise as a stress (1) stimulates the hypothalamus, which (2) stimulates the anterior pituitary to release ACTH, which (3) stimulates the adrenal cortex to release cortisol, which (4) stimulates the body to protect against the systemic anabolism of tissue.' There are multiple experiments to demonstrate that noise may produce these effects, although some are undertaken in such high levels of sound that they are unrealistic, and others draw such gloomy conclusions that their relevance to man is suspect. Part of the problem with all of these experiments as they relate to man is the emotional value placed on the sound, i.e. sounds of equal intensity produced a different reflex muscle tension, and annoyance and disturbance scaling depending upon whether the subject liked the sound or not. These after all are experimental verifications of everyday truisms. A welcome sound, music, a motor purring well, the sound of waves breaking on the rocks, all can be relaxing whereas sounds of a similar intensity—the neighbour's dog barking, somebody else's lawnmower motor, etc. can be aggravating and tension producing. The reader should refer to the papers cited for further details including a book bringing together the proceedings of a conference on the physiological effects of noise, edited by Welch and Welch (1970).

There are certain relevant epidemiological studies of the effect of noise. The report of an increased incidence of mental hospital admission amongst those subjected to high levels of aircraft noise has been widely quoted (Abey-Wickram et al., 1969). They suggest that in those susceptible to mental disease the incidence of mental hospital admission is greater in those living close to high levels of airport noise than in the population at large. They are careful not to infer that the noise *per se* causes mental disease. Knipschild (1976) reported an extensive study of people exposed to intense noise of aircraft at Schipol Airport near Amsterdam, and compared them with people living in similar but quiet areas. He suggests that in areas where there was greater aircraft noise more people were under medical treatment for heart trouble and hypertension and more, particularly women, on cardiovascular drugs. Differences between the populations, he felt, could not be explained by age, sex, smoking habits, or socioeconomic variables. A further investigation in which 20 general practitioners cooperated showed that in areas where aircraft noise was high the visits to general practitioners were significantly higher than in quiet areas, the increased numbers being due to psychological problems and psychosomatic symptoms. There was also an increased incidence of use of sedatives, hypnotics, antacids and cardiovascular drugs. The incidence of use of these drugs increased as the airport noise levels increased, whereas at a control village not exposed to noise the incidence remained constant. This type of work requires urgent validation for the numbers of people involved are high—over 1 million in noise levels considered hazardous by the author in the Netherlands alone.

That the general public believe that noise is an intrusion in their home is reflected in a recent report from Canada which shows that for daytime L eq levels of above 70 dBA house prices dropped by approximately $700/dB, and thus a noise barrier resulting in a 15-dBA reduction might be worth approximately $10 000/housing unit. This Canadian work is preliminary but plausible (Hall, Breston and Taylor, 1978).

Clinical features

The diagnosis of noise-induced permanent threshold shift (NIPTS) is based on a full evaluation of history, physical examination and laboratory tests, including the audiogram. It should be emphasized from the outset that there is neither any one audiometric pattern which is diagnostic of noise-induced hearing loss, nor are there many patterns which are exclusive of the diagnosis.

The diagnosis of NIPTS is usually circumstantial and may be difficult to substantiate in logic, because it ultimately is a diagnosis made by exclusion. When other causes of hearing loss are eliminated, and there had been adequate exposure to noise, the diagnosis of NIPTS is made. The situation would be more satisfactory if there were positive rather than negative diagnostic features. Several temptations must be resisted. The most widespread error and one which is frequently made by those dealing with occupational hearing loss on an epidemiological scale, is to suggest that because hearing loss is present and there has been adequate noise exposure, that the two are causally related. To believe this is to believe that working in noise protects the ear from all other forms of disease which cause hearing loss. In our own series (Alberti and Morgan, 1974) of compensation evaluations, now grown to more than 3000 workmen evaluated for NIPTS, 3.5 per cent have other ear disease as the major cause of hearing loss—diseases such as otosclerosis, chronic otitis media, Menière's disease, congenital hearing loss, and even acoustic neuroma. Conversely, the presence of other diseases does not preclude a diagnosis of NIPTS. The man with a mid-frequency familial hearing loss may have superimposed upon it a noise loss, the well-treated otosclerotic may yet develop NIPTS in the operated ear, and the patient who has worked in high noise levels for 20 years who has had only one episode of Menière's disease, and has a bilateral notched high frequency hearing loss is more likely to have this caused by noise. Many of these factors will be clearer when widespread hearing conservation schemes have been in practice for some time, but at present both in North America and most European countries prior information of the patient's hearing and ear disease is at a premium.

Audiograms will quantify a hearing loss and give some indication of the site of lesion. They will not by themselves provide a diagnosis. This is based upon careful evaluation of history, both personal and familial, and of past and present occupational, recreational and accidental noise exposure. Enquiry must be made of illnesses associated with or known to cause deafness; head injuries and ototoxic drugs; haematological, serological, radiological, and other investigative procedures may be indicated, and a complete examination of the ears, nose and throat must be made. As social and military noise exposure has increased, so has its importance in the history. In the USA there are few young men who have not served in the armed forces and been exposed to the extremely intense sounds of a modern armamentarium. There are many who use guns for recreational purposes, others who ride motorcycles, use outboard motor-boat engines, play in rock bands, etc. It becomes a matter of exquisite judgment to attribute various percentages of loss to current employment, past employment, military service and social events! A history of ototoxic drug use is often difficult to obtain and may require a careful search through old hospital records. Serological investigation is often recommended as a routine, although it must be stated that of 1000 consecutive tests in our patients with presumed NIPTS the positive rate was only 0.2 per cent and even here the cause/effect relationship with hearing loss was questionable. The question of difference in hearing thresholds between the two ears will be discussed further below.

Any history of physical signs, including audiometric findings, suggestive of other cochlear or retrocochlear lesions such as Menière's disease, acoustic neuroma, meningioma, etc. should be investigated fully; the first responsibility of the examining physician is the welfare of the patient. When the results of the history and physical findings, together with laboratory tests and audiograms are evaluated, it is usually possible to make a tentative diagnosis that an individual may be suffering from hearing loss attributable to noise.

It is often stated that in pure NIPTS thresholds must be equal in both ears. The usual exceptions cited to this rule are people using guns fired from the shoulder, in which case the ear closest to the muzzle of the gun often has the worse hearing, for the head shadow protects the opposite ear. Pilots of certain types of aircraft, particularly the older piston planes, such as the DC3, also were cited for they often flew with one ear covered with the headset and the other ear uncovered to listen to the motor through an open window, developing a loss in that ear. However, unequal hearing thresholds in NIPTS, far from being a curiosity, are fairly common.

There are many instances, particularly with impact noise-producing machinery such as rock drills in mines, various types of mobile metal-forming machines, and even such seemingly innocuous devices as a farm tractor—where one ear is chronically exposed to more sound than the other, and where hearing loss develops at different rates in the two ears. In our experience based on the evaluation of more than 1000 hard-rock miners (nickel, silver, gold, uranium), more than 10 per cent have an unexplained difference between the two ears of more than 10 dB, after blast exposure and ear disease have been eliminated. Commonly the shapes of the audiograms are similar, but one has progressed further into the low frequencies than the other. However, even this is not always the case, for there are sufficient examples of quite atypical audiograms with no known explanation even after full investigation, to give considerable food for thought (Alberti *et al.*, 1979). Full investigation is warranted whenever it is indicated on clinical grounds, although the writer has balked at the investigation of all tinnitus in occupational hearing loss patients because of the frequency of the symptom following noise exposure, even though it may be a symptom of acoustic neuroma.

If there is a history of acoustic trauma or blast, such as the use of explosives in mining or construction, a tank or tyre exploding, or exposure to cereal making guns, then one ear may be more affected than the other because of the protection afforded by the head shadow, or even if both are equally affected initially one may recover more fully than the other.

Exaggerated hearing loss (EHL)

Hearing thresholds may be difficult to establish because of genuine problems in undertaking the test or because of the conscious or subconscious wish to elevate the apparent threshold. The cause of the latter range from a desire to use hearing loss to better circumstances (withdrawal from the front line in the military, or from a dangerous job such as mining to a belief that someone owes them something for their handicap, especially if it is associated with financial loss (lack of promotion, demotion, or unemployment). The manifestations range from merely making quite sure a sound is heard to a concerted attempt to deceive.

The incidence varies significantly with the methodology of compensation. Where claims are settled in court, with lawyers in an adversary situation, the rate of inaccurate thresholds is extremely high, and where it is settled by compensation tribunals, much lower. The timing of compensation awards is also important: if hearing loss is only compensated when workers stop employment in noise (retirement or demotion), the incidence is much higher. In our own experience of over 400 claimants with EHL the incidence was 22 per cent as long as awards were only made when the claimant left noisy employment. A recent change in Ontario compensation laws allows payment whilst still working in noise and the incidence has been reduced to 10 per cent of all claims. Where cases are settled in court the incidence may be almost 100 per cent.

Certain clinical, social and audiometric features characterize EHL many of which are extensively reviewed by Ventry and Chaiklin (1965). The claimant is frequently wearing a hearing aid ostentatiously, he exaggerates the listening process, leaning forward, often cupping the ear. However, conversation about an unrelated topic—a recent sports event or the weather, with one's back turned, is answered at normal conversational level. In our experience those with EHL have significantly less education than average and are of lower socioeconomic status. There is frequently a story of job-loss, or inability to obtain employment.

Audiometrically a skilled, suspicious tester will quickly detect the exaggerated body posture and inappropriate test reactions. The responses to speech audiometry are characteristic—wrong answers but related in meaning—schoolboy for schoolgirl, northwest for northeast, etc. The pure-tone audiogram is often flat, and the speech reception threshold out of line with the pure-tone average. A common trick is for the subject to hum during the test, thus masking lower frequencies and dropping the audiogram. A good strategy in compensation work is to start testing with the impedance bridge, preferably attached to a write-out device which the subject can see: the belief that results are obtained requiring no response from him is often enough to prevent further attempts!

It should be emphasized that in claims for NIPTS there are very few EHLs with normal hearing—virtually all have some loss, but less than claimed.

Audiometry

The hearing tests which are undertaken are crucial to the diagnosis and accurate quantification of the hearing loss. The degree of accuracy required if financial compensation is at stake, is much greater than that required for pure diagnostic audiometry. The basis of most compensation assessments for noise-induced hearing loss is the pure-tone audiogram, and thus it must be extremely reliable.

Authorities vary enormously in the period of time for which a worker must be away from noise in order to quantify hearing for medical/legal purposes.

Some insist on a six-month period of freedom from noise, whilst at the other extreme some require only 72 h. In practice in any area where hearing loss from noise is compensated whilst the workman continues to work in noisy surrounding, albeit perhaps wearing ear defenders, it is impractical to ask for his removal from the noisy environment for more than a few days before a judgment is made. There are as many pragmatic adaptations to a local scene as there are variations in methods of compensation!

There are many techniques for obtaining a pure-tone audiogram which include conventional, behavioural threshold audiometry, automatic recording audiometry of discrete and continuous frequency type (Békésy), various forms of electrical response audiometry including late evoked response audiometry (ERA) and more recently brainstem audiometry (BERA) and electrocochleography (EcochG). Of these only ERA is currently in widespread use in threshold determinations in adults. Psychogalvanic skin response audiometry (PGSR) is a further technique which has been favoured. It should not be forgotten that convential pure-tone audiometry is quite a complicated psychoacoustic task which for extreme accuracy requires skills often beyond the experience of the patient, who may be ill-educated, not fluent in the language of the tester, and tired from travelling for his test. It is hardly surprising that inaccurate results frequently occur. The addition of the frank dissembler to these ranks makes this type of hearing testing a considerable challenge. It is our practice never to rely upon the results of one test for pension purposes; we only feel happy if the results of conventional tests match with those of the ERA or with the speech results.

Much has been made in the past of the shape of the audiogram in noise-induced hearing loss, with the suggestion that a notch centred at about 4 kHz with some recovery above this frequency is a prerequisite of the diagnosis. This is just not true. Firstly, notched audiograms may occur in the absence of noise as a response to ototoxic drug exposure or age changes. Secondly, the notch of noise-inducing hearing loss may range between 3 and 6 kHz and after a period of time the recovery above the notch disappears, leaving a complete high frequency loss. The slope may be abrupt—the ski-slope type of loss with normal hearing to 1000 or 1500 Hz followed by a drop of as much as 30 dB/octave. By contrast it may be almost flat, a relatively common finding after many years in drop-forging or high noise exposure. In people working in predominantly low frequency noise, particularly if hearing protection is worn, the major loss may be in the lower frequencies. Thus, although audiometric shape may be a guide, it is certainly not a major diagnostic factor. With so many different types of noise exposure added to ears of different susceptibilities, this should not be surprising.

One feature of the pure-tone audiogram emphasized by Klockhoff *et al.* (1974) and reiterated by ourselves (Alberti, Morgan and Czuba, 1978) is the probability that a hearing loss of 40 dB or greater at 500 Hz is more likely to be due to causes other than noise, organic or non-organic. We place considerable reliance upon this finding and routinely undertake a fairly extensive battery of tests including evoked response audiometry in people whose hearing at 500 Hz is poor. The yield of dissemblers and other ear disease is extremely high.

Speech audiomentry

(A) SPEECH RECEPTION THRESHOLDS

The relationship between pure-tone hearing and speech reception thresholds (SRT) has been widely based on Fletcher's pure-tone average, in which the average pure-tone thresholds at 500, 1000 and 2000 Hz are said to equate with the SRT. This formula only applies if the pure-tone audiogram is relatively flat. In a sloping audiogram the SRT matches well with the pure-tone threshold average of the better two frequencies, 500, 1000 and 2000 Hz and the relationship is a good test for inaccurate pure-tone hearing responses. We recommend the use of another test such as ERA whenever the two are 10 dB or more apart. There have been many fears expressed about accent and dialect of the patient affecting the results of speech audiometry. After several years' experience in a multilingual community it is concluded that the key factor is that the tester can understand the words spoken by the patient, for with widespread radio and television the patient can usually understand the test words.

(B) SPEECH DISCRIMINATION AUDIOMETRY

The first, and perhaps the major handicap experienced in NIPTS is difficulty in discriminating speech, particularly in background noise, i.e. the signal-to-noise ratio required to decode the signal (speech), is elevated. The relationship between this handicap and pure-tone hearing loss is difficult to evaluate, and is relative to the hearing at high, rather than low, frequencies. Unfortunately there are no well accepted standard clinical tests which are sufficiently quantified for pension evaluation. With some of the steeply sloping losses, the frequently practised shortcut of undertaking speech discrimination tests, at a 35–40 dB intensity above the speech reception threshold may give very misleading results because of the steeply falling off audiogram heightening the frequencies required to perceive consonants at a level above sound presentation. In order to get an accurate speech discrimination score it is usually necessary to perform a speech audiogram. Noble (1973) gives a detailed review of the problems concerned in reconciling pure-tone acuity, speech hearing and hearing loss in acoustic trauma, which should be consulted.

ERA

Although ERA was introduced to facilitate early diagnosis of profound childhood hearing loss, it has proved to be a useful tool in accurate quantification of adult hearing loss, particularly in cases with suspected psychogenic loss (exaggerated hearing loss, dissembling, malingering, and the wide range of other pseudonyms under which this masquerades).

It is a valid and accurate technique in neurologically normal adults (Alberti, 1970; Davis *et al.*, 1976). We have found that in cases of doubt it helps to establish the probable hearing threshold and significantly shortens the testing time required to establish it by means of conventional test techniques. A good audiologist can usually detect a dissembling patient and will be able to move him towards the accurate threshold of hearing, but this may take several hours of work. The ERA enables much time to be saved. It should be emphasized that for legal validity it is wise to have results from more than one test coinciding. It is prudent to have the evoked response testing undertaken by a separate tester unaware of the results of the first tester. With modern dedicated equipment the test takes about 1 h.

It is possible that BERA will find a place in the testing of compensation cases, although at the time of writing this has not yet been established.

Other audiometric techniques

Many tests have been applied to the diagnosis of exaggerated hearing loss. Standard audiometric texts give full details of the technique of Béskésy and PGSR audiometry, the Stenger test, etc. Impedance tests, especially stapedius reflex estimations are sometimes useful in detecting EHL, although not of much value in quantifying it. If reflexes to pure tones are detected below the admitted pure-tone thresholds, the latter are wrong! Even a gap between PTT and reflex thresholds of less than 20 dB, particularly at lower frequencies, should be viewed with suspicion. However, in spite of many recent efforts to quantify hearing loss by applying various reflex tests, these are significantly less reliable than other techniques. Clinics tend to use equipment which is available, which frequently reflects the date at which the facility was established. Thus the older American clinics have PGSR equipment and the newer ones ERA equipment.

In the final assessment the accurate establishment of a hearing threshold in industrial hearing loss, as in other forms of hearing loss, is based upon a suspicious tester with good clinical skills.

Therapy for NIPTS

Noise-induced hearing loss is entirely preventable but totally incurable. Nevertheless it can be helped by various rehabilitative manoeuvres. As the early symptoms are largely caused by the loss of ability to inhibit unwanted sound, the remedial efforts are turned to increasing signal-to-noise ratio of various signals. The use of a television amplifier, either a separate loudspeaker, plug-in headset or induction loop, will allow all the family to watch, without deafening the normally hearing or amplifying all the sound in the room as with a hearing aid. A telephone handset amplifier provided by many telephone companies or in portable form available from electronic hobby shops is often helpful, and telephone and doorbells can be made louder. The Bell Telephone system will also install bells with a lower centre frequency to accommodate the high-tone loss of the patient.

As the loss becomes more severe a hearing aid may be indicated and can now frequently be fitted with success, in spite of the difficult audiometric configuration.

Even in those with a 'ski-slope' type of loss, a modern high-frequency-emphasis aid, of low gain, with an open or vented ear mould (which further filters out low frequencies) is often of considerable help.

Hearing conservation programmes

The current emphasis on prevention and compensation of noise-induced hearing loss has led to more and more plants and industries establishing hearing conservation programmes, which often involve an otologist—frequently in a consulting role. The typical hearing conservation programme is a multidisciplinary project requiring engineering, managerial and medical skills.

Sound measurement

The first part of a programme is usually to undertake a sound survey to identify potentially hazardous areas. Much industrial noise is a mixture of impact and steady-state noise, with the steady-state noise often being broad-band. Sound levels frequently fluctuate throughout a work cycle, so it is important to sample a total cycle. In addition workmen move around in their place of work and it is necessary to sample from several typical work positions. The business of noise measurement is a skilled one which requires special equipment and training. Sound level meters are frequently used, although more sophisticated techniques include recording of noise levels on specially calibrated and accurate tape recorders with subsequent analysis of the recordings under laboratory conditions. Whilst many records are made in broad-band noise in the A-scale weighting, it is more accurate to make one-third octave band measurements. An analysis of the results enables a sound profile of a particular plant or process to be established. From this the L eqs can be worked out and thus the risk to the working population is established. In general terms most sound surveys fall short of this ideal and merely indicate whether the levels are above the 90 dBA and if so by how much, and for how long.

Sound control

If it is established that sound levels are hazardous, then steps are taken to control the amount of sound to which workers are exposed, both by engineering and by personal protection. The engineering controls range from redesigning machinery or encasing it, to quite simple modifications. It is usually impractical to make major modifications to an existing machine, although noise specifications can be written into new orders. A frequently practised compromise in recent years has been to separate the operatives from the machines by placing controls in an observation booth similar to an audiometric soundproof booth; this has been used to good effect in the engine room of ships, in the control rooms of generating stations, in metal refineries and in papermaking plants—to give but a few examples. Plant design should include separation, or isolation of noisy machinery: too often a workman is harmed not by his own machine, but by a neighbouring one from which he is not isolated! For further details a noise control manual should be consulted.

Hearing screening

The next feature of a hearing conservation programme is adequate hearing testing. Industrial hearing testing is screening and identification audiometry, it is not diagnostic. The standards required are different from diagnostic or pension evaluation tests and should not be confused. Testers are usually less skilled, frequently industrial nurses whose hearing testing training consists of one three- or four-day course. The function of the hearing test is to identify those with a hearing loss; to identify those whose hearing alters; and to determine whether the hearing conservation programme is effective. New employees should be screened and those with a hearing loss identified. They should be referred for accurate quantification of the loss and diagnosis of its cause. This will limit an employer's liability to any further hearing loss caused whilst the employee is working for him rather than to the total loss, including pre-existing problems. After a relatively short period of time in a new noise level, perhaps three months, the worker's hearing should again be tested for any major change in hearing levels which might suggest that the workman has 'tender' ears. If such a change is found it should be identified both to the workman and to management. One of the typical problems in powerfully unionized industry is to know what to do with people whose hearing has been found to change. The possibility of this arising should be discussed by the supervising physician at the inception of the programme so that management and labour can discuss their strategy before the event. If this is done it is often possible to introduce a probationary period of employment. Thereafter hearing tests should be undertaken at annual intervals. These serve several purposes. If there is great change in hearing—particularly in one ear—it is likely that its cause is ear disease unrelated to employment. The workman should be referred for appropriate diagnosis and therapy if necessary. The writer has seen two patients in whom hearing loss progressed more rapidly in one ear, which was documented in serial audiograms which were not acted upon until years later when the diagnosis of acoustic neuroma was quite clear (*Figure 18.17*). A greater than average decrease in hearing thresholds may also reveal non-use of personal protective devices. The workman should be counselled. Averaging of audiograms of the total work force shows mean changes of hearing which give a good indication of the general effectiveness of hearing conservation measures.

A management which is willing to establish a hearing conservation programme is often understandably naive in knowing how to go about it. They are often unaware of the need for calibration of audiometric equipment or of the limitations of the testing. It may be remarkably difficult to find sufficiently quiet quarters in a plant to undertake hearing testing, and it is usually necessary to install one or more soundproof booths or alternatively to use mobile soundproofed equipment. There are many manufacturers who offer mobile equipment based either in truck bodies, trailers or caravans appropriately modified to attenuate sound. The amount of attenuation required for the enclosures, whether they be permanent or mobile, is dependent upon the ambient noise levels. As only air-conduction hearing tests are undertaken, the attenuating effect of the earphone cushions is a factor so that levels can be higher than

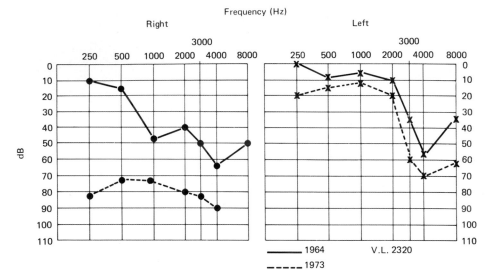

Figure 18.17 Serial audiograms submitted with a pension claim of a man who had been a hard rock miner for 20 years. The asymmetry was investigated, and found to be due to an acoustic neuroma which was successfully removed

if free field or bone tests were also undertaken. The matters are comprehensively dealt with in a paper by Shipton and Robinson (1975).

The type of equipment used has varied from simple manual audiometers to discrete frequency semi-automatic recording audiometers, of which there are several manufacturers. In plants where many are to be examined it is often the custom to have multiple test stations with six employees being tested simultaneously.

Two practical problems of industrial audiometry are the timing of the test and the storage of records. It was originally believed that all tests should be undertaken in a rested ear (16 or preferably 48 h out of noise), and thus before the work starts— preferably on Monday morning after a weekend away. This approach whilst theoretically correct, is quite impractical, leading to long lineups of men waiting for hearing tests, often several hours, and effectively taking them away from work for half a day or more. It is now believed, particularly with the advent of relatively effective personal protection programmes, that the screening testing can take place at any time of the day. If a workman's hearing has changed significantly then he should be brought back for the specially-rested periods, such as Monday morning. There is good evidence to suggest that with relatively effective hearing protection programmes a wait of no more than 15 min is enough to minimize the temporary threshold shift (Anderson *et al.*, 1974).

The question of record storage, particularly in middle-sized plants, has bedevilled hearing conservation programmes and bankrupted many companies offering this service on contract to industry. In small plants manual record keeping is adequate as long as the audiograms are stored in digital form, preferably on one piece of paper, so that changes can be readily appreciated. Anyone who has attempted to compare the results of 20 consecutive annual self-recording audiograms from one patient knows the type of difficulty encountered! Visual scanning and hand-sorting of records is adequate for one visit, but difficult if comparison is to be made; some form of mechanical storage is virtually obligatory. Larger companies usually have their own computers and personnel identification numbers for their workmen. It is a relatively simple matter to enter the results of audiograms each day and to devise programmes which will print out changes in hearing; identify people with abnormal hearing; and also undertake the epidemiological evaluations required. A common practice is to print out the first, the most recent (usually one year old) and the current test. Service companies performing hearing conservation programmes should be prepared to provide this type of record storage themselves, even though it frequently means a two-stage procedure after the audiogram has been obtained. The usual output of the self-recording audiogram must be converted by a trained observer into digital form for each frequency, and the digital form must then be encoded for entry into computer—either directly into a terminal or by producing a punch card. There are signs of tentative steps amongst audiometer manufacturers to produce devices which undertake this transfer automatically, but they are not yet widely available.

The question of which frequencies to test in a hearing screening programme continues to be raised. Conventionally the screening audiogram involves the frequencies 500, 1000, 2000 and 4000 Hz. There are many legislations in which 3000 Hz, and some in which 6000 Hz is compensated. Therefore these may be included. The very minimum initial test should include all the frequencies currently compensated in that particular area, and any which there is reasonable likelihood of being added in the future. Mills (1976b) makes a very appealing argument for limitation of the frequencies at which continuous hearing monitoring audiometry is undertaken. Once a baseline audiogram has been obtained he suggests that the efficiency of monitoring audiometry would be significantly increased if subsequent tests in those with normal audiograms, were only performed at 4 kHz, on the basis that if there is no change at this frequency there will be no change at any other frequency from noise exposure. He suggests that on the other hand after ten years in intense noise when there may already be a significant change at 4 kHz, it is unlikely that a further change will occur there, and the testing should be concentrated at 2 kHz. The only problem with this approach is that the annual test will fail to detect changes due to causes other than noise. It is important to detect these so that employers' liability may be limited to noise-induced hearing loss. This is one of the ways in which monitoring audiometry can be shown to pay for itself—something which is a prime consideration in the eyes of management. Some of the practical problems involved in industrial audiometry and its limitations are well outlined in papers by Robinson, Shipton and Whittle (1973, 1975).

Personal hearing protection

Personal protective devices are the cheapest, although perhaps not the most effective way, of preventing hearing loss from noise. It is likely that where noise levels remain hazardous and the workman cannot be isolated, a programme of personal hearing protection must be embarked upon. These require considerable propaganda to be accepted, although where both labour and management give their full backing, it is surprising how well they are received. There has been a recent tendency in the labour movement in North America and in some European countries, to fight for better health as well as more pay for their members. Where this has taken place, as for example in some Scandinavian shipyards, and amongst United Steelworkers' Union and United Autoworkers' Union in North America, the attitude of labour has changed dramatically in regard to the use of safety measures, including hearing protectors. Whereas even ten years ago the machismo image of the worker was preserved by ignoring safety procedures, at present in many plants the worker who ignores the safety features is himself ignored and considered stupid. Such programmes require full cooperation of management, who must also be seen to comply—including the plant physician. The physician who does not wear hearing protecting devices himself can hardly expect workers under his care to use them. This physician, often an otologist, involved in hearing conservation programmes, must be prepared to talk to management and labour and spend time in explaining the problems and hazards of hearing loss as well as techniques of prevention. In some industries they will be the only form of protection available, and in many others they will be required to complement engineering controls. In more and more jurisdictions employers are obliged to provide *adequate* hearing protective devices if noise levels are considered to be hazardous. A recent count in the USA showed 189 different types of commercially available hearing protectors, plugs or muffs, and that was only a sampling! This is an indication that no single device is perfect. Many factors enter into the choice of the appropriate type of protector including individual preference, the need to wear other protective devices, durability, hygiene, etc. Some of these items will be examined further.

The cheapest and most commonly used type of protector is a prefabricated earplug. They are usually made of soft plastic, and there are two particularly commonly used types—one based upon the wartime V-51R, an asymmetrical single flanged plug which is made in five sizes which adapt well to the vagaries of the human ear canal. The other commonly used soft plastic plug is the so-called 'fircone' or 'Com-fit' which in its various forms has two or three soft flanges which effectively seal the ear canal. Many workers find earplugs uncomfortable, at least initially, and care must be taken to ensure that they use plugs of adequate size, i.e. ones that may be relatively uncomfortable at first fitting. Fortunately the skin of the ear canal usually hardens and what was initially almost an intolerable burden becomes acceptable later on. A modern version of the earplug is the foam polyurethane plug, sold under the trademark 'EAR' or 'Deci-damp.' These cylindrical plugs can be compressed so that they fit easily into the ear canal and over a period of 2 min expand to fit the shape of the canal, sealing it comfortably but tightly. Care must be taken that they are inserted far enough in so that jaw movements do not work them out, and that they are held in place whilst expansion occurs. Whilst effective, they may be difficult to remove. From a hygiene standpoint they are cheap enough to be disposable, although if there is not much dust and dirt around they can be washed. A wide range of non-plastic disposable plugs have been used, of which an old favourite is waxed cotton. This is effective if the plug is well inserted, but tends to loosen with jaw movements; cotton wool is wholly ineffective. A compound which looks like cotton wool, mineral wool, is made up of fine fibreglass down threads and is effective if properly inserted. It is disposable but the conical plugs must be folded accurately to produce maximum effect. There are many people who find the fibreglass irritating to the skin of the ear canal and they have been largely superseded by the polyurethane plugs. A newer version covers the glass down with a thin plastic film.

Individually moulded plugs have had their advocates in North America. They appear like soft hearing aid earmoulds and are made of silicone rubber to which a curing agent has been added. They can be fitted with handles so that they are easy to remove. They are relatively expensive to make and in our experience whilst potentially good, in practice are the least effective of all hearing protectors we have tested (*see below*).

Semi-insert hearing protectors, the so-called 'Glorig' which consists of earplugs on a spring, are used where the plugs are required intermittently and where muffs are unacceptable. Some shipyards and mines have used them for intermittent noise exposure, and they are also in use in the food-handling industry where a muff would be inappropriate because of the need to wear a net over the hair, but where the fear of dropping plugs into food is a real one! They are difficult to fit properly and require considerable spring tension.

Theoretically the most effective type of hearing protector is the earmuff. This consists of a cup worn around the ear filled with a sound absorbing material, sealed to the side of the head by malleable plastic or rubber gasket. Because of the uneven shaping of the head, the gasket is preferably filled with liquid or, nearly as good, with foam rubber. The muffs must be pressed to the side of the head, and are therefore worn with spring bands. There are many types of muff available including ones which are specific to right and left ear, and thus must be fitted with care; as well as ones that fit under hard hats, either by having a separate spring band behind the neck or by being affixed directly to the hard hat. The most sophisticated, effective, and expensive muffs are those built directly into the flying helmets of modern jet fighter pilots. These have attenuation figures close to the theoretical maximum, and in addition may contain intercom units. It is probable that this type of military device will find a role in industry because current muffs and hard hat combinations are interfered with by other safety devices such as safety glasses and respirators.

Anything that breaks the seal between an earmuff and the side of the head reduces the amount of attenuation available. The need to wear safety glasses was originally not a serious drawback because the arms were made of flat metal. However in many industries metal arms are not allowed for fear of electrocution and have been replaced with thick plastic. This immediately reduces the attenuation of the muff. The current fashion of wearing long hair also reduces the seal between the muff and the head and has made the muffs significantly less effective in practice than their optimum attenuation figures suggest.

Theoretical limitations of personal hearing protection are the level at which bone conduction becomes the dominant factor. In sufficiently high sound levels both the earplug and earmuff vibrate and conduct a sound to the ear both by bone and air. In theory it is unlikely that attenuation of more than 25 dB in the lower frequencies and 40 dB in the higher frequencies is possible with a plug, or 30 dB in the lower frequencies and 50 dB in the higher frequencies with a muff. In practice these figures are rarely, if ever, reached. Some of the scientific bases of hearing protection attenuation have been reviewed by Shaw and Thiessen (1976) and should be referred to. The acoustics of circumaural earphones are fully described by Shaw and Thiessen (1962). A detailed review of various problems related to personal hearing protection and hearing conservation is given by Martin (1976b) which is both comprehensive and informative.

How effective are hearing protectors in practice? There is often a large gap between the test laboratory and the factory floor, and this is well exemplified with hearing

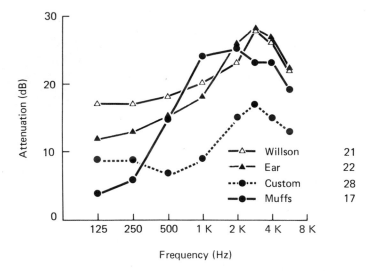

Figure 18.18 Mean attenuation characteristics of three types of earplugs and a group of earmuffs, as issued to industrial workers, and fitted by them. (From Riko, K., Abel, S. M. and Alberti, P. W. *Journal of Otolaryngology*, 1979. In press)

protectors. We have recently carried out a study of the attenuation of hearing protectors issued to men in their place of work, frequently worn for long periods and at the time of study fitted by the men as they would fit it themselves at work. The results are disappointing. *Figure 18.18* shows the mean attenuation characteristics of three types of plug and a group of muffs. It can be seen that the muffs are hardly better than the best plugs, and the personalized protective devices are significantly worse than the others. *Figure 18.19* shows the average attenuation for 102 plugs ± 1 standard deviation. These figures show that the best fitting plugs are extremely effective but that the worst plugs give extremely poor attenuation.

The reasons for this are manifold. The plug may be of the wrong size, or more commonly it is incorrectly inserted. Many men are unwilling to put them fully into the ear and frequently in the case of the custom-moulded plugs merely rest them against the pinna. The custom-moulded plugs shrank with ageing and often had sections cut off where they were uncomfortable! Foam rubber plugs were not inserted far enough or came out with jaw movement, and the same was true of waxed plugs. Muffs had broken seals, and large dents occurred where safety glasses had been applied or springs bent back to relieve pressure on the head. It is thus apparent that in practice the attenuation figures obtained are much less than the theoretical maximum promulgated by the manufacturers. The type of hearing protector required and the effective amount of protection provided for a work force is not to be determined by maximum attenuation figures or even by mean attenuation figures. The effective attenuation for a work force is at best one standard deviation below the mean attenuation. It can readily be appreciated that protectors with large standard deviations of effectiveness are less useful for a population than ones with similar or even lower mean protection, but smaller individual variability in the amount of protection provided. In our experience (although not in all others), the variability of protection afforded by muffs is as great as the better plugs.

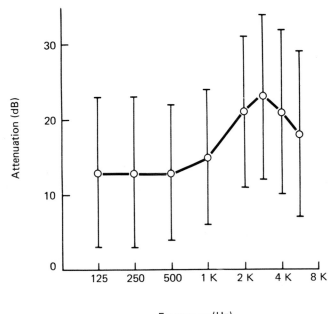

Figure 18.19　Average attenuation of 102 earplugs, ±1 standard deviation. Plugs as issued to workmen and fitted by themselves. (From Riko, K., Abel, S. M. and Alberti, P. W. *Journal of Otolaryngology*, 1979. In press)

Any programme of hearing conservation requires constant education and monitoring of the use of the protective devices. The plant nurse must be skilled in fitting, training, and encouraging workers to use the devices appropriately.

The question of communication in noise is frequently raised. Workers fear that they will be unable to hear warning signals and that they cannot hear conversation when wearing protector devices. Arguments rage but certain studies, and notably those reported by Martin (1976c) who also reviews other work in the field and published work from our own laboratory (Abel *et al.*, 1977), lead to the following conclusions:

(1) Hearing protectors do not remove all sound; they are to be likened to sunglasses which remove some of the brightness from vision without obliterating what the eye is seeing completely.
(2) If the signal is loud enough to be heard above background noise, then it will be heard by those wearing hearing protectors.
(3) A signal of sound spectrum totally different from the background noise may be discernible to the unprotected ear at a low intensity and be masked by hearing protectors.

The question of speech communication is relatively simple. Someone talking above the level of background noise should be heard and understood by a normal-hearing subject wearing hearing protectors. If two normal-hearing persons are conversing each wearing hearing protectors, then because of the speaker's use of protectors his voice will be lowered because he hears less background noise against which to raise it. He may then be inaudible. The matter is more complicated in those with a pre-existing hearing loss, particularly of a high frequency type. *Figures 18.18* and *18.19* demonstrate graphically that maximum attenuation is produced in the higher frequencies. When this is added to a pre-existing high frequency loss it becomes a precipitous drop. Martin's and our own experiments show that speech discrimination in a background of noise is markedly worse when compared with normal-hearing subjects both with and without hearing protection, but is probably worsened by the hearing protector. Thus the person with a pre-existing hearing loss introduced into a hearing protection programme may suffer real degradation in communication.

To be effective hearing protectors must be worn all the time, for even short periods of non-compliance in high noise effectively reduces the protection by considerable amounts. An example given by Martin (1976b) shows that hearing protectors with an effective attenuation of 30 dB worn in an environment of 115 dBA reduce sound levels at the wearer's ears to 85 dBA. If the user fails to wear them for a total of only 10 min he will be exposed to 115 dBA for 10 min, which is equal to L eq of 98 dBA for 8 h, and the effective protection has thus been reduced from 30 dBA–17dBA. Not only must hearing protection be worn—it must be worn continuously.

Medical–legal and social implications

There are many complicated and interrelated questions which confuse the student attempting to understand the practical implications of these problems. What is a safe level of noise at which no hearing loss occurs? What is the probability for any given noise that any particular amount of hearing loss occurs? How should one define social handicap in terms of hearing loss? How can one measure social handicap in hearing? If compensation laws are introduced, what should be compensated? Hearing loss? social handicap? loss of earning power? von Gierke and Johnson (1976) summarize many of these points. Many problems arise from a lack of basic knowledge and major differences in philosophy between various investigators.

It is still not clear how hearing changes throughout life in a completely ear-disease-free and non-noise exposed population. Without this knowledge it is difficult to have a yardstick against which to compare noise-exposed populations. Most major surveys, including the US Public Health Service Survey which is frequently used as a standard, included people with ear disease and noise exposure. Even if this sort of information were available there is no clear answer to the question as to what percentage of the population should be protected. Does the risk to hearing in the population follow a normalized distribution, or are there certain ears that are pathologically sensitive to the effect of noise which should be excluded from general statements? Is the discussion about 100 per cent protection, or 95 per cent protection? What is one trying to protect? All hearing at all frequencies or hearing only in the so-called 'speech frequencies'? What indeed are the speech frequencies? Many of these factors are discussed in detail in a NIOSH criteria document (1973), which gives an extensive background and well-argued conclusions.

The American Academy of Ophthalmology and Otolaryngology (1964) have suggested that all that is important are the frequencies 500–2000 Hz, and their utterances have been inscribed into law in many American states, although the AAOO is re-examining the question. Many other equally prestigious authorities suggest that higher frequencies are important and they are used for compensation assessment in certain American jurisdictions, in various Canadian provinces, in Great Britain, and in Europe. The question of 3000 Hz and/or 4000 Hz highlights one problem. If the hearing *loss* is to be compensated, sensitive 4000 Hz must be included. If hearing *handicap* is being compensated it is probably adequate to include only 3000 Hz.

To prevent any damage to hearing over a 40-year work exposure, noise levels should be below 73 dBA. It has rightly been pointed out that few people work in high noise for 40 years and that it is unrealistic to protect all of the population. It is also apparent that a significant proportion of the population will have some hearing damage in the high frequencies to exposures of 85 dBA for 40 years. This therefore makes a convenient starting point for safety regulations if it is accepted that all frequencies must be protected. This is certainly not accepted in all jurisdictions, and there are cogent arguments that suggest that too much attention has been paid to hearing at 4000 Hz.

The DRC codified in ISO 1999 have also come under attack, so that a separate British standard has been issued (BSI, 1976). Burns *et al.* (1977) give detailed arguments why they believe the British standard is preferable to the International one, which include a critique of American audiological techniques and population selection. In their conclusions they point out one of the major problems experienced in all of this type of work—the relative inaccuracy of audiometric threshold testing.

The equal energy concept has been described earlier, in which it is stated that if sound energy to which a subject is exposed is doubled then the equivalent safe period of exposure should be halved. This has given rise to a 3-dB halving, i.e. whatever sound level is deemed safe for an 8-h exposure, a level of 3 dB higher is safe for a 4-h exposure, although this is not universally accepted. It is possible that the 3 dB is more accurate for higher frequencies and 5 dB for lower frequencies (von Gierke and Johnson, 1976).

It is little wonder that legislators have taken quite empirical attitudes to many of these problems, 5-dB halving is enshrined in most American law, in Britain a 3-dB halving has been adopted. Some jurisdictions use a 4-dB halving, arrived at on the basis of hard bargaining between the various experts! There is a wide range of baselines for a 'safe' 8-h daily exposure. The American EPA have recommended an 80-dBA baseline; NIOSH have recommended an 85-dBA baseline; most American states and Canadian provinces still use 90 dBA!

Compensation

Traumatic hearing loss, i.e. hearing loss caused by head injury or a single traumatic episode, has been compensable in many parts of the world since the early parts of the twentieth century. Hearing loss from prolonged noise exposure became compensable for war veterans in many parts of the western world, although the facilities for testing hearing varied enormously from country to country. As a result of this change in philosophy hearing loss caused by prolonged exposure to industrial noise became compensable in the late 1940s in one American state, and in one Canadian province. Gradually the areas covered increased so that by the mid-1960s many of the American states and all of Canada was covered. European countries also varied in the speed with which hearing loss was compensated. In 1975 hearing loss from noise became a prescribed industrial disease in certain industries in the UK, although for pragmatic reasons it was not open to workers in all noisy industries.

Legislators have faced several problems. How would hearing loss be measured for compensation purposes? How was hearing handicap to be defined, and was hearing loss or handicap to be compensated? Most jurisdictions have opted to compensate hearing handicap, so the concept of a low fence was introduced, a level of hearing beneath which no 'handicap' existed, even though the hearing level itself was not normal. The American Academy of Ophthalmology and Otolaryngology adopted a 25-dB average in the better ear at 500, 1000 and 2000 Hz. The province of Ontario in Canada initially (in 1948) adopted a 25-dB average at 500, 1000 and 2000 Hz at an ASA audiometric standard which is equivalent to approximately a 35-dB low fence in ISO terms. This has recently been amended to include 3000 Hz. In Britain a 40-dB low fence has been adopted for average hearing at 1000, 2000 and 3000 Hz. In California when this matter was being debated there was adamant union pressure to include 4000 Hz, and equally adamant management pressure to exclude it. A compromise was arrived at which averaged 500, 1000, 2000 and 3000 Hz, also with a 25-dB low fence. In Australia a complex weighting system has been adopted which includes many more frequencies in the compensation schedule, but the philosophy in that country is much more to compensate all hearing loss rather than handicap.

At what frequencies to start compensating is only the beginning. There are many schemes to determine how to assess a percentage hearing loss, varying points at which 100 per cent hearing loss is reached ranging from 80 to more than 90 dB, and a variety of methods—both linear and non-linear—for getting there. Presbyacusis corrections of different types are frequently applied. These matters and their effects on a population with noise-induced hearing loss are discussed in some detail in a paper by Alberti *et al.* (1976). The audiograms of 964 patients who had been referred for compensation assessment were compared to see how they would fare under various laws. The mean percentage hearing loss in terms of compensation ranged from a low of 13.8 per cent under a presbyacusis corrected AAOO formula, to a 41 per cent loss in Australia. In addition jurisdictions vary on how 100 per cent hearing loss is converted to handicap. In Britain 100 per cent hearing loss is equivalent to 100 per cent disability; in the Province of British Columbia, Canada, a total hearing loss rates only 15 per cent whole-body disability; whilst other jurisdictions include values of 30, 40 or 50 per cent.

The method of applying a presbyacusis correction also varies widely—some American states correct by 0.5 dB/year above the age of 40, some age 50, in Ontario age 60, and others weight differently at each frequency.

Probably the biggest factor in ultimate economic terms is the time for which a pension is paid, which is dictated by compensation philosophy. Some are prepared to pay whilst a workman is retrained for work requiring less hearing. Examples of this school are the many American states which compensate for a maximum period of 300 weeks. Others compensate for loss of earning power and go on until normal retirement age. Some compensate for loss of quality of life and compensate a handicapped hard-of-hearing person for life; Britain and the Canadian provinces are appropriate examples. An occasional jurisdiction compensates for the loss of hearing and compensates virtually any shift from the normal, whether there is an occupational or social handicap or not. This is best exemplified by the current Australian schemes (Alberti *et al*, 1976).

The actual weekly payment may be related to a basic disability pension and/or to the worker's income, sometimes to a maximum limit, sometimes not. Thus a fixed percentage disability may lead to a wide range of weekly payments and the total amount of money received by a claimant depends not only upon the percentage hearing loss but on his age, and the length of time for which the funds are to be paid— a scheme which appears to compensate in a niggardly manner may in fact be extremely generous in the long term.

So far only the question of compensating a pure-tone hearing loss has been discussed. The relationship between this and hearing handicap exists, but is indirect. Much depends upon the personality and social situation of the hard-of-hearing person; the previously extroverted person whose social life was all talk and whose work was mixing with people and selling may well be more handicapped than the quiet withdrawn scholar happy in libraries and shy with people. There have been attempts to codify social handicap and hearing loss by means of a questionnaire, which for industrial purposes include two prime examples, those of Atherley and Noble (1971) and of Kell and his colleagues (1971). The quite simple scale of Kell relates reasonably well to the results of pure-tone audiometry (Coles, 1975). The Atherley and Noble questionnaire is extremely detailed and time-consuming, and a skilled interviewer is required. The length of time taken to administer the test is however probably no longer than that required for a full audiometric evaluation and the length of training for the tester no greater than that for an audiologist.

However, there are so many variables in the presentation of questionnaires that hearing handicap scales based upon them are only useful for investigational purposes. They are still impractical for compensation use. Handicap questionnaires are much more important in the evaluation of rehabilitation with hearing aids.

The financial aspects of industrial hearing loss cannot be ignored, for they represent vast sums of money. It has been suggested that in the manufacturing industries alone in the USA it would cost 11 billion dollars to comply with a maximum 90 dBA level in the work place, and a further 8 billion dollars to comply with an 85 dBA work place noise level, even if spread over some years. This totally ignores military noise exposure and the resource industries. The cost of compensation for hearing loss is also extremely high, e.g. in Ontario, as was previously described, there are currently approximately 2500 new claims for industrial hearing loss/year in a population of 8 million, of which approximately 1000 are pensioned, the average pension paid/workman over his lifetime is $15,000. As the pensions are charged back to the industries in which the damage occurred, the costs can be very significant. It is against this type of background that hearing conservation programmes must be evaluated, and the cost of personal protective devices is relatively low compared with these figures.

Conclusions

Unwanted sound is very much part of the western world. It must not be concluded however that all sound is bad—indeed the aim of the otologist working with excessive noise is to preserve hearing so that wanted sounds can be heard. The composer and philosopher Murray Schafer (1977) has written a book in which he puts sounds into perspective—good sounds and bad sounds, historical sounds and current sounds, western sounds and third-world sounds. He, a musician, described the importance of sound to man when he describes the soundscape of the world and starts as this chapter ends by quoting Walter Whitman:

> 'Now I will do nothing but listen . . .
> I hear all sounds running together, combined,
>   fused or following,
> Sounds of the city and sounds out of the city,
> Sounds of the day and night . . .'

References

AAOO (1964). 'Guide for conservation of hearing in Noise', *Transactions of American Academy of Ophthalmology and Otolaryngology*, Suppl.

Abel, S. M., Alberti, P. W., Riko, K. and Madsen, R. (1977). *Journal of the Acoustic Society of America*, **62**, Suppl. 1, 575

Abey-Wickram, I., a'Brook, M. F., Gattoni, F. E. G. and Herridge, C. F. (1969). *Lancet*, **2**, 1275

Alberti, P. W. (1970). *Annals of Otology, Rhinology and Laryngology*, St. Louis, **79**, 800

Alberti, P. W. and Morgan, P. P. (1974). *Laryngoscope*, **84**, 1822

Alberti, P. W., Morgan, P. P. and Czuba, I. (1978). *Acta otolaryngologica, Stockholm*, **25**, 328

Alberti, P. W., Morgan, P. P., Fria, T. J. and Leblanc, J. C. (1976). In *Effects of Noise on Hearing*. Ed. by D. Henderson, J. Hamernik *et al.* New York; Raven Press

Alberti, P. W., Symons, F. M. and Hyde, H. L. (1979). *Acta otolaryngologica, Stockholm*, (In press)

Alford, B. R., Jerger, F. J., Coats, A. C., Billingham, J., French, B. O. and McBrayer, R. O. (1966). *Transactions of the American Academy of Ophthalmology*, **70**, 40

Anderson, E. L., Sataloff, J., Vassallo, L. and Menduke, H. (1974). *American Industrial Hygiene Journal*, **35**, 223

Atherley, G. R. C. and Noble, W. G. (1971). In *Occupational Hearing Loss*. Ed. by D. W. Robinson. London; Academic Press

Barr, T. (1886). *Transactions of the Philosophy Society of Glasgow*, **17**, 223

Baughn, W. L. (1966). *International Audiology*, **51**, 331

Baxter, J. D. and Ling, D. (1974). *Canadian Journal of Otology*, **3**, 110

Beagley, H. A. (1965a). *Acta otolaryngologica, Stockholm*, **60**, 437

Beagley, H. A. (1965b). *Acta otolaryngologica, Stockholm*, **60**, 479

Békésy, G. von (1953). *Journal of the Acoustic Society of America*, **25**, 770

Békésy, G. von (1960). *Experiments in Hearing*. New York; McGraw-Hill

Bell, A. (1966). *Noise—An Occupational Hazard and Public Nuisance*. Geneva; WHO

Benjamins, C. E. (1938). *Acta otolaryngologica, Stockholm*, **26**, 249

Bess, F. H. and Powell, R. L. (1972). *Clinical Paediatrics*, **11**, 61

Bess, F. H. and Poyner, R. E. (1974). *Archives of Otolaryngology*, **99**, 45

Bleeker, J. D. and de Vries, H. L. (1949). *Acta otolaryngologica, Stockholm*, **37**, 287

Bohne, B. A. (1976). In *Effects of Noise on Hearing*. Ed. by D. Henderson *et al.* New York; Raven Press

Bohne, B. A., Ward, P. H. and Fernandez, C. (1976). *Transactions of the American Academy of Ophthalmology and Otolaryngology*, **82**, 50

Bohne, B. A., Ward, P. H. and Fernandez, C. (1978). *Audiology and Hearing Education*, **4**, 8

Borg, E. (1976). In *Acoustics Impedance and Admittance*. Ed. by A. S. Feldman and L. A. Wilber. Baltimore; Williams & Wilkins

Bredberg, G. (1967). *Journal of Laryngology*, **81**, 739

Bredberg, G. (1968). *Acta otolaryngologica, Stockholm*, Suppl. 236

Bredberg, G. (1977). *Acta otolaryngologica, Stockholm*, **83**, 71

Bredberg, G. and Hunter-Duvar, I. M. (1975). In *Handbook of Sensory Physiology*. Vol. 5. Part II. Ed. by W. D. Keidl and W. D. Neff. New York; Springer-Verlag

BSI (1976). *Method of estimating the risk of hearing handicap due to noise exposure*. BS5-330, British Standards Institution

Bunch, C. C. (1929). *Archives of Otolaryngology*, **9**, 625

Bunch, C. C. (1937). *Laryngoscope*, **47**, 615

Burns, W., Hinchcliffe, R. and Littler, T. S. (1964). *Annals of occupational Hygiene*, **7**, 323

Burns, W., Hinchcliffe, R. and Littler, T. S. (1968). *Noise and Man*, 1st edn. London; John Murray

Burns, W., Hinchcliffe, R., Littler, T. S. and Robinson, D. W. (1970). *Hearing and Noise in Industry*. London; HMSO

Burns, W., Hinchcliffe, R., Littler, T. S. and Robinson, D. W. (1973). *Noise and Man*, 2nd edn. London; John Murray

Burns, W., Hinchcliffe, R., Littler, T. S., Robinson, D. W., Shipton, M. S. and Sinclair,

A. (1977). *National Physics Laboratory Report* AC80

Camis, M. (1930). *Physiology of the Vestibular Apparatus*. Oxford; Clarendon Press

Cantrell, R. W. (1975a). *Agard Conference Proceedings No. 171*. p. C10.01 France; NATO

Cantrell, R. W. (1975b). *Agard Conference Proceedings No. 171*. p. C11.10. France; NATO

Cawthorne, T. (1949). *Acta otolaryngologica*, Stockholm, Suppl. **78**, 145

Chadwick, D. L. (1966). *Proceedings of the Royal Society of Medicine*, **59**, 957

Chaney, R. B. Jr., McClain, S. E. and Housen, R. (1973). *Journal of the Acoustical Society of America*, **54**, 1219

Chueden, H. and Strauss, P. (1974). *Monatsschrift fur Ohrenheilkunde u. Laryngo-Rhinologie*, **108**, 377

Cody, D. T. R., Simonton, K. M. and Hallberg, O. E. (1967). *Laryngoscope*, **77**, 480

Cohen, A. (1973). *Proceedings of the International Congress on Noise as a Public Health Problem*, Washington, D.C.; US Environmental Protection Agency

Coles, R. R. A. (1963). *Journal of the Royal Naval Medical Services*, **49**, 1

Coles, R. R. A. and Rice, C. G. (1966). *Journal of Sound Vibration*, **4**, 172

Coles, R. R. A. (1968). *Philosophical Transactions of the Royal Society* A, **263**, 289

Coles, R. R. A. (1975). In *Sound Reception in Mammals*. Ed. by R. J. Bench, A. Pye and J. D. Pye. London; Academic Press

Corso, J. F. (1976). In *Effects of Noise on Hearing*. Ed. by D. Henderson *et al*. New York; Raven Press

Darbyshire, J. O. (1976). *British Journal of Audiology*, **10**, 74

Davis, H., Fernandez, C., Covell, W. P., Legouix, J.-P. and McAuliffe, D. R. (1953). *Journal of the Acoustic Society of America*, **25**, 1180

Davis, H., Fernandez, C., Covell, W. P., Legouix, J.-P. and McAuliffe, D. R. (1954). *Proceedings of the Fourth Panamerican Congress on Oto-rhino-laryngology*

Davis, H., Fernandez, C., Covell, W. P., Legouix, J.-P. and McAuliffe, D. T. (1957). *Physiology Review*, **37**, 1

Davis, H., Fernandez, C., Covell, W. P., Legouix, J.-P., McAuliffe, D. R., Deatherage, B. H., Rosenblut, B., Fernandez, C., Kimura, R. and Smith, C. A. (1958). *Laryngoscope*, **68**, 596

Davis, H., Fernandez, C., Covell, W. P., Legouix, J.-P., McAuliffe, D. R. (1976). *Annals of Otology, Rhinology and Laryngology*, St. Louis, Suppl. 28

Dayal, V. S., Kokshanian, A. and Mitchell, D. P. (1971). *Annals of Otology, Rhinology and Laryngology, St. Louis*, **80**, 897

Deetjen, H. (1899). *Zeitschrift fur Biologie*, **39**, 159

Dickson, E. D. D., Ewing, A. W. G. and Littler, T. S. (1939). *Journal of Laryngology*, **54**, 531

Dreschner, D. G. (1976). In *Effects of Noise on Hearing*. Ed. by D. Henderson *et al*. New York; Raven Press

Ducel, G., Suter, T. and Dupont, B. (1976). *Sozial Praventiv Medizin*, **21**, 135

Durant, John D. (1976). In *Effects of Noise on Hearing*. Ed. by D. Henderson *et al*. New York; Raven Press

Duvall, A. J., Sutherland, C. R. and Rhodes, V. T. (1969). *Annals of Otology, Rhinology and Laryngology*, St. Louis, **78**, 432

Duvall, A. J., Sutherland, C. R., Rhodes, V. T., Ward, W. D. and Lauhala, K. E. (1974). *Annals of Otology, Rhinology and Laryngology*, St. Louis, **83**, 498

Eldredge, D. H. and Covell, W. P. (1958). *Laryngoscope*, **68**, 465

Engstrom, H., Ades, J. W. and Andersson, A. (1966). *Structural Pattern of the Organ of Corti*. Baltimore; Williams & Wilkins

Evans, M. (1969). Perception of Sounds— Infrasonic to Ultrasonic. *British Society of Audiology Meeting*

Evans, E. F. (1976). In *Effects of Noise on Hearing*. Ed. by D. Henderson *et al*. New York; Raven Press

Fearn, R. W. (1973). *Journal of Sound Vibration*, **29**, 396

Fife, D. and Rappaport, E. (1976). *American Journal of Public Health*, **66**, 680

Fletcher, J. L. and Gross, C. W. (1977). *Sound & Vibration*, **11**, 26

Fosbroke, J. (1831). *Lancet*, **1**, 645

Fowler, E. P. (1929). *Transactions of the American Otology Society*, **19**, 182

Fowler, E. P. (1939). *Medicine of the Ear*. New York; Nelson

Gavreau, V., Condat, R. and Saul, H. (1966). *Acoustica*, **17**, 1

Gierke, H. E. von (1965). *Archives of Environmental Health*, **11**, 327

Gierke, H. E. von and Johnson, L. (1976). In *Effects of Noise on Hearing*. Ed. by D. Henderson *et al*. New York; Raven Press

Gjaevens, K., Moseng, J. and Nordahl, T. (1975). *Norske Laegeforen*, **95**, 776

Glorig, A. (1958). *Noise and Your Ear*. New York and London; Grune & Stratton

Glorig, A. and Davis, H. (1961). *Annals of Otology, Rhinology and Laryngology*, St. Louis, **70**, 556

Glorig, A. and Wheeler, E. (1955). *Illinois medical Journal*, **107**, 1

Glorig, A. and Ward, W. D. (1961). *Laryngoscope*, **71**, 1590

Goldman, D. E. and von Gierke, H. E. (1961). *Shock and Vibration Handbook*. Ed. by C. M. Harris and C. E. Crede. New York; McGraw-Hill

Habermann, J. (1890). *Archiv fur Ohrenheilkunde*, **30**, 1

Habermann, J. (1906). *Archiv fur Ohrenheilkunde*, **69**, 106

Hall, F. L., Breston, B. E. and Taylor, S. M. (1978). In *Noise Regulation Reporter*, No. 97. Washington, D.C.; Bureau of National Affairs Inc.

Hamernik, R. P. and Henderson, D. (1976). In *Effects of Noise on Hearing*. Ed. by D. Henderson *et al*. New York; Raven Press

Hansen, D. R. and Fern, R. W. (1975). *Lancet*, **2**, 203

Hawkins, J. E., Johnsson, L. G., Stebbins, W. C. *et al.* (1976). *Acta otolaryngologica, Stockholm*, **81**, 337

Henderson, D., Hamernik, R. P., Dosanj, D. S. and Mills, J. H. (1976). *Effects of Noise on Hearing.* New York; Raven Press

Henderson, D., Hamernik, R. P., Dosanj, D. S., Mills, J. H. and Crossley, J. (1974). *Laryngoscope*, **84**, 714

Henderson, D., Hamernik, R. P., Dosanj, D. S., Mills, J. H., Hynson, K. and Hamernik, R. P. (1977). *Journal of the Acoustic Society of America*, Suppl. 1., **62**, S34

Hinchcliffe, R. (1958). *Gerontologica*, **2**, 311

Hinchcliffe, R. (1967). *Proceedings of the Royal Society of Medicine*, **60**, 1111

Hood, J. D. (1950). *Acta laryngologica, Stockholm*, Suppl. 92

Hughes, K. B. (1976). *Journal of Laryngology*, **90**, 803

Huizinga, E. (1934). *Pflügers Archiv fur die gesamnte Physiologie des Menschen und der Tiere*, **234**, 665

Huizinga, E. (1935). *Acta otolaryngologica, Stockholm*, **22**, 359

Huizinga, E. (1936). *Pflügers Archiv fur die gesamnte Physiologie des Menschen und der Tiere*, **145**, 447

Huizinga, E. (1952). *Acta otolaryngologica, Stockholm*, Suppl. **100**, 174

Hunter-Duvar, I. M. (1978). *Proceedings of Fourteenth Workship in Inner Ear Biology, 1977.* Paris; Institut National de la Santé et de la recherche Medicale

Hunter-Duvar, I. M. (1978). *Acta Otolaryngologica*, Suppl. 351

Igarashi, M. Schuknecht, H. F. and Myers, E. N. (1964). *Journal of laryngology*, **78**, 115

ISO Standard 1999. *Acoustics: Assessment of occupational noise exposure for hearing conservation purposes.* International Organization for Standardization. 1975–08–01

Jerger, J. F. and Lewis, N. (1975). *Archives of otolaryngology*, **101**, 480

Johnsson, L.-G., and Hawkins, J. E. (1976). *Annals of Otology, Rhinology and Laryngology*, St. Louis, **85**, 725

Kacker, S. K. and Hinchcliffe, R. (1970). *Journal of Laryngology*, **84**, 155

Kärjä, J. (1968). *Acta otolaryngologica, Stockholm*, Suppl. 241

Kelemen, G. (1962). *Acta otolaryngologica, Stockholm*, **55**, 365

Kell, R. L., Pearson, J. C. G., Acton, W. I. and Taylor, W. (1971). In *Occupational Hearing Loss.* Ed. by D. W. Robinson. London; Academic Press

Kerr, A. G. and Byrne, J. E. T. (1975). *Journal of Laryngology and Otology*, **89**, 131

Kiang, N. Y. S., Liberman, M. C. and Levine, R. A. (1976). *Annals of Otology, Rhinology and Laryngology, St. Louis*, **85**, 752

Klockhoff, I., Drettner, B. and Svedberg, A. (1974). *Audiology*, **13**, 326

Knight, J. J. and Coles, R. R. A. (1960). *Journal of the Acoustic Society of America*, **132**, 800

Knipschild, P. G. (1976). *Medische gevolgen von vliegtuiglawaai.* (M.D. thesis), University of Amsterdam

Koide, Y., Makato, Y., Masaru, K. Nakano, Y., Yoshikawa, Y., Nagaba, M. and Morimoto, M. (1960). *Annals of Otology, Rhinology and Laryngology, St. Louis*, **69**, 661

Konoshi, T., Butler, R. A. and Fernandez, C. (1961). *Journal of the Acoustic Society of America*, **33**, 349

Kryter, K. D. (1970). *Effects of Noise on Man.* New York; Academic Press

Kryter, K. D. (1976). In *Effects of Noise on Hearing.* Ed. by D. Henderson *et al.* New York; Raven Press

Kylin, B. (1960). *Acta otolaryngologica, Stockholm*, Suppl. **152**, 8

Kylen, P. and Arlinger, S. (1976). *Acta otolaryngologica*, **82**, 402

Kylen, P., Stjernvall, J.-E. and Arlinger, S. (1977). *Acta otolaryngologica*, **84**, 252

Land, F. T. (1957). *Journal of Laryngology*, 71

Larsen, B. (1953). *Journal of laryngology*, **67**, 536

League, R., Parker, J., Robertson, M. *et al.* (1972). *Preventive Medicine*, **1**, 231

Lebo, C. P. and Oliphant, E. E. (1968). *Laryngoscope*, **78**, 1211

Lehnhardt, E. (1960). *Acta otolaryngologica, Stockholm*, **52**, 438

Lehnhardt, E. (1965). *Archiv fur Ohren-, Nasen- u. Kehlkopfheilkunde*, **85**, 11

Lim, D. J. (1976). *Annals of Otology, Rhinology and Laryngology*, St. Louis, **85**, 742

Linsday, J. R. (1947). *Archives of otolaryngology*, **66**, 584

Lipscomb, D. M. (1969). *Archives of otolaryngology*, **90**, 545

Littler, T. S. (1966). *Proceedings of the Royal Society of Medicine*, **59**, 963

Lyon, R. H. (1973). *Lectures in Transportation Noise.* Cambridge, Mass; Grozier Publishing

McKenzie, D. (1916). *The City of Din.* London; Adlard

Maguire, N. S. and van Wagoner, R. S. (1977). *Dimensions in Health Services*, **54**, 16

Markides, A. (1971). *Sound*, **5**, 99

Martin, A. M. (1976a). In *Effects of Noise on Hearing.* Ed. by D. Henderson *et al.* New York; Raven Press

Martin, A. M. (1976b). In *Scientific Foundations of Otolaryngology.* Ed. by R. Hinchcliffe and D. Harrison. London; William Heineman Medical Books

Martin, A. M. (1976c). In *Disorders of Auditory Function II.* Ed. by S. D. G. Stevens. London; Academic Press

Melnick, W. (1976). In *Effects of Noise on Hearing.* Ed. by D. Henderson *et al.* New York; Raven Press

Miller, J. D., Watson, C. S. and Cavell, W. P. (1963). *Acta otolaryngologica, Stockholm*, Suppl. 176

Mills, J. H. (1976a). In *Effects of Noise on Hearing.* Ed. by D. Henderson *et al.* New York; Raven Press

Mills, J. H. (1976b). In *Hearing and Deafness*. Ed. by S. K. Hirsh, D. H. Eldridge, I. J. Hirsh and S. R. Silverman. St. Louis; Washington University Press

Mohr, G. C., Cole, J. N., Guild, E. and von Gierke, H. E. (1965). *Aero Space Medicine*, **36**, 817

Morrison, D., Schindler, R. A. and Wersall, J. (1975). *Acta otolaryngologica, Stockholm*, **79**, 11

Moulonguet, A. and Poncet, P. (1947). *Annals of otolaryngology*, **44**, 34

Murray, N. E. and Reid, G. (1946). *Journal of Laryngology*, **61**, 92

Nakamura, S. (1964). *Journal of Otorhinolaryngology Society of Japan*, **67**, 669

Neely, K. K. (1959). *Medical Services Journal of Canada*. **15**, 235

Neiger, M. and Fisch, U. (1967). *Schweizerische Zeitschrift Militarie Medizin*, **44**, 196

NIOSH (1973). *Criteria for recommended standard on occupational exposure to noise*: HSM 73-11001. US National Institute of Occupational Safety and Health

Noble, W. G. (1973). *Audiology*, **12**, 299

Onchi, Y. (1951). *Journal of the Otorhinolaryngology Society of Japan*, **54**, 493

Paparella, M. M., Oda, M., Hiraide, F. and Brady, D. (1972). *Annals of Otology, Rhinology and Laryngology, St. Louis*, **81**, 632

Parrack, H. O. (1966). *International Audiology*, **5**, 294

Paulsen, K. and Vietor, K. (1975a). *Archives of Otology, Rhinology and Laryngology*, **209**, 159

Paulsen, K. and Vietor, K. (1975b). *Laryngologie, Rhinologie und Otology, Grenzgeb*, **54**, 824

Peterson, A. G. P. and Gross, E. E. (1963). *Handbook of Noise Measurement*, West Concord, Mass.; General Radio Co.

Pfander, F. (1965). *HNO (Berlin)*, **13**, 27

Pfander, F. (1975). *Das Knalltrauma*. Berlin; Springer-Verlag

Ramazzini, B. (1713). Translated from the Latin *De Morbis Artificum* by W. C. Wright (1964) p. 438, New York; Hafner

Rice, C. G. (1969). Personal communication quoted by D. Chadwick in *Diseases of the Ear, Nose and Throat*. Ed. by J. Ballantyne & J. Groves, 3rd ed. 1971, London; Butterworth

Riko, K., Akel, S. M. and Alberti, P. W. (1979). *Journal of Otolaryngology* (In press)

Rintelmann, W. F., Lindberg, R. F. and Smitley, E. K. (1971). *Journal of the Acoustic Society of America*, **51**, 1249

Robinson, D. W. and Shipton, M. S. (1973). *National Physics Laboratory Report* AC61

Robinson, D. W., Shipton, M. S. and Whittle, L. S. (1973). *National Physics Laboratory Report* AC64

Robinson, D. W., Shipton, M. S. and Whittle, L. S. (1975). *National Physics Laboratory Report* AC71

Ruedi, L. and Furrer, W. (1947). *Das akustische Traume*. Basel; Karger

Sataloff, J. (1952). *Annals of otology*, **61**, 107

Salmivalli, A. (1967). *Acta otolaryngologica, Stockholm*, Suppl. 222

Schafer, R. Murray (1977). *Tuning of the world*. McClelland & Stewart

Schneider, E.-A. (1974). *Annals of Otology, Rhinology and Laryngology*, St. Louis, **83**, 406

Shaw, E. A. G. and Thiessen, G. J. (1962). *Journal of the Acoustical Society of America*, **34**, 1233

Shaw, E. A. G. and Thiessen, G. J. (1975). *Physics Today*, **28**, 46

Shaw, E. A. G. and Thiessen, G. J. (1976). Paper presented at Symposium on Hearing Protection at the National Physics Laboratory, Teddington, England. Ottawa, Canada; National Research Council

Shipton, M. S. and Robinson, D. W. (1975). *National Physics Laboratory Report* AC69

Smyth, G. D. L. (1977). *Annals of Otology, Rhinology and Laryngology*, St. Louis, **86**, 3

Sokolovski, A. (1969). *International Audiology*, **4**, 585

Spoendlin, H. (1972). *Acta otolaryngologica, Stockholm*, **73**, 235

Spoendlin, H. (1976). In *Effects of Noise on Hearing*. Ed. by D. Henderson *et al*. New York; Raven Press

Taylor, C. F. (1976). 'Hearing loss in new apprentices due to exposure to non-industrial noise'. *Journal of Social and Occupational Medicine*, **26**, 57

Taylor, W., Pearson, J. C. G., Mair, A. and Burns, W. (1965). *Journal of the Acoustic Society of America*, **38**, 113

Thalmann, R. R. (1976). In *Effects of Noise on Hearing*. Ed. by D. Henderson *et al*. New York; Raven Press

Thiessen, G. J. (1976). *Effects of Noise on Man*. Ottawa, Canada; National Research Council of Canada Publ. No. 15383

Titche, L. L., Windrem, E. O. and Starmer, W. T. (1977). *Annals of Otology*, **86**, 357

Tondorf, J. (1960). *Journal of the Acoustic Society of America*, **32**, 238

Tullio, P. (1929). *Das Ohr und die Entstehung der Sprache und Schrift*. Belin und Wien; Urban

Ulrich, R. F. and Pinheiro, M. L. (1974). *Acta otolaryngologica, Stockholm*, **77**, 51

Ventry, I. M. and Chaiklin, J. B. (1965). *Journal of Auditory Research*, **5**, 179

Ward, W. D. (1962). *Journal of the Acoustical Society of America*, **34**, 1230, 1610

Ward, W. D. (1963). In *Modern Developments in Audiology*. Ed. by J. Jerger. New York; Academic Press

Ward, W. D. (1969). *International Audiology*, **5**, 309

Ward, W. D. (1973). In *Modern Developments in Audiology*, 2nd edn. Ed. by J. Jerger. New York; Academic Press

Ward, W. D. (1976a). In *Hearing and Deafness*. Ed. by S. K. Hirsh, D. H. Eldredge *et al*. St. Louis; Washington University Press

Ward, W. D. (1976b). In *Effects of Noise on Hearing*. Ed. by D. Henderson *et al*. New York; Raven Press

Ward, W. D. (1977). In *Handbook of Physiology*, Vol. 9. Ed. by D. H. K. Lee. Baltimore, Md.; American Physiological Society

Weber, H. L., McGovern, F. J. and Zink, D. (1967). *Journal of Speech Hearing Disorders*, **32**, 343

Welch, B. L. and Welch, A. S. (1970). *Physiological effects of Noise.* New York; Plenum Press

Welleschik, B. (1976). *Laryngologie, Rhinologie, Otologie, Grenzgeb.* **55**, 515

Westin, Jerome B. (1975). *Aviation Space and Environmental Medicine,* **46**, 1135

Whittle, L. S. and Robinson, D. W. (1974). 'Discotheques and pop music as a source of noise induced hearing loss. Review and bibliography.' *National Physics Laboratory Acoustics Report* AC66

Yarington, C. T. Jr. (1968). *Laryngoscope,* **78**, 685

Yost, Wm. A. and Neilsen, D. (1977). *Fundamentals of hearing.* New York; Hold, Reinhard & Winston

19 Inflammatory lesions of the labyrinth and auditory nerve
J L W Wright

Inflammatory changes involving the labyrinth and auditory nerve may occur in the course of specific viral and bacterial infections when a particular organism may be implicated, or no overt infection may be apparent and the cause may remain obscure. These changes may give rise to either predominantly cochlear or labyrinthine symptoms, or both structures may be equally involved (Bocca and Giordano, 1956). The onset of the inflammatory process may be rapid with severe vertigo and partial or profound hearing loss, or there may be a gradual deterioration in cochlear and vestibular function.

Viral infections

Upper respiratory tract

Evidence for the role played by the upper respiratory tract viruses in the aetiology of labyrinthitis has come from clinical observation of patients suffering from infections with labyrinthine symptoms, and subsequent examination of the histological features on sectioned temporal bones. Lindsay (1959) described acute vertigo, sudden deafness and tinnitus in four patients who were suffering from acute upper respiratory tract infections. Series of patients with similar upper respiratory infections and vestibular or cochlear symptoms were described by Heller and Lindenberg (1955), and by Lieberman (1957). It appears that about one third of all patients with acute labyrinthine symptoms have an acute upper respiratory tract infection at the time of onset. Infection with the adenovirus Type 3 in a patient with predominantly cochlear symptoms was found by Jaffe and Maassab (1967) to be associated with a rising titre of neutralizing antibodies. Sudden deafness with labyrinthine symptoms has been reported with influenza (Van Dishoeck and Bierman, 1957), in Eaton agent infection (Van Dishoeck, 1963), and after rabies injection (Jaffe, 1967).

Schuknecht, Kimura and Naufal (1973) have reported the histological findings in seven patients with sudden hearing loss of whom five had acute upper respiratory tract infections at the time of onset of symptoms. Two patients had acute coryza, one had acute pharyngitis, and two were suffering with pneumonia. Examination of the temporal bones of these patients showed severe atrophy of the hair-cells of the organ of Corti with changes of decreasing severity from basal to apical end. There was also atrophy of the tectorial membrane and of the stria vascularis, but the spiral ganglion cell population was normal. At present it is not known why similar infections in different patients may lead to relatively more damage in either the cochlea or vestibule.

Mumps

The high incidence of mumps infection in cases of sudden hearing loss was demonstrated by Saunders and Lippy (1959) using the mumps complement fixation test. They found that of nine patients with sudden deafness, six patients had a high mumps antibody titre compared with only 2.5 per cent of a control group of 370 patients. Mumps infection can lead to a rapid unilateral hearing loss which in very young children may escape detection and may only be discovered when the child is older. Bilateral symptoms are rare. Cochlear symptoms predominate and adults affected may complain of tinnitus and hearing loss. However Lindsay (1959) described one case in which there was severe vertigo and this persisted for a period of six weeks from the onset of symptoms.

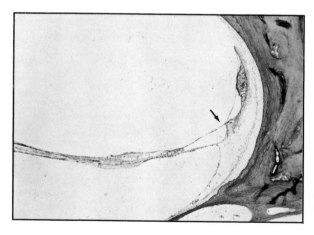

Figure 19.1   Endolymphatic viral labyrinthitis. This patient was severely deaf from an early age, possibly following measles infection. Reissner's membrane is depressed (arrow) towards the basilar membrane narrowing the endolymphatic space. The organ of Corti consists of a few flattened cells

The histological findings in mumps labyrinthitis have been well documented by Lindsay *et al.* (1960). They described the temporal bones of a six-year-old child who had developed severe hearing loss during a mumps infection at the age of 28 months. There was severe atrophy of the organ of Corti and of the stria vascularis in the basal turn with less severe change towards the apex. The tectorial membrane showed severe shrinkage and in places was rolled into a sphere with encapsulation by a single layer of flat cells. There was also some loss of cochlear neurones. Similar changes are seen in *Figure 19.1.*

Measles

Deafness due to measles is less common than that due to mumps but is more commonly bilateral. The histological findings have been described by Lindsay and Hemenway

(1954) as endolymphatic labyrinthitis. They examined the temporal bones of a child who had died aged seven months from measles meningo-encephalitis. Both ears showed severe atrophy of the organ of Corti (*Figure 19.2*), with shrinkage and encapsulation of the tectorial membrane. There was also degenerative change in the stria vascularis indicating a possible viraemia and infection of the inner ear via the blood stream. Mild endolymphatic hydrops was also present. It is possible that there had been direct spread of infection from the subarachnoid space via the cochlear aqueduct.

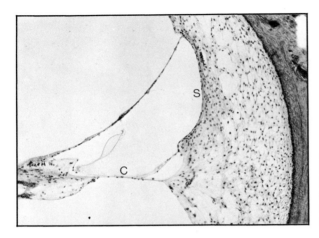

Figure 19.2 Measles labyrinthitis. Section through the basal turn of the cochlea showing severe atrophy of the stria vascularis (S) and absence of the organ of Corti (C)

Schuknecht and Wright (1973) described similar findings in a patient who had suffered profound bilateral hearing loss at an early age. There was atrophy of both the auditory and vestibular membranous labyrinths with hydrops secondary to fibrous obliteration of the vestibular aqueducts. There was also some degeneration of the vestibular nerves and it was felt that this process was due to direct attack by the measles virus.

Herpes zoster

The classic syndrome described by Ramsay Hunt (1907) consists of facial nerve paralysis with herpetic eruption involving the external ear. The close relationship between herpes zoster and chicken pox viral infections was shown at first by common antigen complement fixation tests and later a common virus was isolated. Hope-Simpson (1965) suggested that herpes zoster is a manifestation of latent varicella acquired earlier in life and reactivated by unknown factors after lying dormant in the sensory ganglia for many years.

The clinical manifestations are known as herpes zoster oticus or Ramsay Hunt Syndrome. The patient at first complains of earache, which is followed by a vesicular eruption in the pinna or in the ear canal. There may also be lesions on the palate, fauces, face or trunk. The vesicular eruption is followed by facial palsy, hearing loss and vertigo which may occur singly or together. Herpes zoster oticus accounts for between 2 and 7 per cent of all facial palsies (Schuknecht, 1974). Approximately 50 per cent of patients with facial palsy due to herpes zoster have some degree of permanent motor disability.

Vertigo may vary from mild unsteadiness to severe disequilibrium with nausea and vomiting. There may be an associated sensorineural hearing loss with high pitched tinnitus. Audiometric testing may show a predominantly high-tone loss (Harbert and Young, 1967), and loudness recruitment is usually absent (Welsh and Welsh, 1962). Slight recovery of hearing thresholds may be seen but is unusual.

The histological features of herpes infection were described in detail by Blackley, Friedmann and Wright (1967). They examined the temporal bones of a patient who died at about seven months from the onset of the vesicular eruption. The most prominent feature was marked perineural and intraneural round cell infiltration of the facial nerve (*Figure 19.3*), the auditory nerve, the cochlea (*Figure 19.4*), and the

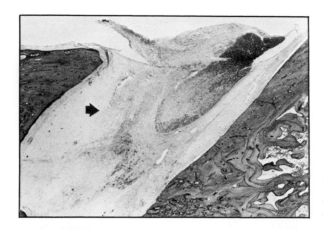

Figure 19.3 Herpes zoster oticus with facial palsy. Marked round cell infiltration along the course of the facial nerve

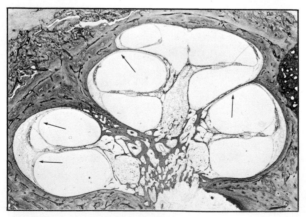

Figure 19.4 Herpes zoster. Mid-modiolar section through the cochlea of a patient who died two months after the onset of herpes zoster oticus. There is a diffuse round cell infiltration of the cochlear tissues and a perilymph precipitate in the basal and middle turns (arrows). A similar precipitate may be seen in toxic bacterial labyrinthitis

mastoid. There was also considerable perivascular cuffing by small lymphocytes in the modiolus (*Figure 19.5*), in the facial nerve, and in the skin of the external-ear canal. The organ of Corti was damaged and the macula of the saccule was infiltrated by lymphocytes. Similar changes were reported earlier by Maybaum and Druss (1934), Denny Brown, Adams and Fitzgerald (1944), Findlay (1952), and Guldberg-Moller, Olsen and Kettel (1959). More recently Zajtchuk, Matz and Lindsay (1972) reported the histological findings in a patient who had suffered severe vertigo due to herpes

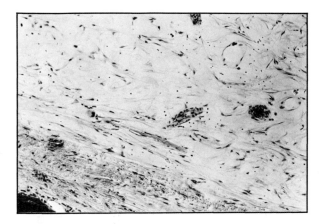

Figure 19.5   Same case as *Figure 19.4.* Perivascular cuffing and round cell infiltration in the modiolus of the cochlea

zoster oticus and found degenerative changes in the sensory and neural elements of the superior and lateral semicircular canals with fibrosis and new bone formation.

There is no satisfactory specific treatment for herpes zoster oticus.

Rubella

The developing ear is particularly at risk during the first trimester of pregnancy in cases of maternal rubella, although defects may occur in the second trimester also (Monif, Hardy and Sever, 1966). Other organs at risk include the eye, heart and brain. Encephalitis is not uncommon and may lead to mental retardation.

The incidence of deafness in maternal rubella has varied widely with different surveys ranging from 8 per cent (Barr and Lundstrom, 1961), to 50 per cent (Rendle-Short, 1963). Fisch (1969) has estimated the incidence of deafness from rubella as 6 per cent per year without an epidemic, and 33 per cent in an epidemic year.

The rubella virus may be isolated from the nose, throat, blood and urine of patients with rubella. From the circulation of the mother it spreads to the placenta and then to the fetus. Infants with congenital rubella may harbour the virus for up to three years and may excrete it in saliva, urine and faeces.

The histopathological findings have been described by Lindsay *et al.* (1953), Hemenway, Sando and McChesney (1969) and by Lindsay (1973). There is a marked cochleosaccular aplasia with flattening of the organ of Corti and absence of hair-cells. There is distortion and encapsulation of the tectorial membrane and collapse of Reissner's membrane. There is degeneration of the macula of the saccule. The hearing loss associated with these changes usually has a flat audiometric pattern (Fisch, 1956), a pattern usually associated with strial atrophy. Friedmann (1970) has described large protruding granulomas in the stria vascularis of the apical and middle turns of the cochlea in rubella.

Other viruses

The labyrinth may be involved in glandular fever. Gregg and Schaeffer (1964) reported the clinical findings in a patient with infectious mononucleosis who suffered severe hearing loss, tinnitus and vertigo. Cytomegalic inclusions in the cochlea have been reported in infants who died as a result of intra-uterine infection with a cytomegalovirus (Davis, 1969).

Attempts have been made to induce viral labyrinthitis in the experimental animal by direct inoculation techniques via the oval window, and these attempts have failed (Karmody, 1975). It appears that a more likely route is via the blood stream (Lindsay and Hemenway, 1954).

Protozoa

Congenital toxoplasmosis may present at birth with encephalitis, choroidoretinitis, jaundice and hepatosplenomegaly. There may also be lesions in the inner ear. Keleman (1958) described calcareous deposits in the stria vascularis and spiral ligament of the cochlea in an infant who died ten days after birth. However Wright (1971) believes that toxoplasmosis is not a significant cause of congenital and infantile deafness.

Deafness has been reported following malaria but this is not well documented (Friedmann, 1974).

Bacterial infections

There have been many classifications of the response of the labyrinth to bacterial infection and the most satisfactory is that used by Schuknecht (1974). He described the four progressive stages as acute toxic, suppurative, chronic, and sclerotic labyrinthitis.

Acute toxic labyrinthitis

This condition has also been referred to as serous labyrinthitis and irritative labyrinthitis in which there is a non-purulent inflammatory reaction in the inner ear. It may occur during infections of the middle-ear space and mastoid when toxins may gain access to the perilymphatic compartment via the oval or round windows. Occasionally a fistula may be present, most commonly in the horizontal semicircular canal but sometimes found in the superior or posterior canals, or in the promontory. Toxic labyrinthitis may also occur as a complication of bacterial meningitis, and it may be seen after ear surgery involving removal of the stapes footplate.

The clinical symptoms in toxic labyrinthitis are indistinguishable from those of acute suppurative labyrinthitis and the diagnosis is made in retrospect after treatment when some cochlear and labyrinthine function remains in the affected ear. The patient complains of vertigo and hearing loss of variable severity. There is at first an irritative nystagmus with the fast component to the side of the lesion which may be followed later by a paralytic nystagmus in the opposite direction. The patient may have a positive fistula sign and this is helpful if positive but a negative fistula test does not necessarily exclude the presence of a fistula. Caloric reactions may be depressed.

The pathological features in toxic labyrinthitis have been described in cases of induced labyrinthitis in experimental animals (Paparella and Sugiura, 1967) and on sectioned human temporal bones by Schuknecht and Montandon (1970). There was a fine fibrinous precipitate in the perilymphatic fluid (*Figure 19.4*) and variable slight endolymphatic hydrops. The two patients described by Schuknecht and Montandon had experienced reversible hearing loss while suffering from pneumococcal meningitis. The management of acute toxic labyrinthitis is early and vigorous treatment of the underlying infection with adequate antibiotic therapy in order to prevent the onset of suppurative labyrinthitis. Surgical drainage of any ear infection should be confined to the middle ear and mastoid, and the labyrinth should not be entered.

Acute suppurative labyrinthitis

Bacterial invasion of the inner ear may occur with either acute or chronic infections of the middle ear and mastoid. In acute infections the pathway may be either the oval or round windows while in chronic infections with bone erosion there may be a fistula into the labyrinth. In cases of meningitis there is bacterial invasion from the subarachnoid space via the internal auditory meatus (*Figure 19.6*) or infection may

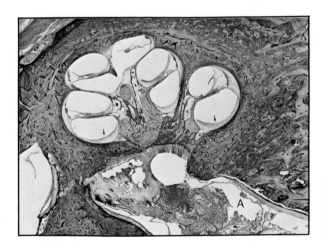

Figure 19.6 Acute suppurative labyrinthitis. There is pus formation in the internal auditory meatus (A), and a purulent exudate in the cochlea (arrows)

occur via the cochlear aqueduct. Bloodstream infection is important in cases of septicaemia, and septic emboli may cause labyrinthine damage from ischaemia in addition to damage from inflammatory causes.

The incidence of suppurative labyrinthitis in reported series is only relevant to their particular place and time as much depends on the availability of medical care and antibiotics. In the pre-antibiotic era the incidence of labyrinthitis in cerebrospinal meningitis was reported as ranging from 4 to 37.5 per cent (Fraser and Dickie, 1920), and 15 per cent in cases of suppurative otitis media (Fraser, 1914). Severe deafness secondary to meningitis was found in 20 per cent of a survey of 5000 deaf children in residential care (Shambaugh *et al.*, 1933). It is significant that in the past 20 years few large series of labyrinthitis and deafness due to meningitis or otitis media have been published. Invasion of the labyrinth by massive cholesteatoma was reported by Wright, Colman and Connor (1976) in nine patients with chronic suppurative otitis media. All had received courses of antibiotics in the past but surgical excision and labyrinthectomy was essential. Wright and Bradshaw (1973), found only five cases of severe deafness due to meningitis in an Oxford survey of 188 deaf children, while Zakzouk (1977) reported 30 cases of severe deafness following meningitis in a survey of 364 deaf children in Saudi Arabia.

The commonest causative organisms in suppurative labyrinthitis are beta haemolytic streptococci, pneumococcus, haemophilus, staphylococcus, proteus and pseudomonas. However the clinical symptoms of severe hearing loss and vertigo are similar whichever organism is involved.

The histological findings are invasion of the perilymphatic space by polymorpho-nuclear leucocytes (*Figure 19.7*) and this is usually heaviest near the site of entry of

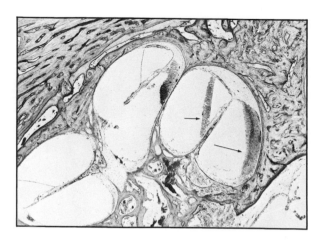

Figure 19.7 Suppurative labyrinthitis in a baby who died aged seven months with meningitis due to haemophilus. There is pus formation in the perilymphatic spaces

infection. This is followed by endolymphatic hydrops and the formation of a fibrinous precipitate. Later there is frank pus formation and necrosis of portions of the membranous labyrinth (*Figure 19.8*).

In the treatment of suppurative labyrinthitis combinations of the appropriate antibiotics should be given in large doses and surgical drainage carried out when indicated on clinical grounds. Drainage of the labyrinth requires wide exposure of the cochlear lumen, the vestibule, and of the three semicircular canals.

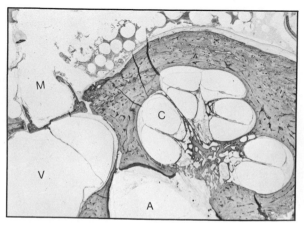

Figure 19.8 Sequel to suppurative labyrinthitis. There is severe degeneration of the membranous labyrinth with hydrops involving the cochlea (C) and the vestibule (V). All the structures of the cochlear duct are atrophic. A is internal auditory meatus. M is middle ear

Chronic labyrinthitis

This condition has also been called paralabyrinthitis, perilabyrinthitis, and circumscribed labyrinthitis in order to describe the clinical syndrome associated with fistula formation into the labyrinth. Pathological fistula is usually secondary to chronic suppurative otitis media where there is bone erosion by rarefying osteitis or by cholesteatoma. Tumours are a rare cause. Surgical fistulae may follow stapedectomy or accidental injury to the bony labyrinth during mastoid surgery. The fenestration operation is now rarely performed.

The patient complains of transient induced vertigo produced by head movement, sneezing, coughing, manipulation of the ear, or by exposure to a cold wind. A positive fistula sign is the presence of nystagmus and a subjective feeling of unsteadiness following rhythmical tragus pressure. Histologically there is at first a thickening of the endosteal lining of the labyrinth but in a progressive disease process this is soon followed by invasion with granulation tissue, squamous epithelium and fibrous tissue (*Figure 19.9*). The appearance of a positive fistula sign in the course of middle-ear or

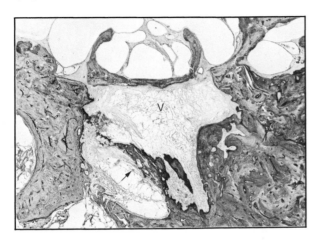

Figure 19.9 Chronic labyrinthitis. The vestibule (V) is partially filled with fibrous tissue which has a loose stroma. There is a spur of new bone (arrow)

mastoid disease is thus an indication for early surgical exploration. Frequently granulation tissue or cholesteatoma can be removed from the fistula without damaging the inner ear, and the deficit closed with a bone chip.

A gradual high-tone sensorineural hearing loss may be found in patients with chronic suppurative otitis media with or without overt signs of fistula formation (Paparella, Brady and Hoel, 1970).

Labyrinthine sclerosis

The healed inactive stage of suppurative labyrinthitis has also been called labyrinthitis ossificans. There is extensive fibrosis and new bone formation in the lumen of the labyrinth. Osteoblastic activity arises in the undifferentiated mesenchymal cells found in the adventitia around capillary networks in the inflammatory granulation tissue (Paparella and Sugiura, 1967). Bone spicules may be found in the vestibule (*Figure 19.9*), and there may be extensive bony obliteration of the cochlea (*Figure 19.10*).

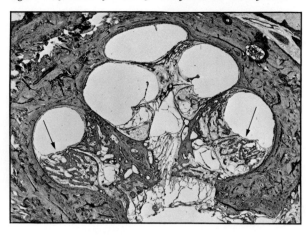

Figure 19.10 Sclerotic labyrinthitis, also called labyrinthitis ossificans. There is osseous replacement of the basal turns of the cochlea

There is permanent loss of auditory and vestibular function but patients are usually well adapted to their disability at this stage.

Syphilis (*see also* Chapter 15)

Both the congenital and acquired forms of the disease may cause inflammatory changes in the inner ear with deafness and vertigo. There may be either sudden or gradual hearing loss with either form. The incidence of inner-ear involvement is approximately 18 per cent in congenital syphilis and 25 per cent in the secondary form. It rises to around 80 per cent in late neurosyphilis (Tamari and Itkin, 1951).

ACQUIRED FORM

Hearing loss usually appears towards the end of the secondary stage or commencement of the tertiary stage of infection and may be accompanied by tinnitus and vertigo. There is rapid progression of the deafness over a few months and both ears are affected. The diagnostic tests for syphilis are important as hearing loss may be the first sign of the disease since the primary stage. The commonly performed tests are the Wasserman, Kahn, Reiter treponema immobilization and the treponemal antibody test. The early pathological changes are an acute syphilitic labyrinthitis and diffuse round cell infiltration. Later there is osteitis of the temporal bone and atrophy of portions of the membranous labyrinth (*Figure 19.11*). In the tertiary stage there may be gummatous destruction of the middle ear, mastoid and petrous bone.

Acquired syphilis should be treated with high doses of penicillin. This should be combined with prednisone 30 mg daily for one week and 25 mg daily for three weeks. If there is no hearing improvement at the end of this period the steroid is curtailed. If however there is an improvement in auditory thresholds then treatment should continue for six months.

CONGENITAL FORM

Infection reaches the fetus from the mother via the placenta and the child is born with active disease. Deafness may become apparent during the first two years of life or later

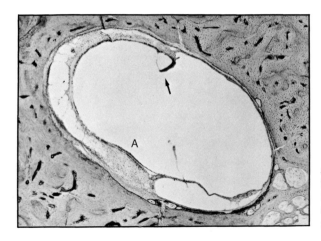

Figure 19.11 Syphilis. Changes in the membranous labyrinth include degeneration of the canal ampullae (A) and membranous ruptures (arrow)

in the second decade. It occurs in approximately 25–38 per cent of patients with congenital syphilis (Karmody and Schuknecht, 1966). The early onset of deafness is usually sudden, severe and bilateral. There may be episodes of vertigo and vomiting with some fluctuation of hearing at first (Perlman and Leek, 1952). The early hearing loss is more severe in the low tones.

Late-onset hearing loss is usually bilateral and progresses rapidly to severe deafness. It may be associated with Hennebert's sign (Hennebert, 1911), in which there is a positive fistula sign without middle-ear disease. The Tullio phenomenon is also common in congenital syphilis and consists of vertigo with nystagmus induced by high intensity noise. Both phenomena may be due to erosion of the bony labyrinth, or to fibrous bands passing from the inner surface of the stapes footplate to the membranous labyrinth (Nadol, 1974).

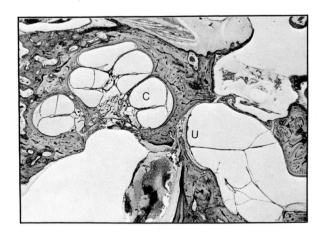

Figure 19.12 Syphilis. There are severe degenerative changes in the cochlea involving the stria vascularis, spiral ligament and the organ of Corti. The utricle (U) is also atrophic

The histological features are a rarefying osteitis with round cell infiltration and endarteritis. There is endolymphatic hydrops and marked atrophy of the organ of Corti. Degenerative changes are also seen in the spiral ligament, basilar membrane, and the cochlear neurones (*Figure 19.12*). The utricle and saccule are also atrophic and there may be similar changes in the canal ampullae.

Acute vestibular neuronitis

This has previously been referred to as epidemic vertigo, epidemic neurolabyrinthitis, acute labyrinthitis, and vestibular paralysis. It is characterized by the sudden onset of vertigo with nausea and vomiting but without hearing loss. There may be a recent history of an upper respiratory tract infection, and several members of a closely related group may be affected at the same time.

Coats (1969) has given a thorough description of the clinical signs and symptoms required for a diagnosis of acute vestibular neuronitis. The patient has spontaneous nystagmus of a paralytic type with the fast component of the nystagmus towards the normal ear. The vertigo and nystagmus subside gradually over a period of weeks but caloric tests show a permanent vestibular deficit on the affected side. There are no cochlear symptoms.

Attempts to prove a virus aetiology have not been successful and the cause is as yet unknown. Similarities between this condition and symptoms in herpes zoster infection have been drawn by Hart (1965). The site of the lesion is thought to be the vestibular nerve (Pfaltz, 1955; Hart, 1965).

Chronic vestibular neuronitis

This condition occurs in middle-aged patients and is characterized by recurring mild attacks of vertigo extending over several years. There are no cochlear symptoms. The attacks are less severe than those seen in the acute form and vomiting is unusual. An occasional severe episode may be followed by a paralytic nystagmus, and there may be a reduced caloric response in the affected ear. Histological examination of the vestibular nerve from a patient who has undergone vestibular neurectomy for this condition has shown nerve swelling and myelin degeneration (Hilding *et al.*, 1968).

Diabetic vestibular neuronitis

Peripheral and central neuropathies are well known in diabetes mellitus and the vestibular neurones may also be affected. Naufal and Schuknecht (1972) described the histological findings in a diabetic patient with recurrent vertigo. They found a loss of vestibular neurones, most severe in the superior division of the nerve (*Figure 19.13*).

Carcinomatous encephalomyelitis

This condition is a motor and sensory neuropathy associated with malignant tumour. There is progressive degeneration of the anterior and posterior horn cells of the cervical spinal cord, and portions of the medulla. The auditory and vestibular nerves may be involved in this degenerative process (*Figure 19.14*). Leukaemia may also be followed by labyrinthine changes (Zechner and Altman, 1969).

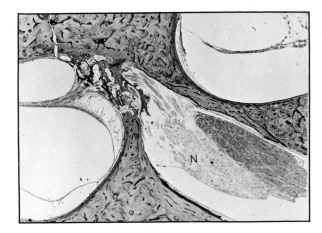

Figure 19.13 Diabetic vestibular neuronitis. The patient had experienced episodes of severe vertigo for several years prior to death. There is severe atrophy of the superior division of the vestibular nerve (N)

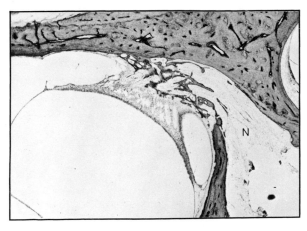

Figure 19.14   Carcinomatous encephalomyelitis. There is severe atrophy of the vestibular nerves (N)

Cogan's syndrome (*see also* Chapters 15 and 24)

This was described by Cogan (1945) as interstitial keratitis of non-syphilitic origin associated with auditory and vestibular symptoms. There may be sudden vertigo with nausea and vomiting, and hearing loss of a sensorineural type which is usually bilateral. Caloric tests show loss of vestibular function.

Vogt-Koyanagi syndrome

This syndrome consists of uveitis with alopecia, vitiligo and deafness. The onset is characterized by severe headache, orbital pain and malaise which progresses over a few weeks to uveitis with vitiligo, poliosis and alopecia. At this stage there may be bilateral hearing loss with tinnitus and vertigo. The ophthalmic lesions may progress to blindness but the hearing loss frequently recovers.

Wegener's granuloma

The necrotizing granulomatous process seen in Wegener's granuloma may invade the inner ear. Blatt and Lawrence (1961) found granulomatous tissue extending from the middle ear through the round window into the labyrinth in a patient who had suffered a sudden severe hearing loss. There was marked destruction of the membranous labyrinth.

Relapsing polychondritis

This is an inflammatory reaction in multiple cartilages characterized by inflammatory infiltration with lymphocytes and plasma cells leading to cartilage destruction. It is similar to rheumatoid arthritis. Patients may complain of unilateral or bilateral hearing loss with vertigo. The hearing loss is gradual and deteriorates over a period of two years (Cody and Sones, 1971). There may be recovery of auditory function following treatment with steroids.

Temporal arteritis

A patient with severe vertigo, absent caloric response and hearing loss was reported by Cody (1971). The caloric response and hearing recovered following treatment with cortisone.

Polyarteritis nodosa

Sensorineural hearing losses in this condition have been reported by Brown and Woolner (1960) and by Toma (1968). Recovery is usual with steroid therapy (Peitersen and Carlsen, 1966).

Multiple sclerosis

Patients with this disorder frequently suffer with attacks of vertigo which may be associated with hearing loss and tinnitus. The nystagmus may be horizontal, vertical or rotatory, and may be in a different direction in each eye. Signs of late disease are Charcot's Triad of intention tremor, scanning speech and nystagmus. Audiometric tests reveal a retrocochlear lesion, and there may be some recovery of hearing levels (Citron *et al.*, 1963). The lesion appears to be a demyelinating process in the brain stem as examination of sectioned temporal bones in patients with multiple sclerosis has revealed no pathological changes in the vestibular nerves or sense organs (Ward, Cannon and Lindsay, 1965).

Balance disorders due to ageing

Schuknecht (1974) has proposed four different types of equilibrium disorder due to age changes in different portions of the labyrinth. Although there is not as yet pathological proof of these conditions they are based on sound theoretical precepts and the symptom groups are readily recognized by experienced otologists who see large numbers of vertiginous subjects.

Cupulolithiasis

This term was introduced to replace names used for the disorder known as postural vertigo, positional vertigo, and benign paroxysmal vertigo. Schuknecht (1969) believes that the disorder is caused by the presence of a deposit on the cupula of the posterior semicircular canal which renders it unduly sensitive to gravitational force and head movement. The patient complains of sudden transient vertigo on head movement and nystagmus can be elicited by positional tests when nystagmus is seen with the affected ear in the dependent position. The vertigo and nystagmus are fatiguable. Similar symptoms may also be seen after head injury and may be due to release of otoconia into the endolymph from a disrupted utricle (Schuknecht, 1962, 1973).

Ampullary disequilibrium

There is momentary vertigo associated with angular head movements. Patients experience rotation of the field of vision which persists after the head movement has ceased. Degenerative change in the ampullary mechanism of the semicircular canals is postulated.

Macular disequilibrium

This occurs when the head position is changed relative to the direction of gravity, mainly when changing from recumbent to upright posture. Degenerative changes in the sensory epithelia of the utricle and saccule are postulated.

Vestibular ataxia

This is a constant unsteadiness on ambulation. Steps are hesitant and broad-based. There appears to be loss of vestibular control over the lower limbs and lesions are postulated in the vestibulospinal tracts, medial longitudinal bundle, and the vestibular nuclei.

All the illustrations in this chapter are by courtesy of Professor H. F. Schuknecht.

References

Barr, B. and Lundstrom, R. (1961) *Acta Otolaryngologica*, **53**, 413

Blackley, B., Friedmann, I. and Wright, I. (1967) *Acta Otolaryngologica*, **63**, 533

Blatt, I. and Lawrence, M. (1961) *Archives of Otolaryngology*, **73**, 639

Bocca, E. and Giordano, R. (1956) *Archivio Italia Otolaryngico*, **67**, 47

Brown, H. and Woolner, L. (1960) *Annals of Otology, Rhinology and Laryngology*, **69**, 810

Citron, L., Dix, M., Hallpike, C. and Hood, J. (1963) *Acta Otolaryngologica*, **56**, 330

Coats, A. (1969) *Transactions American Academy of Ophthalmology and Otolaryngology*, **73**, 395

Cogan, D. (1945) *Archives of Ophthalmology*, **33**, 144

Cody, D. (1971) *Clinical Otology International Symposium*. St. Louis; C. V. Mosby Co.

Cody, D. and Sones, D. (1971) *Laryngoscope*, **81**, 1208

Davis, G. (1969) *Annals of Otology, Rhinology and Laryngology*, **78**, 1179

Denny Brown, D., Adams, R. D. and Fitzgerald, P. J. (1944) *Archives of Neurology and Psychiatry*, **51**, 216

Findlay, J. P. (1952) *Medical Journal of Australia*, **2**, 810

Fisch, L. (1956) *Journal of Laryngology*, **69**, 479

Fisch, L. (1969) *Public Health*, **83**, 168

Fraser, J. (1914) *Journal of Laryngology*, **29**, 284

Fraser, J. and Dickie, J. (1920) *Proceedings of the Royal Society of Medicine*, **13**, 23

Friedmann, I. (1970) *Ciba Foundation Symposium*. London; J. & A. Churchill

Friedmann, I. (1974) *Pathology of the Ear*. Oxford; Blackwell

Gregg, J. and Schaeffer, J. (1964) *South Dakota Journal of Medicine and Pharmacy*, **17**, 22

Gulberg-Moller, J., Olsen, S. and Kettel, K. (1959) *Archives of Otolaryngology*, **69**, 266

Harbert, F. and Young, I. (1967) *Archives of Otolaryngology*, **85**, 632

Hart, C. (1965) *Annals of Otology, Rhinology and Laryngology*, **74**, 33

Heller, M. and Lindenberg, P. (1955) *Annals of Otoloty, Rhinology and Laryngology*, **64**, 931

Hemenway, W., Sando, I. and McChesney, D. (1969) *Archiv für Ohren- Nasen- und Kehlkopfheilkunde*, **193**, 287

Hennebert, C. (1911) *Clinique Bruxelles*, **25**, 545

Hilding, D., Kanda, T. and House, W. (1968) *Otolaryngology Clinic of North America*, Oct., 305

Hope-Simpson, R. E. (1965) *Proceedings of the Royal Society of Medicine*, **58**, 9

Hunt, J. Ramsay (1907) *Archives of Otolaryngology*, **36**, 371

Jaffe, B. F. (1967) *Archives of Otolaryngology*, **86**, 55

Jaffe, B. F. and Maassab, H. F. (1967) *New England Journal of Medicine*, **276**, 1406

Karmody, C. S. (1975) *Annals of Otology, Rhinology and Laryngology*, **84**, 179

Karmody, C. and Schuknecht, H. (1966) *Archives of Otolaryngology*, **83**, 18

Keleman, G. (1958) *Archives of Otolaryngology*, **68**, 547

Lieberman, A. (1957) *Laryngoscope*, **67**, 1237

Lindsay, J. (1959) *Archives of Otolaryngology*, **69**, 13

Lindsay, J. (1973) *Archives of Otolaryngology*, **98**, 258

Lindsay, J., Caruthers, D., Hemenway, W. and Harrison, S. (1953) *Annals of Otology, Rhinology and Laryngology*, **62**, 1201

Lindsay, J., Davey, P. and Ward, P. (1960) *Annals of Otology, Rhinology and Laryngology*, **69**, 918

Lindsay, J. and Hemenway, W. (1954) *Annals of Otology, Rhinology and Laryngology*, **63**, 754

Maybaum, J. L. and Druss, J. G. (1934) *Archives of Otolaryngology*, **19**, 575

Monif, G., Hardy, J. and Sever, J. (1966) *Bulletin of Johns Hopkins Hospital*, **118**, 85

Nadol, J. B. Jr. (1974) *Archives of Otolaryngology*, **100**, 273

Naufal, P. M. and Schuknecht, H. (1972) *Archives of Otolaryngology*, **96**, 468

Paparella, M., Brady, D. and Hoel, R. (1970) *Transactions of the American Academy of Ophthalmology and Otolaryngology*, **74**, 108

Paparella, M. and Sugiura, S. (1967) *Annals of Otology, Rhinology and Laryngology*, **76**, 554

Peitersen, E. and Carlsen, B. (1966) *Acta Otolaryngologica*, **61**, 189

Perlman, H. and Leek, J. (1952) *Laryngoscope*, **62**, 1175

Pfaltz, C. (1955) *Oto-Rhino-Laryngological Journal*, **17**, 454

Saunders, W. and Lippy, W. (1959) *Annals of Otology, Rhinology and Laryngology*, **68**, 830

Schuknecht, H. F. (1962) *Transactions of the American Academy of Ophthalmology and Otolaryngology*, **66**, 319

Schuknecht, H. F. (1969) *Archives of Otolaryngology*, **90**, 765

Schuknecht, H. F. (1974) *Pathology of the Ear*. Harvard University Press

Schuknecht, H., Kimura, R. and Naufal, P. (1973) *Acta Otolaryngologica*, **76**, 75

Schuknecht, H. and Montandon, P. (1970), *Archiv für Klinic experimental Ohren, Nasen und Kehlkopfheilkunde*, **195**, 207

Schuknecht, H. and Ruby, R. (1973) *Advances in Oto-Rhino-Laryngology*, **20**, 434

Schuknecht, H. and Wright, J. L. W. (1973) *Journal of Laryngology*, **87**, 947

Shambaugh, G., Wallner, L., Greene, L. and Shambaugh, G. Jr. (1933) *Archives of Otolaryngology*, **18**, 430

Tamari, M. and Itkin, P. (1951) *Eye, Ear, Nose and Throat Monthly*, **30**, 252

Toma, G. (1968) *Journal of Laryngology*, **82**, 129

Van Dishoeck, H. A. E. (1963) *Acta Otolaryngologica*, **183**, 30

Van Dishoeck, H. A. E. and Bierman, T. A. (1957) *Annals of Otology*, **66**, 963

Ward, P., Cannon, D. and Lindsay, J. (1965) *Laryngoscope*, **75**, 1031

Welsh, L. and Welsh, J. (1962) *Laryngoscope*, **72**, 653

Wright, J. L. W., Colman, B. H. and Connor, A. F. (1976) *Journal of Laryngology*, **90**, 257

Wright, J. L. W. and Bradshaw, R. B. (1973) *Journal of Laryngology*, **87**, 547

Wright, M. I. (1971) *The Pathology of Deafness*. Manchester University Press

Zajtchuk, J., Matz, G. and Lindsay, J. (1972) *Annals of Otology, Rhinology and Laryngology*, **81**, 331

Zakzouk, S. (1977) *Deafness Survey*, Riyadh. Personal communication.

Zechner, G. and Altman, F. (1969) *Annals of Otology*, **78**, 375

20 Acoustic neuroma

J D K Dawes and John Hankinson

Otolaryngologists have always had an interest in acoustic nerve tumours, not only because they arise in the internal auditory meatus but because they should primarily present in ear, nose and throat departments. Although the commonest presenting symptoms are unilateral deafness and tinnitus, Lundborg (1950) commented that only 10 per cent of these tumours were correctly diagnosed by otologists. Great interest had been aroused when Dix, Hallpike and Hood (1948) showed that loudness recruitment was present in cochlear deafness but was absent in cases of acoustic tumour, for it then became possible to suspect the presence of a small tumour on the basis of audiological testing alone. Schuknecht and Woeller (1955) advanced the possibility of earlier diagnosis by recognizing that speech discrimination is relatively poor compared with what would be expected from the pure-tone audiogram. Furthermore, Jerger (1960), using continuous and interrupted signals in conventional and fixed frequency Békésy audiometry, produced a useful analysis for recognition of retrocochlear lesions. Following earlier diagnosis, neuroradiological and otomicro-surgical techniques were developed by House and his colleagues (1961, 1964, 1968) to deal with these smaller acoustic tumours. Quix (1912) had described a case of translabyrinthine removal of an acoustic tumour but it was left to House to reawaken interest in this method.

Acoustic nerve tumour is known as acoustic neuroma, neurinoma, schwannoma, neurilemmoma, neurofibroma and perineural fibroblastoma. It accounts for 8 per cent of all intracranial tumours and about 80 per cent of those occurring in the cerebello-pontine angle. It is commoner in females in the ratio 3 : 2. The true incidence of the lesion in the population is not known. On the basis of autopsy studies by Hardy and Crowe (1936) and Leonard and Talbot (1970), Morrison (1975) calculated a random post-mortem incidence of about 1 per cent. Patients are known to present with manifestations of tumour from adolescence onwards but the majority present between the fourth and sixth decade. The clinical presentation is preceded by a clinical history of deafness of from 1 to 30 years' duration.

Although the tumour is usually solitary it may occur bilaterally and may then be the principal manifestation of familial neurofibromatosis (von Recklinghausen's disease), in which case pigmented naevi, multiple individual nodules or plexiform skin neurofibromas, and neurological signs of tumours of major nerve trunks may be seen.

Pathology

These tumours arise from the Schwann or neurilemmal cells of the auditory nerve. As the cranial nerves leave the brain stem they are covered by a glial stroma for a short distance before acquiring a neurilemmal sheath. In the case of the auditory nerve the glial stroma extends almost to the entrance of the internal auditory meatus before the neurilemmal sheath begins (Henschen, 1915). Therefore almost all acoustic neuromas arise within the internal auditory meatus; the majority arise from the superior vestibular nerve, others from the inferior vestibular and more rarely from the cochlear nerve. Occasionally a schwannoma arises from the facial nerve. Macroscopically the tumour may vary in size from a few millimetres, when it lies within the meatus, to a

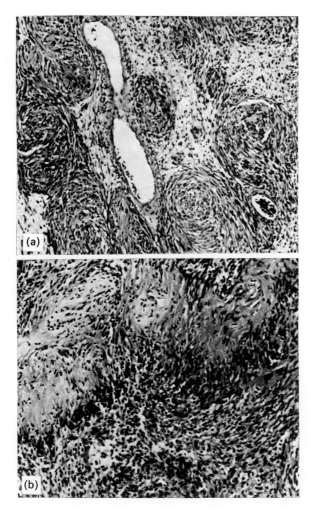

Figure 20.1 Photomicrographs of an acoustic schwannoma: (a) the dense interwoven bundles of elongated cells which constitute the so-called Antoni type A tissue, in this instance forming some whorls; and lying between these spindle-celled areas is the looser, more scantily cellular polymorphic Antoni type B tissue; (b) an area of marked palisading of nuclei, a distinctive histological feature of many schwannomas (Haematoxylin and eosin × 120). (Reproduced by courtesy of Professor B. E. Tomlinson, Newcastle General Hospital)

diameter of 7 cm or more when, at operation or at autopsy, it may be seen to lie at the base of the brain within the cerebello-pontine angle. It then displaces not only the cranial nerves from the fifth to the ninth but the brain stem and cerebellum also. The tumour is flesh-coloured, well circumscribed, encapsulated and nodular in the case of

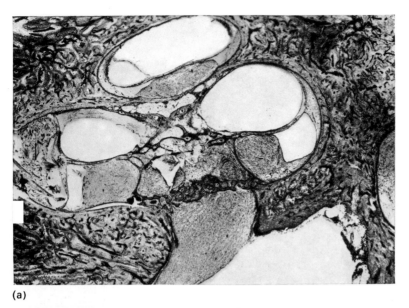

(a)

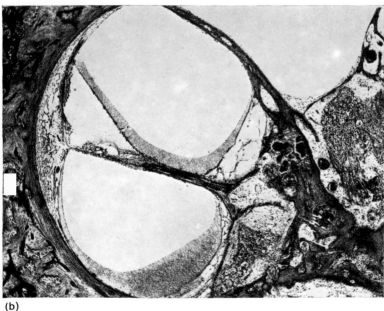

(b)

Figure 20.2 (a) Acoustic nerve tumour; (b) exudate in cochlea. (Ferens Institute)

large ones. Usually its consistency is firm but when large the centre may show hydropic or cystic change. No nerves pass through the tumour; they are displaced by it and may be adherent to its capsule. Thus the tumour, arising from the neurilemmal sheath within the meatus, may slowly fill the meatus and displace the facial nerve anteriorly. With increase in size it bulges into the lateral basal cistern and erodes the walls of the internal auditory meatus and, possibly, the petrous apex also. Here, as it increases in size, it displaces the cerebellum and brain stem and becomes adherent to them. The posterior cranial fossa may not only be encroached upon by tumour bulging from the meatus but also by a large arachnoid cyst surrounding the tumour. Arachnoiditis producing cyst formation is very common and is presumably induced by the tumour itself, for the tumour may be small with a large cyst and vice versa. Occasionally some of the symptoms of a space-occupying lesion within the posterior fossa may arise from the size of the cyst rather than that of the tumour. These tumours have been classified macroscopically into two groups depending upon whether they arise medially or laterally—the former being more in the cerebello-pontine angle, the latter within the petrous bone. This is of more clinical than pathological interest, as the tumour always arises from the neurilemmal sheath, perhaps more medially or laterally in the beginning, but finally occupying the whole meatus. Occasionally the main mass may lie in the cerebello-pontine angle, with little erosion of the meatus, but more commonly the internal auditory meatus is expanded, funnel-shaped and eroded.

Microscopically, two types can be recognized: (a) fasciculated; and (b) reticular. Within the same tumour areas of different pattern may be seen (*Figure 20.1*). In the fasciculated or Antoni A type an orderly arrangement of parallel cells and inter-cellular fibres form interwoven bundles with alternating nuclear and fibrous zones. The cells are fusiform with oval nuclei lying in palisades which are separated by bundles of reticular fibres. Sometimes the cells are grouped in compact whorls of variable size. In the reticular or Antoni B type there is a disorderly, loose meshwork of cells of variable shapes with intercellular vacuoles or microcysts and reticular tissue. There are good reasons to believe that this neurilemmoma is different in nature from the neurofibroma of von Recklinghausen's disease (Willis, 1948).

The tumour may spread throughout the whole pyramid of the petrous bone leading to degeneration of the spiral ganglion cells and often to an albuminous exudate in the labyrinthine space (*Figure 20.2*). Storrs (1974) reports two cases of acoustic neuromas presenting in the middle ear. Silverstein and Schuknecht (1966) showed that the protein of the perilymph is very high in cases of acoustic neuroma and thought that this increase in protein preceded that which occurred in the cerebrospinal fluid. It has also been suggested that pressure on the veins in the internal auditory meatus may be responsible for the endolymphatic hydrops sometimes seen in this condition (Brunner, 1925; Watkyn-Thomas, 1939).

Symptoms and signs

These may begin at any time from the 'teens'. Although the tumour most commonly arises from the vestibular nerve the earliest symptoms are usually auditory. This is not surprising for slowly progressive changes of the vestibular nerve produce little or no disturbance, due to central adaptation, even though the caloric responses are completely absent. Careful questioning may, however, elicit a history of minor imbalance and occasionally true vertigo. Headache and earache are not uncommon in the earlier stages of the natural history of the disease. As the facial nerve also lies within the internal auditory meatus it might be expected that facial nerve paresis would be an early sign but this is not usually the case. An enormous neuroma may fill and erode the meatus, occupy the cerebello-pontine angle producing the symptoms and signs of raised intracranial pressure (viz. headache, vomiting and papilloedema) and other signs in other sensory cranial nerves such as the fifth without the patient showing any facial weakness. It appears that the function of sensory nerve fibres is affected early by pressure whereas motor nerves may be gradually displaced, even stretched and splayed out over the surface of the tumour without loss of function. Altered taste or lacrimation may be the only manifestation of facial nerve displacement.

Auditory function

The earliest symptom is most often a progressive unilateral perceptive deafness, frequently accompanied by tinnitus, which gradually increases over a period of 1–30 years or more until the hearing loss is complete. A progressive perceptive hearing loss is present in almost every case, although it may not be the presenting symptom. Occasionally the hearing loss is of sudden onset and sometimes the patient may not have a demonstrable loss by pure-tone audiometry and yet may notice that hearing in the affected ear is poor for understanding speech. The otologist and audiologist may occasionally mistake the perceptive loss for a conductive loss, but with the use of correct masking this difficulty is overcome. This error commonly occurs when using tuning forks without masking the normal ear, for then the negative Rinne recorded on the affected side is not recognized as a false negative Rinne. With the Weber test the patient will usually lateralize the sound to the good hearing ear and therefore this test should not be excluded from the routine out-patient assessment. Occasionally it will also help to detect a badly recorded, unmasked audiogram in which the recorded air conduction is no more than a shadow curve and the bone conduction a record of the good hearing ear. With proper narrow band masking methods this difficulty in diagnosis is unlikely to arise (Dix and Hallpike, 1958).

The pure-tone audiogram, when recordable, has no characteristic curve. The majority have a high-tone loss, others a flat curve, some a central trough and in others it may be normal. Loudness recruitment, as determined by the binaural alternate loudness balance test of Fowler (1928), is absent in almost every case, its presence thus making the diagnosis unlikely. Complete recruitment can occur, however, in early acoustic tumours and disappear after successful removal (Dix and Hood, 1953; Hood, 1969). This must be due to interference with the blood supply to the inner ear, which can be restored by early removal of the tumour before irreparable changes have occurred in the hair-cells. Loudness reversal, i.e. loudness increasing less rapidly with an increase in intensity, may be seen in retrocochlear lesions even when little or no hearing loss exists (Hood, 1969). Occasionally there is need for a test in bilateral hearing loss when the loudness balance test is not applicable and it is important to exclude a retrocochlear lesion. Reger's mono-aural balance test, in which two loudnesses are compared, as in Fowler's test but using different frequencies in the same ear, is too complex a test for the majority of patients. The difference limen test of Denes and Naunton (1949) may also be of value in distinguishing end-organ deafness from nerve deafness in a patient with bilateral hearing loss. Hood and Poole (1966) studied the loudness discomfort levels (LDL) in patients with end-organ lesions, conductive deafness and retrocochlear lesions. In Menière's disease the LDL was, as in normal ears, at a level of 90–105 dB; but in conductive and retrocochlear lesions it was above 120 dB. Thus, as it is easy to eliminate the conductive lesions by testing bone conduction, measurement of LDL could be a useful diagnostic test in bilateral hearing loss.

Patients with acoustic neuroma are often found to have abnormally poor speech discrimination in relation to pure-tone thresholds, compared with patients having lesions of the organ of Corti (Schuknecht and Woeller, 1955). House's (1964) series showed a poor speech discrimination of 0–30 per cent in 69 per cent of his cases, and another 9 per cent showed marked impairment. Johnson (1968) found a poor discrimination score in 61 per cent of 167 patients tested.

Békésy audiometry provides a useful method of analysis and differentiation from lesions of the cochlea. Adaptation or threshold drift is present in acoustic neuromas. Jerger (1960) compared the Békésy responses of continuous and interrupted tones in conventional and fixed frequency audiometry. His analysis is useful for the recognition of retrocochlear lesions, for the majority of patients have a Type III or Type IV audiogram. In the conventional Békésy audiogram there is either a rapid fall of the continuous tone recording below that of the interrupted tone even at low frequencies (Type III), or the continuous tone falls consistently below that of the interrupted tone even at low frequencies (Type IV). In the fixed frequency audiogram of a Békésy Type III, the interrupted tracing remains unchanged but the continuous frequency falls rapidly to as much as 40–50 dB within 60 s. In Type IV fixed frequency recordings, the continuous frequency tracing is always at a lower level than the interrupted tracing even at frequencies of 500 Hz and lower. In Menière's disease this difference between interrupted and continuous frequencies does not occur in the lower tones. With the SISI (short increment sensitivity index) test a proportion of patients have low scores. A modification of this test as described by Thompson (1963) may also be of value. Tone decay (Carhart, 1957) indicates adaptation in response to a continuous tone. This is never more than 20 dB in Menière's disease but often more than 30 dB in cases of acoustic neuroma. Occasionally the deafness is bilateral and then other signs of von Recklinghausen's disease must be sought. However, bilateral deafness may be evidence of a more centrally placed lesion affecting both nuclei and their connecting fibres.

Brackmann (1975) and King, Gibson and Morrison (1976) suggest that testing the acoustic reflex is the most reliable audiometric screening test of patients with a sensorineural deafness for the detection of eighth nerve tumours. Patients with these tumours rarely demonstrate an acoustic reflex at less than 75 dB above their hearing threshold. Anderson et al. (1970) and King, Gibson and Morrison (1976) showed that in these tumour patients in whom an acoustic reflex was obtained, the reflex showed a rapid decay. Bosotra and Russolo (1976) made an oscilloscopic analysis of the stapedius muscle reflex studying the threshold, latency, amplitude and rise time of the reflex in patients with brain stem experimental and pathological lesions and their findings may be of value in the detection of acoustic neuromas.

Gibson and Beagley (1976) and Beagley et al. (1977) studied the electrocochleograph in patients with acoustic neuromas and their findings are summarized as showing a widened action potential response usually in small tumours; a complete absence of action potential with possible preservation of the cochlear microphonic demonstrating that some cochlear hair-cells are still functioning; the occasional presence of a normal action potential in electrocochleography with a severe or total subjective deafness.

Tinnitus often accompanies the deafness and, although varying in type and severity, it is of itself of no value as a diagnostic sign.

Vestibular function

Dix and Hallpike (1960) stated that the vestibular response to hot or cold water is absent in every case but others do not find this to be absolute, particularly with very small tumours. If all the other physical signs indicate that the patient has a lesion in the cerebello-pontine angle and there is a caloric response, the space-occupying lesion is probably not an acoustic neuroma but a meningioma. Patients complained of vague unsteadiness or imbalance in 80 per cent of House's cases but true vertigo occurred in 15 per cent only. Vertigo, however, may be very severe and lead to a diagnosis of Menière's disease or labyrinthitis (Fraser and Gardiner, 1930). Although nystagmus has been observed in 75 per cent of cases, and is usually of first degree ipsilateral type with quick movement to the affected side, this is not indicative of a lesion confined to the meatus and in many cases it is associated with pressure or displacement of the cerebellum and brain stem. House reported nystagmus in less than 10 per cent of his cases. Jongkees, Maas and Philipzoon (1962) found positional nystagmus with eyes closed in 11 of their 12 cases but only three patients had eye-open sustained nystagmus. Linthicum and Churchill (1968) found positional nystagmus in 22 per cent but latent nystagmus was found by electronystagmography in only 10 per cent of 149 patients tested. Morrison (1975) found spontaneous vestibular nystagmus occasionally in small or medium-sized tumours and latent nystagmus observed after abolition of eye-fixation was found in 60 per cent of medium sized tumours and in 33 per cent of intracanalicular neuromas. Vertical nystagmus is rarely present and is due to central involvement. In the early stages of the lesion, past-pointing defects and Rombergism do not occur but as the lesion enlarges to exert pressure on central structures and cerebellum, these physical signs appear and are accompanied by defects of co-ordination and ataxia. These latter physical signs indicate a large tumour.

Trigeminal nerve involvement

The diminution or absence of the corneal reflex used to be regarded as the earliest confirmatory physical sign and reports always show it to be present. To disturb the corneal reflex the tumour must have eroded the internal auditory meatus and have expanded within the cerebello-pontine angle pressing on the trigeminal nerve. By modern definition this is a relatively large tumour and although a useful physical sign, reduction of the corneal reflex is less likely to be seen when the diagnosis is established early, being present, for example, in only 43 per cent of House's series. More extensive sensory disturbance of the face indicates an even larger tumour.

Facial nerve involvement

A facial tic which precedes paresis may be the presenting symptom of an acoustic neuroma but, as explained above, paralysis is often a very late physical sign unless there has been a sudden rapid increase in size of an intrameatal tumour, possibly due to haemorrhage. It was found in only 15 per cent of the House series whereas previously it had been seen in as many as 50 per cent. Hitselberger and House (1966) noted hypoaesthesia of the posterior wall of the external auditory meatus in 25 cases of surgically confirmed acoustic neuromas. It is thought that this portion of the external auditory canal is supplied by sensory twigs of the facial nerve. Facial involvement may be first noticed by a failure of blinking or a failure to bury the eyelashes on the affected side when the eyelids are closed tightly. A regulated tap on the supra-orbital region shows a delayed blinking reaction. Other aspects of facial nerve function can be demonstrated by tests of taste and tear secretion.

Electrogustometry applied to the anterior two-thirds of the tongue shows a decrease in sensitivity to more than 20 μA stimulation (Pulec and House, 1964). Chemical tests of taste threshold (Hinchcliffe, 1958) are useful, but Hinchcliffe (1969) has met cases where the chemical threshold was normal and there was no response to electrical stimulation of the tongue. Other useful tests for assessing the general visceral efferent fibres of the facial nerve, which are carried by the greater superficial petrosal nerve and the chorda tympani, are the submandibular salivary flow test of Magielski and Blatt (1958) and the quantitative nasolacrimal reflex measurements of Zilstorff-Pederson (1959). Schirmer's test using strips of filter paper hooked over the lower eyelid can be a useful clinical test for measuring lacrimation. The taste threshold is reduced before lacrimation, and is therefore likely to be of greater clinical use.

Cerebellar involvement

When the tumour is large, cerebellar signs of ataxia, nystagmus and ipsilateral limb incoordination are found.

Raised intracranial pressure is usually of late onset. Mistiness of vision is often the first subjective indication of papilloedema. Headache and vomiting may accompany this but are also late manifestations. Bradycardia and nuchal pain are indicative of serious coning of the cerebellum. Finally, stupor, respiratory irregularities and coma terminate events.

Diagnosis

It is hoped by modern methods of investigation that acoustic nerve tumours will be diagnosed while small and preferably still confined to the internal auditory meatus. The most important factor is to be highly suspicious in all cases of unilateral sensorineural hearing loss of gradual or sudden onset or even when superimposed upon a conductive hearing loss due to other causes. Every suspected case should be submitted to intensive audiological study to determine if the lesion is retrocochlear. For this reason, a battery of hearing tests such as loudness balance, speech audiometry, tone decay, Békésy audiometry and the SISI test has been recommended in varied combination for all cases, because no one in itself is absolutely diagnostic. However, there is a danger in the indiscriminate and unplanned use of these tests, for the audiometrician through repeated unnecessary testing may lose interest and may record inaccurately or record what is expected rather than what is true; the patient himself may become bored and his responses inaccurate. With limited audiological facilities the loudness balance test is probably the most reliable; speech discrimination can also be very helpful. Rather than rely upon a battery of tests, Hood (1969) recommends the loudness balance test of Fowler, saying 'Few diagnostic tests can be

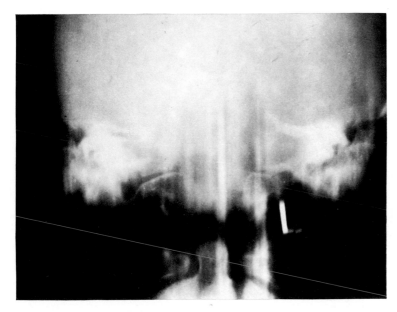

Figure 20.3 Tomogram of bilateral acoustic neuromas. The left internal auditory meatus shows a marked funnel-shaped expansion. The right meatus is expanded in its depths

relied upon to give 100 per cent results. Yet, in some respects, the diagnostic significance of the loudness recruitment test is as high as this. Thus, our own figures, well supported by others, show that the test is positive in 100 per cent of Menière's disease and negative in 90 per cent of cases of acoustic nerve tumours. A negative result, therefore, gives odds approaching the infinite against Menière's disease. A positive result gives odds of 9 to 1 against tumour. There can, we think, be few diagnostic tests which give results more decisive than this'. Nevertheless, patients with small acoustic neuromas may still show evidence of recruitment.

The introduction of more objective tests such as the study of the acoustic reflexes and electrocochleography have added a new dimension to the study of retrocochlear lesions.

The caloric response is always absent in large tumours but with very small tumours it may be present. The presence of spontaneous nystagmus is now regarded as one of the later signs, but positional nystagmus and latent nystagmus may be found with small tumours. In specialized clinics, rotation tests and electronystagmography are being used to analyse this problem further (Greiner, Conraux and Collard, 1969).

Whenever the audiological and caloric tests, or clinical suspicion, suggest the presence of a retrocochlear lesion, tomograms (*Figures 20.3, 20.4* and *20.5*) of the internal auditory meatus should be obtained, as routine views of the internal auditory meatus are not so reliable. Eighty five per cent of House's series of 54 tumours showed an erosion or enlargement of the internal auditory meatus. As little as 1 mm difference between the two sides is regarded as significant and particularly so if this is accompanied by erosion or difference in shape.

When plain x-rays or tomograms suggest the presence of neuroma the next investigation of choice is an EMI scan before and after the intravenous injection of an

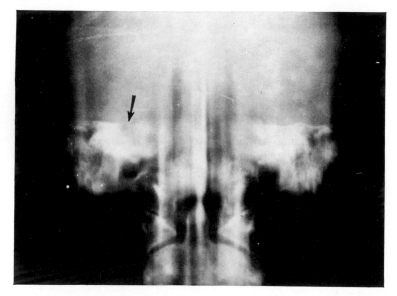

Figure 20.4 Tomogram to show erosion of the right internal auditory meatus. (Reproduced by courtesy of Dr. A. Appleby, Newcastle General Hospital)

iodine-containing contrast medium such as Conray. This examination shows most tumours which are encroaching on the cerebello-pontine angle cistern. It also shows the size of the ventricles of the brain confirming or excluding the presence of hydrocephalus. This is of course invaluable information if lumbar puncture is contemplated.

Lumbar puncture may be of particular value when the physical signs are minimal and it is then a relatively safe procedure. The cerebrospinal fluid may show a high protein content with large tumours but with very small ones it may be normal. However, lumbar puncture is more usefully combined with cisternal myelography. A cisternal myelogram is indicated when there is a suspected retrocochlear lesion with a normal EMI scan or the scan shows only a small projection into the cerebello-pontine angle. Myodil demonstrates the size of the cerebello-pontine projection and has the advantage over air studies in that the internal auditory meatus may be outlined if normal and the opaque material fails to enter the meatus when it is obstructed by tumour.

The presence of a reduced corneal reflex, facial weakness or cerebellar signs, in addition to the characteristic audiological picture are almost diagnostic of a cerebello-pontine angle tumour and these are readily identified by the EMI scan (*Figures 20.6* and *20.7*). In these cases lumbar puncture and cisternal myelography are contraindicated and vertebral angiography is a safer investigation and can be of value in not only demonstrating the tumour but also in assessing its vascularity (*Figure 20.8*).

House and Hitselberger stress the importance of combining hypocycloid tomography of the internal auditory meatus with myelography. The typical findings in a case of a small neuroma are shown in *Figure 20.9*.

The diagnosis of small eighth nerve tumours is dependent upon clinical suspicion and confirmation by neuroradiological techniques.

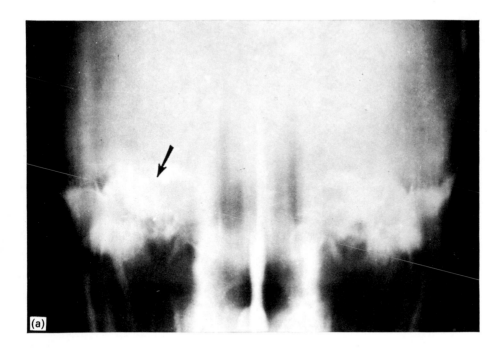

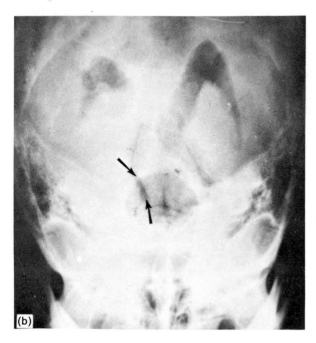

Figure 20.5 (a) Tomogram to show expansion of the right internal auditory meatus; (b) air encephalogram of the same patient to show the extension of the tumour into the cerebello-pontine angle outlined by the arrows. (Reproduced by courtesy of Dr. A. Appleby, Newcastle General Hospital)

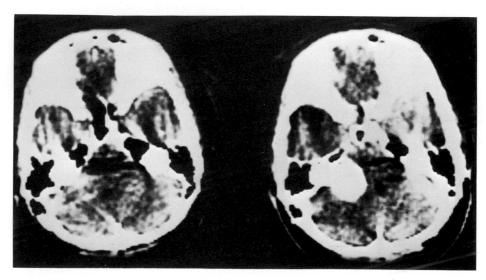

Figure 20.6 EMI scan before Conray (left) and after Conray (right). The enhancing effect on a large left cerebello-pontine angle acoustic neuroma is shown. The fourth ventricle shows some displacement to the right side

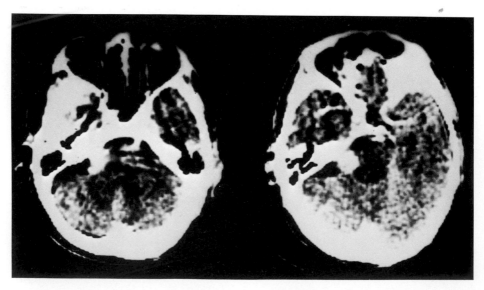

Figure 20.7 EMI scan of a small acoustic neuroma after Conray injection. The dense uptake of the contrast medium by the tumour adjacent to the petrous bone is clearly shown. Even the lobulated shape of the tumour can be detected

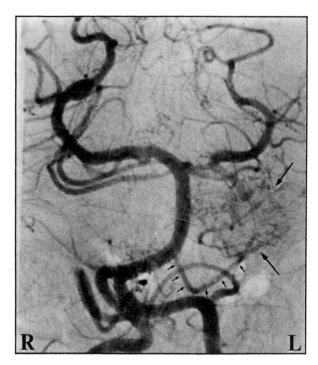

R   L

Figure 20.8 Vertebral angiograph of a patient with a large left acoustic neuroma. The large left anterior inferior cerebellar artery is clearly shown (small arrows) running in relation to the inferior surface of the tumour. The extensive vascularity of the tumour from this artery is shown (large arrows). A normal sized but displaced posterior inferior cerebellar artery is demonstrated.(This illustration is shown by the courtesy of Dr. A. Appleby)

Differential diagnosis

Menière's disease is the condition most frequently confused with acoustic neuroma. However, an acoustic tumour: (1) does not often cause intermittent severe vertigo; (2) very rarely produces recruitment; (3) speech discrimination is often very poor; (4) the loudness discomfort level is frequently raised; (5) tone decay is common; and (6) the Békésy audiometric response is usually different. A normal vestibular response to the caloric tests may exclude acoustic neuroma. If these tests are not decisive then repeated observation, tomography and cerebrospinal fluid examination may be necessary.

Arachnoid cysts occur in the cerebello-pontine angle and may simulate acoustic neuroma. They may be the result of meningitis, possibly otitic in origin, or may be congenital. However, an arachnoid cyst is commonly associated with acoustic nerve tumours and may contribute in part to the symptomatology.

Meningioma of the posterior cranial fossa may cause difficulty in diagnosis, but the chronological order of events may be different, as cranial nerves other than the auditory are affected first. Secondly, a caloric response may be present; and thirdly, tomography does not often show erosion of the internal auditory meatus. However, this differentiation is only of academic interest if the approach to the posterior fossa is suboccipital.

Congenital cholesteatoma frequently produces evidence of facial weakness earlier in the course of the disease; and erosion of the petrous apex, considered together with the clinical history, is almost diagnostic.

Pontine glioma may lead to difficulties if the lesion remains largely unilateral, for the auditory symptoms may be unilateral and produce the audiological abnormalities associated with acoustic tumour. There may be spontaneous nystagmus of horizonto-rotatory type or positional nystagmus, cerebellar incoordination and ataxia, a reduced corneal reflex or even a facial paralysis. Despite these gross physical signs the internal auditory meatus is normal and a ventriculogram shows a normal cerebello-pontine angle and features characteristic of a glioma distorting the pons.

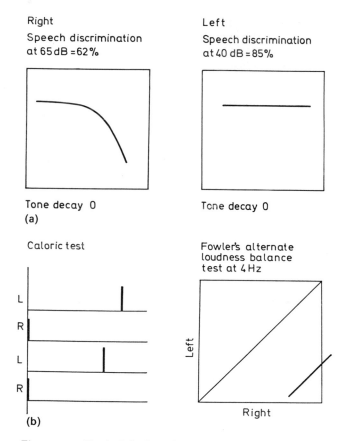

Right

Speech discrimination
at 65 dB = 62%

Left

Speech discrimination
at 40 dB = 85%

Tone decay 0

(a)

Tone decay 0

Caloric test

Fowler's alternate
loudness balance
test at 4 Hz

(b)

Figure 20.9   Typical findings in a patient (aged 52) with a small acoustic neuroma, only 2 cm in diameter. (a) Audiograms. Note reduced speech discrimination in right (affected) ear; (b) absence of caloric response and absence of recruitment in right ear; (c) tomograph shows 2 mm expansion of right internal auditory meatus; (d) myelogram of normal side; (e) myelogram of affected side, showing acoustic neuroma marked by arrow

Multiple sclerosis if presenting as unilateral demyelination in the pons may cause difficulty in differential diagnosis. The distinction is made by the clinical history, neurological examination and, possibly by examination of the cerebrospinal fluid.

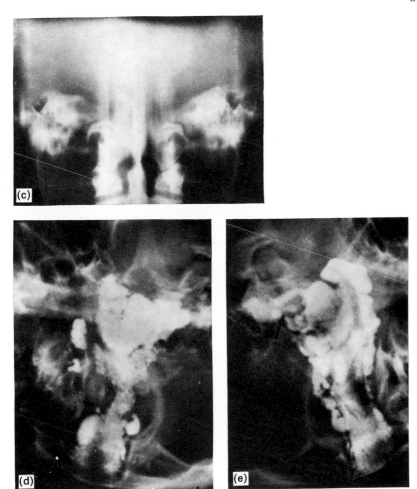

Figure 20.9 (cont.)

Management

It is important to realize that diagnosis, investigation, prognosis and management of the small neuroma is from almost every point of view different from that appropriate for the large tumour. During the past 15 years the development of specialized otoneurological and neuroradiological investigations have led to the diagnosis of an increasing proportion of small neuromas which are either confined to the petrous bone or invade the intracranial cavity to a minimal degree. Furthermore, the increasing use of the operating microscope by otologists and neurosurgeons facilitates the removal of these tumours with preservation of the facial nerve in a greater number of cases and with a reduced morbidity and mortality (Yasargil and Fox, 1974; Morrison and King, 1977). Where such specialized methods of investigation and treatment are available it would seem desirable to remove the tumours when small rather than wait until a greater size is reached. Olivecrona's (1967) figures of 4.1 per cent mortality for small tumours when compared with his 16.5 per cent for medium sized and 22.5 per cent for large tumours emphasizes the fact that for all practical purposes small tumours and large tumours can be regarded as two different diseases. Small tumours can be dealt with efficiently by the suboccipital approach through the posterior fossa or by a translabyrinthine approach. In the case of small tumours confined to the internal auditory meatus either the suboccipital route or the middle fossa route can be used, particularly when cochlear and vestibular function are only partially damaged, although in the majority of cases these functions are so extensively damaged that they are not worth preservation. Large tumours encroaching upon the posterior fossa and distorting cerebral structures are at least 2.5 cm and probably more in diameter and should always be the responsibility of the neurosurgeon with the assistance of the otologist. These are the tumours described in the voluminous literature on the subject. They have always been regarded as technically the most difficult and the most hazardous of the common benign tumours. These have usually been approached by the suboccipital route but more recently Morrison and King (1973) have combined the translabyrinthine and middle fossa routes, whereas House has used the translabyrinthine and suboccipital approaches together as the combined transigmoid approach for these large tumours in the hope of obtaining total excision with preservation of the facial nerve.

Over the years there have been many reports of large series of cases subjected to surgery. These are somewhat complicated by the proportions involving total removal and intracapsular removal, but a few figures from some accounts will indicate the risk attached to the surgery of large acoustic neuroma. Thus Cushing (1932) in 219 cases of intracapsular removal had a mortality of 11.4 per cent. Dandy (Gonzalez-Revilla, 1947) had a mortality of 22 per cent of 140 total removals. In his last 41 cases Dandy's operative mortality dropped to 2.4 per cent. Mortality rates now, due to the improvements in anaesthesia and operative technique are less than they were 20 years ago although they are often still high if the series includes a high proportion of large tumours (House, 1968; Thomsen, 1976). In contrast Yasargil and Fox (1974) quote a figure of 3.3 per cent and Morrison and King (1977) one of 2.2 per cent. The justification for a procedure to remove large tumours which may carry such a risk is the inevitability of a fatal outcome from brain stem distortion and hydrocephalus and the possibility of cure by the removal of a benign tumour. Death after surgical removal of an acoustic neuroma is most frequently caused by infarction of the brain stem due to vascular injury when removing tumour from the side of the pons.

Surgical excision can be either complete, subtotal or intracapsular. At present the majority of neurosurgeons favour complete removal whenever possible but this must be related to the quality of life subsequently enjoyed by survivors. Therefore, particularly in the elderly, some lesser procedure with a diminished risk of neurological deficits may be justified. This would be the object of subtotal removal in which relatively small portions of tumour capsule might be left attached to the side of the pons or anteriorly, attached to the facial nerve. Intracapsular removal, which is usually far from complete, has proved an unsatisfactory procedure because of the high incidence of recurrence requiring further surgery with even greater risk. The occasional largely cystic tumour seems to have the least tendency to recurrence following an incomplete removal. Olivecrona (1967), analysing the results of operation on 415 acoustic neuromas, found that in 58 per cent of patients subjected to total removal working capacity was normal or moderately impaired. In this series 72 per cent of patients who had a total removal were alive five years later.

With a large tumour the facial nerve is often stretched and splayed out over its anterior surface and is very adherent to the tumour capsule. It is then unlikely that the continuity of the nerve can be preserved. Similarly the glossopharyngeal, vagus and accessory nerves may be in contact with the lower pole of the tumour and may suffer some damage when being separated from it. With a small tumour, the only nerve which is displaced is the facial, which may be damaged by traction on the capsule if it has not first been dissected free. A post-operative facial nerve paralysis is a hard penalty for a patient to pay when his complaint was of unilateral deafness, particularly so when the hearing is also made worse, but total removal gives a cure of a potentially lethal condition. With small tumours, apart from surgical morbidity, which could be largely eliminated no matter what the approach, preservation of facial nerve function has become the prominent feature of the modern surgical outlook on acoustic neuroma. Rarely is it possible to preserve auditory function. Accepting that early diagnosis improves the possibility of surgical excision and prognosis, the decision remains as to when to operate and which approach is likely to give the best results.

The small tumour

Without definite confirmatory evidence, many surgeons are reluctant to consider surgery if the only abnormal findings are based on audiological and vestibular tests. Confirmation of the diagnosis is dependent on raised protein in the cerebrospinal fluid, but more so on neuroradiological findings such as enlargement or erosion of the internal auditory meatus, or a failure of filling of the meatus by Myodil. If surgery is not undertaken the patient must be kept under constant surveillance until the diagnosis is more certain. A very small tumour may be within the meatus or just medial to it, depending upon its site of origin from the neurilemmal sheath. Both types can be approached and totally removed by the suboccipital route with a low mortality and a low morbidity (Yasargil and Fox, 1974; Smith, 1977). The medially placed tumour is easily excised with preservation of the adjacent nerves including the facial. If within the meatus, the posterior wall of the internal auditory meatus is lowered so that the whole meatus may be inspected and the tumour removed. House (1961) and Fisch (1970) adapted the technique of exposing the internal auditory meatus devised by House in 1958, for removal of those very small tumours less than 1 cm in diameter, when the patient's hearing is worth preserving. For the somewhat larger ones, which are associated with poor hearing, he developed Quix's translabyrinthine approach. The advantage of the latter method is that the facial nerve is exposed first, the meatus is then opened and finally the tumour is carefully dissected off the facial nerve. Although post-operatively the communication between the mastoid and posterior fossa is sealed by a viable muscle graft and the aditus and epitympanum are occluded also by muscle, the protection provided against infection is not as satisfactory as in the suboccipital approach which does not open the middle-ear cleft. The translabyrinthine approach (House, 1968; Morrison and King, 1977) has given satisfactory results with low morbidity and mortality, but in these small tumours the suboccipital would be expected to provide an equally satisfactory outcome.

The size of the somewhat larger tumours can usually be determined radiologically. Either the suboccipital or translabyrinthine route is suitable but the latter approach is only advisable for those less than 2.5 cm in diameter. The advantage of the suboccipital route is that the whole tumour and its blood supply may be readily seen but the facial nerve is initially hidden from view and may be damaged. The translabyrinthine route alone can be used for total removal of tumours of this size with preservation of the facial nerve; but care must be taken to spare the anterior inferior cerebellar artery from which the internal auditory artery originates. It was shown by Atkinson (1949) that damage to the anterior inferior cerebellar artery led to fatal infarction of the lateral tegmental region of the pons and that this was not an infrequent cause of death following this type of surgery. A further factor was the presence of an unusually small posterior inferior cerebellar artery on the same side, suggesting the interdependence of these vessels in providing an adequate collateral circulation. These features are well demonstrated by vertebral angiography.

The larger tumours

The suboccipital, transmeatal route gives a much better exposure and allows total removal under good vision. The translabyrinthine route alone provides insufficient exposure to obtain total removal and a second-stage suboccipital approach is required for removal of the remnant (which will prove to be the greater part of the tumour). Hitselberger and House (1966) developed a combined suboccipital, petrosal approach which included division of the sigmoid sinus and which permitted a view of the lateral side of the posterior fossa from the foramen magnum to the internal auditory meatus. Even using such a wide exposure they were able to extirpate completely only 50 per cent of these tumours. This approach seems to have no great advantage over the suboccipital route, with removal of the outer third of the cerebellum when the tumour is very large, for in these cases the major concern is to avoid damage to the pontine blood supply while removing the tumour.

Morrison and King (1973) combined the translabyrinthine and middle fossa routes as the translabyrinthine-transtentorial approach. The technique gives ready access to the tumour, a good exposure of the pons and does not injure the cerebellum and therefore the incidence of post-operative cerebellar dysfunction is significantly reduced. However, post-operative temporary dysphasia does occur, if the dominant temporal lobe is retracted, as does epilepsy.

It is not possible to compare the results of the removal of small tumours through the translabyrinthine approach with these larger ones removed by the suboccipital route. The greatest gain with the translabyrinthine approach is a marked reduction in the incidence of post-operative facial paralysis for in House's series permanent weakness occurred in 12 per cent only. Cerebrospinal fluid leakage is rare with the suboccipital approach but is more likely to occur following the translabyrinthine operation, as is meningitis, either early or delayed. Meticulous haemostasis is essential before closure if post-operative haemorrhage is to be avoided, for it must be admitted that reopening of the posterior fossa for haemorrhage in these cases is rarely followed by a successful outcome. With the translabyrinthine approach it may become necessary to open the posterior fossa to deal with post-operative haemorrhage. Therefore, no matter which approach is used, close cooperation with neurosurgical colleagues must be maintained. Occasionally persistent haemorrhage from the superior petrosal sinus may prevent further progress during a translabyrinthine operation. The operation is abandoned and continued a week later.

A patient after the House operation for a very small tumour returns to work in two to four weeks and the incidence of cerebellar ataxia is low. With somewhat larger tumours, using a suboccipital approach, ataxia post-operatively is not severe but the patient is unlikely to return to work after such a short period. Convalescence after the removal of large acoustic neuromas may be protracted and, not infrequently in the elderly, or in patients lacking in determination, there is never a proper recovery of social or economic independence. This is in marked contrast to the results obtained by the removal of small tumours by any of the methods that have been described.

Surgical technique

Middle fossa transtemporal approach (*Plate 2a, facing p. 668*)

A vertical incision beginning in front of the ear at the zygomatic process and extending upwards to the superior temporal line is deepened through the temporal muscle to the bone. A 3 cm craniectomy is made just above the zygomatic arch to open the middle fossa and gain access at floor level. Dura is elevated to the level of the arcuate eminence at first and then gently anteriorly and medially to expose the facial hiatus. Care must be taken as the geniculate ganglion may not have a bony covering. Dural elevation is then continued forwards to expose the middle meningeal artery as it enters the cranium through the foramen spinosum. The greater superficial petrosal nerve is identified at its exit from the facial hiatus and used as a guide for finding the geniculate ganglion which is exposed by drilling with a diamond burr. The facial nerve is then followed medially to the internal auditory meatus. The superior vestibular nerve is identified at its exit and finally the dura along the posterior wall of the internal auditory meatus is incised and the tumour carefully separated from the surrounding structures and excised. The internal auditory artery is preserved. Haemostasis must be meticulous and is probably best obtained by the use of bipolar diathermy. Finally the dural edges are approximated and covered with gel-foam. The middle fossa dura is allowed to sink back over the defect and the wound is closed in layers.

Translabyrinthine approach (*Plate 2b, facing p. 668*)

Through a post-aural wound the mastoid cavity is excavated, outlining the lateral sinus plate, the tegmen typani, the superior petrosal sinus, the semicircular canals and the descending portion of the facial canal. The semicircular canals are opened and removed, so opening the vestibule from its posterosuperior aspect. The superior vestibular nerve, which supplies the ampullae of the superior and horizontal canals and utricle, is then identified where it enters the vestibule and immediately above this the petrous segment of the facial canal is seen where it joins the internal auditory meatus. Bone is removed between the superior petrosal sinus, the lateral sinus and the posterior and inferior margins of the meatus to expose the posterior fossa dura overlying the tumour. The dura is then incised and by careful dissection the tumour is isolated, care being taken not to damage the lateral branch of the anterior inferior cerebellar artery which may loop into the canal. The tumour is then separated from the facial nerve. If the tumour is fairly large an intracapsular removal may be done first, then the posterior part of the capsule is removed and finally the capsule remnant is dissected off the facial nerve. Haemostasis is obtained and the dural edges are approximated and supported by a fascial or viable muscle graft. Finally the aditus is scarified and packed with muscle and the post-aural wound closed.

A careful watch must be maintained throughout the operation for changes in blood pressure, pulse or respiration which would suggest traction on blood vessels supplying the pons. Post-operatively intensive antibiotic therapy is given.

Combined trans-sigmoid sinus approach

Essentially this consists of combining a suboccipital craniectomy with the translaby-rinthine approach. The sigmoid sinus is divided and the dura of the posterior fossa can then be opened from the foramen magnum to the internal auditory meatus giving a wide access for a large tumour.

Translabyrinthine–transtentorial approach (*Figures 20.10–20.15*)

The patient is placed in a supine position with the head rotated away from the side of the tumour. The head of the table is elevated but the patient's head is somewhat

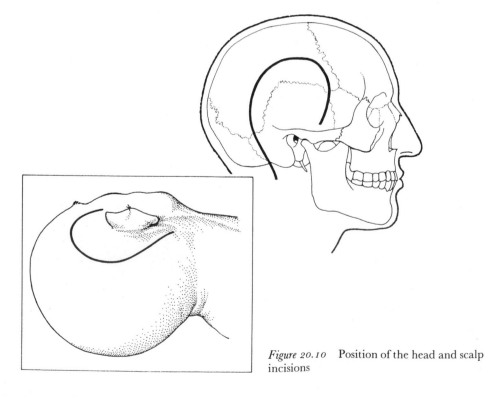

Figure 20.10   Position of the head and scalp incisions

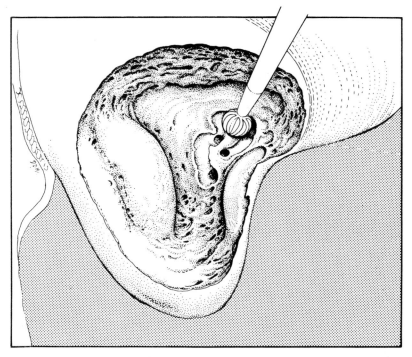

Figure 20.11 Dissection through labyrinth. The facial canal is seen anteriorly
and the sigmoid sinus posteriorly

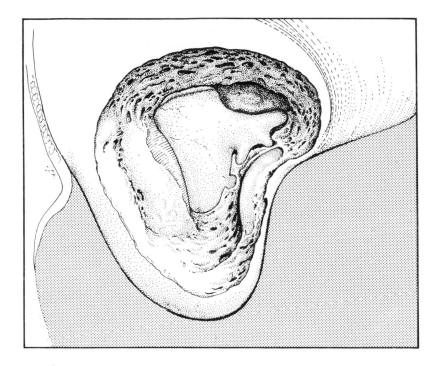

Figure 20.12 Posterior fossa dura exposed including the anterior edge of the sigmoid sinus

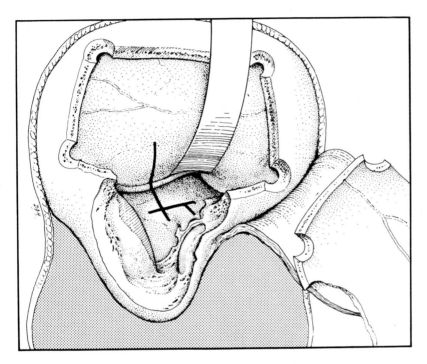

Figure 20.13 Temporal craniotomy and translabyrinthine exposures are now in continuity. The solid line indicates the dural incision crossing the superior petrosal sinus above and opening the internal auditory canal anteriorly

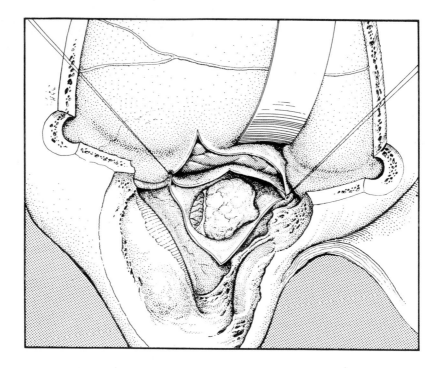

Figure 20.14 Division of the superior petrosal sinus and extension of the incision into the tentorium

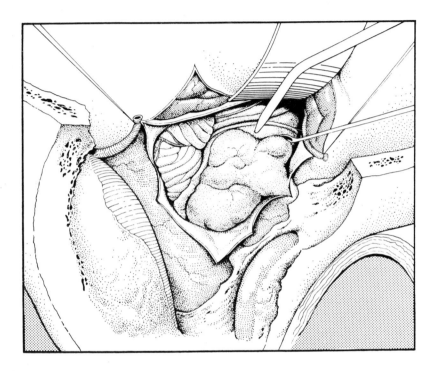

Figure 20.15 The superior aspect of the tumour is seen in its relation to the brain stem and laterally its origin in the internal auditory meatus. Note the very limited cerebellar exposure

extended to lessen the necessity for retraction of the temporal lobe. A large incision (*Figure 20.10*) is made and a temporal bone flap is turned by the neurosurgeon. The standard translabyrinthine approach to the internal auditory meatus is then performed by the otologist (*Figures 20.11* and *20.12*). To join the two surgical fields the tegmen tympani is removed and the dura is opened as illustrated dividing the superior petrosal sinus between ligatures (*Figure 20.13*). The dura is retracted and the temporal lobe elevated as little as possible by an extradural retractor to expose the superior surface of the tumour (*Figure 20.14*). The facial nerve is exposed in the depths of the meatus and the tumour carefully dissected under microscopical control attempting to preserve the facial nerve. The view of the pons is excellent but with a large tumour the lower cranial nerves are not seen until the dissection is complete.

Combined suboccipital and transmeatal operation (*Plate 2d, facing page 668* and *Figures 20.16–20.20*)

POSITION OF PATIENT

Operations on the posterior cranial fossa are more conveniently performed with the patient supported in the sitting position using a chair or an operating table designed for the purpose. The advantages of the sitting position are:

(1) Better vision and convenience of approach for the surgeon with the operative field placed directly in front and at eye level.
(2) Constant drainage, by gravity, of cerebrospinal fluid and blood from the operative field.
(3) Reduction of venous congestion compared with the prone position.

There are two hazards to the anaesthetized patient in the sitting position which must be avoided:

(1) Reduction of blood pressure level can be dangerous and should be prevented by the appropriate anaesthetic techniques and by constant blood pressure monitoring. The patient's legs should be supported by compressive bandages and should not be dependent, so as to reduce 'pooling' of blood.

(2) A lesser risk, if constantly kept in mind and guarded against, is aspiration of air into a dural venous sinus or into a venous channel in the bone. This is heralded by electrocardiographic irregularities and a serious fall in blood pressure. To prevent further aspiration of air and to compensate for change in blood pressure it is essential that the table and the towelling should permit an immediate reversal of the patient's position. It should be possible for the table to rotate backwards through 90° so that the head and body assume a horizontal position with the legs elevated in relation to the trunk. Fortunately this manoeuvre is rarely necessary, but it must be undertaken with the minimum of delay. The proponents of the sitting position maintain that it provides technical advantages which justify a small risk—a view not shared by all neurological surgeons.

The degree of flexion of the patient's head at the atlanto-occipital articulation is important. Flexion is desirable to expose this region and particularly for the removal of the arch of the atlas, but excessive flexion can be dangerous when there is tonsillar impaction. This applies also at ventriculography when the head is positioned conveniently for posterior parietal burr holes.

ANAESTHESIA

Patients with infratentorial lesions are often peculiarly sensitive to drugs causing respiratory depression. Premedication should therefore be minimal—preferably atropine only. General anaesthesia is now usually preferred and typically consists of an intravenous induction, the application of local anaesthetic to the larynx and trachea and orotracheal intubation followed by maintenance with low concentrations of nitrous oxide, trilene and/or halothane. In spite of light premedication and low maintenance concentrations of inhalational agents, respiratory depression is common and blood carbon dioxide levels are frequently above normal. This has led many teams to prefer mechanical ventilation to spontaneous breathing and better operating conditions undoubtedly follow the use of this technique. It must be accepted, however, that in abolishing spontaneous breathing a useful clinical sign is lost and interference with lower brain stem centres may not be so noticeable.

As well as those problems associated with the sitting position already mentioned there are those related to the site of the operation. Alterations in breathing, heart rate, electrocardiogram and blood pressure may all be produced by surgical manipulation of the lower brain stem or contiguous structures. The alterations, which can be almost instantaneous, may be sympathetic or vagal. The most serious are changes in heart rate or rhythm causing a precipitate and sometimes catastrophic fall in blood pressure. For this reason, monitoring is especially important and elaborate systems are justified by the significant increase in protection they provide. Continuous display of the electrocardiogram and blood pressure (from an intra-arterial cannula) gives a continuous contact with the patient that cannot be obtained from intermittent measurements. Early warning of changes can be life saving.

Atropine and propanolol are useful in counteracting the cardiac effects of central vagal and sympathetic stimulation and vasopressors should always be to hand and used, preferably in anticipation, to prevent serious hypotension.

Post-operatively patients may have lower cranial nerve lesions and extubation should be delayed until the patient is awake and cooperative.

INCISION

The incision is either a vertical paramedian or curved 'hockey-stick' incision (*Figure 20.16*). Occipital bone is removed, including the posterolateral part of the foramen magnum and exposing the lower edge of the lateral sinus above and to the medial edge of the sigmoid sinus laterally (*Figure 20.17*). If mastoid air-cells are opened they are closed with Horsley's wax.

If the intracranial pressure is significantly raised, as judged clinically, ventricular drainage for a period of 48 h before operation may be indicated. Otherwise the ventricles can be aspirated during the course of the operation. On opening the dura, cerebrospinal fluid is drained from the cisterna magna and, on elevating the cerebellum, fluid can often be drained from an arachnoid cyst commonly found over the lateral pole of the tumour. The glossopharyngeal, vagus and accessory cranial nerves are then separated from the inferior pole of the tumour and covered with a pattie (*Figure 20.18*). This is facilitated, as is much of the operation, by the use of magnifying spectacles, a binocular loupe (× 2.5) or a microscope.

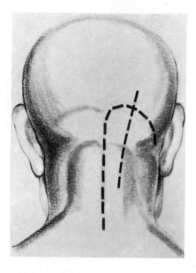

Figure 20.16   The 'hockey-stick' incision and the vertical paramedian incision

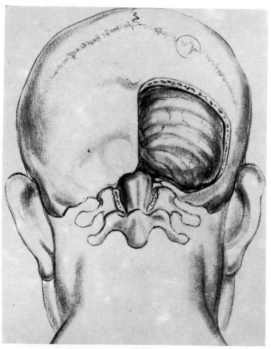

Figure 20.17   The   extent   of   the bone removal

If the cerebellar hemisphere is bulky and obstructing the exposure of the cerebello-pontine angle the outer third can be resected without appreciable effect on function, but this is not often necessary.

DISSECTION AT INTERNAL AUDITORY MEATUS (*Plate 2d, facing page 668*)

This is probably best done by an ear, nose and throat surgeon experienced in the use of the operating microscope and the high speed diamond drill and it necessitates the removal of a variable amount of the petrous bone forming the posterior lip of the internal auditory meatus and the bone lateral to it. The origin of the tumour from the auditory nerve is demonstrated and the nerve is divided laterally. The lateral pole of the tumour is then lifted out of the canal posteriorly showing the flattened facial nerve lying anteriorly.

A circular incision about 1 cm in diameter is made in the capsule of the tumour and intracapsular removal of tumour tissue is done. If the tissue is soft, suction is sufficient but firmer tumour requires the use of a curette or the pituitary rongeurs. Because of the fear of penetrating the capsule anteriorly or medially intracapsular removal is usually far from complete but is sufficient to enable the capsule to be drawn away from the pons. Small arteries running on to the capsule should be divided as close to the capsule as possible and this particularly applies to the anterior inferior cerebellar artery; and here again some degree of magnification is essential. It is possible at this stage to elevate the lower pole of the capsule in order to see this artery and also the flattened band of the facial nerve as it lies on the front of the tumour and on the lateral side of the pons. The superior pole should be carefully separated from the trigeminal nerve which appears as a wide flat bundle arched upwards over it. In large tumours a nubbin of growth may have extended through the tentorial incisura. This can sometimes be withdrawn but occasionally the tentorium must be divided.

The capsule is progressively reduced in size as it is freed from the porus laterally and from the pons medially. If it is not possible to remove the middle portion of the tumour capsule from the splayed facial nerve and, if this structure has so far been identified and preserved, it is justifiable to leave a small portion of capsule. Similarly if a piece of capsule medially is attached to the pons in such a way that traction on it produces disturbance of vital signs, this piece also should be left (*Figures 20.19* and *20.20*).

It is essential to have the field completely dry with the use of peroxide patties, small pieces of gel-foam, bipolar coagulation and clips, with the blood pressure at a normal level. Coagulation and clipping of vessels should be employed with great discretion as

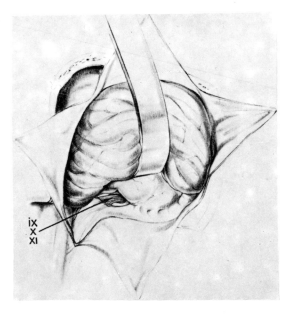

ix
x
xi

Figure 20.18 The relationship of the tumour to the lower cranial nerves (after Drake, 1967)

the commonest cause of death is infarction of brain stem structures. Vessels should be dealt with on the capsule as the dissection proceeds. Oozing can be controlled by gentle packing with cotton wool and by patience. The wound is closed with multiple layers of black silk sutures without drainage.

POST-OPERATIVE CARE

The cornea should be protected until it is possible to judge whether the patient has

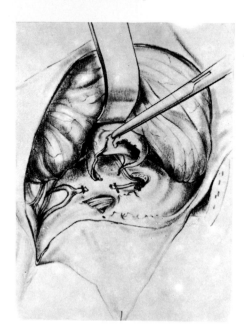

Figure 20.19 Part of the capsule has been removed. The facial nerve, anterior inferior cerebellar artery and the lower cranial nerves can be seen (after Drake, 1967)

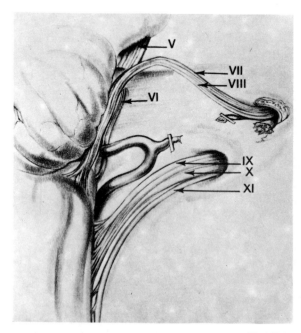

Figure 20.20 A diagrammatic representation of important structures at the end of the tumour removal. A small nubbin of tumour remains in the internal auditory meatus (after Drake, 1967)

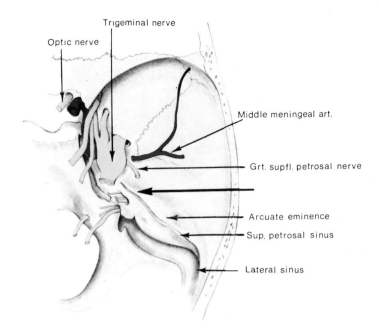

(a)

Optic nerve

Trigeminal nerve

Middle meningeal art.

Grt. supfl. petrosal nerve

Arcuate eminence

Sup. petrosal sinus

Lateral sinus

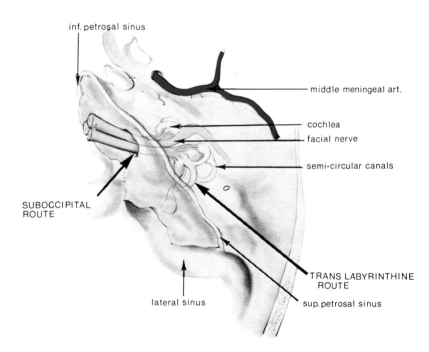

(b)

inf. petrosal sinus

middle meningeal art.

cochlea

facial nerve

semi-circular canals

SUBOCCIPITAL
ROUTE

TRANS LABYRINTHINE
ROUTE

lateral sinus

sup. petrosal sinus

Plate 2 (a) The middle fossa seen from above. The arrow indicates the middle fossa surgical approach to the internal auditory meatus. (b) The temporal bone seen from above to show the translabyrinthine and suboccipital transmeatal approaches (*continued*)

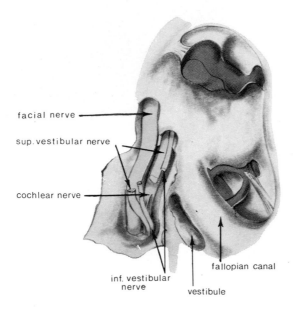

facial nerve

sup. vestibular nerve

cochlear nerve

inf. vestibular nerve

vestibule

fallopian canal

(c)

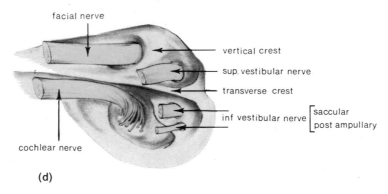

facial nerve

vertical crest

sup. vestibular nerve

transverse crest

inf vestibular nerve $\begin{bmatrix} \text{saccular} \\ \text{post ampullary} \end{bmatrix}$

cochlear nerve

(d)

Plate 2 (continued)   (c) View of the internal auditory canal as seen in the translabyrinthine approach. (d) View of the internal auditory canal as seen in the suboccipital transmeatal approach after removing the posterior wall

suffered any damage to the trigeminal and facial nerves. If both nerves are damaged which sometimes happens, usually temporarily, so that the patient has both an anaesthetic and a dry cornea, lateral third tarsorrhaphy is indicated. Fluids by mouth should not be given until it is certain that the swallowing reflexes are intact. For a period of days, varying according to the patient's condition, post-operative observation and care amounting to 'intensive care' are necessary. This is available in neurosurgical departments as it is the usual practice following major intracranial operations.

Tracheostomy is indicated if there has been disturbance of the swallowing reflexes. It is also often a life saving procedure when the patient is drowsy and there is difficulty in keeping the chest clear. In some units tracheostomy is performed as a routine following the removal of any large acoustic neuroma. The management of a tracheostomy under these circumstances and the decision when it should be discarded require special care and experience.

These views would not be held by all neurosurgeons but they are a description of the average position of those favouring an approach combined with their otological colleagues—an essential attitude in both the diagnosis and treatment of these benign, dangerous and not uncommon tumours.

References

Anderson, H., Barr, B. and Wedenberg, E. (1970) *Acta Otolaryngologica, Suppl.* **263**, 232

Atkinson, W. J. (1949) *Journal of Neurology, Neurosurgery and Psychiatry*, **12**, 137

Beagley, H. A., Legouix, J. P., Teas, D. C. and Remond M. C. (1977) *Clinical Otolaryngology*, **2**, 213

Bosotra, A., Russolo, M. and Poli, P. (1975) *Acta Otolaryngologica*, **80**, 61

Bosotra, A. and Russolo M. (1976) *Archives of Otolaryngology*, **102**, 284

Brackmann, D. (1975) Quoted by King, Gibson and Morrison (1976b)

Brunner, H. (1925). *Monatschrift Ohrenheilkunde und Laryngo-rhinologie*, **59**, 697

Burrows, E. H. (1969) *British Journal of Radiology*, **42**, 902

Carhart, R. (1957) *Archives of Otolaryngology*, **65**, 32

Cawthorne, Sir T. E., Dix, M. R. and Hood, J. D. (1968) *Neuro-ophthalmology*, **4**, 81

Clemis, J. D., Burns, R. O. and Shambaugh, G. E. (1968) *Archives of Otolaryngology*, **87**, 645

Cushing, H. (1917). *Tumours of the Nerves Acusticus and the Syndrome of the Cerebello-pontine angle*. Philadelphia; Saunders

Cushing, H. (1932) *Intracranial Tumours*. Springfield Ill.; Thomas

Dandy, W. E. (1925) *Surgery, Gynaecology and Obstetrics*, **41**, 129

Denes, P. and Naunton, E. F. (1949) *Journal of Laryngology*, **63**, 251

Dix, M. R. (1968) *Annals of Otology, Rhinology and Laryngology, St. Louis*, **77**, 1131

Dix, M. R. and Hallpike, C. S. (1958) *Proceedings of the Royal Society of Medicine*, **51**, 889

Dix, M. R. and Hallpike, C. S. (1960) *Laryngoscope*, **70**, 105

Dix, M. R., Hallpike, C. S. and Hood, J. D. (1948) *Proceedings of the Royal Society of Medicine*, **41**, 516

Dix, M. R., Hallpike, C. S. and Hood, J. D. (1949) *Proceedings of the Royal Society of Medicine*, **42**, 527

Dix, M. R. and Hood, J. D. (1953) *Journal of Laryngology*, **67**, 343

Dix, M. R. and Hood, J. D. (1969) *Acta Otolaryngologica, Stockholm*, **67**, 310

Drake, C. G. (1967) *Journal of Neurosurgery*, **26**, 554

Fisch, U. (1970) *Advances in Oto-rhino-laryngology*, **17**, 202

Fowler, E. P. (1928) *Archives of Otolaryngology*, **8**, 151

Fraser, J. S. and Gardiner, W. T. (1930) *Proceedings of the Royal Society of Medicine*, **23**, 726

Gardner, W. J. and Turner, O. A. (1940) *Archives of Neurology and Psychiatry*, **44**, 76

Gibson, W. P. R. and Beagley, H. H. (1976) *Journal of Laryngology and Otology*

Gonzalez-Revilla, A. (1947) *Bulletin of the Johns Hopkins Hospital*, **80**, 254

Greiner, G. F., Conraux C. and Collard, M. (1969) *Vestibulometrie Clinique*, Paris; Deron et Cie

Hardy, M. and Crowe, S. J. (1936) *Archives of Surgery*, **32**, 292

Henschen, F. (1915) *Archives of Psychiatry*, **56**, 21

Hinchcliffe, R. (1958) *Acta Otolaryngologica, Stockholm*, **49**, 453

Hinchcliffe, R. (1969) Paper read to the Belgian Otolaryngolocical Society, December 1969

Hitselberger, W. E. and House, W. F. (1966) *Archives of Otolaryngology*, **83**, 218

Hitselberger, W. E. and House, W. F. (1966) *Archives of Otolaryngology*, **84**, 267, 286

Hood, H. (1968) *Archives of Otolaryngology*, **87**, 651

Hood, J. D. (1968a) *International Audiology*, **7**, 232

Hood, J. D. (1968b) *Journal of the Acoustical Society of America*, **44**, 959

Hood, J. D. (1969) *Journal of Laryngology*, **83**, 695

Hood, J. D. and Poole, J. P. (1966) *Journal of the Acoustical Society of America*, **40**, 47

House, W. F. (1961) *Laryngoscope*, **71**, 1363

House, W. F. (1964) *Archives of Otolaryngology*, **80**, 599

House, W. F. (1968) *Archives of Otolaryngology*, **88**, 576

Jerger, J. (1960). *Journal of Speech and Hearing Research*, **3**, 275

Johnson, E. W. (1968) *Archives of Otolaryngology*, **88**, 598

Jongkees, L. B. W., Maas, V. P. M., and Philipzoon, J. H. (1962) *Practica otorhinolaryngologica*, **24**, 65

King, T. T., Gibson, W. P. R. and Morrison, A. W. (1976a) *Clinical Otolaryngology*, **1**, 153

King, T. T., Gibson, W. P. R. and Morrison, A. W. (1976b) *British Journal of Hospital Medicine*, 259

Krarup, B. (1958) *Acta Otolaryngologica, Stockholm, Suppl.*, **140**, 195

Krarup, B. (1959) *Neurology*, **9**, 53

Leonard and Talbot (1970) *Archives of Otolaryngology*, **91**, 117

Lidén, G. (1969) *Journal of Laryngology*, **83**, 507

Lierle, D. M. and Reger, S. M. (1955) *Annals of Otolaryngology, Rhinology and Laryngology*, **64**, 263

Linthicum, F. W. and Churchill, D. (1968) *Archives of Otolaryngology*, **88**, 604

Litton, W. B. and McCabe, B. F. (1966) *Laryngoscope*, **76**, 1113

Lundborg, T. (1950) *Nordisk Medicin*, **44**, 1520

Magielski, J. E. and Blatt, I. M. (1958) *Laryngoscope*, **68**, 1770

Montgomery, W. W. and Ojemann, R. G. (1968) *Archives of Otolaryngology*, **83**, 566

Morrison, A. W. (1975) *Management of Sensorineural Deafness*. London; Butterworths

Morrison, A. W. (1976) *Operative Surgery*, 3rd edn, (Rob and Smith). London; Butterworths

Morrison, A. W. and King, T. T. (1973) *Journal of Neurosurgery*, **38**, 382

Morrison, A. W. and King, T. T. (1977) *Proceedings of the Royal Society of Medicine*

Nielson, A. (1942) *Annals of Surgery*, **115**, 849

Ojemann, R. G., Montgomery, W. M. and Weiss, A. D. (1972) *New England Journal Medicine*, **287**, 895

Olivecrona, H. (1967) *Journal of Neurosurgery*, **26**, 6

Pulec, J. L. and House, W. F. (1964) *Archives of Otolaryngology*, **80**, (a) 681; (b) 685

Pulec, J. L. and Hughes, R. L. (1964) *Archives of Otolaryngology*, **80**, 677

Quix, F. H. (1912) *Verhandlungen der Deutschen otologischen Gesellschaft*, **10**, 392

Rand, R. W. (1969) *Microneurosurgery*. St. Louis; Mosby

Rand, R. W. and Kurze, T. L. (1967) *Transactions of the American Academy of Ophthalmology*, **71**, 682

Russell, D. S., Robertson, L. J. and Lumsden, C. E. (1959) *The Pathology of Tumours of the Nervous System*. London; Edward Arnold

Schuknecht, H. F. and Woeller, R. C. (1955) *Journal of Laryngology*, **49**, 75

Silverstein, H. and Schuknecht, H. F. (1966) *Archives of Otolaryngology*, **84**, 395

Smith, M. (1977) *Proceedings of the Royal Society of Medicine*

Stout, A. P. (1935a) *American Journal of Cancer*, **24**, 751

Stout, A. P. (1935b) *American Journal of Cancer*, **25**, 1

Stout, A. P. and Murray, M. R. (1942) *Revue Canadien de Biologie*, **1**, 657

Thompson, G. (1963) *Journal of Speech and Hearing Disorders*, **28**, 299

Thomsen, J. (1976) *Acta Otolaryngologica*, **81**, 406

Turner, O. A. and Gardner, W. J. (1938). *American Journal of Cancer*, **32**, 339

Watkyn-Thomas, F. W. (1939) *Proceedings of the Royal Society of Medicine*, **32**, 487

Willis, R. A. (1948) *Pathology of Tumours*. London; Butterworths

Wilmot, T. J. (1969) *Journal of Laryngology*, **83**, 521

Valvassori, J. (1966) *Laryngoscope*, **76**, 1104

Yasargil, M. G. and Fox, J. L. (1974) *Surgery and Neurology*, **2**, 393

Zilstorff-Pederson, K. (1959). *Acta Otolaryngologica, Stockholm*, **50**, 501

21 Ototoxicity
John Ballantyne

'Ototoxicity may be defined as the tendency of certain therapeutic agents and other chemical substances to cause functional impairment and cellular degeneration of the tissues of the inner ear, and especially of the end-organs and neurons of the cochlear and vestibular divisions of the eighth cranial nerve.' (Hawkins, 1976.)

The list of drugs and other chemical agents is a truly formidable one and, in the massive *Index-Handbook of Ototoxic Agents 1966–1971* (Worthington *et al.*, 1973), the list of ototoxic agents alone occupies no less than two and a half pages of closely-spaced print. Apart from the antibiotics (mainly the aminoglycosides), salicylates (and other analgesics), antimalarial agents and diuretics, which are the most important of them, the list includes analeptics (including caffeine), anaesthetic agents (topical but not general), anticonvulsants, antidepressants, antidiabetic agents (including insulin), antihistamines, anti-inflammatory agents, antineoplastic agents, antituberculous agents (apart from the aminoglycosides), cardiovascular agents, contraceptives, heavy metals, sedatives and tranquillizers (including thalidomide), and no fewer than 13 miscellaneous 'chemical agents' (including nicotine and tobacco); and to these we must add more if we are to bring it up to date.

It was almost 300 years ago when Morton (1696) mentioned the occurrence of temporary deafness in patients being treated for fevers with cinchona bark, and Laveran (1898) noted that tinnitus and hearing impairment could develop at a relatively early stage in the treatment of malaria with quinine. Fourteen years earlier Schwabach (1884) reported deafness from therapeutic doses of salicylates. Fortunately these toxic effects of salicylates and cinchona alkaloids are usually, though not always, reversible; and the same can be said of the diuretic agents, frusemide and ethacrynic acid. But the most important ototoxic drugs are the aminoglycoside antibiotics, whose toxic effects are nearly always permanent and may develop or progress even after their withdrawal.

Quinine and salicylates

Quinine was widely used in the past, both as an antiprotozoal agent in the treatment of malaria and as an abortefacient; and salicylates are extensively used as analgesics.

Tinnitus and/or hearing loss may occur with either or both, but characteristically these effects are reversible. Nevertheless, both symptoms may be permanent (Gignoux, Martin and Cajgfinger, 1966) and on very rare occasions congenital hearing losses have been reported in infants whose mothers had taken high pre-natal doses of quinine in attempts to induce abortion (McKinna, 1966).

The effects of both quinine and salicylates are probably induced by vasoconstriction of the small vessels of the cochlear micro-vasculature, possibly by an inhibitory effect on local prostaglandin synthesis (Ferreira and Vane, 1974).

Diuretics

Ethacrynic acid (Edecrin) and frusemide (Lasix) are two potent diuretic agents which, although quite different in chemical structure, have similar actions on the renal tubules, where they inhibit reabsorption of sodium and water in the proximal portion of the loop of Henle (Hawkins, 1976).

Sensorineural hearing loss following the use of ethacrynic acid was first described by Maher and Schreiner (1965) and in many of their cases it was characterized by immediate onset and reversibility in patients with renal failure. Since that time there have appeared many other reports of transient hearing loss after the administration of this drug, but four years later Pillay and his colleagues (1969) reported permanent losses.

Transient (Venkateswaran, 1971) and permanent (Lloyd-Mostyn and Lord, 1971) hearing losses have also been reported with intravenous frusemide.

Permanent hearing loss may also occur when patients being treated with an aminoglycoside are given either of these diuretics.

Although some authors (Mathog, Thomas and Hudson, 1970; Crifò, 1973) have described some loss of hair-cells after intravenous administration, others have found little or no change in them (Kohonen, Jauhainen and Tarkkanen, 1970; Federspil and Hansen, 1973). Indeed, the main histopathological changes have been found in the stria vascularis, in which extensive oedematous changes have been seen within minutes of an injection (Quick and Duvall, 1970; Quick and Hoppe, 1975).

Antiheparinizing agents

Ransome *et al.* (1966) reported several cases of sensorineural hearing loss due to the drug hexadimethrine bromide (Polybrene). This formerly was used in patients who were being treated for renal failure by haemodialysis, during the course of which heparin was given as an anticoagulant; and Polybrene was given at the end of each dialysis as an antiheparinizing agent. Six out of 14 patients treated with this drug developed various degrees of sensorineural deafness, often very severe.

The histopathological changes in the temporal bones of one patient being so treated included gross degeneration of the organ of Corti, degeneration of the stria vascularis, some degeneration of the spiral ganglion, thickening of Reissner's membrane, rupture and disorganization of the endolymphatic sac, and a fibrin-free exudate in the subepithelial connective tissues of the vestibular maculae and cupulae.

Cytotoxic agents

There have been several reports of sensorineural hearing loss following the regional perfusion of nitrogen mustard (Conrad and Crosby, 1960; Lawrence *et al.*, 1961; Young *et al.*, 1961; Schuknecht, 1964; Cummings, 1968).

Pathological changes were demonstrated in the organs of Corti (Schuknecht, 1964; Cummings, 1968).

Anticonvulsant drugs

Overdosage with certain anticonvulsant drugs, especially phenytoin, may be associated with vestibular disorders (Nozue *et al.*, 1973). These may be acute (when they resemble a 'posterior fossa syndrome') but clear rapidly as soon as the drug is withdrawn; or much more commonly, chronic, when disturbance of balance continues, usually in a young epileptic patient who has had repeated doses of the anticonvulsant over a long period (Ajodhia and Dix, 1974).

Detailed studies of the spontaneous 'rebound nystagmus' which may occur in such cases have shown it to be associated with chronic cerebellar degeneration (Hood, Kayan and Leech, 1973), with loss of Purkinje cells in the cerebellar cortex (Hoffman, 1958).

Other drugs used in the control of epilepsy, such as ethosuximide (Zarontin), may have similar vestibulotoxic effects.

Beta-blocking agents

Beta-adrenoceptor blocking agents have been used for several years in the control of cardiac dysrhythmias and anginal symptoms, and many of them are now available; they include propranolol (Inderal), oxprenolol (Trasicor) and practolol (Eraldin).

All of them may produce adverse reactions but practolol appears to be unique in its ability to cause deafness. In a significant proportion of these cases, the deafness has presented clinically as a mixture of sensorineural loss with conductive deafness, the latter sometimes due to serous otitis media, in one or both ears. Characteristically the deafness has been noticed only months, and sometimes years, after the appearance of other side effects, notably a psoriasiform skin rash and dryness of the eyes; other adverse reactions include bronchitis and pleurisy, 'plastic' peritonitis, and recurrent ulceration in the mouth and nose (McNab Jones *et al.*, 1977).

Up to the middle of 1977 only 94 cases of deafness, out of a total of approximately 1400 adverse reactions, had been reported to the Committee on Safety of Medicines (Inman, 1977); and in only 13 of these 94 cases was deafness the main complaint.

Despite the delayed appearance of adverse reactions to practolol there have been no long-term studies on the ears of animals, and the pathogenesis of this unusual form of mixed deafness is unknown.

The aminoglycoside antibiotics

Very soon after the discovery of streptomycin, the first effective chemotherapeutic agent against tuberculosis, it became evident that it could damage both balance and hearing (Hinshaw and Feldman, 1945), the latter effect usually occurring when the dosage was high, e.g. 3 g daily (Bignall, Crofton and Thomas, 1951); it rarely occurred if the dose did not exceed 0.5 g daily (Cawthorne and Ranger, 1957), or 24 mg/kg body weight (Meyler, 1963). Deafness occurred predominantly in patients who were being treated for tuberculous meningitis and in many instances it may have resulted from the tuberculous process rather than from the drug (Jamieson, 1952).

When dihydrostreptomycin came on the scene, it was found that vestibular disturbances were generally less severe and later in onset than those which occurred with streptomycin and, since its antimicrobial activity was about the same as that of the earlier drug, it was hoped that it would be even more successful than streptomycin in the treatment of tuberculosis. But it soon became evident that it was much more cochleotoxic, and that its effect on hearing was unpredictable, sometimes delayed in onset, and not infrequently progressive. It was not long before it was withdrawn from use altogether, but many other aminoglycosides have followed and in 1962 Leach listed nine antibiotics, most of them aminoglycosides, which were 'known or suspected to be toxic to the labyrinth to a greater or lesser degree when administered parenterally' (Leach, 1962). More recently gentamicin and tobramycin have been added to this formidable list.

These drugs are all closely related to one another in their microbiology, pharmacology and toxicity. But the aminoglycosides neomycin, kanamycin, gentamicin and tobramycin differ from the streptomycins in that they all contain the base deoxystreptamine, instead of streptidine, linked to various aminohexoses; and neomycin consists of three sugar rings, the others two. It is the variations in chemical configuration, including the number and placement of basic groups on the various sugars, that affect the toxicity (as well as the activity) of the different aminoglycosides (Hawkins, 1976).

Kanamycin and neomycin are particularly toxic to the cochlea, rarely to the vestibular system; but gentamicin and tobramycin are more vestibulotoxic in humans, although both of them can show either type of ototoxicity. Most of these toxic effects occur with parenteral administration of the drugs, but sensorineural hearing loss may also follow oral administration, notably of neomycin (Ballantyne, 1970), and even topical application. It has been reported after the injection of joint cavities, the irrigation of surgical wounds, the superficial dressing of burns, rectal or colonic irrigations, and intrabronchial or intrapleural administration. It may also follow the instillation of ear drops, many of which contain either neomycin or gentamicin.

Routes of access to the inner ear

The ototoxic antibiotics are transported to the labyrinthine fluids by way of the blood stream, when given systemically or applied topically to areas other than the ears.

When given intrathecally, they probably reach the inner ear from the cerebrospinal and perilymph fluids. Alternatively they may be secreted into the perilymph from the vessels of the spiral ligament, or directly into the endolymph from the stria vascularis (Hawkins, Beger and Aran, 1967).

When the aminoglycosides are applied topically to the middle ear (Spoendlin, 1966; Kohonen and Tarkkanen, 1969), they may reach the perilymph by passing through either the round window membrane or the annular ligament; and thence to the organ of Corti by passing from the scala vestibuli, through Reissner's membrane, into the endolymphatic space.

These drugs are eliminated from the inner ear by resorption in the stria vascularis (Osteyn and Tyberghein, 1968); and the stria itself may be damaged by their toxic products, thus retarding still further the rate of elimination.

Histopathology

COCHLEOTOXICITY

The histopathological changes which occur in the sensory epithelia of the labyrinth have been extensively studied in animals, notably in guinea-pigs, by the surface preparation technique of Engström (1951). More recently these studies have been extended to the scrutiny of the scanning electron microscope.

The changes have been remarkably consistent, the outer hair-cells of the basal turn being first affected in cases of cochlear toxicity (*Figure 21.1*), the damage later progressing towards the apex. Degeneration of inner hair-cells, which are affected much later, follows in a reverse direction. The extent of damage can be recorded graphically in a cochlear cytogram, or 'cochleogram' (*Figure 21.2*). Degeneration of the hair-cells first affects those which are provided with large granulated (type 2) nerve-endings; after the sensory cells have disappeared, the whole organ of Corti may collapse and the corresponding nerve fibres and ganglion cells degenerate. Even with total disappearance of all hair-cells, however, there is usually survival of 5–10 per cent of the neurons (Spoendlin, 1974).

More recently Johnsson and Hawkins (1972) have demonstrated vascular changes in the cochlea which may precede (and indeed may be responsible for) the degenerative changes in the hair-cells. These include strial atrophy and destruction of the pericapillary spaces in the spiral ligament.

VESTIBULOTOXICITY

In the vestibular neuroepithelium the type 1 hair-cells are usually damaged before the type 2 cells, the stereocilia becoming fused into 'giant' hairs; and Lindeman (1969) has demonstrated that these degenerative changes are more noticeable in the sensory epithelia of the ampullary cristae than in the utricular and saccular maculae.

The vestibular secretory tissues corresponding with the vascular stria of the cochlea are the 'dark cells' which appear on the slopes of the ampullary cristae, and Hawkins and Preston (1975) have demonstrated shrinkage and vacuolization of these cells in the squirrel monkey after streptomycin or gentamicin.

Drug concentrations in the labyrinthine fluids

Stupp *et al.* (1967) have shown that the specific ototoxic effects of the aminoglycoside antibiotics are related to the high concentrations and prolonged presence of these

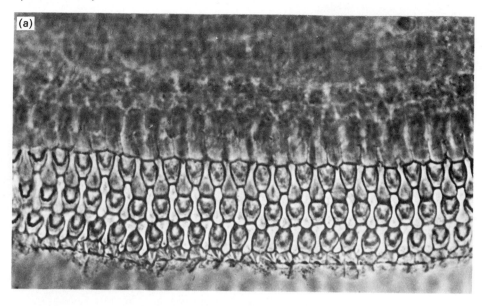

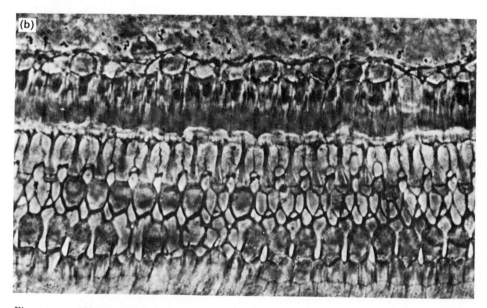

Figure 21.1   Surface preparations of the cochlea: (a) Normal regular pattern; (b) Ototoxic damage to outer hair-cells, showing 'collapse bodies'. (By courtesy of Professor Hans Engström)

substances in the lymphatic fluids of the inner ear. For example, 5 h after a single injection of kanamycin into a guinea-pig, the antibiotic concentration in the perilymph began to exceed the serum level, and so it remained 20 h later; furthermore, during long-term treatment with daily injections, there was a continuous accumulation of toxic substances in the inner ear, but not in the serum or other tissues. This accumulation of ototoxic antibiotics in the labyrinthine fluids and their delayed elimination from them may be accounted for by impaired diffusion due to compression

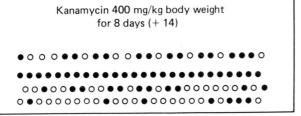

Figure 21.2   Cochleogram ('cochlear cytogram') in ototoxicity

and occlusion of the intercellular gaps in the membranes (Müsebeck, 1964; Kohonen, 1965).

The mechanism of ototoxicity

The precise mechanism by which the aminoglycoside antibiotics exert their toxic effects on the inner ear is uncertain.

In 1973 Hawkins suggested that, in the same way as there is a (highly effective) blood–brain barrier against these drugs, so there may be a (less effective) blood–ear (or haemato–labyrinthine) barrier, which may be able to impede the entrance of undesirable blood-borne substances into the inner-ear fluids; and it may also play an essential part in maintaining the 'micro-homeostasis' (environmental equilibrium) of the inner ear, an equilibrium which is expressed in the near-constancy of the widely different concentrations of sodium and potassium ions in the endolymph and perilymph.

This barrier must presumably depend upon the integrity of the spiral ligament and vascular stria, and their micro-vasculature which is primarily responsible for the elaboration of the labyrinthine fluids; and Hawkins presents evidence that the aminoglycosides can damage these 'secretory' tissues.

However, even though degenerative changes in the stria may precede the progressive loss of hair-cells from the organ of Corti, there is much other evidence that points to a direct toxic action on the hair-cells; and the 'secretory' tissues have powers of recuperation which are not shared by the organ of Corti itself (Quick and Duvall, 1970; Duvall, Ward and Lauhala, 1974).

There is no doubt that the risk of ototoxicity is greatly enhanced by defective renal function, and many of the ototoxic antibiotics are themselves nephrotoxic; ethacrynic acid and frusemide have only been known to damage the hearing in patients with renal failure; and Polybrene may be nephrotoxic as well as ototoxic (Ransome *et al.*, 1966). These facts all serve to emphasize the structural resemblance between the stria vascularis of the cochlea and the glomerular tufts of the kidney; and Haller *et al.* (1962) described a 'constriction of the capillaries within the glomerular tufts' due to hexadimethrine bromide. It is probable that it acted in a similar way on the micro-vasculature of the cochlea, the anoxic degeneration of the stria leading to electrolyte imbalance in the labyrinthine fluids.

The ototoxic action of the aminoglycosides can thus be compared with their nephrotoxic action, which affects membrane function and protein synthesis in tissues actively engaged in transporting water and ions.

'The peculiar toxicity of the aminoglycosides for only two organs of the body, namely, the inner ear and the kidney, has proved more difficult to explain than their mode of action in bacterial cells' (Hawkins, 1976). It has been shown that their antimicrobial effect depends upon the ability to inhibit protein synthesis, but recent work on the cochlea by Schacht (1974, 1976) has demonstrated an interference with the lipids of the cell membranes, rather than with the synthesis of proteins. The same mechanism has been demonstrated in renal tissues.

The clinical features of ototoxicity

The earliest symptom of ototoxicity is often one of high-pitched tinnitus, usually noticed before the onset of any subjective hearing loss. With those drugs which are mainly vestibulotoxic, of course, the main symptom is disturbance of balance, which may sometimes be extremely resistant to treatment.

Not uncommonly deafness appears after a latent period, and it may become progressively worse as treatment is continued.

Characteristically the pure-tone audiogram shows an essentially high-tone loss (*Figure 21.3*) but, at a certain stage of gentamicin toxicity, a Z-shaped audiogram may be seen (Huizing, 1972); recruitment can be demonstrated (Lidén, 1953). The hearing loss may not be evident until some time, even several months, after the drug has been withdrawn (Šupáček, 1972). On occasions it will advance to total loss.

Certain families show an unusual predisposition to aminoglycoside ototoxicity (Podvineć and Stefanović, 1966; Miszke, 1972), and in the very young and the very old, even with ordinary doses, dangerous concentrations of aminoglycosides may appear in the blood. Reports are accumulating of ototoxic damage from small doses of these drugs given to patients who have been previously treated by other ototoxic agents,—e.g. antimalarial drugs (Nilges and Northern, 1971); diuretics (West, Brummett, and Himes, 1973); other ototoxic antibiotics (Frost, Hawkins and Daly, 1960)—or exposed to noise (Darrouzet and de Lima Sobrinho, 1962).

Ototopical ototoxicity

Many substances can enter the perilymph by way of the round window membrane, and there is cause for concern about the potential ototoxicity of a wide variety of topical aural preparations, whether they be instilled as drops or placed in the middle ear during the course of various surgical procedures.

Bellucci and Wolff (1960) have written about the potentially harmful effects of absorbable gelatin sponge (Gel-foam) upon the inner ear, and Shenoi (1973) has described the damage that could be done by another similar preparation (Sterispon), when placed in close proximity to an open oval window. This latter product used to contain small quantities of free formaldehyde, but new manufacturing processes are claimed to have overcome this problem.

Bicknell (1971) reported a high incidence of sensorineural hearing loss after operations for myringoplasty, and the only factor common to all the cases he recorded was that pre-operative sterilization had been done with chlorhexidine (Hibitane) in

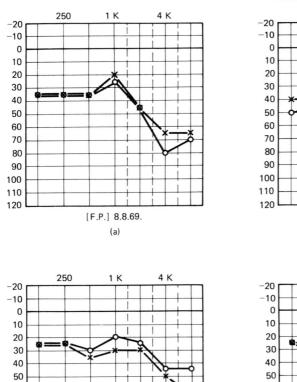

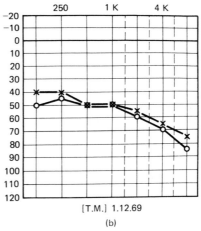

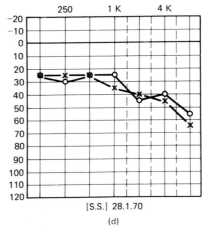

Figure 21.3   Audiograms of patients suffering from ototoxic effects of oral neomycin

spirit. Taylor (1975) has recently reported a case of profound sensorineural deafness following the application of chromic acid to a small posterior perforation of the tympanic membrane.

All the aminoglycoside antibiotics and a number of others (e.g. chloramphenicol, tetracycline and erythromycin) have produced ototoxic effects when placed in the middle ear (Gulick and Patterson, 1964; Koide, Hata and Hando, 1966; D'Angelo, Patterson and Morrow, 1967; Kohonen and Tarkkanen, 1969; Stupp *et al.*, 1973); and ethacrynic acid and frusemide may cause dramatic strial oedema and widespread destruction of the spiral organ when given intratympanically (Hawkins, 1976).

Prevention and treatment of ototoxicity

Although there have been a few reports of spontaneous recovery of hearing in cases of ototoxic deafness (e.g. Moffat and Ramsden, 1977), there is at present no known effective treatment for ototoxicity, once established. Hopes expressed for the reduction of toxicity by vitamins A and B, for mercaptoethylamine (Kluyskens, 1953) and for dimercaptopropanol (Hennebert, 1953) have proved unfounded, and special salts of the various ototoxic antibiotics have been equally unsuccessful. Combinations of 'Ozothine' (an aqueous preparation of oxidative products of oil of turpentine) with streptomycin have been found to reduce the toxicity of the latter (Holz, Hoffman and Beck, 1967; Strange, Socla and Beck, 1967), but they also reduce its antimicrobial activity (Stupp et al., 1973).

Some authors have recommended certain maximum doses of ototoxic drugs (e.g. Ajodhia and Dix, 1974) and others have suggested regular monitoring of serum levels (e.g. Line, Poole and Waterworth, 1970), but it is only in recent times that attempts have been made to calculate 'safe' doses of these drugs in accordance with the patient's renal status. For example, Mawer and his colleagues (1974) have developed a computer programme from which they have constructed 'nomograms' for the calculation of kanamycin and gentamicin dosages. However, 'wild variations in blood levels . . . may occur in renal impairment despite "accurate calculations".' (Quick, 1973).

Hence it behoves the prescribing physician to limit the dosage and duration of any ototoxic drug to the minimum consistent with the clinical control of the condition for which it is required. Ototoxic drugs in general, and the aminoglycoside antibiotics in particular, should be avoided altogether unless they are essential to the survival and future well-being of the patient, especially in cases of renal or hepatic failure, in the very young and the very old, and in pregnant women (Ballantyne, 1976); and they should be used with great caution in those previously treated with other potentially ototoxic agents, in those previously exposed to excessive noise, and in those with a known familial incidence of ototoxicity (Ballantyne, 1973).

Ideally serial audiograms should be done in all patients receiving these drugs, which should be withdrawn if at all possible as soon as any symptoms or signs of ototoxicity develop.

Patients with vestibular symptoms may be helped by a system of graduated exercises, supplemented by labyrinthine sedatives; whilst those with hearing problems may require hearing aids, with or without auditory training and/or instruction in lip-reading.

In those (fortunately) very rare cases where the hearing loss is total, it would seem possible that in the future such subjects may be considered for electrode implants.

References

Ajodhia, J. M. and Dix, M. R. (1974). *Minerva otorinolaringologia*, **25**, 117

Ballantyne, J. C. (1970). *Journal of Laryngology*, **84**, 967

Ballantyne, J. C. (1973). *Audiology*, **12**, 325

Ballantyne, J. C. (1976). 'Ototoxic Drugs'. In *Scientific Foundations of Otolaryngology*. Ed. by Hinchcliffe, R. and Harrison, D. F. N. London; William Heinemann Medical Books Ltd.

Bellucci, R. J. and Wolff, D. (1960). *Annals of Otology (St. Louis)*, **69**, 517

Bicknell, P. G. (1971). *Journal of Laryngology*, **85**, 957

Bignall, J. R., Crofton, J. W. and Thomas, J. A. B. (1951). *British Medical Journal*, **1**, 554

Cawthorne, T. E. and Ranger, D. (1957). *British Medical Journal*, **1**, 1444

Conrad, M. and Crosby, W. H. (1960). *Blood*, **16**, 1089

Crifò, S. (1973). *Archives of Otorhinolaryngology*, **206**, 27

Cummings, C. W. (1968). *Laryngoscope*, **78**, 530

D'Angelo, E. P., Patterson, W. C. and Morrow, R. C. (1967). *Archives of Otolaryngology*, **85**, 682

Darrouzet, J. and de Lima Sobrinho, E. (1962). *Review of Laryngology Otology and Rhinology*, **83**, 781

Duvall, A. J., Ward, W. D. and Lauhala, K. E. (1974). *Annals of Otology (St. Louis)*, **83**, 498

Engström, H. (1951). *Acta oto-laryngologica*, **40**, 5

Federspil, P. and Hansen, H. (1973). *Research in Experimental Medicine*, **161**, 175

Ferreira, S. H. and Vane, J. R. (1974). In *The Prostaglandins*, Vol. 2. Ed. by Ramwell, P. W. New York; Plenum Press.

Frost, J. O., Hawkins, J. E. Jr. and Daly, J. F. (1960). *American Review of Respiratory Diseases*, **82**, 23

Gignoux, M., Martin, H. and Cajgfinger, H. (1966). *Journal français Oto-rhino-laryngologique*, **15**, 631

Gulick, W. L. and Patterson, W. C. (1964). *Annals of Otology (St. Louis)*, **73**, 204

Haller, J. A., Jr., Randsdell, H. J., Jr., Stowens, D. and Rubel, W. F. (1962). *Journal of thoracic and cardiovascular Surgery*, **44**, 486

Hawkins, J. E., Jr., (1973). *Audiology*, **12**, 383

Hawkins, J. E., Jr. (1976). 'Drug Ototoxicity'. In *Handbook of Sensory Physiology*. Vol. V Auditory System. Part 3: Clinical and Special Topics, pp. 707–748. Berlin & Heidelberg; Springer-Verlag

Hawkins, J. E., Jr., Beger, V. and Aran, J. M. (1967). In *Sensorineural Hearing Processes and Disorders*, p. 411. Ed. by Graham, A. B. Boston; Little, Brown & Co.

Hawkins, J. E., Jr., and Preston, J. E. (1975). 'Vestibular Ototoxicity'. In *The Vestibular System*. Ed. by Naunton, R. F. New York; Academic Press

Hennebert, M. P. E. (1953). *Annals of Oto-Laryngology (Paris)*, **70**, 473

Hinshaw, H. C. and Feldman, W. H. (1945). *Proceedings of the Mayo Clinics*, **20**, 313

Hoffman, K. W. (1958). *Neurology (Minneapolis)*, **8**, 210

Holz, E., Hoffman, M. and Beck, C. (1967). *Archiv Klinische experimentelle Ohren-, Nasen-, u. Kehlkopfheilkunde*, **188**, 236

Hood, J. D., Kayan, A. and Leech, J. (1973). *Brain*, **96**, 483

Huizing, E. H. (1972). *Audiology*, **11**, 30

Inman, W. H. N. (1977). Personal communication

Jamieson, S. R. (1952). *British Medical Journal*, **1**, 83

Johnsson, L.-G. and Hawkins, J. E., Jr. (1972). *Laryngoscope*, **82**, 1105

Kluyskens, P. (1953). *Giornale R. Societa Biologica*, **147**, 733

Kohonen, A. (1965). *Acta oto-laryngologica*, suppl. 208

Kohonen, A. and Tarkkanen, J. (1969). *Acta oto-laryngologica*, **68**, 90

Kohonen, A., Jauhainen, T. and Tarkkanen, J. (1970). *Acta oto-laryngologica*, **70**, 187

Koide, Y., Hata, A. and Hando, R. (1966). *Acta oto-laryngologica*, **61**, 332

Laveran, A. (1898). *Traité du paludisme* p. 368. Paris; Masson et Cie

Lawrence, W., Kuehn, P., Masle, E. T. and Miller, D. G. (1961). *Journal of Surgical Research*, **1**, 142

Leach, W. (1962). *Journal of Laryngology*, **76**, 774

Lidén, G. (1953). *Acta oto-laryngologica*, **43**, 551

Lindeman, H. H. (1969). *Journal of Laryngology*, **83**, 1

Line, D. H., Poole, G. W. and Waterworth, P. M. (1970). *Tubercle*, **5**, 76

Lloyd-Mostyn, R. H. and Lord, I. J. (1971). *Lancet*, **2**, 1156

McKinna, A. J. (1966). *Canadian Journal of Ophthalmology*, **1**, 261

McNab Jones, R. F., Hammond, V. T., Wright, D. and Ballantyne, J. C. (1977). *Journal of Laryngology*, **91**, 963

Maher, J. F. and Schreiner, G. E. (1965). *Annals of internal Medicine*, **62**, 15

Mathog, R. H., Thomas, W. G. and Hudson, W. R. (1970). *Archives of Otolaryngology*, **92**, 7

Mawer, G. E., Ahmad, R., Dobbs, S. M., McGouch, J. G., Lucas, S. B. and Tooth, J. A. (1974). *British Journal of Clinical Pharmacology*, **1**, 45

Meyler, L. (1963). *Acta Otolaryngologica*, Suppl. **183**, 92

Miszke, A. (1972). *Audiology*, **11**, 23

Moffat, D. A. and Ramsden, R. T. (1977). *Journal of Laryngology*, **91**, 511

Morton, R. (1696). *Exercitationes de morbis universalibus acutis*. Ed. ult. Venice; Typis Hieronymi Albuzzi

Müsebeck, K. (1964). *Annalen Universitatssternwarte, Sarav.*, **11**, 159

Nilges, T. C. and Northern, J. L. (1971). *Annals of Surgery*, **173**, 281

Nozue, N., Mizuno, M. and Kaga, K. (1973). *Annals of Otology*, **82**, 389

Osteyn, F. and Tyberghein, J. (1968). *Acta oto-laryngologica*, Suppl. 234

Pillay, V. K. G., Schwartz, F. D., Aimi, K. and Kark, R. M. (1969). *Lancet*, **1**, 77

Podvinéc, S. and Stefanović, P. (1966). *Journal français Oto-rhino-laryngologique*, **15**, 61

Quick, C. A. (1973). 'Chemical and Drug Effects on the Inner Ear'. In *Otolaryngology*. Ed. by Paparella, M. M. and Shumrick, D. A. Vol. 2 (The Ear), pp. 397–406, Philadelphia; W. B. Saunders

Quick, C. A. and Duvall, A. J. (1970). *Laryngoscope*, **80**, 954

Quick, C. A. and Hoppe, W. (1975). *Annals of Otology (St. Louis)*, **84**, 94

Ransome, J., Ballantyne, J. C., Shaldon, S., Bosher, S. K. and Hallpike, C. S. (1966). *Journal of Laryngology*, **80**, 651

Schacht, J. (1974). *Annals of Otology (St. Louis)*, **83**, 613

Schacht, J. (1976). *Journal of the acoustic Society of America*, **59**, 940

Schuknecht, H. F. (1964). *Southern medical Journal*, **57**, 1161

Schwabach, D. (1884). *Deutsche medizinische Wochenschrift*, **10**, 163

Shenoi, P. (1973). *Proceedings of the royal Society of Medicine*, **66**, 193

Spoendlin, H. (1966). *Practical oto-rhino-laryngologica* (Basel), **28**, 305

Spoendlin, H. (1974). 'Neuroanatomy of the Cochlea'. In *Electrical Stimulation of the Acoustic Nerve in Man*, pp. 7–23. Ed. by Merzenich, M. M., Schindler, R. A. and Sooy, F. A. San Francisco; Velo-Bind, Inc.

Strange, G., Socla, T. and Beck, C. (1967). *Archiv Klinische experimentalle Ohren-, Nasen- u. Kehlkopfheilkunde*, **188**, 242

Stupp, H. F., Rauch, S., Sous, H., Brun, J. P. and Lagler, F. (1967). *Archives of Otolaryngology*, **86**, 515

Stupp, H. F., Küpper, K., Lagler, F., Sous, H. and Quante, M. (1973). *Audiology*, **12**, 350

Šupáček, I. (1972). *Audiology*, **11**, 29

Taylor, P. H. (1975). *Journal of Laryngology*, **89**, 1075

Venkateswaran, P. S. (1971). *British Medical Journal*, **4**, 113

West, B. A., Brummett, R. E. and Himes, D. L. (1973). *Archives of Otolaryngology*, **98**, 32

Worthington, E. L., Lunin, L. F., Heath, M. and Catlin, F. I. (1973). *Index-Handbook of Ototoxic Agents 1966–1971*. Baltimore and London; Johns Hopkins University Press

Young, W. G., Jr., Lesage, A. M., Dillon, M. L., Lee, J. M., Collaway, H. A., Jr and Reeves, J. W. (1961). *Annals of Surgery*, **154**, 372

The term presbyacusis means deafness of ageing which is the auditory manifestation of a biological process involving all the tissues of the body. The speed of onset of degenerative change in the ear is determined by genetic factors, and by the physical stress to which it is subjected during a normal lifespan.

Aetiology

The deafness is characteristically bilateral and symmetrical with a variable age of onset. Some people may show impairment at the age of 40 while others may reach the age of 80 with excellent hearing. The true sex incidence has not been reliably established.

Surveys of the incidence of hearing loss in age-related urban and rural populations have purported to show that the onset of presbyacusis is earlier in the urban population, presumably due to higher overall noise exposure (Weston, 1964; Rosen *et al.*, 1964). Diet was reported by Rosen (1969) to have an effect on presbyacusis. He found that a high fat content diet was associated with increased cardiovascular disease and worse hearing. Weston (1964) found that 70 per cent of patients with presbyacusis also had arteriosclerosis and that the relative severity of the deafness appeared to increase with the degree of arteriosclerosis. However he found no relationship between tobacco consumption and the age of onset or severity of deafness.

Pathology

Middle-ear changes

There has been much discussion on the importance of age changes in the middle-ear structures and the relationship of these changes to hearing loss. Glorig and Davis (1961) described a consistent high-tone conductive hearing loss in an audiometric study of the elderly deaf. Nixon, Glorig and High (1962) showed that ageing caused a slight impairment of high-frequency sound transmission through the middle ear. The loss averaged around 12 dB at 4000 Hz. They postulated that the tympanic membrane thickens with age and loses elasticity, and that the ligaments of the ossicular joints loosen leading to a diminution of mechanical integrity.

Conductive lesions due to age changes were also suggested by Goodhill (1968). However, Belal and Stewart (1974) in a histological study of the ageing middle ear have shown that the changes in the ossicular joints progress towards fibrosis, calcification and ankylosis with no conductive hearing loss seen on the available audiograms studied.

It appears therefore that presbyacusis is predominantly a phenomenon affecting the sensory and neural structures of the inner ear.

Inner-ear changes

The cells of the inner ear and neural pathways are very highly differentiated and cannot reproduce once a specialized function has been established for them. They undergo degeneration by a process of wear and tear in which the highly differentiated cells are not replaced, by accumulation of products of metabolism in the tissues, and by the accumulation of deleterious genes.

Saxén (1952) described two main types of hearing loss. One type was associated with atrophy of the spiral ganglion with a normal organ of Corti, and the other type was due to atrophy of the stria vascularis and the supporting structures of the organ of Corti on the basilar membrane.

Later Schuknecht (1955) described progressive degeneration of the organ of Corti from the basal to the apical end, and a further type of deafness due to degeneration of the spiral ganglion cells characterized by severe loss of auditory discrimination. The same author described two further types of hearing loss based on audiometric and histological studies (Schuknecht, 1964), and four main types of pathological change in the cochlea are now recognized (Schuknecht, 1974). These types are caused by selective atrophy of different morphological structures in the cochlea which may be involved alone or in combination. The changes are usually bilateral and symmetrical.

Sensory presbyacusis

This condition is associated with abrupt high-tone hearing losses and histologically there is atrophy of the organ of Corti in the basal end of the cochlea. The onset is in middle age and progress of the lesion is slow so that the speech frequencies are affected only late in the process (*Figure 22.1*). At first there is distortion and flattening of the organ of Corti, followed by loss of both the supporting elements and the hair-cells (*Figure 22.2*). In the later stages the organ of Corti may completely disappear leaving a totally denuded basilar membrane. Ishii *et al.* (1967) have described the accumulation of lipofuscin granules in the epithelial cells of the cochlear duct, increasing in quantity as a function of age and have postulated that these are insoluble byproducts of lysosome activity seen more readily in dying cells.

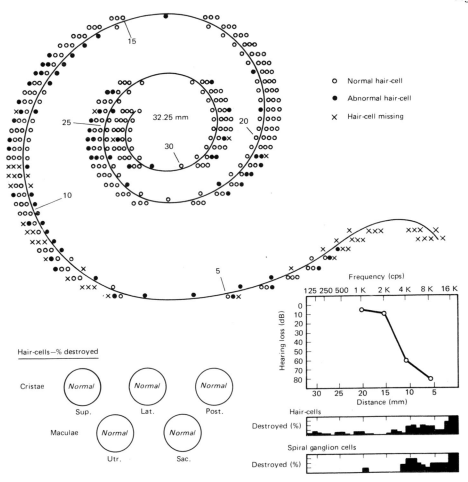

Figure 22.1 Audiogram and cochlear reconstruction of a patient with slowly progressive sensory presbyacusis. The loss of hair-cells is more severe in the basal turn of the cochlea

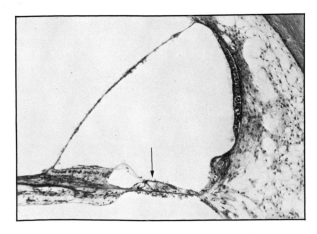

Figure 22.2 Section through the cochlea showing the site of hair-cell loss. The stria vascularis is normal

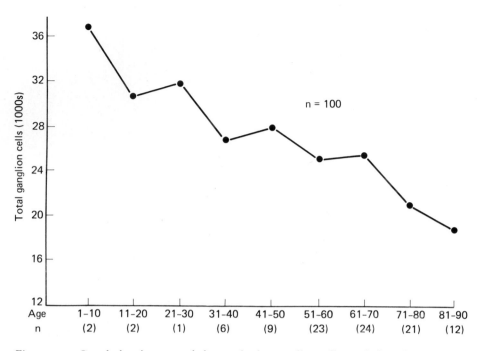

Figure 22.3   Graph showing normal changes in the ganglion-cell population of the cochlea with age. There is a progressive reduction in cell numbers throughout life

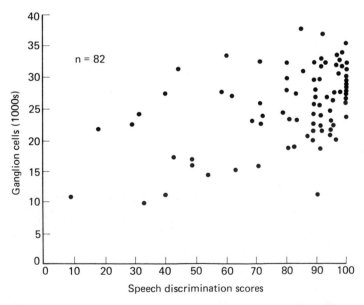

Figure 22.4   Graph showing the relationship between total ganglion-cell count and speech discrimination. The latter is only severely affected when the cell population falls below 20 000

Neural presbyacusis

There is a gradual loss of neurones from the central nervous system throughout life. This change has recently been studied in the ganglion-cells of the cochlea by Otte, Schuknecht and Kerr (1978). It can be seen (*Figures 22.3* and *22.4*) that there is a fall in the ganglion-cell count from an average of 37 000 in the first decade to 20 000 in the ninth decade, but that this fall is compatible with normal speech discrimination. In neural presbyacusis the ganglion-cell count falls well below this level (*Figure 22.5*).

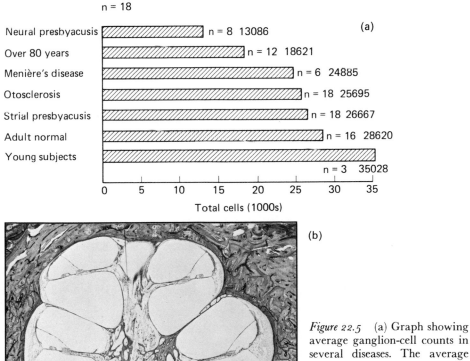

Figure 22.5 (a) Graph showing average ganglion-cell counts in several diseases. The average number is well below 20 000 in neural presbyacusis; (b) neural presbyacusis. There is severe atrophy of the spiral ganglion throughout all turns of the cochlea

The classic clinical picture is of a severe loss of speech discrimination, and histologically there is widespread atrophy of the spiral ganglion (*Figure 22.5a*).

Strial presbyacusis

The function of the stria vascularis is as yet unknown. It has been postulated that it may be the site of endolymph secretion, the source of the positive electrical potential of the scala media (Misrahy *et al.*, 1958), or that it is an energy source for the cells of the basilar membrane.

Strial atrophy may be found after labyrinthitis or following salicylate intoxication

(Myers and Bernstein, 1965). However it is also the most common cause of deafness of ageing. The hearing loss has a slow onset, usually in the fifth and sixth decades. It is characterized by the flat audiometric pattern and this is associated with good speech discrimination (*Figure 22.6*) until the pure-tone levels fall below an average of 50 dB of hearing loss.

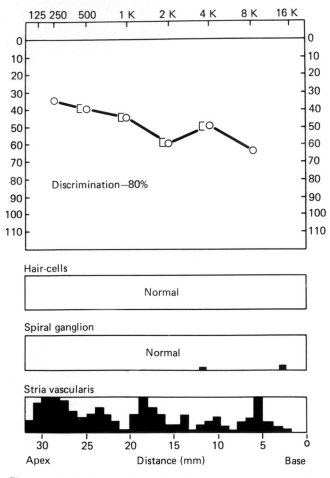

Figure 22.6   Strial atrophy with a flat pure-tone hearing loss and good speech discrimination

The histological findings are a patchy atrophy of the stria vascularis which is more severe in the apical half of the cochlea. There may be loss of all three cell layers of the stria (*Figure 22.7*) and often cystic changes may be seen with associated basophilic deposits (*Figure 22.8*). Loss of hearing for all the frequency range may be due to diffuse endolymph change throughout the cochlear duct.

Cochlear conductive presbyacusis

This is a term used by Schuknecht (1974) to describe a type of deafness found in the elderly and characterized by descending audiometric patterns. Histological studies

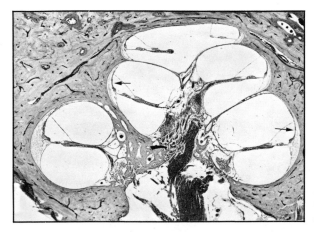

Figure 22.7   Midmodiolar section of the cochlea showing severe strial atrophy

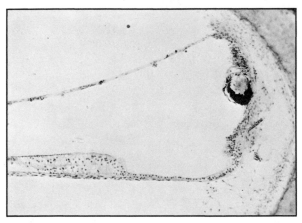

Figure 22.8 There is cystic change in the stria with a large basophilic deposit

usually show no morphological changes in the cochlear structures to explain the hearing loss and it is postulated that there is a disorder in the motion mechanics of the basilar membrane. Changes in the physical response characteristics of the membrane are greater in the basal turn where it is thick, and less severe in the apical turn where it is wider and thinner. Stiffening and calcification of the basilar membrane were described by Mayer (1919) and by Crowe, Guild and Polvogt (1934). More recently Nomura (1970) described fat and cholesterol deposits in the filamentous structure of the pars pectinata of the basilar membrane, and felt that such changes could alter the response characteristics of the membrane.

The only change found consistently in ears with hearing losses having descending patterns is atrophy of the spiral ligament (Wright and Schuknecht, 1972). Atrophic changes commence in the second decade and continue throughout life. At first there is a loss of fibrocytes in the region of the ligament adjacent to the attachment of the basilar membrane followed by the appearance of a zone of acellularity in the midportion of the ligament. With further change two distinct zones become apparent, a thin external zone consisting of densely packed fibrocytes in a fibrillar stroma, and a larger internal zone, largely acellular and containing large cystic spaces (*Figure 22.9*). Similar changes can be found in ears with normal hearing but they are more frequent in ears showing descending audiometric patterns.

Central changes

In many patients there are undoubtedly senile changes in the central auditory pathways. Kirikae, Sato and Shitara (1964) reported atrophy in the central auditory nuclei and concluded that such a change may account for some lowering of speech

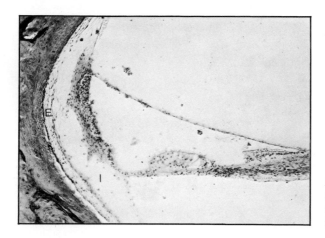

Figure 22.9 Spiral ligament atrophy. A thin external fibrillar zone E is apparent, and a larger internal acellular zone I

discrimination. Hansen and Reske-Nielson (1965) described degeneration of the ganglion cells of the ventral cochlear nucleus, superior olive, inferior colliculus and medial geniculate body in randomly selected senile patients. The importance of these changes in presbyacusis has been stressed by Hinchliffe (1962). They may be responsible for lowering of the upper-tone limit, decreased frequency discrimination, impaired auditory temporal discrimination, decreased sound localization, decreased auditory perceptual judgment, impaired intelligibility of moderately distorted speech, and decreased ability to recall long sentences.

Clinical features

In the majority of patients there is a slow progressive bilateral hearing loss which may be accompanied by continuous high-pitched tinnitus. There may be a family history of similar hearing losses, and this is particularly marked in the strial type of presbyacusis (Schuknecht, 1974). Occasionally there is sudden profound hearing loss in one ear following gradual bilateral deterioration and this may be due to basilar membrane rupture following spiral ligament atrophy (Gacek and Schuknecht, 1969). Gradual hearing loss is at first for the high frequencies then later the clarity of speech is lost. Sibilant and fricative consonants are especially badly heard. There is usually some degree of recruitment leading to intolerance of amplification. On clinical examination the tympanic membranes may be normal and Rinne tests positive with a central Weber. In advanced cases communication with the patient may be difficult but the elderly deaf person is more likely to respond to slow, clear speech with short words spoken near the ear, than to a loud shout. In general male voices are heard better than female or children's voices.

Audiometric tests

Pure-tone audiometry is most frequently used to assess the degree of hearing loss and to establish the pattern of the deficit. These patterns are invariably retained once established (Dayal and Nussbaum, 1971). The commonest single change is that of strial atrophy with a uniform flat loss and good speech discrimination (Schuknecht and Ishii, 1966).

The progressive diminution of hearing acuity with ageing as measured on pure-tone audiometry was first studied by Bunch (1931), who found increasing high-tone hearing loss. Similar findings were reported by Steinberg, Montgomery and Gardner (1940) and by Webster, Himes and Lichtenstein (1950). In 1954 the American Standards Association produced standard curves of average hearing levels for men and women up to the age of 65 years, and the Wisconsin Hearing Survey (1957) established standard presbyacusis curves. These showed the average hearing levels to be expected with age (*Figure 22.10*). Surveys carried out on patients aged between 70 and 90 years have shown very little hearing deterioration for pure tones after the age of 70 (Sataloff and Menduke, 1957; Hinchcliffe, 1959). More recent surveys have also confirmed these findings (Jokinen, 1969 and 1970; Jokinen and Karja, 1971).

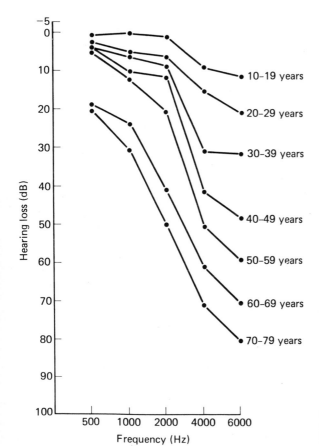

Figure 22.10 Comparison of decade audiograms. (Wisconsin State)

Loudness recruitment is a marked feature of presbyacusis but can only be measured by binaural loudness balance when there is a substantial difference in the two ears at the same frequencies. Where both ears exhibit the same degree of loss then the short increment sensitivity index test may be useful. Tone decay may be marked in mainly neural presbyacusis. All audiometers used for testing should be calibrated to the ISO–64 audiometric standards recommended by the International Standards Association (Davis and Cranz, 1964).

There is a gradual decrease in speech discrimination ability as a function of age, and patients with identical pure-tone hearing losses may have different speech discrimination scores. Goetzinger, Dirks and Embrey (1961) reported that discrimination difficulty arises from atrophic changes involving both peripheral and central portions of the auditory mechanism. There may be a decrease in the intelligibility of distorted speech where the defect is thought to be primarily cortical (Bocca, 1958), or a decreased ability to recall long sentences (Pietrantoni and Arslan, 1956). There may also be impaired auditory perceptual judgment where fewer clicks than normal are reported over a given time, even when presented well above threshold (Weiss and Birren, 1957).

Treatment

There are no effective medications which will influence either the onset or the progress of presbyacusis. All too frequently the only positive benefit is the provision of a hearing aid. Careful clinical examination should be undertaken to exclude an associated conductive loss due to impacted wax or serous otitis media. Relatives should be counselled as to the nature of the disability and the type of voice best heard. Lip-reading is usually not well learnt by the elderly deaf but attempts at tuition should be made if amplification does not lead to an increase in voice intelligibility. The choice of hearing aids is discussed elsewhere in this book (Chapter 28).

Acknowledgement

All the illustrations in this chapter are by courtesy of Dr H. F. Schuknecht, Professor of Otolaryngology, Harvard University Medical School.

References

Belal, A. and Stewart, T. (1974). *Annals of Otology, Rhinology and Laryngology,* **83**, 159

Bocca, E. (1958). *Laryngoscope,* **68**, 301

Bunch, C. C. (1931). *Archives of Otolaryngology,* **13**, 170

Crowe, S., Guild, S. and Polvogt, L. (1934). *Bulletin of the Johns Hopkins Hospital,* **54**, 315

Davis, H. and Cranz, F. (1964). *Journal of Speech Research,* **1**, 7

Dayal, V. and Nussbaum, M. (1971). *Acta Otolaryngologica,* **71**, 382

Gacek, R. and Schuknecht, H. (1969). *International Audiology,* **7**, 199

Glorig, A. and Davis, H. (1961). *Annals of Otology, Rhinology and Laryngology,* **70**, 556

Goetzinger, C., Dirks, D. and Embrey, J. (1961). *Archives of Otolaryngology,* **73**, 662

Goodhill, V. (1968). *Archives of Otolaryngology,* **90**, 759

Hansen, C. and Reske-Nielson, E. (1965). *Archives of Otolaryngology* **82**, 115

Hinchcliffe, R. (1959). *Acoustica,* **9**, 303

Hinchcliffe, R. (1962). *Journal of Speech and Hearing Disorders,* **27**, 301

Ishii, T., Murakami, Y., Kimura, R. and Balogh, K., Jr. (1967). *Acta Otolaryngology,* **64**, 17

Jokinen, K. (1969). *Acta Otolaryngologica*, **68**, 327

Jokinen, K. (1970). *Acta Otolaryngologica*, **69**, 155

Jokinen, K. and Karja, F. (1971). *Acta Otolaryngologica*, **70**, 227

Kirikae, I., Sato, T. and Shitara, T. (1964). *Laryngoscope*, **74**, 205

Mayer, O. (1919). *Archiv fur Ohren-, Nasen- u. Kehlkopfheilkunde*, **105**, 1

Misrahy, G., De Jonge, B., Shinabarger, E. and Arnold, J. (1958). *Journal of the Acoustic Society of America*, **30**, 705

Myers, E. and Bernstein, J. (1965). *Archives of Otolaryngology*, **82**, 483

Nixon, J., Glorig, A. and High, W. (1962). *Journal of Laryngology and Otology*, **76**, 288

Nomura, Y. (1970). *Acta Otolaryngologica*, **69**, 352

Otte, J. Schuknecht, H. and Kerr, A. G. (1978). *Laryngoscope*, **88**, 1231

Pietrantoni, L. and Arslan, M. (1956). *Giornale di Gerontological* Suppl. 10

Rosen, S., Plester, D., El-Mofty, A. and Rosen, H. (1964). *Archives of Otolaryngology*, **79**, 34

Rosen, S. (1969). *International Audiology*, **8**, 260

Sataloff, J. and Menduke, H. (1957). *Archives of Otolaryngology*, **66**, 271

Saxén, A. (1952). *Acta Otolaryngologica*, **41**, 213

Schuknecht, H. (1955). *Laryngoscope*, **65**, 402

Schuknecht, H. (1964). *Archives of Otolaryngology*, **80**, 369

Schuknecht, H. and Ishii, T. (1966). *Japanese Journal of Otology*, **69**, 1825

Schuknecht, H. (1974). *Pathology of the Ear.* Boston; Harvard University Press

Steinberg, J. C., Montgomery, B. C. and Gardner, M. B. (1940). *Journal of the Acoustic Society of America*, **12**, 291

Webster, J. C., Himes, M. W. and Lichtenstein, M. (1950). *Journal of the Acoustic Society of America*, **22**, 473

Weiss, A. D. and Birren, J. E. (1957). *American Psychology*, **12**, 385

Weston, T. E. T. (1964). *Journal of Laryngology*, **78**, 273

Wright, J. L. W. and Schuknecht, H. (1972). *Archives of Otolaryngology*, **96**, 16

23 Vascular lesions of the inner ear
P M Shenoi

Introduction

Earlier literature on this subject appears mainly as a mass of clinical observations in patients presenting as sudden unilateral sensorineural deafness and in whom the diagnosis was presumed to be due to interruption in blood supply. Perhaps one of the earliest systematic studies on the relationship between arteriosclerosis and deafness was reported by Fabinyi (1931). More recently Rosen and Olin (1965) demonstrated a significant hearing loss of sensorineural type in patients with a high incidence of coronary heart disease and arteriosclerosis. Our understanding and knowledge of the changes in the inner ear due to vascular lesions owe much to studies in experimental animals. Recent years have shown a steady flow of publications of carefully controlled experimental vascular lesions and their effects on function, electrophysiological changes within the cochlea, histochemical and biochemical changes, and histopathological changes as seen under the light and electron microscopes. There is a general acceptance amongst otological pioneers in regarding some forms of sensorineural deafness as being due to inner-ear ischaemia as in certain congenital and hereditary losses; acoustic trauma; ototoxic deafness (quinine and salicylates); presbyacusis; Menière's disease; and sudden unilateral deafness.

Vascular anatomy of the inner ear

Internal auditory meatus and porus acousticus

The important anatomical relations within the internal auditory canal are dealt with, in greater detail, elsewhere (Volume 1). Observations on the origin, course and relation to the seventh and eighth cranial nerves of the labyrinthine artery (internal auditory artery) were based on careful post-mortem dissection of the petrous temporal regions, or by contrast medium radiography, with or without subtraction techniques, of the vessels. For further details, the reader is referred to the writings of Mazzoni

(1969, 1970, 1972); Fisch (1968); Smaltino, Bernini and Elefante (1971) and Caillé, Piton and Boussens (1974). Attention is drawn to the loop formed by the anterior inferior cerebellar artery at the porus acousticus.

Internal ear—cochlea

Detailed study of the vascular anatomy within the cochlea has involved both *in vivo* and *in vitro* techniques. The *in vivo* technique essentially involves creating a fenestra in the external bony wall of the cochlea and the method is frequently used in evaluating the cochlear blood flow (Perlman, Kimura and Fernandez, 1959; Lawrence, 1971 and 1973).

In vitro technique has been extensively used for the study of detailed vascular anatomy in the cochlea. Basically, the method involves intravascular injection of a suitable contrast medium—Berlin Blue, Indian Ink, Prussian Blue, intravascular precipitation of Prussian Blue and subsequent histological sections, horseradish peroxidase and benzidine staining techniques, and surface preparation with osmium tetroxide.

(1) LABYRINTHINE ARTERY (INTERNAL AUDITORY ARTERY)

Our detailed knowledge of the vascular anatomy within the cochlea owes much to the painstaking study in various mammals, including humans, by Axelsson (1968, 1971, 1972, 1974) and Axelsson and his associates (1972, 1973, 1974, 1975). The following detailed account of the vessels within the cochlea including the nomenclature was adopted from the description by Axelsson (1968). The labyrinthine artery continues laterally as the common cochlear artery after it has given off the anterior vestibular artery which supplies the vestibular apparatus (*Figure 23.1*). The common cochlear artery soon divides into two terminal branches: (a) the *vestibulo-cochlear artery* which is usually overshadowed by the acoustic nerve and ultimately divides, on arriving at the modiolus, into vestibular and cochlear branches and (b) the *spiral modiolar artery*.

The vestibular branch of the vestibulo-cochlear artery supplies the basal end of the cochlea and the vestibule. The cochlear branch of the vestibulo-cochlear artery, however, takes a course towards the apex of the cochlea in a spiral fashion to supply about a quarter to one half of the basal turn and anastomoses with the basal branches of the spiral modiolar artery (*Figure 23.2*). The main trunk of the spiral modiolar artery runs apically in a coiled fashion, around the acoustic nerve in the modiolus where it lies superior to the spiral ganglion. The spiral modiolar artery supplies the entire cochlea except for the first basal half-turn. Arising from the artery at right angles are the radiating arterioles supplying the capillary regions in the modiolus, the spiral lamina and the external wall. The radiating arterioles connect with each other in the scala vestibuli to form spirally running arcades.

The venous drainage of the cochlea is represented by two separate veins: (a) the vein of the scala tympani and (b) the vein of the scala vestibuli, both of which run spirally around the modiolus. Considerable variation is seen in their course and distribution. The vein of the scala tympani is formed by a series of individual veins draining the scala tympani, the scala media and the spiral ganglion. The vein of the

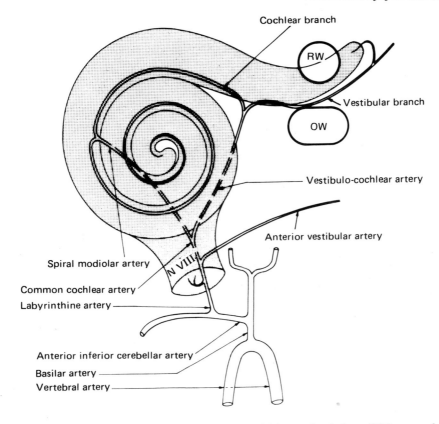

Cochlear branch

RW

Vestibular branch

OW

Vestibulo-cochlear artery

Anterior vestibular artery

Spiral modiolar artery

N VIII

Common cochlear artery

Labyrinthine artery

Anterior inferior cerebellar artery

Basilar artery

Vertebral artery

Figure 23.1 Man, arterial system, schematic. OW = oval window, RW = round window, N VIII = acoustic nerve. (From Axelsson (1968), reproduced by courtesy of the Editor, *Acta Oto-Laryngologica*)

scala vestibuli is similarly formed by individual veins draining both the spiral lamina and scala vestibuli except in the first quarter of the basal turn which is drained by both the vein of the round window and the posterior vestibular vein. Both the vein of the scala tympani and the vein of the scala vestibuli join at about the basal end of the cochlea to form the common modiolar vein which eventually forms the vein of the cochlear aqueduct near the round window after the common modiolar vein receives the vestibulo-cochlear vein.

(2) SPIRAL LAMINA AND SPIRAL LIMBUS (*Figure 23.3*)

In addition to the radiating arterioles and collecting venules, there are two distinct vessels seen consistently, i.e. (a) vessel of the basilar membrane and (b) the vessel of the tympanic lip, both of which have attracted considerable attention and their role in maintenance of the cyto-architecture of the hair-cells in the organ of Corti is the centre of much speculation (Lawrence, 1966). Furthermore the vessel of the basilar membrane or lack of it has been postulated as a possible cause of congenital deafness (Johnsson *et al.*, 1973; Hilding, 1973). The limbus is supplied by the limbus vessel.

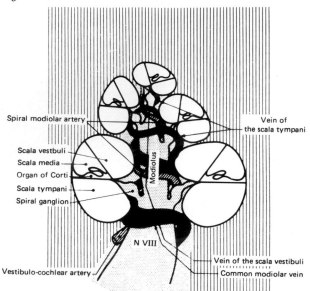

Figure 23.2 Man, modiolus, radial section, schematic. The basal half of the basal turn is supplied by the vestibulo-cochlear artery; the rest of the cochlea by the spiral modiolary artery. In contrast with the guinea-pig, there is double venous drainage, one in the scala vestibuli and one in the scala tympani. (From Axelsson (1968), reproduced by courtesy of the Editor, *Acta Oto-Laryngologica*)

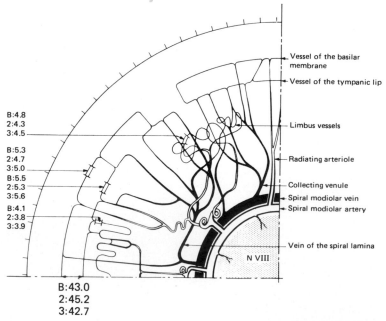

Figure 23.3 Guinea-pig, spiral lamina, transverse section, schematic, measurements. $1 = 1 =$ diameter of vessels. $\leftarrow\rightarrow =$ distance between vessels. (From Axelsson (1968), reproduced by courtesy of the Editor, *Acta Oto-Laryngologica*)

(3) EXTERNAL WALL OF THE MEMBRANOUS COCHLEA (*Figure 23.4*)

(a) *Scala vestibuli*

There are five different types of vessels in the region of scala vestibuli—radiating arterioles, arteriolar arcades, collecting venules, the vessel at the vestibular membrane (Reissner's membrane) and the capillary network above the vestibular membrane.

The radiating arterioles arise at right angles to the spiral modiolar artery and have a spiral course centrally whilst in the periphery they are relatively straight. Arteriolar arcades are formed by connecting arterioles and the radiating arterioles supply all the spiral vessels in the external wall. However, in the basal turn most of the branches from the radiating arterioles join the collecting venules to form arterio-venous anastomoses. Collecting venules drain into the vein of the scala vestibuli in the same turn but may drain, occasionally, into the stria vascularis, and the vessel of the spiral prominence which is an ill-defined capillary network. The vessel at the vestibular membrane (Reissner's membrane) is formed by the capillary network in the scala vestibuli and is seen lying close to the attachment of Reissner's membrane. This vessel connects the arterioles and venules in the scala vestibuli and venules of the scala tympani.

(b) *Scala tympani*

This demonstrates two different types of vessels, i.e. collecting venules and venules at the basilar membrane. Collecting venules drain all the spiral vascular system in the

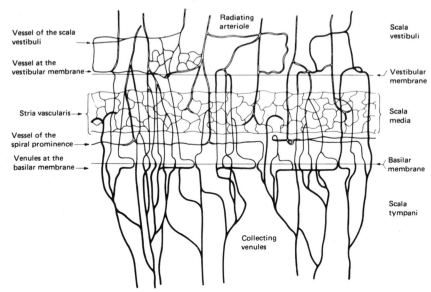

Figure 23.4   Guinea-pig and man, external wall, radial section, schematic. Radiating arterioles predominate in the scala vestibuli and supply spiral vascular systems; the vessel of the scala vestibuli, the vessel at the vestibular membrane, the stria vascularis, and the vessel of the spiral prominence. Collecting venules predominate in the scala tympani and drain spiral capillary vessels and the capillary net in the scala vestibuli. A spiral vessel is formed basally to the basilar membrane by the venules at the basilar membrane. Radiating arterioles and collecting venules connect with one another by arteriovenous anastomoses lying externally to the stria vascularis. (From Axelsson (1968), reproduced by courtesy of the Editor, *Acta Oto-Laryngologica*)

external wall. The collecting venule just below the attachment of the basilar membrane is termed the venule at the basilar membrane. These collecting venules ultimately drain into either the vein of the scala media or common modiolar vein.

(c) Scala media

Principally there are three different vessels, i.e. stria vascularis, the vessel of the spiral prominence, and arterio-venous anastomoses.

Stria vascularis demonstrates a well defined apical and basal marginal vessel and consists of capillaries with differing diameter. It also has connection with the radiating arterioles of the scala media and the collecting venules of both scala vestibuli and tympani. There is no connection between the stria vascularis and the vessel of the spiral prominence. Lateral to the stria vascularis is the arterio-venous anastomosis between the radiating arterioles and collecting venules.

The vascular anatomy of the external wall presents in a much simplified manner in the apical turn compared with the basal portion. This variation, according to Axelsson, probably protects the basal turn from the effects of vascular occlusion.

(4) VASCULAR ANATOMY OF THE BASAL END OF THE COCHLEA (*Figure 23.5*)

The basal end of the cochlea differs from the apical region in being supplied and drained from ante and retrograde directions.

The distribution of the vestibulo-cochlear artery has been referred to earlier. Venous drainage of the basal end of the cochlea is through the vestibulo-cochlear vein which is formed by the vein of the round window and both the anterior and posterior vestibular veins. The posterior vestibular vein drains the spiral lamina and the scala vestibuli whilst the anterior vestibular veins drain parts of the vestibule and the labyrinth. The vein of the round window is seen at the superior aspect of the round window and receives short venules from the scala tympani at the basal end before joining the vestibulo-cochlear vein. The common modiolar vein joins the vestibulo-cochlear veins to form the vein of the cochlear aqueduct which is in close proximity to the round window and runs parallel to the cochlear aqueduct to its destination into the internal jugular vein.

The radiating arterioles in common with the collecting venules have a much more oblique course in the basal end. The stria vascularis demonstrates a marked difference compared to the other regions and is characterized by the presence of a sparse network of capillaries. However, at the extreme basal end the stria is represented by two parallel vessels with inter-communicating branches.

The dimensions of the human cochlear vessels vary from 15–20 μm in the region of the arterio-venous anastomosis to 5–10 μm in the capillaries of the scala vestibuli. A maximum of 20–40 μm diameter is recorded for the radiating arterioles.

There is very little information on the detailed vascular anatomy of the vestibular apparatus.

Ultrastructure of the cochlear blood vessels

Kimura and Ota (1974) observed in the guinea-pig a well-defined morphological difference in the small blood vessels of the modiolus and the lateral wall of the membranous labyrinth. Whilst the modiolar smaller blood vessels had similar smooth muscle cells to the rest of the peripheral vasculature in the human body, those in the radiating arterioles of the spiral ligament had flat smooth muscle cells which are widely spaced and akin to pericytes. Such a difference in the morphology together with a lack of nerve supply suggested to the authors that the capacity for vasomotion in these vessels was limited. These vessels do not respond to cervical sympathetic chain stimulation, nor are they influenced by adrenaline chloride whether applied locally or injected systemically (Perlman and Kimura, 1955a). These results paved the way to the belief that the cochlear blood flow is controlled by the vessels at the modiolus.

The vessels in the modiolar connective tissue, which are branches of the spiral modiolar artery, appear to be fenestrated and probably play an important role in fluid exchange. The fluid surrounding the neural elements within the modiolus is contributed largely by these fenestrated vessels.

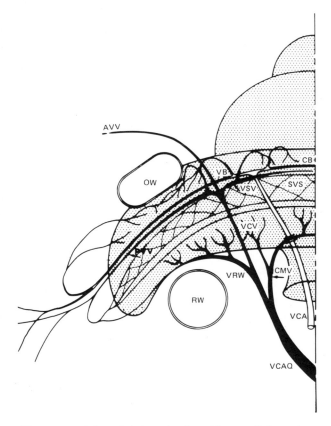

Figure 23.5 Man, basal end of cochlea, radial section, schematic. Note the vessels turning around the basal end of the spiral lamina supplying the external basal end. OW = oval window, RW = round window, VCA = vestibulo-cochlear artery, CB = cochlear branch, VB = vestibular branch, VCAQ = vein of the cochlear aqueduct, CMV = common modiolar vein, VRW = vein of the round window, VSV = vein of the scala vestibuli, PVV = posterior vestibular vein, AVV = anterior vestibular vein. (From Axelsson (1968), reproduced by courtesy of the Editor, *Acta Oto-Laryngologica*)

Stria vascularis

In recent years a good deal of published work has accumulated on the ultrastructure of the stria vascularis. The reader is referred to the following works to mention but a few: Lim (1969); Sugar, Engström and Stahle (1972); Anniko (1976).

Cochlear blood vessel pattern in the human fetus and post-natal period (*Figure 23.6*)

Johnsson (1972) and Johnsson and Hawkins (1972) in an exhaustive study compared the cochlear vasculature in human fetuses of varying weeks of gestation with that in infants and adults. The following features were observed.

(1) SPIRAL LIGAMENT

In all the fetal specimens, the vascular bed was already well differentiated into arterioles which have reached adult size, and capillary plexuses. The important variations in the arterioles are (a) the presence of well defined perivascular spaces around the arterioles in the adult which in the fetus are barely visible, and (b) in many fetuses the arterioles demonstrated a 'Y' shaped pattern above the stria vascularis. The course of the arterioles in the fetus and adults is a straight radial one whilst in the first decade of life many arterioles take a serpentine course towards the stria.

The capillary plexuses are much more dense in the fetus than in infants. The vessel at the vestibular membrane (Reissner's membrane) in the fetus is in the form of a dense capillary plexus.

The veins of the scala vestibuli are not defined in the fetus and appear to be in the form of a capillary plexus.

(2) STRIA VASCULARIS

The stria is mainly composed of light and dark cells in a fetus of 14–19 weeks (dark cell = marginal cell; light cell = intermediate cell), whilst in premature infants there is denser vascularization with numerous shunts.

(3) SCALA TYMPANI

In the spiral ligament of the scala tympani, the vascular architecture is less well developed than in the scala vestibuli. In all the fetuses and premature infants, the basal coil demonstrates single-layered endothelial tubes which form a dense plexus. The middle and apical turns show mature vessels. Several venous capillaries drain into two or three collecting venules which join to form a single venule radiating towards the vein of the scala tympani. In the middle and apical turns the vascular pattern in the scala tympani is much more diffuse and dense.

(4) REISSNER'S MEMBRANE

There is no blood vessel seen in the Reissner's membrane of the fetus.

(5) SPIRAL LAMINA

The vascular pattern is more or less similar to that of adults. The outer spiral vessel (vessel of the basilar membrane) decreases in size in older fetuses and at about 17–24 weeks the inner spiral vessel (vessel of the tympanic lip) is well defined.

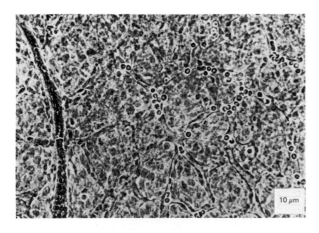

Figure 23.6 Fetal spiral ligament from scala vestibuli of the
basal turn, showing the dense
capillary network above the
stria. A radiating arteriole is seen
at the left. 14 weeks' gestation.
OsO_4 phase—contrast. (From
Johnsson (1972), reproduced by
courtesy of the Editor, *The Annals
of   Otology,   Rhinology   and
Laryngology*)

Perivascular spaces are present in cochlear vessels especially in the spiral ligament, outer spiral vessel, vessels in the modiolus and in bony walls of the cochlea. These spaces have connection with the subarachnoidal spaces and could transport cerebrospinal fluid.

(6) INVOLUTION OF VESSELS

A gradual atrophy of the capillaries is the main feature in the vascular anatomy of the cochlea after birth. The diameters of the arterioles decrease in size during the first decade, to reach adult size. Atrophy of the vessels also occurs in the vestibule. Intravascular strands and avascular channels are the 'tell-tale' features of devascularization in adults, representing remnants of vessel wall and peri-vascular spaces of atrophic vessels respectively.

(7) NEO-VASCULARIZATION

There is no evidence of neo-vascularization (neo-vasculogenesis) within the cochlea.

Thus it would appear from extensive vascular studies that hearing loss resulting from vascular occlusion could either be due to a lesion in the main artery, i.e. labyrinthine or spiral modiolar artery or due to extensive impairment of the cochlear capillary circulation. The presence of numerous anastomoses peripherally confers a greater degree of immunity against physiological damage if the lesion is smaller and placed peripherally in the cochlea (Axelsson, 1968). It would seem that the labyrinthine artery is an end-artery without any communication with the vessels of the otic capsule.

Organ of Corti

The mechanism of continued survival of the spiral organ of Corti has been a subject of much interest and speculation. There appear to be two distinct postulates, both of which are based on experimental findings. Those who maintain that the stria vascularis is mainly concerned in supplying oxygen to the organ of Corti based their findings on loss of hair-cells due to strial atrophy and include Perlman *et al.* (1955a, 1959); Kimura and Perlman (1956, 1958); Alford *et al.* (1965); Igarashi, Alford and Konishi (1969); Johnsson *et al.* (1973). Furthermore Schuknecht and his co-workers (1964 and 1966) have observed a close correlation between hearing loss in humans and histological changes in the stria vascularis. The opponents of such theory include Lawrence (1966) and Lawrence and Clapper (1973) who demonstrated atrophy of the organ of Corti in guinea-pigs by selective interruption of blood supply in the vessels of the basilar membrane. There were no changes in the stria vascularis. Hilding (1973) has corroborated the findings of Lawrence by observing vascular abnormalities in animal inherited deafness. Lawrence (1971) sums up the findings by attributing to the stria vascularis the function of 'maintaining the endolymph and its ionic content presumably to set up the proper environment for the energy conversion properties of the organ of Corti. The vessels of the basilar membrane provide nutrients and oxygen to the sensory cells and supporting structures of the organ of Corti' . . . Although it is tempting to postulate that the stria vascularis is mainly concerned with preservation of physiological function whilst the vessels of the basilar membrane maintain the structural integrity of the organ of Corti, this issue has by no means been fully resolved.

Physiology of microcirculation

The term 'microcirculation' is used to indicate blood flow through the small vessels including the pre-capillary arterioles, capillaries and post-capillary venules. It is concerned primarily with the transfer of nutrients and the removal of metabolic waste by-products. The pre-capillary sphincter controls the flow of blood into the capillaries and is independent of central nervous system. It is, however, controlled by pressure, metabolites and humoral agents.

Bloch (1962) demonstrated by absorption studies and television microscopy techniques that the so-called lamellar flow (axial cellular stream in the centre and peripheral plasma layer) in the vessel does not exist. Erythrocytes were frequently found in close proximity to the vessel wall and seen to deform, readily altering their spherical outline. Furthermore, they were also observed to spin round on their long axes.

Autonomic control of the inner ear

Advances in the techniques of demonstrating the main transmitter substance of the adrenergic fibres by Falck (1962) and Falck *et al.* (1962) have opened up a new horizon for enquiry into the adrenergic nerve supply of the inner ear. The consensus of opinion was summed up by Spoendlin and Lichtensteiger (1966), Spoendlin (1973) and Wersäll, Densert and Lundquist (1973). Essentially the inner ear derives its adrenergic supply in two different ways (*Figure 23.7*). (i) A perivascular route in the form of a dense plexus over both the vertebral and labyrinthine arteries and extending cranially up to the modiolus and the spiral ganglion. No such fibres were observed around the blood vessels of spiral limbus, basilar membrane and the stria vascularis.

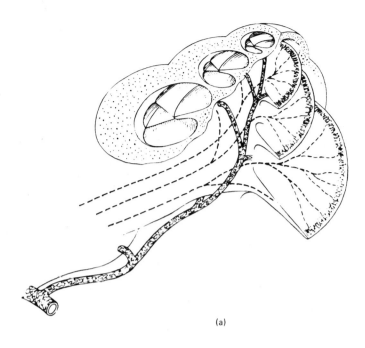

(a)

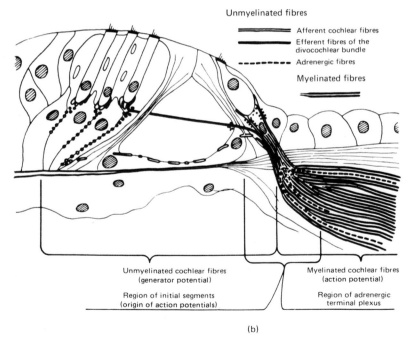

Unmyelinated fibres

Afferent cochlear fibres
Efferent fibres of the
divocochlear bundle
Adrenergic fibres

Myelinated fibres

Unmyelinated cochlear fibres
(generator potential)

Myelinated cochlear fibres
(action potential)

Region of initial segments
(origin of action potentials)

Region of adrenergic
terminal plexus

(b)

Figure 23.7 Schematic representation of the double adrenergic innervation of the cochlea by two different systems. (a) The perivascular system which belongs to the peripheral post-ganglionic sympathetic system. (b) An adrenergic innervation system independent of the blood vessels originating in the central nervous system and reaching the periphery with the cochlear nerve. It is represented with interrupted lines. (From Spoendlin and Lichtensteiger (1966), reproduced by courtesy of the Editor, *Acta Oto-Laryngologica*)

The fibres are thought to originate from the stellate ganglion or the medial cervical ganglion with the plexus representing fibres from both sides of the body. The function of these fibres is thought to be related to regulation of cochlear blood flow. (ii) An extensive network of adrenergic nerve plexus within the bony osseous lamina extending up to the Habenula perforata. These findings were subsequently confirmed by Ross (1971). Similar nerve fibres were identified in the utricular macula and cristae of semicircular canals. All these fibres were independent of blood vessels and thought to arise from the superior cervical ganglion. Their exact course into the inner ear is shrouded with mystery. However, one of the possible routes is by establishing connections between the tympanic plexus and the auricular branches of the tenth and seventh cranial nerves. Although the precise function of these fibres is not known, the possible functions attributed are (a) its effect on the auditory nerve activity at the site of the generator potential, (b) the control of fluid balance. A third possibility that these fibres may chemodynamically influence the sensory neurons cannot be discounted at the present time (Ross, 1971).

The question of parasympathetic nerve supply in the inner ear is still unresolved due to the lack of a specific histochemical method. Wersäll and his associates report having observed cholinergic nerve terminals in the plexus cochlearis. Churchill, Schuknecht and Doron (1956), Schuknecht, Churchill and Doran (1959) and Hilding and Wersäll (1962) demonstrated acetylcholinesterase in the inner ear which implicated the presence of cholinergic innervation.

Control of cochlear blood flow

A good deal of information has accumulated over the years, mostly in experimental animals, on the physiological and pharmacological studies of the autonomic control of cochlear blood flow. Unfortunately the results have been as varied, and at times frankly conflicting, as the methods employed to determine cochlear blood flow. The technique of studying cochlear blood flow varied from earlier workers, who used a simple method of direct observation of vessels over the tympanic membrane and fenestrated semicircular canals to a much more sophisticated technique in recent years, consisting of electrical impedance plethysmography (Suga and Snow, 1969; Snow and Suga, 1973b), radioactive microsphere technique (Todd *et al.*, 1974) and kinetics of production of perilymph (Schnieder, 1974).

Adrenergic control

Perhaps the earliest experimental findings on the adrenergic control of cochlear blood flow were reported by Frazer (1936) who evaluated the effect of stimulation of the stellate and superior cervical sympathetic ganglia by employing a dye injection technique in cats. Frazer demonstrated vasoconstriction of the vessels of not only the internal ear but also that of the outer and middle ear. Seymour (1954) demonstrated vasodilatation in animal stria vascularis following sympathetic block, whilst stimulation of the sympathetic chain caused marked constriction of the vessels of the stria in the same animals.

On the contrary, Rambo, Wolff and Freeman (1953) found no appreciable alteration in the vessels of the labyrinth in monkeys, following denervation of the sympathetic nerve supply to the inner ear. Perlman and Kimura (1955a) observing blood flow under the microscope in cats reported no visible alteration in the blood flow following transection or electrical stimulation of the cervical sympathetic chain. Strong (1957) observed no change in the vessels of the fenestrated lateral semicircular canal in dogs following stimulation of the stellate ganglion and vago-sympathetic trunk. Todd *et al.* (1974) whilst observing changes in the otic blood flow following sympathetic stimulation, came to the conclusion that sympathetic control on the intracranial vasculature has a modulating role rather than a controlling role. The authors postulated a cyclic AMP mediated role in the receptor cells to produce a sympathetic response.

Effect on the animal cochlear microphonics was observed by Seymour and Tappin (1951 and 1953), who reported a decrease on sympathetic stimulation.

Clinical observations on the adrenergic control of otic blood flow were made on patients with known Menière's disease and in sudden sensorineural deafness treated with either cervical or dorsal sympathectomy (Golding-Wood, 1960; Passe, 1951; Strong, 1957) and stellate ganglion block (Wilmot, 1959; Singleton, 1971; Polus, 1972).

Passe (1951) observed vasodilatation over the human tympanic membrane within 60 s of cervical sympathetic chain block; such observation was extended to the vessels over the promontory and lateral semicircular canals.

Effects of sympatho- and parasympatho-mimetic drugs

Alpha and beta sympathetic receptors have different functions. Thus stimulation of α receptors leads to vasoconstriction and that of β receptors to vasodilatation. Cerebral vasculature is under the influence of α receptors (Goodman and Gillman, 1965).

(1) *α receptor stimulators.* Noradrenaline (Lavertenol), phenylephrine hydrochloride, methoxamine hydrochloride, ephedrine.
(2) *α receptor blocking agents.* Phenoxybenzamine, ergotamine tartrate, dihydroergotamine mesylate, tolazoline hydrochloride.
(3) *β receptor stimulators.* Isoproterenol hydrochloride and isoxsuprine hydrochloride.
(4) *β receptor blocking agents.* Dihydroisoproterenol.
(5) *Antiadrenergic agents.* Guanethidine sulphate.
(6) *Cholinergic*
    (a) *Choliomemetic agents.* Acetylcholine, bethanechol chloride and pilocarpine.
    (b) *Anticholinesterase agents.* Neostigmine, edrophonium chloride.
    (c) *Cholinolytic agents.* Atropine and scopolamine.

(1) ALPHA RECEPTOR STIMULANTS AND THEIR EFFECTS

Mygind and Falbe-Hansen (1948) reported dilatation of the cochlear blood vessels following subcutaneous injection of adrenaline. Morimitsu (1960) observed transient decrease followed by an increase in cochlear blood flow in animals receiving adrenaline and noradrenaline. Nomura (1961) reported increased cochlear blood flow in animals with large doses of adrenaline and noradrenaline and these observations were largely confirmed by Perlman, Tsunoo and Spence (1963), using a different technique. Snow and Suga (1973a) reported increased cochlear blood flow with adrenaline and ephedrine sulphate whilst Lavertenol, phenylephrine hydrochloride and methoxamine hydrochloride caused transient decrease followed by subsequent increase in cochlear blood flow. Schnieder (1974) using perilymphatic kinetics to estimate cochlear blood flow reported an increase in both cochlear and cerebral blood flow with smaller doses of adrenaline whilst larger doses caused a decrease in flow.

(2) ALPHA RECEPTOR BLOCKING AGENTS AND THEIR EFFECTS

Snow and Suga (1973a) demonstrated an increase in cochlear blood flow with phenoxybenzamine, ergotamine tartrate, dihydroergotamine mesylate and tolazoline hydrochloride.

(3) BETA RECEPTOR STIMULANTS AND THEIR EFFECTS

Snow and Suga (1973a) reported weak vasodilatation although cochlear blood flow readily decreased with a fall in systemic blood pressure with larger doses of isoproterenol hydrochloride and isoxsuprine hydrochloride.

(4) BETA RECEPTOR BLOCKING AGENTS AND THEIR EFFECTS

Snow and Suga (1973a) reported a decrease in cochlear blood flow with dihydroisoproterenol.

(5) ANTI-ADRENERGIC AGENTS AND THEIR EFFECTS

Guanethidine sulphate caused an initial increase and subsequent decrease (Snow and Suga, 1973a).

(6) CHOLINERGIC

(a) *Choliomemetic*

Acetylcholine was shown to increase cochlear blood flow by Morimitsu (1960), whilst pilocarpine dilated vessels; Snow and Suga (1973a) demonstrated dilatation of cochlear blood vessels following administration of acetylcholine, bethanechol chloride and pilocarpine.

(b) *Anticholinesterase*

Smaller increase in cochlear blood flow was observed following injection of neostigmine and edrophonium chloride (Snow and Suga, 1973a).

(c) *Cholinolytic*

Morimitsu (1960) reported decrease in cochlear blood flow with atropine sulphate, these findings being confirmed by Suga and Snow (1973a) with both atropine and scopolamine hypobromide.

Vasodilators and their effects

Papaverine hydrochloride was shown to increase cochlear blood flow by Morimitsu (1960), Snow and Suga (1973a) and Schnieder (1975). Amyl nitrite caused an increase in cochlear blood flow although the systemic blood pressure showed a drop in its level (Morimitsu, 1960, and Snow and Suga, 1973a). Histamine hydrochloride was shown to increase cochlear blood flow with a concomitant drop in systemic blood pressure by Snow and Suga (1973a). However, Mygind and Falbe-Hansen (1948) demonstrated constriction of blood vessels in the inner ear whilst Schnieder (1975) reported a reduction in cochlear blood flow. No marked change in cochlear blood flow was noted with niacin, nicotinyl alcohol tartarate (Snow and Suga, 1973a). Hydralazine hydrochloride was shown to increase cochlear blood flow with a decrease in systemic blood pressure (Snow and Suga, 1973a).

Betahistine hydrochloride (SERC) has been shown to increase cochlear blood flow in guinea-pigs and chinchillas following topical, intravenous and intragastric administration (Martinez, 1972).

Effect of hypertonic glucose

Hypertonic glucose produced an increase in cochlear blood flow in animals (Morimitsu, 1960; Snow and Suga, 1973a). The increase is attributed to an expansion in intravascular space.

Effect of sodium carbonate

Administration of a 7 per cent solution caused increased cochlear blood flow, probably from its effect on the blood carbon dioxide tension (Snow and Suga, 1973a).

Gaseous control of cochlear blood flow

(1) EXPERIMENTAL STUDIES

Carbon dioxide, 10 or 5 per cent, mixed in oxygen when inhaled produced a marked and significant increase in both the cerebral and cochlear blood flow (Morimitsu, 1960; Snow and Suga, 1973a; Pollock *et al.*, 1974; Schnieder, 1975); the 10 per cent carbon dioxide mixture, however, showing a much more marked effect when compared with a 5 per cent mixture. Eckenhoff, Hafkenschiel and Landmesser (1947) demonstrated in dogs a lack of adverse reaction on coronary flow following inhalation of 5–7 per cent carbon dioxide. Inhalation of 100 per cent oxygen produced a distinct reduction in cochlear blood flow (Snow and Suga, 1973a).

(2) HUMAN STUDIES

Fisch, Murata and Hossli (1976) in a well-controlled human study, demonstrated the effects of inhalation of carbon dioxide on the oxygen tension in the perilymph. The results of the study have an important clinical application. They selected five patients undergoing stapedectomy for otosclerosis and six patients with sudden deafness of a week's duration and in both groups of patients the oxygen tension in the perilymph was measured by inserting a silver-silver chloride microelectrode through the footplate of the stapes. The procedure was carried out under general anaesthetic with monitoring of blood pressure, P_{O_2}, P_{CO_2} and ECG. The results of the investigation showed a 200 per cent increase in perilymphatic oxygen tension within 3–6 min of inhaling 5 per cent carbon dioxide in 95 per cent oxygen and reaching a peak recording between 16 and 33 min. Patients receiving low molecular weight dextran and eupaverine showed no change in the perilymphatic oxygen tension (*Figures 23.8 and 23.9*).

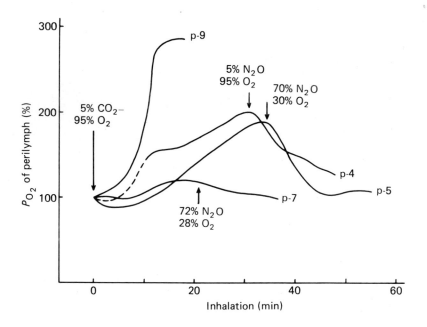

Figure 23.8 P_{O_2} of perilymph during inhalation of 5 per cent carbon dioxide in 95 per cent oxygen in patients with ostosclerosis. (From Fisch *et al.* (1976), reproduced by courtesy of the Editor, *Acta Oto-Laryngologica*)

An important contribution to our understanding of the effects of carbon dioxide on the cerebral blood flow in healthy volunteers was made by Kety and Schmidt (1948) who reported a striking and consistent increase in the cerebral blood flow (average of 75 per cent increase) following inhalation of 5 and 7 per cent carbon dioxide. The increased cerebral blood flow was associated with decreased cerebrovascular resistance. However, one pertinent observation was the significant rise in systolic blood pressure without any alteration in cardiac output. Inhalation of 85–100 per cent oxygen resulted in a significant decrease in the cerebral blood flow.

Gibson, Ramsden and Moffat (1977) in evaluating the benefits of intravenous naftidrofuryl (Praxiline) in Menière's disease, attributed the changes in cochlear microphonics and summating potential, as shown in electrocochleography, to increased perfusion of the stria vascularis.

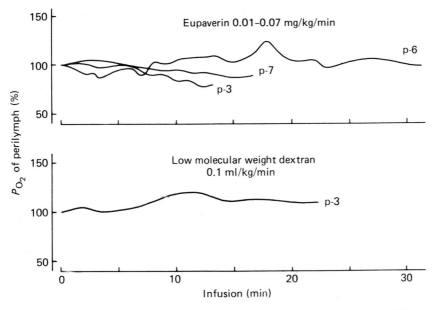

Figure 23.9 Response of oxygen tension of the human perilymph to vasodilating drugs. (From Fisch *et al.* (1976), reproduced by courtesy of the Editor, *Acta Oto-Laryngologica*)

Patho-physiology of vascular occlusion

Our detailed understanding of the alterations in function—changes in endocochlear potentials, changes in oxygen tension and biochemical disturbances, and changes in cyto-architecture within the inner ear as a result of vascular occlusion—has been entirely due to systematic observations in experimental animals. Understandably such detailed study in humans is virtually non-existent.

Histological changes

Changes within the internal ear may be due to either arterial or venous obstruction. In experimental animals different histological changes are observed following arterial obstruction and it depends whether the blood flow is interrupted suddenly and completely or gradually and incompletely.

(1) VENOUS OBSTRUCTION

Perlman (1952) from his observations on the occlusion of the inferior cochlear vein in guinea-pigs concluded that the absence of gross changes within the cochlea and vestibular apparatus must have been due to the extensive collaterals existing through the vein of the vestibular aqueduct. However, in animals with extensive venous obstruction of the labyrinth, there were widespread cochleo-saccular changes (Kimura and Perlman, 1956a, b). The outer hair-cells were more prone to degeneration in the basal part of the cochlea than the apical. Stria vascularis demonstrated degeneration.

The cristae and utricle were less frequently affected. There was a varying degree of haemorrhage in the labyrinthine spaces.

(2) ARTERIAL OBSTRUCTION—COMPLETE

Obstruction to the anterior inferior cerebellar artery causes extensive damage throughout the cochlea affecting various compartments. A definite sequence of events could be observed histologically commencing with changes in the inner hair-cells within half an hour of obstruction followed by rapid detachment of supporting cells from the basilar membrane. The spiral ganglion and spiral ligament also shared the rapid damage. In extreme degrees of obstruction, the hair-cells were replaced by fibrosis and later by ossification (Kimura and Perlman, 1958). Bernstein and Silverstein (1966) demonstrated lesions in the apical region of the cochlea following ligation of the anterior inferior cerebellar artery and postulated the possibility of similar vascular lesions in syphilitic deafness in humans.

(3) ARTERIAL OBSTRUCTION—TEMPORARY

Perlman, Kimura and Fernandez (1959) recorded cessation of blood flow in the animal stria vascularis (up to 30–60 min obstruction) almost immediately after obstruction of the artery. With the release of obstruction, fast blood flow returned presumably due to accumulation of acid metabolites. There were no alterations either in the vessel wall or in the cells.

Histologically changes were observed much more commonly in the basal turn of the cochlea. In shorter periods of obstruction (15 min) the outer hair-cells were the first to show degeneration followed by the inner hair-cells, pillar cells, and supporting cells with longer periods of occlusion. No hydrops of the endolymphatic duct was observed.

(4) MICROEMBOLIZATION

Alford *et al.* (1965) demonstrated, for the first time, the effects of microembolization (Polystyrene emboli) in a series of animal experiments. There was degeneration of the hair-cells in the organ of Corti with frequent degeneration of the stria vascularis, although in some degeneration of the hair-cells was independent of the strial atrophy. There were changes in the vestibular apparatus also. Thus histological changes in the end-organs might well, according to the authors, account for the deafness and vertigo arising from vascular lesions in humans.

Suga and his associates (1970) used barium sulphate to produce microembolization in guinea-pig cochleas and demonstrated variable changes ranging from atrophy of the stria and degeneration of the organ of Corti to dilatation of the cochlear duct. Reflex vasospasm in response to microembolization has been postulated as the possible mechanism of damage to the cochlea. The vestibular apparatus appears to be relatively resistant to vascular damage.

Alteration in inner-ear function due to arterial occlusion

Effect on endo-cochlear potentials

The maintenance of resting endo-cochlear potential at approximately $+80–100$ mV is supposed to be related to the 'Potassium pump', probably located within the stria vascularis, and it is dependent on ATP utilization. A decrease in the normal endo-cochlear potential has been observed during vascular insufficiency in the inner ear. Perlman, Kimura and Fernandez (1959) made exhaustive studies of changes in the endo-cochlear potential during temporary obstruction to the internal auditory artery in guinea-pigs. There was usually an interval of about 10 s from the commencement of the occlusion to the disappearance of cochlear responses. The obliteration of neural components (N1 and N2) preceded that of cochlear microphonics (CM). This phenomenon, according to the author, indicates the extreme degree of sensitivity of cochlear neurons to lack of oxygen and that the delay in cochlear microphonics was possibly due to damage to the stria vascularis and generally reflects on the precarious oxygen reserve. The recovery time (interval from the end of occlusion to the first sign of recovery of responses) was shorter for occlusion of less than 5 min duration and as the length of occlusion was prolonged there was a proportional increase in the recovery time. However, beyond 30 min of occlusion neither the cochlear microphonics nor N1 seemed to reach 50 per cent of the reference amplitude. The maximum duration of occlusion was about 60–65 min for CM and about 50–55 min for AP.

Loss of both endo-cochlear and action potential was also observed following microembolic obstruction of the smaller cochlear vessels (Alford *et al.*, 1965; Sugar *et al.*, 1972). The later authors also observed the beneficial effects of phenoxybenzamine hydrochloride (α adrenergic blocking agent) by inhibiting the decrease in cochlear potential. However, isoproterenol hydrochloride and 10 per cent carbon dioxide failed to show similar beneficial effects.

Effect on oxygen tension

Endolymph oxygen tension was determined by Misrahy *et al.* (1958) in guinea-pigs in whom they recorded a level of 55–70 mmHg nearer the stria vascularis with a gradual decrease in the oxygen tension in the scala media. Anoxia produced a rapid drop in oxygen tension in the scala media within seconds of breathing pure nitrogen. Inhalation of 10 per cent carbon dioxide in air increased the oxygen tension in the endolymph, and a similar increase in perilymph oxygen tension was observed in humans by Fisch, Murata and Hossli (1976), although breathing of pure oxygen could result in vasoconstriction of cochlear vessels in animals.

The effect of sudden but temporary arterial obstruction on endo-cochlear oxygen tension was investigated in guinea-pigs by Tsunoo and Perlman (1969), who reported a drop in oxygen reserve in the cochlea within a few seconds from the onset of obstruction in the artery and was exhausted in about 100 s. Thus the oxygen reserve in the cochlea is sufficient to maintain normal function for only a few seconds following cessation of blood flow and the function recovers much more rapidly in comparison with the oxygen tension which recovers in a linear fashion on recovery of normal blood flow. The author concluded that the function can be maintained even after 6 min of obstruction to the internal auditory artery.

Biochemical changes in the cochlea

Oxidative phosphorylation is the main source of energy supply within the cochlea and requires the presence of oxygen. Biochemical changes resulting from anoxia in the cochlea are mainly due to altered glucose metabolism. Anaerobic metabolism leads to the accumulation of lactate and is responsible for lactic acidosis. Following anoxia there is a rapid change in the phosphorylase activity within the stria vascularis although the endolymphatic levels of lactate have not yet been determined. However, perilymphatic concentration of lactate rises to fourfold within 30 min and to sixfold within 1 h of anoxia (Thalmann, Miyoshi and Rauchbach, 1973).

Studies on the 'Potassium pump', thought to be sited in the stria vascularis, indicate that the maintenance of a potassium gradient in the scala media requires the active use of ATP and oxidative phosphorylation. Bosher and Warren (1968), using a flame spectrophotometer to measure endolymphatic sodium and potassium ion concentration during anoxia in animals, observed a decrease in potassium ions with a concomitant increase in sodium ions within the scala media. The results reflect the measure of damage to the active transport mechanism dependent on oxidative phosphorylation. Similar results were reported by Suga, Nakashima and Snow (1970), in common with findings in acoustic trauma. Matschinsky and Thalmann (1967) were responsible for demonstrating ample stores of glycogen and glucose in the organ of Corti and the stria vascularis. Within 30 min of onset of ischaemia, the creatine-P content together with ATP showed a drop in level in the stria vascularis. However, in the organ of Corti the breakdown was rather slow and hardly altered even after 3 min of anoxia.

The rate of degradation of glycogen in the organ of Corti revealed a maximum rate of degradation in the basal turn (Thalmann, Miyoshi and Rauchbach, 1973) which might help to explain the location of maximum damage during vascular occlusion in the basal coil, as reported by Perlman, Kimura and Fernandez (1959). It would thus appear that the organ of Corti is unique in resisting a certain degree of damage through vascular insufficiency by virtue of its ample glucose and glycogen content, efficient glycolytic mechanism and relatively low energy requirement (Thalmann, Miyoshi and Rauchbach, 1973).

Microcirculatory pathology

Most of the observations on rheology (science dealing with the shape and behaviour of blood cells and plasma) of blood in low-flow states have been based on *in vitro* studies, involving investigations at low microscopic resolution levels. Brånemark (1968) observed changes in human microcirculation recorded through a special observation chamber inserted in a pedicled skin tube. The change in the plasma was labelled as a 'skimming phenomenon', consisting of a flow of plasma only in the capillaries during reduction in the amount of blood per unit of time. The changes in the cells were strikingly different to that observed hitherto and for the first time established non-adherence of erythrocytes to the capillary endothelium even in long-standing stasis although they did form rouleaux during low flow velocity. During normal flow, however, there was absence of adherence of erythrocytes, granulocytes and platelets. The granulocytes and platelets failed to show any change in structure or function during low-flow state. Stasis *per se* is not adequate to induce intravascular clotting and would require the help of vascular endothelial damage to trigger the clotting mechanism. The microvascular system of man was found to withstand several hours of diminished or total blockage in the flow and still return to normal function on restoration of flow.

General circulatory disturbances

Arterial embolism

Secondary to valvular disease of the heart, atrial fibrillation, following myocardial infarction.

Arterial thrombosis

Thrombosis superimposed on an arteriosclerotic plaque and formed by agglutination of erythrocytes and platelets. It can occur in a larger vessel of the neck such as the bifurcation of the common carotid or in a medium-size vessel such as the posterior inferior cerebellar artery.

Small blood vessel disease (arterial)

Such as that seen in diabetes mellitus.

Venous thrombo-embolism

Due to venous stasis in the post-operative period and changes in platelet behaviour.

Altered blood rheology

Hypercoagulable state such as observed in polycythaemia, macroglobulinaemia; haemoconcentration such as seen in dehydration, leukaemia and sickle-cell disease.

Low molecular weight dextran

Experimental observations in shock have revealed the presence of sludging in the smaller vessels resulting from sluggish flow and consequent increase in blood viscosity amongst other factors. Dextran is basically a carbohydrate having a specific affinity for water and a capacity to bind it. Studies on experimental hypovolaemic shock have shown the invaluable help of low molecular weight dextran (molecular weight 40 000) in restoring the plasma volume. The beneficial action of low molecular weight dextran on microcirculation is due to (a) a plasma dilution property, (b) prevention of sludging, (c) in some instances a cell-dispersing property (Charm and Kurland, 1974).

Clinical disorders

During ischaemia preservation of tissue function largely depends upon the nature of vascular obstruction, i.e. whether or not complete and the presence of collateral circulation. Since the inner ear lacks any collateral circulation between the labyrinthine artery and the vessels of the otic capsule, the final outcome of residual function therefore rests upon the site and duration of ischaemia. Peripheral vascular patterns within the cochlea can probably accommodate any obstruction to the flow if the obstruction is situated in the terminal branches of the main labyrinthine artery (Axelsson, 1968). Ischaemia may be caused by arterial thrombosis or embolism with superadded spasm and from haemorrhage. Disturbances in function likewise may vary from a transient bilateral tinnitus during a vasovagal attack to that of severe sensorineural deafness and vertigo in main arterial obstruction. Vascular lesions within the inner ear may broadly be classified and discussed under the following headings.

(a) Congenital: (1) Hereditary deafness.
                          (2) Cochlear otosclerosis.
(b) Traumatic: Cochlear or vestibular component involved either singly
                              or in combination.
                          (1) Blow on the head, with or without fractured skull.
                          (2) Blast injury.
                          (3) Acoustic trauma.
(c) Infective: (1) Viral—rubella.
                          (2) Bacterial—syphilis.
(d) Metabolic: Diabetes mellitus.
(e) Degenerative: Presbyacusis.
(f) Vascular accident: (1) Sudden deafness.
                          (2) Menière's disease.
                          (3) Lermoyez syndrome.
                          (4) Leukaemia.
                          (5) Subarachnoid haemorrhage.
                          (6) Radiation exposure.
                          (7) Benign positional nystagmus.
                          (8) Occlusion of the anterior inferior cerebellar artery.
(g) Ototoxic: (1) Quinine.
                          (2) Salicylates.
                          (3) Aminoglycosides
                          (4) Ethacrynic acid.
(h) Miscellaneous: (1) Paget's disease.
                          (2) Von-Recklinghausen's disease.

(a) Congenital

(1) HEREDITARY DEAFNESS
Evidence of vascular insufficiency as a possible mechanism of loss of hair-cells in inherited deafness largely stems from experimental data. The controversy surrounding the role of the stria vascularis and the vessel of the basilar membrane in the preservation of the organ of Corti has already been referred to. Hilding (1973)

concluded from his study in Shaker-1 mice, Hedland mink, and Ames Waltzer mice that the premature involution of the outer spiral vessel (vessel of the basilar membrane) was an important factor in the aetiology of degeneration in the organ of Corti. Johnsson *et al.* (1973) found strial atrophy in the cochlea of deaf Dalmation dogs. A systematic study of such vascular abnormalities in hereditary and congenital deafness in humans is lacking and, pending such a study, the role of vascular insufficiency remains unresolved. Johnsson *et al.* (1973) did, however, report that in the fetus the outer spiral vessel (vessel of the basilar membrane) is larger than the adult vessel.

(2) COCHLEAR OTOSCLEROSIS

Rüedi and Spocndlin (1968) drew attention to vascular shunts within the inner ear of patients with cochlear otosclerosis, and suggested that these shunts were responsible for sensorineural deafness. Normally, there is no evidence of any anastomosis between the vessels of the membranous and bony labyrinths. However, an actively growing otosclerotic focus can break through the endosteal layer and establish contact with the spiral ligament, where new channels form between the vessels in the otosclerotic bone and veins in the spiral ligament—such changes were observed in ten temporal bones with cochlear otosclerosis. The congestion in the spiral ligament, as a result of blood shunting from the otosclerotic focus into the inferior cochlear vein, causes damage to the sensory structures within the inner ear (the reader is referred to the earlier section on the effects of venous obstruction in animals (Perlman, 1952)). The findings of Rüedi and Spoendlin have been confirmed by Nager (1966), Linthicum (1966) and Johnsson (1973). However, Schuknecht and Gross (1966), Lindsey and Beal (1966), Altman, Kornfield and Shea (1966) were unable to confirm Rüedi's findings.

Gussen (1975) examined four temporal bones with extensive labyrinthine otosclerosis and observed loss of capillaries and pericapillary spaces in the spiral ligament. Gussen suggests that the vascular shunts observed by Rüedi in labyrinthine otosclerosis might well represent a by-pass of blood flow from the sparse capillary network in the spiral ligament into the rich vascular spaces of an otosclerotic focus.

Differential diagnosis includes deafness due to heredodegenerative disease, cochlear hydrops, acoustic tumour. Tomography and polytomography usually help to clear the diagnosis.

Treatment

Recently sodium fluoride therapy has been advocated in an attempt to arrest the disease process. The reader is referred to Chapter 14 for further details.

(b) Traumatic

(1) BLOW ON THE HEAD

Sensorineural deafness resulting from a blow on the head may be due to concussion injury to the inner ear or to disruption and intracochlear haemorrhage when the fracture line extends into the bony labyrinth (Schuknecht, 1969). Sensorineural deafness following intracochlear haemorrhage is more likely to be permanent (*see* Chapter 24 for details of symptoms, diagnosis and treatment).

(2) BLAST INJURY

Inner-ear damage from exposure to blast is well documented and is often associated with a torn tympanic membrane. Sensorineural deafness following exposure to such injury appears to be confined to the higher frequencies (Kerr and Byrne, 1975) and is often accompanied by tinnitus though not by vestibular disturbances. Kellerhals (1972) found severe capillary damage in the cochleas of guinea-pigs exposed to pressure waves from blank cartridge fire. The second coil of the cochlea was worse affected. In the same study Kellerhals was impressed by the cellular protection from damage in a group of animals receiving prophylactic infusion of Dextran 40. Diagnosis presents little problem in the wake of a history of sudden exposure to a blast injury. Vestibular disturbance is non-existent.

Treatment

Experimental observations prompted Kellerhals (1972) to evaluate the effects of Dextran 40 in a clinical trial on male workers who were exposed to a chemical explosion in Switzerland. One group (selected at random) of five patients received immediate 10 per cent Dextran 40; the regime consisted of rapid infusion of 500 ml within 1–2 h followed by a series of 500 ml slow intravenous infusion on the first, second, fourth, sixth and the eighth day. The control group of five patients did not receive any specific treatment. Comparison of the hearing tests at intervals demonstrated a statistically significant improvement in the hearing of patients receiving Dextran 40.

It is perhaps pertinent to recall that Fisch, Murata and Hossli (1976) found no increase in the perilymph oxygen tension in humans during intravenous infusion of low molecular weight dextran. However, 5 per cent carbon dioxide in 95 per cent oxygen when inhaled showed considerable increase in the perilymph oxygen tension presumably from improved capillary perfusion and such a regime is worth a trial in patients suffering from sensorineural deafness following exposure to blast injury.

(3) ACOUSTIC TRAUMA

Whilst detailed information on this subject appears elsewhere (Chapter 18), in this chapter only information relevant to blood flow and acoustic trauma will be examined.

There have been several reports, in recent years, of the adverse effects of high intensity sound on both the microcirculation and the respiratory enzymes within the cochlea. Misrahy *et al.* (1958) were able to demonstrate in guinea-pigs exposed to a pure tone of 4000 Hz for 20 s a diminished oxygen tension in the scala media and concluded that the damage to the hair-cells from intense sound must be through its adverse action on the microcirculation in the cochlea. These findings were subsequently confirmed by Koide, Yoshida and Konno (1960), working with guinea-pigs and rabbits exposed to 15 min of sound at 4000 Hz and intensity of 105 phon. Hawkins (1971) conclusively showed, in guinea-pigs, constriction of strial vessels in animals exposed to wide band noise of 118–120 dB SPL for 8–110 h. The capillary constriction appeared to be due to swollen endothelial cells and together with adjacent pericytes produced an effective blockage for the escape of red blood corpuscles (*Figures 23.10* and *23.11*). The changes were pronounced in animals exposed for 30 h or more, where outer hair-cell damage was observed in the third row and to a lesser extent in the second row. Narrowing of the vessels was not observed in the spiral ligament or spiral

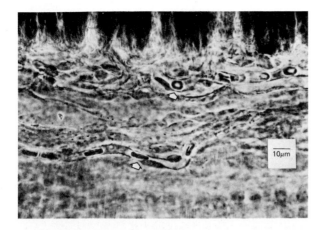

Figure 23.10 Capillary vaso-constriction with endothelial swellings and trapped red blood cells (arrows) in inner and spiral vessels. Second turn. Noise exposure 118–120 dB for 30 h continuously. (From Hawkins (1971), reproduced by courtesy of the Editor, *The Annals of Otology, Rhinology and Laryngology*)

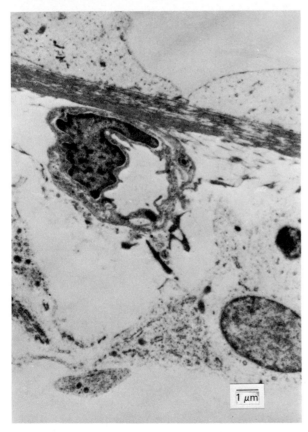

Figure 23.11 Electron micrograph of swollen endothelial cell encroaching on the lumen of the outer spiral vessel beneath the tunnel of Corti in the second upper turn. Noise exposure 118–120 dB for 110 h in all. (From Hawkins (1971), reproduced by courtesy of the Editor, *The Annals of Otology, Rhinology and Laryngology*)

prominence. Lipscomb and Roettger (1973) observed constriction of the vessels in the cristae and to a lesser extent in the capillaries of the saccule in rats exposed to 110 dB SPL broad spectrum noise for 48 h. Similar vasoconstriction was seen in the capillaries of the cochlear tissue. Duvall, Ward and Lauhala (1974) reported, in chinchillas exposed to 700–2800 Hz noise of 123 dB for 15 min, collapsed vessels in the stria containing distorted red blood corpuscles, when examined under light microscopy. There were changes in ultrastructure of the stria vascularis also. Furthermore, these authors also observed by using horseradish peroxidase staining technique alteration in cellular transport in the stria, changes being maximum in those areas correspondingly showing severe strial damage.

Koide, Yoshida and Konno (1960) noted an increase in the glucose content of the perilymph in guinea-pigs and rabbits exposed to white noise. These authors concluded that the biochemical changes were entirely due to reduced blood flow in the cochlea affecting directly the oxidative phosphorylation. Furthermore, electron microscopic examination of the specimen led them to believe that the damage was mainly felt at the apex of the outer hair-cells within the structure of the mitochondrion. Conti and Borgo (1964), whilst investigating in guinea-pigs the effects of high intensity sound (100 dB for 3 h) on respiratory enzyme, observed a reduction in the concentration of cytochrome oxidase in the stria vascularis, external spiral sulcus and the organ of Corti.

It would appear from a brief review of the reports that vasoconstriction is the main pathological feature in the animal cochlea exposed to intense noise and these observations could well have an important application in the future management of patients exposed to intense sound.

(c) Infective

(1) VIRAL—RUBELLA DEAFNESS
Sensorineural deafness due to *in vitro* rubella infection is a well known entity. The damage to the inner ear is thought to be mediated through a direct action of the virus on the vessels. Temporal bone studies have shown extravasation of blood in the inner ear and similar changes are also observed in the middle and external ears (Kelemen, 1966).

(2) SPIROCHAETAL—SYPHILITIC DEAFNESS
Bernstein and Silverstein (1966) examined temporal bones from two patients, one with acquired and one with congenital syphilis. In the first patient, changes were confined to loss of ganglion cells with a normal organ of Corti. The temporal bones from the congenital syphilitic patient showed hair-cell changes in the apical region of the cochlea and the semicircular canals, presumed to be due to vascular obliteration. Audiometric information is not available in these patients. Vascular involvement in other parts of the body is well documented in patients with congenital and late acquired syphilis.

For details on symptoms, diagnosis, treatment, see Chapter 15.

(d) Metabolic

DEAFNESS IN DIABETES MELLITUS
Although recorded in diabetic patients, the incidence of sensorineural deafness is by no means clear due to conflicting reports. The hearing loss may be sudden in onset thus resembling a vascular accident and two such cases were described by Jørgensen (1960). Audiograms in these patients showed losses at 2, 4 and 8 kHz and both patients had severe diabetic retinopathy. One of the patients developed sudden sensorineural deafness in the right ear, associated with a left-sided retinal haemorrhage. The hearing

improved subsequently. Two years later the same patient developed sudden contralateral hearing loss.

In a carefully researched study of 69 diabetic patients, Jørgensen and Buch (1961) found sensorineural deafness in 28 patients due to diabetes, having excluded other forms of deafness due to age, noise and ototoxicity. The hearing loss was characteristically bilateral being confined to higher frequencies and insiduous in onset. Occasionally there was some discrepancy between the thresholds on the two sides. In some even the lower frequencies were involved. Vestibular symptoms were present in only 9 out of 69 patients.

Rosen and Davis (1971) examined the relationship between microangiopathy and hearing loss in 130 diabetic patients. In the younger age group of up to 24 years, both hearing loss and microangiopathy were rare. The incidence of hearing loss showed a steady increase in the older age group coinciding with a concomitant rise in the incidence of microangiopathy in the vessels of the bulbar conjunctivae and nail bed. Audiometric findings allowed the authors to separate the findings into two distinct groups, i.e. a high frequency hearing loss in relatively younger patients and a flat type of curve in older groups. Capillary fragility was definitely increased in nine patients.

In a controlled study of 33 diabetic patients, Axelsson and Fagerberg (1968) failed to observe any significant difference in the hearing levels of diabetic patients when compared with that of the normal population. In a few, however, there was definite indication of retrocochlear hearing loss.

Histopathological findings in the inner ear of diabetic patients
Microscopic changes characteristic of diabetic angiopathy elsewhere in the body notably the vessels of the lower extremities, kidneys and the retina include (a) periodic Acid-Schiff positive substance in the vessel wall, (b) endothelial proliferation (Goldenberg *et al.*, 1959). Such lesions were absent in arteriosclerosis.

Periodic Acid-Schiff positive staining was seen in the capillary walls within the stria of diabetic patients' temporal bones (Jørgensen, 1961a). Furthermore, the walls of modiolar vessels (arterioles and venules) and the vessels in the internal auditory canal were thickened, whilst the spiral ligament and vestibular apparatus were unaffected. Jørgensen, whilst finding a good correlation between the duration of diabetes and strial changes, not least of all the correlation between the strial changes and changes in the retinal vessels, was convinced that the hearing loss in diabetic patients was due to diabetic angiopathy. Sudden hearing loss was attributed to haemorrhage. Similar changes were confirmed within the vessels of the internal auditory artery in four temporal bones from diabetic patients by Makishima and Tanaka (1971). Axelsson (1961) was not convinced of such changes within the smaller vessels in the cochlea and postulated the possibility of diabetic angiopathy at the level of the brain stem.

Diagnosis
Hearing loss in diabetes does not differ from that due to noise, ageing and ototoxicity. Diagnosis is confirmed by glycosuria and other biochemical tests routinely carried out in diabetic patients. If the patient is a known diabetic and is receiving medical treatment, the patient may volunteer the information, failing which a good history will provide the necessary clue.

Treatment

It would appear that if the diabetes is adequately controlled, the hearing loss is no greater than that of the normal population within a range of 11–50 years of age (Axelsson and Fagerberg, 1968).

(e) Degenerative: presbyacusis

In this section vascular insufficiency in presbyacusis will be considered and the reader is advised to turn to Chapter 22 for other details.

Schuknecht (1964) classified presbyacusis into (a) sensory presbyacusis in which there is atrophy of the organ of Corti and auditory nerve at the basal end of the cochlea, (b) neural presbyacusis due to loss of neural population in the auditory pathways and cochlea (sensory cells least affected), (c) metabolic presbyacusis due to atrophy of stria vascularis only, (d) mechanical presbyacusis due to changes in the sensory cells or ganglion cells.

There are conflicting views on the relationship between presbyacusis and arteriosclerosis. Fabinyi (1931) discovered a great variety of lesions within the inner ears of 26 patients aged between 41 and 78 years, involving both the hair and ganglion cells. Although there was no certain evidence of correlation between changes in the internal auditory artery and presbyacusis, Fabinyi's guarded conclusion included a possible relationship between high-tone deafness and some degree of cerebral arteriosclerosis. Hansen and Reske-Nielsen (1965) compared histological changes in 12 patients with their ante-mortem audiograms; all patients being over 80 years of age except two (60 and 69 years respectively). These authors observed changes in the vessels of the internal auditory canal, circle of Willis and peripheral cerebral vessels more marked than those in the stria vascularis and modiolus. The causes of sensory degenerative changes were attributed to a combination of arteriosclerosis and senile atrophy.

Those who observed changes in the smaller blood vessels of the cochlea include Saxén (1952) and Jørgensen (1961b). The material examined by Saxén demonstrated a close correlation between angiosclerotic changes in the blood vessels of the cochlea, especially smaller vessels, pre-capillaries and capillaries, and sensory tissue in the cochlear duct. The vessels in the internal auditory canal and base of the brain were unaffected. Jørgensen (1961b) examined 25 temporal bones of patients ranging from 2 months to 85 years and found typical angiosclerotic changes in the elderly patients confined to the vestibular apparatus and capillary walls of the stria vascularis. The reduction in the ganglion cells at the basal end of the cochlea was in no way related to pathological changes in the vessels. Johnsson and Hawkins (1972) and Johnsson (1973) in a systematic study consisting of surface preparation examination of temporal bones from newborn to 99 years of age observed the following changes.

(a) Spiral ligament and stria vascularis: capillaries of the scalae vestibuli and tympani had been replaced by intervascular strands representing atrophy with ageing. Similar changes were seen in arterioles, though not changes typical of arteriosclerosis.

(b) Atrophy of spiral ligament in older patients.

(c) Good correlation between the strial atrophy, in older patients, and hair-cell loss in the extreme basal and apical turns.

(d) In general strial atrophy was most severe in the middle and apical turns, although the basal turn showed pronounced changes in the organ of Corti.

(e) Spiral vessels showed marked thickening in the outer spiral vessel wall (vessel of the basilar membrane), without any correlation between those changes and hair-cell loss.

(f) Devascularization was considerably less obvious in the vestibular system. In conclusion the authors summarize that the reduction in local blood supply, so common in other parts of the body during the process of ageing, results from a gradual disappearance of capillaries and probably is a key factor in the loss of function in the cochlea of older patients. It would appear that the normal process of involution seen in post-natal vessels is continued throughout life.

Krmpotic--Nemanic (1971) suggested a new concept of dense connective tissue, osteoid or bone, deposited at the lateral end of the auditory canal, which could compress the neural tract and possibly even the blood vessels causing atrophy of sensory ganglion, cells and stria vascularis respectively.

Takahashi (1971) looked at the ultrastructural changes, which included transmission electron microscopy and phase contrast studies, in human temporal bones and discovered atrophy of the stria being the commonest change in the apical and basal coils of the over-sixties group. Atrophy of the spiral prominence and blood vessels was also typical in the older age group.

Clinical correlation between presbyacusis and generalized arterial disease; dietary factors

Rosen and Olin (1965) compared the hearing loss in healthy aged persons in the United States with the Mabbans in Sudan. Whilst in Americans there was a good correlation between hearing loss and increased blood pressure, in the Mabbans there was no such correlation. The authors were convinced that it was probably the arteriosclerosis that was reponsible for both the hearing loss and high blood pressure. In a comparison of hearing levels of patients receiving different types of dietary fat, Rosen and Olin (1965) reported that in Finns from the Eastern regions of Finland there was a significant increase in hearing loss concomitant with an increase in coronary heart disease. Conversely, there is a low incidence of hearing loss in Yugoslavians from the Dalmation Coast, in whom coronary heart disease is the lowest in Europe and whose dietary habits include a predominantly polyunsaturated fat intake. Despite such a significant clinical study, it would seem that dietary precautions must be observed from a very young age to avoid hearing loss due to arteriosclerosis.

In a later study Rosen, Olin and Rosen (1970) compared the effects of saturated dietary fat with polyunsaturated fat on hearing in a controlled group of patients in a Finnish mental hospital. Hearing was significantly worse in patients receiving a diet rich in saturated fats. Following cross-over of the patients in the trial, those now receiving polyunsaturated fats instead of saturated showed a significant fall in their hearing. The authors conclude that diet plays an important part in prevention of hearing loss.

Symptoms, diagnosis, differential diagnosis and treatment are discussed in Chapter 22.

(f) Vascular accident

(1) SUDDEN DEAFNESS

Sudden loss of cochlear function has often been attributed to vascular origins. Because of the difficulty of identifying the exact role of inadequate vascular supply by conventional methods such as angiography, the exact incidence of sudden sensorineural deafness due to vascular insufficiency is unknown.

Symptoms

Sudden hearing loss is likely to be more noticeable than the insiduous hearing loss of many other diseases. Often the hearing loss is preceded by roaring tinnitus, which may accompany, or develop after the hearing loss. Occasionally the deafness is noticed on waking up in the morning. There may be a recent history of upper respiratory tract infection. There does not appear to be a definitive predilection to any side but occasionally both ears may be involved. Vertigo may be absent, but if present it may vary from dizziness (momentary loss of balance) to a true rotational vertigo. Male preponderance is noticeable.

Aetiology

The exact mechanism of vascular insufficiency in sudden sensorineural deafness is said to vary from thrombosis and embolism in the labyrinthine artery, to spasm and sludging either through vasomotor imbalance, viral infection or sickle-cell crisis. Disorders of coagulation with subsequent thrombosis are seen in polycythaemia and macroglobulinaemia. Hypoxia due to severe anaemia and carbon monoxide poisoning, and arterial spasm in vertebrobasilar migraine have also been incriminated.

Fowler (1950, 1956) described a definite correlation between emotional stress in 23 patients out of 26 with sudden sensorineural deafness and ascribed the cause to sludging in the vessels, although in only five patients was sludging noted in the conjunctival vessels. Most of the patients were below 40 years of age. Wilmot (1959) came to similar conclusions.

Svane-Knudsen (1957) found a slightly higher incidence in the over-40 year age group in a series of 21 patients. Audiometry revealed two distinct types of curves, i.e. (a) a very steep drop for 1, 2, 4 and 8 kHz and (b) involving all frequencies but with a tendency to fall considerably to higher ones. Nineteen patients had spontaneous nystagmus although only two had complete loss of response on caloric test. An alternative theory of neuritis due to vascular disturbance was suggested as the mechanism.

Rasmussen (1949) having identified a majority of patients with sudden sensorineural deafness in the over-40 year age group, firmly believed that haemorrhage in the inner ear due to arteriosclerosis was the most likely cause of deafness. Hallberg (1956) in a large series of 178 patients with sudden sensorineural deafness, concluded that 89 patients were arteriosclerotic and had their deafness directly as a result of it.

Lindsey and Zuidema (1950) suggested a vasomotor imbalance in a younger age group of 16 patients with sudden deafness. Jerger *et al.* (1961) examined for the first time the possibility of a neural loss in addition to an end-organ lesion and were able to separate the patients with sudden deafness into two separate groups following completion of a battery of audiological tests. The results inevitably led them to postulate different aetiological backgrounds.

Jaffe (1973) discovered a 'hypercoagulation state' in 24 out of 37 patients with sudden deafness. Interestingly a majority of the hypercoagulable patients recovered their hearing loss, whilst those with normal blood coagulation showed a poor recovery. Viral-induced hypercoagulable state was suggested as the mechanism of altered blood flow. In an earlier publication Jaffe (1967) described hearing loss due to carbon monoxide poisoning. Welsh and Welsh (1963) described sudden deafness in polyarteritis nodosa.

Morrison and Booth (1970) described a total of 94 patients with multi-aetiological sudden sensorineural deafness and considered that in 10 patients the deafness was vascular in origin, including one with sickle-cell trait and two with anaemia.

Dubs (1956) documented three patients with traumatic embolus of the internal auditory artery. Arenberg, Allen and Deboer (1972) for the first time recorded a single case of sudden deafness due to emboli following cardiopulmonary by-pass operation. The hearing did improve over a period of months and the embolic nature of the onset was established by subsequent cerebral emboli. Wright and Saunders (1975) reported similar micro-embolization following cardiopulmonary by-pass surgery. Recently the author has seen two patients with sudden vertigo and deafness following cessation of warfarin therapy for deep vein thrombosis. Higgs (1973) reported four patients with acoustic tumour (an incidence of 10 per cent in the series) in whom the only presenting symptom was sudden deafness. Higgs postulated the likely cause as being compression of the internal auditory artery by the tumour or possibly even haemorrhage into the intracanalicular tumour.

Investigations

Every case of sudden sensorineural deafness constitutes an otological emergency and immediate admission to an ENT department is necessary for proper evaluation and immediate treatment. More often than not there is a delay in referral and successive generations of medical students and house officers should be informed of the urgency of instituting treatment if the hearing is to be salvaged.

Investigations should include a full range of cochlear and vestibular function tests. Cochlear function tests should include tests to identify the level of the lesion, i.e. cochlear or retro-cochlear, and include a pure-tone audiogram, speech discrimination score, loudness balance test, Békésy audiometry, tympanometry and acoustic reflex delay. Where available electrocochleography would be useful not only to record the initial response but to monitor progress with treatment. A negative serum Wasserman reaction and VDRL test exclude syphilis. Hypercoaguable state should be investigated by coagulation screening. Serum proteins with electrophoresis and cryoglubulin estimation is helpful. Haemoglobin C and S is estimated in negroid races to exclude sickle-cell trait. Full blood count and ESR are helpful in excluding polycythaemia, anaemia and leukaemia. Radiological survey of temporal bones including tomography is advisable to exclude an eighth nerve tumour.

Diagnosis

This must be from all other causes of sudden sensorineural deafness which includes traumatic, infective, toxic, Menière's disease, psychogenic deafness and acoustic tumour.

Treatment

If the hearing loss is shown to be an end-organ type from the investigations, the following therapies should be considered.

Vestibular sedatives   As a supportive therapy to overcome crippling effects of vertigo. In some, relevant audiological assessment may have to wait until the vertigo is adequately controlled. Prochlorperazine maleate (Stemetil) 12.5 mg intra-muscularly is given if there is gastrointestinal disturbance. If vertigo is mild, prochlorperazine maleate 5 mg three times a day or even double the dose is helpful. Cinnarizine (Stugeron) is a powerful peripheral vestibular sedative and can be administered in 15 mg tablets three to four times a day. There are several other preparations available such as dimenhydrinate (Dramamine), Spansule, prochlorperazine maleate (Vertigon), thiethylperazine maleate (Torecan).

Vasodilators   Vasodilator therapy has been extensively used for the treatment of vascular insufficiency in the inner ear. There is no conclusive evidence that such therapy helps to improve the microcirculation in the inner ear. Various preparations are available.

(1) Nicotinic acid 100 mg twice daily to be increased to four times a day. Patient should be warned of the flushing accompanying such treatment.
(2) Buphenine hydrochloride C (Perdilatal forte) 6 mg tablets—two tablets three times a day.
(3) Drugs that improve cerebral circulation.
    (i) Cyclandelate (Cyclospasmol) 100 mg tablets, two tablets four times a day.
    (ii) Isoxsuprine (Duvadilan Retard) 40 mg twice daily.
    (iii) Naftidrofuryl (Praxilene) 100 mg three times a day; 40 mg ampoules for intramuscular use.
    (iv) Histamine phosphate 2.75 mg in 250 ml normal saline to be given as infusion over 1.5–2 h for the first three days (Sheehy, 1960).

Improving microcirculation   Reference has already been made to the pharmacological properties and its effect on microcirculation of low molecular weight Dextran 40.

Svane-Knudsen (1957) used dextran 10 per cent (molecular weight 150 000) in one to three infusions of 0.5 litre each or 1 litre of 6 per cent dextran (molecular weight 110 000 in normal saline). Although there was definite improvement in the hearing in patients following exposure to blast injury, the number of patients was too small to draw any conclusions. Fisch, Murata and Hossli (1976) demonstrated no improvement in the human perilymph oxygen tension following administration of low molecular weight dextran.

Gaseous inhalation   Fisch, Murata and Hossli (1976) treated patients with sudden sensorineural deafness by inhalation of 5 per cent carbon dioxide in 95 per cent oxygen for 30 min in each hour. Of six patients exposed to such a regime, two showed an increase in the perilymph oxygen tension whilst no such increase was realized in the other two patients. The authors are tempted to suggest that those showing an increased perilymph oxygen tension probably had vascular disturbance which was corrected by the accompanying vasodilatation. Inhalation of 10 per cent carbon dioxide in 90 per cent oxygen caused a dangerous increase in systolic blood pressure although 5 per cent carbon dioxide failed to show any such increase in blood pressure. A careful recording of blood pressure should be maintained during such a regime.

Shea and Kitbach (1973) have advocated inhalation of 5 per cent carbon dioxide in 95 per cent oxygen for 30 min four times a day for fluctuating deafness, as a means of improving cochlear blood flow.

Hyperbaric oxygen therapy   It would be tempting to imagine that hyperbaric oxygen therapy as used for treatment of frost-bite and gangrene in the lower extremities might be beneficial in sudden deafness. However, there is ample experimental evidence that breathing pure oxygen in animals reduces the cochlear blood flow (Snow and Suga, 1973) and causes cerebral vasoconstriction in humans (Kety and Schmidt, 1948).

Gaudin (1972) treated 18 patients with inner-ear complications, mainly vestibular symptoms, and tinnitus, following stapedectomy and myringoplasty (etc.) with 60 per cent oxygen inhalation, and the results showed an improvement in symptoms. There are many variables in the evaluation of Gaudin's results and caution should be exercised in administering oxygen to improve cochlear blood flow.

Surgical treatment   Stellate ganglion block performed soon after the onset of deafness has been practised by Wilmot (1959), Golding-Wood (1960) and Singleton (1971).

Cervical sympathectomy in patients responding favourably to stellate block has been suggested in some quarters although its value needs to be properly evaluated.

Recent advances in microsurgery of the vessels at the base of the brain (Donaghy and Yasargil, 1967) could well pave the way to new horizons in future surgical management.

Suggested therapy   If the sensorineural hearing loss is considered to be an end-organ lesion, the following regime is suggested as a guide line.

  (i) Smoking is discouraged.
 (ii) Vestibular sedation to control vestibular disturbances.
(iii) Inhalation of 5 per cent carbon dioxide in 95 per cent oxygen for 30 min in each hour for the first 12 h. Blood pressure and blood gases monitored carefully.
 (iv) At the same time 10 per cent low molecular weight Dextran 40 intravenous infusion is commenced allowing the infusion to run between 1 and 2 h, followed by 500 ml of 10 per cent Dextran 40 as a slow intravenous infusion for 4–8 h on the first, second, fourth, sixth and eighth days.
  (v) Vasodilatation achieved by the use of cerebral vasodilators such as naftidrofuryl 100 mg three times a day from the second to the 15th days.
 (vi) Where appropriate stellate block may be considered.

(2) MENIÈRE'S DISEASE
A detailed discussion on Menière's disease appears in a separate chapter in this book. In this section only evidence of vascular insufficiency in relation to Menière's disease will be discussed.

Although the exact cause of Menière's disease is still unknown, traditionally the pathogenesis of the disease has been attributed to vasoconstriction in the inner ear and in particular in the stria vascularis. Seymour and Tappin (1953) observed strial vaso-constriction in experimental animals on stimulation of the cervical sympathetic chain. Vasoconstriction leads to vascular stasis and retention of acid metabolites within the stria results in leakage of protein into the scala media. The ensuing increase in osmotic pressure attracts fluid from the perilymph causing excessive accumulation of fluid in the endolymphatic space. Relief from acute vertiginous symptoms by stellate block has further added support to the vascular theory in Menière's, and reference has already been made to the rich adrenergic innervation of the inner ear. Encouraged by the success of cervical sympathectomy in one patient (Mogan and Baumgartner, 1945) together with the remarkable effect of stellate ganglion block, Passe and Seymour (1948) first reported in the British literature 12 patients with Menière's disease treated by 'stellectomy' and division of dorsal pre-ganglionic nerve fibres. All but one had relief from vertigo, and all but two showed hearing improvement during the short term follow-up. In a subsequent report Passe (1951) treated 88 cases of Menière's disease by cervical sympathectomy and showed that up to 82 per cent had relief from vertigo, in some up to ten years, following surgery. However, 17 per cent showed recurrence of varying degrees of vertigo. In a much later publication, Passe (1957) observed relief of vertigo in 28 (62 per cent) out of 45 patients treated with cervical sympathectomy. Hearing improved in 32 patients (71 per cent).

Golding-Wood (1960) in his short study of the effects of removing the stellate and the first two thoracic ganglia showed a 60 per cent improvement in vertigo, whilst the hearing improved only in 23 per cent. Five cases showed a relapse of vertigo 2–3 years after surgery. In a much larger series of 229 patients, Golding-Wood (1969) evaluated the long-term results of bilateral cervical sympathectomy. Sixty-three per cent had not had any vertigo in the first 12 months after the operation whilst the figure dropped to 50 per cent in patients reviewed four years or over. Recurrence of vertigo was usually seen within 2–2.5 years after surgery and occurred in 11 per cent. Such recurrence was attributed to renewed sympathetic activity which was absent in those patients seen three years from surgery. Hearing was difficult to assess due to fluctuation in threshold; 30 per cent however, showed improvement by the end of the second year. In a more recent publication, Golding-Wood (1973) examined the results in 247 patients following cervical sympathectomy. The following was the distribution between the total numbers and time elapsed from surgery: 73 for 12 years, 131 for nine years, 152 for seven years, 187 for five years, 236 for three years. Fifty per cent were free from vertigo three years following surgery. Twelve per cent had recurrence of vertigo in 2–2.5 years after surgery. Hearing improvement was demonstrated in 30 per cent of patients.

Cervical sympathectomy is eminently suited to patients having had destruction of one end-organ for advanced Menière's disease who later develop the disease in the contralateral ear. It should also be considered in bilateral advanced disease resistant to medical treatment and in cases where the risk from hearing loss due to saccus decompression procedures is unacceptable.

(3) LERMOYEZ'S SYNDROME

Some consider this as a variant of Menière's disease in which the hearing improves following an attack of tinnitus and vertigo. Several theories have been put forward to explain the syndrome and include (1) spasm of the internal auditory artery, (2) the result of abnormal metabolism and (3) due to allergic manifestations.

(4) LEUKAEMIA AND WEGENER'S GRANULOMA

Haemorrhage in the inner ear was the finding at post-mortem in an 11 year old girl with leukaemia who developed sudden unilateral sensorineural deafness (Schuknecht, Igarashi and Chasin, 1965). The perilymphatic space contained blood and to a lesser degree there was blood in the endolymphatic space in the saccule and posterior semicircular canal. Sensory organ and ganglion cells were normal in appearance. Schuknecht (1974) reports an organizing blood clot in the vestibular apparatus of a 69 year old patient with Wegener's granulomatosis who had severe vertigo before death.

(5) SUBARACHNOID HAEMORRHAGE

Holden and Schuknecht (1968) examined 12 temporal bones of seven patients who died as a result of spontaneous subarachnoid haemorrhage and observed the presence of erythrocytes in the cochlear aqueduct in six. Blood was present in the internal auditory meatuses in all specimens; there was extension of blood into Rosenthal's canal in seven, and osseous spiral lamina in three specimens. In several specimens blood cells had extended up to the macula of the saccule and the cristae of the posterior semicircular canal. Such a finding could suggest that vertigo in subarachnoid haemorrhage in some patients at least is due to peripheral end-organ involvement.

(6) RADIATION DAMAGE

Kelemen (1963) in a controlled study exposed rats to radiation by x-rays and radium, and observed intracochlear haemorrhages, destruction of stria vascularis, and extensive damage to both the organ of Corti and vestibular apparatus. Gamble and Chandler (1968) confirmed the above findings in guinea-pigs.

Sensorineural deafness has been reported in humans following radiotherapy of the ear or an adjacent structure such as the parotid gland and nasopharynx (Leach, 1965; Dias, 1966; Gamble and Chandler, 1968). It would be advisable to warn the patients of such a possibility for medico-legal reasons.

(7) BENIGN POSITIONAL NYSTAGMUS

Experimental animal study has demonstrated the relative resistance of the vestibular apparatus to ischaemia, compared with the cochlea.

In benign positional nystagmus, typically the patient complains of sudden bouts of rotational vertigo accompanied by gastrointestinal symptoms on placing the head in a critical position. Occasionally it may simply be momentary loss of balance without nausea. Bárány (1921) gave an accurate description of the disease and Dix and Hallpike (1952) made a careful and in-depth study of 100 patients. The symptoms can be precipitated by quickly placing the patient from an upright position on the couch to a supine head hanging position with the head rotated to the side to which symptoms are referred. A brisk rotary nystagmus directed to the undermost ear appears after 1–5 s latent period. Frequently the nystagmus has a horizontal component and once again directed to the undermost ear. Nystagmus is associated with nausea and vertigo lasting for a period of 5–6 s and sometimes longer. Repeating the test procedure only succeeds in producing a few transient nystagmic beats due to fatigue. Hearing is not affected and caloric test demonstrates normal end-organ response.

Aetiology

Dix and Hallpike (1952) recorded degeneration of the utricular and saccular maculae together with degeneration in the subepithelial connective tissue of the utricular macula and suggested that changes were probably secondary to chronic infection, trauma and *ischaemia*. Cawthorne and Hallpike (1957) in addition to the utricular and saccular changes also observed degeneration of the horizontal semicircular canal cristae. These changes were attributed to *arteriosclerosis*.

Lindsay and Hemenway (1956) described a group of seven patients in their fifth to seventh decades of life presenting with acute vertigo and normal hearing. Subsequently these patients developed benign positional nystagmus which persisted for several weeks. Histological examination of temporal bones from one such patient showed degeneration of not only vestibular nerve fibres from Scarpa's ganglion to utricle, but also in the ampullae of horizontal and superior semicircular canals. Saccule and posterior semicircular canal were normal. The authors suggested sudden obstruction to the anterior vestibular artery. Diagnosis and treatment of benign positional vertigo cupulolithiasis are described in Chapter 26.

(8) OCCLUSION OF THE ANTERIOR INFERIOR CEREBELLAR ARTERY

The syndrome is characterized by sudden vertigo, hearing loss, cerebellar disturbances, facial paralysis, loss of sensation to pain and temperature on the ipsilateral side of the face and partial loss of pain and temperature on the contralateral side of the body. In addition to damage to the vestibular and cochlear nuclei in the brain stem, vascular insufficiency in the inner ear leads to changes in the membranous labyrinth (Schuknecht, 1974).

(g) Ototoxic deafness

For full details on this subject, the reader is advised to refer to Chapter 21. Only ototoxic agents which cause damage to the inner ear through vascular insufficiency will be examined in this section.

(1) QUININE

Deafness from administration of this antimalarial agent is rare nowadays. The sensorineural hearing loss confined to higher frequencies can result from idiosyncrasy to the drug, although tinnitus is said to be severer than the deafness. Schuknecht (1974) examined the possibility of quinine deafness in the newborn following ingestion of the drug by the mother. Experimental studies have revealed the profound effect of quinine on the spiral vessels (Rüedi, 1951; Hawkins, 1967). The vessels demonstrate constriction due to swelling of endothelial cells. Lawrence (1971) confirmed the vascular changes by cineradiography of the blood flow in the spiral vessels of the basilar membrane and tympanic lip, in animals receiving quinine hydrochloride.

(2) SALICYLATES

Salicylates are used for relief of symptoms in various types of arthritis. Deafness from salicylates is rare except in those with idiosyncracy or perhaps in aspirin poisoning, although the hearing loss does tend to improve over a period of a few days. Tinnitus is much more distressing than deafness. Hawkins (1967) has demonstrated vaso-constriction due to endothelial swelling in spiral vessels of animals.

(3) AMINOGLYCOSIDES: STREPTOMYCIN, NEOMYCIN AND GENTAMICIN
The role of aminoglycosides in ototoxic deafness is discussed fully in Chapter 21.

Rüedi (1951) demonstrated vascular changes in guinea-pigs poisoned by streptomycin. Ostyn and Tyberghein (1968) reported strial atrophy in guinea-pigs treated with streptomycin.

Riskaer *et al.* (1972) treated two groups of guinea-pigs with neomycin 100 mg/kg body weight for 30 days and 150 mg/kg body weight for 60 days. In both groups of animals there were identical light microscopical changes within the cochlea. The strial vessels were of small calibre and the entire stria was narrower in depth. Johnsson and Hawkins (1972) demonstrated, by surface preparation in cats treated with neomycin sulphate 50 mg/kg body weight for 14–16 days, severe strial atrophy. The changes were more pronounced in the lower basal turn and to a lesser extent in the apical turn. In addition, both the inner and outer hair-cells were damaged. Animals sacrificed immediately after receiving the drug, showed narrow capillaries in the stria vascularis containing distorted erythrocytes. In places showing extreme strial damage, the vessels were represented by mere strands.

Johnsson and Hawkins (1972) also examined the damage caused by gentamicin in the inner ear of guinea-pigs receiving 100 mg/kg body weight for 16–20 days and found damage to the outer hair-cells together with changes in the stria vascularis. However there is no mention of a direct effect on the strial capillaries.

(4) ETHACRYNIC ACID
Ethacrynic acid is a potent diuretic and was extensively used until its side effect on hearing had been uncovered. Surface preparation examination of the inner ears of cats receiving 75–200 mg/kg body weight of ethacrynic acid showed mild to severe strial atrophy, and the changes appeared to be dose-related (Johnsson and Hawkins, 1972). Strial changes appeared to be confined to the cells rather than any direct effect on the capillaries and changes were pronounced in the basal turn and apical turns.

(f) Miscellaneous: Paget's and Recklinghausen's disease

In these two conditions, Paget's osteitis deformans and Recklinghausen's osteitis fibrosa, Rüedi (1968) has demonstrated (eight temporal bones) vascular shunts between the basal coil of the cochlea and the abnormal bony labyrinth. In a further 15 temporal bones of patients with Paget's disease, Rüedi observed shunts between internal auditory vein and abnormal bone. These shunts may well give rise to venous stasis and consequent sensorineural deafness.

References

Alford, B. R., Shaver, E. F., Rosenberg, J. J. and Guilford, F. R. (1965) 'Physiological and histopathological effects of micro-embolism of the internal auditory artery', *Annals of Otology*, **74**, 728

Altman, F., Kornfield, M. and Shea, J. J. (1966) 'Inner ear changes in otosclerosis', *Annals of Otology*, **75**, 5

Anniko, M. (1976) 'Surface structure of stria vascularis in the guinea pig cochlea', *Acta Otolaryngologica, Stockholm*, **82**, 343

Arenberg, K., Allen, G. W. and Deboer, A. (1972) 'Sudden deafness immediately following cardiopulmonary by-pass', *Journal of Laryngology*, **86**, 73

Axelsson, A. (1968) 'The vascular anatomy of the cochlea in the guinea pig and man', *Acta Otolaryngologica, Stockholm*, Suppl., 243

Axelsson, A. (1971) 'The cochlear blood vessels in guinea pigs of different ages', *Acta Otolaryngologica, Stockholm*, **72**, 172

Axelsson, A. (1972) 'The demonstration of the cochlear vessels in the guinea pig by contrast injection', *Journal of Laryngology*, **86**, 121

Axelsson, A. (1974) 'The vascular anatomy of the Rhesus monkey cochlea', *Acta Otolaryngologica, Stockholm*, **77**, 381

Axelsson, A. and Ernston, S. (1972) 'Cochlear vascular anatomy in a strain of the Waltzing guinea pig', *Acta Otolaryngologica, Stockholm*, **74**, 172

Axelsson, A. and Fagerberg, S. E. (1968) 'Auditory function in diabetes', *Acta Otolaryngologica, Stockholm*, **66**, 49–64

Axelsson, A. and Lind, A. (1973) 'The capillary area in the rabbit cochlea', *Acta Otolaryngologica, Stockholm*, **76**, 254

Axelsson, A. and Lipscomb, D. (1975) 'The vascular pattern of the chinchilla cochlea', *Acta Otolaryngologica, Stockholm*, **79**, 352

Axelsson, A., Miller, J. and Holmquist, J. (1974) 'Studies of cochlear vasculature and sensory structures', *Annals of Otology*, **83**, 537

Bárány, R. (1921) 'Diagnose Von Krankheitserscheinungen im Bereisch des otolithenapparatus', *Acta Otolaryngologica, Stockholm*, **2**, 434

Bernstein, J. M. and Silverstein, H. (1966) 'Anterior cerebellar and labyrinthine arteries', *Archives of Otolaryngology*, **83**, 422

Bloch, E. (1962) 'A quantitative study of the haemodynamics in the living microvascular system', *American Journal of Anatomy*, **110** (2), 125

Bosher, S. K. and Warren, R. C. (1968) 'Observations on the electrochemistry of the cochlear endolymph of the rat: a quantitative study of its electrical potential and ionic composition as determined by means of flame spectrophotometry', *Proceedings of the Royal Society*, B, **171**, 227

Brånemark, P. I. (1968) 'Rheological aspects of low flow states', pp. 161–180. In *Microcirculation as Related to Shock*. Ed. by Shepro, D. and Fulton, G. P. New York; Academic Press

Caillé, J. M., Piton, J. and Boussens, J. (1974) 'Anatomic-radiological study of the cerebello-labyrinthine arterial system', *Fortschr. Hals-nas-ohrenheilk*, **21**, 47

Cawthorne, T. E. and Hallpike, C. S. (1957) 'A study of the clinical features and pathological changes within the temporal bones, brain stem and cerebellum of an early case of positional nystagmus of the so-called benign paroxysmal type', *Acta Otolaryngologica, Stockholm*, **48**, 89

Charm, S. E. and Kurland, G. S. (1974) *Blood Flow and Microcirculation*. New York, London, Sydney and Toronto; John Wiley.

Churchill, J. A., Schuknecht, H. F. and Doron, R. (1956) 'Acetylcholinesterase activity in the cochlea', *Laryngoscope*, **66**, 1

Conti, A. and Borgo, M. (1964) 'Behaviour of cytochrome oxidase activity in the cochlea of the guinea pig following acoustic stimulation', *Acta Otolaryngologica, Stockholm*, **58**, 321

Dias, A. (1966) 'Effects on the hearing of patients treated by irradiation in the head and neck area', *Journal of Laryngology*, **80**, 276

Dix, M. R. and Hallpike, C. S. (1952) 'The pathology, symptomatology and diagnosis of certain common disorders of the vestibular system', *Proceedings of the Royal Society of Medicine*, **45**, 341

Donaghy, R. M. P. and Yasargil, M. G. (1967) *Microvascular surgery*. Report of the first conference. St. Louis; The C.V. Mosby Company; Stuttgart; George Thieme Verlag

Dubs, R. (1956) 'Traumatic embolus', *Practica Oto-Rhino-Laryngologica, Basel*, **18**, 1334

Duvall, A. J., Ward, W. D. and Lauhala, K. E. (1974) 'Strial ultrastructure and vessel transport in acoustic trauma'. *Annals of Otology*, **83**, 498

Eastcott, H. H. G. (1969) *Arterial Disease*. London; Pitman Medical

Eckenhoff, J. E., Hafkenschiel, J. H. and Landmesser, C. M. (1947) 'The coronary circulation in the dog', *American Journal of Physiology*, **148**, 582

Fabinyi, G. (1931) 'Regarding morphological and functional changes of the internal ear in arteriosclerosis', *Laryngoscope*, **41**, 663

Falck, B. (1962) 'Observations on the possibilities of the cellular localization of monoamines by a fluorescence method', *Acta Physiologica, Scandinavica*, Suppl., 197

Falck, B., Hillarp, N-A., Thieme, G. and Torp, A. (1962) 'Fluorescence of catecholamines and related compounds condensed with formaldehyde', *Journal of Histochemistry and Cytochemistry*, **10**, 348

Fisch, U. (1968) 'The surgical anatomy of the so-called internal auditory artery'. In *Disorders of* the *Skull Base Region—Proceedings of the Xth (10th) Nobel symposium held in Stockholm, 1964*, pp. 121–130. Stockholm; Almqvist and Wiksell

Fisch, U., Murata, K. and Hossli, G. (1976) 'Measurement of oxygen tension in human perilymph', *Acta Otolaryngologica, Stockholm*, **81**, 278

Fowler, E. P. (1950) 'Sudden deafness', *Annals of Otology*, **59**, 980

Fowler, E. P. (1956) 'Intravascular agglutination of the blood: a factor in certain diseases and disorders of the ear', *Annals of Otology*, **65**, 535

Frazer, P. (1936) 'The vasomotor control of the ear', *Journal of Laryngology*, **51**, 579

Gamble, J. E. and Chandler, J. R. (1968) 'Radiation effects on the inner ear', *Archives of Otolaryngology, Stockholm*, **88**, 156

Gaudin, E. P. (1972) 'Oxygen treatment of inner ear disorders', *Journal of Laryngology*, **86**, 721

Gibson, W. P. R., Ramsden, R. T. and Moffat, D. A. (1977) 'The immediate effects of Naftidrofuryl on the human electrocochleogram in Menière's disorder', *Journal of Laryngology*, **91**, 679

Goldenberg, S., Morris, A., Joshi, R. A. and Blumenthal, H. J. (1959) 'Non-atheromatous peripheral vascular disease in the lower extremity in diabetes mellitus', *Diabetes*, **8**, 261

Golding-Wood, P. H. (1960) 'Observations on sympathectomy in the treatment of Menière's disease', *Journal of Laryngology*, **74**, 951

Golding-Wood, P. H. (1969) 'The role of sympathectomy in the treatment of Menière's disease', *Journal of Laryngology*, **83**, 741

Golding-Wood, P. H. (1973) 'Cervical sympathectomy in Menière's disease', *Archives of Otolaryngology*, **97**, 391

Goodman, L. S. and Gilman, A. (1970) *The Pharmacological Basis of Therapeutics*, IVth Ed. New York, London, Toronto; The Macmillan Company

Gussen, R. (1975) 'Labyrinthine otosclerosis and sensori-neural deafness. Pathologic findings of the spiral ligament', *Archives of Otolaryngology*, **101**, 438

Hallberg, O. E. (1956) 'Sudden deafness of obscure origin', *Laryngoscope*, **66**, 1237

Hansen, C. C. and Reske-Nielsen, E. (1965) 'Pathological studies in presbyacusis', *Archives of Otolaryngology*, **82**, 115

Hawkins, J. E. Jr. (1967) 'Vascular patterns of the membranous labyrinth'. In *Third Symposium on the Role of Vestibular Organs in Space Exploration*, pp. 241–258. Ed. by Graybiel, A. Washington, D.C.; NASA

Hawkins, J. E. Jr. (1971) 'The role of vasoconstriction in noise-induced hearing loss', *Annals of Otology*, **80**, 903

Higgs, W. A. (1973) 'Sudden deafness as the presenting symptom of an acoustic neuroma', *Archives of Otolaryngology*, **98**, 73

Hilding, D. (1973) 'Vascular abnormalities in animal inherited deafness'. In *Vascular Disorders and Hearing Defects*, pp. 297–305. Ed. by deLorenzo, A. J. D. Baltimore; University Park Press

Hilding, D. and Wersäll, J. (1962) 'Cholinesterase and its relation to the nerve endings in the inner ear', *Acta Otolaryngologica, Stockholm*, **55**, 205

Holden, H. B. and Schucknecht, H. F. (1968) 'Distribution pattern of blood in the inner ear following spontaneous subarachnoid haemorrhage', *Journal of Laryngology*, **82**, 321

Igarashi, M., Alford, B. R. and Konishi, S. (1969) 'Functional and histopathological correlations after microembolism of the peripheral labyrinthine artery in dogs', *Laryngoscope*, **79**, 603

Jaffe, B. F. (1967) 'Sudden deafness: an otological emergency', *Archives of Otolaryngology*, **86**, 55

Jaffe, B. F. (1973) 'Clinical studies in sudden deafness', *Fortschr. Hals-nas-ohrenheilk*, **20**, 221

Jerger, J., Allen, G., Robertson, D. and Harford, E. (1961) 'Hearing loss of sudden onset', *Archives of Otolaryngology*, **73**, 350

Johnsson, L-G. (1972) 'Cochlear blood vessel pattern in the human fetus and post-natal vascular involution', *Annals of Otology*, **81**, 22

Johnsson, L-G. (1973) 'Vascular pathology in the human inner ear', *Fortschr. Hals-nas-ohrenheilk*, **20**, 197

Johnsson, L-G. and Hawkins, J. E. Jr. (1972) 'Vascular changes in the human inner ear associated with ageing', *Annals of Otology*, **81**, 364

Johnsson, L-G. and Hawkins, J. E. Jr. (1972) 'Symposium on basic ear research: II strial atrophy in clinical and experimental deafness', *Laryngoscope*, **82**, 1105

Johnsson, L-G., Hawkins, J. E. Jr., Muraski, A. A. and Preston, R. E. (1973) 'Vascular anatomy and pathology of the cochlea in Dalmation dogs'. In *Vascular Disorders and Hearing Defects*, pp. 249–295. Ed. by deLorenzo, A. J. D. Baltimore, London, Tokyo; University Park Press

Jørgensen, M. B. (1960) 'Sudden loss of inner ear function in the course of long-standing diabetes mellitus', *Acta Otolaryngologica, Stockholm*, **51**, 579

Jørgensen, M. B. (1961a) 'The inner ear in diabetes mellitus', *Archives of Otolaryngology*, **74**, 373

Jørgensen, M. B. (1961b) 'Changes of ageing in the inner ear: histological studies', *Archives of Otolaryngology*, **74**, 164

Jørgensen, M. B. and Buch, N. H. (1961) 'Studies of inner ear function and cranial nerves in diabetes mellitus', *Acta Otolaryngologica, Stockholm*, **53**, 350

Kelemen, G. (1963) 'Radiation and ear', *Acta Otolaryngologica, Stockholm*, Suppl., 184

Kelemen, G. (1966) 'Rubella and deafness', *Archives of Otolaryngology*, **83**, 520

Kellerhals, B. (1972) 'Acoustic trauma and cochlear microcirculation', *Fortschr. Hals-nas-ohrenheilk*, **18**, 91

Kerr, A. G. and Byrne, J. E. T. (1975) 'Concussion effects of bomb blast on the ear', *Journal of Laryngology*, **89**, 131

Kety, S. S. and Schmidt, C. F. (1948) 'The effect of altered arterial tensions of carbon dioxide and oxygen on cerebral blood flow and cerebral oxygen consumption of normal young men', *Journal of Clinical Investigation*, **27**, 484

Kimura, R. and Perlman, H. B. (1956a) 'Extensive venous obstruction of the labyrinth. A. Cochlear changes', *Annals of Otology*, **65**, 332

Kimura, R. and Perlmann, H. B. (1956b) 'Extensive venous obstruction of the labyrinth. B. Vestibular changes', *Annals of Otology*, **65**, 620

Kimura, R. and Perlmann, H. B. (1958) 'Arterial obstruction of labyrinth,' *Annals of Otology*, **67**, 5

Kimura, R. S. and Ota, C. Y. (1974) 'Ultrastructure of the cochlear blood vessels', *Acta Otolaryngologica, Stockholm*, **77**, 231

Koide, Y., Yoshida, M. and Konno, M. (1960) 'Some aspects of the biochemistry of acoustic trauma', *Annals of Otology*, **69**, 661

Krmpotic-Nemanic, J. (1971) 'A new concept of the pathogenesis of presbyacusis', *Archives of Otolaryngology*, **93**, 161

Lawrence, M. (1966) 'Effects of interference with terminal blood supply on organ of Corti', *Laryngoscope*, **76**, 1318

Lawrence, M. (1971) 'Blood flow through the basilar membrane capillaries', *Acta Otolaryngologica, Stockholm*, **71**, 106

Lawrence, M. (1973) 'In-vitro studies of the microcirculation', *Fortschr. Hals-nas-ohrenheilk*, **20**, 244

Lawrence, M. and Clapper, M. (1973) 'Cine studies of organ of Corti blood supply'. In *Vascular Disorders and Hearing Defects*, pp. 130–148. Ed. by deLorenzo, A. J. D. Baltimore, London, Tokyo; University Park Press

Leach, W. (1965) 'Irradiation of the ear', *Journal of Laryngology*, **79**, 870

Lim, D. J. (1969) 'Three-dimensional observation of the inner ear with the scanning electron microscope', *Acta Otolaryngologica, Stockholm*, Suppl., 255

Lindsey, J. R. and Beal, D. D. (1966) 'Sensorineural deafness in otosclerosis', *Annals of Otology*, **75**, 436

Lindsey, J. R. and Hemenway, W. G. (1956) 'Positional vertigo due to unilateral sudden partial loss of vestibular function', *Annals of Otology*, **65**, 692

Lindsey, J. R. and Zuidema, J. J. (1950) 'Inner ear deafness of sudden onset', *Laryngoscope*, **60**, 238

Linthicum, F. H. Jr. (1966) 'Correlation of sensori-neural hearing impairment and otosclerosis', *Annals of Otology*, **75**, 512

Lipscomb, D. M. and Roettger, R. L. (1973) 'Capillary constriction in cochlear and vestibular tissue during intense noise stimulation', *Laryngoscope*, **83**, 259

Makishima, K. and Tanaka, K. (1971) 'Pathological changes of the inner ear and central auditory pathway in diabetes', *Annals of Otology*, **80**, 218

Martinez, D. M. (1972) 'The effect of "SERC" (Betahistine hydrochloride) on the circulation of the inner ear in experimental animals', *Acta Otolaryngologica, Stockholm*, Suppl., **305**, 29

Matschinsky, F. M. and Thalmann, R. (1967) 'Quantitative histochemistry of microscopic structures of the cochlea, II Ischaemic alterations of levels of glycolytic intermediates and co-factors in the organ of Corti and stria vascularis', *Annals of Otology*, **76**, 638

Mazzoni, A. (1969) 'Internal auditory canal. Arterial relations at the porus acousticus', *Annals of Otology*, **78**, 797

Mazzoni, A. and Hansen, C. C. (1970) 'Surgical anatomy of the arteries of the internal auditory canal', *Archives of Otolaryngology*, **91**, 128

Mazzoni, A. (1972) 'Internal auditory artery supply to the petrous bone', *Annals of Otology*, **81**, 13

Misrahy, G. A., Hildreth, K. M., Shinbarger, E. W., Clark, L. C. and Rice, E. A. (1958) 'Endolymphatic oxygen tension in the cochlea of the guinea pig', *Journal of the Acoustical Society of America*, **30**, 247

Mogan, R. F. and Baumgartner, C. J. (1945) 'Menière's disease', *Archives of Otolaryngology*, **41**, 113

Morimitsu, T. (1960) 'Observations of the cochlear blood circulation in guinea pigs by impedance plethysmography', *Otologia Fukuoka*, **6**, (Suppl. 7), 437

Morrison, A. W. and Booth, J. B. (1970) 'Sudden deafness: an otological emergency', *British Journal of Hospital Medicine*, Sept. 1970, 287

Mygind, S. H. and Falbe-Hansen, J. (1948) 'Experimental histological studies on the labyrinth', *Acta Otolaryngologica, Stockholm*, **34**, 59

Nager, G. T. (1966) 'Sensori-neural deafness and otosclerosis', *Annals of Otology*, **75**, 481

Nomura, Y. (1961) 'Observations on the microcirculation of the cochlea: An experimental study', *Annals of Otology*, **70**, 1037

Ostyn, F. and Tyberghein, J. (1968) 'Influence of some streptomyces antibiotics on the inner ear of the guinea pig', *Acta Otolaryngologica, Stockholm*, B, Suppl., 234

Passe, E. R. G. and Seymour, J. S. (1948) 'Menière's syndrome', *British Medical Journal*, **2**, 812

Passe, E. R. G. (1951) 'Sympathectomy in relation to Menière's disease, nerve deafness and tinnitus', *Proceedings of the Royal Society of Medicine*, **44**, 760

Passe, E. R. G. (1953) 'Surgery of the sympathetic for Menière's disease, tinnitus and nerve deafness', *Archives of Otolaryngology*, **57**, 257

Perlman, H. B. (1952) 'Experimental occlusion of the inferior cochlear vein', *Annals of Otology*, **61**, 33

Perlman, H. B. and Kimura, R. S. (1955a) 'Observations on the living blood vessels of the cochlea', *Annals of Otology*, **64**, 1176

Perlman, H. B., Kimura, R. and Fernandez, C. (1959) 'Experiments on temporary obstruction of the internal auditory artery', *Laryngoscope*, **69**, 591

Perlman, H. B., Tsunoo, M. and Spence, A. (1963) 'Cochlear blood flow and function: Effect of pressor agents', *Acta Otolaryngologica, Stockholm*, **56**, 587

Polus, K. (1972) 'The problem of vascular deafness', *Laryngoscope*, **82**, 24

Rambo, J. H. T., Wolff, D. and Freeman, G. (1953) 'A vascular study of the effects of autonomic nervous system on the internal ear', *Annals of Otology*, **62**, 1149

Rasmussen, H. (1949) 'Sudden deafness', *Acta Otolaryngologica, Stockholm*, **37**, 65

Riskaer, N., Christensen, E., Petersen, P. V. and Weidman, H. (1972) 'The ototoxicity of Neomycin', *Acta Otolaryngologica, Stockholm*, **46**, 137

Rosen, Z. and Davis, E. (1971) 'Microangiopathy in diabetes with hearing disorders', *Eye, Ear, Nose and Throat Monthly*, **50**, 479

Rosen, S. and Olin, P. (1965) 'Hearing loss and coronary heart disease', *Archives of Otolaryngology*, **82**, 236

Rosen, S., Olin, P. and Rosen, H. V. (1970) 'Dietary preservation of hearing loss', *Acta Otolaryngologica, Stockholm*, **70**, 242

Ross, M. D. (1971) 'Fluorescence and electron microscopic observations of the general visceral, efferent innervation of the inner ear', *Acta Otolaryngologica, Stockholm*, Suppl., 286

Rüedi, L. (1951) 'Some experimental findings on the functions of the inner ear', *Annals of Otology*, **60**, 993

Rüedi, L. (1968) 'Are there cochlear shunts in Paget's and Recklinghausen's disease?' *Acta Otolaryngologica, Stockholm*, **65**, 13

Rüedi, L. and Spoendlin, H. (1968) 'Pathogenesis of sensori-neural deafness in otosclerosis', *Annals of Otology*, **75**, 525

Saxén, O. (1952) 'Inner ear in presbyacusis', *Acta Otolaryngologica, Stockholm*, **41**, 213

Schneider, E. A. (1974) 'A contribution to the physiology of the perilymph, Part II Cochlear and cerebral blood flow', *Annals of Otology*, **83**, 247

Schnieder, E. A. (1975) 'A contribution to the physiology of the perilymph. Part IV Effect of histamine on the cochlear microcirculation', *Annals of Otology*, **84**, 228

Schuknecht, H. F. (1964) 'Further observations on the pathology of presbyacusis', *Archives of Otolaryngology*, **80**, 369

Schuknecht, H. F. (1969) 'Mechanism of inner ear injury from blows to the head', *Annals of Otology*, **78**, 253

Schuknecht, H. F. (1969) 'Cupulolithiasis', *Archives of Otolaryngology*, **90**, 765

Schuknecht, H. F. (1974) *Pathology of the Ear.* Cambridge, Mass.; Harvard University Press

Schuknecht, H. F. and Gross, C. W. (1966) 'Otosclerosis and the inner ear', *Annals of Otology*, **75**, 423

Schuknecht, H. F. and Igarashi, M. (1964) 'Pathology of slowly progressive sensori-neural deafness', *Transactions of the American Academy of Ophthalmology and Otolaryngology*, **68**, 222

Schuknecht, H. F. and Ishii, T. (1966) 'Hearing loss caused by atrophy of the stria vascularis', *Japan Journal of Otology, Tokyo*, **69**, 1825

Schuknecht, H. F., Churchill, J. A. and Doran, R. (1959) 'The localization of acetylcholinesterase in the cochlea', *Archives of Otolaryngology*, **69**, 549

Schuknecht, H. F., Igarashi, M. and Chasin, W. E. (1965) 'Inner ear haemorrhage in leukaemia', *Laryngoscope*, **75**, 662

Seymour, J. C. (1954) 'Observations on the circulation in the cochlea', *Journal of Laryngology*, **68**, 689

Seymour, J. C. and Tappin, J. W. (1951) 'The effect of sympathetic stimulation upon the cochlear microphonic potentials', *Proceedings of the Royal Society of Medicine*, **44**, 755

Seymour, J. C. and Tappin, J. W. (1953) 'Some aspects of the sympathetic nervous system in relation to the inner ear', *Acta Otolaryngologica, Stockholm*, **XLIII**, 618

Shea, J. J. and Kitbach, A-E. (1973) 'Management of fluctuant hearing loss', *Archives of Otolaryngology*, **97**, 108

Sheehy, J. L. (1960) 'Vasodilator therapy in sensorineural hearing loss', *Laryngoscope*, **70**, 885

Singleton, G. T. (1971) 'Clinical sympathetic chain block in sudden deafness', *Laryngoscope*, **81**, 734

Smaltino, F., Bernini, F. P. and Elefante, R. (1971) 'Normal and pathological findings of the angiographic examination of the internal auditory artery', *Neuroradiology*, **2**, 216

Snow, J. B. Jr. and Suga, F. (1973a) 'Labyrinthine vasodilators', *Archives of Otolaryngology*, **97**, 365

Snow, J. B. Jr. and Suga, F. (1973b) 'Control of cochlear blood flow'. In *Vascular Disorders and Hearing Defects*, pp. 167–183. Ed. by deLorenzo, A. J. D. Baltimore, London, Tokyo; University Park Press

Spoendlin, H. and Lichtensteiger, W. (1966) 'The adrenergic innervation of the labyrinth', *Acta Otolaryngologica, Stockholm*, **61**, 423

Spoendlin, H. (1973) 'Automatic nerve supply to the inner ear'. In *Vascular Disorders and Hearing Defects*, pp. 94–111. Ed. by deLorenzo, A. J. D. Baltimore, London, Tokyo; University Park Press

Strong, M. S. (1957) 'Dorsal sympathectomy in labyrinthine disease', *Archives of Otolaryngology*, **65**, 340

Suga, F. and Snow, J. B. Jr. (1969) 'Adrenergic control of cochlear blood flow', *Annals of Otology*, **78**, 1081

Suga, F., Nakashima, T. and Snow, J. B. Jr. (1970) 'Sodium and potassium ions in endolymph', *Archives of Otolaryngology*, **91**, 37

Suga, F., Preston, J. and Snow, J. B. Jr. (1970) 'Experimental microembolization of cochlear vessels', *Archives of Otolaryngology*, **92**, 213

Sugar, J. O., Engström, H. and Stahle, J. (1972) 'Stria vascularis', *Acta Otolaryngologica, Stockholm*, Suppl., **301**, 61

Svane-Knudsen, V. (1957) 'Sudden "spontaneous" lesion of aural function', *Acta Otolaryngologica, Stockholm*, **47**, 270

Takahashi, T. (1971) 'The ultrastructure of the pathologic stria vascularis and spiral prominence in man', *Annals of Otology*, **80**, 721

Thalmann, R., Miyoshi, T. and Rauchbach, E. (1973) 'Biochemical correlations of inner ear ischaemia'. In *Vascular Disorders and Hearing Defects*, pp. 219–248. Ed. by deLorenzo, A. J. D. Baltimore, London, Tokyo; University Park Press

Todd, N. W., Clairmont, A. A., Dennard, J. E. and Jackson, R. J. (1974) 'Sympathetic stimulation and otic blood flow', *Annals of Otology*, **83**, 84

Tsunoo, M. and Perlman, H. B. (1969) 'Temporary arterial obstruction', *Acta Otolaryngologica, Stockholm*, **67**, 460

Weideman, M. P. (1974) *Microcirculation.* Stroudsburg, Pennsylvania; Dowden, Hutchinson and Ross, Inc.

Welsh, L. W. and Welsh, J. J. (1963) 'Unilateral sensorineural deafness', *Annals of Otology*, **72**, 113

Wende, S., Nakayama, N. and Schwerdtfeger, P. (1975) 'The internal auditory artery', *Journal of Neurology, Bruxelles*, **210**, 21

Wersäll, J., Densert, O. and Lundquist, P. G. (1973) 'Studies of fine structure of inner ear vessels'. In *Vascular Disorders and Hearing Defects*, pp. 43–73. Ed. by deLorenzo, A. J. D. Baltimore, London, Tokyo; University Park Press

Wilmot, T. (1959) 'Sudden perceptive deafness in young people', *Journal of Laryngology*, **73**, 466

Wright, J. W. L. and Saunders, S. H. (1975) 'Sudden deafness following cardiopulmonary by-pass surgery', *Journal of Laryngology*, **89**, 757

24 Diagnosis and management of sudden and fluctuant sensorineural hearing loss
J B Booth

Ten years ago, the literature contained only occasional articles on sudden or fluctuating hearing loss, and very few quoted experience of treating a series of patients. Since then symposia have been held and even special editions of journals have been filled, but for all this academic effort, it is doubtful if many additional patients have benefited. There are two reasons for this. First, many of the causes are in themselves extremely rare, not only in otological practice, but still more so to the general family practitioner. Many too, are associated with other symptoms which will initially, and rightly, command much greater attention even when the patient may have been admitted to hospital. These will often come within the specific causes listed in *Table 24.1*. Second, for the patient to obtain diagnosis and treatment he has to present to the doctor either in his local surgery or office, and the family practitioner must then decide to refer him to the specialist immediately if much of the treatment advocated is to be beneficial. Sudden deafness is an emergency but *all* concerned have to realize this. Balanced against the serious causes needing immediate help, come the vast majority never seen by a doctor, yet alone a zealous otologist, and who may think that the hearing loss this time will recover as it did previously when they 'had a cold'. Fortunately the presentation in many cases of sudden deafness does show a difference which alerts both the doctor and the patient.

It should be appreciated at the outset that much of what has been written on this subject contains two ingredients—the case report(s) followed by the theory of causation. Here an attempt will be made to distil the facts so far established and to guide the newcomer or clinician meeting the occasional case to a pragmatic approach.

The incidence of sudden and fluctuant hearing loss is unknown and estimates vary, but in the largest series Shaia and Sheehy (1976) found slightly over 2 per cent in their new patient load at the Otologic Medical Group. Another estimate of the incidence is 10.7 cases/100 000 (Byl, 1977). In the USA a national registry for idiopathic sudden hearing loss has been set up and this should not only lead to a more accurate assessment of the incidence, but also place the subject on a sounder footing both academically and clinically (Siegel, 1973). In the meantime it is certain that the conditions provide a continuing diagnostic and intellectual challenge embracing the whole of sensorineural hearing loss.

Table 24.1   Some causes of sudden or fluctuating sensorineural hearing loss

Cochlear
  (i) Inflammatory—e.g. viral, bacterial, spirochaetal
  (ii) Traumatic
  (iii) Vascular
  (iv) Haematological—e.g. anaemia, embolism, coagulation disorders
  (v) Collagen diseases—e.g. polyarteritis nodosa, Cogan's syndrome
  (vi) Endolymphatic hydrops, including Menière's disease
  (vii) Metabolic disorders
  (viii) Ototoxicity
  (ix) Skeletal system—otic capsule

Retrocochlear and central nervous system
  (i) Meningitis—all forms
  (ii) Disseminated sclerosis
  (iii) Sarcoidosis
  (iv) Vogt–Koyanagi–Harada syndrome
  (v) Xeroderma pigmentosa
  (vi) Tumours—e.g. acoustic neuroma, carcinomatous neuropathy
  (vii) Central deafness

Idiopathic

It is important to recognize that the above classification cannot be rigidly applied. Often two or more conditions may co-exist in the one patient, whilst some of the diseases listed may damage hearing at more than one anatomical level. The review of *specific causes* which follows must therefore seem somewhat diffuse, and it must include some material which is also mentioned in Chapters 15, 17, 19 and 21–23.

Specific causes

Many of the cases reported seem only like isolated incidences. What can we learn from these widely varying aetiologies? In many the incidence is statistically no greater than chance, but in some the clinical and audiometric pattern, together with temporal bone findings, are of great importance. In addition, many 'specific' causes seem to be copied from an earlier author's 'classification' and thereby come to assume an apparently much greater 'incidence' than examination of the records seems to bear. It should also be remembered that in several of the causes hearing loss is but one manifestation of a systemic disease, from which the patient may also have a generalized toxaemia, metabolic or other major disturbance. In some of these, the deafness occurs when the disease is at its height and is noticed only later when the patient's health improves sufficiently for him to be aware of his misfortune.

Cochlear causes

Inflammatory

VIRAL

Mumps

The first person to note the occurrence of deafness accompanying epidemic parotitis was Hintz in 1803. Toynbee in 1860 confirmed this; he described a complete disorganization of the nervous apparatus and dark fluid in the vestibule and the cochlea in a temporal bone from a patient who died from the condition.

Patients with mumps infection may have a benign, complicated or even lethal course. The disease is usually more severe in adults. Hearing loss is uncommon, occurring in less than 0.1 per cent of cases, but adolescents and adults are more likely to be affected. Vuori, Lahikainen and Peltonen (1962) examined almost 300 male patients with mumps, average age 20 years, and one was left with a severe hearing defect. Saunders and Lippy (1959) noted that one of their patients with raised mumps antibody titres, had parotitis and in all nine the deafness was unilateral. Although encephalitis occurs in less than 0.1 per cent of patients, up to 23 per cent are said to develop clinical meningitis. Most reported cases of sensonineural hearing loss are unilateral.

Temporal bone studies (*see* Chapter 19) are reported by Lindsay, Davey and Ward (1960) and Smith and Gussen (1976).

Measles

It has long been known that measles can cause inner-ear deafness and estimates vary widely but in post-war years it seems to be between 5 and 10 per cent of cases. It has also been reported as producing congenital deafness in a child whose mother had the disease in pregnancy; immunization against measles in pregnancy has been implicated in two other congenital cases.

Temporal bone studies in two cases are reported by Bordley and Kapur (1977) and by Lindsay and Hemenway (1954) in another.

Varicella zoster virus

Herpes zoster oticus is well known by all otologists, and sudden deafness with facial palsy forms part of the Ramsay Hunt syndrome. Temporal bone studies of patients with cochlear and/or vestibular symptoms are few. Two well-documented cases died with relatively acute changes (Blackley, Friedmann and Wright, 1967; Maybaum and Druss, 1934). The first died from carbon monoxide poisoning 214 days after the onset of the herpes and the second also had periarteritis nodosa.

From a clinical standpoint, many patients afflicted by this virus present early because of their symptoms. In zoster deafness the site is sometimes neural, sometimes sensory but most often mixed. Steroid therapy has been tried in this group with excellent results; the risks of disseminating the virus seems to be more theoretical than real.

Chlamydia

The genus Chlamydiaceae comprises two species—*C. trachomatis* and *C. psittaci.* The first is well known and causes a variety of ocular and genital infections in man, the best known being trachoma. The second is less often encountered in man but causes several infections in animals, e.g. psittacosis, ornithosis. In recent years *C. psittaci* has been shown to cause endocarditis in man and is well recognized though infrequently as a cause of ocular infections.

Darougar *et al.* (1978) have reported a case with long-standing interstitial keratitis and uveitis associated with a marked otological syndrome and fatal cardiovascular lesions. The girl had a sudden bilateral hearing loss, tinnitus and imbalance. The deafness was initially moderate, sensorineural and symmetrical, with poor speech discrimination. Treatment with prednisolone failed to do anything for the hearing loss which fluctuated, but always relapsed leading ultimately to almost total loss. Later *C. psittaci* was isolated from the eye and she received two courses of doxycycline, which helped the kerato-uveitis but otherwise after treatment, there was a definite increase in the intensity of the clinical signs and the number of recurrences. Just over three years from the first eye symptoms and ten months after the initial sudden hearing loss, she died suddenly. She had a coroner's post mortem and no temporal bone studies were possible.

Infectious mononucleosis
Only two cases seem to be on record of this infection causing sudden hearing loss (Gregg and Shaeffer, 1964; Jaffe, 1967). Both cases were unilateral; no details of the second are given. In the first, the infection had already been in progress for 27 days before the boy noticed the tinnitus and the marked hearing loss. Eleven days before the deafness he had received Type III oral polio vaccine; 20 days later when he was examined, his audiogram showed a total loss of hearing and vestibular function on the affected side. The heterophil antibody titre was positive 1:14. He received oral vasodilator therapy; after one year there was a very slight return of hearing but no vestibular improvement.

BACTERIAL

Chronic otitis media
The possibility of a fistula, with chronic suppurative otitis media, is always present both clinically and at operation. A recent review by Dawes and Watson (1978) illustrates well many of the relevant points. *Figure 24.1* shows the site of the fistula in their 66 cases, occurring over a 12-year period. They emphasize that it is the rate of change of the inflammatory process rather than the size of the fistula which will determine whether or not vertigo occurs (*see* Chapter 12).

Syphilis (*see* Chapter 15)
Either in the congenital or the acquired form, this all-invasive disease can cause sudden deafness. Karmody and Schuknecht (1966) reported congenital syphilis as a cause resulting in a profound and usually bilateral loss, especially in younger patients.

They also emphasized that the deafness is usually very sudden and may be partially asymmetric possibly with fluctuation. In the milder case the hearing loss may be more marked in the low and high frequencies rather than the more conventional flat pattern. It is frequently accompanied by a poor speech discrimination. About 5 per cent of patients with late syphilis of the temporal bone present with sudden deafness, while sudden deteriorations in one or both ears occur at later stages of the disease in

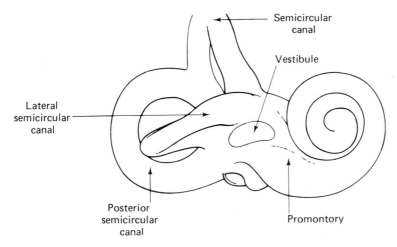

Semicircular
canal

Vestibule

Lateral
semicircular
canal

Posterior
semicircular
canal

Promontory

Figure 24.1 Diagram to show the sites of fistulae in 66 cases produced by chronic suppurative otitis media. (Reproduced by permission of the authors and Editor of the *Journal of Laryngology and Otology*)

a further 15 per cent. Sudden bilateral loss in the patients with acquired deafness is unusual (Morrison, 1975).

The otological symptoms of late congenital syphilis may be almost indistinguishable from those of Menière's disease.

Electrocochleography may be helpful in diagnosis (Ramsden, Moffat and Gibson, 1977). A diphasic action potential with a large negative summating potential on the descending limb was found in 78 per cent of ears from which an action potential was recorded. The cochlear microphonic is consistently small (*see Figure 24.2*). It should be noted that these findings are not pathognomonic of syphilis and may be seen in several

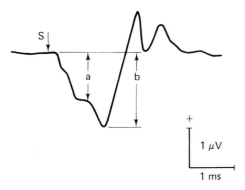

Figure 24.2 Characteristic waveform in congenital syphilis showing the negative SP on the descending limb of the AP. a = parameter for measuring SP; b = parameter for measuring AP; S = stimulus onset. Band pass 250 Hz–3.2 kHz, 100 μs click 110 dB HL. (Reproduced by permission of the authors and Editor of the *Annals of Otology*)

other pathologies. In syphilis, where few hair-cells remain, the duration of the summating potential is reduced so that it is only evident on the descending limb. The pattern after treatment has so far not been analysed in detail or related to the audiometric result; all that can be said at this stage is that a proportion do revert to the normal pattern: such an analysis is presently being made (Moffat, 1978).

Traumatic

ELECTRICITY

It is generally considered that individuals unlucky enough to be struck by lightning are either killed or suffer no untoward effects. Whilst reports are few, lightning may affect the ear in two ways—rupture of a tympanic membrane, which is almost always the case, and occasionally a sensorineural loss. Although the perforation would be unilateral, the sensorineural loss may be bilateral. The sensorineural hearing loss may be transient or for a longer period, but none has so far been reported as permanent (Wright and Silk, 1974).

RADIOTHERAPY

Radiotherapy given to head and neck tumours regularly involves its application to the ear and organ of Corti. For many years it was considered that the cochlea was resistant to radiotherapeutic injury.

Dias (1966) reviewed 29 cases and commented on the conductive changes which could occur during radiotherapy in this area. He noted it to be most apparent in the 4000-Hz range and that 2000 Hz was least affected. Such conductive changes are easily appreciated either in terms of the treatment on the eustachian tube or the middle ear. Oedema or fibrosis will affect the former and may well interfere with the levator palati muscle and inflammation may be expected to some degree in the latter. A tympanic effusion may also affect fenestral function and lead to the false impression of a sensorineural loss. Otherwise Dias was unable to find any evidence of inner-ear damage.

However, this has been strongly challenged, first by Leach (1965) and more recently by Moretti (1976). Leach showed that no less than 36 per cent of 56 cases suffered a hearing deficit. Of the 11 affected, eight had impairment during treatment and the other three showed late changes; three sustained losses which lasted from 3–9 months after cessation of treatment. Two patients developed total hearing loss in one ear, one three months following therapy and the other gradually over seven years.

Moretti obtained similar results and found that no less than seven out of 13 patients developed a sensorineural loss. He noted that all the profound losses were related to doses, some of which were large (20 300 rad over four years!). Moretti also noticed that although small sensorineural hearing losses were noted during the first few years, the onset of the severe hearing loss was gradual and occurred over 3–6 years following cessation of radiotherapy. The more profound losses had a descending pattern (high-tone losses) and the lesser losses had flat patterns. Older patients seemed to be more susceptible.

Otherwise the degree to which an ear may be affected is unpredictable as is the time of onset. It is possible also to suffer labyrinthine loss, even years after the irradiation. One case reported by Leach, a carcinoma of the nasopharynx in a 55 year old who had received 4000 rad came to post mortem. The temporal bone findings (sides unspecified) showed the organ of Corti to be absent, the spiral ganglion and nerve to be atrophic and no maculae or cristae were seen in the vestibular apparatus.

The commoner (and less spectacular) traumatic causes of sudden cochlear deafness are fully discussed in Chapter 23.

Vascular

In considering the possibility of a vascular cause for sudden deafness, attention must be paid to the arterial supply to the inner ear and therein the cochlea. Although this is dealt with in detail in Chapter 23 the simplest or most gross arrangement is worth recapitulation. The arterial loop at the internal auditory meatus gives rise to the internal auditory artery. The loop is the main trunk or branch of the anterior inferior cerebellar artery in 80 per cent of cases, the accessory inferior cerebellar artery in 17 per cent and a branch of the inferior cerebellar artery in 3 per cent. Furthermore, in 5 per cent the left vertebral artery arises directly from the aortic arch between the left common cartoid and subclavian arteries. The vertebral arteries are unequal in size and in about 10 per cent, one vertebral artery supplies all the blood to the brain stem, the other terminating in the neck (Berkowitz and Stroud, 1973). It is likely, therefore, that any single individual occlusion or spasm may vary in its effects depending on the anatomical variant of this supply, but so far no particular symptoms or pathology have been found to be related to any specific anatomical variation.

In the experimental work of Kimura and Perlman (1958) they obstructed the flow of the anterior inferior cerebellar artery (in guinea-pigs). Three combinations of end-organ involvement occurred. The most common was involvement of all the cochlear and vestibular end-organs, a second combination involved only the cochlea, saccule and posterior ampulla, and a third involved the utricle, horizontal and superior canals and part of the saccule, but with no cochlear involvement. They explain these variations in extent of damage by variations in the arterial branches occluded. The anterior vestibular artery is often a direct branch of the anterior inferior cerebellar and supplies the utricle and superior and horizontal ampullae, while the posterior vestibular artery is a branch of the common cochlear artery and supplies the saccule and posterior ampulla. Study of injected material indicated that collaterals existed beyond the point of obstruction that would further the maintenance of blood-flow in the anterior vestibular artery to the utricle and superior and horizontal ampullae. In the study of seven patients with sudden unilateral partial vestibular loss, described by Lindsay and Hemenway (1956), one case showed changes involving the utricle, and superior and horizontal ampullae, sparing the cochlea, saccule and posterior ampulla. This combination corresponds to the description by Kimura and Perlman in two of 65 of their experimental animals, and implies involvement primarily of the anterior vestibular artery.

Gussen (1976) has reported a case of a 57 year old man who had sudden onset of dizziness and unilateral deafness two months before death. The patient suffered from hypertension and congestive and renal failure. At autopsy, subarachnoid haemorrhage with punctate cortical haemorrhages and arteriolar thickening involved the right superior cerebellar hemisphere. The pathological changes involved primarily the right cochlea, saccule and posterior ampulla, and were consistent with vascular embarrassment of the temporal bone of two months duration. The cochlea demonstrated total loss of the organ of Corti and severe degenerative changes of the stria vascularis, spiral ligament, outer sulcus cells and distal cochlear nerve fibres. The saccule demonstrated loss of its macula and nerve fibres. The posterior ampulla showed evidence of previous rupture of its membranous wall with fibrosis and the beginnings of bone formation. Fresh haemorrhage, present in some areas of both temporal bones, was related to the patient's terminal subarachnoid haemorrhage. Comparing this case with one of the six cases reported by Schuknecht, Kimura and Naufal (1973) and the changes in the experimental animals, Gussen concludes that there is a more diffuse degeneration of the membranous structures associated with the vascular lesion. This includes loss of the organ of Corti, atrophy of the stria vascularis, ischaemic necrosis of the spiral ligament, loss of outer sulcus cells, and varying degrees of atrophy of spiral ganglion-cells and peripheral nerve fibres. In addition, fibrous and bony proliferation within the inner ear occurred in the vascular lesion, whereas no such fibrous or bony proliferation has been reported in viral labyrinthitis. (Finally, it should be added that the patient had been maintained on corticosteroid therapy for 16 years for rheumatoid arthritis!)

Amongst the earliest to relate sudden deafness to vascular disease and possible atherosclerosis was Hallberg (1957). He would also seem to be the first to notice raised lipids and only occasionally has this factor been mentioned since (Schiff and Brown, 1975—case 3). It is currently part of the routine investigation regime by Hinchcliffe (1978).

BUERGER'S DISEASE (THROMBOANGIITIS OBLITERANS CEREBRI)

Cerebral involvement in patients with Buerger's disease is rare. It has been estimated as less than 0.5 per cent. Kirikae *et al*, (1962) have reported a single case. A moderate smoker, after developing intermittent claudication, noted a hearing loss on the same side. Whilst an injection of vasodilator drugs improved the leg, there was no improvement in the hearing loss. Five years later the radial artery of the opposite side became slowly occluded over two months. At surgery, part of the artery was excised and the diagnosis was confirmed histologically. Seven months after the operation, the patient became suddenly deaf on the same side (i.e. the opposite side to the earlier loss). Both sides showed a sensorineural loss with absence of recruitment. (*See also* Polyarteritis Nodosa.)

Haematological

HAEMOPOIETIC SYSTEM

Anaemia, as such, has rarely been reported as being associated with deafness, sensorineural or otherwise. Morrison and Booth (1970) reported two patients with profound anaemia (haemoglobin levels of 29 and 31 per cent) associated with iron deficiency–both had a sudden bilateral total loss and neither showed any improvement following transfusion (*see also* Malnutrition).

More recently, Morrison (1978) has reported a 58 year old lady who awoke with sudden total bilateral deafness whose EcochG confirmed that there was no action potential or cochlear microphonic on either side. She was found to have some megaloblastic change in the bone marrow and a plentiful supply of iron; she had a moderate anaemia due to folic acid deficiency. No recovery has taken place in the hearing.

POLYCYTHAEMIA VERA

In polycythaemia vera the viscosity of the blood is increased five to eight times normal; the total red cell count becomes elevated by 20–50 per cent and the total blood volume is increased to two to three times normal. These alterations affect the peripheral blood by causing engorgement of the capillaries, venules and arterioles with high viscosity, slowly circulating oxygen-deficient blood. When Vaques first described polycythaemia in 1892, he noticed tinnitus and vertigo among the primary symptoms. The first person to record a pure-tone air-conduction threshold shift was Magni in 1961. Davis and Nilo (1965) have reported an interesting case in which they found that the pure-tone thresholds and speech discrimination scores reflected the clinical disease. In this condition, the loss is a bilateral sensorineural type. They noted that as the viscosity etc. increased, the hearing fell; after phlebotomy, the hearing improved and then remitted after three to six weeks. They observed this fluctuation over two such episodes. Jaffe (1967) has also reported a single case.

SICKLE-CELL DISEASE

Whilst sickle-cell disease is not generally considered as a cause of deafness, it has been shown by Todd, Sergeant and Larson (1973) that sensorineural hearing loss of apparently gradual onset can occur. This loss is only reported in the homozygous disease (abnormal haemoglobin S). Both ends of the audiometric range may be affected but more often the higher tones. The sickling phenomena occur and crisis develops when certain intermolecular hydrophobic bonds form with subsequent polymerization. Any decrease in the P_{O_2} with associated hypoxaemia can initiate the process and the concomitant stasis, hyperviscosity, or acidosis significantly increases the likelihood of sickling. The end effect is tissue hypoxia. In the inner ear it is considered that the sickling and impaired blood flow in the cochlear venous system with secondary anoxia of the hair-cells and striae vascularis are the most likely cause of the sensorineural hearing loss. Todd, Sergeant and Larsen (1973) found sensorineural loss in 22 per cent of their 83 patients. They considered two possible pathological causes—anaemia and thrombosis. The haemoglobin level in SS disease was considered unlikely to reflect the oxygen carrying capacity since the decreased oxygen affinity of Hb S allows greater oxygen release/g Hb than in Hb A. Furthermore, the oxygen affinity is lower in cases with lower haemoglobin levels. The pattern of hearing loss in SS disease is similar to that in certain animal studies which show a low-grade continuous venous thrombotic process. However, they were unable to find a correlation between the irreversibly sickled cells and the hearing loss in their small group.

The haemolytic process characteristic of sickle-cell disease is associated with increase of bone-marrow activity. Active bone marrow is present in the petrous temporal bone in SS disease but Serjeant, Norman and Todd (1975) failed to find evidence that this caused any narrowing of the internal auditory canal or compression of the eighth cranial nerve. It is most important to realize that sickle-cell crises can cause sudden sensorineural hearing loss. Although only two such cases are on record, both were bilateral (Morganstein and Mannace, 1969; Urban, 1973).

Morrison and Booth (1970) have reported one case of bilateral deafness in sickle-cell trait (haemoglobin S and C) which they presumed to be thrombotic.

WALDENSTROM'S MACROGLOBULINAEMIA

This condition, which tends to occur in elderly males, is characterized by retinal changes, an abnormal bleeding tendency from mucous membranes, generalized weakness and dyspnoea. Fundamental to the diagnosis is a raised sedimentation rate and marked increase of serum globulin level, in the form of a narrow, dense band in the B2 region. The abnormal macroglobulin coats the platelets and reduces their adhesiveness; it also interferes with fibrin polymerization.

It is most often met in otolaryngological practice as a cause of epistaxis or bleeding from the gums, but a few cases of sudden deafness have been recorded although vertigo may be the earliest symptom (Coyle *et al.*, 1961, Afifi and Tawfeek, 1971). Immediate diagnosis is essential if the patient is to be protected against probable permanent bilateral deafness. The optic fundus must be examined and may reveal gross retinal haemorrhages or central vein thrombosis. Ruben *et al.* (1969) reported a case developing first in one ear and ten months later in the other. Subsequently both ears deteriorated to an almost total loss and, whilst vestibular function was lost in the second ear, that on the original side remained normal. Wilkinson, Davidson and Sommaripa (1966) reported another bilateral case.

Multiple myeloma and leukaemia must be excluded and also certain collagen diseases (especially lupus erythematosus and rheumatoid arthritis), which are associated with secondary macroglobulinaemia. Primary cryoglobulinaemia and subacute bacterial endocarditis must also be excluded.

HYPERCOAGULATION

In addition to the clinical syndromes with known haematological characteristics, a further, less well-defined group exists whose common feature can best be described as 'hypercoagulation'. Jaffe (1970, 1975) has investigated hypercoagulation in great depth as a possible cause of sudden deafness. The clinical diagnosis of hypercoagulation is characterized by recurring episodes of thrombophlebitis and sometimes pulmonary embolism. Jaffe carried out highly specialized tests and emphasizes how important it is that these should be carried out on site and not sent away to a laboratory elsewhere. By such attention to detail, he found a much higher degree of accuracy in the results. He believes that the two-stage prothrombin technique measuring the prothrombin consumption rate to be the most accurate test (1968, 1975). Jaffe found that no less than 54 per cent (of 37 patients) had accelerated prothrombin consumption values. In 13 patients with sudden hearing loss and normal coagulation, only 16 per cent recovered good hearing; when the coagulation was abnormal 66 per cent recovered. Furthermore, it is known that the stria vascularis has a slow blood flow with a high haematocrit value. It is suggested that stasis of blood flow and accelerated coagulation may be the twin interrelated factors responsible. Temporal-bone studies in two patients have shown possible intravascular plugs in the spiral ligament in one and in the stria vascularis in both (Jaffe, 1970).

Whilst there is no difficulty in accepting that sudden hearing loss may be caused by viruses or by vascular disease, in their myriad forms, the 'arranged marriage' between the two by describing the effects of viruses on the cardiovascular and haemopoietic systems, seems contrived beyond the bounds of reason at this time. It is known that viruses can become attached to erythrocytes and cause haemagglutination and that they can cause oedema of capillary endothelial cells. It is also known that they can damage the vessel wall, releasing collagen, which causes platelet agglutination. Viruses are also known to adhere to the platelet surface and cause lysis of platelets, releasing at least three factors: serotonin, ADP (causing an increased platelet agglutination) and platelet factor 3 which is a stimulus for clotting. (Platelet factor 3 is the most important factor in causing an increase in prothrombin consumption.)

Viruses may also destroy erythrocytes, releasing the procoagulants of the first stage to accelerate coagulation. However, in spite of all the theory, Jaffe was unable to demonstrate any of these pathways in his patients with sudden deafness. It should also be noted that, whilst viral diseases may cause haematological conditions, e.g. haemolytic anaemia, there is no evidence of hypercoagulability in such patients except perhaps when their illness is at its most extreme.

Fat embolism has also been reported as a cause of sudden deafness in two cases following the manipulation of fractures (Jaffe, 1970).

Psychosomatic factors or emotional episodes were considered by Fowler (1950) to be significant but no proper assessment such as those done in Menière's disease has ever been published. Such work on sudden deafness is in progress (Hinchcliffe, 1978)and work in relation to hyperlipidaemia which will also be published shortly (Moffat, Booth and Morrison, 1979).

LEUKAEMIA

The first account of leukaemia of the inner ear was presented by Politzer in 1884; the patient experienced bilateral, severe deafness one year prior to death. The various forms of leukaemia may affect the ear but it is usually the middle ear that is involved. Otological complications occur almost invariably in those patients with the acute forms, particularly acute lymphocytic leukaemia. The changes seen in the temporal bone fall into three categories: leukaemic infiltration, haemorrhage, and infection.

Leukaemic infiltration may occur in the muco-periosteum of the middle ear following the mucous membrane folds but this may extend on to the ossicles and the sheaths of the tendons of the intratympanic muscles. Infiltration into the bone marrow spaces of the petrous apex frequently occurs and also, to a lesser extent, within the ossicles. Infiltration into the inner ear is uncommon. Haemorrhage into the inner ear is also uncommon.

Sudden deafness and/or vertigo is reported in acute leukaemia and seems to occur most often in the acute stem-cell type. As a general rule, the otological symptoms appear to be more associated with infiltration and seem to be based on the degree.

Haemorrhagic changes in the temporal bone are more frequently seen in patients with acute lymphocytic leukaemia than the other forms. Patients with acute leukaemia suffer from a bone-marrow failure with a resultant thrombocytopenia, and other coagulation defects such as hypofibrinogenaemia may occur. Disseminated intravascular coagulation and secondary fibrinolysis may also occur.

The histopathological findings of the temporal bones in acute leukaemia do not show a more specific pattern than the above. However, it must be admitted that the otologist's role is barely more than academic and limited to treating the middle-ear infection etc. The main treatment lies in the condition and type itself (Schuknecht, Igarashi and Chasin, 1965; Paparella *et al.*, 1973; Sklansky, Jafek and Wiernik, 1974).

Collagen diseases

POLYARTERITIS NODOSA (PAN)

Deafness in this condition is itself unusual and only on rare occasions has it been the presenting symptom. The deafness is sensorineural. Lake-Bakaar and Gibbs (1978) have reported a case with profound bilateral deafness and sudden tinnitus; electrocochleography pointed to an end-organ impairment. Before treatment the patient's hearing improved to within normal limits; subsequently her PAN was treated with prednisolone and there has been no recurrence of deafness. Peitersen and Carlsen (1966) reported a case, also with bilateral, and almost symmetrical, gradually deteriorating hearing loss. Subsequently the hearing fluctuated. After an interval of more than six months, PAN seemed the most likely diagnosis and she was treated with prednisolone and this brought about a considerable hearing improvement. (Interestingly, they also show the audiogram of a case of fluctuant hearing loss in a confirmed case of temporal arteritis—but no commentary.)

The remaining reported cases total only approximately a dozen; the only common features would seem to be that the deafness is sensorineural and bilateral. In most of the early reports, minimal details are available. Later in the disease, or perhaps already present, other lesions of polyarteritis nodosa will be found in the body and it is by these that the diagnosis is made.

In 1934, Druss and Maybaum reported two cases in two separate articles (in the same journal)—the first, of a 33 year old man with no symptoms referrable to the ears who died ten weeks after an operation but whose temporal bones were nevertheless examined! The smaller arterioles in the bone marrow of the petrous pyramid showed changes which were reported as characteristic of PAN in the acute stages. The second (Maybaum and Druss, 1934), was of a 51 year old man with herpes zoster oticus from which he died (referred to elsewhere in this chapter) who showed no signs of PAN in the temporal bone, but did elsewhere in the body. Since then and including the above mentioned cases, Rossle (1937) described the characteristic changes of PAN in an artery in the middle-ear mucosa. McNeil, Berke and Reingold (1952) added a case causing bilateral deafness but without renal involvement; autopsy did not include the temporal bones. Rose and Spencer (1957) included one case of acute mastoiditis in their monograph. Welsh and Welsh (1963) mentioned one case causing unilateral sudden deafness.

Wing and Bulteau (1967) reported a case with unilateral loss accompanied by pain in the left temple; audiometry showed a moderate conductive loss and the renal biopsy showed PAN. He was treated with prednisone and chlorambucil; after two weeks all symptoms had disappeared. Per-Lee and Parsons (1969) reported a case which personifies the continued difficulty in deciding, particularly during life, whether a case is classified as PAN or Wegener's granuloma. To many PAN would seem more likely but, like Wing and Bulteau, the case is reported as a Wegener's.

Recently Gussen (1977) reported the most authentic case. She examined the temporal bone of a 66 year old woman with PAN who became deaf seven months before death. PAN of the left internal auditory artery was demonstrated with fibrosis and bone formation involving the cochlear and vestibular systems. Endolymphatic hydrops of the basal turn of the cochlea was also present, as well as a chronic perforation of the free wall of the saccule. Gussen feels that this adds further clinical evidence of vascular lesions causing the three patterns of end-organ involvement described by Kimura and Perlman in their guinea-pig experiments.

WEGENER'S GRANULOMATOSIS

Whilst pathologically there may be difficulties in differentiating this from PAN, clinically they are usually quite different in their presentation. Cases of PAN seldom present to an ENT surgeon, whilst most will see Wegener's granulomatosis in their career and it will frequently present because of nasal symptoms. Similarly, whilst clinically it is different from lethal midline granuloma, pathologically these two may also present problems; the latter is considered by some to be another variant of PAN. Indeed Wegener himself in 1939, stated that PAN was a common finding in patients with lethal granulomata of the midline facial tissues (quoted by Duvall, Nelms and Williams, 1969).

Wegener's granulomatosis has three principle components:

(1) Necrotizing granulomatous lesions in the upper or lower respiratory tract or both.
(2) Generalized focal necrotizing vasculitis involving both arteries and veins, almost always present in the lungs and more or less widely disseminated in other sites.
(3) Glomerulitis, characterized by necrosis and thrombosis of loops or lobes of the capillary tuft, capsular adhesions, and evolution as a granulomatous lesion.

Otorrhoea is quoted as being present in 38 per cent of those with invasion of the nasal complex; blockage of the eustachian tube is a common otological manifestation and probably the cause of the otorrhoea. Antral disease, spreading to the middle ear itself, is very rare. Friedmann and Bauer (1973) have reviewed the cases associated with deafness, together with many of those with PAN. They report two new cases, the first presenting with deafness. She was a 44 year old female whose sudden facial pain and deafness led to operation and it was from the mastoidectomy granulations that the diagnosis was made. The second was a 41 year old male who eight days after an operation for a lumbar intervertebral disc protrusion, but at which instead only granulomatous thickening of the dura was found, noticed a loss of hearing (bilateral); examination showed both ears to be discharging. He remained extremely ill and died just under three weeks from the 'laminectomy' operation. Friedmann carried out temporal bone studies; he was able to compare this with his own earlier case and that reported by Blatt and Lawrence (1961). He found abundant evidence of giant cellular granulomatous tissue occupying the tympanic cavity. The ossicles were damaged and the stapes footplate bogged down by this tissue (a finding similar to the case described by Densert, Rausing and Toremalm, 1969). The inner-ear structures appeared to be only moderately affected.

Ear symptoms are mentioned in several of the six cases reported by Brown and Woolner (1960). In Case 6, after earlier otorrhoea, the patient developed a rapid hearing loss in one side, accompanied by vertigo, vomiting and spontaneous nystagmus to the opposite side. The patient had presented four months before with bilateral tinnitus without apparent cause at that time.

In the case of Blatt and Lawrence, the main lesion was in the nasopharynx, but there is no mention clinically or at autopsy of any renal involvement or other lesions. In the recent case of Friedmann, the nose shows a large haemorrhagic lesion at the tip, but this only occurred four days before death (the histology of the nose is not stated). Schuknecht, Allam and Murakami (1968) (Case 10) have examined the temporal bone of a 31 year old female who died of non-healing midline granuloma of the palate and nasal cavities, which also invaded the petrous bone and destroyed the bone in the peritubal area.

It is of interest that the second case reported by Toma (1968) was initially thought after removing a leg nodule to show changes of PAN, but a year later went on to develop further lesions in the eyes, lung and kidneys from which she died. This case again typifies the difficulty in differentiating pathologically between PAN and Wegener's granulomatosis.

COGAN'S SYNDROME

In 1945, Cogan reported four cases of non-syphilitic keratitis characterized by vestibular and auditory disorders. He noted that in syphilitic keratitis only 4 per cent of the patients developed deafness, and that this did not occur until months or even years after the keratitis. He saw his first four cases all within one year and was impressed that whilst the corneal changes progressed relatively little, the vertigo became incapacitating and the deafness progressive and ultimately profound.

Norton and Cogan reviewed the cases again in 1959. They confirmed the ocular signs of patchy, deep corneal infiltrates which tend to fluctuate in intensity and distribution, usually located in the periphery, and accompanied by deep corneal vascularization if they persist long enough. No evidence of syphilitic infection, by the tests then available, could be found. However, the sensorineural hearing loss is progressive, often sudden in onset, and always associated with tinnitus and vertigo. Very occasionally, the vestibular/auditory symptoms have preceded the eye changes but only by a few weeks or a month or so in all reported cases. More than three quarters of the cases have occurred in patients under 30; two have been associated with pregnancy (one developed the bilateral interstitial keratitis during the latter part of gestation and the hearing loss 21 months later, the second started with tinnitus in the first month and the bilateral hearing loss did not develop until 12 days after delivery (Cody and Williams, 1960).

Other cases have been associated with vaccination, particularly for smallpox. Some have been treated with steroids, e.g. triamcinolone or cortisone, but whilst this remains advocated, there is no evidence that it has been beneficial (Bellucci, Grobeisen and Sah, 1974). The youngest case on record was a five year old girl, the oldest 64 with rheumatoid arthritis.

At present, there is much debate whether the condition exists in isolation or forms part of the condition—polyarteritis nodosa (PAN). Clinically it has to be differentiated from syphilis in the usual way, and thereafter is diagnosed by the pattern of symptoms as already outlined. The hearing loss is bilateral and should be suspected particularly in those under 30. Laboratory findings are a leucocytosis and occasionally an eosinophilia. So far it would appear that only one case has been tested for syphilis by the fluorescein treponema antibody (FTA Abs) test (Belluci, Grobeisen and Sah, 1974).

Temporal-bone studies by Wolff *et al.* (1965) have stressed the presence of fibrous tissue and new bone growth in the perilymphatic spaces, and hydrops involving the saccule and cochlear duct.

This finding of 'hydrops' led Beckman and Trotsky (1970) to treat a case with oral glycerine using it as a hyperosmolar agent. (The patient was simultaneously being treated with triamcinolone and acetazolamide.) On the two occasions in which they tried this regime, it resulted in a marked hearing improvement.

At present it is quite undecided if Cogan's syndrome is a separate entity. Cases with systemic involvement tend to be labelled PAN and cases with rheumatoid arthritis (Smith, 1970), temporal arteritis and sarcoidosis with similar features have all been described. There are at least four cases reported as Cogan's syndrome associated with PAN. Oliner *et al.* (1953) reported one case and mentioned an earlier report quoting the incidence of 'nerve deafness' as 3 per cent in 65 cases of PAN with neurological signs. Crawford (1957) and Boyd (1957) each reported two cases and possibly another; Fisher and Hellstrom reported another case in 1961. Hallberg (1956) reported one case which presented with sudden unilateral deafness.

Endolymphatic hydrops

Hallberg (1956) thought that no more than 5 per cent of all cases of sudden hearing loss eventually developed Menière's disease. He found only 57 such cases in his review of 1270 patients. Morrison (1978) confirms this suggestion but anticipates that the figure may increase with improved diagnostic procedures such as electrocochleography. Two cases of sudden hearing loss which have shown endolymphatic hydrops at autopsy, have now been reported. Takahara *et al.* (1974) reported a case of an 80 year old man who developed unilateral sudden sensorineural hearing loss when he suffered from acute nephritis. He never experienced any vertigo, nausea or vomiting. He died of rupture of a dissecting aneurysm 21 years after the episode of deafness. The temporal bone showed a combination of the idiopathic endolymphatic hydrops and neural and metabolic type presbyacusis. Sando *et al.* (1977) reported a 63 year old man who at the age of 26 woke with a sudden total hearing loss in one ear. There were no associated symptoms of vertigo or tinnitus; 37 years later he had a lymphosarcoma— right cervical mass (on the opposite side to the earlier deafness). He received 3000 rad during which he noted a hearing loss on the right side—but again no associated vertigo or tinnitus. Three months later audiometry confirmed the earlier total hearing loss on the left and a high-tone sensorineural hearing loss on the right—both ears had normal caloric responses. Two months later he died—autopsy showed severe endolymphatic hydrops, mostly in the basal turn (*see Figure 24.3*). Sando *et al.* also reported the history and temporal-bone findings on a second case with recurring bouts of sudden hearing loss which occurred in both ears on several occasions.

MENIÈRE'S DISEASE

Menière's disease, as opposed to conditions producing a Menière-like disorder due to endolymphatic hydrops, displays a characteristic pattern (*see also* Chapter 25). It is well known that it may fail to oblige by producing its three principal symptoms simultaneously and therein lies some of the fascination and challenge in diagnosis. If the criteria suggested by Wilmot (1974) are adhered to, then a more accurate diagnosis is likely. He listed eight positive and eight negative criteria and they cannot be too highly recommended or reiterated often enough (*Table 24.2*).

More recently criteria 7 and 8 in the positive list seem to be in danger of becoming overlooked. It has been known to many otologists and particularly to their predecessors who practised mainly as physicians, that inflation of the middle ear, could help many patients with vertigo and occasionally tinnitus—they may well not have understood in the most scientific terms 'why' and we know now that very small differences in middle-ear pressure may produce changes in subjective acuity which are hardly measurable either by acoustic impedance or audiometry. If continued sessions of inflation become required then the insertion of a 'grommet tube' may have a place (if carried out, the post-nasal space should always be examined and probably biopsied if there is the slightest doubt).

In a recent study Hall and Brackmann (1977) showed intermittent mild eustachian tube blockage in nearly one-third of their cases of Menière's disease; they noted the negative pressure was greatest when the symptoms were most severe. The fundamental question however remains unanswered. 'Why do these patients have reduced middle-ear pressures?' Is there, for example a change in vasomotor factors affecting tubal function, as happens in the adjacent nasal mucous membrane under other conditions? Recently also, immediate relief of symptoms in the acute attack of Menière's disease

Table 24.2

Positive	Negative
1. A peripheral fluctuating recruiting cochlear (sensorineural) hearing loss is or has been present in one or both ears.	The hearing loss is not equal or approximately equal in the two ears.
2. Tinnitus (usually of low tone) is or has been present in the affected ear or ears.	The hearing loss is not of the falling 'senile' type.
3. Rotational vertigo is or has been present.	The imbalance experienced has not been confined to postural or positional giddiness or to a false sensation of movements of objects or of the patient.
4. The central nervous system is normal.	The blood pressure has not been raised significantly at the time of the vestibular examination, or in the past.
5. The neck movements are full and normal.	There is no evidence of, or strong suspicion of, atherosclerotic disease in the cardiovascular system generally.
6. The carotid artery impulses are equal and normal.	There is no history of previous head or neck trauma of any severity.
7. The tympanic membranes, middle ears and conductive hearing mechanism are normal on both sides.	There is no history of the taking of known ototoxic drugs or of imbalance following the taking of any drug.
8. Eustachian tube function in both ears is normal.	There is no history of chronic ill health and no evidence of such on clinical examination.

Menière's disease has been claimed by decompressing the whole patient in a pressure chamber (Ingelstedt, Ivarsson and Tjernstrom, 1976). They lowered the ambient pressure, maintaining it at certain levels, e.g. -50 and/or -70 cm H_2O, for varying periods of time. At such levels, the eustachian tube opens passively thereby reducing the relative overpressure in the middle ear (as on ascent in flying). They postulate that the relative middle-ear overpressure becomes transmitted via the oval window and round window membrane to the inner ear, causing an increased intralabyrinthine pressure! This increased pressure is then supposed to flush the excess endolymphatic fluid into the expandable saccus! Such a suggestion seems incompatible with the appearance of the inside of the sac at surgery which is almost routinely observed by surgeons to have no lumen whatsoever.

Glycerol dehydration test
In the diagnosis of fluctuant hearing loss, this test is of particular interest. When it was originally introduced by Klockhoff and Lindblom in 1966, it was hoped by this means to select those cases of Menière's disease whose hearing etc. would be improved by diuretic therapy—the chosen drug was chlorthalidone which promotes sodium excretion without great potassium loss. More recently they have taken as significant, a rise of at least 10 dB in three adjacent octave bands or speech discrimination improvement exceeding 12 per cent. No effect was seen in more advanced Menière's cases where a non-fluctuating hearing loss was present or in sensorineural deafness of less specific types (Klockhoff and Lindblom, 1966). Snyder (1974) felt that a pure-tone threshold improvement of 15 dB was more likely to be significant; he also noticed

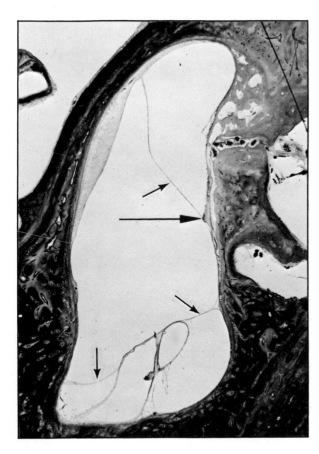

Figure 24.3 Left ear. Severe endolymphatic hydrops is seen at the extreme basal end of the cochlear duct (small arrows). Large arrow demonstrates collapsed ductus reuniens (× 23). (Reproduced by permission of the authors and Editor of the *Annals of Otology*)

that the changes were more marked in the low tones and the significant change in the speech discrimination score.

Recently the glycerol dehydration test has been carried out in patients during continuous electrocochleographic recording (by the transtympanic route). This appears to be a more sensitive indication of alterations occurring within the cochlea than the other two (Moffat *et al.*, 1978). Gibson, Ramsden and Moffat (1977) had shown by the same method in 65 per cent of patients, under investigation for Menière's disorder, that a large DC potential was recorded which caused an apparent widening of the summating potential/action potential (SP/AP) waveform. This potential was thought to be an SP which was enhanced relative to the AP component and to be directly related to the presence of endolymphatic hydrops. During glycerol dehydration the marked negative SP was seen to decrease. A dose of 1.2 g/kg body weight of iced, lemon-flavoured glycerol was used and patients were excluded if their plasma osmolality change was less than 10 mmol/kg; the mean change in plasma osmolality was 18.2, with a range of 10–40 mmol/kg. One third of their patients failed to show any change in the AP/SP complex and just under 50 per cent showed a definite increase (greater than 1 ms) (*see Figure 24.4*).

Another dehydration test using intravenous frusemide (20 mg) has also been advocated. It is claimed that whereas the effects of glycerol only occur in early Menière's, frusemide can reduce the endolymphatic hydrops and improve the caloric

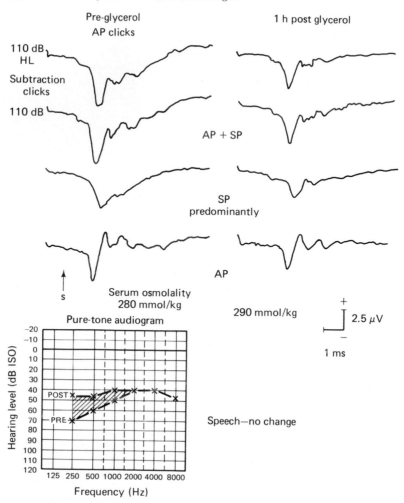

Figure 24.4 Electrocochleography during glycerol dehydration test, together with changes in pure-tone audiogram. The marked negative SP which is thought to be responsible for the wide AP/SP waveform commonly observed in Menière's disease is seen to decrease after dehydration. In this case there was no change in speech discrimination. (Reproduced by permission of the authors and Editor of the *Journal of Laryngology and Otology*)

response not only in Menière's (positive in 80 per cent of typical cases) but also in labyrinthine syphilis (42 per cent) and sudden deafness (27 per cent). Frusemide depresses the reabsorption of sodium, water and chloride in both the proximal and distal tubules, including the ascending limb of the loop of Henle. It also causes a reduction in blood pressure, a decrease in the flow of CSF and a diminution of the pressure of CSF and chamber pressure in the eye (Futaki, Kitahara and Morimoto, 1975, 1977).

Recently also urea by mouth, 20 g has been used as an alternative to glycerol (Angelborg, Klockhoff and Stahle, 1977).

Acoustic impedance measurements have also been carried out during the glycerol test but contrary to an earlier suggestion by other authors, Herman, Carver and Arenberg (1977) were unable to find any change in compliance.

Finally, electrocochleography in a clinical case of Lermoyez's syndrome has been reported by Schmidt *et al.* (1975). They found changes compatible with those in a large group of Menière's patients and concluded that as far as the cochlea is concerned, the syndrome is closely related to Menière's disease.

Metabolic disorders

RENAL FAILURE

The analogy between the nephron and the organ of Corti is one which has become more frequent. Associated and coincident with this renewed interest in renal failure and its treatment by haemodialysis, has also become an interest with further impetus in relation to ototoxic drugs, many of which of necessity have to be given to patients in renal failure.

Certain recent studies, therefore, are not only of interest but helpful to the otologist who may expect to become more frequently involved with the management of such cases. Oda *et al.* (1974) have shown that in a study of 290 patients with chronic renal failure, 43 developed a significant hearing loss which could be attributed to the therapy of the kidney problem. None of the patients complained of hearing impairment before the kidney treatment was started. Many of such patients received ototoxic drugs but the temporal bone findings in eight of the patients showed changes unrelated to this exposure. In seven of these, abnormal blue concretions in the stria vascularis and/or vestibular receptors were found. The severity of the clinical and histopathological findings were directly proportional to the number of haemodialyses and transplants the patients had undergone. It must be remembered that during haemodialysis frequent and intense osmotic pressure changes occur.

Yassin, Badry and Fatt-Hi (1970) found that the degree of hearing loss was directly related to the degree of hyponatraemia irrespective of the level of the blood urea. Urea by itself was non-toxic to the cochlear end-organs and the cochlear affections were greatly improved by correcting the renal failure and restoring the serum sodium. Eighty per cent of the cases with acute renal failure were improved by treatment but only 52.4 per cent in those with chronic forms.

It may be remembered that when hexadimethrine bromide (Polybrene) was used as an anti-heparinizing agent in haemodialysis for renal failure, and used in a dose in excess of 5 mg/kg body weight, it caused an immediate decrease in urinary output. The drug caused sensorineural hearing loss in five of the 14 patients reported by Ransome *et al.* (1966). The drug when used after open heart surgery was not followed by any such complications; it was the association when used in renal insufficiency which led to the ototoxicity.

Occasionally Alport's syndrome has been mentioned in relation to sudden hearing loss. Alport (1927) himself reported a relationship between nephritis and deafness and noted a familial occurrence. The aetiology of the hearing loss has never been clearly defined. Characteristically it varies in severity with the family, is slowly progressive and the high frequencies are those most severely affected. Myers and Tyler (1972) suggest that there may be as many as five variants—renal disease with organ of Corti damage, renal disease with spiral ganglion cochlear neurone loss, renal disease and deafness but no histological ear lesion, renal disease without deafness and finally deafness without renal disease. Hearing loss with normal or only mild renal changes is especially typical of female members of affected families.

RENAL TRANSPLANTATION

Hearing improvement in sensorineural deafness has been reported in two papers. Mitschke *et al.* (1975) noted this in eight out of ten patients with a cochlear loss; the two who had Alport's syndrome failed to improve. Paradoxically McDonald *et al.* (1978) have reported six cases with this syndrome who have undergone transplantation; of these one patient who received a cadaver kidney had a substantial improvement, the remainder (two received allograft kidneys from living, related donors) obtained stabilization of hearing (follow-up period—three years).

MALNUTRITION

In conditions leading to malnutrition, e.g. malabsorption defects etc. peripheral neuropathy is well recognized and usually involves the extremities but may also involve the cranial nerves. In the early stages, segmental demyelination occurs and later, both myelin and axon are involved. When deafness occurs its onset is gradual and occurs months or years after the other symptoms. Whilst tinnitus is usual, vertigo is not reported. Surprisingly in beri-beri (thiamine deficiency) deafness is not seen but has been described in nicotinic acid deficiency and also in hyperemesis gravidarum (Ironside, 1939). In a recent case described by Gussen (1974) the absence of other neurological involvement is inexplicable but the deafness was rapidly progressive. At post mortem, both temporal bones demonstrated segmental demyelination of the vestibular and cochlear nerves; this was not recent in origin and a very fine interstitial fibrosis had occurred.

PREGNANCY

Welsh and Welsh (1963) reported one case of sudden deafness occurring during a sudden hypertensive crisis in toxaemia of pregnancy. After delivery, whilst the blood pressure reverted to normal, the hearing loss remained unchanged. Morrison (1975) reports two cases, one during the third month and the other during the fourth; one produced a retrocochlear loss and the other a high-tone sensorineural loss. Neither, of course, received treatment and none showed any spontaneous recovery. Jaffe (1967) reported five cases, who became suddenly deaf either during or after pregnancy. One became deaf and gave birth to a deaf child, the second gave birth to a stillborn child and developed a unilateral deafness, the third had a normal delivery but became deaf in the post-partum period (her mother had experienced an identical sequence herself) and another had a total loss in one ear after her first child and a total loss, both permanent in the other ear after delivery of her second child.

Svane-Knudsen (1957) reported one case in the eighth month, Sacher (1952) another in the fourth month—both normal pregnancies and Lindsay and Zuidema (1950) reported one case a month after delivery. (Sacher also reports two cases of deafness after excessive physical effort and another case was a diabetic.)

Conversely, Ironside (1939) thought nerve deafness and nystagmus worthy of special mention in the polyneuritis which he observed as a complication of hyperemesis gravidarum, which often led to starvation, in the first or second month of pregnancy.

However, even in those days the condition was uncommon and is most unlikely to exist today. It would be interesting to know if it occurs in anorexia nervosa!

POST-OPERATIVE

Several cases of deafness following surgery have been reported. It seems most generally accepted that these are due to microembolism involving the cochlear division of the internal auditory pathway (Jaffe, 1967). It is interesting, therefore, that two cases have followed cardiopulmonary bypass surgery, a procedure in which anticoagulation is employed (Arenberg, Allen and DeBoer, 1972; Wright and Saunders, 1975). In the second of these, the deafness was indicated by the patient within 24 h and anticoagulation was commenced intially with subcutaneous heparin and continued with oral warfarin. In neither case did the hearing recover and in both it was the left ear that was affected. The operations were to replace the aortic valve only in the first, and the mitral and aortic valves in the second. It should be added that microembolism following the use of pump oxygenator systems is well known. The emboli consist of platelet aggregates, damaged erythrocytes, denatured proteins and fibrin.

Other operations of widely differing nature have on occasion been reported as being followed by sudden hearing loss; one case followed a spinal anaesthetic. The cases are mentioned usually only by title and no details are published to allow any real comparison.

ANAESTHESIA

Investigations on patients receiving nitrous oxide anaesthesia have shown that because of its much greater solubility in blood than nitrogen (34 times), the gas is carried to the middle ear in much greater volumes than the volume of nitrogen that can be carried away. This is the cause of the marked increase in middle-ear pressure during nitrous oxide anaesthesia. This rise occurs very rapidly, e.g. within 15 min and may reach levels of over 300 mmH$_2$O (Thomsen, Terkildsen and Amfred, 1965). The pressure continues to rise in fact until the eustachian tube opens passively and then a sudden fall in middle-ear pressure occurs. When the gas is terminated the nitrous oxide leaves the ear at a much more rapid rate than it can be replaced by nitrogen and subsequently for a period a negative pressure exists. Peacock (1977) has suggested that these factors may be of importance in children, in sero-mucinous otitis media. Waun, Sweitzer and Hamilton (1967) reported pressure changes sufficient to affect drum compliance and transient hearing losses in patients during adenoidectomy. Using the Zwislocki acoustic bridge before, during and after nitrous oxide anaesthesia, they observed a decreased compliance and increased resistance. Shaw, Stark and Gannaway (1978) have also reported on the effect of nitrous oxide (50 per cent), by using the oto-admittance meter before and during anaesthesia. They found that in 49 of the 59 ears, the gas made no difference to the tympanogram; ten possibly (17 per cent) were affected, indicating that the middle-ear pressure might have caused evacuation of the fluid.

Patterson and Bartlett (1976) have reported four cases of hearing impairment after anaesthesia, three receiving ear surgery and a fourth who underwent an orthopaedic operation but already was suspected of having a perilymph leak from a previous stapedectomy (which was subsequently confirmed at operation and closed). In all four, the hearing returned.

DIABETES MELLITUS

The relationship between diabetes and sensorineural hearing loss was first reported by Jordao in 1857. An excellent recent review by Taylor and Irwin (1978) endeavours to put this into perspective and they make the following points from their own initial survey and from the literature. The incidence of sensorineural hearing loss in diabetes will very largely depend on the limits of 'normality' and therein the statistical methodology. Second, nearly all the work has naturally been carried out in the group of diabetics most likely to be affected i.e. those on insulin. They have been careful to limit their upper age limit to 50, thereby reducing the effect of presbyacusis. They noted that a diabetic with a family history had significantly better hearing thresholds than those without. They found that the diabetics, as a whole, were deafer particularly in the lower frequencies and gradually approached each other in the middle range (1–4 kHz) and were similar at 8 kHz. They also quote Dietziel (1964) who so far, has been the only worker to try to relate insulin requirements and hearing level but no such relationship could be found.

Pathogenesis

In a study of the temporal bones of 32 diabetic patients, Jørgensen (1961) found severe PAS-positive thickening of the capillary walls of the stria vascularis. In his series these changes showed a distinct correlation with diabetic retinopathy, nephropathy and angiopathy of the lower limbs, with, of course, late diabetic complications. The spread of diabetic angiopathy has a predilection for certain capillary systems; in the inner ear only the stria vascularis is affected. (Similar changes, though less marked, may also be encountered in severe atherosclerosis.) Jørgensen and Buch (1961) in a series of 28 diabetic patients, found that in the 14 under 40 years of age there was an unmistakable correlation between nephropathy and hearing loss, but in those over 40 this correlation was not found. Neither could they find any correlation between hearing impairment and diabetic neuropathy or blood pressure value.

More recently Friedman and Schulman (1975) have studied 20 diabetic patients with peripheral neuropathy: 55 per cent had a symmetrical hearing loss of the sensorineural type, involving at least one frequency, though none gave a history of hearing loss or ear disease; the hearing loss was unrelated to age, and the impairment was similar at low and high frequencies, with maximum deficiency between 750 and 2000 Hz. Makashima and Tanaka (1971) have described atrophy of neurones in the spiral ganglion and demyelination of the auditory nerve in four diabetic patients.

In interpreting the incidence of diabetes and its effect on hearing, one other fundamental fact must be mentioned—that is the way by which the diagnosis of diabetes mellitus is made, i.e. the glucose tolerance test itself. There has been a longstanding difference between the British and American Diabetic Associations. In the UK the standard test is a 50-g load, given to a patient starved for the 12 h prior to the test and consuming a normal diet for the previous three days; half-hourly venous blood samples over 2.5 h, plus hourly urine analysis, forms the standard test. In the USA a 100-g load is given to a similarly fasted patient and sampling is carried out over 5 h. Both tests pick up the frankly diabetic patients but the American test is otherwise considered to be non-physiological because of the high load and it is argued that this is the reason for the higher incidence of reactive hypoglycaemia. Our own preliminary findings in Menière's disease (Moffat *et al.*, 1979) using the British test, failed to find any diabetic GTT curves, as against an incidence of 3 per cent in the general population, no fasting hypoglycaemia ($<$ 40 mg/100 ml) and possible reactive hypoglycaemia in only 11 per cent, but still within the normal range as 20 per cent of patients over the age of 40 have 2-h blood glucose levels in excess of 150 mg/100 ml.

HYPERLIPIDAEMIA

When considering this condition as a cause of fluctuating hearing loss, it is important to stress at the outset the difference between primary and secondary hyperlipidaemia (Chait, 1974). There are a large number of conditions causing secondary hyperlipidaemia, the most common of which are diabetes, alcoholism, chronic renal failure and gout. Pregnancy may also cause it and oral contraceptives have been shown to elevate the plasma triglyceride in most subjects taking them. It is therefore essential to exclude these secondary causes, if not at the time of the original sampling, at least when the fasting lipids are being checked.

The next factor to be taken into account is the incidence of hyperlipidaemia, not in populations elsewhere in the world, but in the same part of the same country. Cholesterol levels have been shown to vary widely between countries, e.g. Finland and Yugoslavia, and between different parts of the same country. A survey in the north-east of London of 276 carefully screened men and women, aged 20–69 years, showed that 4.3 per cent of men and 4.8 per cent of women (aged 40–69) had serum cholesterol values exceeding 300 mg/100 ml (7.8 mmol/l); 14 per cent of men and 3 per cent of women had triglyceride levels, greater than 2.0 mmol/l (180 mg/100 ml). By these definitions, 17 per cent of men and 8 per cent of women had hyperlipidaemia (Lewis *et al.*, 1974).

It cannot be stressed enough that great care is required in carrying out these investigations and relating them to statistics of 'normal controls' in the same geographical area and to the normal levels for the individual laboratory and the methods adopted.

Booth (1977) investigated 44 patients with premature bilateral sensorineural hearing loss, without vertigo, and failed to find any incidence of hyperlipidaemia greater than in the local general population or any patient requiring treatment other than by a modification of diet.

Further cases seem to confirm this finding and none has shown any significant improvement in hearing so far; conversely there has also been no progression.

A small number of known primary hyperlipidaemic patients have also been examined audiometrically; so far all have proved normal, though they have only been tested in the range of 250–8000 Hz.

The work of Spencer stemmed from his own progressive, non-fluctuating hearing loss during the previous five or six years, with isolated periods of vertigo. This prompted him to have a glucose tolerance test and the technician noted the marked turbidity of his serum. A repeat fasted examination showed a serum cholesterol of 250 mg/100 ml and triglyceride of 170 mg/100 ml, thereby indicating a Type IV pattern; lipoprotein electrophoresis showed a raised pre-beta fraction of 40 per cent. Changes in his diet over a three-month period resulted in his regaining 87 per cent of the lost hearing. This simple but important observation in a fertile and inquisitive mind led him to carry out lipid studies in many other types of hearing loss in his own practice in Charleston, West Virginia (Spencer, 1973).

In his most recent report, Spencer (1975) has investigated 444 cases; he has found that symptoms of inner-ear disease were cochlear or vestibular, and were often associated with cranial symptoms. The configuration of the pure-tone audiograms frequently showed a fluctuating low-tone slant or a rising curve with a non-fluctuating high-tone slant above 2000 Hz. Spencer found that 46.6 per cent of his patients had hyperlipoprotinaemia and a further 10.3 per cent were borderline. An elevated glucose tolerance curve was demonstrable in 87 per cent of the hyperlipidaemic patients. Obesity was present in over 80 per cent of cases. Two-thirds of the nonhyperlipidaemic patients showed a decreased glucose tolerance. (Also investigated were 16 patients with Bell's palsy, nine of whom were hyperlipidaemic and two diabetic.) Of the 207 hyperlipidaemic patients, 34 were Type IIa, 16 Type IIb and 164 Type IV.

Whilst diabetes mellitus and hyperlipidaemia should both be excluded, they do not so far seem likely to provide help except for a minority. Finally it should be emphasized that blood for lipid studies should be taken after eating a normal diet, followed by a 12–14 h fast, lying fully recumbent for 30–45 min, and withdrawn without venous stasis—otherwise the results are valueless; if abnormal, they should be repeated in association with GTT if not already done and a full work-up to exclude other secondary causes.

HYPOTHYROIDISM

Schuknecht (1974) found the literature up to that time unconvincing on the relationship between acquired idiopathic hypothyroidism and sensorineural hearing loss, though commented that clinicians seemed to have the impression that there probably was such an association. Post (1964) investigated 42 patients—7 with spontaneous primary hypothyroidism and 35 hypothyroid patients with treated carcinoma of the thyroid. He noted that slow mentation while hypothyroid may be interpreted by the patient as a subjective hearing loss. None of the patients with a sensorineural loss attained entirely normal hearing when euthyroid. He was unable to demonstrate any specific correlation between age, degree of hypothyroidism and resulting deafness. He was also unable to determine the time required for patients to remain hypothyroid before experiencing a hearing loss. Stephens and Hinchcliffe (1968) found a significant correlation between the diagnosis of myxoedema, and fatigue or temporary threshold drift measured at 8000 Hz by the Carhart technique. Stephens (1970) later confirmed that this was not an artefact relating to age etc., but a true finding. He suggested that the sensorineural lesion in myxoedema lies proximal to the hair-cells. Meyerhoff (1976) reviewed the possible relationship between all forms of reduced thyroid function and hearing loss; under the heading 'non-genetic acquired' he reiterated the claims made up to that time, i.e. that there was no definite association.

A recent investigation by Bhatia *et al.* (1977) on 66 cases of idiopathic hypothyroidism, showed that whilst only 25 patients complained of hearing impairment, audiometry showed it to be present in 43 per cent. They considered that the degree of hearing loss was related to the severity of the hypothyroidism. Tinnitus was only present in 7 per cent, all of whom had a moderate or severe degree of hypothyroidism (serum PBI below 3 µg/100 ml). The hearing loss was always bilateral and symmetrical and mainly progressive and sensorineural. They considered the cochlea to be the site of the lesion. There was no audiometric improvement but definite subjective improvement on becoming euthyroid.

So far as can be ascertained, no temporal bones of a patient with myxoedema have been reported, nor have they been in Pendred's syndrome. It is of interest that in the latter, the deafness also is bilateral, sensorineural in type with a greater loss in the high frequencies associated with recruitment.

Ototoxicity

This subject is more fully and lucidly dealt with in Chapter 21, but the site of action and the pharmacology of certain of the drugs are relevant here also. Several cause sudden hearing loss, and as they appear to do so by differing means, a brief examination may help in the elucidation in the pathogenesis of the sensorineural pattern they produce.

ANTIBIOTICS

Whilst all antibiotics. in the 'allergic' subject may produce an antigen–antibody response, this has seldom been reported as a cause of sudden deafness. Morrison and Booth (1970) reported a single case of a severe penicillin hypersensitivity reaction which caused a sudden bilateral neural loss. Morrison (1975) reported one case of hypersensitivity to ampicillin which produced bilateral blindness and bilateral retrocochlear deafness with vertigo; large doses of steroids resulted in a good recovery.

The aminoglycoside group of antibiotics are notorious, even infamous, for their otoxicity. Without exception, they may cause damage to the neuroepithelium of the inner ear, either of the cochlea or of the vestibular labyrinth, depending on the individual antibiotic. It is also known that certain families have an unusual predisposition to the toxic effects and also even in ordinary doses they may achieve dangerous concentration in the blood in the elderly. The danger from the group is their concentration and retention in the inner-ear fluids. This concentration both in the inner ear and the kidney exceeds that of all other organs, even of the blood, many times over.

Dihydrostreptomycin, kanamycin, neomycin and tobramycin have a predilection for the spiral organ of Corti. Streptomycin and gentamicin are more likely to affect the vestibular neuroepithelium. It should be remembered that previous aminoglycoside drug administration followed by treatment with ethacrynic acid predisposes towards ototoxicity.

Neomycin

Temporal bone studies in a patient who died of renal failure after receiving 8 g of neomycin intramuscularly and causing total deafness, showed inner and outer hair-cell degeneration and a normal spiral ganglion count. Some changes in the stria vascularis were noted in the basal turn (Lowry, May and Pastore, 1973). Lindsay, Davey and Ward (1960) examined the bones of a patient who had received 18 g in 19 days (and earlier small doses of streptomycin and polymyxin B).

Tobramycin

This factor six of an aminoglycoside complex named nebramycin is known to be capable of producing hair-cell damage in the cochlea. A recent study is of considerable interest (Wilson and Ramsden, 1977). They used electrocochleography to monitor the intravenous administration of tobramycin. When peak serum drug levels exceeded 8–10 μg/ml, an immediate dramatic reduction in cochlear output was observed, which recovered fully as serum levels fell. The patients experienced no auditory or vestibular symptoms either during or after treatment. There was a rapid decrease in amplitude of both the whole nerve action potential (AP) and cochlear microphonic (CM). These changes were evident as soon as peak antibiotic blood levels were obtained (*see Figure 24.5.*) (The n_1 component is thought to originate from the basal coil and to provide the largest negative deflection in the normal EcochG at high sound intensities; n_2 is much smaller and originates from further up the cochlea. In basal turn damage, n_2 may become relatively larger due to the disappearance of n_1). In two (of the three) of the patients, the EcochG changes were more dramatic on the occasion of the second test; this may imply that the cochlea becomes more susceptible to the harmful effects of the drug towards the end of a course of treatment. Finally, it should be noted that

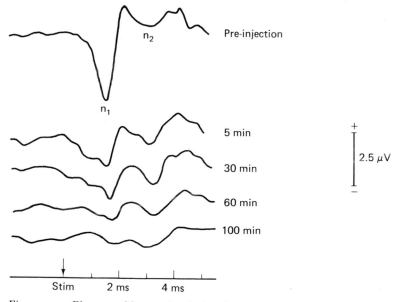

Figure 24.5   Electrocochleography during intravenous tobramycin administration, during mid-treatment. The changes shown are those in click-induced AP after 80 mg tobramycin (wideband click 95-dB hearing level). (Reproduced by permission of the authors and Editor of the *British Medical Journal*)

most of the EcochG changes occurred above everyday frequencies, i.e. above 8 kHz. The speed of the effect suggests a direct action at a site in the cochlea, involving a temporary metabolic block. What is therefore of particular interest and surprising is that, by electrocochleography, such changes could be detected without the patient realizing them and that they were temporary, and also that this fact could be recorded in this way. Electrocochleography after treatment (on the 12th day in the case shown in *Figure 24.2* and five days after the second course) showed a complete reversion to normal.

(Conversely, kanamycin, not under discussion here, is known to have its effect in the basal turn where the oxygen consumption is greatest.)

Gentamicin

This drug falls into the second group of aminoglycosides—those having a more likely effect on the vestibular neuroepithelium. The incidence of this ototoxicity is low (2.3

per cent). Moffat and Ramsden (1977) failed to find any change either in the size of the AP or CM or in the shape of the AP waveform, as compared with their tobramycin findings. It should never be forgotten that the above aminoglycoside antibiotics are seldom if ever given in patients other than when they are desperately ill. Certain aids to prescribing in the form of a nomogram and a digital computer to match the dose according to the individual patient (Mawer *et al.*, 1974) may be found helpful.

Erythromycin

Erythromycin would not generally be regarded as ototoxic but six cases have been recorded with certain common and therefore interesting features. Erythromycin works by inhibiting protein synthesis, particularly of the highly polymerized homopeptides. There are no reports of the drug affecting other parts of the nervous system. All developed a sensorineural hearing loss, but of the six cases, five received the drug intravenously as erythromycin lactobionate—in all six, the deafness was transient. Another patient treated with erythromycin gluceptate intravenously failed to develop any sensorineural hearing loss. All those developing the deafness were females, and the significant change of the acid radical and its temporary malfunction of the cochlea remains unclear (Karmody and Weinstein, 1977).

DIURETICS

Ethacrynic acid

It is no surprise that this drug which is used as a diuretic, is administered as one form of treatment for renal failure. It is an unsaturated ketone derivative of aryloxacetic acid; after intravenous injection, one third is excreted by the liver in the bile, and two thirds by the kidney. The drug's ototoxicity is thought to be due to a cystine metabolite and the conjugation of the drug probably in the liver would explain its toxicity in the cochlea.

Most cases of ototoxicity occur either when ethacrynic acid is given in patients with renal disease, or intravenously. It is rare after oral administration in normal doses in those without renal disease. The sensorineural hearing loss may be permanent or temporary and this will depend upon the above factors.

Temporal bone findings showed changes in the stria vascularis, the semicircular canals and the saccule (Matz, Beal and Krames, 1969; Matz, 1976). In this case, the hearing loss was bilateral and occurred 20 min after an intravenous injection of 50 mg of the drug (the patient had also received 18 g of neomycin orally in seven days before this). It is perhaps important to add that a study on guinea-pigs, in which the stria vascularis has been examined using the scanning electron microscope, showed a different pattern. Instead of the human findings, they found large intercellular spaces in the intermediate region of the stria due to acute separation of these cells rather than atrophy (Horn, Langley and Gates, 1977).

Frusemide (Furosemide)

Frusemide acts mainly on the distal convoluted tubule and loop of Henle of the kidney. Although clinically dissimilar, the pharmacological action of frusemide is not unlike that of ethacrynic acid. Both transient and permanent deafness have been noted following the use of frusemide. Experimental studies in animals show identical results to those of ethacrynic acid and produce changes in the stria vascularis.

The types of case are also similar—they are patients with poor renal function on dialysis or after transplantation. Intravenous use also appears to be more dangerous. With frusemide the onset of deafness appears insidious and gradually progresses up to six months after the suspected administration. The audiograms show a flat, slightly sloping sensorineural loss in almost all cases with poorer than expected speech discrimination scores. In the six cases reported by Quick and Hoppe (1975) five were children.

Sudden deafness has also been produced after 240 mg intravenously on two consecutive days; the patient had a total permanent deafness in one ear and a severe loss in the other which improved over six weeks (Lloyd-Mostyn and Lord, 1971). The drug had been given for oliguria (urea 8mg/100ml). In another case, 500 mg was given as a single dose to a patient with chronic renal failure; sudden hearing loss was noted but returned to normal in 4 h. The same pattern occurred the next day when the dose was repeated! (Venkateswaran, 1971).

DEPOPROGESTERONE

Oral contraception is in widespread use by women all over the world, but it seems that there are only three reported cases of sudden deafness, all of which are presumed to be 'thrombotic', i.e. vascular. Sellars (1971) reported a case following the intramuscular injection of depoprogesterone (150 mg); the deafness developed in one ear, seven days later together with tinnitus and vertigo. She had previously taken Norgestryl (ethinyl oestradiol) for three months earlier the same year and this had produced dizziness and she was then changed to Lynestrenol (methoxy-ethinyl-oestradiol) for one month which also produced dizziness. After the depoprogesterone she became totally deaf with depressed labyrinthine function.

Gonzales, Istre and Rubin (1968) reported two cases, both considered to be cochlear losses in whom the labyrinthine caloric responses were reduced. The first developed a unilateral loss on norethindrone with mestranol (2 mg daily after three months) and had partial recovery (after treatment) of the hearing loss which was thought to lie in the end-organ; the second, after taking Ortho-novum for two years. The pill was discontinued because of feelings of dizziness. Four days later she had an abrupt hearing loss (which was associated with withdrawal bleeding). She had a mild loss on one side and an almost complete loss on the other; the former returned to normal and a moderate loss remained on the latter (no treatment was given).

PROPYLTHIOURACIL

A single case is on record of a young girl who developed hyperthyroidism with a diffuse goitre. She received propylthiouracil for ten months before complaining of tinnitus and a fluctuating hearing loss in the left ear (cochlea). After discontinuing medication, she underwent a subtotal thyroidectomy followed by a complete return of the hearing to normal after two weeks, but the mild tinnitus persisted (Smith and Spaulding, 1972). (Hypersensitivity to iodine, thiouracil and propylthiouracil have all been reported as causing PAN; each preparation was followed by pyrexia soon after administration; none showed any evidence or complaints of deafness.)

MARIJUANA *(Cannabis sativa L.)*

Marijuana minimally affects the sensory acuity (Caldwell *et al.*, 1969) but in chronic users significantly changes vestibular functions (Spector, 1974). The first only occurs whilst under the influence of the drug, and so far there is no evidence that either produces a long-term effect.

CARBON MONOXIDE INTOXICATION

It will be a considerable surprise to most otolaryngologists to learn that probably more than 300 cases of hearing loss from carbon monoxide intoxication are on record. The gas by its combination with haemoglobin to form carboxyhaemoglobin may thereby deprive vital organs of oxygen. It is little wonder, therefore, that this may affect the inner ear, causing hearing loss, tinnitus, nystagmus and ataxia. The vestibular impairment is considered to be directly related to the duration of exposure, but there is argument as to whether the predominant lesion is central or peripheral. The intoxication may be chronic or acute. Chronic intoxication usually results in a permanent, symmetrical, high-frequency hearing loss. In one series, no less than 78 per cent of 263 patients were affected and only 27 per cent showed slight improvement (Lumio, 1948).

Acute intoxication is much less common and hearing loss is quite unpredictable, though when it occurs, some improvement may be expected; it is usually bilateral and may be asymmetric. U-shaped audiograms have also been reported (Baker and Lilly, 1977). Post-mortem histological evidence of carbon monoxide victims has shown haemorrhage and cellular degeneration in the cochlear nuclei, vestibular nuclei, spiral ganglion and in various parts of the cochlea itself.

VACCINATION

Sudden deafness following vaccination has now been reported in at least nine cases. These have recently been collected and analysed as a group (Mair and Elverland, 1977). The majority of these cases (eight) have occurred following the administration of tetanus antitoxin but also one following tetanus toxoid. The deafness occurred from two days after the toxoid, up to ten days. In all but three cases, the vaccine was given as a prophylaxis or re-vaccination, not as treatment. The sensorineural deafness appears to affect the cochlear nerve and only two cases have subsequently improved. Peripheral neuropathies following administration of antitetanus serum and tetanus toxoid are well documented. Hearing loss has also been reported following vaccination for whooping cough (including a booster), rabies injections, and possibly subsequent re-vaccination against smallpox. No case has been reported following diphtheria vaccination or oral polio immunization (*see* Infectious Mononucleosis). These cases are presumed to be due to either a local hypersensitivity or antigen–antibody reaction and it is highly likely that many other cases have gone unnoticed or unreported. Even one reported case seems to have been caused by a bee sting! A case is also reported of a young doctor who received 'orthobiotic serum'; the mode, the contents and the reason are not stated. It produced sudden deafness; four days later he received an intravenous injection of sodium nicotinate with return of hearing to normal in 3 h (Moulonguet and Bouche, 1951).

Skeletal system and otic capsule

Cochlear otosclerosis, Paget's disease (osteitis deformans), metastic carcinoma, and relapsing polychrondritis may all rarely cause sudden cochlear hearing loss. They are discussed in other chapters and are only mentioned here for completeness.

Retrocochlear (eighth nerve) and central nervous system

Meningitis

Leptomeningitis still causes a few cases of sudden deafness—it is typically bilateral, and total or subtotal. It may occur as a complication of acute otitis media, and is usually pneumococcal in origin. Tuberculous menigitis may still rarely be encountered and the cranial nerves may still be involved by the arachnoiditis and adhesions in spite of modern therapy; as in other bacterial forms of meningitis both the cochlear and vestibular nerves may be affected (McCabe, 1975).

Acute meningovascular syphilis still occurs and may present to the otologist.

Viral disease may also cause meningitis, although it is infrequently the cause of sudden deafness. Morrison (1978) has reported a case of mumps meningitis causing unilateral deafness in a 14 year old boy; steroid therapy was unhelpful and there was no subsequent recovery.

Disseminated sclerosis

Sudden deafness, usually bilateral, is well documented in disseminated sclerosis but it is more commonly seen in the well-established case. It is uncommon for it to be the presenting symptom but it can and does occur, as a retrocochlear type loss. Episodes of sudden vestibular failure are a more common form of presentation and are recorded in 5 per cent of cases.

The deafness is usually of a moderate low-tone transitory type with vestibular involvement. It is important to realize that it may improve spontaneously and not to attribute this to any steroid therapy! Conversely, the otologist can reassure the patient with known disseminated sclerosis that the hearing will usually improve. As there is no advantage at this time in making a more definite diagnosis, lumbar puncture is unnecessary but other causes should be excluded as already outlined. The CSF may show a rise in immunoglobulin IgG but this has not so far been related to any particular stage in the disease and a failure to find a raised level does not by any means eliminate the diagnosis. What can be said is that a level above 15 per cent, makes the diagnosis likely and above 25 per cent above normal very probable. (The CSF IgG however may also be raised in neurosyphilis, carcinomatous meningitis, connective tissue disorders, Guillan–Barré syndrome and some encephalitides.) The question which needs to be asked prior to lumbar puncture is to what practical use the results, even if positive, will be put. From a topographical point of view, the lesion is considered to be distal to the cochlear nuclei in disseminated sclerosis, but central to the neurilemmal–neuroglial junction (Dix, 1965).

From a diagnostic viewpoint, the only other test within the ambit of the otologist is the heat test. In the first instance the body temperature is raised, ideally by using a heat cradle (Jestico and Ellis, 1976). Electronystagmography allows the nystagmus to be readily seen and recorded. In disseminated sclerosis, this may be increased in frequency and amplitude in those in whom it is already present, or provoked in the suspected case. The nystagmus which is the central type, is characteristically multidirectional and is not enhanced by loss of fixation. This induced 'deterioration' in the clinical state is, it should be emphasized, merely transient.

Sarcoidosis

Sarcoidosis in otolaryngological practice is uncommon but when it occurs it is usually observed involving the parotid gland and facial nerve, nasal cavity and larynx. The nervous system is affected in only 5 per cent of cases though this rises to 50 per cent if uveo–parotid fever is present. Any of the cranial nerves may be involved but the facial is the most common. Mucous membrane lesions occur in approximately 2 per cent of all sarcoid patients and in the tonsil and larynx 2.4 and 1.4 per cent respectively. No case of sarcoidosis has yet been described which is confined only to the nervous system but occasionally a case may present first to the otolaryngologist and he should be aware of such a possibility (Hybels and Rice, 1976).

Twenty-nine cases of sarcoidosis have been reported affecting the ear and the mechanism of the deafness is undecided. The deafness may be unilateral or bilateral, minimal to profound, and there is no characteristic audiometric pattern; it may be progressive or fluctuant. Vertigo and tinnitus may occur and vestibular function may be diminished or abolished.

No patient has come to post mortem for temporal bone study but patients with deafness and vertigo have been shown to have adhesive arachnoiditis of the posterior fossa. In the 28 patients reviewed by Kane (1976), 80 per cent showed eye changes and 40 per cent had facial nerve palsies—one third of these were bilateral; 20 per cent were seen to have parotid swelling. The trigeminal nerve may be involved in its sensory distribution. Treatment is by steroids in substantial dosage, e.g. prednisolone 60 mg daily.

Vogt–Koyanagi–Harada syndrome

In 1926, Harada described what he believed to be a distinct entity comprising bilateral detachment of the retina, uveitis, mild meningeal irritation and 'dysacousia'. It is now generally considered that this 'disease' forms part of the now combined syndrome. Vogt in 1906, noted the association between bilateral uveitis, alopecia, vitiligo, poliosis (whitening of the hair) and 'dysacousia'. (Koyanagi described his variant in 1929— this brought the vitiligo and the deafness together.) Most of the reported cases have occurred in people of pigmented race. The principle feature is the prolonged bilateral uveitis, causing blindness. The hearing loss develops at or near the time the blindness occurs; it is also usually bilateral, of varying degree, frequently associated with tinnitus and vertigo. The ear symptoms begin to improve after 1–3 weeks as the tinnitus and vertigo subside, gradually returning to normal. Vision often returns to normal in 2–6 months but glaucoma and cataract may continue as complications. The vitiligo, poliosis and alopecia usually appear when the uveitis begins to improve. Rosen (1945) reported one case and reviewed those then in the literature—a total of 45; Maxwell has reported another (1963). Schuknecht (1974) notes that ordinarily three stages may be recognized in the disease: the meningeal, the ophthalmic and the convalescent. The meningeal stage is present in at least 50 per cent of the patients and may last from 2–4 weeks. The hearing loss may occasionally be unilateral and does not always recover. The cause remains unknown.

Xeroderma pigmentosa

This skin disorder may present to otolaryngologists either because of facial neoplasia or deafness. Whilst the latter has been recognized for many years as part of the neurological component of this disease, very little attention has been paid to it. The condition is inherited as a Mendelian recessive characteristic but the causes which initiate the neurological abnormalities or the malignant changes in the skin, remain unexplained.

The hearing loss is of the sensorineural type and is usually accompanied by other progressive neurological abnormalities. The deafness seems most likely to be due to a systemic degeneration involving the higher auditory pathways. Occasionally, there may be no skin involvement in this condition (Longridge, 1976).

Tumours

ACOUSTIC NEUROMA

Few would regard this as a common tumour and in relation to the vast number of cases of all forms of unilateral sensorineural hearing loss investigated in clinics, the number of confirmed cases is infinitesimal. However, its clinical interest makes every clinician feel this effort to be well worthwhile and the satisfactory surgical removal rewarding thereby entirely vindicating the investigative time involved. Those who see these tumours but infrequently or rarely, will be surprised to learn that they may present as sudden deafness. It is of the greatest importance that this should be thoroughly understood and, even though the deafness may no longer seem worth treating, it is always worth investigating as thoroughly as circumstances allow.

It is interesting to note that Cushing in 1914 mentioned that two cases had sudden hearing loss as a manifestation of cerebello–pontine angle tumour, but it was not described as the presenting symptom in the English literature until 1956 by Hallberg (*see also* Hallberg, Vihlein and Siekert, 1959). In addition, Edwards and Paterson (1951) mentioned five patients whose hearing loss was described as abrupt in their review of 157 cases. Higgs (1973) reported that 10 per cent in his series of 44 patients presented with sudden deafness. Morrison (1975) showed that no less than 17 per cent of his patients presented in this way. Conversely, in the series of more than 1200 cases of sudden deafness reported by Shaia and Sheehy (1976) almost 1 per cent had an acoustic tumour. They found nothing to distinguish these cases from the group as a whole, other than the fact that 50 per cent had a profound or total loss of hearing; 70 per cent had a reduced vestibular response and all had an enlarged internal auditory canal.

Many clinicians will remember the days when tumours were seldom seen in their early stages, but now, when improved diagnostic facilities allow much greater numbers to be diagnosed, the specialist otologist recognizes that many cases are successfully brought to surgery on what is initially the slenderest of investigative evidence. Experience gradually raises the index of suspicion. Conversely, in the 16 cases who presented with sudden idiopathic deafness reported by Morrison (1975) and who proceeded to advanced meatal studies, five were shown to have slight enlargement of the internal meatus but no tumour! More recently, he has found three cases (out of 178) with fluctuant hearing loss (Morrison, 1979). It should also be noted that steroid therapy in acoustic neuromas may result in a slight improvement.

Besides acoustic neuroma, other 'tumours' of the petrous bone or posterior cranial fossa must be borne in mind, including cysts and so-called primary cholesteatoma.

CARCINOMATOUS NEUROPATHY

The highest incidence of this condition has been found in patients with carcinoma of the lung, ovary and stomach, and lowest in the rectum, cervix and uterus. Other malignant diseases may also have an associated involvement—progressive multifocal leuco-encephalopathy is linked with Hodgkin's disease, lymphosarcoma and some other reticuloses. There is also an unusual form of encephalomyelitis nearly always associated with oat-cell bronchial carcinoma (Henson, 1970). Peripheral neuropathy caused by malignant disease ranks second to the Guillan–Barré syndrome. Conversely, unexplained peripheral neuropathy should be the signal to search for malignant disease.

No particular association with either branch of the eighth nerve has so far been shown and whilst sudden deafness may occur, it is obviously of no more than academic interest. Hearing loss has been reported in carcinomatous meningitis and five such cases have been seen in which the hearing loss was the presenting symptom (Alberts and Terrence, 1978).

Central deafness

'Central' deafness may be unilateral or bilateral but it is the latter type that seems to yield the most helpful information so far. It should be stressed that cases are rare, autopsy reports are few and that there is no uniform pattern of hearing loss. However, certain features appear to give some diagnostic and investigative guide.

Jerger *et al.* (1969) and Jerger, Lovering and Wertz, (1972) have reported two cases in great detail. Both were cases of bilateral temporal lobe damage, both males, the first aged 21 and the second 62—the first ambidextrous, using his left hand for writing but his right for eating and bowling, the second right-handed. Both experienced transient aphasia but no hearing problems after the first side (left) episode. Both reported severe hearing loss after the second (right) episode. In both, the presumed sensitivity loss had essentially recovered within three months of the second episode; both showed marked inability to recognize either single words or sentences. However, there was one significant difference and that was in their ability to localize sound; in the younger case this was impaired but not in the older. The younger had interaural imbalance in the relation between loudness and signal duration which was so marked that it prevented effective localization; in the older there was no such imbalance and localization was accurate.

The first (younger) patient had a mild receptive aphasia and some paraphasia after the first attack. After the second attack, seven months later he noticed the world had become 'strangely silent'. He had no tinnitus or vertigo and no other CNS symptoms. (Caloric tests were also normal.) After the second admission he was able to carry out pure-tone audiometry which showed sensorineural loss; Békésy audiometry however proved impossible. The patient's course was characteristic of cerebral infarction but the aetiology remained obscure. It was concluded that he had experienced occlusion of the terminal branches of the middle cerebral artery on each side at different points in time, resulting in bilateral partial cerebral hemisphere infarction, maximal in the temporal lobes, and producing the clinical picture of cortical deafness. In the second case, at his second admission, he could initially hear quite well but during the examination he lost his ability to understand speech; this returned to normal two days later. A pure-tone audiogram later that same year (two months) showed a bilateral sensorineural hearing loss of equal severity and no greater than might have been expected from a test done six and a half years before.

Angiography showed occlusion of the major middle cerebral trunk with anastomotic filling in a retrograde manner from the parieto–occipital branch of the right posterior cerebral artery.

This patient had a third and final admission, six months later for acute cerebral infarction with right hemiplegia and aphasia; he died one week later of an acute

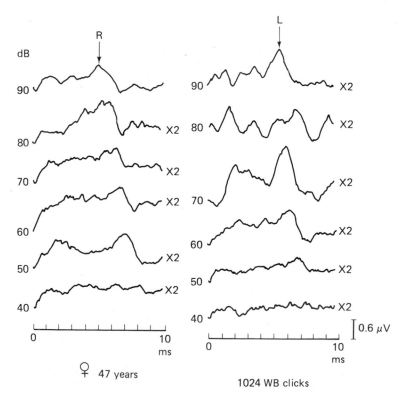

BSER

Figure 24.6 Brain-stem evoked response—shows psychonormal responses with the usual five peaks and normal latencies; the fifth peak is shown by the arrow (case of central deafness). (Reproduced by kind permission of Dr. C. J. Earl, Consultant Neurologist, Middlesex Hospital, Mr. H. A. Beagley and Mr. J. M. Graham, Nuffield Speech and Hearing Centre)

myocardial infarct. Examination of the brain revealed bilateral and symmetrical areas of softening of the posterior segments of the superior temporal gyri, these were caused by cystic infarcts; the major arteries displayed moderate atherosclerosis but there was no evidence of embolism.

More recently, Earnest, Monroe and Yarnell (1977) have reported a case of a man who subsequently had bilateral cerebral infarcts that caused a nonfluent aphasia, oral apraxia, and deafness and who at the age of 27 (left-handed) had a mitral valve prosthesis fitted and received subsequent anticoagulation. During each of the following two years he had cerebral episodes but no mention of deafness. Five years after surgery, he had multiple right-sided symptoms and evaluation of hearing confirmed that he could follow neither written nor spoken commands. The anticoagulant was temporarily discontinued. Pure-tone audiometry in this case showed apparent total deafness but acoustic impedance measurements including stapedius reflex testing were normal. Over two years the patient progressively improved but remained essentially deaf. Two and a half years after the above incidence, a CT scan showed symmetrical, well-defined, bilateral temporo–parietal, low absorption defects with mild ventricular enlargement; a further scan a year later was unchanged. The defects were considered to be due to old infarctions.

Earnest, Monroe and Yarnell expressed the view that the cortical clinical syndrome

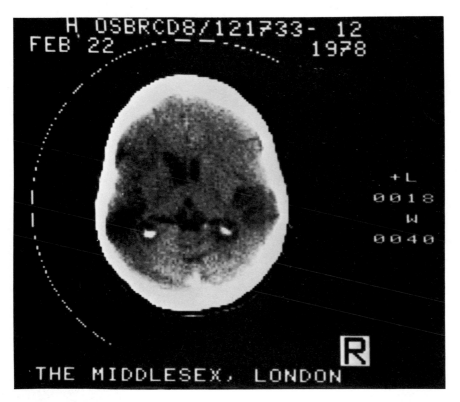

Figure 24.7 CT scan with contrast (same patient as in *Figure 24.6*), showing bilateral opacities in the temporo–parietal areas. (Reproduced by kind permission of Dr. C. J. Earl, Consultant Neurologist, Middlesex Hospital, Mr. H. A. Beagley and Mr. J. M. Graham, Nuffield Speech and Hearing Centre)

of pure word deafness in many cases is probably a less severe form of cortical deafness and is due to less extensive bilateral temporal grey matter lesions. Strictly white matter lesions may produce cases of either syndrome.

Graham (1978, personal communication) has recently carried out brain stem evoked responses (BSER) (*Figure 24.6*) on a 48 year old lady (right-handed) who three years before had a mitral valve replacement. Later that year she had a right brachial artery embolus followed six months later by an episode of dysphasia (an isotope scan at that time showed a left temporal defect). She suffered a series of epileptic fits commencing nine months later and the most recent a month prior to the BSER. At that time she showed an almost total deafness with some evidence of dysphasia. A CT scan and isotope scan showed bilateral temporal infarction and a right occipital infarct (*see Figure 24.7*). Galvanic responses were negative. No cortical ERA responses could be obtained but stapedial (acoustic) and post-auricular myogenic responses were both present. A similar diagnosis to the other cases reported has been made, i.e. bilateral temporal lobe infarction of embolic origin.

CORTICAL ENCEPHALITIS

Diffuse cortical encephalitis causes an auditory aphasia, when both temporal lobes are involved; the patients have normal pure-tone audiograms but no understanding of speech. The diagnosis is confirmed by EEG and the condition may develop over weeks or months with periods of fluctuation and acute episodes. Morrison (1975) reports three cases, all adult females, in all of whom the sudden hearing loss occurred relatively late in the disease but all made good recoveries with steroids followed by ACTH. However one has continued to have occasional episodes of auditory aphasia.

Idiopathic

Pathogenesis

There are two 'rival' theories as to the causation of the idiopathic case—viral and vascular. It has been known for so long that certain viruses, e.g. mumps, measles, rubella, cause sensorineural deafness, that the finding of a preceding 'viral' infection in many cases of sudden loss, varying in incidence from 30–40 per cent according to the author, made the association of ideas, if not of facts, irresistible (e.g. Dishoeck and Bierman, 1957). Conversely, the suddenness of onset made the analogy with similar events in the cardiovascular system equally attractive to the opposing school (e.g. Hallberg, 1956). As many of the cases occurred in patients over 40 years of age, the association looked even more tempting. Attempts have been made to reconcile these view-points, as already mentioned in the section of specific causes under 'Hypercoagulation'.

It is traditional in otology to try to match the clinical picture with the findings from the temporal bone laboratory, wherever possible. As in many other otological conditions, few patients die of their disease, so the interval between the event, in this case sudden deafness, and autopsy may be long, and reparative processes will have been at work. Alternatively, the end may come very rapidly from overwhelming disease, which in itself may complicate the histological picture. However, all this is familiar and expected by temporal bone experts. Perhaps one illustrative case may be permitted (Schuknecht, Kimura and Naufal, 1973—case 6). A 57 year old man developed left-sided Menière's disease. One year later, he experienced sudden deafness of the contralateral (right) side. He was hospitalized and treated immediately with heparin and intravenous histamine. After five days the histamine therapy was discontinued but the heparin was continued. Two days later he had severe pain in the left leg and an immediate left femoral embolectomy and left lumbar sympathectomy were performed. Two days later (i.e. nine days after the onset of sudden deafness) he died. Autopsy revealed a bilateral bronchopneumonia, thrombosis of the splenic artery, and severe endolymphatic hydrops in the left ear. The changes in the right temporal bone were considered to be compatible with a viral aetiology and the slight head cold he had felt three days before the onset of the deafness.

Only very few such temporal bones have become available (Schuknecht, Kimura and Naufal, 1973). The changes are greatest in the organ of Corti and always most severe at the basal end of the cochlea. The severity of the change varies from loss of part of the hair-cell population, to total loss of the organ. Varying degrees of atrophy (from partial to total) of the stria vascularis may be found and the tectorial membrane may be distorted, shrunken or missing. These are essentially also the findings in viral labyrinthitis, as seen in temporal bones from cases of mumps, measles and rubella. There is no apparent difference between RNA or DNA viruses e.g. measles and mumps are both RNA viruses, whilst varicella zoster virus is a DNA virus.

There are three potential routes by which a virus can gain entrance to the inner ear, a circulatory route, a meningeal route, or possibly directly from the middle ear. Initial cochlear contact is believed to be via the stria vascularis and structures bathed by endolymph when the circulatory route is involved, and via the perilymphatic system when the meningeal system is the portal (Beal, Hemenway and Lindsay, 1967; Sando *et al.*, 1977). When the route is circulatory (haematogenous) during the viraemic stage, the pathological process is limited primarily to the stria vascularis, the tectorial membrane and the organ of Corti. When the process is caused by spread of infection from encephalitis or meningoencephalitis, degeneration in the neural elements in Rosenthal's canal and the osseous spiral lamina is a prominent feature. The inflammatory process infiltrates along the nerves and vessels from the internal auditory meatus through the modiolus into the scala tympani and scala vestibuli. The cochlear duct may become secondarily dilated and degenerative changes may occur in the organ of Corti, tectorial membrane and stria vascularis (Lindsay, 1973).

Recently, Nomura and Hiraide (1976) reviewed and summarized 12 cases, adding one of their own. They reviewed the history, and the clinical and histopathological findings. They formed the opinion that in some cases the site of the lesion was the tectorial membrane and in spite of the technical difficulties associated with preserving the ante-mortem state of tissue in the temporal bone, considered that either detachment or ultrastructural pathology at the junction of the sensor hairs and the tectorial membrane should be regarded as significant—the 'roll up', shrunken, and droplet states of the membrane being the final stages of a morphological succession.

Symptomatology

'Sudden hearing loss is a symptom in search of a diagnosis'. (Simmons, 1973). It will be readily apparent that many of the causes of sudden hearing loss are in themselves rare. Many of them are discussed in other chapters. The preceding section is devoted to excluding the specific causes, thereby leaving the so-called 'idiopathic' losses—still the largest single group and constituting the everyday case—for treatment according to 'site-of-loss'.

For the purist, 'sudden' hearing loss means an instantaneous event; 'rapid' hearing loss means deafness occurring over a short period of time, e.g. hours. If the loss subsequently improves, either spontaneously or as a result of treatment, then some would label this 'fluctuant'! It should be appreciated that cases may present in any of these ways and the distinction between them from a diagnostic viewpoint is frequently somewhat artificial. It will become apparent that such divisions should not be interpreted too rigidly.

AGE AND SEX DISTRIBUTION

In the 1220 cases reported by Shaia and Sheehy (1976) age at onset of the symptoms was as follows:

Under 30	13 per cent
30–39	13 per cent
40–49	21 per cent
50–59	22 per cent
60–69	18 per cent
70 years +	13 per cent

Three-quarters of the patients therefore were over the age of 40, but 1.4 per cent dated the onset of their sudden hearing loss below the age of ten. Four per cent had a sudden bilateral loss, and a half of these were simultaneous. Only a quarter of the 1220 patients were seen within one month of onset. As all series show that the best results are obtained in those receiving their treatment within 15 days of onset, it will be immediately appreciated how vast is the wastage of untreated cases. In all series, the sex distribution is approximately equal at all age groups.

PRECIPITATING FACTORS

Many published series state an incidence of a preceding viral infection in 30–40 per cent. Almost every virus has been reported or implicated as a causative factor in a proportion of these cases, but certain facts should be considered before such an aetiology is too readily accepted.

The viruses which have been suggested as causing sudden hearing loss may be divided into three groups. The first of these consists of viruses causing acute respiratory diseases such as influenza, para-influenza and rhinoviruses. Such infections are very common. Adults suffer on average four to five respiratory infections a year, so that about a third of any group of adults will give a history of a respiratory infection within the preceding four weeks. There is no confirmed evidence of a seasonal incidence as might be expected for the respiratory viruses and none following an epidemic such as might be expected after influenza. Although a high incidence might be expected in children because they sustain more infections than adults none such has been reported (Rowson, Hinchcliffe and Gamble, 1976).

The second group includes poliovirus, Coxsackie virus, rubella, Epstein–Barr virus, adenovirus Type 3 and herpes simplex virus. Following such infections, occasional cases of sudden hearing loss have been reported, but they are very uncommon. The third group comprises three viruses—mumps, measles and varicella zoster, all of which are known to produce sudden deafness.

OTHER SYMPTOMS

Many patients with sudden hearing loss can state the day, date and time that it occurred, or that they awoke with it. It is a dramatic, well-remembered event. *Pain* or a feeling of pressure may be present in the affected ear but so far no particular prognostic significance has been found to be attached to this. *Tinnitus* occurs in approximately 80 per cent of cases usually starting with, and alarmingly as, the deafness. In approximately 25 per cent the tinnitus may precede the deafness by minutes or hours, very occasionaly by some days. *Vertigo* is commonest in those with a probable vascular aetiology. It carries a poorer prognosis for hearing recovery, whilst tinnitus apparently does not affect the outcome.

In the series of Shaia and Sheehy (1976), 60 per cent had no vestibular symptoms, 22 per cent had them initially, and 18 per cent persistently.

Vertigo of any duration associated with the hearing loss is an indication to investigate the patient very thoroughly, and the possibility of an acoustic neuroma should never completely leave the mind.

There is a series of reports of patients who after developing sudden deafness, subsequently go on to develop episodic vertigo characteristic of endolymphatic hydrops. Wolfson and Leiberman (1975) recorded five such cases. The interval in their cases ranges from 6–10 years. After long observation, destructive labyrinthectomy was carried out with complete relief of the vertigo. Of their five cases, four were young when the vertigo presented; one 10 years, two aged 11, and one 16 (the fifth was 59). The children had become suddenly deaf in early childhood, one from the age of 3, one from 4 and one from 10; two cases were caused by mumps. Nadol, Weiss and Parker (1975) reported 12 cases, with vertigo developing from 1–68 years later! They found the long interval particularly puzzling. Few of the 12 had any coincidental vestibular symptoms at the time of onset of the sudden deafness. Again labyrinthectomy was curative. Both groups of authors question whether the cause could be Menière's disease. Wolfson and Leiberman argue against this, on the grounds that total hearing loss as the initial symptom in Menière's disease is extremely rare, and that as four of their five patients developed the vertigo in childhood, Menière's disease is again rare, though not unknown, in such an age group. Nadol, Weiss and Parker on the other hand are opposed to the possibility of two diagnoses, preferring a single aetiology of endolymphatic hydrops and regarding this as yet another variant.

Investigation of sudden or fluctuant sensorineural hearing loss may require:

Haematology
Haemoglobin, full blood count, ESR, prothrombin time
Paul Bunnell screening test and titre
(Blood for viral studies—repeat specimen will be required after 2–3 weeks to assess change in titre)

Syphilis serology (full—including FTA (Abs) and TPHA)

Sickle-cell test (if appropriate and Hb electrophoresis)

Fasting serum lipids (after 12–14 h complete fast and $\frac{3}{4}$ h total body rest; no stasis during blood withdrawal, i.e. no sphygmomanometer or other occluding cuff)

Glucose tolerance test
(Serum electrolytes including urea, calcium, phosphorus, phosphate, uric acid etc.)

Electrocardiogram
Radiology
Chest x-ray
Mastoids (plain films)
Internal auditory meatus (tomography, preferably by hypocycloidal poly-tomography)
CT scan ('EMISCAN')
Myodil cisternography

Audiometry
Pure-tone audiogram

Tone decay test (Carhart)

Speech audiometry

Acoustic impedance measurements including stapedial reflex thresholds.

Electrocochleography

Lumbar Puncture—for routine CSF examination, serology, Lange curve and immunoglobulins

It must be remembered that when a patient with sudden hearing loss presents, within the early stages, i.e. under 15 days, everyone carrying out investigations wants to help simultaneously. At the receiving end of this investigative enthusiasm and energy, lies a patient! Many of these investigations are time-consuming (e.g. glucose tolerance tests) and as they yield the least urgent information they should be left until last. Those conditions encompassed by the taking of blood on a rested, fasted patient can all be accomplished in a single venepuncture the morning after admission. Lumbar puncture if considered necessary (which is seldom now the case) should be left until last, as after this the patient may have much discomfort in the back and the head. To follow this with any procedure requiring mobility, mental attention and cooperation or the maintenance of a prolonged position is cruel.

AUDIOMETRY
A patient with sudden hearing loss needs first the simplest tests, of pure-tone thresholds, acoustic impedance measurements (except in cases of suspected oval or round window rupture or perilymphatic fistula); stapedial (acoustic) reflex thresholds and tone decay (e.g. Carhart). Tests of longer duration can be more conveniently carried out later on. It should be remembered that tones above 85 dB can cause temporary threshold shift even in a normal ear. In an already damaged cochlea the possibility of further damage by test tones at high intensities is very real (Simmons, 1973).

From the simple pure-tone test two most interesting prognostic factors have been reported (Mattox and Simmons, 1977). First, the less obvious, is the significance of the test frequency of 8 kHz, and second is the shape of the audiogram. In their series they noted that all but one patient with an upward-sloping audiogram had complete or good recovery. Conversely all but two patients with a severe downward slope had a fair or poor recovery. Flat and less severe down-sloping patterns fell between the two extremes. Expressed in another way, if the threshold loss, going from the apex to the base of the cochlea was either improving or stable at 8 kHz, the prognosis for a good or complete recovery was 78 per cent. If there was no hearing at 8 kHz, regardless of the hearing at other frequencies, the same prognosis was only 29 per cent. Recovery was always better at the apex of the cochlea, than at the base. This seemed independent of the contour or the severity of the loss on the initial threshold audiogram. It should be remembered that these findings were noted on *untreated* patients.

In the series reported by Shaia and Sheehy (1976) 12 per cent showed a low-tone loss, 32 per cent a flat loss and 31 per cent a high-tone loss. However 25 per cent showed a profound or total loss. It is this last group which deserves special mention and again they may be sub-divided—first into those with a severe loss and second those with a total loss.

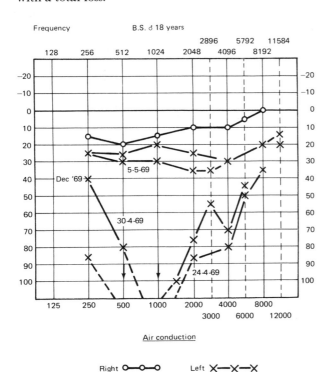

Figure 24.8 Retrocochlear lesion. The pure-tone audiogram shows the low level of hearing in the left ear when first seen on 24-4-69 and the improvement after treatment at one week, at two weeks, and the final result at eight months. (Reproduced by kind permission of the Editor of the *British Journal of Hospital Medicine*)

In the same series, of the ten patients who were found to have acoustic tumours, five had a total loss. Those with severe losses may show some hearing at both low and high frequencies but none in the mid-range (*see Figure 24.8*).

Audiometry in sudden hearing loss serves two purposes—first, to assess the day-to-day level of the loss by the level of the pure-tone threshold, and second to determine the site of the lesion. The site is of particular importance in determining the treatment.

Many of the patients showing a retrocochlear pattern have the contour shown in *Figure 24.8* and frequently they will be in the younger age group, i.e. below 40.

In the group with a total loss, the primary audiometric tests will be of no avail in helping the worried clinician or patient, but electrocochleography has a useful part to play. Graham *et al.* (1978), used transtympanic electrocochleography (EcochG) to test 70 patients with sudden hearing loss. Of particular interest are the 24 per cent where threshold audiometry was impossible. Of these 17 patients, a result was obtained, indicating a retrocochlear pattern in seven. In the remaining ten patients, neither a cochlear microphonic (CM) nor an action potential (AP) was found, suggesting a cochlear loss, with or without retrocochlear involvement. In two of these patients, the promontory electrode was used to provide direct stimulation to the cochlea and this evoked a subjective sensation of sound, suggesting that the cochlear nerve was intact to some extent (House and Brackmann, 1974; Graham and Hazell, 1977).

A study by Nishida, Kumagami and Dohi (1976) attempted to use electrocochleographic findings as a prognostic guide. However they did not compare their results with any conventional audiometric pattern and indeed these are not mentioned. The cochlear microphonic was not recorded at any stage in the study and the results are similar to those found in Menière's disease.

VESTIBULAR TESTS

These have a particular place in those patients with sudden hearing loss which has been accompanied by vertigo but in most instances such tests can be deferred until all the necessary audiometric tests have been completed, and the patient's morale is beginning to improve. They are never urgent.

Electronystagmography is often helpful; it is of special benefit in diagnosing vertebro–basilar insufficiency or other possible vascular causes of positional nystagmus.

Management

It has been stated earlier that at least two prognostic factors are known—the shape of the audiogram with involvement at 8 kHz, and the presence of vertigo. Almost every conceivable treatment has been given and two things are common to all of the reports—first that the regimes, whether of a single preparation or a complicated sequence of therapies, were all successful, and second that better results were obtained if started within 15 days of the onset of the hearing loss. The deep cynicism of this discussion may gladden those who have hitherto thrown up their hands and told their patients that nothing can be done, but such an attitude will not only lead to many cases of neglected diagnosis but also to dismissal of many treatable patients. There are many excellent reviews (Saunders, 1972) and many regimes from which to choose.

The following is intended as a guide—those whose investigations have otherwise been negative and are found to have a purely cochlear (sensory) type of loss should have daily pure-tone threshold audiometry under identical test conditions. Speech audiometry and discrimination scores should also be carried out daily. Those who fail to show spontaneous improvement under observation by the tenth or twelfth day, should be offered treatment. Conventional therapy is to give vasodilators but their action on the microvasculature of the cochlea is unproven. Betahistine dihydrochloride has been shown in animals to cause a significant increase in capillary flow in the inner ear by relaxing the precapillary sphincters in this region. This causes an increase in the flow in the stria vascularis. The drug is widely advocated in the treatment of Menière's disease. More recently Gibson, Ramsden and Moffat (1977) administered naftidrofuryl intravenously (40 mg) to patients with suspected Menière's disease, during investigation by transtympanic electrocochleography. They found an increase in the cochlear microphonic within 2 min, reaching maximum at 10 min. The summating potential (SP) decreased gradually and reached a minimum after approximately 20 min. It should be added that this has not been a consistent finding, nor has a similar investigation been carried out on patients with sudden hearing loss.

Among the many proposed or associated aetiological factors in producing sudden deafness, is hypercoagulability of the blood. Because of this alleged association, low molecular weight dextran by intravenous infusion has been recommended. This preparation (Rheomacrodex) with a molecular weight of 40 000 is available as a 10 per cent solution either in 5 per cent dextrose or in normal saline. It is contraindicated in patients with cardiac failure and bleeding disorders (Gluckman, Quenelle and Thomas, 1976). This can be combined with oral vasodilator therapy but in the author's hands has been disappointing and discontinued.

Oral vasodilator drugs are usually given on an empty stomach to promote maximum and rapid absorption. The dose should be sufficient to maintain the flushing effect without side effects. They should be administered for one month in the first instance and if they appear to have been helpful, should be continued for a total of three months. There are no clinical trials of such drugs in this condition, but the patient's psychology may be improved by the facial flushing and the satisfaction that the clinician is trying. It may be appropriate here to add the reminder that nicotinic acid also reduces the blood cholesterol. If an intravenous histamine regime is preferred a solution of 2.75 mg in 250 ml saline is given intravenously on three consecutive days after a full meal at the rate 50–60 drops/min; time for administration 60–90 min (Shaia and Sheehy, 1976). Alternatively, by using a serial dilution intracutaneous test for histamine, the optimum dose may be determined for each individual as suggested for Menière's disease (Wilson, 1973).

A mode of treatment which must also be mentioned when considering vasodilatation is stellate ganglion block. However, as might be expected with a treatment designed to produce an immediate response, and in common with all other similar therapies, no benefit has been reported after two weeks from the onset of sudden deafness.

Those who have favoured the viral aetiology have frequently advocated the use of steroids. It has been the experience of Morrison and Booth (1970), and remains so, that they are the treatment of choice when the loss is retrocochlear and are the only effective treatment in the severe case of this type. Recently it has been suggested by Graham *et al.* (1978) that promontory stimulation might assist in the selection of patients with retrocochlear loss. They have proposed that if stimulation remains positive seven days after the onset, degeneration has not occurred in the nerve and that there is reasonable hope of recovery. This interesting proposal is certainly worthy of further study. Steroids in all forms have been used and selection should probably depend on personal experience. They are used in the synthetic form which means that oral administration is easily possible for out-patients. Corticotrophin as ACTH gel necessitates intramuscular injections (Schiff and Brown, 1975).

For clinicians without an established or familiar scheme, prednisone may be recommended—60 mg on the first day in divided doses (every 6 h), 50 mg on the second day, 40 mg daily for three days, 30 mg daily for three days and then the regime may be tailed off, so that the patient ends medication in approximately three weeks.

ANTICOAGULANTS

Many patients with the cochlear pattern of loss are in the older age groups. Their cardiovascular system should be properly assessed and appropriate treatment prescribed; only then should anticoagulants be considered. It should be remembered that they will require to be maintained regularly and this must be impressed upon the patients so they do not default.

Heparin may be chosen in the initial stages, and it may be appropriate to add that this also has an effect in reducing the serum lipid, by stimulating lipoprotein lipase formation. (It also binds with histamine.)

VITAMINS

These are frequently given either singly, e.g. niacin, or in widely varying combinations. Lipoflavanoid probably remains the most favoured. Perhaps the most surprising result is that reported by Shaia and Sheehy (1976), that even three months after the onset of sudden hearing loss they were able to report an improvement in 10 per cent of patients on their histamine regime. Sadly this has not been the experience of others, with any other form of treatment. It is more usual at that late stage only to investigate the patients, to exclude the possibility of other disease and to reassure them if none is found.

References

Afifi, A. M. and Tawfeek, S. (1971). *Journal of Laryngology*, **85**, 275

Alberts, M. C. and Terrence, C. F. (1978). *Journal of Laryngology*, **92**, 233

Alport, A. C. (1927). *British medical Journal*, **1**, 504

Angelborg, C., Klockhoff, I. and Stahle (1977). *Scandinavian Audiology*, **6**, 143

Arenberg, I. K., Allen, G. W. and DeBoer, A. (1972). *Journal of Laryngology*, **86**, 73

Baker, S. R. and Lilly, D. J. (1977). *Annals of Otology*, **86**, 323

Ballantyne, J. C. (1976).'Ototoxic Drugs'. In *Scientific Foundations of Otolaryngology*, p. 849. Ed. by R. Hinchcliffe and D. Harrison, London; Heinemann

Beal, D. D., Hemenway, W. G. and Lindsay, J. R. (1967). *Archives of Otolaryngology*, **85**, 591

Beckman, H. and Trotsky, M. B. (1970). *Annals of Otology*, **91**, 179

Bellucci, R. J., Grobeisen, B. and Sah, B. C. (1974). *Bulletin of the New York Academy of Medicine*, **50**, 672

Berkowitz, W. P. and Stroud. M. H. (1973). *Laryngoscope*, **83**, 1084

Bhatia, P. L., Gupta, O. P., Agrawal, M. K. and Mishr, S. K. (1977). *Laryngoscope*, **87**, 2082

Blackley, B., Friedmann, I. and Wright, I. (1967). *Acta Otolaryngologica*, **63**, 533

Blatt, I. M. and Lawrence, M. (1961). *Archives of Otolaryngology*, **73**, 639

Booth, J. B. (1977). *Proceedings of the Royal Society of Medicine*, **70**, 642

Bordley, J. E. and Kapur, Y. P. (1977). *Archives of Otolaryngology*, **103**, 162

Boyd, G. G. (1957). *Archives of Otolaryngology*, **65**, 24

Brown, H. A. and Woolner, L. B. (1960). *Annals of Otology*, **69**, 810

Byl, F. M. (1977). *Laryngoscope*, **87**, 817

Caldwell, D. F., Myers, S. A., Domino, F. F. and Merriam, P. E. (1969). *Perceptual and Motor Skills*, **29**, 755

Chait, A. (1974). *Journal of clinical Pathology*, **26** (Suppl. 5) 68

Cody, D. T. R. and Williams, H. L. (1960). *Laryngoscope*, **70**, 447

Cogan, D. G. (1945). *Archives of Ophthalmology*, **33**, 144

Coyle, J. T., Frank, P. E., Leonard, A. L. and Weiner, A. (1961). *Archives of Ophthalmology*, **4**, 75

Crawford, W. J. (1957). *Pennsylvanian medical Journal*, **60**, 835

Darougar, S., John, A. C., Viswalingam, M., Cornell, L. and Jones, B. R. (1978). *British Journal of Ophthalmology*, in press

Davis, E. C. and Nilo, E. R. (1965). *Laryngoscope*, **75**, 1847

Davis, H., Morgan, C. T., Hawkins, J. E., Galambos, R. and Smith, F. W. (1952). *Acta Otolaryngologica* (Suppl.), **88**

Dawes, J. D. K. and Watson, R. T. (1978). *Journal of Laryngology*, **92**, 83

Densert, O., Rausing, A. and Toremalm, N. G. (1969). *Archives of Otolaryngology*, **89**, 826

Dias, A. (1966). *Journal of Laryngology*, **80**, 276

Dietzel, K. (1964). *International Symposium Uben. Diabetes Fragen*, 1–3 Oct. 1962, Berlin; Academie Berleg

Dishoeck, H. A. E. van and Bierman, Th. A. (1957). *Annals of Otology*, **66**, 963

Dix, M. R. (1965). *Journal of Laryngology*, **79**, 695

Druss, J. B. and Maybaum, J. L. (1934). *Archives of Otolaryngology*, **19**, 502

Duvall, A. J., Nelms, C. R. and Williams, H. L. (1969). *Transactions of the American Academy of Ophthalmology and Otology*, **73**, 1187

Earnest, M. P., Monroe, P. A. and Yarnell, P. R. (1977). *Neurology*, **27**, 1172

Edwards, C. H. and Paterson, J. H. (1951). *Brain*, **74**, 144

Fisher, E. R. and Hellstrom, H. R. (1961). *Archives of Pathology*, **72**, 572

Fowler, E. P. (1950). *Annals of Otology*, **59**, 980

Friedmann, I. and Bauer, F. (1973). *Journal of Laryngology*, **87**, 449

Futaki, T., Kitahara, M. and Morimoto, M. (1975). *Acta Otolaryngologica*, **79**, 419

Futaki, T., Kitahara, M. and Morimoto, M. (1977). *Acta Otolaryngologica*, **83**, 272

Gibson, W. P. R., Ramsden, R. T. and Moffat, D. A. (1977). *Journal of Laryngology*, **91**, 679

Gibson, W. P. R., Moffat, D. A. and Ramsden, R. T. (1977). *Audiology*, **16**, 389

Gluckman, J. L., Quenelle, D. J. and Thomas, J. N. (1976). *South African medical Journal*, **50**, 15

Gonzalez, G., Istre, C. and Rubin, W. (1968). *Journal of the Louisiana State medical Society*, **120**, 487

Goodhill, V. (1976). *Proceedings of the Royal Society of Medicine*, **69**, 565

Graham, J. M. and Hazell, J. W. (1977). *British Journal of Audiology*, **11**, 59

Graham, J. M., Ramsden, R. T., Gibson, W. P. R. and Moffat, D. A. (1978). *Journal of Laryngology*. **92**, 581

Gregg, J. B. and Shaeffer, J. H. (1964). *South Dakota Journal of Medicine*, **17**, 22

Gussen, R. (1974). *Journal of Laryngology*, **88**, 523

Gussen, R. (1976). *Annals of Otology*, **85**, 94

Gussen, R. (1977). *Archives of Oto-Rhino-Laryngology*, **217**, 263

Hall, C. M. and Brackmann, D. E. (1977). *Acta Otolaryngologica*, **103**, 355

Hallberg, O. E. (1956). *Laryngoscope*, **66**, 1237

Hallberg, O. E. (1957). *Journal of the American medical Association*, **165**, 1649

Hallberg, O. E., Vihlein, A. and Siekert, R. G. (1959). *Archives of Otolaryngology*, **69**, 160

Harada, E. (1926). *Acta Societatis Ophthalmologicale Japonicale*, **30**, 359

Henson, R. A. (1970). *Modern Trends in Neurology— 5*, p. 209. London; Butterworths

Herman, L. H., Carver, W. F. and Arenberg, I. K. (1977). *Archives of Otolaryngology*, **103**, 84

Higgs, W. A. (1973). *Archives of Otolaryngology*, **98**, 73

Hinchcliffe, R. (1978). Personal communication

Horn, K. L., Langley, L. R. and Gates, G. A. (1977). *Archives of Otolaryngology*, **103**, 539

House, W. F. and Brackmann, D. E. (1974). *Laryngoscope*, **84**, 2163

Hybels, R. L. and Rice, D. H. (1976). *Laryngoscope*, **86**, 1873

Ingelstedt, S., Ivarsson, A. and Tjernstrom, O. (1976). *Acta Otolaryngologica*, **82**, 368

Ironside, R. (1939). *Proceedings of the Royal Society of Medicine*, **32**, 588

Jaffe, B. F. (1967). *Archives of Otolaryngology*, **86**, 55

Jaffe, B. F. (1970). *Laryngoscope*, **80**, 788

Jaffe, B. F. (1975). *Otology Clinics of North America*, **8**, 395

Jaffe, B. F. and Penner, J. A. (1968). *Transactions of the American Academy of Ophthalmology and Otolaryngology*, **72**, 774

Jerger, J., Weikers, N. J., Sharbrough, F. W. and Jerger, S. (1969). *Acta Otolaryngologica* (Suppl.) 258

Jerger, J., Lovering, L. and Wertz, M. (1972). *Journal of Speech Hearing Disorders*, **37**, 523

Jestico, J. V. and Ellis, P. D. M. (1976). *British medical Journal*, **2**, 970

Jørgensen, M. B. (1961). *Archives of Otolaryngology*, **74**, 373

Jørgensen, M. B. and Buch, N. H. (1961). *Acta Otolaryngologica*, **53**, 350

Kane, K. (1976). *Journal of Laryngology*, **90**, 537

Karmody, C. S. and Schuknecht, H. F. (1966). *Archives of Otolaryngology*, **83**, 18

Karmondy, C. S. and Weinstein, L. (1977). *Annals of Otology*, **86**, 9

Kimura, R. and Perlman, H. B. (1958). *Annals of Otology*, **67**, 5

Kirikae, I., Nomura, Y., Shitara, T. and Kobayashi, T. (1962). *Archives of Otolaryngology*, **75**, 502

Klockhoff, I. and Lindblom, U. (1966) *Acta Otolaryngologica*, **61**, 459

Klockhoff, I. and Lindblom, U. (1967), *Acta Otolaryngologica* Suppl. **224**, 450

Lake-Bakaar, G. and Gibbs, D. D. (1978). *Journal of the Royal Society of Medicine*, **71**, 144

Leach, W. (1965). *Journal of Laryngology*, **79**, 870

Lewis, B., Wootton, I. D. P., Krikler, D. M., February, A., Chait, A., Oakley, C. M., Sigurdsson, G., Maurer, B. and Birkhead, J. (1974). *Lancet*, **1**, 141

Lindsay, J. R. (1973). *Annals of Otology*, **82** (Suppl.) 5

Lindsay, J. R., Davey, P. R. and Ward, P. H. (1960). *Annals of Otology*, **69**, 918

Lindsay, J. R. and Hemenway, W. G. (1954). *Annals of Otology*, **63**, 754

Lindsay, J. R. and Hemenway, W. G. (1956). *Annals of Otology*, **65**, 692

Lindsay, J. R., Proctor, L. R. and Work, W. P. (1960). *Laryngoscope*, **70**, 382

Lindsay, J. R. and Suga, F. (1976). *Laryngoscope*, **86**, 1029

Lindsay, J. R. and Zuidema, J. J. (1950). *Laryngoscope*, **60**, 238

Lloyd-Mostyn, R. H. and Lord, I. J. (1971). *Lancet*, **2**, 1156

Longridge, N. S. (1976). *Journal of Laryngology and Otology*, **90**, 539

Lowry, L. D., May, M. and Pastore, P. (1973). *Annals of Otology*, **82**, 876

Lumio, J. S. (1948). *Acta Otolaryngologica* (Suppl.) 71

McCabe, B. F. (1975). 'Diseases of the End Organ and Vestibular Nerve'. In *The Vestibular System*. p. 299. Ed. by R. F. Naunton, New York, San Francisco, London; Academic Press

McDonald, T. J., Zincke, H., Anderson, C. F. and Ott, N. T. (1978). *Laryngoscope*, **88**, 38

McNeil, N. F., Berke, M. and Reingold, I. M. (1952). *Annals of internal Medicine*, **37**, 1253

Mair, I. W. S. and Elverland, H. H. (1977). *Journal of Laryngology*, **91**, 323

Makashima, K. and Tanaka, K. (1971). *Annals of Otology*, **80**, 218

Mattox, D. E. and Simmons, F. B. (1977). *Annals of Otology*, **86**, 463

Matz, G. J. (1976). *Laryngoscope*, **86**, 1065

Matz, G. J., Beal, D. D. and Krames, L. (1969). *Archives of Otolaryngology*, **90**, 152

Mawer, G. E., Ahmad, R., Dobbs, S. M., McGough, J. G., Lucas, S. B. and Tooth, J. A. (1974). *British Journal of Clinical Pharmocology*, **1**, 45

Maxwell, O. N. (1963). *Archives of Otolaryngology*, **78**, 138

Maybaum, J. L. and Druss, J. G. (1934). *Archives of Otolaryngology*, **19**, 575

Meyerhoff, W. L. (1976). *Laryngoscope*, **86**, 38

Mitschke, H., Schmidt, P., Kopsa, H. and Zazgornik, J. (1975). *New England Journal of Medicine*, **292**, 1062

Moffat, D. A. (1978). Personal communication

Moffat, D. A., Booth, J. B. and Morrison, A. W. (1979). *Journal of Laryngology*, in press

Moffat, D. A., Gibson, W. P. R., Ramsden, R. T., Morrison, A. W. and Booth, J. B. (1978). *Acta Otolaryngologica*, **85**, 158

Moffat, D. A. and Ramsden, R. T. (1977) *Journal of Laryngology and Otology*, **91**, 511

Moretti, J. A. (1976). *Laryngoscope*, **86**, 598

Morganstein, K. M. and Mannace, E. D. (1969). *Laryngoscope*, **79**, 2172

Morrison, A. W. (1975). *Management of Sensorineural Deafness*, London & Boston; Butterworth

Morrison, A. W. (1978). Personal communication

Morrison, A. W. (1979). *British Journal of hospital Medicine*, **19**, 237

Morrison, A. W. and Booth, J. B. (1970). *British Journal of hospital Medicine*, **4**, 287

Moulonguet, A. and Bouche, J. (1951). *Annales d'Otolaryngologie*, **69**, 71

Myers, G. J. and Tyler, H. R. (1972). *Acta Otolaryngologica*, **96**, 333

Nadol, J. B., Weiss, A. D. and Parker, S. W. (1975). *Annals of Otology*, **84**, 841

Nishida, H., Kumagami, H. and Dohi, K. (1976). *Archives of Otolaryngology*, **102**, 601

Nomura, Y. and Hiraide, F. (1976). *Journal of Laryngology*, **90**, 1121

Norton, F. W. D. and Cogan, D. G. (1959). *Archives of Ophthalmology*, **61**, 695

Oda, M., Preciado, M. C., Quick, C. A. and Paparella, M. M. (1974). *Laryngoscope*, **84**, 1489

Oliner, L., Taubenhaus, M., Shapira, T. M. and Leshin, N. (1953). *New England Journal of Medicine*, **248**, 24

Paparella, M. M., Berlinger, N. T., Oda, M. and El Fiky, F. (1973). *Laryngoscope*, **83**, 1510

Patterson, M. D. and Bartlett, P. C. (1976). *Laryngoscope*, **86**, 399

Peacock, M. R. (1977). *Journal of Laryngology*, **91**, 81

Peitersen, E. and Carlsen, B. J. (1966). *Acta Otolaryngologica*, **61**, 189

Per-Lee, J. H. and Parsons, R. C. (1969) *Southern Medical Journal*, **62**, 161

Post, J. T. (1964). *Laryngoscope*, **74**, 221

Quick, C. A. and Hoppe, W. E. (1975). *Annals of Otology*, **84**, 94

Ramsden, R. T., Moffat, D. A. and Gibson, W. P. R. (1977). *Annals of Otology*, **86**, 827

Ramsden, R. T., Wilson, P. and Gibson, W. P. R. (1978). *Annals of Otology*, in press

Ransome, J., Ballantyne, J. C., Shaldon, S., Bosher, S. K. and Hallpi, C. S. (1966). *Journal of Laryngology*, **80**, 651

Rose, G. A. and Spencer, H. (1957). *Quarterly Journal of Medicine*, **26**, 43

Rosen, E. (1945). *Archives of Ophthalmology*, **33**, 281

Rossle, R. (1937), *Archiv fur Ohren-, Nasen-, und Kehlkopfheilkunde*, **142**, 193

Rowson, K. E. K., Hinchcliffe, R. and Gamble, D. R. (1976). *British Journal of Audiology*, **10**, 107

Ruben, R. J., Distenfeld, A., Berg, P. and Carr, R. (1969). *Journal of the American medical Association*, **209**, 1364

Sacher, H. (1952). *Harefuah*, **43**, 129

Sando, I., Harada, T., Loehr, A. and Sobeli, J. H. (1977). *Annals of Otology*, **86**, 269

Saunders, W. H. (1972). *Laryngoscope*, **82**, 1206

Saunders, W. H. and Lippy, W. H. (1959). *Annals of Otology*, **68**, 830

Schafier, I. A., Scrivier, C. R. and Efron, M. L. (1962). *New England Journal of Medicine*, **267**, 51

Schiff, M. and Brown, M. (1975). *Laryngoscope*, **84**, 1959

Schmidt, H., Odenthal, D. W., Eggermont, L. J. and Spoor, A. (1975). *Acta Otolaryngologica*, **79**, 287

Schuknecht, H. F. (1974). *Pathology of the Ear*. Cambridge, Mass.; Harvard University Press

Schuknecht, H. F., Allam, A. A. and Murakami, Y. (1968). *Annals of Otology*, **77**, 5

Schuknecht, H. F., Igarashi, M. and Chasin, W. D. (1965). *Laryngoscope*, **75**, 662

Schuknecht, H. F., Kimura, R. S. and Naufal, P. M. (1973). *Acta Otolaryngologica*, **76**, 75

Sellars, S. L. (1971). *Journal of Laryngology*, **85**, 281

Serjeant, G. R., Norman, W. and Todd, G. B. (1975). *Journal of Laryngology*, **89**, 453

Shaia, F. T. and Sheehy, J. L. (1976). *Laryngoscope*, **86**, 389

Shaw, J. O., Stark, E. W. and Gannaway, S. D. (1978). *Journal of Laryngology*, **92**, 131

Siegel, L. G. (1973). 'A national registry for idiopathic sudden deafness.' In *Vascular Disorders and Hearing Defects*, p. 307. Ed. by A. D. Darin de Lorenzo, Baltimore, London, Tokyo; University Park Press

Simmons, F. B. (1973). *Laryngoscope*, **83**, 1221

Sklansky, B. D., Jafek, B. W. and Wiernik, P. H. (1974). *Laryngoscope*, **84**, 210

Smith, G. A. and Gussen, R. (1976). *Archives of Otolaryngology*, **102**, 108

Smith, J. L. (1970). *Laryngoscope*, **80**, 121

Smith, K. E. and Spaulding, J. S. (1972). *Archives of Otolaryngology*, **96**, 368

Snyder, J. M. (1974). *Archives Otolaryngology*, **100**, 360

Spector, M. (1974). *Laryngoscope*, **84**, 816

Spencer, J. T. (1973) *Laryngoscope*, **83**, 639

Spencer, J. T. (1975). *Otology Clinics of North America*, **8** (2), 483

Stephens, S. D. G. (1970). *Journal of Laryngology*, **84**, 317

Stephens, S. D. G. and Hinchcliffe, R. (1968). *International Audiology*, **7**, 267

Suane-Knudsen, V. (1957). *Acta Otolaryngologica*, **47**, 270

Takahara, S., Saito, R., Konishi, S. and Igarashi, M. (1974). *Japanese Journal of ORL*, **77**, 959

Taylor, I. G. and Irwin, J. (1978). *Journal of Laryngology*, **92**, 99

Thomsen, K. A., Terkildsen, K. and Arnfred, I. (1965). *Archives of Otolaryngology*, **82**, 609

Todd, G. B., Serjeant, G. R. and Larson, M. R. (1973). *Acta Otolaryngologica*, **76**, 268

Toma, G. A. (1968). *Journal of Laryngologica*, **82**, 129

Toynbee, J. (1860). *The Diseases of the Ear*, London; Churchill

Urban, G. E. (1973). *Laryngoscope*, **83**, 633

Venkateswaran, P. S. (1971). *British medical Journal*, **4**, 113

Vogt, A. (1906), *Kiln. Mbl. Augenheilk.*, **44**, 228

Vuori, M., Lahikainen, E. A. and Peltonen, T. (1962). *Acta Otolaryngologica*, **55**, 231

Waun, J. E., Sweitzer, R. S. and Hamilton, W. K. (1967). *Anesthesiology*, **28**, 846

Welsh, L. W. and Welsh, J. J. (1963). *Annals of Otology*, **72**, 113

Wilkinson, P., Davidson, W. and Sommaripa, A. (1966). *Annals of internal Medicine*, **65**, 308

Wilmot, T. K. (1974). *Proceedings of the Royal Society of Medicine*, **67**, 331

Wilson, P. and Ramsden, R. T. (1977). *British medical Journal*, **1**, 259

Wilson, W. H. (1973). *Archives of Otolaryngology*, **97**, 139

Wing, L. and Bulteau, V. (1967). *Journal of the Oto-Laryngological Society of Australia*, **2**, 91

Wolff, D., Bernhard, W. G., Tsutsumi, S., Ross, J. S. and Nussbaum, H. E. (1965). *Annals of Otology*, **74**, 507

Wolfson, R. J. and Leiberman, A. (1975). *Laryngoscope*, **85**, 1762

Wright J. L. and Silk, K. L. (1974). *Laryngoscope*, **84**, 1378

Wright, J. L. W. and Saunders, S. H. (1975). *Journal of Laryngology*, **89**, 757

Yassin, A., Badry, A. and Fatt-Hi, A. (1970). *Journal of Laryngology*, **84**, 429 and 437

Zajtchuk, J. T., Matz. and Kindsay, J. R. (1972). *Annals of Otology*, **81**, 331

25 Menière's disease
B H Colman

Definition

Menière's disease is a disorder of unknown aetiology, the symptoms of which originate in the labyrinth and typically present as a triad consisting of fluctuating deafness, tinnitus and episodes of vertigo. Often there is also a sensation of fullness. A varying degree of permanent impairment of cochlear and vestibular function eventually supervenes in most cases. Distension of the endolymphatic system is a very frequent outstanding pathological feature, though this appearance is not specific to Menière's disease and its exact significance and relation to the symptoms is not fully understood.

Synonyms

The term *Menière's syndrome or symptom complex* could imply that the condition is merely a collection of symptoms without a known pathological basis. For this reason the term 'disease' is generally preferred, since the clinical and histological features are sufficiently constant to indicate the presence of a definite abnormality.

The expression 'atypical Menière's disease' is to be condemned. *Labyrinthine hydrops* is not recommended because it could indicate distension of both endolymphatic and perilymphatic compartments. The expression *endolymphatic hydrops* is often used and is acceptable because of the outstanding histopathological feature of the disease. Such hydrops, however, does occur in a number of other disorders, including congenital syphilitic labyrinthitis and viral infections. In syphilis the progressive endolymphatic hydrops is characterized, as Carmody (1966) points out, by attacks of vertigo and fluctuating hearing which can be identical to the acute episodes of Menière's disease.

The spelling of the eponym should be that used by Prosper Menière himself. His name was sometimes misspelt by his contemporaries and others have copied their error in the century since. Atkinson (1961) has commented on this matter.

Menière's contribution

In 1861 Prosper Menière (1799–1861), successor to Itard as Physician-in-Chief at the Imperial Institute for Deaf Mutes in Paris, published a description of the clinical entity that was soon designated 'Maladie de Menière'.

His account was so complete and accurate that virtually no addition could improve the picture he gave. In brief, Menière described a condition characterized by sudden and recurring attacks of vertigo, often associated with nausea and vomiting, together with deafness and tinnitus affecting patients with previously healthy ears. He stressed that these patients, beyond having some degree of impaired hearing and tinnitus, were in good health between attacks.

Menière correlated the vertigo with the experimental work of Flourens (1842) on the physiology of the labyrinth. He appreciated the significance of the association of deafness with vertigo and, as a result, became the first to show that this group of symptoms had its origin in the labyrinth.

The current opinion was that the attacks were due to cerebral apoplexy but Menière had observed that they were not followed by paralyses and therefore refuted this view.

Incidence

Menière's disease is not a particularly uncommon disorder, though the criteria for diagnosis employed by various clinicians vary tremendously and so accordingly does the apparent frequency of the disease. Cawthorne (1956) in an analysis of over 2000 cases of vertigo considered that almost 60 per cent were due to Menière's disease. This series might be selective in favour of cases of vertigo of labyrinthine origin as they had been referred for an otological opinion. Matsunaga (1976) gives an average incidence of 0.5 per cent for the disease in patients attending ear, nose and throat clinics in various hospitals in different countries. Drachman and Hart (1972) and Wilmot (1974) both quote a 5 per cent incidence of Menière's disease in a clinic dealing with balancing disorders.

Age of onset

The experience of most otologists is that symptoms generally start before the age of 50 in most patients. In *Table 25.1* are presented figures found in a series of patients of Cawthorne (1947), Golding-Wood (1960a), Hedgecock (1968) and Haye and Quist-Hanssen (1976).

Bilateral involvement

Menière emphasized that the disorder was more often unilateral than bilateral. Dederding (1929) was inclined to rate more than half her patients as being bilaterally affected on account of bilateral tinnitus and indicated that in many early cases the symptoms in the apparently healthy ear are minimal and therefore ignored. Golding-Wood (1960a) found sufficient evidence to incriminate the second ear in 44 per cent of his 314 patients with another 5 per cent becoming affected in the second ear later.

Table 25.1   Ménière's disease and the age at onset of symptoms

Age group	Cawthorne	Golding-Wood	Hedgecock	Haye and Quist-Hanssen
0–10	6	6	—	2
10–20	27	24	—	10
21–30	99	75	6	24
31–40	135	97	24	30
41–50	92	84	44	26
51–60	52	25	71	15
61–70	12	3	46	3
71–80	1	—	14	1
81–			—	—
Total	424	314	205	111

Stahle (1968) stated that of 334 patients seen, 14 per cent were affected bilaterally and in patients affected for ten years or more the figure rose to 25 per cent. Cawthorne (1969) quoted an incidence of 10 per cent, Hedgecock (1968) quotes 9 per cent and Haye and Quist-Hanssen (1976) quote 37 per cent of their 111 patients as having bilateral involvement. The incidence appears to depend upon the length of time patients are kept under observation and on the criteria used in diagnosing involvement of the second ear. It is also to be noted that Greven and Oosterveld (1975) in a study of the contralateral ear in 292 patients with Ménière's disease noted that 73 per cent had tinnitus or hearing loss or recruitment, and that 10 per cent had all three of these symptoms.

Predisposing factors

No definite predisposing factors are known. According to Matsunaga (1976) in his statistical survey the disease is commoner in developed countries and in urban populations. It is rarer in cold countries and commoner in the male than the female. The disease seemed to reach a peak incidence in the late 1950s and early 1960s. Racial or familial tendencies do not appear to exist. Exacerbations sometimes tend to follow emotional stress and the pre-menstrual period. Later stages of pregnancy are also found to increase the number of attacks in some patients with Ménière's disease.

Clinical features

In order to improve the accuracy of the diagnosis and to establish uniform standards the criteria to be used should be those laid down by the Committee on Hearing and Equilibrium of the American Academy of Ophthalmology and Otolaryngology (AAOO) under the chairmanship of Alford (1972).

Various positive and negative criteria which should be applied in accurate diagnosis of Ménière's disease have also been emphasized by Wilmot (1974). Episodic paroxysms of vertigo with deafness and tinnitus constitute the acute phase of the disease between which periods of quiescence or remission of varying duration occur. During these remissions hearing may return to normal in the earlier stages of the disease. Although the symptoms conform to a general pattern, there is considerable variation in their intensity and duration and in their sequence and time of appearance. The pattern of the attacks and the type of vertigo may also sometimes vary. The cycle of activity and remission in Menière's disease is characteristically irregular and capricious and makes the assessment of treatment difficult.

The acute attack

The dramatic symptom of vertigo dominates the clinical picture in the acute phases, or 'crises' as Menière termed them. The deafness and tinnitus assume greater importance to the patient as the vertigo subsides. Unless the attack is of minor degree it is accompanied by nausea and often vomiting and other symptoms of vagal disturbance. Although an attack may strike at any time about half of the patients are warned of its approach by prodromal symptoms. Most frequently the warning is described as a muffled or heavy feeling in the ear which may increase to become a dull ache, particularly behind the ear, or as a sensation of warmth around the ear.

The prodromal phase may start with tinnitus or produce a change in the character or intensity of an existing one. Discordant hearing sometimes heralds the attack. In others the warning is a vague sense of uneasiness which the patient has learnt to recognize.

The acute phase may consist of a single attack, especially in the early stages of the disorder, but more usually there are several which recur at varying intervals over a period of days or a week or two. This cluster formation of attacks often exhibits a tendency for the first one to be the most severe or to build up to a climax and then decline in intensity and frequency.

The remission phase

After the paroxysm of vertigo has subsided some gradual improvement of the hearing and lessening of the tinnitus may follow, but sooner or later a cumulative hearing defect appears after successive attacks. The tinnitus, likewise, tends to become permanent and may be the most distressing symptom in this phase.

The vestibular apparatus, like the cochlea, is capable of varying degrees of recovery after an acute attack. In the remission phase the reduction of vestibular function in the affected ear is not subjectively evident because of the excellent compensation which generally occurs in the vestibular system. Nevertheless, brief imbalance often continues to be experienced on sudden head movements.

The interval between single attacks or clusters of attacks may extend for months and not uncommonly for years, so that the patient may assume, especially if the residual cochlear symptoms are mild, that recovery has taken place.

The duration of the remission between acute episodes found by Golding-Wood (1960a) in a series of 119 cases and by Haye and Quist-Hanssen (1976) in 111 patients is shown in *Table 25.2*.

Table 25.2   Duration of remission phase

	< 3 mths	*3 mths–1 yr*	*1–2 yr*	*2–3 yr*	*3–5 yr*	*5–10 yr*	*> 10 yr*	*Total*
Golding-Wood	—	61	21	7	17	10	3	119
Haye and Quist-Hanssen	11	24	7	9	12	18	12	93

Cardinal symptoms

The cardinal symptoms of Menière's disease are those of recurring vestibular and cochlear failure. The nature of the onset varies slightly. The commonest, according to Stahle (1968) is for deafness to occur at the same time as the vertigo. This was the pattern in 41 per cent of his patients. Vertigo was the first symptom in 37 per cent. The disease began with hearing loss in 22 per cent and in some of his patients the time lapse amounted to over five years.

VERTIGO

Menière described four variations of the manner in which vertigo could occur:

(1) A rotatory sensation during which the room appears to whirl around when the eyes are open, or of the patient himself being rotated when the eyes are closed. This is the most common form.

(2) A sensation of unsteadiness which causes the patient to veer to one side when attempting to walk.

(3) A sensation of to-and-fro or up-and-down motion 'as experienced when being on the bridge of a ship at the mercy of a stormy sea'.

(4) Vertigo of such sudden onset and violence that the patient is thrown to the ground as though having been struck on the head. These are sometimes known as 'drop-attacks' or 'utricular crises' and are uncommon.

The prodromal symptoms may allow some patients to take precautionary measures before the disequilibrium develops. In a moderate attack the patient may be able to accommodate himself by lying or sitting down until it diminishes sufficiently for him to get home, but if the attack is severe and sudden the patient is completely disabled until the symptoms abate. Head movements during the attack exacerbate the vertigo so that the victim tends to lie rigid, the eyes closed, and gripping the bed as he feels himself gyrating through space.

The paroxysms come on at any time and may even waken the patient so that he sees the room whirling round. These definitive attacks are often accompanied by nausea and sometimes vomiting and persist for a prolonged period of time (from 20 min to no more than 24 h). The patient is fully orientated and conscious throughout the attack and there are no neurological accompaniments, or sequelae to the attack except those referrable to the labyrinth. End-organ type vestibular nystagmus is always present during the attack. During and briefly before a definitive attack hearing in the affected ear may decrease and tinnitus increase, remaining so for a variable time after the attack. Some patients, however, noticed no subjective change in the hearing during an attack and occasionally hearing increases during an attack.

Between the definitive attacks there may be various types of adjunctive attacks, such as motion intolerance, positional vertigo, drop attacks and momentary ataxia when changing direction. Between attacks there is no nystagmus with the eyes open (though there may be eyes-closed nystagmus detected on electronystagmography). The diagnosis of Menière's disease is not acceptable unless the patient is in normal health between attacks.

DEAFNESS

Menière recorded the deafness as being of 'nerve type' and had noted that there was a greater inability to hear bass voices than treble. The sensorineural deafness is in fact of end-organ type, though late in the disease when the deafness is severe the audiometric features of hair-cell dysfunction may be lost. The hearing loss tends to affect at first the lower frequencies and this feature is peculiar to deafness in this disorder. Although fluctuating hearing is a character of the disease, the low frequency deafness of the early case is particularly prone to recovery so that hearing sometimes returns entirely to normal during a remission. Improvement after attacks may be experienced for years or this tendency may disappear rapidly. Usually, there is a gradual deterioration of hearing after successive attacks, each of which is followed by incomplete recovery. Sometimes the loss is so severe and sudden that a patient is seen in whom permanent and severe deafness has supervened after only one or two attacks. Total deafness occurs but is rare.

Distortion is another feature of the deafness in Menière's disease. The patient may complain that sounds are heard at a different pitch in the affected ear (diplacusis) and that there is an increased sensitivity to loud noises (recruitment). Speech discrimination is reduced but not severely as in retrocochlear lesions. The reduction in speech discrimination is such that in bilaterally affected patients a hearing aid is often difficult to utilize satisfactorily.

TINNITUS

Tinnitus is almost always present to some degree. It is subjective, often being described as humming like a dynamo. It is exacerbated during or just before a paroxysm when it may become a loud roaring, whistling or banging sound. Like the deafness it may be present for a long time before the full manifestations of Menière's disease become apparent.

Additional clinical features

VAGAL SYMPTOMS

Nausea and vomiting are common features in the paroxysms and are accompanied by sweating, pallor and a slowing of the pulse.

These may lead to transient faintness. Unconsciousness is not a feature. Colicky abdominal pain and diarrhoea are occasionally encountered. The symptoms of gastric and intestinal disturbance have often led patients to assume the illness to be a stomach upset or a bilious attack. Ipsilateral rhinorrhoea and nasal congestion (unilateral vasomotor rhinitis) have been seen as rare additional features of parasympathetic motivation.

FULLNESS AND HEADACHE

A feeling of fullness or aching or bursting sensation in or behind the ear is not uncommon before or during the definitive attack. The exact explanation is not known. It has been suggested that it is caused by the build-up of endolymph.

Many observers have noted the association of clearcut migraine occurring with the vertigo. Atkinson (1943) found headache in some form in 58 per cent of 108 cases of Menière's disease and considered that 20 per cent of the series had properly defined migraine. Golding-Wood (1960a) gives 7 per cent as having unequivocal migraine.

NYSTAGMUS

Although nystagmus may be difficult to observe during a violent attack it has been seen to occur in different directions in different attacks in the same patient and even to vary its direction in the same attack. The nystagmus quickly disappears as the vertigo subsides.

ANXIETY STATE

As may be expected, the nature of the symptoms is such that a significant number of patients develop an overlying anxiety state. This must not be permitted to mask the organic nature of their basic disorder and must be taken into account in the management of it.

Variations of the clinical picture

These arise owing to variations in the timing, sequence and even absence of one or more of the main features that together constitute a typical case.

MENIÈRE'S DISEASE WITHOUT VERTIGO

In this form the patient exhibits a deafness with the characteristics of that typically found in Menière's disease and it is thought that in these patients the endolymphatic hydrops is localized to the cochlea. As already noted the complete picture of Menière's disease may develop only after a lapse of several years and until the full symptoms are present the synonym should not be applied. The term 'cochlear hydrops' may be employed and has been described histologically by Lindsay and Schulthess (1958).

MENIÈRE'S DISEASE WITHOUT DEAFNESS

Some cases of vertigo unaccompanied by deafness later develop Menière's disease. The pathological basis of this form has not yet been shown and only the natural history of the condition will clarify the diagnosis. Occasionally accurate audiological examination, especially by speech audiometry, demonstrates the presence of a hearing loss of which the patient was unaware. Clearly, the label of Menière's disease without deafness can very readily become a convenient dumping ground for cases of vertigo of unknown origin.

THE LERMOYEZ SYNDROME

In this rare variant the hearing loss and tinnitus become worse over a period of a couple of hours to a couple of days. Vertigo then occurs, often suddenly, and with it hearing and tinnitus improve.

MENIÈRE'S DISEASE IN COMBINATION WITH OTHER EAR DISEASES

The most important of these is chronic middle-ear suppuration co-existing with Menière's disease. This may lead to a diagnosis of erosion of the labyrinth capsule or serous labyrinthitis when in fact no such complication is present. Likewise, in otosclerosis, a disorder in which vertigo is occasionally quite a prominent feature, the combination with true Menière's disease can present a confusing picture. Menière's disease, otosclerosis and chronic suppuration are all common disorders and so sometimes will occur together. Altmann and Kornfeldt (1965) have produced histological evidence of otosclerosis and endolymphatic hydrops co-existing in the same ear in two temporal bone studies. Schuknecht (1969) has also produced evidence of these diseases co-existing (*Figure 25.1*).

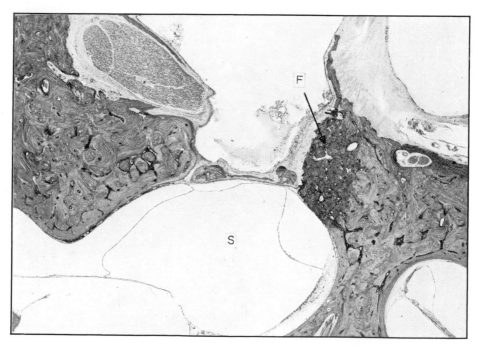

Figure 25.1   Menière's disease in association with otosclerosis. The grossly distended saccule (S) lies against the stapes footplate. An otosclerotic focus (F) is present anteriorly. (Reproduced by courtesy of Professor H. F. Schuknecht)

Investigation

General assessment

Obviously the patient's general medical state must be assessed in detail. The cardiovascular system must be healthy, carotid pulses equal and normal and the blood pressure within normal limits when taken in both arms. The central nervous system will be healthy and neuro-otological examination will be negative apart from the findings relating to the labyrinth. Neck movements will be unimpaired. In the course of his assessment the otologist will have taken note of his patient's psychological adjustment to his symptoms.

History

An accurate history which includes a detailed description of each relevant symptom can lead to a correct provisional diagnosis in most cases, but it is essential to carry out a full routine examination in every case. A search for incidents, either of vertigo, deafness or tinnitus, even in the distant past, should be made as these may have been forgotten if recovery has apparently taken place. Headache and other migrainous symptoms should be sought while a past history of ear disease and operations may be relevant to the differential diagnosis. There will be no history of ototoxic drugs having been used.

Preliminary otological examination

This is undertaken to exclude any evidence of pathological conditions past or present in the middle-ear cleft. The condition of the tympanic membranes must be ascertained, the patency of the eustachian tubes confirmed and the presence of fluid in the tympanic cavity excluded. The fistula test should always be applied, a positive Hennebert sign will be found in approximately 50 per cent of patients according to Schuknecht (1975) who attributes this to the formation of adhesions between the distended saccule and the inner surface of the stapes footplate.

Audiological investigation

Preliminary tuning-fork tests will confirm the sensorineural nature of the deafness, though a false negative Rinne may be present in patients with a severe unilateral deafness. The tuning-fork tests may also demonstrate diplacusis. Complete audiometric investigation follows and is an essential step towards diagnosis. The tests involved have been reviewed by Schuknecht (1963), by Holmgren (1964) and by Hedgecock (1968).

PURE-TONE AUDIOMETRY

Establishment of air- and bone-conduction thresholds is the first step. The audiogram in patients with Menière's disease will confirm the sensorineural nature of the deafness and provides a base-line with which future fluctuations can be compared.

The audiometric pattern may be flat (55 per cent) or low frequency (27 per cent) early in the disease. Only late in the disease may a falling curve be found, although this is disputed. In older patients, of course, a pre-existing high frequency loss, which may also be seen in the unaffected ear, may be superimposed. Serial audiometry is essential in order to document the fluctuations accurately and often shows the partial recovery of hearing between attacks, especially for the lower frequencies. But as the disease progresses the curve is seen to flatten out and the threshold, although it may halt its progress at any point (*Figure 25.2*), is increasingly raised.

In his long-term study of hearing in 356 patients, Stahle (1976a) noted that hearing tended to deteriorate more rapidly in the early stages of the disease and then frequently become relatively stable. Even within three years he found that the mean value for hearing in these patients had deteriorated to 55 dB on pure-tone audiometry. In respect of speech audiometry he found that the mean value after three years of the disease was 62 dB for the speech reception threshold, and 52 per cent for the discrimination score and that at this time further deterioration was frequently arrested.

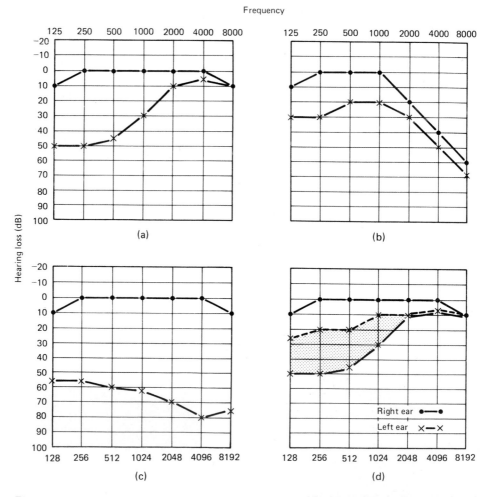

Figure 25.2   Air conduction audiograms of patients with Menière's disease affecting the left ear: (a) hearing loss maximal in low tones; (b) hearing loss maximal in high tones with a pre-existing high-tone loss also shown in the unaffected ear; (c) hearing loss of high and low tones, i.e. a flat type of curve; (d) hatched area shows the recovery possible after an acute episode

Speech audiometry is an important means of differentiating between sensory and neural deafness. In patients with Menière's disease the pure-tone threshold matches the speech and reception threshold very closely in over 90 per cent of patients. Although discrimination is impaired, it is much less severely affected than in patients with a neural type of lesion.

Other tests may also help identify an end-organ lesion. Loudness recruitment should be complete in patients with Menière's disease, there is a lowered loudness discomfort level and also a lowered difference limen for intensity. A high score is generally obtained in the short increment sensitivity index (SISI) test. Tone decay can be expected to be near normal. Békésy audiometry will generally show a type 2 tracing (*Figure 25.3*). It must be remembered that atypical and conflicting results are not unusual. Moreover, these are subjective tests. Objective methods, such as stapedius reflex testing and electrocochleography are therefore of greater reliability. The former is regarded by Morrison (1975) as a most reliable guide to the presence of recruitment even if the hearing loss is bilateral and either symmetrical or asymmetrical. Electrocochleography will often show an alteration in the action potential scan and delayed conductivity depending on the type of lesion present.

In audiometric testing, good equipment and conditions and a competent examiner are essential. It should also be remembered that although the various test results are usually in agreement they sometimes are not, even though Menière's disease is definitely thought to be present. In contrast the audiometric patterns described above are occasionally found in patients with neural lesions, such as cerebello–pontine angle tumours. Careful clinical judgment is thus of the highest importance at all times.

Investigation of vestibular function

PRELIMINARY EXAMINATION

A preliminary examination includes walking, turning and standing with eyes open and shut (Romberg test) and the past pointing test. These tests are usually performed without difficulty in the remission phase of Menière's disease. Spontaneous nystagmus is absent except in an attack. During an attack nystagmus is always present. Both spontaneous and positional types may be found. From ENG studies it is known that the nystagmus may even alternate between these types, or even change direction in a single attack. It is advisable to examine routinely the pupils and fundi, to test for areas of facial anaesthesia and loss of the corneal reflex, and to examine the patient for positionally induced nystagmus.

VESTIBULAR ANALYSIS

The differential caloric test of Fitzgerald and Hallpike (1942) is well known and still often employed (*Figure 25.4*). The commonest response in Menière's disease is to find a hypoactive labyrinth with the calorogram showing a pattern of a canal paresis. Some patients show a pattern indicating a directional preponderance of the nystagmus to one or other side and in a minority a pattern of a canal paresis and a directional preponderance may be combined. It is furthermore to be emphasized that a normal response is by no means uncommon and does not rule out the presence of Menière's disease. This may be explained by either the labyrinth recovering between acute attacks or by the phenomenon of recruitment. A comprehensive account of the clinical, caloric and rotational test findings has been given by Wilmot (1974).

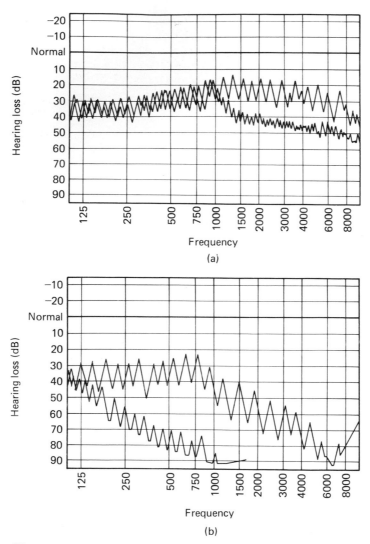

Figure 25.3 Békésy audiograms: (a) Type 2 recording typically found in Menière's disease. The tracings are superimposed up to 1000 Hz. Above this frequency the tracing for the continuous tone (thick line) drops below the tracing for the interrupted tone and its swing is of reduced amplitude; (b) Type 3 recording, such as found in a retrocochlear lesion. The tracing for the interrupted tone follows that obtained in a conventional audiogram, but the tracing for the continuous tone (thick line) falls away rapidly as the frequency increases. Its swings remain of wide amplitude. (Reproduced by courtesy of CIBA, from the collection by Dr. Frank Netter)

Electronystagmography is essential for detailed investigation of vestibular function. During remission the patient with Menière's disease seldom shows a spontaneous or positional nystagmus with ENG testing. After an acute attack, however, ENG may show nystagmus for several days despite apparent complete recovery. It has not yet been possible to relate any particular type of ENG recording to any specific internal ear abnormality. The use of ENG in caloric testing has been discussed by Colman

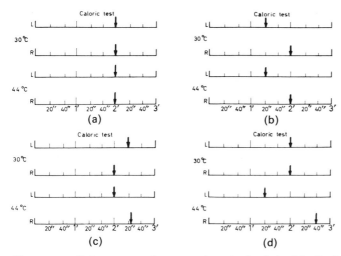

Figure 25.4 Calorograms that may be obtained in Menière's disease: (a) normal response; (b) left canal paresis; (c) right directional preponderance; (d) left canal paresis with right directional preponderance

(1969a) and by Hinchcliffe (1969) in patients with Menière's disease. ENG was also the method used by Stahle (1976a) in his detailed analysis of 356 patients with severe Menière's disease.

Stahle assessed the responses by measuring the speed of the slow phase of the nystagmus during a 10-s period sampled at the peak of the caloric reaction and calculated the percentage difference between the two ears by the method of Jongkees and Philipszoon (1964). Stahle found that in 59 per cent of his patients the caloric response was reduced. It was exaggerated in 1 per cent, and was normal in 40 per cent. It is to be noted, however, that 'normal' means no significant difference between the responses in the two sides. Phenomena such as directional preponderance were not taken into consideration in his investigation. He found a parallelism between acoustic and vestibular response in his patients. The greatest deterioration was in the first five years although a reduction was observed in the first two years. His figure of 59 per cent for reduced caloric response is to be compared with the figure of 80 per cent quoted by Thomas and Harrison (1971). The discrepancy is probably accounted for by the use of different criteria of normality.

A simple screening test which can be done rapidly and conveniently in a busy out-patient clinic consists of injecting 2 ml of iced water against the posterosuperior quadrant of the drum, with the head extended 60 degrees. The injection is made under direct vision using a speculum, and the nystagmus is timed in the usual way. Canal paresis is readily demonstrated. Alternatively, the minimal caloric test can be employed in which 0.2 ml of iced water is injected. If no response is obtained it is increased to 0.4 ml, and if need be to 0.8 ml.

An important refinement in vestibular analysis, though not one which is as yet in general use is the employment of *galvanic stimulation* as described by Pfaltz (1976). This method provides an important means of differentiating an end-organ from a neural type of lesion. The reliability of the method has received experimental support from Swaak and Oosterveld (1976) who working with rabbits also concluded that it was an accurate means of identifying the site of the lesion.

Radiographic investigation

Routine radiographic investigation of the temporal bone should be made and will frequently call for polytomography. According to House (1975), a search should be made for narrowing of the internal auditory meatus as well as dilatation and, the possibility of otosclerosis of the otic capsule should also be borne in mind. Every otologist will be fully aware of the importance of an expanded meatus, and the need to carry out further studies, but not many have accepted the concept of meatal stenosis. Many aspects of otosclerosis of the labyrinthine capsule and its relationship to sensorineural hearing loss are likewise still debated, but the report of Cole and Funkhauser (1972) is of interest. They found that 25 of their 250 patients on whom polytomography was done with symptoms of Menière's disease had evidence of otosclerosis of the labyrinthine capsule. In all 25 the findings were bilateral, and seven siblings had been diagnosed as having Menière's disease or a conductive deafness.

Other special investigations

These may include various laboratory tests such as the glycerol test. Internal ear fluid analysis may be helpful in patients with particularly difficult diagnostic problems.

Laboratory tests

Although the aetiology of endolymphatic hydrops has never been established, the possibility of various contributing factors has been emphasized by Powers (1972), Pulec (1973), Glasscock and Miller (1977) and Pulec (1977). The latter found that careful evaluation revealed a specific aetiology in 55 per cent of patients whom he studied. Accordingly, one should consider the need for a 5-h glucose tolerance test, endocrinal studies for adrenal/pituitary insufficiency and hypothyroidism. Powers (1975) in addition has drawn attention to the need for adequate allergy evaluation in certain selected patients. Serological tests are essential and should include the treponemal immobilization test, the fluorescent treponemal antibody test and the fluorescent treponemal antibody absorption test.

Glycerol test

The glycerol test has been described by Klockhoff and Lindblom (1967) and by Klockhoff (1975) and has proved itself to be a valuable diagnostic tool in patients with fluctuant sensorineural loss due to endolymphatic hydrops. The glycerol is given orally in a calculated dose, together with an equal volume of physiological saline. In a positive test improved hearing thresholds occur for pure-tone and for speech tests and reach a maximum about 3 h after the administration of glycerol. If the patient is in spontaneous remission and has good hearing then a poor response or even a negative result may be obtained. A negative result may also be obtained in patients with advanced endolymphatic hydrops with non-fluctuant hearing. Preliminary salt loading lessens the number of patients coming to test in remission and so, accordingly, increases the value of the procedure as shown by Arenberg and his co-workers (1974). The test is not only useful in diagnosis, it is also of value in identifying the patient who may be suitable for either long-term diuretic therapy or, alternatively, who may be considered suitable for a saccus operation. The test is highly reliable and very rarely indeed gives a false-positive result in patients with other types of sensorineural hearing loss. The experimental work on guinea-pigs carried out by Angelborg and Ågerup (1975) has demonstrated that the diuresis occurring after glycerol administration produces a lowering of CSF and internal ear pressures and confirms the scientific validity of the test.

Futaki and his co-workers (1977) have used frusemide as a basis for similar tests and found it gave greater diuresis than glycerol. Instead of measuring improvement in hearing function they measured their results by electronystagmographic assessment of the caloric response. They found that the frusemide test was more likely to be positive even with patients in remission or with very advanced hearing loss. It was equally specific for endolymphatic hydrops, but in their hands was more sensitive than the glycerol test and had fewer side effects, such as nausea or headache.

Internal ear fluid analysis

This has been described by Silverstein and Schuknecht (1966) and by Schuknecht (1974). Diagnostic permeatal labyrinthotomy was performed under local anaesthesia and a micropipette used to obtain fluid through the perforated stapes footplate. In Menière's disease, fluid with the biochemical features of normal endolymph was obtained. In patients with eighth nerve tumour, fluid with a very high protein content resulted. The procedure is not without danger of cochlear damage. It seems likely that the investigation may have application (1) in labyrinthectomy to confirm the clinical diagnosis of Menière's disease and to exclude an overlooked eighth nerve tumour and (2) in those rare instances in which the diagnosis between Menière's disease and eighth nerve tumour cannot be established beyond doubt by conventional methods.

Differential diagnosis

A vast number of clinical conditions enter into the differential diagnosis of vertigo. Fortunately, the pattern of the acute phase, the succeeding interval of quiescence in which there is an absence of other signs in the central nervous system, and the characteristic nature of the deafness, make the diagnosis of typical Menière's disease relatively easy in most cases.

With the variants of the disease it is more difficult, since in these one or more of the components of the triadic syndrome is absent and the classic clinical picture may develop only after a long period.

The conditions from which Menière's disease must be distinguished fall into the following four groups.

Other disorders affecting the labyrinth

EXTERNALLY INDUCED PRESSURE CHANGES

It is said that vertigo may be produced by wax or a foreign body pressing on the tympanic membrane, though the mechanism is not clear. Effusions into the middle-ear cleft can have a similar effect. Cholesteatoma, neoplasms and fenestration operations may cause vertigo by pressure transmissions through a fistula in the semicircular canal directly into the labyrinth: the experienced otologist will have little difficulty in identifying these conditions.

TRAUMA

Vertigo very often complicates head injuries. The more serious the head injury the more likely is vertigo to be present. It is often positional in character, gradually improving. It is most important to examine for positionally induced nystagmus in patients giving a history of head injury. The characteristics of the nystagmus are generally those associated with the so-called benign peripheral type of disorder, but sometimes a nystagmus of the central, non-fatiguable type will be observed. According to Proctor, Gurdjian and Webster (1956) about 47 per cent of patients with longitudinal fractures of the petrous bone had a positional nystagmus. In patients with transverse fractures, the injury to the labyrinth is much more severe and generally total destruction occurs with all the symptoms and signs of unilateral labyrinthine failure. Whatever the type of injury there will nearly always be a sensorineural deafness as in Menière's disease.

INFECTION

Labyrinthitis arising from any type of otitis media may occur. Virus labyrinthitis causing labyrinthine failure is an occasional complication of some of the infective fevers, including influenza.

DRUG TOXICITY

Labyrinthine failure due to ototoxicity is most commonly seen as a result of administration of the aminoglycoside group of antibiotics. A non-specific effect on the vestibular system can arise from a variety of drugs, more generally producing a less well-defined dizziness as Alberti and Black (1968) point out in their excellent review of iatrogenic problems in otolaryngology.

BENIGN POSITIONAL VERTIGO

Not all cases are the result of head injury, but as in the traumatic type the characteristic vertigo and nystagmus only occur when the head is placed in the critical position. Hearing is normal and so are the caloric responses.

PERILYMPH FISTULA

The possibility of perilymph leakage through the oval window is always to be considered in a patient who after stapedectomy demonstrates fluctuant hearing, especially if some disequilibrium co-exists as Harrison and his colleagues (1967) emphasized. Similar symptoms may also occur from so-called spontaneous perilymph fistula at either the round or oval window as pointed out by Goodhill (1976).

COGAN'S DISEASE

A rare disease, possibly a collagen disorder, generally affecting young adults, in which non-specific inflammatory and degenerative changes are found in the inner ear and in the vestibular and spiral ganglia. The symptoms are those of Menière's disease to which are added a burning and redness of the eyes and the blurring of vision which attend a patchy and fluctuating interstitial keratitis. As the deafness increases, the vertigo, nausea and vomiting disappear. The deafness generally progresses to a very severe degree through a sequence of exacerbations and remissions (Serrins, Harrison and Chandler, 1963).

Disorders of the vestibular nerve and its central connections

EIGHTH NERVE TUMOUR

Difficulty occasionally arises in differential diagnosis when the tumour is small enough to produce otological symptoms and signs alone. Later, as the tumour expands outside the internal acoustic meatus to cause other neurological and brain-stem signs there is usually no problem in diagnosis. The main symptom of eighth nerve tumour is usually hearing loss, because although the tumour generally originates on the vestibular division of the nerve its rate of growth is so slow that excellent vestibular compensation occurs. Atypical cases occur, however, the fluctuating symptoms of which are very similar to Menière's disease. There is progressive unilateral sensorineural deafness, usually with tinnitus and impaired caloric responses. Audiometric testing in this condition should indicate the presence of a retro–cochlear lesion, but it is emphasized that audiometric patterns are often atypical and can be misleading. In doubtful cases, therefore, an EMI scan, and possibly contrast studies of the internal auditory meatus will be needed.

VESTIBULAR NEURONITIS

This is characterized by the sudden onset of vertigo without hearing loss. It occasionally occurs in small epidemics often with a history of upper respiratory tract infection. The condition may affect one or both vestibular nerves. The caloric responses are diminished, hearing tests show no abnormality. The vertigo and vomiting gradually settle and further attacks do not usually occur.

DISSEMINATED SCLEROSIS

The characteristic pathological changes in the area of the vestibular nuclei and tracts may cause either paroxysmal vertigo and vomiting or just a persistent dizziness. As the changes are unlikely to be limited to this area there are usually other signs of central nervous system involvement, such as transient weakness of the limbs, diplopia and spontaneous nystagmus but a hearing loss and tinnitus are unusual.

EPILEPSY

Epilepsy may have a vertiginous aura, but the diagnosis is manifest from the loss of consciousness and the fit. There are no auditory symptoms and the caloric and positional tests are normal.

MIGRAINE

The association of migraine and Menière's disease has been discussed. Migraine may be preceded by a vertiginous aura which sometimes continues throughout the period of the headache and vomiting. Sometimes the vertigo becomes the predominant feature and replaces the headaches (migraine equivalent). Prior attacks of typical migraine and the possible presence of ocular symptoms point to the diagnosis.

SYPHILIS

Syphilis, the great but almost forgotten imitator, can affect the cochleo–vestibular apparatus and its connections either as a basal meningoneuritis or less frequently by gumma formation. In some cases the onset of vestibular failure is acute, the attacks recurring at frequent intervals but becoming less severe as the patient becomes permanently deaf. Serological tests for syphilis are necessary when any difficulty exists in the diagnosis of labyrinthine failure.

DISORDERS OF THE CARDIOVASCULAR SYSTEM

Anoxia for any reason can affect the vestibular nuclei and the peripheral end-organs. The anoxia may be due to cardiac insufficiency, anaemia or a fault of the peripheral circulation.

Labyrinthine vasospasm as a possible cause of Menière's disease is discussed under pathogenesis.

CHRONIC ISCHAEMIA OF BRAIN STEM

The patient, usually elderly, complains of a mild vertigo of varying duration generally described as a 'swimming' sensation. Whilst occurring at any time it is most frequently observed on rising suddenly from the sitting position, or on getting out of bed. Bilateral sensorineural deafness and tinnitus commonly co-exist in these patients.

In young patients a fleeting imbalance on assuming the erect position is often experienced as a result of postural hypotension. In these patients no auditory symptoms are present.

ACUTE ISCHAEMIA OF BRAIN STEM

In the presence of pronounced cervical spondylosis a vertebral artery may be compressed by movements of the head and neck, especially if there is a co-existing atherosclerosis in the artery. The vertigo may be brief, and the patient sometimes falls to the ground in what is termed the 'drop attack'. Any deafness and tinnitus that may be present are probably derived from an associated presbyacusis.

THROMBOSIS OF POSTERIOR INFERIOR CEREBELLAR ARTERY (LATERAL MEDULLARY SYNDROME)

The severe paroxysmal vertigo with vomiting in this condition may be as dramatic as in Menière's disease but is followed immediately by an array of neurological signs due to medullary infarction. Deafness is present only if the lesion extends beyond the point of entry of the eighth nerve into the brain stem.

Other disorders

VERTIGO OF CERVICAL ORIGIN

An ill-defined giddiness occasionally complicates whiplash, i.e. flexion–extension, injuries of the neck. It can be particularly difficult to exclude functional causes,

especially when matters of legal compensation arise. Dizziness associated with neck pain, stiff neck, or a suboccipital headache sometimes is produced by disturbance of the neck proprioceptive mechanisms. It is interesting to note that the pathological nystagmus which can be demonstrated by electronystagmography in such patients will disappear with the symptoms after local treatment with short-wave diathermy and, if necessary, traction. More severe neck injuries may affect the vertebral artery and so interfere with the blood supply to the brain stem, especially if the artery is involved in atheromatous changes. Comprehensive reviews of vertigo complicating injuries of the neck have been made by Sandler (1967) and by Toglia, Rosenberg and Ronis (1969), to which reference should be made.

PSYCHOGENIC DIZZINESS
The neurotic patient generally describes his dizziness in such a vague manner, but in such flowery terms that the diagnosis is often self-evident. The absence of any abnormality on repeated audiometric, vestibular and neurological examination helps towards the diagnosis in doubtful cases. Without electronystagmography, however, it is easy to make the mistake of labelling as neurotic those patients who have a definite abnormality even though it cannot be exactly identified on a topographical or pathological basis.

Pathology

Menière's disease is a non-fatal disorder, and it has not yet been reproduced in experimental animals. Consequently, material for histological study is difficult to obtain and the appearances are often confused by post-mortem changes and by preparation artefact.

Although it was long suspected that endolymphatic hydrops was associated with Menière's disease this was only confirmed by Hallpike and Cairns in 1938. Many others have since reported similar findings. Their various accounts have been collected by Altmann and Kornfeldt (1965) who reviewed all the known temporal-bone studies and added five of their own.

The most comprehensive description at present available is that of Schuknecht (1974, 1975) based on material in his own collection. The most obvious abnormality is the distension of the endolymph spaces. This mainly affects the cochlea and the saccule. The utricle is involved to a lesser degree and the semicircular canals only slightly and that in the region of their ampullae. Dilatation of the endolymphatic sac has not been found. The distension of the scala media of the cochlea is seen as a bulging Reissner's membrane into the scala vestibuli, often leading to obliteration of this part of the perilymph compartment. Reissner's membrane is frequently observed to bulge through the helicotrema into the apical part of the scala tympani. In places, Reissner's membrane appears to be adherent to the osseous wall of the scala vestibuli. Distension limited to the cochlea in a case having the characteristic auditory symptoms of Menière's disease, but without vertigo, has been reported by Lindsay and Schulthess (1958), thus providing a pathological basis for this clinical variant.

A second feature in Menière's disease concerns herniation or rupture of the membranous labyrinth. These herniations have been described by Lawrence and McCabe (1959) and by Schuknecht (1963, 1968). They can occur at any site in

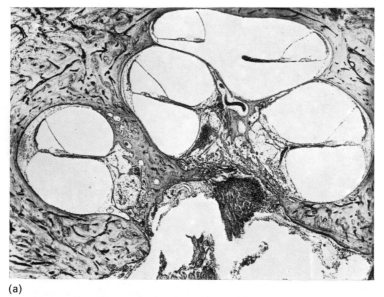

(a)

(b)

Figure 25.5   (a) Normal cochlea (the unaffected side of a case of Menière's disease); (b) left cochlea affected by Menière's disease showing gross dilatation of the scala media with displacement of Reissner's membrane through the helicotrema. (Reproduced by courtesy of the Royal Society of Medicine)

Reissner's membrane or in the saccule, utricle or ampullae. That rupture can occur implies that healing can occur. Accordingly, it has been suggested that these ruptures are vital phenomena and are related to the exacerbations and remissions which characterize Menière's disease (*Figures 25.6* and *25.7*). This concept, however, is not accepted by Lindsay (1968, 1969). He had previously described an actual defect in the wall of the saccule, though later doubted if his previous interpretation was correct. He suggested that the lesion could have been present before fixation of the tissues was

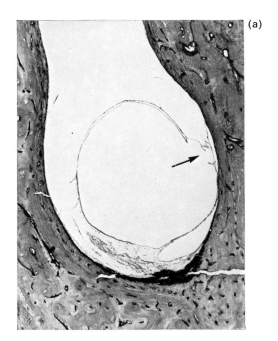

(a)

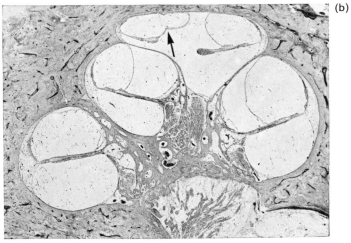

(b)

Figure 25.6 (a) Herniation of posterior semicircular canal in region of the ampulla. Either healing has occurred, or the rupture has never been complete; (b) rupture healed or incomplete at the apex of the cochlear duct. (Reproduced by courtesy of Professor H. F. Schuknecht)

completed and might indeed be artefact (*Figure 25.8*).

A third feature described by Schuknecht is collapse of the membranous labyrinth which presumably occurs when a break in the membranous labyrinth fails to heal as in *Figure 25.7*. It may be that a permanent break of this kind is the situation which occurs in 'burnt out' Menière's disease.

The fourth point of interest concerning the membranous labyrinth is the proliferation of fibrous tissue in the vestibule which occasionally occurs. Fibrous bands form between the footplate and the wall of the utricle and the saccule, and are thought

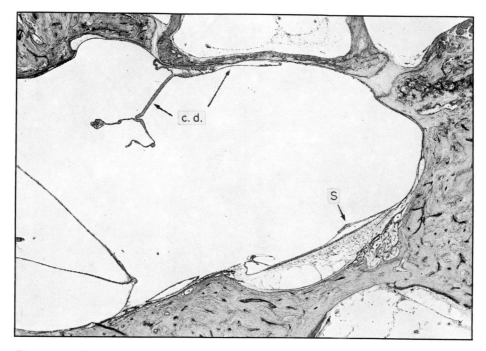

Figure 25.7   Region of vestibule from an ear with endolymphatic hydrops. The saccule (S) has collapsed onto its macula, the collapsed membranous sac (c.d.) represents herniation from the vestibular end of the cochlear duct. (Reproduced by courtesy of Professor H. F. Schuknecht)

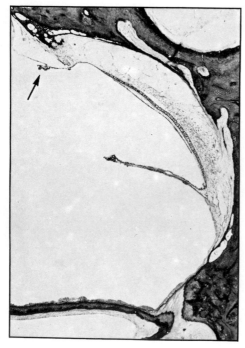

Figure 25.8   The reinforced segment retains its normal position. The posterior pàrt of the saccule wall is everted (arrow). There is no attempt at healing and the appearance may be due to preparation artefact. (Reproduced by courtesy of Dr. John Lindsay)

to account for the presence of Hennebert's sign in some patients with Menière's disease (momentary giddiness and nystagmus when alternating positive and negative pressures are applied in the external meatus).

The fifth point of interest concerns the hair-cell and ganglion-cell population of the ear affected by Menière's disease. Schuknecht, Benitez and Beekhuis (1962) were able to achieve early fixation of the labyrinthine structures in three temporal bones from patients with Menière's disease and found normal hair-cell populations in the organ of Corti, the maculae of the saccule and utricle and of the cristae of the three semicircular canals. The neurone populations of the spiral and vestibular ganglia were also normal. Schuknecht (1968) confirmed these findings in a further paper and concluded that degenerative changes only occur in exceptional cases. Such exceptions have been presented by Lindsay, Cohurt and Sciarra (1967) and also by two cases now in the Schuknecht collection. In these cases the loss of hair-cells and of ganglion cells is confined to the apical region of the cochlea. Schuknecht (1975) reports that the same features are sometimes seen in animal ears following experimentally produced hydrops, and suggests that this may be due to the accumulation of toxic or metabolic products in this area. It may well be that degenerative changes in the receptors are not gross enough to be shown by light microscopy in the majority of human temporal bones studied, as Lindsay (1968) has pointed out.

Pathological investigations employing the electron microscope in Menière's disease have been carried out on the avulsed semicircular canal and its ampullary portion obtained from patients subjected to partial labyrinthectomy. The significance of the changes so far described must remain *sub judice* as some of them have been seen in the cells of apparently normal inner ears of the guinea-pig, according to Friedmann (1963). Stria vascularis obtained from a similar source and examined by the electron microscope has been described by Kimura and Schuknecht (1970). They reported features all of which showed close similarity to those of the normal stria from healthy animals and did not relate any particular findings to the disease process. Electron microscopic findings have also been reported by Fisch (1970) and by Colman, Friedmann and Wright (1975) who examined the vestibular nerve and other material in patients undergoing neurectomy in Menière's disease. Again, it is difficult to know whether the features described are those of Menière's disease or are the result of other processes, such as ageing.

Tissue taken from the wall of the saccus during the course of operation has been described by Saito and his colleagues (1977) who reported subepithelial deposits of deep brown pigmented material, the nature of which could not be determined, as well as the very frequent occurrence of fibrosis around the sac.

Biochemical analysis of the labyrinthine fluids has been undertaken in three cases of Menière's disease by Wullstein and Rauch (1961) and they concluded that the endolymph had a normal potassium and probably normal sodium concentration. Further biochemical studies on 52 patients with Menière's disease were reported by Rauch (1968). They confirmed him in the opinion that the endolymphatic hydrops was not caused by any sodium or potassium disturbance and that even in the more advanced cases of Menière's disease the sodium and potassium values were near normal. This has been the generally accepted view, but it is interesting to note that Silverstein and Takeda (1977) working with experimental hydrops in animals found an increase of sodium in the endolymph and suggest that in spite of previous evidence this may also occur in humans with Menière's disease.

Pathogenesis

Despite much experimental work and speculation on the pathogenesis of Menière's disease the cause of the condition remains unexplained.

Menière considered the condition to be a functional disorder of the internal ear and he is said to have been engaged on a paper relating it to certain types of migraine at the time of his death.

Confusion has arisen following Menière's reference in his famous paper of 1861, to the post-mortem finding of a serosanguineous exudate in the semicircular canals of a young woman who had died five days after the onset of continuous vertigo, vomiting and deafness. When Menière first recorded this case as an addendum to the chapter on nerve deafness in his translation of Kramer's textbook of otology in 1848, he did not mention the vertigo and described the exudate as filling the labyrinth. Williams (1952) has pointed out that Menière quoted this case some 13 years after the event, merely to illustrate that the symptoms could arise from a labyrinthine lesion and his intention was not to identify such a haemorrhagic lesion as the cause of the non-fatal syndrome he had described. Lack of appreciation of Menière's objective in presenting this evidence, together with misquotation, has led to the long-lasting misbelief that he had ascribed haemorrhage into the labyrinth as the cause of the syndrome.

It has been assumed for many years that some disturbance of the blood supply to the labyrinth could be the cause of Menière's disease. Lermoyez (1929) who compared Menière's disease with Raynaud's disease, put forward the theory that an ischaemia of the labyrinth due to spasm of the internal auditory artery or its branches could be the cause of the vestibular and cochlear symptoms.

Later, this presumed spasm of the internal auditory artery or its branches, or both, was widely conceived as being part of a generalized imbalance of the vasoconstrictor and vasodilator functions of the autonomic nervous system. Under normal circumstances the sympathetic and parasympathetic parts of the autonomic nervous system are coordinated to resist environmental changes in the organism and so to contribute to homeostasis. Support to the idea of a vasospasm of the labyrinthine vessels as a result of a predominating sympathetic action was given by Morgan and Baumgartner (1934) and by Passe and Seymour (1948) when they recorded relief of vertigo by sympathectomy. In this respect it is significant that a severe acute episode of Menière's disease can be dramatically halted by a stellate ganglion block.

Although the predominance of vasoconstriction rather than vasodilatation has been favoured in attempts to explain the pathogenesis of Menière's disease, oscillations between these states in the labyrinth have also been suggested as the basis of crises. Furthermore, there is a body of opinion which regards vasodilatation as the basic cause of the abnormalities occurring in the disorder, as in migraine.

The endolymphatic distension

The various theories of the cause of the endolymphatic hydrops have been reviewed by Lawrence (1968) though he emphasizes that he does not necessarily accept the view that over-accumulation of endolymph *per se* is the cause of clinical symptoms. As he points out, the hydrops may be a concomitant and incidental occurrence along with the other features of the disease, all arising from some basic underlying disturbance such as alteration in ionic concentrations or osmotic pressure relationships. Most otologists, however, accept the hydrops as the basic feature, even though there is difficulty in explaining its cause and in correlating it with the symptomatology.

Generally, theories of causation of the endolymphatic hydrops can be grouped as follows:

(1) Those based on disturbance of fluid formation. These are mainly dependent on the principle of radial flow of internal ear fluids, described by Naftalin and Harrison (1958).
(2) Those concerned with mechanical blockage and disturbed reabsorption. These are mainly dependent on the theory of longitudinal flow of endolymph as described by Guild (1927), i.e. with disturbance of the saccus endolymphaticus.

It should not be thought that these two theories are incompatible or conflicting and it may well be that both types of flow are necessary in the normal internal ear. The work of Johnstone (1975) should also be noted. He put forward electrophysiological and physicochemical evidence which supports the possibility of two fairly independent circulations, one mainly confined to the cochlea and the saccule and the other confined to the utricle and canals. This may suggest a lesser role for the absorptive function of the endolymph sac than has been formerly supposed.

Lundquist (1976) has also put forward evidence in favour of radial flow (combined with longitudinal flow) in that radial flow provides for energy metabolism and ion exchange and is the only satisfactory way in which the high energy demands of the organ of Corti can be met.

The possibility of excess fluid in the labyrinth was envisaged by Knapp in 1871 and he suggested that Menière's disease could be the counterpart of ocular glaucoma. Mygind and Dederding (1938) considered that the labyrinthine symptoms were part of a more generalized vasomotor disturbance which in the labyrinth affected the stria vascularis. They suggested that this produced arteriolar spasm and capillary atony leading to deficient oxygenation of the essential tissues and consequently an increased permeability of the strial capillaries. Indeed, the strial circulation has since come increasingly under suspicion as the real site of the lesion in Menière's disease.

Working with cats, Seymour (1954) was able to provide *in vivo* photographic evidence of vasomotor activity in the capillary fields of the spiral ligament, caused by electrical stimulation of the cervical sympathetic trunk. In a further communication Seymour (1960) offered the hypothesis that reduced blood flow in the stria vascularis from vasospasm resulted in anoxia of the sensory apparatus of the end-organs and in a diminished secretion of endolymph which became qualitatively abnormal as metabolites accumulated in it. The consequent rise in the osmotic pressure within the scala media caused a transference of fluid from the perilymphatic and vascular compartments so that distension occurred. He also demonstrated that in Menière's disease a high local concentration of histamine in the stria was capable of producing prolonged dilatation of arterioles and venules so that the capillaries drained of blood. This, however, might be expected to produce a fall in hydrostatic pressure and thus a transfer of fluid from endolymph to capillaries.

When considering theories of autonomic dysfunction producing a vasospasm in the strial capillaries with the resultant increasing permeability and hydrops, it has to be remembered that no nerve fibres have ever been seen in this situation. Perlman and

Kimura (1955) were unable to find any change in capillary diameters in various experiments, neither were they able to confirm the results of Seymour. Moreover, they felt that vasoconstriction would be expected to reduce hydrostatic pressure in the stria so that with a small osmotic pressure in the endolymph, fluid absorption from the endolymph would occur.

Williams (1965) has adopted the suggestion of Seymour in respect of excessive histamine being present in the stria and postulates that toxic amounts of histamine cause vasodilatation of the capillaries rather than vasoconstriction. He suggests that in this situation increased permeability of damaged vessel walls would cause an excess capillary fluid to be produced, so resulting in hydrops.

In their theory of radial flow of endolymph, Naftalin and Harrison (1958) suggest that secretion and absorption occur in the same radial area of the cochlea. Their theory deals with ionic exchanges in the internal ear, and they suggest that fluid in the internal ear passes from perilymph to endolymph and that the function of the stria is to absorb endolymph. They postulate that the function of Reissner's membrane is to retain potassium ions in the endolymph and to prevent protein from entering endolymph by being impermeable to large molecules. The stria, like the tubular cell of the kidney, extracts sodium and inserts potassium to maintain a high endolymph concentration of the latter. They emphasize that according to their theory, ionic transport against gradients is done by the stria vascularis, the only structure in this area capable of doing so. Potassium and sodium exchange across Reissner's membrane is in the direction of concentration gradients and therefore requires no energy.

They go on to state that perilymph is formed by ultrafiltration from vascular tissues of the perilymph space and that in Menière's disease there is decreased perilymph production. This leads to an apparent increase in endolymph and later is followed by a true increase of endolymph due to gradual increase of potassium as flow through Reissner's membrane diminishes.

According to Rauch (1968) various types of haemodynamic dysfunction could theoretically produce the endolymphatic hydrops. Occurring in the internal ear, these could take the following forms:

(1) Decline of capillary pressure arising from vasodilatation and causing less perilymph to be formed.
(2) Local disturbance of capillary permeability.
(3) Colloid osmotic disturbances.
(4) Venous obstruction.

Like Naftalin and Harrison he sees the primary defect as being in the production of perilymph. He submits that this is qualitatively abnormal and also is produced in deficient quantity. He points out that the flow from perilymph to endolymph is dependent on electrolyte rather than protein concentrations so that with Reissner's membrane functioning normally there occurs an increased flow across Reissner's membrane and consequently an excessive amount of endolymph. It will be noted that the theories of Naftalin and Harrison and of Rauch have much in common and are both based on sound pathophysiological principles.

In the theories so far mentioned the endolymphatic distension has been attributed to over-production of fluid, but there is also evidence that such an excess could be due to deficient absorption by the saccus endolymphaticus.

The earlier animal experiments reported by Lindsay (1947) and later by Schuknecht (1963) in which the saccus endolymphaticus was obstructed or destroyed, suggested that this organ was not essential for the maintenance of normal endolymph volume. Prolonged experimental blockage of the cochlear aqueduct (perilymph aqueduct) also failed to produce any inner-ear changes. Thus, defects in these structures might be considered to be not responsible for any significant failure of endolymph absorption. More recent work, however, has been described and discussed by Kimura and Schuknecht (1965) and by Kimura (1967, 1968) who carried out a series of important and careful experiments. The results indicated that obliteration of the endolymphatic duct and sac resulted in development of gross endolymphatic hydrops in guinea-pigs and moderate hydrops in cats and chinchillas. Hydrops did not occur in squirrel monkeys, though in these animals a fistula was frequently seen in the saccule wall posterior to the reinforced area. The appearance of these fistulae in a primate is perhaps related to the controversy concerning the observation of herniations and ruptures which was referred to under the heading of 'Pathology' earlier in this chapter. In the guinea-pig, inner-ear hydrops occurred whenever attempts were made to seal the opened endolymphatic duct. Partial blockage of the sac by insertion of foreign material or by surgical trauma of the open sac resulted in hydrops only in a few instances. The conclusion was that the endolymphatic sac and duct of the guinea-pig have a function, probably that of endolymph resorption. It must be clearly emphasized, however, that the production of experimental hydrops by these or similar surgical methods in animals is no indication that human Menière's disease arises from similarly situated lesions.

The theory that the saccus endolymphaticus may have a resorptive function finds additional support from other observations in animals, in addition to those described above. Histochemical studies by Ishii, Silverstein and Balogh (1966) as well as electron microscopic studies by Lundquist, Kimura and Wersäll (1964) and by Lundquist (1965) reveal that its epithelium has high metabolic activity and that it has morphological characteristics which one sees in systems associated with fluid transport. Injection of foreign particles into the cochlear duct also provides evidence of major resorptive and phagocytic functions in the endolymph sac. The work of Adlington (1967) likewise suggests a resorptive function.

Bast and Anson (1950) have also drawn attention to the fact that the structure of the saccus is ideally constructed for fluid resorption. Anson and colleagues (1965) were led to similar conclusions as a result of their anatomical studies. More recently Lundquist (1976) whose views on radial flow have already been mentioned, has put forward further evidence to show that the main function of the saccus is to act as a reabsorptive and defence mechanism for the internal ear. According to him the light and dark epithelial cells of the intermediate part of the saccus can reabsorb endolymph and digest cellular debris respectively whilst the complex capillary network around the saccus has endothelial characteristics indicative of active fluid transport.

Radiological evidence has been put forward by Clemis and Valvassori (1968) which suggests that in patients with Menière's disease there may be an obstruction to flow in the endolymphatic duct caused by occlusion of the surrounding osseous vestibular aqueduct. Their work has not received general acceptance, although some support has been provided by Stahle and Wilbrand (1974). Öigarrd and his colleagues (1976) were able to demonstrate the patency of the aqueduct in 95 per cent of controls. Again it was visible in only 50 per cent of patients with Menière's disease. But it was visible in only 50 per cent of patients with other ear disorders and they were forced to conclude therefore that a narrow or invisible aqueduct is a non-specific radiological sign in a variety of diseases. Arenberg (1977) and his co-workers accept that non-visualization of the vestibular aqueduct correlates to some extent with the occurrence of Menière's disease, but emphasize that failure to demonstrate the aqueduct on polytomography does not necessarily indicate that it is obliterated anatomically. The disparity may be for either technical or morphological reasons and it is clear that the final decision on the clinical validity of this possible relationship must await more accurate analysis of results obtained by operations on the saccus. It must also be noted that Sze Sun Yuen and Schuknecht (1972), in a series of temporal bone studies, found no evidence whatever of aqueduct stenosis in patients with Menière's disease when compared with an equal number of controls. They did, however, find that the endolymph duct itself was somewhat smaller in patients with Menière's disease, but felt this seemed the result rather than the cause of the disorder.

Observations on the saccus made in human patients may also be relevant. Thus Shambaugh (1969) has commented on the ischaemic appearance of the sac in patients with Menière's disease. The lumen of the sac was also found to be much reduced by adhesions or even entirely obliterated in 73 per cent of his patients. These observations suggested to him that at least in some cases endolymphatic hydrops was due to deficient resorption by an abnormal and avascular endolymphatic sac. The results of the various operations on the saccus for the relief of idiopathic endolymphatic hydrops also lend some indirect support to the idea that it has a resorptive function.

It is now increasingly thought that the circulatory defect is in the stria vascularis. Whatever the nature of the local circulatory abnormality, Pulec (1977) and others have emphasized the importance of searching for an underlying systemic disturbance as mentioned in an earlier paragraph. Pulec found that if a proper search is made as many as 55 per cent of patients diagnosed as having Menière's disease can be found to have some kind of predisposing abnormality.

Other causes of the hydrops based on focal sepsis and avitaminosis have been suggested, but they lack clinical or scientific support. Likewise, there is no evidence to support the possibility of sodium retention being primarily responsible for the excess fluid in the labyrinth as proposed by Furstenberg, Lashmet and Lathrop (1934). Neither do antigen–antibody theories enjoy wide acceptance.

Correlation of pathology with symptoms

Attempts have been made to explain the symptoms partly on a mechanical basis and partly on a biochemical one. It has also been suggested that the early and variable symptoms may be caused by mechanical factors whilst the later irreversible symptoms are due to permanent biochemical effects.

MECHANICAL FACTORS IN THE PRODUCTION OF SYMPTOMS

Animal experiments by McCabe and Wolsk (1961) have supported the notion that endolymphatic hydrops causes a hearing loss mechanically. They raised the endolymphatic pressure by injecting very small amounts of an endolymph-like (high potassium–low sodium) solution into the scala media and obtained a rapid decrease of the cochlear alternating current potentials. The normal activity returned when the pressure was released by withdrawal of the fluid.

The assumption that the early and reversible low-tone hearing loss in Menière's disease could be explained on a mechanical basis by the greater distortion of the broad part of the basilar membrane has been supported by the use of models of the cochlea constructed by Tonndorf (1957). In his experiments on cochlear models Tonndorf has assumed that Reissner's membrane has elastic properties and retains such properties during acute episodes of Menière's disease though it loses some of this elasticity later. Experiments on animals by Henriksson (1968) indicate that in the pressure studies he carried out the membranous labyrinth does indeed possess elastic properties. Henriksson also concluded that a higher level of pressure did not in itself alter vestibular activity though the actual change in pressure (from injecting fluid) did so. This he regarded purely as a mechanical effect resulting from changes in the size and shape of the membranous labyrinth. Tonndorf (1968) expanded his original theory as a result of further work on mechanical cochlear models and concluded that several of the auditory changes seen in Menière's disease could be explained on the basis of altered response characteristics of the cochlea resulting from the hydrops. He concluded that during the acute and short-lasting attacks the cochlear duct distended in the direction of both scala vestibuli and scala tympani. Due to the nature of the stiffness gradient of the basilar membrane, the degree of distension (he suggested) increased with the distance from the stapes in an exponential manner. This form of distension results in: (1) an increase in stiffness and mass of the partition; and (2) a mechanical biasing of the basilar membrane. These changes he found to be more pronounced at the apical end so that there was a lessening of the stiffness gradient. He concluded that these changes, acting alone or in combination, could be responsible for phenomena that appear to be the underlying causes of the low frequency hearing loss, the diplacusis and harmonic distortion. During prolonged episodes, or in the chronic stages of the disease, he presumed that Reissner's membrane became flaccid so that the distension of the cochlear duct was confined to this structure and produced a uniform increase in the mass of the partition. He submitted that this was the underlying cause of the flat hearing loss and the diplacusis often seen in the remission stage of the disease.

A mechanical explanation of the sudden onset of vertigo is rather difficult. Lindsay (1960) emphasized the frequency with which out-pouchings of the membranous labyrinth could be found at certain points of weakness in the presence of hydrops, especially in the saccule and at the junctions of the canal ampullae with the utricle. He suggested that such out-pouchings near the canal ampullae would interfere mechanically with the contained crista. Lawrence and McCabe (1959) and Schuknecht, Benitez and Beekhuis (1962) have expressed the view that the formation of a fistula in the membranous labyrinth initiates the abrupt attacks of vertigo as the collapsing ampullary wall displaces or interferes with the movement of the cupulae. They point out that leakage of potassium into the perilymph space would have a paralytic effect on the vestibular nerve fibres, a theory first advanced by Dohlman (1965). House (1968a) accepts the phenomenon of rupture and permanent fistula formation between endolymph and perilymph, but in contrast to Lawrence and McCabe, and Schuknecht, he holds the opinion that rupture is associated with relief of an attack of vertigo, not its onset. Schuknecht and colleagues (1962) point out that the exact site of the rupture and the competence of the utriculo-endolymphatic valve were factors influencing the association and sequence of the vestibular and cochlear symptoms.

BIOCHEMICAL FACTORS IN PRODUCTION OF SYMPTOMS

Although mechanical factors provide some explanation of the vestibular and cochlear symptoms there is increasing evidence of additional biochemical factors. Much has been written on the biochemical and electrophysical effects consequent upon mixing of endolymph and perilymph following rupture of some part of the membranous labyrinth, or alternatively consequent upon experimental introduction of artificial endolymph into the perilymph spaces. As long ago as 1954 it was demonstrated by Tasaki and his collaborators that cochlear microphonics and action potentials in the cochlear nerve were impaired by the substitution of an endolymph-like solution in the scala tympani. This also happened when injection was made into the scala vestibuli although there was some delay in the onset of impairment in the latter case. From what we know nowadays about the communications between the scala tympani and the Corti-lymph (*see below*) the delay may be due to the time taken for the injected fluid to pass from the scala vestibuli through the helicotrema into the scala tympani and from there into the Corti-lymph. Tasaki and his colleagues found that Ringer's solution (which has perilymph-like characteristics) injected either into the scala tympani or scala vestibuli had no effect, but it diminished the cochlear output when injected into the scala media. It is also to be noted that Schuknecht and Seifi (1963) found that a small mechanically-produced fistula of Reissner's membrane produced only a localized hearing loss and had little effect on cochlear function in regions separated from the fistula by only a few millimetres. It is of interest that as a result of vital dye experiments in guinea-pigs, Tonndorf, Duvall and Reneau (1962) claimed to confirm that the spaces within the organs of Corti and the tissues of the spiral ligament and limbus were perilymphatic spaces and 'perilymphatic tissues' with free communications between them. This free communication through the spiral ligament seemed to explain the passage of a dye from the scala vestibuli to the scala tympani without traversing the helicotrema.

A perilymph pathway connecting the scala tympani with the tunnel of the organ of Corti has been demonstrated by Schuknecht and Seifi (1963) in the cat. Several hundred minute openings in the inferior shelf of the osseus spiral lamina lead to bundles of nerve fibres, along which the perilymph seeps to reach the habenula perforata and organ of Corti, so providing a suitable fluid environment (so-called Corti-lymph) for neural excitation and transmission. The exact role of these perilymphatic pathways in normal and abnormal situations has yet to be clarified, but it may be that in Menière's disease perilymph, which has become contaminated with an increased level of potassium, reaches the organ of Corti through them. They have been further described by Lim (1970) and by Schuknecht (1974).

Certain vestibular symptoms were reproduced in experiments carried out by Silverstein (1970a). He perfused the perilymph spaces with artificial endolymph and thus produced a nystagmus which he thought was probably caused by alteration of the neural and sensory cell excitability of the vestibular labyrinth. The artificial endolymph itself washed out in about 45–60min and he observed that this exchange took place even in the presence of an accidental fistula between the endolymphatic and perilymphatic spaces. His work offers further support to the theory which explains some of the symptoms of Menière's disease by a sudden increase of the potassium concentration in the perilymph. It would appear that sodium and potassium ions in artificial endolymph can be exchanged in the perilymphatic space, diffusion involving the perilymphatic capillary blood circulation.

Perhaps the formation of permanent fistulae which allow the continuous contamination of the fluids may be the significant feature in the pathology of the so-called 'burnt-out' cases and in the loss of labyrinthine function after membranous labyrinthectomy. The inactivation of the sensorineural apparatus may result from the establishment of an unsuitable fluid environment while not causing any degenerative changes of the neurosensory structures (*see* Schuknecht, Benitez and Beekhuis, 1962). However, evidence of significant chemical contamination is not yet definitely established.

It is not yet agreed how important are these biochemical factors as compared with the mechanical ones in the pathogenesis of Menière's disease and the correlation between electrolyte content and bioelectric potentials requires further clarification.

Verification or otherwise of the conjectures set out in this section is needed. The answer may lie in the better understanding of the biochemical and electrophysical aspects of the physiology of the inner ear and its fluids.

Two points must be constantly borne in mind when considering these theories.

(1) No abnormality of perilymph or endolymph in respect of their potassium or sodium content has ever been demonstrated in patients with Menière's disease. Indeed, the evidence is that these ionic concentrations are normal.

(2) Although experimental alteration of electrolyte concentrations in endolymph and perilymph produces profound changes in the electrical activity of the cochlea, neither perilymph nor endolymph has direct contact with the hair-cells or non-medulated nerve fibres of the organ of Corti. In any case, according to the classic membrane theory it would be physiologically impossible for action potentials to be generated in high potassium fluid surroundings, such as endolymph.

Rauch (1960) demonstrated that the fluid environment in the spaces of the organ of Corti (i.e. the spaces of Nuel and the tunnel of Corti) has extracellular properties and resembles perilymph (i.e. is poor in potassium). It thus provides an appropriate medium for neural excitation and transmission. Colman (1969b) has suggested that only at this site can electrolyte disturbance produce its effects. Such disturbances would be compatible with the normal ionic concentrations which have been reported for potassium and sodium in endolymph and perilymph in patients with Menière's disease, and increase of potassium in the cortilymph could result from direct or indirect leakage from the endolymph compartment.

Treatment

Because our knowledge of the basic pathology is so inadequate it is difficult to design any satisfactory medical or surgical treatment for Menière's disease. Schuknecht (1976) recently summed up the situation regarding medical treatment in the following words.

'I think if we sit as a jury of honest judges looking on the results I doubt that we could approve one single drug in the treatment of Menière's disease.'

The situation seems to have improved very little since Furstenburg and his co-workers (1934) commented on the 'bewildered and futile state of medical therapy in the Menière's syndrome complex'. Indeed, one might reasonably ask whether medical treatment has improved to any significant extent since Menière first described the disease. Many treatments are designed to influence endolymph production or absorption, even though the exact significance of the endolymphatic hydrops has never been determined. Changing views on the pathogenesis of Menière's disease have brought about different lines of treatment. Various forms of medical treatment employing dietetic measures and medication, the latter mainly consisting of vitamins, antihistamines, vasodilators and diuretics, have all had their protagonists.

A variety of surgical procedures has been designed to relieve suspected vasospasm in the labyrinth or to decompress the labyrinth or to sever its nervous connections or to destroy the labyrinthine end-organs wholly or in part. Any success claimed for these different methods of treatment, both medical and surgical (with the exception of total destruction or total denervation) must always be weighed against the widely varying periods of remission that occur naturally in this disorder. Indeed, there is evidence which suggests that most medical treatment and certain surgical procedures are only effective through their placebo effect, and that the 'improvement rate' is merely what one would expect from the natural history of the disease.

The situation is unlikely to be clarified until more medical treatments have been adequately tested with double-blind cross-over trial techniques, and until medical and surgical results have been reported on a commonly agreed standard such as that prepared by the Alford Committee of the AAOO (1972). At present few authors follow its recommendations and so confusion is as rampant as ever in respect of results.

General management

The relief of the tense and anxious state resulting from the dread of unpredictable attacks of vertigo is of prime importance. An unrelenting tinnitus and the frustration due to deafness, especially in those bilateral cases to whom a hearing aid is unhelpful, can produce great depression which requires alleviation. Some patients have the ability to adjust themselves to these symptoms with remarkable success whilst others sometimes appear near to suicide. An understanding and sympathetic approach to the patient's problems is essential. Strong reassurance, stressing the non-fatal nature of the disorder, is necessary and should be coupled with some explanation as to its cause, for example, 'an excess of fluid in the balance organ' or 'some disorder of the blood supply to the inner ear'. The patient must be told that the condition can be ameliorated even if it cannot be completely cured. It must be pointed out that it is necessary to adopt as relaxed a life as possible and that recurrence of symptoms sometimes follows excessive strain or emotional stress. It is probably wise to tell the patient that relapses may occur occasionally and that if need be management may be altered from time to time. Otherwise the patient will inevitably suffer loss of confidence sooner or later.

Fortunately, many patients have either long natural remissions, sometimes halting spontaneously for life after but one or two attacks, or they appear to be controlled by medical treatment sufficiently to lead an ordinary active life. Although some relief or even control of the symptoms may appear to have been achieved, the capricious nature of Menière's disease renders attempts to assess the value of any medical treatment uncertain. Too much must not be expected from the short-term use of medical treatment and this certainly cannot be expected to abolish the disease.

Patients should be warned against exposure to cold temperatures, especially when tired, as there is some evidence that exacerbations are likely under such circumstances. It is sometimes difficult to give advice about car driving and the following of certain employments in which an attack of vertigo might constitute a special hazard. An assessment is necessary of the frequency and severity of the attacks and of the amount of warning given by any prodromal symptoms before the vertigo begins. When doubt exists it is better to advise against such activities at least on a temporary basis.

Despite the not uncommonly lowered speech discrimination for amplified speech in the deafness of Menière's disease, an adequate trial with a hearing aid should always be given in bilateral cases. Tinnitus may be very upsetting and is particularly difficult to alleviate, although some masking effect may be provided by a suitable hearing aid.

Treatment in the remission phase

Before going on to discuss various points in medical management it should be emphasized that apart from streptomycin and those medications which give some suppression of the sensation of vertigo a lot of medical treatment is on an empirical basis. With a few exceptions there is little statistical evidence that medication alters the natural history of the disease or confers any special benefit. Nevertheless, most otologists provide some kind of medical treatment, even though they may be unconvinced that it gives real benefit. It can be reasonably said, however, that some form of medical regimen provides the patient with reassurance and a feeling that something is being done. Indeed, there is some evidence that supervision of this kind, special testing, and involvement in the machinery of a big hospital, has a significant placebo effect. If the patient is seen regularly it also gives the opportunity of offering suitable surgical treatment at the appropriate time if deterioration is occurring.

As mentioned in a previous paragraph, it is important to search for any underlying or predisposing cause as emphasized by Pulec and to provide specific treatment for any abnormality discovered such as thyroid dysfunction, pituitary/adrenal insufficiency, glucose intolerance and similar problems.

DIETETIC THERAPY

A regime based on low sodium intake, combined with the use of ammonium chloride as a diuretic, was first introduced by Furstenburg and his colleagues in 1934. Although Boles and his co-workers (1975) working from the same clinic reported satisfactory results and few operations in a series of 500 consecutive patients treated on similar lines, these regimes have been questioned and their value has become increasingly doubted as a result of our improved knowledge of fluid electrolyte concentrations. There is little evidence that labyrinthine or serum electrolyte concentration can be altered by ordinary dietetic measures. Golding-Wood (1960a) and others who have carried out clinical experiments on patients with Menière's disease have been led to the conclusion that fluid and salt restriction is probably valueless and unjustified, but on the other hand Harrison and Naftalin (1963), as a result of experiments to induce vertigo by biochemical means, considered that sodium diuresis, the state in which they believed that vertigo was most likely to occur, could not take place on a low salt diet.

VASODILATORS

The use of vasodilators is a natural corollary to the theory of labyrinthine ischaemia and of circulatory abnormalities in the stria vascularis. Experiments by Snow and Suga (1975) on the effects of various drugs on the micro-circulation of the internal ear are of interest in this respect. They found that the cochlear flow was greatly increased by carbon dioxide, amyl nitrite and betahistine. A substantial increase resulted from papaverine, a smaller increase after administration of histamine and no increase at all after nicotinic acid. Accordingly, there may be some experimental basis for the use of the drugs first mentioned, although none at all for the use of nicotinic acid, even though it is so frequently prescribed. Although good results have been claimed for carbon dioxide inhalation and for histamine injection there are no satisfactory controlled studies.

Several investigators, however, including Betrand (1972) and Wilmot (1972) in carefully controlled double-blind trials on betahistine (Serc) have found this drug to be of benefit.

ANTIHISTAMINES

Various phenothiazine drugs with antihistamine properties have been reported to be useful in the management of Menière's including drugs such as cinnarizine (Stugeron) and diphenidol. For the latter-mentioned a double-blind trial carried out by Futaki, Kitahara and Morimoto (1975) gave statistically significant results. Various other antihistamines and piperazines have also been recommended because of their sedative and vestibular suppressant effects. Droperidol has also been used on account of its profound suppression of vestibular activity.

DIURETICS

The use of diuretic agents such as hydrochlorothiazide and chlorthalidone, is based on the diuretic/osmotic effect of glycerol which has been discussed earlier in this chapter. Klockhoff and Lindblom (1967) used hydrochlorothiazide in a particularly careful double-blind study and found it to be a considerable benefit in the short term. Klockhoff and his co-workers (1974) obtained very similar results with the latter drug also. With both drugs, however, longer follow-up led them to conclude that there was no indication present of a change in the long-term course of the disease. Hearing loss continued to progress and vertigo remained a problem in a number of patients.

OTHER DRUGS

Lithium carbonate was introduced in the hope that it might favourably alter the transport of fluid and ions across the membranes of the internal ear and good results were reported from initial pilot studies. Recently, however, a double-blind cross-over trial carried out by Thomsen and his colleagues (1976) demonstrated no more than a placebo effect. The same would doubtless apply to most other drugs if similarly tested. Lemon bioflavinoid derivatives have not been shown to have any effect and vitamin therapy today has few supporters. On the other hand sedatives and tranquillizers in small dosage often appear helpful, especially in those patients who are aware that attacks tend to occur during periods of stress and preparations such as prochlorperazine (Stemetil) and thyethylperazine (Torecan) are useful to suppress nausea and vomiting, as well as the unsteadiness which sometimes follows an acute exacerbation.

Treatment of the acute attack

Unless the attack is mild and recovery seems to take place quickly the best thing is for the patient to go to bed and stay there with the head firmly supported by pillows. In the first attack especially the frightened patient must be appropriately reassured. Various preparations are available which help to suppress symptoms and if necessary they must be given by injection. The following drugs are commonly used: promethazine (Avomine), dimenhydrinate (Dramamine), perphenazine (Fentazin), promethazine (Phenergan), or chlorpromazine (Largactil). In a severe and prolonged attack the latter is probably the drug of choice given intramuscularly in a dosage of 75 mg. As the vertigo subsides the sedation can gradually be lessened.

The symptoms of the acute attack can also be relieved according to Gejrot (1976) by an intravenous infusion of Xylocaine in a dosage of 1 mg/kg body weight given at a rate of 6 mg/min

Densert and his colleagues (1975) observed that the symptoms could be rapidly relieved by treatment in a pressure chamber and lowering the pressure. Tjernström (1977) also reported that hypobaric treatment could produce rapid relief of symptoms in an acute attack and observed it in 60 per cent of his 46 patients. This is a facility, however, that is not always readily available.

Stellate ganglion block in the experience of many otologists can give rapid relief from an acute attack. The patient lies supine with the neck extended. A small bleb of local anaesthetic is injected into the skin. The great vessels are then retracted laterally by the first three fingers, the lowest being just above the clavicle. A lumbar puncture needle resting against the central fingertip is passed downwards between the trachea and the great vessels in a vertical direction until it strikes the transverse process of the seventh cervical vertebra. The needle is slightly withdrawn in order to clear the longus cervicis muscle and then an injection is made of approximately 10 ml of 1 per cent lignocaine or procaine. Hyaluronidase may be used to help to spread the anaesthetic. It is important to aspirate before the injection is made in order to ensure that no vessel has been accidentally entered.

Streptomycin therapy

Streptomycin therapy was first recommended by Fowler (1948) taking advantage of the selective ototoxic effect of the drug. It acts, of course, bilaterally, and accordingly an indication for using it may be severe vertigo from bilateral disease. It is necessary to emphasize that there is the risk of cochlear injury and, as with any ototoxic drug, the effect can be delayed. It is also necessary to emphasize that bilateral labyrinthectomy whether induced by surgical or by medical means can itself produce some disability. The symptoms have been described by Martin (1967) and by Golding-Wood (1969a).

Eight patients were initially reported by Schuknecht (1957). The same patients and more recent ones were reviewed by Singleton and Schuknecht (1968). All patients were somewhat ataxic for several months after treatment and the average length of time for return of the patient to full activity was four months. In no case was it considered that the symptoms from the bilateral loss of vestibular function were as severe and certainly never so incapacitating as the previous episodes of Menière's disease.

Streptomycin was injected locally into the middle ear by Lange (1972) in 38 patients with severe unilateral Menière's disease. He reported that 34 of them were free of vertigo and that the remaining four were substantially improved. Hearing was preserved in three-quarters of them.

Surgical treatment

Surgical treatment must be considered for those patients in whom disabling symptoms are continuing to occur without evidence of adequate remission. It is customary to provide for about six months of medical treatment before making any decision but this will depend upon individual circumstances. If a patient is getting worse rather than better, and if he is unable to follow his normal activities then surgical treatment may be indicated. In the past the severity of the vertigo has been the main criterion used in reaching a decision. However, with increasing realization that even the best medical treatment does little to conserve hearing, combined with the knowledge that the progressive nature of the disorder will almost inevitably lead to increasing hearing damage, there is now a greater tendency to operate earlier in an attempt to conserve hearing (albeit in the knowledge that surgical treatment is also uncertain and unproven from this point of view).

Most surgical procedures can be considered under the following main headings:

(1) Procedures designed to influence endolymph production (e.g. sympathectomy).
(2) Procedures designed to influence endolymph absorption (e.g. operations on the endolymphatic sac).
(3) Selective denervation of the vestibular labyrinth (i.e. vestibular nerve resection).
(4) Labyrinth destruction.
   (a) Selective destruction of the vestibular labyrinth (by ultrasound or cryosurgery).
   (b) Total destruction of the labyrinth (i.e. labyrinthectomy) combined perhaps with total denervation (i.e. translabyrinthine cochleo–vestibular neurectomy).

The exact procedure will mainly depend on the level of hearing present and whether the disease is unilateral or bilateral. All of the operations except the last in the list aim to preserve hearing. Operations in the last group offer no possibility of retention of hearing after operation and accordingly are only suitable if it is felt the residual hearing in the affected ear can safely be sacrificed, and that the other ear is healthy.

As with medical treatment there is great difficulty in assessing results accurately and few authors, as yet, follow the standardized criteria recommended by the Alford Committee of the AAOO (1972) for reporting results.

CERVICAL SYMPATHECTOMY

Mogan and Baumgartner in 1934 performed bilateral cervical ganglionectomy on a case of 'Menière's disease associated with interstitial keratitis' (Cogan's disease) and relieved the vertigo. The chain is removed from below upwards to just above the stellate ganglion and 2.5 cm or so of the trunk below it. Golding-Wood (1969b) emphasizes that the resection should be from C8 to T3 inclusive, and that ligation division of the internal mammary artery is not necessary for adequate exposure.

Supporters of sympathectomy point out that it is especially suited to patients with severe deafness. The operation should be carried out bilaterally. It is thought that in some way as yet undetermined sympathectomy helps to correct the microcirculatory fault in the stria vascularis.

Golding-Wood (1973) and Wilmot (1977) both report satisfactory results from the operation. The former gives a long-term follow-up in 247 patients treated by bilateral sympathectomy. All his operations were on patients with uncontrollable symptoms from bilateral disease, or disease affecting an only remaining or only useful ear. He found that after operation attacks of vertigo generally ceased abruptly but that some degree of activity recurred after two years and that this correlated with a partial relapse of vertigo amounting to 12 per cent at this time. Nevertheless 50 per cent of the patients retained complete, long-term relief from vertigo. Hearing and tinnitus were improved to a lesser degree but for those patients in whom deteriorating hearing was the main concern he still felt that a sympathectomy was the best procedure. The risk of further hearing deterioration with the Portmann or House operations on the saccus seemed to him to be too great for saccus operations to be the treatment of choice. An important point to remember about sympathectomy is that it is an operation which is remote from the ear and therefore totally free of any risk to hearing. Accordingly perhaps it is especially suitable for those patients having Menière's disease in an only remaining ear. According to Wilmot (1977) it may be considered as one of the alternative procedures available when a previous saccus operation has failed.

OPERATIONS ON THE SACCUS ENDOLYMPHATICUS

In 1897 Cheatle, in accordance with the analogy between Menière's disease and ocular glaucoma, suggested decompression of the labyrinth by making an opening into the perilymphatic space to relieve the 'hypertension' of the endolymph. His suggestion was not acted upon until 1904 when Lake and Milligan independently performed operations based on this concept but these operations were, in fact, labyrinthine destructions.

G. Portmann (1927) believed that Menière's disease was due to a hypertension of the endolymph and successfully drained the endolymph by opening the endolymphatic sac 12 years before Hallpike and Cairns presented their first description of the histopathology of Menière's disease. The patient was still living at the age of 75 in 1966, never having experienced a return of the vertigo (M. Portmann, 1969).

The mastoid is opened and the sinus plate exposed. If possible this is done without entering the antrum in order to avoid a wide communication with the middle ear. The saccus is uncovered in that area of dura which lies between the sinus plate and the lower half of the posterior semicircular canal.

If further separation of the dura is made anteriorly it becomes more adherent to the bone at the point where the ductus emerges from the vestibular aqueduct, and frequently there is a small bony projection at this point where the dura tents upwards into the bone. The operation can be completed at this point having done a simple decompression. Alternatively the saccus can be opened and a Silastic drain inserted between its lumen and the mastoid (the area then being covered by free muscle graft), or pedicled muscle graft can be brought in according to the method of Fisch in the hope of improving the blood supply to the area. The operation can proceed to the opening of the dura of the medial wall of the sac to create a fistula into the adjacent subarachnoid space. To maintain the patency of the shunt so created either a strip of Silastic or some kind of drain can be inserted after which the outer wall of the sac is reconstituted and reinforced by a piece of free muscle. The surgical anatomy of the endolymphatic sac has been described in detail in a beautifully illustrated paper by Arenberg and his co-workers in (1977) to which reference should be made.

The results reported by various surgeons employing different techniques are illustrated in *Table 25.3*. Palva and his colleagues (1976) found their results were somewhat less satisfactory than those in most published series, but nevertheless were in accordance with the experience of many others. Many otologists with interest and experience in this field will find themselves in sympathy with Palva's observations.

Shambaugh (1968) in reviewing reported results of various surgeons was struck by the similarity of results regardless of whether the sac was merely exposed, exposed and incised, incised and drained, or had a shunt inserted into the subarachnoid space. He suggested that the one common factor in all operations was that the sac had been exposed, and suggested that the benefit from all of these procedures might be simply the result from uncovering the sac wall. Indeed, at the present time there seems to be a tendency away from the more complex procedures, especially those requiring insertion of a subarachnoid shunt, back towards simple decompression. Morrison (1976) and Smyth, Houlihan and Hassard (1977) support this trend in favour of decompression. The author's experience has been that decompression, drainage and subarachnoid shunt procedures yield approximately equal results and are frequently equally disappointing and unpredictable.

There is evidence that the better results in saccus surgery are obtained in the earlier and reversible stage of the disease, i.e. when hearing is fluctuating. Preferably hearing should be normal or near-normal during remissions. There is also evidence that better results are obtained in patients who give a positive glycerol test. It should be noted, however, that good results can be obtained later in the disease, as Smyth, Houlihan and Hassard (1977) have indicated. The work of Clemis and Valvassori (1968) relating to the tomographic demonstration of the vestibular aqueduct has been referred to in a previous paragraph. Although the matter remains controversial, some surgeons regard preliminary radiological demonstration of the aqueduct to be important in the selection of patients for operations on the saccus.

Saccus decompression and saccus drainage are both relatively straightforward procedures without any great risk of complications. Fisch (1976), however, has quoted a risk (4 per cent) producing a sensorineural hearing loss. This is often said to be due to accidental injury of the posterior semicircular canal, but the complication can undoubtedly occur in the absence of such an accident, especially in patients in whom the sac has been opened. The insertion of a saccus–subarachnoid shunt risks other complications, including those of CSF leakage, as reported by Gardner (1975) as well as meningitis. Although these serious complications are extremely unusual in experienced hands it is the existence of them (in the absence of any statistically proven advantage) that is partly responsible for the move away from subarachnoid shunt procedures.

Table 25.3

	House and Owens (1973)	Paparella and Hanson (1976)	Morrison (1976)	Fisch (1976)	Smyth, Houlihan and Hassard (1977)	Pulec (1977)
Operation	CSF shunt	Drain into mastoid	Drain into mastoid	Synangiosis	Decompression	CSF shunt
Number	172	43	87	52	22	251
Hearing better or stabilized	66%	30%	69%	48%	77%	50%
Vertigo absent or significantly improved	62%	94%	79%	48%	73%	64%
Follow-up period	1–8 years	1–8 years	1–4½ years	5 years	2–11 years	2½ years

Results obtained by various types of operation on the endolymphatic sac.

ENDOLYMPH-PERILYMPH SHUNTS

Shunts created inside the labyrinth have been suggested by Fick, and by Cody to help promote endolymph absorption. Decompression of the saccule as described by Fick (1964) is based on the assumption that in most cases of Menière's disease the distended saccule comes into contact with the vestibular surface of the stapes footplate. He described excellent results from sacculotomy in respect of relief of vertigo and preservation of hearing, but the experience of nearly all other otologists has been that the operation carries a dangerously high incidence of very severe sensorineural deafness and the operation should perhaps be regarded as a destructive one. It serves as a useful alternative to labyrinthectomy in old patients with extremely poor hearing in the affected ear. It is a relatively minor operation and if need be can be done under local anaesthetic. There is a high likelihood of relieving the acute episodes of vertigo, and the more gradual loss of function compared to a conventional labyrinthectomy allows for easier compensation. If sufficient improvement is not obtained a labyrinthectomy can still be offered subsequently.

Cody, Simonton and Hallberg (1967) and Cody (1968) described a modification of the Fick operation. They inserted a stainless steel tack which was left permanently in position in the stapes footplate so that the distending saccule could be automatically and repetitively decompressed by contact against it. Cody (1974) has reported a long-term follow-up of 140 such operations. He found that vertigo could be satisfactorily controlled in 80 per cent of his patients and that there had been a hearing improvement in 24 per cent, but in spite of these encouraging results the operation has not become generally accepted because of the high risk to hearing.

House (1968a) used a cryosurgical probe on the promontory to try and create a small endolymph–perilymph fistula in the wall of the membranous labyrinth. Whatever the effects of cryosurgery there seems to be no experimental evidence that a fistula is produced. An otic/periotic shunt operation has been described by Pulec (1968) who inserted a small tube through the basilar membrane using a round window approach. From our knowledge of the hazards of producing direct communication between the endolymph and perilymph spaces in Menière's disease it seems unlikely that any useful hearing would survive these procedures.

INTRACRANIAL DIVISION OF THE EIGHTH NERVE

The eighth nerve was first divided by Parry in 1904. McKenzie (1931) limited the operation to section of the vestibular portion and Dandy (1941) was able to report a series of 401 operations with only one death utilizing a posterior fossa approach.

More recently a middle-fossa micro-surgical approach has been described by House (1968b). The technique is now well known and has been further modified and described by Fisch (1970, 1973) (*Figure 25.9*). Through a middle-fossa craniotomy and working extradurally the superior semicircular canal is identified and blue-lined. Using this as a landmark, bone is then removed from the meatal plane until the internal auditory meatus is exposed in its entire length and entire transverse diameter, its dural sleeve is incised and after division of the vestibulo–facial anastomosis the meatal segment of the vestibular nerve is removed, using fine micro-neurectomy scissors. Great care is taken to avoid injury to the facial nerve and cochlear nerve as well as the arterial and venous blood supply to the internal ear.

The operation demands a high degree of surgical skill and it potentially carries the

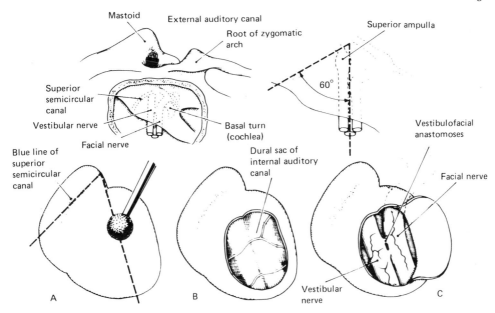

Figure 25.9   Resection of the vestibular part of the eighth nerve through the middle-fossa approach. The superior surface of the left petrous bone is illustrated through the craniotomy, the surgeon sitting at the head of the table. The superior semicircular canal is blue-lined, the internal auditory meatus lies at an angle of approximately 60 degrees. Bone is removed over this area until the dura of the internal meatus is exposed. The dura is then incised posteriorly away from the facial nerve. The vestibular nerve is separated from the facial nerve and its various component parts are removed. (By courtesy of Professor Ugo Fisch)

various complications and risk of morbidity which are associated with intracranial surgery in the middle fossa.

There has now been considerable experience with the operation and in experienced hands it has shown itself to be highly predictable in the relief of vertigo and in preservation of hearing. The effect on hearing in the long term and any influence on the disease itself remain to be determined. The results obtained by Fisch (1970, 1976) are probably representative. He quotes 94 per cent of patients relieved of vertigo, 80 per cent with preservation of hearing. Sixty-six per cent had their tinnitus relieved and 63 per cent had the sensation of pressure relieved. His complications include a severe sensorineural hearing loss in about 4 per cent (this may occur from accidental injury to the superior semicircular canal, or basal turn of the cochlea, or interference with blood supply in the internal meatus), as well as a 3 per cent incidence of temporary reversible facial palsy.

Bauer (1974) has suggested that there may be less risk to hearing if only the superior vestibular nerve is divided. Pulec (1977) agrees this lessens the risk to hearing, but increases the possibility of a post-operative positional vertigo.

Vestibular neurectomy is followed by powerful bilateral suppression of vestibular activity, as emphasized by Fisch (1973), which makes for a more rapid compensation compared to that after labyrinthectomy. There is also some evidence that the natural history of the disease may be altered by operation with consequent control of any further hearing deterioration. This is probably due to division of the efferent fibres to the labyrinth as discussed by Chouard (1973).

Although interest in the last decade has centred mainly upon the middle fossa route for this operation it is possible that attention may again turn to the posterior fossa approach with the application of micro-surgical techniques to the original Dandy operation to achieve selective eighth nerve resection. Indeed, Bryan and Bucy (1973) reported on 17 patients using this route, although with substantially less satisfactory results than those obtainable by using the middle-fossa approach.

SELECTIVE DESTRUCTION OF THE VESTIBULAR LABYRINTH

This may be accomplished either by ultrasound or by cryosurgery.

Ultrasonic vibrations were first employed to destroy the human labyrinth by Krejci (1952) followed by Arslan in 1953. Since then many other surgeons have used this particular therapy, especially for unilateral cases in which the hearing remains at a serviceable level, or in bilateral cases where any residual hearing must be conserved.

The nerves and sensorineural elements of the ear appear to be most affected by ultrasound. These effects are brought about by the rupture of their cell membranes and possibly by acting on the sodium–potassium pump which is normally responsible for maintaining a potential difference between the interior and exterior of living cells. Experiments by Angell-James and his colleagues (1963) have shown that the endolymph in the irradiated ears of guinea-pigs has increased sodium and decreased potassium ionic concentration. The histological changes in cells damaged by ultrasound are not immediate as Brain and colleagues (1960) demonstrated.

Suggestions have been made at various times that part of the effect of ultrasound treatment arises from the creation of an endolymph–perilymph fistula in the membranous labyrinth. Although the idea is frequently repeated there is no scientific evidence whatever to support this concept, even from electron microscopic studies.

In this country the technique developed by Angell-James (1963) has been generally employed. The operation is normally done under local anaesthesia in order to observe the behaviour of the nystagmus and also to enable the facial nerve function to be continually observed. The mastoid antrum is opened through a post-aural incision after which the lateral semicircular canal is identified and burred down until the blue-line is evident. The applicator is applied to the canal and an irritative nystagmus appears. The power is gradually increased at a rate at which the patient can tolerate it and application continues for a few minutes after irritation has ceased. The mildness of the post-operative disturbance is in contrast to the quite severe vertigo which generally follows conventional labyrinthine destruction. Angell-James (1969a) reviewed results on 232 patients treated between 1963 and 1967 and they are summarized in *Table 25.4*. Angell-James (1969b) feels that ultrasound treatment must remain the most generally applicable surgical treatment for the patient with Menière's disease and regards it as especially valuable for patients with bilateral disease, for disease in one remaining ear and after previous unsuccessful labyrinthectomy (though the operation of choice for the latter would probably now, in 1979, be translabyrinthine neurectomy).

Stahle (1976b) reported his experience with 356 patients extending over a 12-year period. His initial techniques were very similar to those of Angell-James, but since 1963 he has also directed the ultrasonic beam towards the thinned-out otic capsule in the junction between the lateral and the superior canals. In the last two years, if anatomy has allowed, the posterior semicircular canal has also been irradiated.

Table 25.4 **Results obtained by ultrasound treatment by Angell-James and by Stahle (semicircular canal application)**

	Angell-James— 232 patients	*Stahle—356 patients*
Vertigo		
ceased	85%	52%
improved	15%	45%
Hearing improved or unchanged	56%	50%
Hearing worse	42%	40%
Tinnitus		
ceased	30%	40%
improved	42%	

According to his evaluation 71 per cent of patients had been improved by operation; 42 patients in the entire series received further surgical treatment in some form (half of them further ultrasound application). The best results in respect of relief from vertigo were obtained in those patients who were given a marked depression of the caloric response. His results are given in *Table 25.4*. Somewhat similar figures have been quoted by Sørensen (1970) and by Dionne, Barker and Bryant (1972).

The operation is not without hazard to the facial nerve and severe hearing deterioration can occur if accidental cracking of the thinned semicircular canal occurs. Some of the hearing deterioration after treatment will be attributed to the progressive nature of the uncontrolled disease. Stahle's view, however, was that at least some of the loss must be attributed to the direct effect of ultrasound upon the cochlea. In 43 patients with bilateral disease on whom ultrasound had been applied just to one ear he found hearing had deteriorated in 53 per cent of patients on the operated side as opposed to only 30 per cent on the non-operated side.

Attempts to protect the cochlea from possible damage by ultrasound were employed by Kossoff and his co-workers (1967) by using a special applicator applied to the round window and directing the applicator towards the areas of vestibular sensorineural epithelium. Barnett and Kossoff (1977) give a detailed account of the technique, which has remained virtually unchanged. The dosage was increased to 100 mW after 1970 for a series of 32 patients and appears to give rather better results.

Table 25.5 **Barnett and Kossoff—32 patients**

No vertigo, no hearing loss	50%
No vertigo, some hearing loss	22%
Recurrence of vertigo, no hearing loss	9%
Recurrence of vertigo, hearing loss	19%

Results obtained by Barnett and Kossoff by ultrasound (round window application)

With a minimum follow-up of four years the results are indicated in *Table 25.5* for these 32 patients. Only one patient had a hearing improvement after treatment—this was three months after irradiation. No patients treated with the round window method received any relief from tinnitus. These authors emphasize the importance of correctly aiming the probe in order to avoid hearing damage. When correctly aimed, the measurements indicated that only the first 4 mm of the basal turn were in the direct path of the ultrasonic beam, i.e. hearing frequencies above 16 kHz.

Cryosurgical methods have also been used for selective destruction in attempts to control Menière's disease. In animal experiments Cutt and his colleagues (1968) found it was possible to destroy the end-organs in monkeys satisfactorily without injury to the cochlea or the facial nerve. Further studies by Lundquist, Igarashi and Wersall (1972) demonstrated that in guinea-pigs electron microscopy showed the earliest changes, in the form of intracellular damage which was later followed by epithelial disintegration, presumably due to blocking of cell metabolism. Destruction by ice-crystal formation was seen in the cristae, utricle and saccular maculae, although the cochlea was undisturbed. Ishiyama, Myers and Wolfson (1972) reported somewhat similar findings from electron microscopy and correlated their observations with the degree of freezing. They found that a temperature of at least − 70 °C was essential to ensure adequate destruction.

In clinical use the probe can be placed on the lateral semicircular canal, or on the promontory as described by House (1968c). Wolfson and Cutt (1971) reported a 1–4-year follow-up on 72 patients and found that vertigo was eliminated or greatly reduced in 76 per cent of them. Hearing was unchanged, it either fluctuated or was stable, as pre-operatively. Facial palsy occasionally occurred, but was never permanent. Tabor, La Var and Donohoe (1972) also reported satisfactory results after cryosurgery in 47 patients who had previously been resistant to treatment. An initial freeze at − 160 °C for 2 min was provided and this was repeated a second or maybe a third time depending upon the vestibular and auditory monitoring changes recorded during the application. A significant improvement of vertiginous symptoms was obtained in nearly 80 per cent of patients although hearing loss and temporary facial palsy occurred in 10 per cent.

DESTRUCTION OF THE LABYRINTH

The first attacks upon the bony semicircular canals were undertaken independently by Lake and Milligan in 1904. These were made via a radical mastoidectomy approach, but the fear of a spreading infection in the labyrinth soon restricted the use of such operations to provide drainage in the treatment of suppurative labyrinthitis. Mollison (1931) opened the bony external semicircular canal via a cortical mastoidectomy and injected alcohol into it.

If it is decided that the residual hearing in the ear can be sacrificed safely the labyrinth can be destroyed by various methods.

(1) The post-aural lateral semicircular canal approach.
(2) An extension of this with complete exenteration of all three canals and of the vestibule (and perhaps with neurectomy).
(3) A permeatal transtympanic window approach (which can also include a neurectomy).

Post-aural membranous labyrinthectomy was described by Cawthorne. The lateral bony semicircular canal is exposed, the canal is opened and the membranous canal lifted from the bony tunnel by means of a small hook so that it can be avulsed with its ampullary portion. No vestibular or cochlear function remained in 346 patients operated on by Cawthorne. Tinnitus was generally unchanged.

Appropriate exercises help to establish full compensation. The results are generally excellent and the loss of distorted hearing in the ear is a benefit. Labyrinthectomy done this way is probably the simplest operation available and highly reliable.

The operation is rendered more complete and more certain by opening and exenterating all three semicircular canals and removing the contents of the vestibule through the access thereby created (the so-called three-canal labyrinthectomy).

This procedure is particularly suitable if there has been a previous, failed labyrinthectomy. In this case it should be taken further by continuing the operation until the internal auditory meatus is exposed (translabyrinthine neurectomy). The internal meatus is exposed in its complete length, the dura is opened and the whole of the vestibular nerve is resected as described by Pulec (1968). The cochlear nerve may also be divided in an attempt to help the tinnitus of these patients. Extending the operation in this way makes it a more major procedure and calls for considerable skill, but it makes totally certain of destruction and enables the vestibular nerve to degenerate backwards to the brain stem. It is an operation that can be used after a previous failed labyrinthectomy (provided there is no radical mastoid cavity). The effect on the tinnitus is variable and initial reports on this have probably been too optimistic. A further advantage that is claimed for the procedure is that it allows the surgeon to inspect the internal auditory meatus and to exclude with certainty the presence of a small unsuspected vestibular schwannoma. The advantages of opening the dura have to be balanced against the extra danger to the seventh nerve as well as the possibility even of a CSF leak and possibly consequent meningitis.

Permeatal transtympanic labyrinthectomy was described by Schuknecht (1956) and by Cawthorne (1957) as an alternative to destruction through the lateral semicircular canal. The stapes is exposed by the tympanotomy approach and either removed or turned aside, still attached to the stapedius tendon, so that the edge of the utricle is seen protruding from the facial border of the oval window. The utricle is drawn down by a hook and avulsed with forceps.

A sucker can be introduced into the vestibule and the round window membrane can be broken through. Very small pledgets of gel-foam soaked in 90 per cent alcohol introduced into the internal ear help to ensure that all function is destroyed. Insertion of alcohol on gel-foam in this way carries less danger to the facial nerve than injection of alcohol through a needle with consequent risk of flooding of the area. The stapes can be replaced to seal the oval window again.

Silverstein (1976) has described a technique to extend permeatal labyrinthectomy to include a cochleo–vestibular neurectomy by going through the promontory. He found that the operation was quick, that total ablation was assured, that tinnitus was likely to be relieved, that it gave the opportunity of examining the internal auditory meatus, and that for patients with Menière's disease it gave 100 per cent likelihood of giving excellent relief of the vertigo. It may be considered, however, that the access is somewhat awkward and the hazard to the facial nerve too great for general use.

Although labyrinthectomy generally succeeds in avoiding the acute episodes of disabling vertigo it is sometimes followed by incomplete compensation (especially in older patients) associated with fairly constant, although mild, ill-defined unsteadiness. Palva (1976) comments on this. About half of his patients after three months still showed some uncertainty in walking, especially in the dark, but all were able to resume their previous work. The patients of Pedersen and Sørensen (1970) were perhaps less well motivated: half of 32 patients whom they were able to trace with an average follow-up of seven years still complained of persistent imbalance that was bad enough to incapacitate them and prevent return to full-time work.

OTHER OPERATIONS

Two other forms of operation should be mentioned. Their precise status is still far from being determined.

(1) Insertion of a ventilating grommet through the tympanic membrane has been recommended by Tumarkin (1966) on the assumption that in Menière's disease the internal ear disturbance is a manifestation of abnormal middle-ear pressures secondary to eustachian tube insufficiency. Scientific support for this assumption has been lacking, though it is interesting to note that Hall and Brackmann (1977) found an abnormal negative middle-ear pressure in about a third of their patients with Menière's disease. They concluded that although intermittent eustachian tube blockage frequently accompanies Menière's disease it was not necessarily the cause of it. Although dramatic improvements have been reported following this minor operation it is difficult to discover any scientific basis for it and it seems likely that the effect is purely a placebo one.

(2) Arslan (1971) endeavoured to control endolymphatic hydrops by osmotic means and for this purpose placed sodium chloride crystals on the round window membrane after having elevated the tympano–meatal flap. It has again been difficult to understand the precise rationale of the operation and even more difficult to understand how any long-term benefit can be brought about. The method has not found general acceptance and Palva (1976) as well as others have reported severe sensorineural deafness from the procedure.

Choice of operation

Operation is to be considered when there is failure to control symptoms by so-called medical treatment, or if there is absence of prolonged spontaneous remissions. It is always an individual decision and depends mainly on the degree to which attacks of vertigo are interfering with the patient's normal life. If the symptoms are disabling then operation should be offered. Usually, the severity of the vertigo has been the main factor in reaching a decision. But in recent years, and in spite of the unpredictability of hearing-conservation operations, there has been a tendency to operate earlier in the disease in the hope of controlling the progressive hearing loss. However, the relief of tinnitus and improvement of hearing by surgery although sometimes obtained cannot be relied upon. It seems that the best results in this last respect occur probably in younger patients and in early cases where the degree of permanent cochlear damage is not too great.

The type of operation is generally determined by the level of hearing in the affected ear. If hearing in the affected ear is useless and the other ear is healthy then a destructive operation can be carried out. One will generally be less willing to carry out a destructive procedure in a younger patient who has many years ahead of him in which he may develop bilateral disease. If hearing in the affected ear is still at a useful level, or if the patient has only one hearing ear, or if the patient has bilateral disease, or if he shows any evidence whatever that may suggest early signs of trouble in the apparently healthy ear, then any operation to be offered must clearly be of hearing-conservation type.

Generally speaking, the hearing-destructive operations are straightforward and give a very high probability of relief from the acute attacks. Although they may leave some imbalance they probably are the best method available to restore full working capability to the patient. The hearing-destructive operations include the various types of labyrinthectomy and translabyrinthine neurectomy, and must also include the Fick and Cody operations on the saccule, as well as the salt osmosis method of Arslan.

The hearing-conservation operations are generally more complex procedures. They have a high probability of doing no damage to hearing but offer less certain relief of the vertigo compared to destructive operations (except for middle-fossa vestibular neurectomy). These operations include the various procedures on the endolymphatic sac as well as ultrasound and cryosurgical methods, and sympathectomy. Middle-fossa vestibular neurectomy is also to be included in this category as may posterior fossa neurectomy and perhaps insertion of a ventilating grommet.

Labyrinthectomy in some form will be the operation of choice when disease is clearly unilateral and the hearing is so diminished or distorted as to be useless, but it is again emphasized that apparently minor transient symptoms in the opposite ear are sometimes the first indication of major involvement which may only become manifest after a prolonged interval and, accordingly, in a younger patient are especially to be regarded with apprehension. Labyrinthectomy by either a permeatal or mastoid approach is highly effective in the unilateral case, and in younger well-motivated patients is followed by rapid vestibular compensation. Furthermore, the patient is often relieved of hearing which is so distorted as to interfere with reception on the normal side. The advantages of proceeding to a translabyrinthine resection of the vestibular nerve and maybe the cochlear nerve also must be weighed against its potential further difficulties and complications and should perhaps only be undertaken by a surgeon who has some familiarity with the internal auditory meatus.

The Fick and Cody trans-footplate operations on the saccule must be regarded as destructive procedures: even their main protagonists have failed to demonstrate that hearing can be stabilized or improved. The majority of surgeons who have performed these operations have reported an extremely high incidence of total hearing loss in the ear. Nevertheless, they can be useful operations for the elderly, fragile, or ill patient who can only tolerate a minor operation, done if necessary with local anaesthesia.

Of the operations designed for hearing-conservation there has been increasing interest in operations involving the saccus endolymphaticus. But there is no satisfactory evidence to indicate that any one operation is superior to any other. The best results seem to be obtained in the earlier (therefore reversible) stages of Menière's disease in which hearing is normal or near-normal during remissions. A positive test with glycerol or frusemide may be helpful in making a decision, although the value of demonstrating radiologically the patency of the bony vestibular aqueduct is doubtful. A saccus procedure can nevertheless sometimes give a good result in the later stages of the disease in spite of a negative glycerol test. Ultrasound treatment offers a satisfactory alternative in those departments where the necessary equipment and skills are available and the same may apply to cryosurgery, although there have been far fewer reports relating to the results. Sympathectomy is an operation away from the ear and therefore is the only procedure available which carries no risk to hearing. It should be especially considered in those patients with either bilateral disease or only one functioning ear. Its exact mode of action is likely to remain uncertain until the efferent innervation to the ear is clarified.

Selective resection of the eighth nerve through a middle-fossa approach, although a major procedure, has now established itself as a highly predictable one for vertigo relief. It is associated with an acceptably low risk of further hearing damage in skilled and experienced hands. Its long-term effect upon the natural history of the disease remains to be proven. The precise indications for the operation are still debated. Fisch (1976) regards it as the surgical treatment of choice in those patients with irreversible Menière's disease, i.e. those who have a hearing loss which is stable or a hearing loss which fluctuates but is never normal. Palva (1976) uses the operation if hearing is at a level of 70 dB or better on pure-tone testing with a discrimination score of at least 50 per cent. He also regards it as the treatment of choice if there is a possibility of bilateral disease. The operation is a major one and an intracranial one which should perhaps be regarded not as a primary procedure but one which should be utilized when an earlier operation, such as a saccus operation, has failed in a particular patient. Like trans-labyrinthine neurectomy it is an operation which calls for an advanced degree of surgical skill.

Wider experience is required to clarify with certainty the choice of operation available and for the time being it is to some extent one of personal preference. Unfortunately, the criteria used by different authors to assess the results of treatment fail to conform to the recommendations of the Alford Committee of the AAOO (1972) and this makes comparisons of results very difficult. Until these or similar criteria for assessing results are more widely employed, it will continue to be impossible to compare directly the effects of one treatment with those of another and the management of Menière's disease will remain somewhat haphazard. Until better understanding of the pathogenesis of Menière's disease becomes available and provides some basis for improved medical treatment or preventative measures, future progress seems to lie along the lines of early conservative operation before irreversible damage to the internal ear occurs.

References

Adlington, P. (1967). *Journal of Laryngology*, **81**, 759

Alberti, P. W. R. M. and Munro Black, J. I. (1968). *Journal of Laryngology*, **82**, 731

Alford, B. R. (1972). *Transactions of the American Academy of Ophthalmology*, **76**, 1462

Altmann, F. and Kornfeldt, M. (1965). *Annals of Otology*, **74**, 915

Angelborg, C. and Ågerup, B. (1975). *Acta otolaryngologica*, **79**, 81

Angell-James, J. (1963). *Annals of the Royal College of Surgeons, England*, **33**, 226

Angell-James, J. (1969a). *Archives of Otolaryngology*, **89**, 95

Angell-James, J. (1969b). *Journal of Laryngology*, **83**, 771

Arenberg, I. K., Rask-Andersen, H., Wilbrand, H. and Stahle, J. (1977). *Archives of Otolaryngology*, **103**, 1

Arenberg, I. K. and Spector, G. J. (1977). *Archives of Otolaryngology*, **103**, 268

Arenberg, I. K., Stroud, M. H. and Spector, G. J. (1974). *Revue Laryngologie (Bordeaux)*, **95**, 709

Arslan, M. (1953). *Minerva Otorhinolaryngology*, **3**, 141

Arslan, M. (1971). *H.N.O.* (Berlin), **19:3**, 81

Atkinson, M. (1943). *Annals of internal Medicine*, **18**, 797

Atkinson, M. (1961). *Acta otolaryngologica*, Suppl. 162

Barnett, S. B. and Kosoff, G. (1977). *Archives of Otolaryngology*, **103**, 124

Bauer, M. (1974). *Ful-orr-gegegyogica*, **20**, 113

Bertrand, R. A. (1972). *Acta otolaryngologica*. Suppl. **305**, 48

Boles, R., Rice, D. H., Hybels, R. and Work, W. P. (1975). *Annals of Otology*, **84**, 513

Brain, D. J., Colman, B. H., Lumsden, R. B. and Ogilvie, R. F. (1960). *Journal of Laryngology*, **74**, 628

Bryan, V. and Bucy, P. C. (1973). *Archives of Otolaryngology*, **97**, 115

Carmody, C. (1966). *Archives of Otolaryngology*, **83**, 18

Cawthorne, T. (1947). *Annals of Otology*, **56**, 18

Cawthorne, T. (1956). *Journal of Laryngology*, **70**, 695

Cawthorne, T. (1957). *Journal of Laryngology*, **71**, 524

Cawthorne, T. (1969). *Archives of Otolaryngology*, **89**, 108

Chouard, C. H. (1973). *Revue Laryngologie*, **94**, 51

Clemis, J. D. and Valvassori, G. E. (1968). *Otolaryngology Clinic of North America* (Oct.) 339

Cody, D. T. R. (1968). *Otolaryngology Clinic of North America*, (Oct.), 637

Cody, D. T. R. (1974). *Canadian Journal of Otolaryngology*, **3** (3) 271

Cody, D. T. R., Simonton, K. M. and Hallberg, O. E. (1967). *Laryngoscope*, **77**, 1480

Cole, J. M. and Funkhauser, G. (1972). *Laryngoscope*, **82**, 1027

Colman, B. H. (1969a). *Sound*, **3**, 98

Colman, B. H. (1969b). *Journal of Laryngology*, **83**, 309

Colman, B. H., Friedmann, I. and Wright, J. L. W. (1975). *Acta otolaryngologica*, **79**, 189

Cutt, R. A., Rothwarf, F., Wolfson, R. J., Ishiyama, E., Amatyakul, P. and Myers, D. (1968). *Otolaryngology Clinic of North America*, (Oct.), 649

Dandy, W. E. (1941). *Surgery of Gynecology and Obstetrics*, **72**, 421

Dederding, D. (1929). *Acta otolaryngologica*, Suppl., **10**, 4

Densert, O., Ingelstedt, A., Ivarsson, A. and Pedersen, K. (1975). *Acta otolaryngologica*, **80**, 93

Dionne, J., Barber, H. and Bryant, T. D. R. (1972). *Canadian Journal of Laryngology*, **1**, 6

Dohlman, G. (1965). *Acta otolaryngologica*, **59**, 275

Drachman, D. A. and Hart, C. W. (1972). *Neurology (Minneapolis)*, **22**, 323

Fick, I. A. van N. (1964). *Archives of Otolaryngology*, **79**, 447

Fisch, U. (1970). *Advances in ORL*, **17**, 203

Fisch, U. (1973). *Acta otolaryngologica*, **76**, 229

Fisch, U. (1976). *Journal of Laryngology*, **90**, 75

Fitzgerald, G. and Hallpike, C. S. (1942). *Brain*, **65**, 115

Flourens, M. J. P. (1842). *Recherches experimentales sur les proprietés et les fonctions du systeme nerveux, dans les animaux vertebres* (2nd ed., p. 516). Paris; Baillière

Fowler, E. P. (1948). *Transactions of the American Academy of Ophthalmology*, **52**, 293

Friedmann, I. (1963). *Scientific Basis and Medical Review*, 302

Furstenberg, A. C., Lashmet, F. H. and Lathrop, F. (1934). *Annals of Otology*, **43**, 1035

Futaki, T., Kitahara, M. and Morimoto, M. (1975). *Acta otolaryngologica*, Suppl. 330

Futaki, T., Kitahara, M. and Morimoto, M. (1977). *Acta otolaryngologica*, **83**, 272

Gardner, G. (1975). *Transactions of the American Academy of Ophthalmology*, **80**, 306

Gejrot, T. (1976). *Acta otolaryngologica*, **82**, 301

Glasscock, M. E. and Miller, G. W. (1977). *Laryngoscope*, **87**, 198

Golding-Wood, P. H. (1960a). *Journal of Laryngology*, **74**, 480

Golding-Wood, P. H. (1960b). *Journal of Laryngology*, **74**, 803

Golding-Wood, P. H. (1969a). *Journal of Laryngology*, **83**, 741

Golding-Wood, P. H. (1969b). Personal communication

Golding-Wood, P. H. (1973). *Archives of Otolaryngology*, **97**, 391

Goodhill, V. (1976). *Proceedings of the Royal Society of Medicine*, **69**, 8, 565

Greven, A. J. and Oosterveld, W. J. (1975). *Archives of Otolaryngology*, **101**, 608

Guild, S. R. (1927). *American Journal of Anatomy*, **39**, 57

Hallpike, C. S. and Cairns, H. (1938). *Journal of Laryngology*, **53**, 625

Hall, C. M. and Brackmann, D. E. (1977). *Archives of Otolaryngology*, **103**, 355

Harrison, M. S. and Naftalin, L. (1963). *Journal of Laryngology*, **77**, 832

Harrison, W. H., Shambaugh, G. E., Derlacki, D. L. and Clemis, J. D. (1967). *Laryngoscope*, **77**, 836

Haye, R. and Quist-Hanssen, S. (1976). *Acta otolaryngologica*, **82**, 289

Hedgecock, L. D. (1968). *Otolaryngology Clinic of North America*, (Oct.), 489

Henriksson, N. G. (1968). *Otolaryngology Clinic of North America*, (Oct.), 363

Hinchcliffe, R. (1969). *Sound*, **3**, 92

Holmgren, L. (1964). *Acta otolaryngologica*, Suppl. **192**, 115

House, W. F. (1968a). *Otolaryngology Clinic of North America*, (Oct.), 441

House, W. F. (1968b). *Otolaryngology Clinic of North America*, (Oct.), 587

House, W. F. (1968c). *Otolaryngology Clinic of North America*, (Oct.), 669

House, W. F. (1975). *Otolaryngology Clinic of North America*, **8** (2), 515

House, W. F. and Owens, F. D. (1973). *Journal of Laryngology*, **87**, 521

Igarashi, M. (1965). *Laryngoscope*, **75**, 1048

Ingelstedt, A., Ivarsson, A. and Tjernström, Ö. (1976). *Acta otolaryngologica*, **82**, 368

Ishii, T., Silverstein, H. and Balogh, K. (1966). *Acta otolaryngologica*, **62**, 61

Ishiyama, E., Myers, E. N. and Wolfson, R. J. (1972). *Acta otolaryngologica*, **74**, 80

Johnstone, B. (1975). *Otolaryngology Clinic of North America*, **8** (2), 271

Jongkees, L. B. W. and Philipszoon, A. J. (1964). *Acta otolaryngologica* Suppl. 192

Kimura, R. S. (1967). *Annals of Otology*, **76**, 664

Kimura, R. S. (1968). *Otolaryngology Clinic of North America* (Oct.), 457

Kimura, R. S. and Schuknecht, H. F. (1965). *Practical Otorhinolaryngology*, **27**, 343

Kimura, R. S. and Schuknecht, H. F. (1970). *Acta otolaryngologica*, **69**, 415

Klockhoff, I. (1975). *Otolaryngology Clinic of North America*, **8** (2), 345

Klockhoff, L. and Lindblom, V. (1967). *Acta otolaryngologica*, Suppl., **224**, 449

Klockhoff, I. and Lindblom, U. (1967). *Acta otolaryngologica*, **63**, 347

Klockhoff, I., Lindblom, U. and Stahle, J. (1974). *Archives of Otolaryngology*, **100**, 262

Knapp, H. (1871). *Archives of Ophthalmology, New York*, **2**, 204

Kossoff, G., Wadsworth, J. and Dudley, P. (1967). *Archives of Otolaryngology*, **86**, 535

Lange, G. (1972). *Archiw Klinische Experimentalle Ohren-, Nasen-, u. Kehlkopfheilkunde* (1972), **203**, 16

Lawrence, M. (1968). *Otolaryngology Clinic of North America*, (Oct.), 353

Lawrence, M. and McCabe, B. F. (1959). *Journal of the American Medical Association*, **171**, 1927

Lermoyez, M. (1929). Oreille Larynx, **48**, 542

Lim, D. (1970). *Journal of Laryngology*, **84**, 413

Lindsay, J. R. (1946). *Laryngoscope*, **56**, 325

Lindsay, J. R. (1947). *Archives of Otolaryngology*, **45**, 1

Lindsay, J. R. (1960). *Archives of Otolaryngology*, **71**, 500

Lindsay, J. R. (1968). *Otolaryngology Clinic of North America*, (Oct.), 319

Lindsay, J. R. (1969). Personal communication

Lindsay, J. R. and Schulthess, G. von (1958). *Acta otolaryngologica*, **49**, 315

Lindsay, J. R., Cohurt, R. T. and Sciarra, P. A. (1967). *Annals of Otology*, **76**, 5

Lundquist, P-G. (1965). *Acta otolaryngologica*, Suppl., **201**

Lundquist, P. G. (1976). *Archives of Otolaryngology*, **212**, 231

Lundquist, P. G., Igarashi, M. and Wersall, J. (1972). *Archives of Otolaryngology*, **95**, 530

Lundquist, P. G., Kimura, R. and Wersäll, J. (1964). *Acta otolaryngologica*, **57**, 65

Martin, J. P. (1967). In *Myotatic, Kinesthetic and Other Mechanisms*. Ed. by A. V. S. de Reuck and Julie Knight. London; J. & A. Churchill

Matsunaga, T. (1976). *Otolaryngology (Tokyo)*, **48**, 65

McCabe, E. F. and Wolsk, O. (1961). *Annals of Otology*, **70**, 541

Menière, P. (1861). *Gazette of Medicine, Paris*, **16**, 88

Mogan, R. F. and Baumgartner, C. J. (1934). *Western Journal of Surgery*, **42**, 628

Morrison, A. W. (1975). *Management of Sensorineural Deafness*, Chapter 1. London; Butterworths

Morrison, A. W. (1976). *Journal of Laryngology*, **90**, 87

Mygind, S. H. and Dederding, D. (1938). *Annals of Otology*, **47**, 938

Nadol, J. B. (1977). *Archives of Otolaryngology*, **103**, 524

Naftalin, L. and Harrison, M. S. (1958). *Journal of Laryngology*, **72**, 118

Öigarrd, A., Thomsen, J., Jensen, J. and Dorph, S. (1976). *Acta otolaryngologica*, **82**, 279

Palva, T., Kärja, J. and Palva, A. (1976). *Acta otolaryngologica*, **82**, 303

Paparella, M. M. and Hanson, D. G. (1976). *Laryngoscope*, **86**, 697

Passe, E. R. G. and Seymour, J. C. (1948). *British Medical Journal*, **2**, 812

Pedersen, C. B. and Sørensen, H. (1970). *Archives of Otolaryngology*, **92**, 307

Perlman, H. B. and Kimura, R. S. (1955). *Annals of Otology*, **64**, 1176

Pfaltz, C. R. (1976). *Archives of Otorhinolaryngology*, **212**, 321

Portmann, G. (1927). *Archives of Otolaryngology*, **6**, 309

Portmann, M. (1969). Personal communication

Powers, W. H. (1972). *Laryngoscope*, **82**, 1716

Powers, W. H. (1975). *Otolaryngology Clinic of North America*, **8** (2), 493

Proctor, B., Gurdjian, E. S. and Webster, J. E. (1956). *Laryngoscope*, **66**, 16

Pulec, J. L. (1968). *Otolaryngology Clinic of North America*, (Oct.), 563

Pulec, J. L. (1972). *Laryngoscope*, **82**, 1703

Pulec, J. L. (1973). *Otolaryngology Clinic of North America*, **6** (1), 25

Pulec, J. L. (1977). *Laryngoscope*, **87**, 542

Rauch, S. (1960). *Zeitschrift fur Laryngologie, Rhinologie, Otologie u. ihre Grenzgebiete*, **39**, 16

Rauch, S. (1968). *Otolaryngology Clinic of North America*, (Oct.), 369

Rauchbach, E. and Arenberg, I. K. (1973). *Revue Laryngologie*, **94**, 193

Saito, H., Kitahara, M., Yazaway, Matsumoto, M. (1977). *Acta otolaryngologica*, **83**, 465

Sandler, B. (1967). 'Lesions of the neck and vertigo'. In *Dizziness and Vertigo, Diagnosis and Treatment*, p. 219. New York; Grune & Stratton

Schuknecht, H. F. (1956). *Laryngoscope*, **66**, 859

Schuknecht, H. F. (1957). *Acta otolaryngologica*, Suppl., **132**

Schuknecht, H. F. (1963). *Laryngoscope*, **73**, 651

Schuknecht, H. F. (1968). *Otolaryngology Clinic of North America*, (Oct.), 331

Schuknecht, H. F. (1969). Personal communication

Schuknecht, H. F. (1974). *Pathology of the Ear*. Harvard University Press

Schuknecht, H. F. (1975). *Otolaryngology Clinic of North America*, **8** (2), 507

Schuknecht, H. F. (1976). *Archives of Otorhinolaryngology*, **212**, 384

Schuknecht, H. F. and Seifi, A. E. (1963). *Annals of Otology*, **72**, 687

Schuknecht, H. F., Benitez, J. T. and Beekhuis, J. (1962). *Annals of Otology*, **71**, 1039

Schuknecht, H. F., Griffin, W. L., Davies, G. and Silverstein, H. (1968). *Acta Otolaryngologica*, **65**, 169

Serrins, A. J., Harrison, R. S. and Chandler, J. R. (1963). *Archives of Otolaryngology*, **78**, 785

Seymour, J. C. (1954). *Journal of Laryngology*, **68**, 689

Seymour, J. C. (1960). *Journal of Laryngology*, **74**, 599

Shambaugh, G. E. (1968). *Otolaryngology Clinic of North America*, (Oct.), 607

Shambaugh, G. E. (1969). *Archives of Otolaryngology*, **89**, 98

Silverstein, H. and Schuknecht, H. F. (1966). *Archives of Otolaryngology*, **84**, 395

Silverstein, H. (1970a). *Annals of Otology*, **79**, 754

Silverstein, H. (1970). *Transactions of the American Academy of Ophthalmology*, **58**, 141

Silverstein, H. (1976). *Laryngoscope*, **86**, 1777

Silverstein, H. and Takeda, T. (1977). *Annals of Otology*, **86**, 493

Singleton, E. F. and Schuknecht, H. F. (1968). *Otolaryngology Clinic of North America*, (Oct.), 531

Smyth, G. D. L., Houlihan, F. P. and Hassard, T. (1977). *Journal of Laryngology*, **91**, 1013

Snow, J. B. and Suga, F. (1975). *Otolaryngology Clinic of North America*, **8** (2), 455

Sørensen, H. (1970). In *Vestibular function on earth and in space*. Ed. by J. Stahle. Wenner-Gren Symposium Series No. 15, p. 135. Oxford and New York; Pergamon Press

Stahle, J. (1968). *Otolaryngology Clinic of North America*, (Oct.), 509

Stahle, J. (1976a). *Acta otolaryngologica*, **81**, 113

Stahle, J. (1976b). *Acta otolaryngologica*, **81**, 120

Stahle, J. and Wilbrand, H. (1974). *Acta otolaryngologica*, **78**, 36

Swaak, A. J. G. and Oosterveld, W. J. (1976). *ORL*, **38**, 276

Sze Sun Yuen and Schuknecht, H. F. (1972). *Archives of Otolaryngology*, **96**, 553

Tabor, J. R., LaVar, B. and Donohoe, R. W. (1972). *Laryngoscope*, **82**, 1431

Tasaki, I., Davis, H. and Eldredge, P. G. (1954). *Journal of the Acoustical Society of America*, **26**, 765

Thomas, K. and Harrison, M. S. (1971). *Proceedings of the Royal Society of Medicine*, **64**, 853

Thomsen, J., Bech, P., Geisler, A., Balselv Jørgensen, M., Rafaelsen, O. J. Terkildsen, K., Udsen, J. and Zilstorff, K. (1974). *Acta otolaryngologica*, **78**, 59

Thomsen, J., Beck, B., Geisler, A., Prytz, S., Rafaelson, O. J., Vendsborg, P. and Zillsdorff, K. (1976). *Acta otolaryngologica*, **82**, 294

Tjernström, Ö. (1977). *Acta otolaryngologica*, **83**, 11

Toglia, J. U., Rosenberg, P. E. and Ronis, M. L. (1969). *Journal of forensic Science*, **14**, 219

Tonndorf, J. (1957). *Annals of Otology*, **66**, 766

Tonndorf, J. (1968). *Otolaryngology Clinic of North America*, (Oct.), 375

Tonndorf, J., Duvall, A. J. and Reneau, J. P. (1962). *Annals of Otology*, **71**, 801

Tumarkin, A. (1966). *Journal of Laryngology*, **80**, 1041

Williams, H. L. (1952). *Menière's Disease*. Springfield, Ill.; Thomas

Williams, H. L. (1965). *Laryngoscope*, **75**, 1661

Wilmot, T. J. (1961). *Journal of Laryngology*, **75**, 259

Wilmot, T. J. (1972). *Acta otolaryngologica*, Suppl., 305

Wilmot, T. J. (1974). *Journal of Laryngology*, **88**, 295

Wilmot, T. J. (1977). Personal communication

Wolfson, R. J., Cutt, R. A., Ishiyama, E. and Myers, D. (1968). *Otolaryngology Clinic of North America*, (Oct.), 661

Wolfson, R. J. and Cutt, R. A. (1971). *Archives of Otolaryngology*, **93**, 483

Wullstein, H. L. and Rauch, S. (1961). *Archives of Otolaryngology*, **73**, 262

26 Neurologic aspects of vertigo

Frank M Yatsu and James D Smith

Introduction

Vertigo or dizziness caused by neurological disorders is usually readily distinguished from inner-ear or 'end-organ' diseases because of the prominence of other neurological symptoms. On occasion, this separation cannot be easily made, and to assist in making this distinction, this chapter on the neurologic aspects of vertigo will review the neuro-anatomic and neurophysiologic bases for vertigo and provide a practical clinical approach to distinguish central and peripheral aetiologies.

Anatomy and physiology

The vestibular system is a complex *in vivo* computer system with multiple interconnections between the vestibular labyrinth, brain stem, cerebellum, vestibulo-spinal tracts, optical system, and cerebrum.

The non-auditory portion of the labyrinth is made up of three semicircular canals, the utricle, and saccule. The semicircular canals are the lateral (horizontal) canal, anterior (superior) canal, and the posterior (inferior) canal. The thin-walled membranous labyrinth filled with endolymph is separated from the bony labyrinth by the perilymph. Sensory epithelium is located in the semicircular canals at the widened ampullary end and consists of a transverse crest of supporting and sensory hair-cells. The hair-cells are covered by a gelatinous mass, the cupula. The sensory epithelium of the utricle is located in the macula, and lies in a plane corresponding to the lateral semicircular canal, with the anterior one-third turned up slightly. The sensory epithelium of the saccule is roughly the same size but lies in a vertical plane, perpendicular to the utricular macula. In both maculae the hair-cells are covered by a gelatinous mass which contains small prisms of calcium carbonate. The otolithic organs induce different stimuli with various positions of the head and are subject to linear acceleration, including gravity. These organs are stable (static) receptors in contrast to the semicircular canals which are dynamic receptors. Although the structure of the macula of the saccule is similar to that of the utricle, the nature of its function is still not clear. Because of its orientation, the saccule is thought to be sensitive to linear acceleration in the plane of gravity, such as going up and down in an elevator. Electrophysiological confirmation has not been accomplished (Best, 1973).

The three semicircular canals on each side are oriented in planes perpendicular to each other. This permits response to angular motion about any axis of motion in a three dimensional space. With the head held erect, the lateral canal lies in a plane inclined downward and posterior 30°. The anterior canal on one side will be parallel to the posterior canal of the opposite side, which results in maximal stimulation for both around a common axis. The mechanism of action is bending of the cupula caused by inertia of the endolymph. As the head undergoes angular acceleration the endolymph remains stationary which produces bending of the cupula and either excitation or inhibition of the normal resting discharge level. With bending of the stereocilia and kinocilium of the hair-cells, impulses are transmitted from the respective cupulae or maculae to the primitive bipolar ganglion cells. These cell bodies which form the vestibular or Scarpa's ganglion are located in the internal auditory meatus. The proximal roots of the vestibular nerve exit from the internal auditory meatus, crossing the posterior fossa to enter the brain stem at the inferior border of the pons. They travel behind the facial nerve and are separated from it by the nervus intermedius and the cochlear nerve. The fibres then pierce the medulla passing between the restiform body and the spinal tract of the trigeminal nerve and divide into an ascending and descending branch.

In the medulla there are four large or main vestibular nuclei (*Figure 26.1*). They are the superior (nucleus of Bechterew), the lateral (nucleus of Deiters), the medial (triangular nucleus), and the inferior (descending or spinal) nuclei. Several minor cell groups have been mapped out in the cat and man (Sodjadpour and Brodal, 1968), but the anatomical and functional organization is so complex that it has not been fully agreed upon. Most of the primary fibres enter the lateral vestibular nucleus, and from there the ascending fibres pass to the superior nucleus. The descending fibres pass to the inferior and medial vestibular nuclei.

The vestibular nuclei connections, including both afferent and efferent fibres, connect the spinal cord, the cerebellum, certain nuclei of the brain stem, and the reticular formation. The cells of the superior vestibular nucleus project in ascending fashion to the nuclei of the extraocular muscles (III, IV, VI) via the medial longitudinal fasciculus. Most fibres pass to the ipsilateral eye nuclei.

The lateral vestibular nuclei have been shown to be the sole source of fibres to the vestibulospinal tract (Brodal, 1960). Thus, the lateral vestibular nucleus is primarily concerned with spinal cord mechanisms affecting myotatic reflexes and muscle tone. Because a large portion of the afferent fibres in the lateral vestibular nucleus originates in the utricle, it is clear that the utricle is very involved in cervical cord mechanisms.

The inferior vestibular nucleus is the most intimately related to the cerebellum. Its major outflow is via the primary vestibulocerebellar fibres to the flocculus, nodulus, uvula, and fastigial nucleus.

The medial vestibular nucleus is the least specialized of the vestibular nuclei. It receives afferent fibres from the semicircular canals and utricle and projects ascending

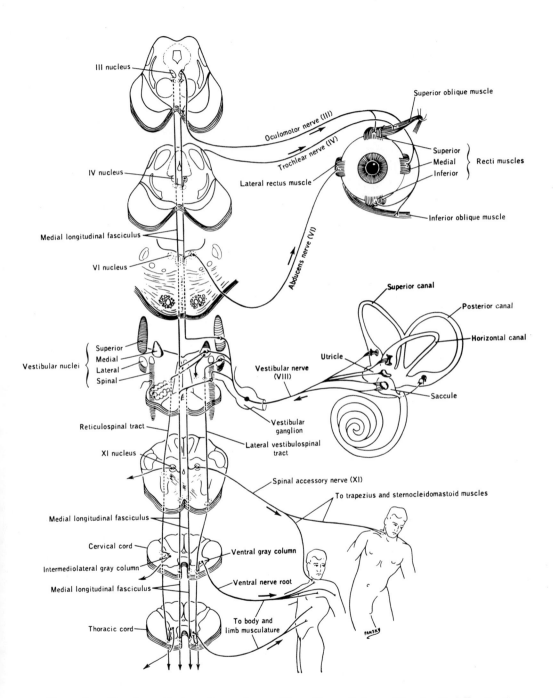

Figure 26.1 Simple vestibular reflex pathways. (From House, E. L., and Pansky, B. *A Functional Approach to Neuro-anatomy*, 2nd ed. New York; McGraw-Hill, 1967)

and descending connections in the medial longitudinal fasciculus. The ascending ones course bilaterally to the extraocular eye muscles and the descending to the cervical segments of the cord. Thus, it has function similar to both the lateral and superior vestibular nuclei (Gacek, 1968).

Vestibular connections to the reticular system are complex and are different for each vestibular nucleus. The lateral vestibular nucleus gives off fibres to the lateral reticular nucleus which are then projected back to the cerebellum. It is assumed that the vestibular-reticular connections elicit vegetative symptoms, such as vomiting, sweating, and cardiovascular reactions.

The correlation of vestibulo-ocular motor responses has been reviewed by Szentagothai (1964). It was his conclusion that the vestibulo-ocular motor fibres in the medial longitudinal fasciculus are links in the elementary three neuron reflex arcs (primary sensory neuron, ascending vestibular neuron, peripheral motor neuron).

It is recognized that pathways from the vestibular nuclei to the cerebral cortex exist, but the exact regions of cortex involved and pathways are controversial. It had been assumed that the cortical vestibular area was situated in the temporal lobe, but recent studies indicate that there is also a small region in the first somatosensory area corresponding to area II of Brodman (Brodal, 1969). These cortical projections appear to be almost exclusively contralateral.

The two vestibular organs work together in a synchronous and harmonious manner. Each side has a resting action potential which has an equal and opposite effect upon the eye and skeletal muscles. With cupula deflection toward the utricle, the frequency of action potentials is increased. There is a corresponding decreased output from the opposite paired cupula (which is deflected away from the utricle). The patient perceives this as angular acceleration. The lateral vestibular nuclei send impulses down the vestibulospinal tract which contracts certain muscles that serve as the righting responses that maintain posture while the superior vestibular nucleus affects the oculomotor nuclei (III, IV, and VI) to produce eye movement. After approximately 20 s of sustained constant angular motion, the cupulae will return to their original position and a resting action potential. With cessation of angular rotation, the opposite reaction occurs. Again the cupular deflection will last about 20 s.

In the diseased state, the normal resting symmetric action potentials of the vestibular system are disrupted. With an imbalance of the two vestibular organs, the patient perceives the same vertiginous sensation as he would with angular acceleration. An excellent clinical example is the patient who has undergone a total vestibular labyrinthectomy on the right side. The vestibular nuclei and central pathways interpret the absence of resting potentials from the right ear and normal resting potential from the the left ear as angular motion or rotation to the left resulting in a nystagmus with the fast component to the left. Animal experiments show that after several hours the cerebellum acts to decrease the resting potential of the remaining normal vestibular system. When this occurs the patient no longer is vertiginous as long as he lies quietly with a minimum of head motion. In young normal individuals, this 'cerebellar clamp' on the vestibular nuclei will gradually be released as central compensation takes place. This process requires approximately three weeks, although sudden motion may continue to give the patient a sensation of disequilibrium. If a patient should lose both labyrinths simultaneously, as in bilateral temporal bone fractures, there is no vertigo or nystagmus, but ataxia occurs as the patient now depends entirely on visual and perceptive cues for his spatial orientation.

Definition and clinical assessment of dizziness and vertigo

In evaluating patients with dizziness and vertigo, a systematic approach is necessary, the most important aspect of which is the history separating and classifying the complaint into one of four categories as proposed by Drachman and Hart (1972). From their experience of over 100 patients in a 'Dizziness Clinic' at the Northwestern University Medical School in Chicago, Illinois (USA), Drachman and Hart (1972) identified four varieties of dizzy patients based upon their functional impairment, which provides an operationally practical and useful approach to dizziness and vertigo. The four varieties of dizziness defined by Drachman and Hart were as follows: (1) a definite rotational sensation or vertigo, (2) a sensation of faintness or impending loss of consciousness, (3) disequilibrium or a sense of imbalance, and (4) an ill-defined sense of dizziness or 'light headedness'. Specific distinguishing clinical features such as precipitating factors, time and rapidity of onset, duration, frequency, associated symptoms, and any relationship to position should be explored. For the last, it is important to know if lying down, rolling to one side, leaning over, sitting up, or turning the head or body will precipitate symptoms. Additional history appropriate to the type of dizziness should be pursued as it relates to neurological, otological, cardiac, psychiatric, gastrointestinal, visual, or other aetiologies.

For the first variety of dizziness, vertigo, associated symptoms and signs assist in distinguishing the more common diseases afflicting either inner ear or central nervous system. For example, vertigo associated with impairment of cochlear function with tinnitus, hearing loss and reduced caloric responses usually implicates pathology at or near the end-organ, while the occurrence of severe, positionally-induced vertigo, though of no localizing value itself, usually suggests end-organ disease. 'Faintness' generally indicates haemodynamic factors causing brain ischaemia. Supportive clinical evidence includes conditions influencing cardiac rhythm (bradycardia, tachycardia, and carotid sinus sensitivity), factors impairing venous return to the heart (hypovolaemia, neuropathies, and myopathies), and orthostatic hypotension. 'Disequilibrium' refers to a sense of unsteadiness or imbalance and occurs during ambulation, particularly when stressed, such as rapid turning, in the dark or on an incline, and suggests cerebellar incoordination, muscle weakness or peripheral sensory impairment. The ill-defined sense of 'light-headedness' is frequently a neurotic complaint and may have no stereotyped conditions for its precipitation or aggravation other than emotional stresses and tensions, and the light-headedness may be reproduced with hyperventilation. While assessment of the patient's neurological history frequently helps identify the specific nature of 'dizziness' and also the underlying pathology, the Nylén-Bárány manoeuvre, detailed below, is frequently crucial in distinguishing central from end-organ aetiologies of vertigo, particularly in patients with posturally-induced vertigo. Other bedside tests used to clarify the nature of dizziness and vertigo may be individualized to the patient's complaints; the selective use of the nine manoeuvres recommended by Drachman and Hart (1972) is helpful. These nine manoeuvres are as follows: (1) blood pressure determinations in the lying and then immediately standing positions and after 3 min of standing; (2) a Valsalva manoeuvre accomplished by forced expiration at 40 mmHg for 15 s; (3) carotid sinus stimulation for 10 s (this manoeuvre is, of course, potentially hazardous and must be performed with cardiac monitoring for the occurrence of asystole); (4) head turning manoeuvres while sitting and standing and performed with eyes both open and closed; (5) abrupt turning while walking; (6) hyperventilation for 3 min; (7) Nylén-Bárány test, for positional vertigo and nystagmus; (8) a standard Bárány rotation and (9) any manoeuvre which reproduces his own dizziness. In addition to these specific manoeuvres, general medical and neurological examinations, neuro-otological studies and laboratory tests, which will be described in greater detail below, will help to establish or suggest a specific pathological process.

Physical examination

As indicated above, the physical examination should be tailored to the specific variety of dizziness or vertigo, but special attention to the head, neck, and neurological aspects should be given. The complete neurological examination includes mental status, cranial nerve, motor, reflex, sensory, and cerebellar testing including Romberg test, heel-to-shin, past-pointing, gait, and tandem gait. The heart rate and rhythm, blood pressure, carotid pulses, and great vessel bruits must be evaluated.

Neuro-otological studies

Thorough evaluation of the labyrinthine system (*see* Chapter 2) is obviously one of the keys to distinguishing peripheral from central aetiologies of vertigo. The cochlear portion of the labyrinth is evaluated with a battery of hearing tests regardless of the presence or absence of auditory complaints. Some discretion may be used if patients have an obvious aetiology for their dizziness. The audiological assessment battery should include pure-tone air and bone conduction thresholds, speech reception threshold (SRT), speech discrimination, threshold decay, and short increment sensitivity index (SISI). In certain circumstances other specialized studies such as Békésy audiometry, alternate binaural loudness balancing, stapedial reflex, and stapedial reflex decay tests may be employed.

The vestibular portion of the labyrinth is best tested by electronystagmography (ENG). The simple office procedure using 5 ml of iced water in the external ear canal is a good screening procedure, but an ENG will give more detailed information as well as a permanent record for future comparison. The ENG should evaluate latent spontaneous nystagmus, positional nystagmus, optokinetic nystagmus, optical tracking, and the bithermal caloric test.

Amongst the most important evaluations of the vestibular system in distinguishing between peripheral and central aetiologies are the positional tests. Nylén (1931) first classified positional nystagmus on the basis of direction-fixed or direction-changing nystagmus. Aschan (1956) modified this classification to make it more clinically practical. Aschan's classification is:

Type I. Nystagmus persistent, direction-changing (commonly reversing in opposite head positions).

Type II. Nystagmus persistent, direction-fixed irrespective of head position.

Type III. Nystagmus transitory. The most common form is the benign paroxysmal type of Dix and Hallpike (1952).

Aschan's classification is particularly useful when testing for nystagmus with eyes open or with Frenzel glasses. This is especially true for Type III where the nystagmus is frequently rotatory in character which will not be detected by ENG. When using ENG to test for positional nystagmus with eyes closed, one must use caution in interpreting the results and Aschan's classification is less useful (Barber, 1973).

Positional testing is done in a variety of ways. One of the simplest methods is to position the patient sitting on an examination table with eyes open, with or without Frenzel glasses in place. The patient's trunk, neck, and head are moved briskly in one unit into a right lateral lying position for at least 30 s, always watching for nystagmus. The patient is then moved back to a sitting position for 30 s. The test is repeated in the left lateral position and head-hanging position (patient supine and the head back 30° from the horizontal). For distinguishing features see *Table 26.1*. Direction-fixed

Table 26.1   Characteristics of peripheral and central positional nystagmus

	Peripheral	*Central*
Latency	2–10 s	None
Duration	Stops in 30 s or less	Continuous for more than 1 min
Fatiguability	Disappears in repetition	Repeatable
Adaptation	Disappears in 50 s	Persists
Position	Present in only one position	Present in multiple positions
Vertigo	Always present, severe	May be mild or absent
Direction	Only to one side	Changes direction with changes of position
Incidence	85–90 per cent of total cases	10–15 per cent of total cases

positional nystagmus (Aschan Type II) is virtually always end-organ in origin. Direction-changing positional nystagmus (Aschan Type I) will usually be end-organ, but a significant percentage will be central in origin and should raise one's index of suspicion. Aschan Type III is always end-organ in origin.

Laboratory studies

Routine laboratory studies should include a complete blood count, blood chemistry, T_4 and TSH, FTA-ABS and urine studies (*Table 26.2*). Radiological studies include mastoid and internal auditory canal (IAC) views if suspicious for ear disease or an acoustic neuroma. It is now felt that screening computed tomography (CT scan) will give a higher diagnostic yield than routine skull x-rays when central nervous system disease is suspected (Weinstein, Alfidi and Duchesneau, 1977). Cervical spine films are indicated if there is a suspicion of cervical vertigo or neck injuries.

Other optional tests which may be indicated are a 5-h glucose tolerance test for hypoglycaemia or diabetes, polycyclic tomograms of the petrous bone if routine IAC views are suspicious, electrocardiogram with rhythm strip or Holter monitoring for one, two, or more days with a diary kept for the timing of symptoms for cardiac diseases, electroencephalogram (EEG) for epilepsy, and psychometric testing for psychophysiological disease.

Of the total of 104 patients with dizziness evaluated using similar techniques by

Table 26.2

Haematology, blood chemistry and urinalysis
  1. Complete blood count
  2. Chemical screen (to include at least FBS, BUN, albumin and globulin)
  3. T$_4$ and TSH
  4. FTA-ABS
  5. Urinalysis

Radiologic studies
  1. Mastoid and internal auditory canal views (if suspicious for acoustic neuroma or ear disease)
  2. CT scan (computed tomography)
  3. Skull x-rays (if indicated)
  4. Cervical spine (if indicated by history)

Optional tests
  1. Five-hour glucose tolerance test
  2. Polycyclic tomograms of the petrous bone
  3. Electrocardiogram with a rhythm strip or Holter monitoring
  4. Electroencephalogram
  5. Psychometric testing

Table 26.3

	Percentage
Peripheral vestibular disorders	38
Hyperventilation syndrome	23
Multiple sensory deficits	13
Psychiatric disorders	9
Uncertain diagnosis	9
Brain stem cerebrovascular accident	5
Neurological disorders, other	4
Cardiovascular disorders	4
Other	
Multiple sclerosis	2
Visual disorders	2
Endocrine disorders	1
Excessive awareness of normal sensation	1
Cervicogenic disorder	0
Seizure	0

Drachman and Hart (1972), the major aetiologies for dizziness are listed in *Table 26.3*. It is noteworthy that a large percentage of patients referred for dizziness had a psychological basis.

Differential diagnosis

The major pathological processes which cause 'central vertigo' can be conveniently discussed and remembered with the mnemonic VERTIGO, *Table 26.4*. The diseases will be discussed according to this scheme, with a final section discussing peripheral positional vertigo to complement the central causes.

Table 26.4   Differential diagnosis of vertigo

VERTIGO

Central or neurologic

Peripheral or 'end-organ'

V- *Vascular or vasogenic*

Stroke	Cerebral
	Brain stem
	Cerebellum

Menière's
Labyrinthitis
Vestibular neuropathy
BPPV
Trauma

Vertebrobasilar insufficiency
Migraine
Vasculitis
Vascular elements

Haemodynamic (reduced cardiac output)
Orthostatic hypotension
Anaemia
Hypoxia–hypocarbia (hyperventilation)
Hypoglycaemia

E- *Epilepsy*   'Vertiginous epilepsy'

R- *Rx*   Antibiotics
Cardiac drugs
Antihypersensitive agents
Hypnotic-sedative drugs
Tranquillizers
Aspirin
Quinine

T- *Tumour*   Primary tumours (acoustic neuroma, gliomas, intraventricular tumours)
Metastatic tumours (primarily meningeal carcinomatosis)

   Trauma   Brain stem
'Cervical vertigo'

   Thyroid   Hypofunction

I- *Infections*   Viral
Syphilis
Vestibular neuronitis

G- *Glial diseases*   Multiple sclerosis

O- *Ocular pathology or imbalance*

V- Vascular or vasogenic (*see also* Chapter 23)

The sensation of vertigo or rotation can result from any destructive or irritative stroke lesion which affects the vestibular pathway, from inner ear to cerebral cortex. As a rule vertigo is more likely to be experienced the closer a lesion is to the vestibular nuclei in the brain stem. Because of the spatial proximity and compactness of neural pathways and connections within the brain stem, strokes causing vertigo in that location also produce other signs and symptoms of brain stem dysfunction. Thus, although vertigo may be an initial or prominent symptom of strokes, vertigo is never a solitary expression of strokes.

Strokes—cerebral cortex

Strokes involving the cerebral cortex due to middle cerebral artery occlusion cause vertigo due presumably to impairment of cortical representations or projections of subcortical vestibular nuclei. Dramatic detailing of such an occurrence is the personal observation of the well-known anatomist, Brodal (1973). With cerebral cortical lesions involving the vestibular projections, the proximity of motor, sensory and visual pathways will produce associated hemiparesis, hemisensory impairment, and homonymous visual field defects. In addition, if the dominant hemisphere is affected, aphasic disorders are expected. Thus, for patients with strokes of the cerebral cortex, vertiginous sensations without other symptoms of inner-ear dysfunction, such as tinnitus or hearing loss, indicate central vertigo. As in the case of Brodal, these vertiginous sensations are transitory.

Stroke—brain stem

Proximal occlusion of the posterior inferior cerebellar artery (PICA), typically arising from the vertebral artery, will cause dysfunction of the area fed by that vessel, namely, the lateral medullary region of the brain stem. Signs and symptoms resulting from PICA occlusion or so-called Wallenberg's syndrome include the frequent occurrence of severe vertigo as a presenting symptom resulting from vestibular nuclear involvement. Because of the proximity of other neural structures, the patients display a variety of neurological signs: with involvement of the nucleus ambiguous of the tenth cranial nerve, hoarseness, and dysphagia; with the descending tract of the trigeminal nerve, homolateral reduction of pain and temperature appreciation; with the descending sympathetic tracts, a Horner's syndrome; with the restiform body and cerebellum, ataxia of the homolateral arm and leg; with the spinothalamic tract, impaired pain and temperature appreciation on the contralateral half of the body; and with the vestibular nuclei, nystagmus, in addition to vertigo. Thus, although direct vascular involvement of the vestibular nuclei can produce profound and prominent symptoms of vertigo, the finding of other brain stem impairment substantiates central vertigo.

Stroke—cerebellum

Strokes, due to emboli or thrombosis, can involve the distal portions of the posterior inferior cerebellar artery (PICA) and cause ischaemic infarction of the cerebellum without producing impairment of the more proximally fed medulla oblongata. These patients present with dramatic symptoms of rotatory dizziness, nausea, vomiting, and an inability to stand or walk unaided, which symptom complex can be confused with an acute labyrinthine disorder or with brain stem ischaemia. Duncan, Parker and

Fisher, (1975) report three patients with cerebellar infarction and discuss the differential diagnostic features distinguishing this disorder from labyrinthine impairment. Cerebellar infarction with associated oedema can be life-threatening because of medullary compression necessitating early recognition and treatment with surgical decompression which can be life-saving. The cardinal features of medullary compression from cerebellar infarction or haemorrhage are those mentioned above plus depressed sensorium and a gaze-palsy, fixed to both caloric stimulation and oculocephalic manoeuvres (Fisher *et al.*, 1965; Fisher, 1967; Lehrich, Winkler and Ojemann, 1970; Sypert and Alvord, 1975).

In Duncan *et al.*'s report (1975), two patients had emboli to the PICA from cardiac sources: one with atrial fibrillation and the other with an aortic prosthesis, while the third had probable thrombosis of the PICA in association with hypertension and diabetes mellitus. Distinguishing findings on examination which excluded labyrinthine dysfunction were the presence of direction-changing nystagmus and brisk symmetrical caloric responses. The pathological findings show infarction of the flocculo–nodular complex of the cerebellum to which they attribute the patients' symptoms, a conclusion bolstered by the experimental studies of Fernandez and Fredrickson (1964), Igarashi, *et al.* (1973), and Aschoff and Cohen (1973).

Vertebrobasilar insufficiency

Vertebrobasilar insufficiency refers to transient episodes of ischaemia in the vertebrobasilar artery distribution, and the pathogenesis is believed to be similar to transient ischaemic attacks (TIAs) of the carotid or anterior cerebral circulation. These TIAs are due primarily to platelet aggregates which form on atheromatous lesions and subsequently dislodge and shower distally to occlude small arterioles. The occlusion causes ischaemia to the area fed by the vessel, while deaggregation of the platelet embolus results in a resolution of symptoms. The exclusive role of platelet aggregates in causing TIAs is, however, disputed since vasospasm and haemodynamic factors may be contributory factors. As originally described by Millikan and Siekert (1955), vertigo and tinnitus are the two most common symptoms observed with vertebrobasilar insufficiency. These two symptoms alone do not, however, constitute sufficient evidence for vertebrobasilar insufficiency since end-organ disease unrelated to the vertebrobasilar system may cause similar symptoms (Barber and Dionne, 1971). Thus, in addition to tinnitus and vertigo, symptoms or signs indicating focal deficits in the distribution of the vertebrobasilar circulation are required. Focal signs include diplopia, facial paralysis, ipsilateral ataxia, or homonymous hemianopia. If focal neurological deficits are not present, it is virtually impossible to distinguish the possibility of platelet emboli from haemodynamic causes resulting from reduced cardiac output or hypotension. For these latter disorders, the triad of vertigo, tinnitus, and faintness to overt syncope without focal neurological signs, is the most common symptom complex resulting from a generalized reduction in cerebral blood flow. Haemodynamic causes of vertebrobasilar insufficiency will be discussed below under 'Vascular Elements'. In patients with vertebrobasilar insufficiency due to platelet emboli rather than haemodynamic causes, the presence of bruits over the vertebral arteries, such as the supraclavicular areas, are helpful but not diagnostic. Frequently, cardiac monitoring is required in cases with uncertain symptoms, and when cardiac causes are excluded, the diagnosis of vertebrobasilar insufficiency due to platelet emboli is made by exclusion. Despite uncertainties in establishing this diagnosis, the minimum criteria require vertigo plus other focal signs and symptoms of brain stem involvement. For vertebrobasilar insufficiency due to platelet emboli, therapy is aimed at reducing the formation of platelet aggregates with aspirin and other antiplatelet aggregation drugs, such as dipyramidole, and in averting thrombosis with anticoagulants (Yatsu, 1977).

Migraine

Migraine is a well-characterized headache syndrome of incompletely understood aetiology but recognized to be multifactorial, including genetic, personality, biochemical, and exogenous factors such as dietary intake of vasoactive compounds, particularly tyramine found in cheddar cheese and citrus foods. Several atypical clinical manifestations of migraine are recognized and include hemiplegic, ophthalmoplegic, and basilar artery migraines. Symptoms of 'basilar artery migraine', a term coined by Bickerstaff (1961), are due to vertebrobasilar ischaemia resulting from vasospasm and impaired blood flow. These patients experience symptoms identical to vertebrobasilar insufficiency discussed above including vertigo, tinnitus, dysarthria, bilateral visual changes (either visual loss or scintillations), and bilateral paraesthesias. Of diagnostic importance, however, is the presence of throbbing headaches, particularly in the occipital area, with nausea and vomiting, plus their predilection in adolescent women. Treatment of basilar artery migraine is aimed at either prophylaxis with mild ergot alkaloids such as ergonovine maleate, beta-adrenergic blockers such as propranolol, antiserotonin agents such as methysergide, and tranquillizing drugs, or acute therapy of an episode of vasospasm, best treated with vasodilators such as amyl nitrite or sublingual nitroglycerin.

Vasculitis

In the differential diagnosis of diseases causing strokes, vasculitides must be considered. In the older population, over 55–60 years of age, cranial or temporal arteritis should be excluded in particular since the potential hazard of blindness can be averted with steroids. Occasionally, these patients may present with symptoms of vertebrobasilar insufficiency, including dizziness, vertigo, and lateral medullary infarction, similar to those seen with atherosclerotic vascular disease (Wilkinson and Russell, 1972). Typically, patients with cranial arteritis present with severe headaches or head pains, although the jaw, neck, and proximal muscles of the extremities may be tender and painful. The temporal artery is frequently firm, non-pulsatile, and tender, and histological examination displays a granulomatous inflammatory reaction, hence the original designation 'temporal arteritis'. The 'arteritis' is seen, however, in arteries elsewhere, and the entity of polymyalgia rheumatica is now recognized to be a similar disease but at one end of a continuum. An elevated sedimentation rate of over 50 mm/h is virtually diagnostic of cranial arteritis. Other arteritides, such as polyarteritis nodosa, systemic lupus erythematosis, and granulomatous angiitis of the brain may similarly present with stroke syndromes and vertigo, but other typical features for each of these diseases are customary and are helpful in establishing the diagnosis.

Vascular elements

Various pathological processes affecting the vascular elements or circulation can cause vertigo by impairing the supply of obligate nutrients to the brain stem. The most prominent vasogenic cause of vertigo is diminished cerebral blood flow due to reduced cardiac output caused by trachycardia, bradycardia, or transient asystole. As a rule, cardiac rates above 150/min, bradycardia under 40/min, or asystoles lasting 4 s or more are sufficient to produce a significant, generally 50 per cent, reduction of cerebral blood flow (Jonas *et al.,* 1977).

Reduced effective cerebral blood flow may also occur with orthostatic hypotension resulting in cerebral ischaemia and vertigo as a prominent symptom. The causes of orthostatic hypotension, usually 30 systolic and 20 diastolic mmHg blood pressure reduction, are multiple and include primary or degenerative diseases of the central nervous system affecting the autonomic system, such as the Shy-Drager syndrome, and conditions which impair venous return such as peripheral neuropathies, myopathies, and spinal cord transections. The most common cause of orthostatic hypotension is hypovolaemia due to blood loss or anaemia.

In addition to the variety of causes which impair effective blood flow to the brain, conditions causing reduced amounts of brain substrates, namely oxygen and glucose, may similarly give rise to vertigo, although dizziness or faintness is more common. Aside from faintness, significant reduction of blood oxygen or glucose will provoke other symptoms of central nervous system impairment such as confusion, disorientation, as well as staggering gait, unsteadiness, and slurred speech.

E- Epilepsy, epileptic vertigo

Vertigo is infrequently an accompaniment of epilepsy (Smith, 1960). Behrman (1955) classified these cases of 'vertiginous epilepsy' into three groups of patients experiencing vertigo: (a) following a seizure; (b) preceding a seizure; and (c) between seizures and temporally unrelated to epileptic spells. Of practical importance clinically are only the first two groups in which vertigo occurs either just prior to or after a seizure. Since post-ictal vertigo may be related to hypoxia, haemodynamic changes, and post-ictal hyperventilation, they cause no diagnostic difficulty within the context of a patient recovering from a grand mal seizure. Of particular interest are patients experiencing vertigo just preceding a seizure. For these cases, two possibilities exist: a cortical lesion may exist in the area of the temporal lobe where projections for vestibular functions exist or, alternatively, the vestibular apparatus within the inner ear may 'drive' the vestibular cortex and initiate seizure discharges, similar to other sensory-induced seizures. Both mechanisms appear to operate in different patients, and the use of EEG telemetry should assist in separating these two entities. To control seizures, regardless of which of the two mechanisms are operative, anticonvulsants are indicated. Behrman (1955) suggests that vertiginous spells preceding a seizure and originating from the cortex can be identified as 'epileptic vertigo' while those being driven from the vestibular apparatus in the inner ear should be called 'vertiginous epilepsy'.

R- Rx

'Rx' or therapies of various kinds, by their predominant action upon the vestibular or circulatory systems, can cause vertigo or dizziness. A careful history of drug intake or abuse in patients with vertigo is, therefore, essential. The variety of drugs responsible include cardiac medications which can impair cardiac output; antihypertensive therapies, particularly ganglionic blockers with an associated tendency to cause orthostatic hypotension; hallucinogenic drugs which cause distortions of visual and auditory input; tranquillizing medications, including phenothiazines, tricyclics, and benzodiazepines; and hypnotic-sedative drugs, such as phenytoin, barbiturates, and alcohol, which affect the vestibular system and also impair psychomotor and co-ordination functions (Goodman and Gilman, 1975). The majority of drugs causing vertigo affect the inner ear and include aspirin (sodium acetylsalicylate), quinine, ethacrynic acid, frusemide and antibiotics such as the aminoglycosides. The aminoglycosides (streptomycin, neomycin, kanamycin, gentamicin and tobramycin) impair the hair-cells of the cochlea and vestibular systems. The effect on the vestibular system may be unilateral (Meyers, 1970; Dayal, Smith and McCain, 1974) which will upset the balance between the two labyrinths and thereby produce vertigo. The combined use of aminoglycosides with certain diuretics, especially ethacrynic acid and frusemide, will potentiate the ototoxic effects.

T- Tumour, trauma, and toxins

Tumour

Tumours of the central nervous system infrequently present with vertigo as a solitary or prominent initial symptom. More commonly vertigo occurs during the course of the tumours' growth in addition to other neurological signs and symptoms indicating focal and generalized brain impairment. Brain tumours most likely to cause vertigo are in close proximity to the vestibular nerve or nuclei and include tumours of the cerebello-pontine angle (CPA), brain stem, cerebellum, IVth ventricle, and cerebral cortex. Positional nystagmus is seen more frequently with brain tumours but the finding is usually of no localizing value, as Nylén (1939) exclusively documented in 673 patients with brain tumours. In his study, the following tumours were analysed for types I and II nystagmus as well as spontaneous nystagmus: acoustic tumours; gliomas of the pons and medulla oblongata; gliomas of the cerebellum including medulloblastomas and astrocytomas; other tumours of the cerebellum, particularly involving the hemisphere and vermis separately; gliomas of the corpora quadrigemina and pineal gland; gliomas of the temporal lobe; and gliomas of the frontal lobe. In 70 cases of glioma of the temporal lobe, vertigo in association with reduced hearing, tinnitus, and disturbed equilibrium occurred in approximately one-third. Twenty-six of these 70 (37 per cent) displayed nystagmus; two were positional or type I; 21 (81 per cent) were type II; while three were spontaneous. In these cases of temporal lobe tumours, other neurological findings such as visual field defects localized the pathology, while the neuro-otological tests did not. In 70 cases of gliomas of the frontal lobe, 15 patients complained of vertigo, six having disturbed sense of equilibrium. A few complained of tinnitus or hearing loss as well. Of the 70, 28 (40 per cent) displayed nystagmus: three (11 per cent) with type I; 22 (79 per cent) with type II; and three were spontaneous.

Brain tumours are customarily divided into those which are primary or arise *de novo* and secondary or metastatic neoplasms, although neurological symptoms for each group are frequently indistinguishable.

Tumours of the central nervous system present in a variety of ways clinically, but typically with relentless progression of neurological deficits over a subacute period of time. The variety of symptoms or signs can be divided into four: (1) paralysis, which is progressive, most commonly of contralateral arm and leg; (2) symptoms of increased intracranial pressure, namely, headache, nausea, vomiting, and blurred vision with associated papilloedema; (3) seizures, either focal or generalized; and (4) an organic brain syndrome characterized as a confusional state, memory loss, or psychomotor retardation.

As noted above in Nylén's (1939) study, nystagmus may be observed with brain tumours in any location, but vertigo is most prominent with posterior fossa tumours. Of the primary tumours causing vertigo, the best known are the acoustic neuromas of which 10–15 per cent may present with vertigo as an initial symptom. (The topic of 'acoustic neuromas' is discussed in Chapter 20.) Other than cerebello-pontine angle tumours, the other posterior fossa neoplasms are of brain stem, cerebellum, and the fourth ventricle. Supratentorial tumours may, as noted in Nylén's series, cause vertigo, usually if the cortical vestibular projections are compromised or intracranial pressure is raised. With primary tumours of the brain stem, White (1963) reported vertigo in nine of 44 patients or 20 per cent incidence, while seven experienced dizziness. These symptoms were not presenting complaints and, as a rule, cranial nerve palsies or corticospinal tract involvement were the initial neurological deficits. Similarly Barnett and Hyland (1952) reported eight of 90 patients (9 per cent) with vertigo due to either brain stem or fourth ventricular tumours. Of posterior fossa meningiomas, Russell and Bucy (1953) reviewed the world's literature and their own experience and found 81 of 137 (54 per cent) incidence of vertigo, but the majority of these meningiomas were at or near the vestibular nerve, behaving like acoustic neuromas.

Secondary or metastatic tumours to the brain present as mass lesions or as meningeal carcinomatosis. As mass lesions, tumour nodules produce symptoms of dizziness similar to primary tumours. With meningeal carcinomatosis, tumour cells proliferate, spread along the subarachnoid space, and compress exiting peripheral nerves, such as the vestibular-cochlear nerve complex. As a result, patients may develop vertigo, tinnitus, and hearing loss, but because of its diffuse involvement, meningeal carcinomatosis will display other cranial nerve palsies, nuchal rigidity, and frequently an organic brain syndrome. If the brunt of meningeal infiltrates is, however, on the spinal cord, back pain, occasionally radicular in nature, weakness, areflexia, and sphincter disturbances are common symptoms. With metastatic brain tumours, vertigo may be an early or initial symptom in 24 per cent of the patients (Störtebecker, 1954), and positional nystagmus may be the only neurological sign of brain tumours (Nylén, 1939). Cawthorne and Hinchcliffe (1961) found that four patients with vertigo, who displayed positional nystagmus of central type, had unsuspected carcinoma of the bronchus with subtentorial metastases. The metastases responsible were primarily to the cerebellum; vertigo with positional nystagmus has not been documented with supratentorial metastases.

The neoplasms liable to metastasize to the brain are carcinomas of bronchus and breast, sarcomas, chorionepitheliomas, melanomas, and hypernephromas. In general, these solid tumours respond poorly to irradiation or chemotherapy, although steroids may be temporarily beneficial in reducing tumour mass and brain oedema. Lymphoproliferative tumours such as Hodgkin's disease and leukaemia respond more favourably to irradiation, steroids, and chemotherapy such as intrathecal methotrexate.

Trauma

Direct head trauma or flexion–extension ('whiplash') injury to the neck is a common cause of vertigo and dizziness and usually impairs inner-ear function or occasionally the brain stem (Biemond and DeJong, 1969). Barber (1971) found that of patients with and without temporal bone fractures, 47 per cent and 20 per cent, respectively, experienced positional vertigo of paroxysmal type. In their assessment of patients with paroxysmal positional vertigo, Harrison and Ozsahinoglu (1975) noted that 24 per cent had a history of head trauma. Typically, vertigo and positional nystagmus are induced with the injured ear in the down position and the rapid component of nystagmus towards the affected ear. The mechanism for producing vertigo may be a direct disruption of the otolithic otoconia with release into the endolymph.

With flexion–extension injury to the neck, severe neck pain can be associated with vertigo and positional nystagmus (Rubin, 1973). In 309 patients with dizziness following flexion–extension neck injury studied by Toglia (1976), latent nystagmus was present in 29 per cent, caloric tests were abnormal in 57 per cent, and rotatory tests were abnormal in 51 per cent, while the routine neurological examinations were normal. Latent nystagmus utilized positional changes to provoke nystagmus which was both direction-fixed and direction-changing, indicating both end-organ and central nervous system causes for nystagmus. As noted by Toglia (1976), following injury, neck pain appears early and is associated with neck tenderness, occipital pains, pain and numbness of the arms, visual disturbances, tinnitus, dizziness, disordered equilibrium, dysphagia, hoarseness, memory deficits, concentrating impairment, sleep disturbances, and emotional lability. Vertigo, dizziness, and tinnitus usually occur days or weeks after injury, and the constellation of cervical pain with vertigo has been termed 'cervical vertigo' (Biemond and DeJong, 1969). The pathogenetic mechanisms explaining the occurrence of cervical pain and vertigo are complex, and frequently are due to massive sensory bombardment centrally disrupting vestibular function. Other mechanisms thought to play a contributory role are cervical sympathetic stimulation and vertebrobasilar artery insufficiency (Toglia, 1976).

Toxic-metabolic disorders

The association of vertigo and various metabolic disorders is recorded in the literature, but documentation with good clinical studies is lacking. Most metabolic disorders have been associated with peripheral pathology and produce both hearing loss and vertigo. The triad of episodic vertigo, tinnitus, and fluctuating hearing loss is most frequently encountered, simulating Menière's disease, and is discussed elsewhere under that topic. For a metabolic screen to exclude such causes of vertigo, Powers (1972) recommends the following tests in patient's with symptoms simulating Menière's disease: thyroid studies (T_4 serum bound test of Murphy-Pattee and T_4 free index test), 5-h glucose tolerance test, adrenal and pituitary tests (ACTH plasma cortisol stimulation test and the insulin stimulation test).

Hypothyroidism

Vertigo occurs occasionally with hypothyroidism and is frequently associated with sensorineural hearing loss and endolymphatic hydrops (Moehling, 1927; Post, 1964; Ritter, 1967; Powers, 1972; Pulec, 1972; Bhatia *et al.*, 1977). Pulec (1972) found in a group of 120 patients with classic Menière's disease that 3 per cent had hypothyroidism. In other series of patients with hypothyroidism, the incidence of vertigo varies widely from a low of 0 per cent (Post, 1964) to 29.1 per cent (Bhatia *et al.*, 1977). Vestibular function tests do not reveal a functional deficit. The symptoms of hypothyroidism include cold intolerance, fatigue, dry skin, mental dullness, deafness, bradycardia, myalgia, neuralgia, and menstrual disorders. Occasionally, ataxia or unsteadiness of gait is a prominent presenting complaint as Cremer, Goldstein and Paris (1969) detailed in 24 patients. The diagnosis is confirmed by laboratory studies using the T_4 serum bond test of Murphy-Pattee and the T_4 free index test. These tests are more accurate and less affected by drugs than basal metabolic rate (BMR), protein bound iodine test (PBI), or tri-iodothyronine resin uptake test (T_3).

The treatment of hypothyroidism is by synthetic thyroid preparations which are readily absorbed from the intestinal tract and have a uniform potency. Powers (1972) found in 17 patients with hypothyroidism that only three responded to thyroid replacement alone while for the rest he purports the necessity of using a combination of endocrine, allergic, and thyroid management.

Hypoglycaemia and hyperglycaemia may result in inner-ear dysfunction. Hypoglycaemia is frequently over-diagnosed by clinical symptoms alone and requires a 5-h glucose tolerance test to establish its presence, particularly since a 3-h test will frequently miss the low point of the curve. Symptoms may occur if the blood sugar drops to 50 mg per cent or less, but occasionally a precipitious drop to levels of 60–70 mg per cent may produce vestibular symptoms. In addition to vestibular symptoms, patients may exhibit neurological symptoms of headache, visual disturbances, muscle spasms, thick speech and, rarely, convulsions. With rapid decline in blood glucose, symptoms of hyperadrenalinaemia occur, including anxiety, tachycardia, sweating, pallor, and tremulousness. Treatment for hypoglycaemia is a high protein, low carbohydrate, and low fat diet. For patients with diabetes mellitus, appropriate drug or dietary therapy should be instituted and managed by an internist.

I- Infections

Infections of the central nervous system such as viral encephalitis and bacterial meningitis frequently cause a sensation of vertigo or dizziness, most likely due to involvement of the vestibular apparatus, possibly by toxins or suppurative labyrinthitis. In these patients, however, the suspicion and diagnosis of infection in the central nervous system can be readily made because of the presence of fever, nuchal rigidity, a depressed sensorium, and characteristic findings of infection on lumbar puncture.

Syphilis

It has been known from ancient times that syphilis produces ear symptoms. Syphilis has been shown to have a peripheral effect producing endolymphatic hydrops and osteitis of the otic capsule. The usual symptoms are vertigo, low tone hearing loss with fluctuation, fullness, tinnitus, and progressive deterioration of speech discrimination. The symptoms occur usually in the fifth decade of life, and the patients usually demonstrate depressed caloric responses bilaterally. Sudden hearing loss requires prompt treatment. Diagnosis is confirmed with a reactive fluorescent treponemea antibody absorption (FTA-ABS) test. Patients may frequently have a non-reactive VDRL. Treatment is described in Chapter 15.

Vestibular neuronitis

Dix and Hallpike (1952) first identified patients with vestibular complaints but with normal hearing which distinguished them from Menière's disease, and they reported on 100 of these cases exhibiting a variety of single and multiple vertiginous attacks, plus sensations of blacking out and disequilibrium, but with normal hearing. All of the patients displayed changes in bithermal caloric responses, and a large number (46 per cent) had evidence of systemic infections, such as chronic sinusitis, dental infections, or upper respiratory infections. Dix and Hallpike called this syndrome 'vestibular neuronitis', the pathology of which they localized to the peripheral vestibular system or nerve pathways to and including the vestibular nuclei. Although theirs was the first large series reported, Clemis and Becker (1973) found several case reports in the earlier literature which fit the same clinical picture. DeWeese (1954) described a similar clinical syndrome but used the term 'acute toxic labyrinthitis'. Hart (1965) described a more homogeneous group with single attacks of sudden vertigo and unilateral vestibular weakness following an upper respiratory infection. He separated these from Dix and Hallpike's vestibular neuronitis patients with multiple attacks and referred to this as 'sudden vestibular paralysis of probable viral etiology'. Coates (1969) described a similar homogeneous group of younger patients who had the same symptoms and findings as Hart's group but preferred the term 'vestibular neuronitis'.

Clemis and Becker (1973) summarized the literature on vestibular neuronitis and found it more common in the 20–60 year age group with no sex predilection. Forty-three per cent of the patients had an antecedent or concomitant 'flu'-like syndrome or upper respiratory infection. The association with sinusitis or dental infections noted by Dix and Hallpike (1952) is poorly substantiated in the literature, but two of Coates' (1969) patients had definite exacerbation of symptoms with recurrent sinusitis.

Patients with vestibular neuronitis present with a rapid or occasionally gradual (few hours) onset of rotatory vertigo, usually accompanied by nausea and vomiting. Occasionally patients may complain of tinnitus or fullness, but hearing loss is rare. Vertigo, nausea, and vomiting may last three to seven days, and characteristically patients lie in bed perfectly still since movement of any kind will aggravate their symptoms. After the first week symptoms gradually improve, but mild vertigo is experienced, especially with rapid motion. By the end of three to four weeks patients will be relatively asymptomatic except for mild instability with quick turns. Early, patients display horizontal or horizonto-rotary nystagmus with the fast component to the unaffected ear. These findings will persist for one to four weeks. Positional nystagmus may be present, especially later in the course of the disease, and still later many will show the typical benign paroxysmal positional vertigo of Dix and Hallpike. Dayal, Smith and McCain (1974) propose that this spectrum of symptoms may represent a continuum of events resulting from central compensation similar to that seen after unilateral labyrinthectomy. Characteristically, spontaneous nystagmus is first observed away from the involved ear, later to become a persistent, direction-fixed positional nystagmus (Aschan Type II), and finally a paroxysmal, positional nystagmus (Aschan Type III).

The frequency of depressed caloric responses is uncertain in vestibular neuronitis, although in Dix and Hallpike's (1952) experience, bilateral or unilateral vestibular paresis or directional preponderance to the normal ear was characteristic. Coates (1969) found more severe vestibular paresis in younger patients with single attacks than in those with multiple attacks.

In long-term follow-up, 58 per cent of patients had no further attacks, 29 per cent continued to be troubled with vertigo and 13 per cent experienced disequilibrium (Clemis and Becker, 1973). Disability will usually last 3–12 weeks with an average of four. These patients are very susceptible to an aggravation of symptoms when working near moving machinery, belts, or wheels which elicit an optokinetic effect. A sensation of instability or frank vertigo with nausea is experienced. A small, homogenous group of younger individuals can be identified who have single attacks and markedly depressed caloric responses for whom the prognosis is excellent for complete recovery with minimal chance for recurrence.

Another group best classified with vestibular neuronitis is 'benign paroxysmal vertigo of childhood'. This terminology is unfortunate as the name may be easily confused with 'benign paroxysmal positional vertigo' of Dix and Hallpike. Dunn and Snyder (1976) presented 33 cases in children 1–5 years of age. A typical episode of acute vertigo unassociated with positional changes lasts 1–10 min and is accompanied by pallor, vomiting, sweating, and instability. Occasionally a child will display torticollis with head tilting, and ataxia may last from several hours to a few days. Between attacks the child is asymptomatic and the neurological examination is normal, including hearing. The caloric examination was abnormal in 21 of 23 patients tested. This condition is self-limiting and lasts a few months to four years. In children it is important to differentiate 'benign paroxysmal vertigo of childhood' from epilepsy and brain tumours.

The treatment of vestibular neuronitis is mainly supportive with vestibular suppressant drugs. The majority of patients will be symptomatic for 4–6 weeks, following which the symptoms will resolve, with central compensation. Some patients may have a recurrence of symptoms with a similar time course for improvement. Younger patients who have a recovery course similar to those patients with unilateral labyrinthine destruction, will rarely experience a second attack. The use of drugs such as diazepam, meclizine, anticholinergics, or anti-emetic drugs may be helpful for early symptomatic relief in the acute stages of vertigo. If patients have severe nausea and vomiting for several days, hospitalization and intravenous fluids may be required. In patients with residual symptoms which are slow to abate, labyrinthine exercises (Hecker *et al.*, 1974) may be helpful. Surgery is not indicated unless a definite peripheral aetiology can be established.

G- Glial diseases: multiple sclerosis or disseminated sclerosis

Vertigo can be a presenting and dominant symptom of multiple sclerosis, but other symptoms and signs indicating multiple lesions are characteristic and frequently diagnostic. In 46 autopsy-proven cases of multiple sclerosis investigated by Carter, Sciarra and Merritt (1950), 7 per cent developed vertigo as an initial symptom while another 11 per cent developed it during the course of their illness. In addition to symptoms indicating multiplicity of lesions, their temporal separation, with remissions and exacerbations, is usual (McAlpine, Lumsden and Acheson, 1972). Multiple sclerosis is typically a chronic neurological disease with variable clinical expressions, some benign, others malignant, with the majority causing moderate to severe impairment of the patient's ability to perform activities of daily living. The aetiology of multiple sclerosis is not yet established, but the roles of slow viruses and of immunological factors are the most popular and receiving the greatest amount of research attention. The possible contributions of dietary fats, nutrition, and other factors such as environment have been postulated. The theories regarding slow viruses and immunological mechanisms propose that a single or a variety of viruses trigger the demyelinating process which in turn provokes an immunologic reaction which in concert fosters the demyelinating process. Epidemiologic studies show a higher incidence of multiple sclerosis in colder, temperate climates than the warmer tropics, and the susceptibility to multiple sclerosis remains even if individuals move to warmer climates after reaching teenage, apparently not before. The prevalence rate of multiple sclerosis in temperate climates such as England, the United States of America, Canada, and the continent is estimated as high as 60/100 000 population. Pathologically, the characteristic lesions are areas of demyelination appearing as hardened or sclerotic lesions in white matter, particularly in the periventricular area. Multiple sclerosis occurs primarily in the third decade of life, and the most common, though not diagnostic, symptom is generalized weakness or loss of energy. Typical symptoms of multiple sclerosis which patients may display indicating the presence of multiple lesions are the following: transient blindness—retrobulbar neuritis; imperative micturition or incontinence—autonomic fibres or corticospinal tracts in the spinal cord; slurred speech—either cerebellar tracts or posterior columns; emotional lability—frontobulbar tracts; and weakness or spasticity—corticospinal tracts. Other neurological symptoms include: diplopia; oscillopsia or the bouncing of visual images associated with vertical nystagmus, a frequent sign of intramedullary pathology; convulsions, both generalized and myoclonic; paraesthesias, including Lhermitte's sign or the occurrence of electric-like shocks down the back, brought on typically by neck flexion; and mental disturbances, especially an organic mental syndrome, the hallmark of which is memory loss.

No laboratory test is diagnostic of multiple sclerosis although elevation of leukocytes and immunoglobulin G in the cerebrospinal fluid occurs in over half of the patients, particularly during exacerbation. The occurrence of rosettes or the clumping of monocytes around virus-infected or myelin basic-protein coated cells is still experimental, but may provide a diagnostic test for multiple sclerosis. In otherwise visually asymptomatic patients suspected of multiple sclerosis, an abnormal visual evoked response (VER) has gained popularity in establishing the presence of multiple lesions and thereby securing the diagnosis of multiple sclerosis. Computerized tomographic (CT) scans have also identified multiple hypodense lesions compatible with demyelinating lesions.

As yet, no satisfactory or proven treatment for multiple sclerosis exists. Steroids, immunosuppressive drugs, and dietary restriction of fats have been used, among at least several hundred treatments, but these therapies remain unproven. Physiotherapy remains an important component of treatment in order to maximize the patient's ability to perform activities of daily living, avoid complications such as bed sores and contractures, and provide a positive psychological attitude.

O- Ocular pathology

Vertigo and a sensation of unsteadiness with spatial disorientation can occur with ocular imbalance resulting in altered spatial information processing through the visual system. Refractive errors, perceptual distortions, diplopia, impairment of pursuit and of refixation, focusing, stroboscopic effects, and optokinetic manoeuvres can be responsible. In 1941, Adler used the term 'ocular vertigo' and specifically noted that vertigo can arise from the following five causes: (1) abnormalities of the dioptric apparatus so that individuals wearing glasses for the first time will develop vertigo resulting from an alteration and distortion of images; (2) extra-ocular muscle weakness causing diplopia in gaze toward the paretic muscle; (3) optokinetic nystagmus, an involuntary pursuit and centrally refixed ocular movement, brought on by rapidly moving objects or motion; (4) looking down from heights causing an abolition of the customary vanishing point as well as from associated psychic factors; and (5) effects of accelerations of the body resulting in conflicting sensory input from two or more organs of equilibrium, including eyes, and producing clashing sensory impressions, as in pilots experiencing sudden acceleration. As a rule, vertigo associated with ocular causes is mild.

Peripheral or benign paroxysmal positional vertigo (BPPV)

Benign paroxysmal positional vertigo is the most common type of all positional vertigo and is the prototype for peripheral causes (Aschan Type III positional nystagmus). Bárány (1921) first drew attention to this disorder and felt the pathology was related to a disorder of the otolith organ. Dix and Hallpike (1952) coined the term benign positional vertigo. They reported a case with autopsy and proposed a vascular lesion affecting the otolithic organ. Schuknecht (1969) reported temporal bone sections showing amorphous basophilic debris on the posterior canal cupula. This was thought to be degenerated otoconia and was referred to as cupulolithiasis.

Aetiology

IDIOPATHIC

The majority of patients with benign paroxysmal positional vertigo will have no history of associated disease. Harrison and Ozsahinoglu (1975) in reviewing 365 cases found 60 per cent were idiopathic. It is most common in the fifth, sixth, and seventh decade (Schuknecht, 1974). In a small series Barber (1973) found women more often affected than men, but Dix and Hallpike (1952) found no sexual predominance in 100 cases.

TRAUMA

Trauma is the second most common cause of peripheral positional vertigo. Barber (1964) found that 47 per cent of patients with longitudinal temporal bone fractures were associated with positional vertigo of the paroxysmal type. In patients with a head injury without fracture, 20 per cent had positional vertigo. Harrison and Ozsahinoglu (1975) found that 24 per cent of their patients with benign paroxysmal positional vertigo had a history of head trauma. Rubin (1973) reported positional nystagmus on ENG in association with whiplash injuries.

OTITIS MEDIA

Dix and Hallpike (1952) first called attention to the association of positional vertigo and suppurative otitis media. They found in a series of 100 patients with otitis media a 26 per cent incidence of positional nystagmus. If asked specifically, many patients with suppurative otitis media will admit to a feeling of vertigo when turning quickly or in specific positions.

OTOLOGIC SURGERY

Positional vertigo may be an occasional complication after stapes surgery. Schuknecht (1974) feels that this is usually associated with excessive trauma within the vestibule at the time of surgery. It may also occur with other surgical procedures such as fenestration, mastoidectomy, or tympanoplasty. The symptoms are usually self-limiting but may persist for several months.

OCCLUSION OF THE ANTERIOR VESTIBULAR ARTERY

Lindsay and Hemenway (1956) felt that partial loss of vestibular function from a vascular or inflammatory lesion would produce positional nystagmus. Occasionally one may see positional nystagmus with vertebrobasilar artery insufficiency (Barber, 1973).

MISCELLANEOUS

Keim and Sachs (1975) reported paroxysmal positional vertigo in three out of five patients with macroglobulinaemia. The pathophysiology was felt to be due to a precipitate of gamma globulin particles on the cupula making it sensitive to gravitational effects. This pathophysiology would be similar to Schuknecht's cupulolithiasis, but they did not present pathological confirmation of their hypothesis.

Money, Johnson and Cerlett (1965) described a peripheral mechanism for alcoholic positional nystagmus. They hypothesized that since the specific gravity of the cupula and endolymph is precisely matched, alcohol may make the cupula less dense than the endolymph making it sensitive to gravitational changes. Money and Myles (1973) reported the effect of deuterium oxide ingestion on man. Thirty minutes to six hours after ingesting deuterium oxide or 'heavy water' a vigorous horizontal nystagmus was produced to the most upward ear on positional testing. It was felt that the deuterium oxide moved from the blood stream to the cupula and then later to the endolymph producing a specific gravity difference. The cupula became heavier than the endolymph, so changes of head position would produce gravitational pull and result in positional nystagmus.

Rahko and Aantaa (1977) found that 50 per cent of the profoundly deaf children tested wearing high gain aids in the range of 120–130 dB sound pressure level, would show ENG evidence of positional nystagmus with loud noises. They felt that hearing aids should not be worn by workers where loss of equilibrium would be dangerous. We have seen one profoundly deaf patient who would have intermittent episodes of instability and vertigo when exposed to loud noises. At times it was so severe that he could not wear the hearing aid for 2–3 months at a time even though it was necessary for communication and his education.

Pathophysiology

Dix and Hallpike (1952), Lindsay and Hemenway (1956) and Cawthorne and Hallpike (1957) reported the pathological findings in the temporal bones of patients with benign paroxysmal positional vertigo. All three cases showed degeneration of the superior vestibular nerve, the utricular macula, and the cristae of the superior and lateral semicircular canals. The inferior vestibular nerve and the crista of the posterior semicircular canal appeared intact. Schuknecht (1974) in reviewing these cases found that post-mortem changes and autolysis precluded evaluation of the cupulae, but agreed that these cases represented occlusion of the anterior vestibular artery.

Schuknecht (1969) reported two patients with benign paroxysmal positional vertigo which he called cupulolithiasis, presumed to be caused by spontaneous degeneration in the vestibular labyrinth. Histological studies showed basophilic deposits on the cupulae of the posterior canal in the affected ear and a layer of granular material in the most inferior part of the posterior canal. He proposed that this material was the degenerated products of otoconia which became loosened from the utricular macula. Schuknecht (1969) also found that stimulation of the isolated posterior semicircular canal produced pure rotary nystagmus. Other animal experiments have confirmed that trauma can disrupt the utricular macula and loosen the otoconia. Schuknecht (1974) has hypothesized that this debris has a specific gravity greater than endolymph and, thus, either floats in the endolymph or due to gravitational forces settles out and becomes attached to the cupula of the posterior canal. The canal is in the most dependent position with the head erect. In the supine, head hanging, or ear-down position, the gravitational force on the cupular deposit produces a strong utriculofugal displacement of the posterior canal. The latency of vertigo in the offending position may be caused by the time required to get the mass in motion. The intense vertiginous sensation may be due to the magnitude of the cupular displacement and the limited duration due to the particles leaving the cupula. Fatiguability may be due to dispersement of the particles in the endolymph after repeated head positionings. After a period of rest the debris once again settled out on the posterior canal ampulla. Lim (1973) has shown that otoconia separated from the gelatinous layer of the macula will dissolve. This may explain the self-limiting character of benign paroxysmal positional vertigo. It could further be proposed that recurrence of the disease much later may be the result of further loss of otoconia from the macula of the utricle and setting up the whole cycle once again. Perhaps the success of Cawthorne's labyrinthine exercises may be on the basis of speeding up degeneration of the otoconia rather than habituation.

Symptoms

Patients with benign paroxysmal positional vertigo will complain of frequent recurring attacks of vertigo precipitated by change in position. These are short-lived attacks accompanied by intense whirling vertigo and usually nausea and/or vomiting. The attack lasts a few seconds as the patient will immediately change position. Frequently symptoms will be noted when first lying down in bed or rolling to one side. Occasionally a patient will be awakened with intense vertigo after having rolled into the offending position in his sleep. The intensity of the vertigo is such that patients will be alarmed and will avoid the offending position at all costs. On careful questioning, one can usually determine that it is the position the patient is in and not the act of moving to that position which precipitates the attack. In most patients the attacks will gradually decrease in frequency and intensity and eventually disappear completely over a period of a few weeks to months. In a few patients the symptoms may persist for several years and become at least partially incapacitating. In patients with a history of trauma, the attacks usually begin 7–10 days after the injury and tend to gradually diminish over a period of 3–6 months. Some may have persistent symptoms for many years. Rubin (1973) has ENG confirmation of findings as long as three years later. However, once a patient with trauma recovers, it is very unusual for the symptoms to return at a later date. In those cases of idiopathic aetiology, there may be intermittent recurrence of symptoms many months or years later. Most patients will not have associated cochlear symptoms, unless the symptoms are related to ear disease or otologic surgery.

Examination

The head and neck examination will be normal unless the patient has ear disease or previous otologic surgery. The neurological examination including gait, Romberg, and cerebellar testing will be normal. The hearing will be unaffected except in those patients who may be in the older age group and have associated hearing losses secondary to noise trauma or presbyacusis. Caloric examination in one-half of the cases will be normal and symmetrical bilaterally. If there is a diminished caloric response, it will usually be in the downmost ear when nystagmus occurs. There is no spontaneous nystagmus. The only consistent physical findings will be those observed during positional testing. When placed in the offending position, there will be a horizontal and rotatory nystagmus toward the downmost ear with intense vertigo after a delay (latency) of 2–10 s. Usually the patient will be quite agitated and request to be moved out of the position. If held in the position, the nystagmus and vertigo will subside and cease in 10–30 s. When the patient is returned to the upright position, the nystagmus may sometimes recur but in the opposite direction. With repeated movement to the offending position the nystagmus and vertigo become less each time until after three or four times it can no longer be detected. This adaptation will usually last only a few minutes. The nystagmus will usually occur in only one position and in one direction. Occasionally a patient may present with a classic history, but physical findings cannot be demonstrated. This does not necessarily mean the patient has been cured or that it will not be demonstrated on a subsequent examination. In this case the patient should be followed and repeat examinations carried out at a later date.

Treatment

The initial treatment in most patients with benign paroxysmal positional vertigo should be supportive. In the majority of patients an explanation of the symptoms and pathophysiology with reassurance that the symptoms will gradually improve is all that is needed.

If this is not enough, the next step is to help the patient with home relaxation hints to prevent the tension which frequently builds up when attempting to avoid the provocative position. With this Cawthorne–Cooksey vestibular exercises or some variant may be helpful in developing habituation. Hecker, Haug and Herndon (1974) describe this as reprogramming the human vestibular system as one would reprogram a computer. The simplest method is to have the patient deliberately move into the provocative position, staying there until the vertigo subsides and repeating it until habituation takes place. This should be performed three to four times a day for at least two months before giving it up. Hecker, Haug and Herndon (1974) present a more elaborate set of exercises which may be necessary in difficult cases. Simmons and Goode (1972) used the same principle but had patients self-administer cold water calorics at home to develop habituation.

With these exercises, patients may be helped initially with some type of vestibular suppressant drug. McCabe (1973) found in cats that diazepam (Valium) was more effective than dimenhydrinate (Dramamine), scopolamine, or atropine in reducing semicircular canal activity. It was felt that this was mediated through blocking of the reticular activating fibres that discharge upon the vestibular nuclei. Clinically, diazepam (Valium) has proven valuable as a vestibular suppressant in doses of 2–5 mg three times daily. One must keep in mind the possibility of psychological and physical dependence that patients may develop with long-term use of any of these drugs. Herndon *et al.*, (1975) found in a double-blind clinical study that a combination of pentylenetetrazol 25 mg, pheneramine maleate 12.5 mg, and nicotinic acid 50 mg (Ru-Vert) clinically and statistically reduced the symptoms of vertigo in patients with positional vertigo. They recommended this in combination with Cawthorne–Cooksey vestibular exercises.

Surgery may be indicated in selected patients who have intractable symptoms and who have significant disability from their disease. Schuknecht (1969) reported two such cases who had no usable hearing in the diseased ear. These patients had total relief of their symptoms after a labyrinthectomy. Gacek (1974) has developed a technique for selective sectioning of the posterior ampullary nerve. This was approached transcanal and the nerve sectioned just posterior and superior to the round window. He presented five cases all with relief of symptoms of positional vertigo.

References

Adler, F. H. (1941) 'Ocular vertigo'. In Symposium on Vertigo, *Transactions of the American Academy of Ophthalmology and Otolaryngology*, **46**, 27

Alpers, B. J. and Yaskin, H. E. (1944) 'The Brun's syndrome', *Journal of Nervous and Mental Diseases*, **100**, 115

Aschan, G. (1956) 'Nystagmography', *Acta Otolaryngologica Suppl.*, **129**, 1

Aschoff, J. C. and Cohen, B. (1973) 'Oculomotor deficiency after cerebellar cortical lesions', *Advances in Otorhinolaryngology*, **19**, 232

Bárány, R. (1921) 'Diagnose von Kraubeitserscheinungen im Berusche des Otolithenappates', *Acta Otolaryngologica, Stockholm*, **2**, 434

Barber, H. O. (1964) 'Positional nystagmus especially after head injury', *Laryngoscope*, **74**, 891

Barber, H. O. (1971) 'The diagnosis and treatment of auditory and vestibular disorders after head injury,' *Clinical Neurology*, **19**, 355

Barber, H. O. (1973) 'Positional vertigo and nystagmus', *Otolaryngology Clinics of North America*, **6**, 169

Barber, H. O. and Dionne, J. (1971) 'Vestibular findings in vertebrobasilar ischemia', *Annals of Otology*, **80**, 805

Barber, H. O. and Morrison, M. D. (1973) 'Clinical manifestations of otolithic dysfunction', *Advances in Otorhinolaryngology*, **20**, 396. Basel; Karger

Barnett, A. J. and Hyland, H. H. (1952) 'Tumours involving the brainstem', *Quarterly Journal of Medicine*, **21**, 265

Behrman, S. (1955) 'Vestibular epilepsy', *Brain*, **78**, 471

Best, T. (1973) 'Sensory systems—vestibular function'. In *Physiological Basis of Medical Practice*, pp 40–62. Ed. by Best, C. H. 9th edn. Baltimore; Williams and Wilkins Co.

Bhatia, P. L., Gupta, O. P., Agrawal, M. K. and Mishr, S. K. (1977) 'Audiological and vestibular function tests in hypothyroidism', *Laryngoscope*, **87**, 2082

Bickerstaff, E. R. (1961) 'Basilar artery migraine', *Lancet*, **1**, 15

Biemond, A. and DeJong, J. M. B. V. (1969) 'On cervical nystagmus and related disorders', *Brain*, **92**, 437

Brodal, A. (1960) 'Fiber connections of the vestibular nuclei'. In *Neural Mechanisms of the Auditory and Vestibular Systems*. Ed. by Rasmussen, G. L. and Windle, W. Springfield; Charles C. Thomas

Brodal, A. (1969) *Neurological Anatomy in Relation to Clinical Medicine*, pp. 374–394. Oxford; The University Press

Brodal, A. (1973) 'Self-observations and neuro-anatomical considerations after a stroke', *Brain*, **96**, 675

Carmichael, E. A., Dix, M. R. and Hallpike, R. W. (1954) 'Lesions of the cerebral hemispheres and their effects upon optokinetic and caloric nystagmus', *Brain*, **77**, 345

Carter, S., Sciarra, D. and Merritt, H. H. (1950) 'The course of multiple sclerosis as determined by autopsy proven cases', *Association for the Research into Nervous and Mental Disease*, **28**, 471

Cawthorne, T. and Hallpike, C. (1957) 'A study of the clinical features and pathological changes within the temporal bones, brain stem and cerebellum of an early case of positional nystagmus of the so-called benign paroxysmal type', *Acta Otolaryngologica*, **48**, 89

Cawthorne, T. and Hinchcliffe, R. (1961) 'Positional nystagmus of the central type as evidence of subtentorial metastases', *Brain*, **84**, 415

Clemis, J. D. and Becker, G. W. (1973) 'Vestibular neuronitis', *Otolaryngology Clinics of North America*, **6**(1), 139

Coates, A. C. (1969) 'Vestibular neuronitis', *Acta Otolaryngologica*, Supp., **251**, 1

Cremer, G. M., Goldstein, N. P. and Paris, J. (1969) 'Myxedema and ataxia', *Neurology*, **19**, 37

Dayal, V. S., Smith, E. L. and McCain, W. G. (1974) 'Cochlear and vestibular gentamicin toxicity: a clinical study of systemic and topical usage', *Archives of Otolaryngology*, **100**, 338

Dayal, V. S., Tarantino, L., Farkashidy, J. and Paradisgarten, A. (1974) 'Spontaneous and positional nystagmus: a reassessment of clinical significance', *Laryngoscope*, **84**, 2033

DeWeese, D. D. (1954) *Dizziness: An Evaluation and Classification.* Springfield, Ill.; Charles C. Thomas

Dix, M. R. and Hallpike, C. S. (1952) 'The pathology, symptomatology and diagnosis of certain common disorders of the vestibular system', *Annals of Otology, Rhinology and Laryngology*, **61**, 987

Drachman, D. A. and Hart, C. W. (1972) 'An approach to the dizzy patient', *Neurology*, **22**, 323

Duncan, G. W., Parker S. W. and Fisher, C. M. (1975) 'Acute cerebellar infarction in the PICA territory', *Archives of Neurology*, **32**, 364

Dunn, D. W. and Snyder, C. H. (1976) 'Benign paroxysmal vertigo in childhood', *American Journal of the Diseases of Childhood*, **130**, 1099

Fernandez, C. and Frederickson, S. M. (1964) 'Experimental cerebellar lesions and their effect on vestibular function', *Acta Otolaryngologica, Suppl.* **192**, 52

Fisher, C. M., Picard, E. M., Polack, A. *et al.* (1965) 'Acute hypertensive cerebellar hemorrhage', *Journal of Nervous and Mental Diseases*, **140**, 38

Fisher, C. M. (1967) 'Some neuro-ophthalmological observations', *Journal of Neurology, Neurosurgery and Psychiatry*, **30**, 383

Gacek, R. R. (1968) 'Neuroanatomical pathways of the vestibular system', *Annals of Otology, Rhinology, and Laryngology*, **77**, 210

Gacek, R. R. (1974) 'Transection of the posterior ampullary nerve for the relief of benign paroxysmal positional vertigo', *Annals of Otology*, **83**, 596

Goodman, L. S. and Gilman, A. (1975) *The Pharmacological Basis of Therapeutics*, 5th edn. New York; Macmillan Co.

Gowers, W. R. (1907) *The Border-land of Epilepsy: Faints, Vagal Attacks, Vertigo, Migraine, Sleep Symptoms and Their Treatment.* London; Churchill

Harrison, M. S. and Ozsahinoglu, C. (1975) 'Positional vertigo', *Archives of Otolaryngology*, **101**, 675

Hart, C. (1965) 'Vestibular paralysis of sudden onset and probably viral etiology', *Annals of Otolaryngology*, **74**, 33

Hecker, H. C., Haug, C. O. and Herndon, J. W. (1974) 'Treatment of the vertiginous patient using Cawthorne's vestibular exercises', *Laryngoscope*, **84**, 2065

Herndon, J. W., Haug, O., Horowitz, N. J. and Lynes, T. E. (1975) 'Benign paroxysmal positional vertigo: a clinical study', *Annals of Otolaryngology*, **84**, 218

Igarashi, M., Miyata, H., Alford, B. R. and Wright, W. K. (1973) 'Experimental cerebellar urulonodular lesions in the squirrel monkey', *Advances in Otolaryngology*, **19**, 220

Jonas, S. *et al.* (1977) 'Importance of Holter monitoring in patients with periodic cerebral symptoms', *Annals of Neurology*, **1**, 470

Keim, R. J. and Sachs, G. B. (1975) 'Positional nystagmus in association with macroglobulinemia', *Annals of Otolaryngology*, **84**, 223

Lehrich, J. R., Winkler, G. F. and Ojemann, R. G. (1970) 'Cerebellar infarction with brainstem compression: diagnosis and surgical treatment', *Archives of Neurology*, **22**, 490

Lim, D. (1973) 'Formation and fate of otoconia: scanning and transmission electron microscopy', *Annals of Otology, Rhinology, and Laryngology*, **82**, 23

Lindsay, J. R. and Hemenway, W. G. (1956) 'Postural vertigo due to unilateral sudden partial loss of vestibular function', *Annals of Otolaryngology*, **65**, 692

McAlpine, D., Lumsden, C. E. and Acheson, E. D. (1972) *Multiple Sclerosis: A Reappraisal*, 2nd edn. Baltimore; Williams and Wilkins

McCabe, B. F. (1973) 'Central aspects of drugs for motion sickness and vertigo', *Advances in Otorhinolaryngology*, **20**, 458. Basel; Karger

Meyers, R. M. (1970) 'Ototoxic effects of gentamicin', *Archives of Otolaryngology*, **92**, 160

Millikan, C. H. and Siekert, R. G. (1955) 'Studies in cerebrovascular disease', *Proceedings of Staff Meetings at Mayo Clinic*, **30**, 61

Moehling, R. C. (1927) 'Vertigo and deafness associated with hypothyroidism', *Endocrinology*, **11**, 229

Money, K. E., Johnson, W. H. and Cerlett, B. M. A. (1965) 'Role of semicircular canals in positional alcoholic nystagmus', *American Journal of Physiology*, **208**, 1065

Money, K. E. and Myles, W. S. (1973) 'Motion sickness and other vestibulogastric illnesses'. Presented at a Symposium: *The Vestibular System*, University of Chicago, Chicago, Illinois, April 27

Nylén, C. O. (1931) 'A clinical study in positional nystagmus in cases of brain tumor', *Acta Otolaryngologica*, Supp., **15**, 1

Nylén, C. O. (1939) 'The oto-neurological diagnosis of tumors in the brain', *Acta Otolaryngologica*, Supp., **33**, 1

Pearson, B. W. and Barber, H. O. (1973) 'Head injury: some otoneurological sequelae', *Archives of Otolaryngology*, **97**, 81

Post, J. T. (1964) 'Hypothyroid deafness: a clinical study of sensori-neural deafness associated with hypothyroidism', *Laryngoscope*, **74**, 221

Powers, W. H. (1972) 'Metabolic aspects of Meniere's disease', *Laryngoscope*, **82**, 1716

Pulec, J. L. (1972) 'I. Meniere's disease: results of a two and one-half-year study of etiology, natural history and results of treatment', *Laryngoscope*, **82**, 1703

Rahko, T. and Aantaa, E. (1977) 'Equilibrial disturbances caused by hearing aids in hard of hearing children', *Journal of Laryngology and Otology*, **91**(4), 357

Ritter, F. N. (1967) 'The effects of hypothyroidism upon the ear, nose and throat', *Laryngoscope*, **77**, 1427

Rubin, W. (1973) 'Whiplash with vestibular involvement', *Archives of Otolaryngology*, **97**, 85

Russell, J. R. and Bucy, P. C. (1953) 'Meningiomas of the posterior fossa', *Surgery, Gynaecology and Obstetrics*, **96**, 183

Schuknecht, H. F. (1969) 'Cupolithiasis', *Archives of Otolaryngology*, **90**, 765

Schuknecht, H. F. (1974) *Pathology of the Ear.* Cambridge; The University Press

Simmons, F. B. and Goode, R. L. (1972) 'Deliberate dizziness therapy (DDT)', *Archives of Otolaryngology*, **95**, 221

Smith, B. H. (1960) 'Vestibular disturbances in epilepsy', *Neurology*, **10**, 465

Sodjadpour, K. and Brodal, A. (1968) 'The vestibular nuclei in man: a morphological study in the light of experimental findings in the cat', *Journal für Hirnforschung*, **10**, 299

Störtebecker, T. P. (1954) 'Metastatic tumors of the brain from a neurosurgical point of view: a follow-up of 158 cases', *Journal of Neurosurgery*, **11**, 84

Sypert, G. W. and Alvord, E. C., Jr. (1975) 'Cerebellar infarction', *Archives of Neurology*, **32**, 357

Szentagothai, J. (1964) 'Pathways and synaptic articulation patterns connecting vestibular receptors and oculomotor nuclei'. In *The Oculomotor System*. Ed. by Bender, M. B. New York; Hoeber Medical Division, Harper & Row

Toglia, J. U. (1976) 'Acute flexion-extension injury of the neck: electronystagmographic study of 309 patients', *Neurology*, **26**, 808

Weinstein, M. A., Alfidi, R. J. and Duchesneau, P. M. (1977) 'Guest Editorial, computed tomography versus skull radiography', *American Journal of Roentgenology*, **128**, 873

White, H. H. (1963) 'Brain stem tumours occurring in adults', *Neurology*, **13**, 292

Wilkinson, I. M. S. and Russell, R. W. R. (1972) 'Arteries in the head and neck in giant cell arteritis: a pathological study to show the pattern of arterial involvement', *Archives of Neurology*, **27**, 378

Yatsu, F. M. (1977) 'Pharmacological basis of acute stroke therapy'. In *Clinical Neuropharmacology*, Vol. 2, pp. 113–150. Ed. by Klawans, H. L. New York; Raven Press

27 Facial paralysis
John Groves

General considerations

Facial paralysis is by far the most common of all peripheral nerve lesions. Its effects upon voluntary and emotional facial expression, upon the mechanisms of mastication and speech, upon the sense of taste, and upon the protective mechanisms of the eye are grave enough in themselves. Added to the often gross cosmetic deformity these constitute a major calamity in the life of the sufferer and those near to him. Otologists have the care of, and the responsibility for, this cranial nerve and major contributions in this field have been made by otological pioneers such as Ballance and Duel (1932), Collier (1963), Cawthorne (1963), Kettel (1959) and Sullivan (1963), to name but a few.

Anatomy of the facial nerve

The facial is the nerve of the second branchial arch, a fact which explains its complex and intimate relationships with the middle-ear cleft and ossicular chain (*Figure 27.1*). It contains about 10 000 fibres in the human. They include:

(1) Motor fibres, numbering about 7000, to the muscles of facial expression, and the buccinator, stapedius, digastric and stylohyoid muscles.
(2) Secretomotor parasympathetic fibres, to the lacrimal and nasal glands, and to the submandibular and sublingual salivary glands.
(3) Taste fibres, from the taste-buds of the palate and the anterior two-thirds of the tongue.

In addition, some evidence suggests that there may be cutaneous sensory fibres from a small area of the external ear, accounting for the distribution of the vesication in herpes oticus.

The motor fibres have their cell bodies in the facial nucleus in the pons. The nucleus receives pyramidal fibres from the contralateral motor cortex and a smaller number from the homolateral side. In addition, fibres from the spinal tract of the trigeminal nerve and fibres from the corpus trapezoideum play upon the facial nucleus. The

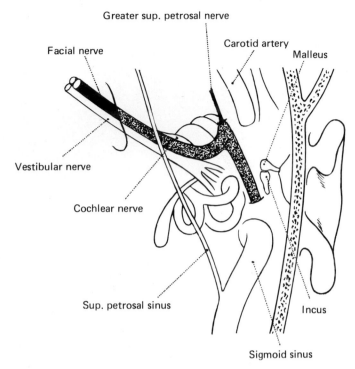

Figure 27.1   The facial nerve seen from above in the floor of the middle cranial fossa

motor fibres sweep around the nucleus of the sixth cranial nerve and emerge from the brain stem at the lower border of the pons. Crossing the cerebellopontine angle in a lateral and forward direction, the nerve is closely related to the two divisions of the auditory nerve, the nervus intermedius and posteriorly the anterior inferior cerebellar artery. The nerve enters the temporal bone through the internal auditory meatus together with the auditory nerve, nervus intermedius, and the internal auditory vessels, all these structures being sheathed in a prolongation of the subarachnoid space with its meninges.

At the lateral extremity of the internal auditory meatus the nerve is above the crista falciformis and anterior to the vertical bony crest ('Bill's Bar'). It continues, with the nervus intermedius, into the bony fallopian canal, which runs above the labyrinth, separated from the middle cranial fossa by a thin layer of bone (*Figure 27.2*). After a few millimetres the nerve makes a U-turn backwards. This bend is the *genu*, and it is marked by a rounded swelling, the geniculate ganglion. In some cases the bony roof of the canal is absent here, so that the ganglion is directly related to the dura mater.

From the genu the nerve runs backwards and slightly downwards in the medial wall of the tympanum. Here the bony fallopian canal wall forms a cylindrical ridge familiar to the operating otologist as the tympanic course of the nerve, lying below the horizontal semicircular canal and above the oval window and promontory. The anterior limit of this part of the nerve is marked by the processus cochleariformis with its emerging tensor tympani tendon, a valuable landmark.

In the bony floor of the aditus the nerve makes a somewhat gradual bend, turning downwards 1 or 2 mm behind the pyramid to the commencement of the vertical or

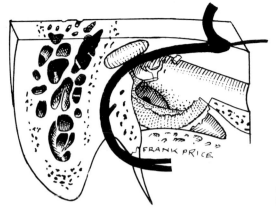

Figure 27.2   The intratemporal course and relations of the facial nerve

mastoid segment. This final part of the intratemporal course of the facial nerve runs directly downwards to the stylomastoid foramen, and is surrounded by mastoid air-cells. It lies at a great depth, rarely less than 2 cm from the outer mastoid surface in the adult.

From the stylomastoid foramen the nerve turns forwards, passes lateral to the base of the styloid process, and enters the parotid gland (*Figure 27.3*). Within the gland subdivision begins, usually first into upper and lower branches, and then again into the six peripheral branches. These branches run forwards in the plane between the superficial part of the parotid gland, and the ramus of the mandible and masseter muscle.

COMPOSITION AND DISTRIBUTION OF THE NERVE
Microscopic studies indicate that, like other peripheral nerves, the facial contains medullated axons of varying size, and presumably of varying conductivity speeds.

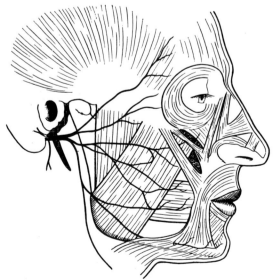

Figure 27.3   The course and relations of the seventh cranial nerve in the face, omitting the parotid gland. Note that the trunk lies on the base of the styloid process, and the first major subdivisions are related to the neck and ascending ramus of the mandible

It seems possible that the larger fibres which have the faster conduction rates, are concerned with voluntary movement, while the smaller diameter 'slow' fibres may be responsible for emotional and reflex movements. The question of maintenance of facial 'tonus' is a little obscure. Muscle spindles—the essential stretch receptors—have been demonstrated in the facial muscles, but it is thought that their proprioceptive nerve fibres probably travel centrally in the trigeminal nerve.

May (1977), and White and Verna (1973) have described the spatial arrangement of the motor fibres in the intra-temporal course of the nerve.

Each medullated nerve fibre branches near its termination into fibrils distributed to the motor end-plates of its own motor unit. In the face, motor units have a comparatively small number of muscle fibres, so that the patterns of muscular activity which are possible are correspondingly large in number, and refined in detail and complexity.

The parasympathetic nerve fibres originate in the superior salivary nucleus and leave the brain stem in the nervus intermedius. At the geniculate ganglion these fibres mingle with those of the motor nerve trunk. Those destined to innervate the submandibular and sublingual glands continue in the facial nerve (*Figure 27.4*) as far as the chorda tympani. They finally reach the submandibular ganglion by way of the chorda and the lingual nerve. Parasympathetic motor fibres for the lacrimal gland leave the geniculate ganglion in the greater superficial petrosal nerve, and reach their destination by way of the vidian nerve, the maxillary nerve, and its zygomatic branch. The secretomotor fibres for the nasal mucosa leave the facial nerve by the same route.

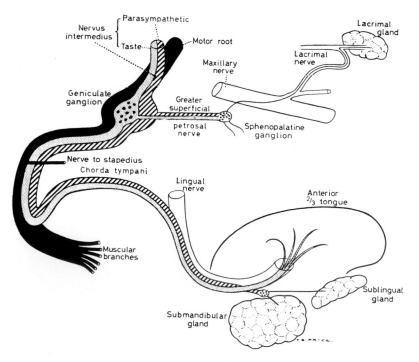

Figure 27.4 Plan of the facial nerve showing its constituent fibres, their relay stations, and destinations

The taste fibres from the anterior two-thirds of the tongue travel in the lingual nerve, and then join the facial nerve by way of the chorda tympani. After ascending the facial nerve, the taste fibres have their cell bodies in the geniculate ganglion. From the palate taste fibres first follow the palatine nerves, and then pass through the sphenopalatine ganglion, vidian nerve and greater superficial petrosal nerve to reach the geniculate ganglion. The central axons of all these taste neurones continue in the nervus intermedius to the brain stem. Their final destination is the tractus solitarius.

BRANCHES OF THE FACIAL NERVE

From above downwards these are:

(1) The greater superficial petrosal nerve, at the geniculate ganglion.
(2) A twig to the tympanic plexus.
(3) The nerve to stapedius, which passes upwards and forwards, from the commencement of the vertical segment of the facial nerve.
(4) There is much variation in the exact level of origin of the chorda tympani which may be anywhere from 1 or 2 mm below the nerve to stapedius to the stylo–mastoid foramen or even lower. Furthermore, the chorda may spring from the front, lateral, or posterior aspect of the nerve trunk. These variables can create difficulties in operations on the nerve if the chorda is used as a landmark for the main trunk.
(5) Below the stylomastoid foramen are the branches to the stylohyoid and digastric muscles and the post-auricular branch to the occipitofrontalis and external auricular muscles.
(6) The final fanwise branching of the nerve in the face has six main subdivisions; (*a*) temporal; (*b*) upper zygomatic; (*c*) lower zygomatic; (*d*) buccal; (*e*) mandibular; (*f*) cervical. These form a complex branching and anastomosing network (*see Figure 27.3*) in which extensive interconnections with the finer branches of the trigeminal nerve are found. There are also many small branches which cross the midline and innervate a limited muscular field on the opposite side of the face.

ANATOMICAL VARIATIONS

It has often been supposed that the intratemporal course of the facial nerve is quite constant. While in most cases the classic description holds good there are anomalies, well described in the literature, which would endanger the nerve during operations within the temporal bone (*Figure 27.5*).

At the so-called 'second bend' or pyramidal segment, instead of turning more or less directly downwards, the nerve may swing rather widely backwards and a little laterally below the level of the lateral semicircular canal before finally descending to the stylomastoid foramen.

Many instances of atypical branching of the vertical segment into two, or even three, main trunks, each leaving a bone through a separate foramen, have been described. In cases of extreme congenital abnormality of the middle ear the tympanic part of the nerve may pass down on the promontory below the oval window, or, after bifurcating, lie partly above and partly below it.

Congenital dehiscences in the bony wall of the fallopian canal are comparatively common in the horizontal or tympanic segment. In the vertical segment pneumatization may proceed to an extent which opens the bony fallopian canal to the air–cell

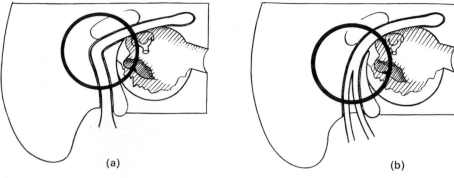

(a)   (b)

Figure 27.5   Anatomical abnormalities of the facial nerve: (a) the 'second bend' is acutely angled lying more superficially, higher, and more posteriorly than is normal; (b) intratemporal branching of the vertical part of the nerve

system. Dehiscences of either kind expose the nerve within to additional pathological and surgical hazards.

In children the plan of the nerve resembles that of the adult, on a slightly reduced scale, but in the infant the absence of the mastoid process and the rudimentary state of the tympanic ring cause the nerve to emerge almost directly laterally behind the tympanic membrane. It is here very vulnerable to the pressure of obstetrical forceps, or to the surgical knife in a post-auricular incision.

BLOOD SUPPLY OF THE FACIAL NERVE

Within the confined space of the fallopian canal special attention to the blood supply of the nerve is necessary; a detailed account is given by Blunt (1954). The stylomastoid artery, a branch of the occipital artery, enters the foramen and runs upwards anterior and slightly medial to the nerve, sending short branches at intervals around and into it. At the geniculate ganglion the petrosal branch of the middle meningeal artery enters the canal and runs distally to anastomose with the stylomastoid artery. Within the internal auditory meatus the nerve is supplied by the internal auditory artery (or arteries, Fisch, 1969) and in the posterior cranial fossa by the anterior inferior cerebellar artery. The veins form a plexus around the nerve from which efferent vessels run obliquely, first between the sheath and the nerve and then through the sheath to lie on its outer surface. Apart from small veins accompanying the chorda tympani, the venous drainage leaves the canal mainly at the stylomastoid foramen and at the genu. Sympathetic nervous control of vasomotor tonus is presumed to be effective through the cervical sympathetic fibres distributed around the branches of the external carotid artery.

THE FACIAL NERVE SHEATH

Throughout the fallopian canal the nerve (and its two infrageniculate branches) are enclosed in a fibrous sheath. As exposed during surgical procedures this sheath consists from without inwards of:

(1) A tough, shiny, grey periosteal layer.
(2) A vascular plane of arteries and venous plexus, embedded in loose connective tissue.

(3) A firm fibrous layer perforated by the vessels and on its deep surface in contact with the perineural connective tissues.

Although a clear plane of dissection is found between the sheath and the nerve, this plane is crossed by innumerable connective tissue strands which require careful division and separation if a length of the nerve is to be uncovered.

Distal to the internal auditory meatus the sheath blends with the dural coverings of the nerve, while at the stylomastoid foramen it fuses with the periosteum and with the adjacent fascial layers covering the digastric muscle, the parotid gland and carotid vessels.

The sheath is easily recognized under the dissecting microscope and it is a valuable barrier against mechanical injury and infection. It should be opened only if there are proper surgical indications for doing so.

RADIOLOGICAL ANATOMY

Although the fallopian canal is not always easy to demonstrate clearly in a radiograph, the funnel-shaped infundibulum can be followed upwards into the vertical segment in the routine views of the mastoid. The stylomastoid foramen itself can always be clearly identified in the submentovertical view of the skull base, while the internal auditory meatus is routinely well shown in Townes' and Stenver's projections, among others.

In cases where it is particularly important to define the fallopian canal itself tomography should always be employed. The projection and depth of 'cut' will vary according to whether the vertical or the horizontal segment of the nerve is to be studied (*see* Volume 1).

Surgical approaches to the facial nerve

Any portion of the facial nerve can be surgically exposed (*Figure 27.6*). The principles are described below, but the operations must be learned by cadaver dissection and under expert tutelage in the operating theatre.

NECK AND FACE

In the neck and face the parotid segments of the nerve are exposed by means of the classic parotidectomy incision. Dissection below the external auditory meatus between the mastoid and the parotid gland defines (at a very deep level) the nerve trunk running forward from the stylomastoid foramen. From this point the nerve is followed into the parotid and its branches are identified in turn. If necessary, partial or complete parotidectomy can then be carried out without injury to the nerve, or appropriate nerve suturing or grafting (*see below*) can be performed. The post-auricular part of the incision can be extended and the nerve can be followed proximally in its endotemporal course if this is necessary to find a healthy central stump.

VERTICAL OR MASTOID SEGMENT

The vertical or mastoid segment is exposed through a post-auricular incision. Sufficient bone is removed to expose the sinus plate, mastoid antrum and lateral semicircular canal. The mastoid air-cells are then cleared leaving the cortical shell

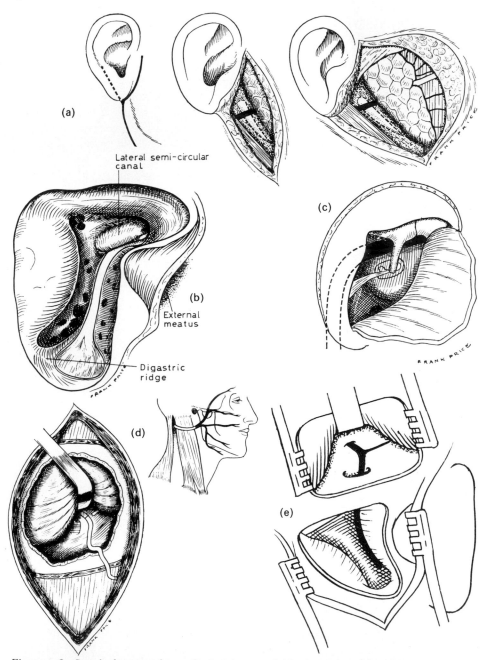

Figure 27.6 Surgical approaches to the facial nerve: (a) in the neck and face. Note the position of the styloid process, which is a palpable landmark although it is not actually exposed to view in the course of the dissection; (b) transmastoid exposure of the vertical part of the nerve. The digastric ridge below and the lateral semicircular canal above are the essential landmarks. It is not necessary to remove the tip of the mastoid process. The tympanic part of the nerve can be followed forwards below the incus; (c) permeatal tympanotomy exposes part of the tympanic portion of the nerve; (d) posterior fossa craniotomy (after Dott), the diagrams show the principle of Dott's operation for facial nerve grafting, bypassing the temporal bone; (e) whole nerve exposure of the facial nerve, combining the transmastoid and middle fossa techniques

undisturbed below and in front. With the electric burr the periosteum on the medial surface of the mastoid process is then uncovered and followed upwards and medially until the entrance to the fallopian canal is defined. This is a few millimetres behind the plane of the deep posterior bony meatal wall, on a level with the digastric ridge of bone (*Figure 27.6b*). Some experience is required, when seeking the fallopian canal near its lower end, to avoid mistaking for the nerve the dense fibrous bands which run vertically into the bone from the vicinity of the digastric groove. The smaller, more laterally placed, chorda tympani may be mistaken for its deeper and much larger parent.

The line of the nerve is thus established from the lateral canal above to the stylomastoid foramen below. Bone is drilled away along this line with the aid of irrigation and suction until only a paper-thin layer remains over the nerve. The sheath is then uncovered, under the operating microscope, with a fine hook or curette. If the sheath is to be opened, it is incised with an extremely fine-pointed knife by cutting outwards away from the nerve, and following its posterolateral aspect where least damage will be done to the vascular system.

TYMPANIC OR HORIZONTAL SEGMENT

The tympanic or horizontal segment can be approached (as in posterior tympanotomy) by an oblique alignment of the dissecting microscope and burr after exposure of the vertical segment as described above. This re-alignment enables the operator to work forwards in a narrow crevice bounded by: (1) the lateral canal above and medially; (2) the fossa incudis and short process of incus above and laterally; (3) the tympanic annulus below and laterally.

The thin shell-like bony covering of this part of the nerve is soon reached and can be followed and removed anteriorly towards the processus cochleariformis without disturbance of the ossicles or tympanic membrane. The writer has not attempted nerve grafting at so high a level in a previously intact ear, but there is certainly no doubt that this approach permits any desired procedure on the nerve if the sacrifice of the incus is permissible. The avoidance of an open mastoidectomy cavity is a very worthwhile advantage, for which a little additional difficulty is a small price to pay. Exposure of the tympanic segment, of course, presents no problem of access when the ear has already been explored by a radical or modified radical mastoidectomy approach.

In the intact ear limited but perhaps useful access to this segment of the nerve may be gained by means of ordinary permeatal tympanotomy.

PETROUS PORTION

The petrous portion of the nerve can be approached by a method described by House (1963). The middle cranial fossa is opened by a vertical incision which splits the temporalis muscle, and partial removal of the squamous temporal bone. The middle fossa dura is lifted from the upper surface of the petrous bone and, with an electric burr under the dissecting microscope, the geniculate ganglion is exposed. Further bone removal in a medial direction uncovers the facial and auditory nerves as far as the medial end of the internal auditory meatus. This technique is applicable when it is necessary to avoid surgical injury to the middle and inner ear.

A translabyrinthine approach can be used if the ear is surgically 'expendable'; for example, because of irreversible total cochlear deafness. It is then permissible to expose the petrous part of the nerve by way of a post-auricular mastoidectomy. The semicircular canals and upper part of the vestibule are removed with the burr, and further dissection upwards and medially opens the fallopian canal and internal auditory meatus. Because this technique opens the subarachnoid space to the middle-ear cleft the site of the labyrinthectomy must be sealed off with a free muscle graft when the operation is concluded.

INTRACRANIAL PORTION

The intracranial part of the nerve is accessible by way of classic posterior fossa craniotomy. A vertical incision 4 cm from the midline and centred on the superior nuchal line is carried down to the bone and the insertion of the posterior nuchal muscles. The latter are detached from the under-surface of the occipital bone which is then opened with a burr and rongeur forceps. A flap is cut in the dura, and the cerebellum is elevated while the cerebrospinal fluid drains away. Careful retraction of the brain will then permit access to the cerebellopontine angle—where not only the facial, but also the trigeminal, glossopharyngeal, vagus, and accessory nerves can be reached.

Dott's operation

Dott (1963) utilized this approach (*Figure 27.6*) to secure a central stump of facial nerve when paralysis is due to irremediable lesions at or distal to the internal auditory meatus. A long free nerve graft (from the sural nerve) is joined to the central stump in the cerebellopontine angle and brought out through the craniotomy opening. This distal end of the graft is passed forward deep to the nuchal muscles and superficial to the upper end of the sternomastoid muscle. At a second operation several weeks later the distal end of the graft is anastomosed to the peripheral facial nerve at the posterior border of the parotid gland (*Figure 27.6d*).

Fisch (1977) has proposed a new application of this principle, effecting a graft from the internal auditory canal (by way of the *middle* fossa approach). The graft is brought out through the temporal craniotomy directly into the parotid region for anastomosis as a one-stage procedure.

Pathology of peripheral nerve lesions

Interruption of nerve function can be caused by any type of mechanical insult—compression, crushing, stretching, or section of the nerve, damage by excessive cold, heat from electrocautery, ultrasonic energy, and application of toxic substances such as local anaesthetics—the list is long and is of obvious surgical interest. The nature, and hence the prognosis, of the injury can be classified in terms of neurapraxia (reversible conduction block) or Wallerian degeneration. In practice many peripheral nerve lesions are 'mixed', having some neurapraxic and some degenerated fibres.

Neurapraxia results from minor degrees of injury. The conductivity of the nerve fibres is blocked at the site of the lesion, but if the nerve is stimulated distal to the lesion a normal nerve action potential is evoked and the muscles concerned are made to contract. If a nerve is merely neurapraxic, removal of the cause is promptly followed by a complete restoration of function.

Degeneration results from more severe lesions, the classic experimental example being complete transection. After such lesions no immediate changes occur apart from the total loss of conductivity at the site of injury. The distal segment of the cut nerve remains normally excitable for 48–72 h. After this time, however, nerve stimulation becomes ineffective, and histological changes within the nerve become evident. The axon itself breaks up and disappears while the myelin sheath disintegrates with the appearance of fatty droplets. These changes occur in the entire nerve distal to the lesion, and proximally also up to the nearest node of Ranvier.

The neurilemma sheath remains intact except where it is damaged or destroyed by the original lesion. Within the neurilemmal tubes the detritus of degeneration is removed by macrophages.

REGENERATION AFTER NERVE INJURY

After the neurilemmal tubes have been cleared the proximal end of each axon cylinder grows downward towards the site of injury. If there is continuity of the tubes with those in the distal part of the nerve most of the growing fibres will penetrate successfully and continue at an approximate rate of 1 mm/day until eventually some at least of the motor end plates are re-innervated. Some fibres may be misdirected so that they innervate muscles different from those they served before the injury. If there is a breach in the continuity of the neurilemmal tubes at the site of the lesion the regenerating axons emerge from the proximal stump of the nerve, and are obliged to 'grope' for their way. They proliferate to form a bulbous swelling ('neuroma') and only a comparatively small number of them succeed in entering the distal part of the nerve and continuing on to the end plates. The greater the gap between the two parts of the nerve, the smaller will be the percentage of successful fibres. This type of repair also results in a much greater degree of misdirection of those fibres which do succeed in bridging the gap.

In the facial nerve the rate of repair is such that a lapse of 10–14 weeks is usually required, after a lesion in the temporal bone, before any voluntary movement returns to the paralysed muscles. Any recovery that occurs sooner than this can only be attributed to the relief of conduction block in fibres which have suffered merely from neurapraxia.

Clinical assessment of facial paralysis

It is necessary in a case of facial paralysis to determine the level of the lesion as well as its pathological basis. In addition, the motor function of the nerve must be ascertained in detail. From an appraisal of all these factors a prognosis can be given and treatment can be planned.

A distinction between upper and lower motor neurone facial palsies can usually be made at first examination. In upper motor neurone palsy the upper half of the face is less involved, and voluntary movements show greater impairment than involuntary or emotional facial expression. These classic rules can sometimes be misleading in partial paralyses of the lower motor neurone type, and the final decision as to whether a case is of central or peripheral type should only be made after the history, and the presence of other symptoms and signs have been considered. Thus in cases of upper motor neurone paralysis other pyramidal tract signs may be present, while in peripheral paralysis disturbances of taste, hearing, balance and lacrimation will provide clues.

ASSESSMENT OF MOTOR FUNCTION

Peripheral facial paralysis may have any grade of severity between minimal and total, depending upon the percentage of nerve fibres affected, and their peripheral distribution in the various areas of the face. Complete paralysis is usually defined as an absence of *all* visible voluntary movement in *all* areas. Lesser degrees of paralysis cannot be accurately defined in such terms as mild or severe. The term *partial* requires to be qualified, in scientific work, by details of the muscular power (normal, weak or absent) in each of the following areas: frontalis, orbicularis oculi, orbicularis oris, levators of the mouth and nostril. Even then the assessment remains a somewhat subjective and personalized process and this often makes the comparison of cases and results of treatment rather difficult. Standardization of assessment has been attempted by many workers (Adour *et al.*, 1977).

The two sides of the face should be compared for symmetry, at rest (as a guide to 'tonus') and during voluntary movement. The patient is then asked to raise his eyebrows, close his eyes, wrinkle his nose, show his teeth, and to attempt to whistle. All these movements are then repeated while the examiner presses his hand firmly on the patient's face near the middle to prevent spurious movements being transmitted from the sound side. Without this precaution a complete paralysis is often mistaken for a partial one.

ELECTRODIAGNOSIS

Electrodiagnostic tests are of the greatest value in the assessment of the functional condition of the nerve. They help to fill the gaps left by ordinary clinical examination, although electrical tests themselves have many limitations which must be understood by those who interpret them.

A *partial* paralysis is irrefutable evidence that the nerve is in continuity. A partial paralysis of more than ten weeks' duration with evident synkinesia ('cross re-innervation') shows clearly that some fibres at least have degenerated and at least some of these have succeeded in regenerating.

The clinician, unaided, cannot deduce in complete facial palsy whether the nerve is neurapraxic, has degenerated, or even whether it is structurally in continuity. He cannot deduce, in complete paralysis, whether spontaneous recovery is to be expected at any early date, and in very long-standing cases he cannot know from clinical examination whether the denervated muscles have irretrievably wasted away.

It will be evident, therefore, that while the results of electrodiagnostic tests are interesting in every case of facial palsy, it is chiefly in cases of *complete* paralysis that they are of crucial importance to the clinician concerned with prognosis and treatment. Their value is as great in avoiding unnecessary treatment as it is in defining the need for active measures. In papers by Collier (1963) and Richardson (1957, 1962, 1963) the reader will find detailed discussions of the application of electrodiagnosis in facial paralysis.

Quantitative nerve excitability tests, as described by Campbell (1963), Richardson (1962, 1963), Taverner (1955) and Laumans and Jongkees (1963), vary in details of technique and sophistication. When the nerve is stimulated percutaneously at the level of the stylomastoid foramen (that is, below the lesion) neurapraxic fibres respond with a visible muscle twitch, while a degenerated nerve is electrically unresponsive.

The technique described by Campbell and Richardson, and used by the present writer, utilizes a unipolar electrode over the nerve trunk and an indifferent electrode

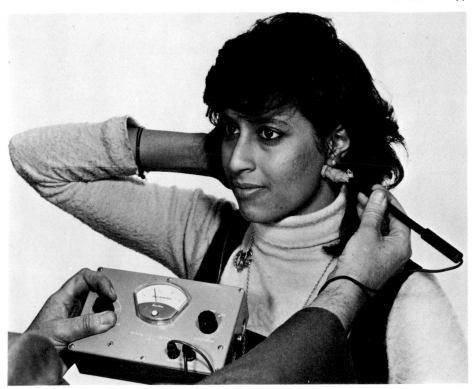

Figure 27.7   Quantitative test of nerve excitability. The patient holds the earth electrode against the back of the neck. The examiner applies the stimulating electrode over the trunk of the facial nerve immediately beneath the external auditory meatus. The smallest current required to induce muscular activity in the face is then determined. The 'end point' is the smallest observable twitch

on the back of the patient's neck (*Figure 27.7*). A square-wave pulse lasting for 1 ms is applied at intervals of 1 s, and the smallest intensity of the stimulus (in mA) which will evoke a visible muscle twitch in any part of the face is determined. The test is done on the normal and again on the paralysed side, and the nerve excitability in mA is recorded. Normal figures range from 3–10 mA—the important figure is not the absolute measure, but the *difference* between the two sides.

Gilliatt and Taylor (1959) showed that after complete nerve section nerve excitability is lost at between two and four days later. Such tests therefore have a time-lag which means they will not indicate when treatment might prevent degeneration—they can only show that it has begun and is inevitable. Nevertheless, their prognostic value is very great. If the causative lesion is self-limiting, and nerve excitability is preserved, spontaneous recovery without treatment is likely. Similarly, if a surgically operable lesion is treated promptly in the presence of normal nerve excitability the paralysis will probably recover quickly and completely.

Strength–duration measurements, now somewhat outmoded, are basically an extended test of nerve excitability in which the intensities required for electrical stimuli of differing durations to evoke muscle contraction are plotted graphically (*Figure 27.8*). Such an examination gives an approximate estimation of the proportion of neurapraxic to degenerated fibres. Both the nerve excitability and strength–duration

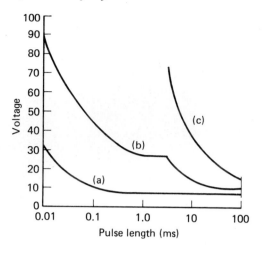

Figure 27.8 Strength–duration tests in facial paralysis: (a) neurapraxia only: (b) mixed lesion—some fibres neurapraxic, others degenerated; (c) complete denervation—all fibres degenerated

tests (if done more than three days after the onset of complete paralysis) can be accepted as evidence of gross continuity in the nerve, if any fibres show neurapraxia only.

Electroneurography (Esslen, 1977)

This test consists of percutaneous nerve stimulation below the mastoid, and the recording of the muscle action potentials by skin electrodes at the periphery. Esslen finds that the combined action potential (CAP) on the paralysed side, expressed as a percentage of the CAP on the normal side, is a reliable indication of prognosis in acute facial palsies. If the CAP is no less than 10 per cent of the normal side, spontaneous recovery will, it is claimed, be satisfactory.

Electromyography

A needle-electrode inserted into a muscle and connected to an oscilloscope will indicate the electrical activity in the motor units with which its point is in contact. The method has the limitation, however, that only a few motor units out of many thousands can be sampled. Interpretation must therefore be wary.

Normal motor units are electrically silent at rest. If the subject carries out voluntary movement a burst of muscle action potentials appears. Even if apparently complete paralysis is present, this simple test may still show that a few fibres are conducting voluntary impulses and this can provide invaluable evidence that the nerve is physically in continuity.

Denervation potentials appear in the muscle fibres if the motor nerve supply has degenerated. These are also known as fibrillation potentials. They are not usually present until about the tenth day after onset of the paralysis, but occasionally are seen earlier. They show that degeneration of nerve fibres has occurred, but unfortunately do not indicate in what percentage of the whole. With diligence some fibrillation can be found in most facial palsies, even when overall nerve excitability shows that most of the fibres are neurapraxic and subsequently recovery is fast and complete, without synkinesis. Absence of fibrillation is perhaps more informative—in early cases (2–10 weeks) it indicates that degeneration is negligible. Around 10–12 weeks it is often a favourable sign that re-innervation of previously denervated motor units is imminent.

After a year or more absence of fibrillation potentials in paralysed muscles suggests that the muscle fibres have wasted and are replaced by fibrous tissue—a finding which is confirmed by loss of response of the muscles to galvanic stimulation.

Polyphasic motor unit potentials

During re-innervation of motor units following Wallerian degeneration characteristic potentials are seen on electromyography. These so-called polyphasic potentials appear when an attempt is made by the patient to move the part of the face being explored, and they are found a week or two before clinical evidence of returning movement is detectable. In complete paralysis of more than, say, ten weeks' duration these potentials must be carefully sought as they indicate that nerve continuity is present, and that regeneration of some fibres at least is assured.

Figure 27.9 shows schematically the basis of electromyography in facial paralysis.

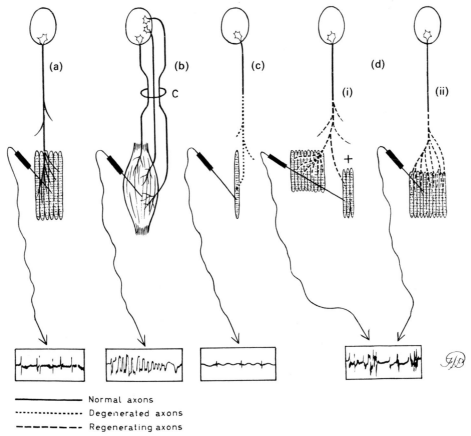

Normal axons
Degenerated axons
Regenerating axons

Figure 27.9 The theoretical basis of electromyography in facial paralysis. Several motor units are illustrated, in different states of innervation, with the characteristic electrical patterns of activity as sampled by the needle electrode: (a) a normal motor unit, during voluntary movement; (b) grouped motor potentials in the presence of compression (C); (c) spontaneous fibrillation potentials due to denervation; (d) polyphasic (recovery) potentials. These occur during re-innervation and may arise by: (i) *spatial* dispersion of electrical activity due to peripheral branching of the regenerating axon which thus re-innervates a larger complement of muscle fibres, (ii) *temporal* dispersion of the electrical activity due to unequal conduction rates in the regenerated branches of the axon. (Reproduced by courtesy of Dr. A. T. Richardson)

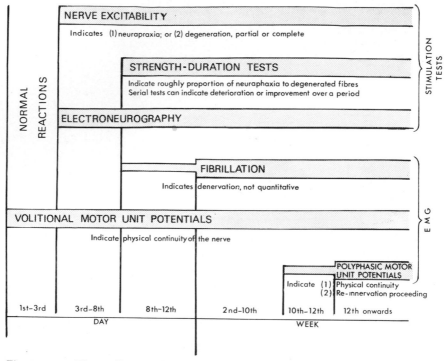

Figure 27.10   Electrodiagnosis in cases of *complete* facial paralysis. The chart indicates the approximate times after onset of paralysis when the various tests may be expected to give helpful information

Figure 27.10 indicates the intervals after onset of paralysis after which the various tests may give useful information.

ANATOMICAL DIAGNOSIS

The level of the lesion in lower motor neurone paralysis can be deduced from:

(1) The causative disease, when this is known, as for instance in cases of neoplasm, destructive middle-ear disease or localized injuries of the nerve.

(2) Tests for lacrimation, hyperacusis (phonophobia), and taste function. These tests will often indicate that the lesion lies above the affected branches of the nerve and below those whose function is intact. Such deductions must be made with care, especially in cases of incomplete facial palsy, and it must be remembered that all of these tests are in reality rather crude.

Lacrimation

In Schirmer's test (*Figure 27.11*) a strip of filter paper 2–3 cm by 5 mm is bent over at one end and hooked over the lower eyelid (any pooling of tears in the eye is first removed to prevent flooding of the test strip). Another test strip is hooked over the lower lid on the unparalysed side. Impaired lacrimation is evident if the wetting of the test strip on the affected side is markedly less than on the other side. Only a gross difference is significant, and if observed should be confirmed in the presence of a strong lacrimatory stimulus (for example, by making the subject sniff the fumes from

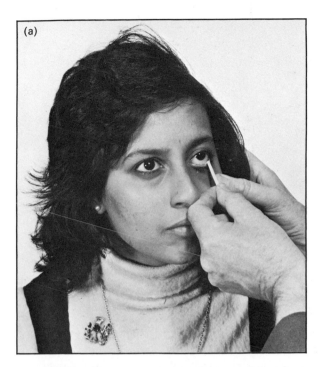

Figure 27.11 Schirmer's test: (a) hooking the folded end of the paper strip over the lower lid. As soon as a strip has been placed in each conjunctiva the eyes are closed throughout the test; (b) prepacked sterile paper strips

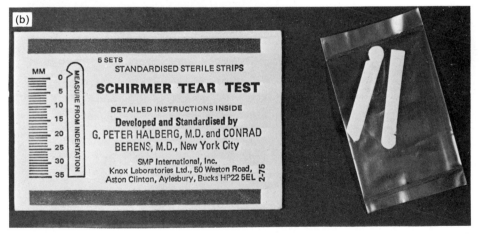

a bottle of ammonia). Definite reduction of lacrimation suggests that the lesion involves the geniculate ganglion (that is, the point of origin of the greater superficial petrosal nerve), or the nervus intermedius.

Hyperacusis or phonophobia
Paralysis of the stapedius muscle results in undue sensitivity to loud sounds which would normally elicit the protective muscle reflex. If present this symptom is a reliable index of stapedius paralysis (provided the patient does not suffer also from inner-ear deafness with recruitment). Even if the symptom of phonophobia is absent, objective testing often reveals stapedius paralysis. Fowler's loudness balance test can be used to show apparent increased loudness at high sound intensities in the affected ear as

compared with the normal one. Changes in the acoustic impedance give a more sensitive index, however, for the intratympanic muscle reflex, and impedance measurements should always be employed for confirmation of stapedius paralysis. The diagnosis of stapedius paralysis is discussed in detail by Jepsen (1955).

Taste

The classic tests may reveal ageusia even in patients who have noticed nothing abnormal in this respect. Unfortunately, many patients fail to distinguish the test substances (for example, salt, sugar, acid) even on the normal side of the anterior two-thirds of the tongue. Quantitative electrogustometry (ELG) determines the minimum direct current in μA required to evoke a metallic or acidic sensation when the anode of an electrical supply is placed on the anterolateral border of the tongue (*Figure 27.12*). The method is described in detail by Krarup (1958) and by Peiris and Miles (1965). When a definite increase of threshold (as compared with the unaffected side) is observed a lesion of the chorda tympani or its more central continuation within the facial nerve may be inferred. Inaccurate results occur with some patients, especially in older people, and in smokers. At present we can only regard tests for taste in facial paralysis as interesting, and sometimes useful. They should never be relied upon heavily.

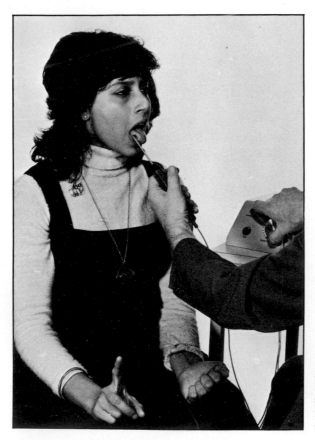

Figure 27.12 A simple technique for electrogustometry. The subject indicates by raising the forefinger that an acidic sensation is perceived

Salivation

Measurement of the submandibular salivary flow by cannulation of the submandibular salivary ducts is a test of parasympathetic function in the facial nerve and chorda tympani which is difficult to perform but is claimed to give a sound prognostic indication by some workers.

Submandibular salivary secretory activity can also be measured by computerized technetium 99^{M} radioactive scanning, before and after salivatory stimulation. Direct correlations with prognosis have not as yet been established.

General management of peripheral facial paralysis

The details of specific treatment for each of the causative diseases are considered elsewhere, but there are many important points in therapy common to all cases.

Reassurance of the patient

The nature of his illness must first be explained. Many patients believe they have had a stroke and are consumed by fear of the future. The likely prognosis must be outlined sympathetically and the patient must be seen frequently throughout the period of incapacity if his morale is to be sustained. If he has pain this must be assessed and adequately suppressed.

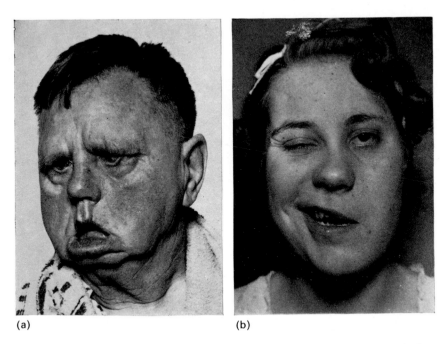

(a)   (b)

Figure 27.13   The deformity of facial paralysis: (a) bilateral complete paralysis due to head injury, causing total loss of facial expression (bilateral tarsorrhaphies were done to protect the eyes); (b) complete left facial paralysis: the patient is trying to smile

Care of the paralysed muscles

Most authorities now agree that electrical stimulation ('galvanism') to the paralysed muscle fibres has no therapeutic value in terms of the eventual quality of recovery.

It has often been recommended that if there is gross sagging of the paralysed side of the face it should be supported by means of adhesive strapping or by a hook in the angle of the mouth attached to an elastic loop around the pinna. Such measures are an additional disfigurement and do no good.

A small plastic hook-shaped support can be cemented to the upper teeth, so that it supports the weight of the paralysed upper lip, at a point a few millimetres medial to the angle of the mouth (*Figure 27.14*). The author favours this method in cases with severe loss of tone, but only when the prognosis indicates that recovery is certain to be long delayed. A widely used alternative is the so-called 'plumping bar', an acrylic bar fixed to the upper teeth or denture. It fills the buccal sulcus and supports the cheek, thus improving appearance, and making mastication easier. It has the disadvantage of somewhat stretching the paralysed muscles which lie over it. None of these dental supports need be considered in the early stages if the nerve remains merely neurapraxic.

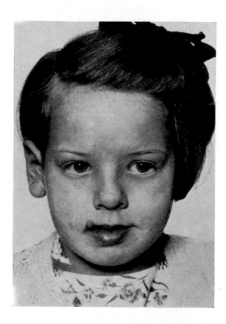

Figure 27.14   Use of a support cemented to the upper teeth to prevent gross sagging and stretching of the paralysed muscles (a case of complete paralysis with total denervation after operation for a large cholesteatoma)

Massage of the muscles probably has no useful effect.

During recovery active exercises before a mirror for a few minutes each day will help the patient to control his face and disguise his disability more successfully. If synkinesis develops, as it usually does after regeneration of nerve fibres, such exercises can teach the patient to avoid its worst effects by refraining from the movements which elicit this defect.

Care of the eye

From the first onset of the paralysis the loss of effective eye closure and reflex blinking render the cornea and conjunctival sac vulnerable to external injury and foreign bodies. Methyl-cellulose eyedrops ('artificial tears') are very helpful if the eye is dry. In the presence of dust, especially if the weather is windy, the patient should cover his eye with his hand. He should report immediately if the eye becomes painful or red. If conjunctivitis occurs and persists, and early recovery of the paralysis cannot be expected, a tarsorrhaphy operation is urgently indicated. In long-standing cases Muhlbauer, Segeth and Viessman (1973) recommend the implantation of permanent magnets in the eyelids. Good tissue tolerance is claimed, and the magnetic strength is carefully adjusted *after* implantation to permit firm closure when required and still allow open vision (by the effort of the levator palpebrae superioris) at will.

TREATMENT OF LONG-TERM SEQUELAE

Permanent paralysis due to gross failure of regeneration of the nerve can be alleviated by plastic surgical treatment. Sagging facial contours can be improved by standard face-lift operations. Assymetry at rest and during movement is reduced by the insertion of slings of fascia lata. These secure the paralysed lips against the disfiguring sideways traction of the muscles of the sound side. Reanimation techniques restore a measure of voluntary (though not emotional) movement. The usual method is to transplant the insertion of the temporal muscle (with its trigeminal motor supply intact) from the mandible to the cheek, where it is joined to fascial slings supporting the corner of the mouth.

Previously denervated muscles (e.g. palmaris longus, or extensor digitorum brevis) may be transplanted into the *normal* side of the face. Here they become innervated, and thus, on contraction, transmit synchronous movement to the paralysed side through their tendons, surgically inserted into the eyelids and mouth sphincter.

Free nerve–muscle transplants have been reported (Thompson, 1976). In these techniques, the transplanted muscle is placed in the paralysed area of the face, and its nerve supply is 'tunnelled' across the midline and anastomosed to a peripheral facial nerve branch on the normal side.

'Cross-face' nerve grafting is also currently under trial. A long nerve graft (from the sural nerve) is used to effect anastomosis between the normal and the paralysed sides. As always, selection of cases is a serious problem, and long-term evaluation of results is hard without comparable control cases.

Faciohypoglossal nerve anastomosis is not nowadays considered an acceptable technique for this type of case although there may rarely be occasions when it should be considered.

None of these surgical measures should be undertaken until all hope of spontaneous facial nerve recovery has been abandoned, and it is clear that there is no hope of direct nerve repair being successful. In practice this means that plastic operations can rarely be justified less than 12–18 months after the onset of paralysis.

Associated movements

Recovery after degenerative facial nerve lesions is invariably marred by the effects of cross re-innervation. Muscles normally capable of independent action appear to receive a common nerve supply. For example, the patient may be unable to close the eye without gross displacement of the angle of the mouth (*Figure 27.15*). Such associated movements may be grotesque, but are often slight, represent no disfigurement, and merely betray to the knowledgeable observer that the nerve at

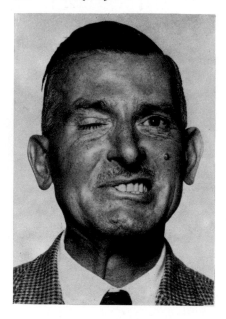

Figure 27.15   Associated movements (synkinesis) after recovery from facial paralysis by regeneration. The right eye closes involuntarily when the patient tries to show his teeth

some time past has regenerated after Wallerian degeneration. Whether slight or severe, the defect is not amenable to any form of treatment.

Contractures

After re-innervation following degenerative lesions it is common to find some degree of fixed contraction in one or more muscle groups. This most usually exaggerates the nasolabial fold. Whether it is due to fibrosis in denervated muscle or a fixed exaggeration of muscle tonus remains undecided. Fortunately, it is in most cases a cosmetic advantage. It confers a degree of symmetry at rest and is only unmasked as a paretic contracture when active movements occur on the sound side. No treatment is required, or indeed possible.

Facial tics and spasms

Spasmodic involuntary movements of the face occasionally follow recovery after denervation, and persist indefinitely. The severity varies from a slight twitching movement of the eyelids to a violent clonic spasm of the entire affected half of the face. The cause is not known and there is no effective treatment

Crocodile tears

Months after recovery of paralysis due to lesions in the geniculate region the distressing condition of excessive lacrimation during meals may appear. This affects the eye on the paralysed side only, is fortunately rather uncommon, and is thought to be due to misdirection of parasympathetic secretory nerve impulses intended for the salivary glands. Golding-Wood (1962) states that the misdirection of impulses is due to sprouting of fibres which establish physiological connection between the tympanic plexus and the greater superficial petrosal nerve. The symptom is abolished by section of the tympanic nerve, which is easily found on the promontory, by way of a simple

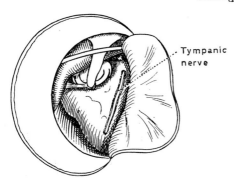

Figure 27.16 Tympanic neurectomy, for the relief of crocodile tearing. The tympanic nerve may be found in a groove on the promontory as shown, or it may be covered by a thin layer of bone

tympanotomy approach (*Figure 27.16*). Without treatment the disability persists indefinitely. Tympanic neurectomy is a minor procedure and should therefore be given a trial, although the present author has had the disappointment of finding that the initial success of the operation is not always maintained. In the event of failure, greater superficial petrosal neurectomy in the floor of the middle cranial fossa may still succeed. It deserves consideration if the patient is sufficiently motivated to jusify such a major intervention.

Direct treatment of the paralysed nerve

The main purpose of any proposed treatment must be clear in the mind of the clinician. He must decide whether his therapy is aimed at: (1) relief of neurapraxia; (2) prevention of degeneration; or (3) promotion of regeneration. He must also decide in the light of his knowledge of the cause and natural history of the paralysis, whether each individual case is likely to do better with or without active surgical intervention. There is no golden rule and often decisions have to be made on the basis of probabilities rather than facts.

Aetiology and management of individual facial paralyses

Aetiology of peripheral facial paralysis

The relative frequency of the numerous causes of facial palsy is hard to discover because of unavoidable 'self-selection' of cases in the series of various authors. The idiopathic group is by far the largest, and to it is attached the name of Sir Charles Bell, who was the first to describe the facial nerve as the nerve of facial expression. The following classification is based on the anatomical site of the causative lesion.

INTRACRANIAL LESIONS
Tumours, multiple sclerosis, poliomyelitis or vascular thrombosis may involve the nerve in the brain stem. In the cerebellopontine angle acoustic neuroma, cysts, primary cholesteatoma or meningitis may cause paralysis.

These conditions are not discussed in this chapter but the otologist must take steps to exclude them before accepting that a case of facial palsy is of intratemporal origin, and a full neurological examination should always be made.

INTRATEMPORAL LESIONS

These include: otitis media, acute or chronic; cholesteatoma; trauma, both surgical and accidental; and tumours.

MISCELLANEOUS DISEASES

Geniculate herpes (Ramsay Hunt syndrome), idiopathic (Bell's) palsy, sarcoidosis, Melkersson's syndrome, polyneuritis, and glandular fever are among the many 'non-surgical' conditions causing facial paralysis.

In this last group the level of the lesion is uncertain, although the great length of the long fallopian canal is considered by many authorities to account for the prevalence of facial neuropathies, compared with other cranial nerve palsies.

Intratemporal lesions

Facial palsy complicating otitis media

Acute inflammation of the middle-ear cavity involves the nerve sheath if there is a dehiscence in the bony canal of the nerve in its tympanic part. Similarly, in acute mastoiditis the sheath becomes involved if an infected air-cell lies directly upon it with no intervening bone.

The paralysis is often of gradual onset, usually partial, and gross nerve fibre degeneration is rare. Nevertheless the condition calls for energetic treatment of the causative infection. Full dosage of antibiotics must be given, preferably parenterally. Early myringotomy is advisable, and cortical mastoidectomy should be done if clinical mastoiditis is present. No attempt need be made to explore the nerve, and early complete recovery follows successful treatment of the otitis.

Chronic middle-ear disease causes facial paralysis if bone destruction by an expanding cholesteatoma involves the fallopian canal. Rarely, proliferation of granulation tissue may, without the presence of cholesteatoma, have the same effect, as for example in neglected cases of aural polypus.

Often the onset of facial paralysis is precipitated by acute infection in an ear already the seat of chronic destructive disease.

The onset of paralysis may be sudden or insidious. At first the cause may be neglected if pain is absent, or if a mistaken diagnosis of idiopathic Bell's palsy is made. A particularly treacherous presentation occurs in the rare retrolabyrinthine (or 'primary') cholesteatoma, in which slow and painless onset of facial paralysis may precede by weeks or months the otological events of deafness, vertigo, discharge, and otoscopic abnormalities. Tomography is essential (*Figure 27.17*).

Without treatment total interruption of nerve continuity is certain to occur. Early treatment may avert degeneration of nerve fibres. Late treatment may facilitate spontaneous regeneration. Too late treatment may still permit successful nerve

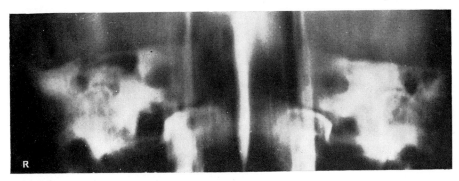

Figure 27.17 Anteroposterior tomograph showing gross retrolabyrinthine bone destruction by cholesteatoma (right ear). Facial paralysis preceded other otological symptoms and signs by a period of six months

grafting, but the results can never be as good as the recovery obtained when the nerve has been preserved by timely operation.

As soon as the cause of the paralysis is recognized the ear must be surgically explored and the appropriate procedure for eradicating the disease and making the ear safe must be completed. The lesion of the nerve is most likely to be in the horizontal (tympanic) portion and cholesteatoma or granulation tissue must be most carefully examined and removed from this region. Nerve sheath exposed by disease is gently defined under the microscope and necrotic bone edges are lifted away from it. If the bony covering is intact here, and there is extensive disease in the mastoid, then the vertical portion of the nerve must be approached and, if necessary, exposed. If any swelling or abnormality of the nerve sheath is found the bony canal should be opened proximally and distally until healthy nerve sheath is exposed in both directions.

In early cases, and especially if pre-operative assessment showed incomplete paralysis or a mere neurapraxia, no more need be done. Whenever possible in the presence of infection it is preferable not to open the nerve sheath because infection is liable to result in intraneural fibrosis with a consequently poor functional result.

In cases of complete paralysis with electrical evidence of gross degeneration it may be necessary to explore the nerve from the stylomastoid foramen to the geniculate ganglion, and to open the sheath freely from below upwards until the entire problem can be exposed and assessed. Unless this is done, the possible need for insertion of a nerve graft may be overlooked. In a neglected case the gross continuity of the nerve may be destroyed, and in a mass of fibrous tissue there is no chance of spontaneous regeneration. The prospects of successful grafting depend finally upon whether the central stump of the nerve can be reached and properly 'freshened' for apposition of the graft. Usually, because of the extent of disease in the middle ear, considerations of preservation of hearing do not hinder the surgeon. The ossicular chain is not worth preserving, and the nerve can be followed as far forward as the genu, or even the internal auditory canal if cochlear function has already been lost.

Surgical decisions whether or not to open the nerve sheath or to excise and graft a segment, or merely to 'decompress' can be difficult. Except in the very early cases, and in cases with partial paralysis it is most unwise to embark upon operation without the most careful electrodiagnostic assessment beforehand. Correlation of the information thus obtained with the appearances found at operation can often resolve the surgeon's dilemma of whether to go on or leave off at a given stage of exploration.

Post-operative facial paralysis

There are many different ways in which the nerve may be injured in operations upon the ear, but such misfortunes are rare today. Micro-surgical precision techniques, the growing tendency towards otological specialization within the specialty of otorhinolaryngology, and present-day awareness of anatomical variations are all contributing to this improvement.

SURGICAL HAZARDS AND THEIR AVOIDANCE

In the infant a standard post-auricular incision may divide the nerve at its exit from the stylomastoid foramen. In opening the antrum one must place the incision at a much higher level in these very young patients. This not only avoids the nerve, but also allows for the fact that the mastoid antrum itself lies above, as well as behind, the external meatus (*Figure 27.18*).

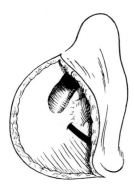

Figure 27.18   The superficial position of the stylomastoid foramen in infancy. An incision as low as that shown would divide the nerve

During a classic cortical mastoidectomy, especially if pneumatization is very extensive, the nerve is in danger in its vertical and pyramidal portions. The only safe rule is to identify the plane of the lateral semicircular canal at the earliest possible stage. If the surgeon then refrains from working at any level more medial than this the nerve will not be endangered. As soon as the compact bone of the digastric ridge is identified the plane of the stylomastoid foramen becomes known. Subsequent gouge or drill work in the known vicinity of the nerve must be along the line of the nerve and not across it, and must be gentle and under clear visibility. In this way if nerve is encountered, it will be uncovered and recognized without being cut or contused.

Apart from the risks of direct injury from bone-cutting instruments, the nerve may also be crushed by detachment and inward displacement of a fragment of the bony wall of the fallopian canal. This injury is more likely to occur during gouging or curetting and it can happen without the surgeon knowing it. The electrically driven burr is a far safer instrument. It removes bone cleanly without any danger of cracking or splitting what lies beneath. If gouges must be used they must be sharp and handled so as to shave away bone rather than crack it. If uncertain of the landmarks, the surgeon must be content to leave a few cells, relying upon drainage and antibiotics, rather than to proceed rashly.

During radical operations the same precautions are necessary and, in addition, special hazards arising in relation to the tympanic part of the nerve must be avoided. During removal of the outer attic wall and bony 'bridge', a bone fragment may be driven across the tympanum against the nerve or, even worse, a gouge may slip off the bone and be driven into the nerve. The risk to the nerve is greater if it is exposed by disease or congenital bony dehiscence. Again, the burr is much safer than the gouge, especially if used under the operating microscope.

When the attic is filled with granulation tissue, or cholesteatoma, the position of the nerve cannot be seen, nor can it be known whether it still has the protection of its bony cover. In this situation, the medial bony wall of the attic must be followed forwards (under the microscope) from the lateral semicircular canal. As the diseased tissue is raised from the bone the horizontal part of the nerve comes into view. This stage is crucial, because if the bony covering has been destroyed the nerve sheath is vulnerable, and it has even been known to be removed, complete with the nerve, in the mass of diseased tissues.

To avoid damage to the nerve in the radical operation, no curettage is permissible in front of the plane of the lateral canal. Bone under the drill must be kept cool by irrigation.

In the final lowering of the posterior meatal wall, sometimes regarded by the novice with apprehension, the risk to the nerve is small. By this time the landmarks are clearly defined. Provided that all bone cutting is parallel to the line of the nerve, a well-sculptured cavity can safely be made.

Treatment of Menière's disease by ultrasound energy applied to the lateral canal has caused a number of facial paralyses, fortunately not permanent. The greatest care is necessary in placement of the instrument, and in preventing over-heating of the tissues.

Permeatal tympanotomy may be complicated by facial palsy in the following ways:

(1) Diffusion of local anaesthetic from the tissues of the external auditory meatus. Such palsies recover completely in an hour or two.
(2) Backward displacement of a wedge of bone during curettage of the posterosuperior meatal wall and tympanic annulus. Such a wedge, if it forms part of the fallopian canal wall, may compress the nerve directly, or indirectly by causing bleeding within the canal.
(3) Above the oval window the nerve is reasonably safe during ordinary procedures on the stapes. 'Drill-out' operations in obliterative otosclerosis or congenital abnormalities of the oval window are specially hazardous, however. Extraordinary care must be taken in cases where the nerve has no bony covering and overhangs the oval window niche.

The removal of bony exostoses of the deep meatal canal has in the past been a cause of paralysis, due to a surgical fracture running backwards and medially from the point of impact of the gouge. This operation is much safer with modern burrs and magnification.

MANAGEMENT OF POST-OPERATIVE FACIAL PARALYSIS

Every patient subjected to an ear operation should be examined immediately after recovery from the anaesthetic, and the presence of normal facial movements should be noted in the case records. This observation is essential proof that the nerve is in continuity. If facial paralysis develops later, and this observation has not been made, erroneous decisions may be taken concerning prognosis and treatment.

Delayed onset of paralysis may be due to pressure of too-tight packing in the ear, or to mild contusion of the nerve. It is implicit that the nerve is exposed, either by the surgeon or by disease, and the surgeon will be aware of this in most cases. Because it is known that the nerve is in gross continuity no active intervention is indicated, other than the prompt removal of the packing from the ear. Paralysis is usually incomplete, with negligible or no degeneration, and recovery occurs in 1–3 weeks. Rarely, delayed paralysis may progress until it is complete. If this progression is rapid it may be due to bleeding in the fallopian canal. In such a case prompt operative decompression of the nerve may prevent degeneration, and will certainly facilitate the regeneration of those fibres which succumb. These cases are rare, and careful judgment must be exercised in deciding whether to operate for this indication.

The surgeon will be guided by his original operative findings, and by his first-hand knowledge of every manoeuvre which was executed in the vicinity of the nerve. In many cases he will be quite sure that no major accident to the nerve has occurred. If his grounds for this conviction are objective, and not based upon wishful thinking he is likely to be right. If he thinks he knows how and where the nerve might have been injured during the operation he would be wise to re-explore and expose the relevant segment. A delayed but progressive paralysis may be due to a fine splinter of bone driven into the nerve, and unless it is removed the eventual outcome may be poor as a result of intraneural fibrosis.

Immediate paralysis, noted as soon as the patient recovers from anaesthesia, indicates that the nerve has been severely injured. If the paralysis is complete, and if electromyography reveals no residual functioning motor units, the nerve may be completely severed. There is no difficulty here in deciding that the nerve must be explored and the sooner the better.

The surgical approach adopted will usually be that used for the first operation—for example, a simple reopening of a radical mastoidectomy. In the case of paralysis after a permeatal tympanotomy however a separate post-auricular approach is probably the best, so that the entire exposure of the nerve may be done through a clean field, and without disturbing the meatus or creating a permanent cavity. The site of the lesion must be examined and if this is not readily apparent, the nerve must be followed from the stylomastoid foramen until the injury is found. Decompression by removal of an impacted bone chip or the release of a haematoma may suffice. If the nerve is cut or torn it should be exposed by incision of the sheath above and below the lesion. The damaged ends are cut squarely across and a nerve graft (from the lateral cutaneous nerve of the thigh or the great auricular nerve) is laid in position (*Figure 27.19*). Location of the graft is easier if the bony canal walls are preserved to form a gutter in which the repair lies snugly. The graft should be a little longer than the gap it is required to bridge, to allow for shrinkage, and it is 'splinted' in the required position by a film of fibrin. The latter is precipitated *in situ* by dropping on to the repair, alternately from separate syringes, drop by drop, a solution of human fibrinogen and a solution of thrombin.

Late cases

Advice is sometimes sought after a lapse of weeks or months in cases of severe or complete paralysis. These have been managed conservatively, in the expectation that recovery will occur. The best time for surgical treatment may have been missed but a heavy responsibility remains, to decide whether operation could still improve the final result. *Until about eight weeks* the preference must be in favour of exploration without further delay. This view is reinforced if paralysis is complete, and was of immediate onset. Electrical evidence of complete denervation likewise argues strongly for active intervention.

After the lapse of two months, however, it is justifiable to postpone a decision for a few more weeks. If reinnervation is going to occur spontaneously, electromyography is likely to give an indication of impending recovery during the third or fourth months. Polyphasic action potentials should be sought at weekly or fortnightly intervals, and if found they will encourage a further period of conservative management. If there is no clinical or electrical evidence of recovery after four months, or if after slight return of movement no further progress is made, the nerve should be explored.

Results

Appropriate action to relieve pressure on a neurapraxic nerve will result in full recovery. If the nerve degenerates re-innervation will be successful provided there is no obstruction such as a displaced bone fragment or dense fibrosis in the nerve. The degree of synkinesis is variable and unpredictable. If the nerve is divided recovery will be negligible unless a successful grafting operation is done. Following a nerve graft, recovery is usually very slow. First signs of returning tonus and voluntary movement may not appear until 4–8 months have elapsed. Continuing improvement may be seen for up to two years, but synkinesis, contractures, clonic spasm, and dissociation of

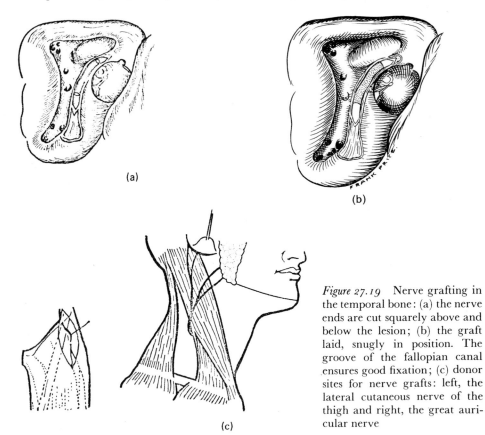

(a)

(b)

(c)

Figure 27.19 Nerve grafting in the temporal bone: (a) the nerve ends are cut squarely above and below the lesion; (b) the graft laid, snugly in position. The groove of the fallopian canal ensures good fixation; (c) donor sites for nerve grafts: left, the lateral cutaneous nerve of the thigh and right, the great auricular nerve

emotional and voluntary movement may all mar the final result to some degree. Nevertheless, as first shown by Ballance and Duel (1932), nerve grafting is far superior in its results to any other technique for injuries with gross loss of continuity. Even in the worst cases, facial symmetry at rest and ability to close the eye are ample rewards for surgical effort. In fact many patients achieve results much better than this.

Facial paralysis due to head injury

PATHOLOGY

Severe head injury causing brain stem damage may result in facial paralysis of central type, but this is rare and most traumatic facial palsies are due to temporal bone fracture. The fracture line may cross the canal for the facial nerve at any point between the internal auditory meatus and the stylomastoid foramen. Bleeding into the canal, and swelling and bruising of the nerve sheath result in paralysis. Often the fracture is comminuted, with many small fragments, one or more of which may be displaced into the fallopian canal. At the moment of fracture the nerve may be sheared across, or 'nipped', by displacement of adjacent segments of bone. The line of the canal for the nerve may be restored if the fragments are re-aligned by the elasticity of the tissues, but permanent obliteration of the canal may result if gross displacement persists. Probably about 90 per cent of such facial palsies are due to injury at or above the geniculate ganglion.

Fractures of the temporal bone are classified (*Figure 27.20*) as longitudinal or transverse with respect to the axis of the petrous. Occasionally both types are seen combined.

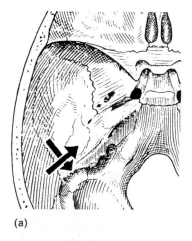

(a)

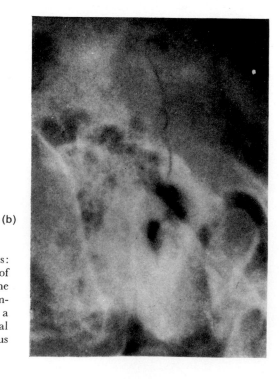

(b)

Figure 27.20 Temporal bone fractures: (a) base of skull, showing the direction of transverse and longitudinal petrous bone fractures; (b) radiograph showing a temporal bone fracture. The patient had a conductive deafness, and a partial facial paralysis of delayed onset. Spontaneous recovery was early and complete

DIAGNOSIS

Apart from the paralysis, other otological signs are usually present.

Conductive deafness is generally due to bleeding into the tympanum, less often to dislocation of the ossicular chain. Until the haemotympanum has resolved, ossicular dislocation is very difficult to diagnose.

A fracture involving the bony meatus usually causes bleeding from the ear and a tear of the tympanic membrane.

Sensorineural deafness is usually due to injury of the labyrinth. In some cases this results from so-called 'concussion' of the labyrinth, but more usually the cause is intralabyrinthine bleeding. The auditory nerve itself may be damaged if the fracture involves the internal auditory meatus. Giddiness and nystagmus are usually present if the inner ear is injured.

X-ray examination can by no means be relied upon to demonstrate the fracture satisfactorily. More often than not the presence of a fracture will be shown, but its full extent and the point at which it involves the facial nerve, are seldom indicated even with polytomography.

Despite the numerous otological symptoms and signs it is all too common for the otologist to be called to the cases only after an interval of days or weeks have passed.

MANAGEMENT

Briggs and Potter (1967) suggested that the incidence of facial paralysis complicating skull fracture may be reduced by administration of ACTH on a prophylactic basis in all cases having bleeding from an ear and radiographic evidence of petrous bone fracture. It has since become a fairly common practice to give high doses of steroids (for example, dexamethasone 4 mg thrice daily) for a few days before 'tapering' the drug when *severe* paralysis complicates a head injury. It is hoped that traumatic oedema of the nerve may be thus reduced—so-called 'medical decompression'.

When paralysis occurs the main principles of management are those given above for post-operative facial palsy. Certain additional problems arise, however.

It is often not known whether the paralysis was of immediate or delayed onset. The situation is obscured if the patient is in coma and several days may elapse before voluntary movement of the face can be examined. In other cases facial palsy may be concealed by gross facial injuries. Whilst the patient is dangerously ill no investigations or treatment of the facial palsy can be considered other than daily nerve excitability testing. This can be done at the bedside, even on the comatose patient, and can give data of great value in the *subsequent* management of the facial nerve.

As soon as the patient can cooperate the otologist will make a full assessment which includes an attempt to fix the level of the lesion.

Cases of partial paralysis, especially if known to be of delayed onset, nearly always recover satisfactorily without active treatment. As Robson and Dawes (1960) emphasized, however, these cases require close observation in the first few days because rapid worsening of the paralysis may be due to progressive bleeding into the fallopian canal. If a case follows this course exploration of the nerve should not be delayed—without operation final recovery will be poor.

Complete paralysis of immediate onset requires operation on the nerve as soon as the patient's general condition permits. The near certainty of gross injury to the nerve justifies this action. The lapse of two or three days after the accident allows time for nerve excitability to disappear, a further indication of a bad prognosis which urges active measures.

If the nerve lesion is considered to be 'high'—that is, in the labyrinthine or geniculate regions, and if there is good cochlear function, then the middle fossa route must be used to expose, decompress or graft the nerve.

If the lesion is tympanic or mastoid in level, or if the inner ear is already destroyed, the transmastoid (post-aural) approach is correct, and allows full access to all levels of the nerve.

RESULTS

The great majority of facial palsies due to head injury do so well that surgical treatment is seldom called for (Potter, 1964). Special vigilance is required to select at the right time those cases requiring operation. The eventual quality of recovery in this small group is good in so far as treatment may prevent fibre degeneration, and less satisfactory in proportion to the extent and severity of loss of nerve substance. The worst results of all are in cases denied (through ill-founded optimism) the benefit of timely decompression or operative restoration of nerve continuity.

Facial paralysis due to tumours within the temporal bone

When facial paralysis complicates carcinoma of the middle ear or glomus tumour (chemodectoma) the cause is usually evident and the desire to conserve the facial nerve cannot be allowed to influence curative treatment. In late cases the nerve will be past saving, while in early cases successful radiotherapy may permit some degree of facial nerve recovery. If total paralysis persists after apparent cure of the growth, consideration can later be given to the insertion of a long graft bypassing the temporal bone according to Dott's technique.

Occasionally facial palsy is caused by temporal bone metastases from malignant disease elsewhere (for example, breast or colon). Diagnosis may be difficult if the primary growth is undiscovered, or if there are no radiographic changes in the affected temporal bone. If there is any suspicion of fluid in the middle ear, it should be aspirated and examined for malignant cells. Any patient with a slowly progressive unexplained facial palsy should have a very thorough general examination to exclude malignant disease as far as possible.

Reports of primary tumours of the nerve itself in its intratemporal course have been reviewed by Kettel (1959b). Several cases of neurofibroma, mostly treated by excision and nerve-grafting, and a few cases of fibrosarcoma, haemangioma, and meningioma (Fisch and Rüttner, 1977; Portmann, 1977; House et al., 1977) have been described. The essential features in such cases are a slowly progressive facial paralysis, in which other symptoms or signs do not appear for weeks or months and with no evidence of malignant disease elsewhere. When the tumour is large enough radiographic evidence of bone erosion appears. If the tumour arises from the tympanic part of the nerve it will, in late cases, cause deafness and abnormal appearances on otoscopy. With these comparative rarities in mind the otologist must be very suspicious about any case of spontaneous facial paralysis which does not conform to the regular pattern of Bell's palsy.

Infratemporal lesions

For practical purposes this group comprises the following.

Maligant disease of the parotid gland

Parotidectomy in cases with an already established facial paralysis must be radical, and the nerve within the gland is removed with no attempt at preservation. Conley (1961), Lathrop (1963) and others stress that immediate repair by nerve grafting should be done. A suitable branching graft is available in the great auricular nerve. The stem of this nerve is sutured to the proximal stump of the divided facial nerve, and its branches are joined one by one to the distal cut subdivisions of the facial (*Figure 27.21*). Excellent results are reported and this technique should always be attempted.

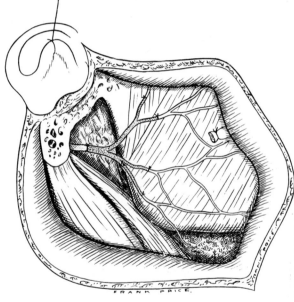

Figure 27.21 Use of a branching graft for nerve repair in the parotid region. If necessary to obtain a healthy central stump the proximal anastomosis may be made in the fallopian canal, after exposure of the vertical segment as in *Figure 27.6*

It is not satisfactory to omit repair of the nerve, and merely to rely upon the re-innervation described by Martin and Helsper (1960) as arising from sprouting motor fibres of the trigeminal nerve. Kettel (1961) denies that this happens, and the weight of the evidence favours his view.

Accidental injury

This should usually be avoidable in parotidectomy operations if no paralysis is present beforehand. Should it occur immediate nerve repair is indicated.

Accidental injury due to facial lacerations (for example, razor fights and windscreen injuries) calls for immediate nerve repair if the trunk or major subdivisions are involved. If repair of the facial nerve or any of its branches is necessary, but for any reason not practicable at the time of initial operation, the cut ends of the nerve should be marked with coloured non-absorbable sutures, or silver clips to facilitate elective nerve grafting at a later date. Near the periphery, in front of the anterior border of the parotid gland, the ramifications of the nerve are very small and also very numerous. Here direct repair is often not practicable and fortunately the denervated area is usually rather small. Spontaneous re-innervation is adequate, in most cases.

In the newborn, partial facial paralysis due to the pressure of obstetrical forceps over the stylomastoid foramen is transitory and requires no active treatment.

Miscellaneous causes of facial paralysis

Agenesis

Agenesis of the facial nerve is extremely rare. From birth there is a facial palsy, partial or complete. No change occurs in the condition over the years, and treatment can only be by plastic surgery if the paralysis is sufficiently severe to justify it. In the neonate it may be difficult to distinguish this condition from birth injury.

Melkersson's syndrome

Melkersson's syndrome, well known in Scandinavia, receives little attention in the English literature. The features are recurring attacks of facial palsy and swelling of the lips. In many cases there is a congenital furrowing of the tongue. The cause is unknown. The paralysis recovers in most cases and in this respect the disease follows a course very like that of Bell's palsy.

Sarcoidosis

Sarcoidosis, among its many otolaryngological manifestations, may cause facial paralysis. This may be in association with the well-known uveoparotid fever (*Figure 27.22*), but more often it is unilateral and without parotid swelling. According to Colover (1948) about 50 per cent of a series of 115 cases of sarcoidosis had facial nerve involvement. The neuropathy is said to be due to involvement of the leptomeninges in sarcoid deposits. In 15 cases seen personally by the author most patients had previously had other symptoms of sarcoidosis (uveitis, cough, pains in the limbs, skin lesions, and so on), so that the significance of the paralysis could usually be correctly assessed when a full history was taken. The course and quality of recovery are indistinguishable from Bell's palsy. Recurrences, however, on the same or the opposite side, are not uncommon. Treatment is symptomatic. Although steroid therapy may be desirable for the general disease, the author has known facial paralysis to occur in a patient already receiving large doses of these drugs for sarcoidosis.

Infective neuritis

Like any other peripheral nerve the facial may take part in an infective polyneuritis. Involvement of other nerves, paraesthesiae, polymyalgia, systemic upset and malaise,

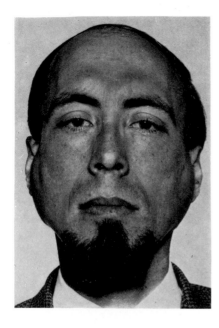

Figure 27.22   Heerfordt's syndrome. Bilateral parotid enlargement in a patient with uveitis and transient facial paralysis due to sarcoidosis

and changes in the cerebrospinal fluid will point towards the diagnosis. Complete absence of any peripheral sensory disturbances in such cases will arouse suspicion of poliomyelitis. Glandular fever and mumps are further examples of virus infections causing facial paralysis.

Facial paralysis due to herpes oticus

PATHOLOGY

There is ample evidence that this condition is due to the herpes zoster–chicken-pox virus. It is classified by tradition among the intratemporal causes of facial palsy because of its frequent association with an auditory nerve lesion, and because of its long-established alternative name, geniculate herpes (Ramsay Hunt). The published histological studies show that the entire length of the facial nerve is involved in an intense lymphocytic inflammatory process. The geniculate ganglion bears no special brunt of the disease, though Fisch (Fisch and Esslen, 1972), exploring these cases by the middle fossa route has confirmed that the labyrinthine and genicular parts are dramatically inflamed and swollen.

CLINICAL FEATURES

The patient feels unwell and often headache with pain in or around the ear will be noticed for a few days before the appearance of facial paralysis and vesication. The nerve is usually tender to palpation below and in front of the ear. Herpetic vesicles may erupt in the external auditory meatus or in the hollow of the concha (*Figure 27.23, see also Plate 1d, facing p. 108*), sometimes giving rise to a bloodstained ear discharge. In many cases vesication lies in the distribution of the second or third cervical nerves as well as, or in place of, the classic situation of the ear. Less commonly,

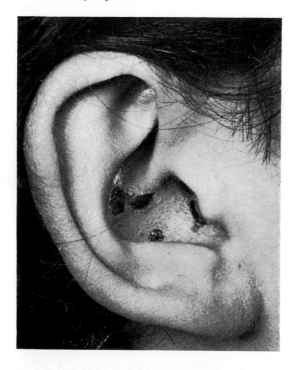

Figure 27.23   Vesication in herpes oticus

vesicles may appear only in the trigeminal nerve area (face, mouth or palate) or in the distribution of the glossopharyngeal or vagus nerves.

Usually the pain is greatest in the affected area, but cases occur in which pain is only slight, and the vesication very transitory, healing in a day or two and leaving no trace. The diagnosis may be missed, therefore, unless a thorough daily search is made in the ear, mouth and throat. It must be remembered that the onset of paralysis and vesication may be separated by a week or more, and either may precede the other.

DIAGNOSIS

Diagnosis is made easier if cochlear or vestibular signs, or both, appear, giving the classic Ramsay Hunt syndrome (Hunt, 1910). Involvement of other cranial nerves (fifth, sixth, ninth, tenth, eleventh and twelfth) may occur, although not commonly. The patient looks and feels ill, and in the more severe cases fever may be marked. The erythrocyte sedimentation rate is usually raised, and there is a lymphocytosis. A rising titre of herpes zoster antibodies is found, although unfortunately this investigation takes too long to be of more than retrospective value.

COURSE OF THE PARALYSIS

Although seldom complete at the first onset, the paralysis usually increases in severity over a period of a few days, and may become total on the affected side. In a few cases deterioration proceeds in 'steps', spread out over two or three weeks. Pure neurapraxia is rare, and most patients show clear evidence of fibre degeneration on electrical testing. The eventual quality of recovery depends upon the proportion of the total fibres which degenerate. Complete permanent paralysis is very rare and the patient can be re-assured that a degree of recovery will eventually be achieved. Clinical improvement may still continue for up to a year or longer after the initial illness.

TREATMENT

Treatment is 'symptomatic', and must include the relief of pain, re-assurance, and the general measures described at the beginning of this chapter. Certainly there are no grounds to justify surgical decompression of the nerve. Such a step would be logical only if the entire course in the temporal bone were uncovered, if there were definite evidence that the paralysis were due to compression, and if the eventual quality of recovery were known to be improved by the relief of that compression. Steroid therapy (for example, prednisone 60 mg/day), once thought to be hazardous, is now considered justifiable in the hope of reducing post-herpetic neuralgia and of protecting the hearing. It is of course necessary to begin this treatment within a day or two of the onset of paralysis.

Idiopathic facial paralysis (Bell's palsy)

There are many theories regarding the aetiology of this condition, but none will bear close examination at the present time. Quite possibly a proportion of cases should be classified as due to the herpes virus (Tomita, 1977). Transitory vesication is easily missed by patient and doctor. A further group possibly belongs to the autoimmune diseases, of which sarcoidosis may be an example. There may be viruses other than herpes, and other autoimmune diseases, which in the years to come will permit us to diagnose and classify Bell's palsies, and the idiopathic group will become smaller and smaller.

PATHOLOGY

For obvious reasons we have little useful information about the histological appearances of the nerve in Bell's palsy. Fragmentary data are available from operative and post-mortem material (Jongkees, 1954; Reddy and Balshi, 1966; Proctor, Corgill and Proud, 1975; Blatt and Freeman, 1969; Fowler, 1963). The appearances are those of classic Wallerian degeneration in the nerve trunk and chorda tympani. Vascular engorgement has been noted, but no changes indicative of inflammation, either in the nerve or its sheath. In late cases fibrotic change is described in the perineural tissues of the region of the stylomastoid foramen. Many experienced facial nerve surgeons have described the macroscopic appearances found at decompression operations. In the vertical (mastoid) segment the nerve sheath is hyperaemic and when it is incised the nerve itself bulges laterally out of the sheath, until it has swollen to two or three times its normal diameter. The appearance suggests an oedema of the nerve which usually extends from the stylomastoid foramen up to about the level of the pyramidal segment, but seldom higher. Purple-coloured streaks, possibly due to haemorrhage, have sometimes been noticed on the nerve trunk.

Surgeons performing 'whole-nerve' decompressions have reported variously upon the level of swelling of the nerve. Fisch (1977) for example finds that in the majority of cases it is at or *above* the labyrinthine segment. Pulec (1974), on the other hand, finds the swelling is mainly in the mastoid segment, and only infrequently extends as high as the tympanic part.

Many authors have believed that this swelling of the nerve is caused by ischaemia. It is suggested that intense vasospasm causes tissue damage within the fallopian canal (primary ischaemia). The resulting swelling of the soft tissues within this narrow space with rigid walls causes a secondary ischaemia which intensifies and prolongs the neural dysfunction. The experimental work of Blunt (1962) is of great interest in this connection. It must be said, however, that these theories appear to be losing favour, and increasingly there is support for proposed virus and immunological theories of pathogenesis.

The theory of vasospasm however has encouraged those who maintain that exposure to cold plays a part in the causation of Bell's palsy (paralysis a frigore). It also provides a basis for treatment by vasodilator methods.

Kettel (1959) has described bone necrosis in the mastoid in some cases of Bell's palsy. The significance of this is uncertain and it is more usual to find the bone and the surrounding air-cells quite normal.

CLINICAL FEATURES

Paralysis often begins without warning. It may first be noticed by a friend or relative of the patient, but within a few hours it becomes severe enough to alarm the sufferer. In many cases paralysis develops during the night and is first noticed next morning during shaving. Sometimes there is pain behind the ear for a few hours before the paralysis. The severity and duration of pain is extremely variable from case to case and many patients have none at all. The paretic disability is, in some cases, most conspicuous as a dysarthria and the writer has had cases in which the paralysis of the face had at first been overlooked, while pharyngeal signs of bulbar palsy were sought in vain. Another fairly common error arises from the fact that loss of facial muscle tone may give a false impression of swelling of the cheek. If there is also pain in the face these patients may be referred to the dentist on suspicion of a dental abscess. More than a few of the writer's own cases have been referred on by dental colleagues. These minor, and mainly unimportant, diagnostic errors are made in the first few hours of the illness. By the time the patient reaches an otologist a few hours later the paralysis has increased and diagnosis is easy.

Watering of the eye is due to impaired drainage of normal tears, while the loss of the blink reflex leaves on the cornea a puddle of tears which intermittently blurs vision by altering the focal length of the refracting system.

Loss of taste, or in some cases the feeling of a metallic taste in the mouth, is a variable symptom, but if spontaneously volunteered by the patient is a reliable sign of involvement of the chorda tympani. Often it is noticed some hours before the facial paralysis begins.

Phonophobia indicating stapedius paralysis is common.

In addition to the facial nerve involvement, nystagmus, trigeminal sensory impairment, and minor (subclinical) *contralateral* facial nerve disorders have been reported.

COURSE AND PROGNOSIS OF THE PARALYSIS

In the vast majority of cases the pattern of nerve injury is laid down within the first few days; by this is meant that paralysis remaining incomplete up to the end of the first week is unlikely to get worse. A nerve that is mainly neurapraxic after the first three days (the earliest time at which degeneration can be predicted) is not likely to go on to severe degeneration later. It is true that late progression (in the second or third week) is occasionally seen but in so-called idiopathic facial palsy it is unusual.

Patients having merely neurapraxia (some 75 per cent of all cases), whether paralysis is partial or complete, are likely to make a full recovery within 2–3 weeks (group A).

A much smaller group (about 10 per cent) have a mixed lesion (neurapraxia in some fibres, degeneration in others). Again, the paralysis may be partial or complete. These cases recover slowly—first by 'unblocking' of neurapraxic fibres and later (ten weeks onward) by regeneration. The stigmata of recovery by regeneration are usually detectable, although often so slight that only a very experienced clinician can detect them. Most, if not all, of these patients are satisfied with the end result, although it is less than perfect (group B).

The last group (some 10–15 per cent) have complete or virtually complete paralysis, with all or nearly all fibres destined to degenerate. The final standard of recovery in this group is often very poor (group C).

There have been striking variations in the many published series giving the prognosis of untreated Bell's palsy, and the percentage figures given above for groups A, B and C are offered only as a representative summary. Tavener, Kemble and Cohen (1967), Campbell (1963), Groves (1968) and Pietersen and Andersen (1966) reported figures as shown in *Table 27.1*.

Table 27.1   Incidence of denervation in hospital series of Bell's palsy

Author	*Groups B and C* (Denervation percentage)
Groves	22
Pietersen and Andersen	19
Taverner	40
Campbell (complete paralysis in all cases)	40

It was pointed out by Groves and by Campbell that the outcome in a series of Bell's palsies is heavily dependent upon the reasons (e.g. severity and duration of paralysis, availability of treatment, etc.) for referral to hospital. Since these reasons tend to determine whether, and how early or late, cases are referred it is not permissible to compare different hospital series with each other, as *Table 27.2* shows.

Table 27.2   Incidence of denervation in relation to time of first referral to hospital

Time first seen	*No. of cases*	*Percentage incidence of denervation, however slight*
Campbell (all cases of *complete* paralysis)		
Within 5 days	39	13
,, 7 ,,	51	20
,, 14 ,,	93	29
,, 21 ,,	113	33
,, 28 ,,	128	40
Groves (consecutive cases, *partial* and *complete*)		
Within 5 days	54	11
,, 14 ,,	97	22

Tavener (1968) stated that of 110 cases seen within five days of onset denervation, however slight, was observable in 47 (group A, 57 per cent; groups B and C, 43 per cent). This brief discussion shows that because hospital series are influenced by selection outside the control of the observer, the true prognosis of this condition still remains unknown. Clinical trials can only achieve statistical validity, therefore, if comparable concurrent control cases, either untreated or differently treated, are compared with the treated group.

TREATMENT

It is clear that patients who fall into groups A and B do not require active treatment and that it would be wrong for these patients to receive any form of treatment which could conceivably cause harm, either to the nerve or to the individual. In group C reasonable therapeutic hazards could be accepted provided that the treatment is of proven value, and that it can be given in time to be effective.

Unfortunately, none of these criteria can be satisfied. Let us consider first the efficacy of the many different forms of treatment, bearing in mind that the primary object is to prevent degeneration of fibres.

Vasodilator therapy

Nicotinic acid by mouth is harmless and could be given to all groups. There is no statistical evidence that it does good. Intravenous histamine or procaine has been widely recommended, without the support of controlled scientific trial. These two drugs have pharmacological hazards, which though these may be small, make it difficult to justify their use in groups A and B at the present time.

Stellate or cervical sympathetic block with local anaesthetic has been urged by Swan (1952) and by Korkis (1961). Although it appears to be a comparatively safe procedure, serious accidents can occur regardless of the skill of the operator, while its efficacy has not been convincingly proved by its advocates. Fearnley and his colleagues (1964) reported a controlled study showing that this treatment is without benefit.

Surgical decompression of the nerve

For more than 40 years controversy has waxed and waned regarding the benefits of decompression of the vertical part of the nerve for Bell's palsy. All are agreed that such treatment could be worthwhile only in the small group of cases who would otherwise do badly. Down the years the recommended time of operation has been advanced from three months to three weeks, or even earlier, with indications based upon various combinations of clinical and electrodiagnostic data. In any event, if operation is deferred until three weeks or more have passed its only hope of creating a favourable effect lies in improving conditions for regeneration. This is a secondary objective, because the primary aim should be to prevent degeneration. Unfortunately the complexity of the problem has so far defeated sincere efforts to prove scientifically whether decompression may be beneficial and, if so, in what particular circumstances. It is impossible to accept as proof of benefit the mere fact of recovery after operation. The information required is a comparison of treated and untreated cases, identical in all other respects, and strictly comparable with regard to the pre-operative functional and electrical state of the nerve.

Properly controlled ethical trial of decompression has been reported by Mechelse *et al.* (1971), and by May and Hawkins (1972) and both teams concluded that the conventional operation done promptly on the basis of lost nerve excitability showed no benefit. Adour and Swanson (1971) reached the same conclusion. Alford, Sessions and Weber (1971) observed better results in cases decompressed, but nonetheless they emphasized that legitimate problems of selection remained unsolved. Later efforts are exemplarized by May and Hawkins who performed decompressions, with apparent benefit, *before* the loss of nerve excitability. Selection was based upon impaired salivary flow. Fisch (1977), Fisch and Esslen (1972), Pulec (1974) and others practise total exposure of the nerve from the internal meatus to the stylomastoid foramen, but as yet there appears to be no proof that this major intervention improves the statistical prognosis. The observation by Fisch of swelling and conduction block of the suprageniculate part of the nerve is of enormous interest but we are discussing treatment, and to observe, even to 'decompress', is not necessarily to cure.

A few authors have mentioned mishaps in facial nerve decompressions, quite apart from the obvious possibility that the nerve itself could be damaged. The present writer has knowledge of a 'dead ear' due to injury of the horizontal canal. Multanen and Holopainen (1963) and others experienced accidental injuries to the ossicular chain. Olson *et al.* (1973) refer to cochlear and vestibular sequelae in some cases. The natural hazards of surgery, and, in 'total nerve exposures', of craniotomy, must further be measured against the overall good prognosis of Bell's palsy. Even the advocates of decompression do not often operate. In a recent discussion Jongkees (1973) stated that he decompressed fewer cases than McGovern, who operated in 'probably less than 5 per cent' of his cases.

Steroid therapy

It has been widely assumed that steroid therapy is appropriate in Bell's palsy, and for some years cortisone derivatives have been given, usually in small dosage, without satisfactory evidence in favour. For a period of 20 years Taverner and his colleagues sought to establish scientifically in controlled trials the efficacy or otherwise of steroid therapy. A trial by Taverner (1954) in which early cases treated with cortisone by mouth were compared with untreated randomly selected control cases showed no difference in the incidence of denervation in the two groups. He and his associates then went on to investigate the effect of ACTH gel injections (Taverner *et al.*, 1966; Taverner, Kemble and Cohen, 1967), first in a controlled sequential-analysis trial which failed to reach statistical significance, and then in a large series (383 cases) in which the final incidence of denervation was 13 per cent. Concurrent controls were not used, however, and the author compared his results with earlier series of untreated cases, unfortunately not similarly selected. The present author's view is that the value of ACTH was not satisfactorily proved.

More recently Taverner and his associates (1971) compared the effects of intramuscular corticotrophin with oral prednisolone in 186 successive cases of Bell's palsy who were allocated at random to one or the other therapy. They concluded from a comparison of the results that oral prednisolone is the treatment of choice. The dose was 80 mg daily in divided doses for five days, followed by a diminishing dose for a further four days. They further concluded that the trial of oral cortisone in 1954 had been inadequate because of low dosage, starting treatment too late, and small numbers of patients. In this latest work the authors scrupulously matched the comparability of the clinical material in the two groups of cases and their conclusion that prednisolone gave better results than ACTH appears statistically unassailable. Doubts remain, however. Hamberger (1977) recommends no treatment in *any* case of Bell's palsy, holding the view that there is no known effective treatment. Adour *et al.* (1972) reported benefit from steroids in a controlled trial, whereas May *et al.* (1976) found no statistically beneficial effect.

SELECTION OF CASES FOR TREATMENT

Given that high-dose steroid therapy, commenced preferably within the first two days of the disease, might be beneficial, there are decisions which must still be matters of clinical judgment. One may elect to treat all cases, discounting the possibility of side effects, or one may consider for treatment only cases with a presumed bad prognosis. Whereas the benefit of steroids was demonstrated by Taverner when commenced in the first four days, it will often be necessary to consider starting treatment in cases presenting later. It is not known whether or not steroids could help if begun in the second or third week. Another problem remains, that of recognizing and evaluating contraindications. Very early pregnancy is the most difficult and potentially most serious, but tuberculosis, diabetes, hypertension, psychosis, epilepsy, cardiac conditions, concomitant infections, and peptic ulcer all require exclusion.

Total paralysis (with stapedius paralysis) is not in itself indicative of a poor end-result. If it is associated with *severe pain*, and/or a grossly raised ELG (electrogustometric) threshold (100 μA or more) the prognosis without treatment is probably poor (Groves, 1973). Marked impairment of lacrimation is probably also a bad sign.

In the present state of knowledge it must be admitted that only general and non-specific therapy should be advised, especially since most cases still only reach the otologist after several days. It must be appreciated that any new forms of treatment can be satisfactorily tested only if they are applied at the beginning, before the nerve injury pattern has become fixed. The need of the future is that cases should automatically be seen by the otologist on the day of onset of paralysis.

Facial hemispasm—clonic spasm

This condition is distinct from the involuntary twitching and spasm sometimes seen as a sequel of a facial paralysis. It is fortunately rare, occurs chiefly in older patients, and is characterized by violent hemifacial muscular contractions without actual paralysis. These occur almost incessantly and are not due to any demonstrable cause. In severe cases the disease is almost unbearable, but none of the methods of treatment which have been tried have proved effective, short of complete section of the facial nerve. In the very worst cases patients may prefer complete facial palsy to the original complaint, but no surgeon could contemplate this drastic treatment as a suitable permanent solution. The problem remains unsolved, but in the most severe cases consideration should be given to selective nerve section of the worst affected peripheral branches. Facial nerve–trunk section with faciohypoglossal anastomosis has been practised, but would scarcely seem justifiable.

References

Adour, K. K., Millesi, A., Tato, J. M., Yanagihara, N., May, M., Jongkees, L. B. W. and Stennert, E. (1977). In *Facial Nerve Surgery*, Ed. by Fisch, U. Amstelveen, The Netherlands; Kugler Medical Publications

Adour, K. K. and Swanson, P. J. (1971). 'Facial paralysis in 403 consecutive patients', *Transactions of the American Academy of Ophthalmology and Otolaryngology*, **75**, 1284, 1301

Adour, K. K., Wingerd, L., Bell, D. N., Manning, J. J. and Hurley, J. P. (1972). 'Prednisone treatment for Idiopathic Facial Paralysis (Bell's Palsy)', *New England Journal of Medicine*, **287**, 1268

Alford, B. R., Sessions, R. B. and Weber, S. C. (1971). 'Indications for surgical decompression of the facial nerve', *The Laryngoscope*, **81**, 620

Ballance, C. A. and Duel, A. B. (1932). *Archives of Otolaryngology*, **15**, 1

Blatt, I. M. and Freeman, J. A. (1969). 'Bell's Palsy, III: Further observations on the pathogenesis of Bell's Palsy and the results of chorda tympani neurectomy', *Transactions of the American Academy of Ophthalmology and Otolaryngology*, **73**, 420

Blunt, M. J. (1954). *Journal of Anatomy*, **88**, 520

Blunt, M. J. (1962). *Medical Journal of Australia*, **1**, 74

Briggs, M. and Potter, J. M. (1967). *British Medical Journal*, **2**, 465

Campbell, E. D. R. (1963). *Journal of Laryngology*, **77**, 462

Cawthorne, T. (1963). *Archives of Otolaryngology*, **78**, 429

Collier, J. (1963). *Archives of Otolaryngology*, **78**, 421

Colover, J. (1948). 'Sarcoidosis with involvement of the nervous system', *Brain*, **71**, 451

Conley, J. J. (1961). *Archives of Otolaryngology*, **73**, 322

Dott, N. M. (1963). *Archives of Otolaryngology*, **78**, 426

Esslen, E. (1977). 'Electromyography and Electroneurography'. In *Facial Nerve Surgery*. Ed. by Fisch, U. Amstelveen, The Netherlands; Kugler Medical Publications

Fearnley, M. E., Rainer, E. H., Taverner, D., Boyle, T. M. and Miles, D. W. (1964). *Lancet*, **2**, 725

Fisch, U. (1969). In *Disorders of the Skull Base Region*. Ed. by Hamberger, C. and Wersäll, J. Stockholm; Almqvist and Wiksell

Fisch, U (1977). Personal communication

Fisch, U. (1977). Panel Discussion. In *Facial Nerve Surgery*, p. 393. Ed. by Fisch, U. Amstelveen, The Netherlands; Kugler Medical Publications

Fisch, U. and Esslen, E. (1972). 'Total Intratemporal Exposure of the Facial Nerve', *Archives of Otolaryngology*, **95**, 335

Fisch, U. and Ruttner, J. (1977). 'Pathology of intracranial tumours involving the facial nerve'. In *Facial Nerve Surgery*. Ed. by Fisch, U.

Amstelveen, The Netherlands; Kugler Medical Publications

Fowler, E. P. (1963). 'The Pathologic findings in a case of Facial Paralysis', *Transactions of the American Academy of Ophthalmology and Otolaryngology*, **67**, 187

Gilliatt, R. W. and Taylor, J. C. (1959). *Proceedings of the Royal Society of Medicine*, **52**, 1080

Golding-Wood, P. H. (1962). *Journal of Laryngology*, **76**, 683

Groves, J. (1968). *British Medical Journal*, **1**, 508

Groves, J. (1973). 'Facial Palsies: Selection of cases for treatment', *Proceedings of The Royal Society of Medicine*, **66**, 545

Hamberger, C. A. (1977). Incidence and management of Bell's palsy according to geographic distribution'. In *Facial Nerve Surgery*. Ed. by Fisch, U. Amstelveen, The Netherlands; Kugler Medical Publications

House, W. F. (1963). 'Surgery of the petrous portion of the VIIIth nerve; *Annals of Otology, Rhinology and Laryngology*, **72**, 802

House, W. F., Pulec, J., Fisch, U., Castro, D., Portmann, M. and Cerny, L. (1977). Panel Discussion 'Management of Intratemporal tumours'. In *Facial Nerve Surgery*. Ed. by Fisch, U. Amstelveen, The Netherlands; Kugler Medical Publications

Hunt, J. R. (1910). *Archives of internal Medicine*, **5**, 631

Jepsen, O. (1955). (Thesis) University of Aarhus; Denmark

Jongkees, L. B. W. (1954). *Acta otolaryngologica, Stockholm*, **44**, 336

Jongkees, L. B. W. (1973). 'Practical Application of Clinical Tests for Facial Paralysis', *Archives of Otolaryngology*, **97**, 220

Kettel, K. (1959a). *Peripheral Facial Palsy*. Copenhagen; Munksgaard

Kettel, K. (1959b). *Archives of Otolaryngology*, **69**, 276

Kettel, K. (1961). *Archives of Otolaryngology*, **74**, 134

Korkis, B. (1961). *Lancet*, **1**, 255

Krarup, B. (1958). *Acta otolaryngologica, Stockholm*, **49**, 389

Lathrop, F. D. (1963). *Annals of Otology*, **72**, 780

Laumans, E. P. J. and Jongkees, L. B. W. (1963). *Annals of Otology*, **72**, 307

Martin, H. and Helsper, J. T. (1960). *Annals of Surgery*, **151**, 538

May, M. (1977). 'Anatomy of cross-section of facial nerve in the temporal bone: Clinical application'. In *Facial Nerve Surgery*. Ed. by Fisch, U. Amstelveen, The Netherlands; Kugler Medical Publications

May, M. and Hawkins, C. D. (1972). 'Bell's Palsy: results of surgery: salivation test versus nerve excitability test as a basis of treatment', *The Laryngoscope*, **82**, 1337

May, M., Welte, R., Hardin, W. B. and Sullivan, J. (1976). 'The use of steroids in Bell's palsy. A prospective controlled study', *Laryngoscope,* **86,** 1111

Mechelse, K., Goor, G., Huizing, E. H., Hammelburg, E., Van Bolhuis, A. H., Staal, A. and Verjaal, A. (1971). 'Bell's Palsy: Prognostic criteria and evaluation of surgical decompression', *Lancet,* **2,** 57

Multanen, I. and Holopainen, E. (1963). 'Operative results in Bell's Palsy', *Acta Otolaryngologica,* Suppl. **188,** 402

Muhlbauer, W. D., Segeth, H. and Viessman, A. (1973). 'Restoration of lid function in facial palsy with permanent magnets', *Chirurgia Plastica (Berlin),* **1,** 295

Olson, N. R., Goin, D. W., Nichols, R. D. and Makim, B. (1973). 'Adverse effects of facial nerve decompression for Bell's Palsy', *Transactions of the American Academy of Ophthalmology and Otolaryngology,* **77,** 67

Peiris, O. A. and Miles, D. W. (1965). *British Medical Journal,* **2,** 1162

Pietersen, E. and Andersen, P. (1966). *Acta orolaryngologica, Stockholm,* Suppl. **224,** 296

Portmann, M (1977). 'Clinical features and diagnosis of facial nerve paralysis caused by intratemporal tumours'. In *Facial Nerve Surgery.* Ed. by Fisch, U. Amstelveen, The Netherlands; Kugler Medical Publications

Potter, J. M. (1964). *Journal of Laryngology,* **78,** 654

Proctor, B., Corgill, D. A. and Proud, G. (1975). 'The pathology of Bell's Palsy'. *Transactions of the Academy of Ophthalmology and Otology,* **82,** 70

Pulec, J. L. (1974). 'Bell's palsy, diagnosis, management and results of treatment', *Laryngoscope,* **84,** 2119

Reddy, J. B. and Balshi, J. F. (1966). *Eye Ear Nose Throat Monthly,* **45,** 62

Richardson, A. T. (1962). *Proceedings of the Royal Society of Medicine,* **55,** 897

Richardson, A. T. (1963). *Annals of Otology,* **72,** 569

Richardson, A. T. and Wynn Parry, C. B. (1957). *Annals of physical Medicine,* **4,** 3, 41

Robson, F. C. and Dawes, J. D. K. (1960). *Journal of Laryngology,* **74,** 275

Swan, D. M. (1952). *Journal of the American Medical Association,* **150,** 32

Sullivan, J. A. (1963). *Archives of Otolaryngology,* **78,** 344

Taverner, D. (1954). *Lancet,* **2,** 1052

Taverner, D. (1955). *Brain,* **78,** 209

Taverner, D. (1968). *British Medical Journal,* **1,** 828

Taverner, D., Cohen, S. B. and Hutchinson, B. C. (1971). 'Comparison of corticotrophin and prednisone in treatment of idiopathic facial paralysis (Bell's palsy)', *British Medical Journal,* **4,** 20

Taverner, D., Kemble, F. and Cohen, S. B. (1967). *British Medical Journal,* **2,** 581

Taverner, D., Fearnley, M. E., Kemble, F., Miles, D. W. and Peiris, O. A. (1966). *British Medical Journal,* **1,** 391

Thompson, N. (1976). 'The use of neuromuscular free autografts with microneural anastomosis to restore elevation of the mouth in cases of unilateral facial paralysis', *Chirurgica Plastica,* **3,** 165

Tomita, H. (1977). In *Facial Nerve Surgery.* Ed. by U. Fisch. Amsterdam; Kugler Medical publications

White, A. and Verma, P. L. (1973). 'Spatial arrangement of facial nerve fibres', *Journal of Laryngology,* **87,** 952

28 Hearing aids
M C Martin

The electronic aid has now been with us for some 50 or more years, but probably because of the simplicity of the concept and the device itself, i.e. hearing aids amplify sound, it has not assumed the importance in the wide range of knowledge available in otology and audiology that it deserves.

Figure 28.1a shows a block diagram of the functional parts of a basic hearing aid which represents the majority of hearing aids that are constructed today. *Figure 28.1b* illustrates the three types of aid currently available, i.e. post-aural, spectacle and in-the-ear aids.

The manner in which the overall performance of an aid is achieved can be observed by taking the performance of each functional part and combining them together, i.e.

microphone performance + amplifier performance
   + earphone performance = overall performance

Hearing aid microphones

Hearing aid microphones are normally built into the case of the aid with amplifier and battery. There are, however, considerable advantages to be gained in reducing the effect of distance between the speaker and the listener by having the microphone on a long lead and plugging it into the aid. This facility is not widely available at the present time.

Microphones used in current aids can be divided into three main types:

(1) Electromagnetic.
(2) Crystal or ceramic.
(3) Electret.

All of these types are made in the very small size needed to fit into present-day aids. *Figure 28.2* shows typical microphone frequency response while *Figure 28.3* indicates the overall size. The electromagnetic microphone has the most limited frequency response, particularly at low frequencies. The crystal microphone was used in most early valve aids and has a good low frequency response but a rather irregular high

(a)

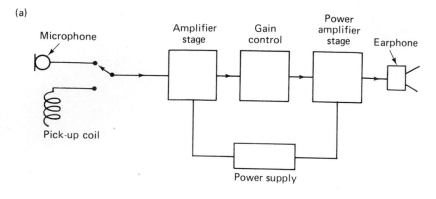

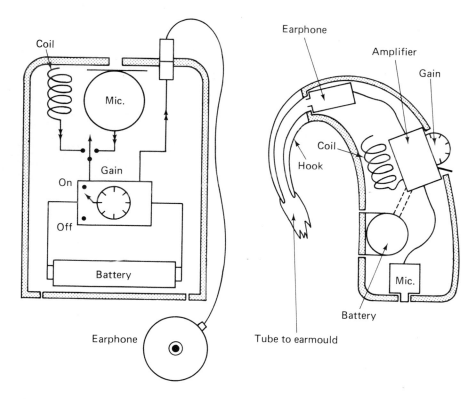

Figure 28.1   (a) A functional block diagram of a hearing aid with a microphone and pick-up coil input. Below are representations of how these parts are laid out in a bodyworn and a post-aural aid

frequency response. The ceramic microphone used the same piezo-electric principle but in place of the natural crystal new materials such as barium titanate which can be moulded are used. This type of microphone is of the high impedance type and therefore a field effect transistor (FET) is built into the housing of the microphone to allow a lower output impedance to be achieved. Such microphones require a power supply to operate the FET.

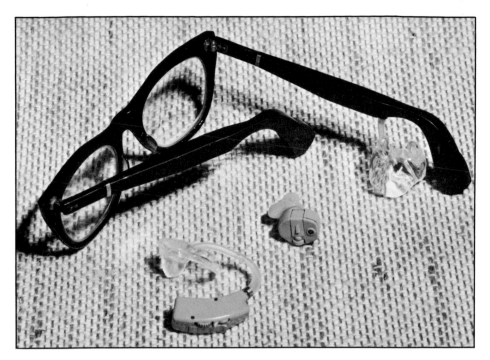

Figure 28.1 (b) Typical head-worn aids of the post-aural, spectacle and in-the-ear types

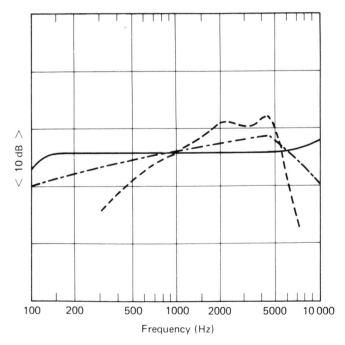

Figure 28.2 The frequency response of three different types of hearing aid microphones for a constant sound pressure level input. ———— Electret microphone; — · — · — Ceramic microphone; — — — Electromagnetic microphone

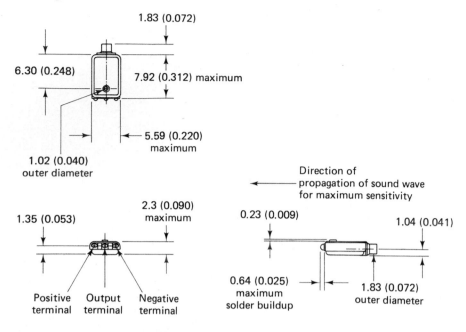

BW-1784 dimensions in mm (inches)

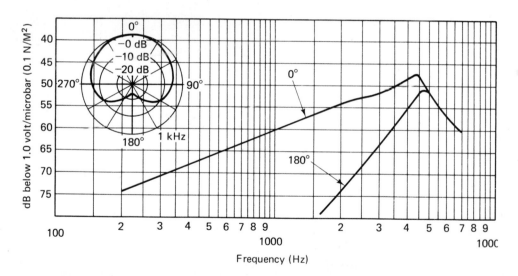

Frequency (Hz)

Figure 28.3   Diagram of directional microphone showing opening for sound at the top and a second hole (1.02 mm) at the back, upper drawing. Lower drawing shows three connection points for power supply for FET and signal output and side view. The size of this microphone is typical of those used in *Figure 28.2*. Lower diagram shows directional characteristic at 1 kHz and the frequency response at 0° and 180° incidence. (Courtesy Knowles Electronics)

The electret microphone can be considered as a capacitor type but with the electric charge being supplied, not by a high voltage across the plates as in a normal capacitor microphone but by an electret material that holds a charge with no external voltage being applied. This charge does decrease with time and therefore the electret microphone does have a finite life measured in years. The main advantage of the electret microphone is that it can have a very wide frequency response in a very small size and will only produce a small electrical output when vibrated, compared to the piezo-electric or electromagnetic microphone. The advantage therefore becomes apparent in post-aural aids, where mechanical vibrations are fed back through the structure of the aid by the earphone and then picked up by the microphone causing feedback to occur. Soft mountings are normally used to minimize this effect, but with an electret microphone the quality of the mounting is not as critical as with other types of microphone where an inadequate mounting will cause mechanical feedback and produce a whistling sound from the aid.

Most hearing aid microphones respond equally to sound from all directions but with the two port microphone (*Figure 28.3*) it is possible to achieve a directional effect. While the microphone has a directional effect it must be remembered that if the speech and noise are coming from the same area then of course there can be no improvement in signal-to noise ratio. However if the speech is from the front and noise from the back there is likely to be an improvement. A further user difficulty with directional microphones is that the directional effect is considerably modified when the aid is on a real head.

Hearing aid amplifiers

The performance of a hearing aid amplifier can be described in terms of its degree of amplification in decibels (dB), the frequency range over which it amplifies and the amount of power that it can deliver into a specified earphone. Other factors are the electrical noise that the amplifier generates in its early stages and the degree of harmonic and intermodulation distortion that is produced. In general the amplifier imposes no limitation on the performance of the aid; it does however determine the current taken from the battery.

Although the majority of aids still use simple amplifier circuits, in recent years the degree of sophistication in amplifiers has increased dramatically, particularly due to the introduction of circuits for controlling the dynamic range of the output signal. Circuits of this type may be given names such as AGC (Automatic Gain Control), AVC (Automatic Volume Control), LDC (Linear Dynamic Compression), etc., and their actions are described in detail later. AGC is the preferred generic term.

Tone control is normally achieved in the amplifier, although it can be achieved acoustically in the earmould and tubing, and in most cases consists of simple high and low frequency cuts. It is important to note that on hearing aids the letters H, N and L are used to denote High Frequency emphasis (low frequency cut), Normal (the widest frequency response that the aid can produce) and Low frequency emphasis (high frequency cut).

Low frequency cut is often useful as a means of reducing the effects of ambient noise and improving speech intelligibility. It must be remembered, however, that a reduction in low frequency response will also result in reduction of loudness. This may be beneficial in cases with severe high frequency loss, where the low frequency energy causes loudness discomfort.

In any amplifier the degree of amplification is described by the difference in

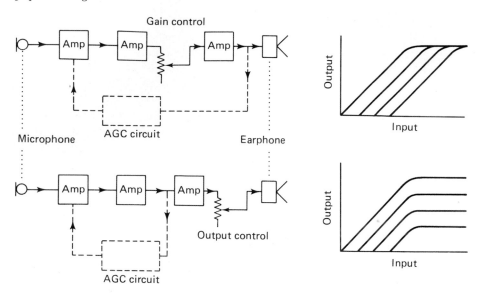

Figure 28.4 Upper diagram shows basic hearing aid with gain control before output stage; the input/output characteristic is shown which results from turning the gain control from maximum to minimum. An AGC circuit is shown dotted (see section on AGC). Lower diagram shows a basic hearing aid with the control on the output; input/output characteristic for different settings of the control can be seen to be constant. This type of control reduces the maximum output whereas the gain control in the upper circuit does not

amplitude between the input and output signals. As the input signal increases the output signal also increases; however, a point will be reached where the output signal will not increase any further, due to the maximum available power output of the amplifier being exceeded. At this point distortion will occur and however large the input signal the output will not increase any further. In hearing aids two of the most important parameters are amplification and maximum output power. Amplification and maximum output power are largely independent in theory, i.e. high gain can be associated with high or low output and vice versa.

The position of the volume control in the amplifier circuit greatly affects the mode of operation of the aid. If the control is connected between the amplifying stages it functions as a control of amplification and should properly be called a gain control. With the gain control on the output of the aid the control acts as an output attenuator and perhaps more properly can be called a volume control. *Figure 28.4* illustrates the differences.

Earphones

Earphones for bodyworn aids, often called receivers or more correctly insert earphones, are of a circular design whereas those in headworn aids are of a rectangular construction. The earphone of a bodyworn aid can be easily changed and it is imperative that the correct earphone for the aid be used. The type of earphone will determine the frequency response, degree of amplification and the maximum acoustic output of the aid. The low frequency response of insert earphones will normally go down to 20 Hz but the high frequency response is usually limited to 3 kHz for outputs in excess of 120 dB and 5 kHz for outputs of 110 dB or less (*see Figure 28.5*).

Earphones for headworn aids have a more limited low frequency range, i.e. 100 Hz but are better at high frequencies, i.e. 4 kHz for outputs of 125 dB and 5 kHz for 120 dB.

Bone conduction aids, i.e. bodyworn or spectacle aids have a vibrator in place of the earphone. The bone conduction vibrator requires considerably more power than an

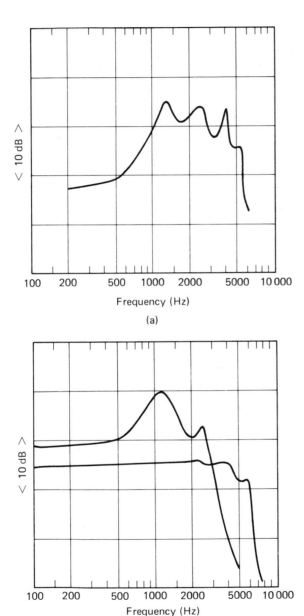

(a)

(b)

Figure 28.5 (a) Typical frequency response of earphone used in post-aural aid. (b) Upper curve indicates typical frequency response curve for high output earphone of the button type used with body-worn aids. Lower curve shows response of wide range earphone. Wide range earphones are not able to give high outputs at high frequencies

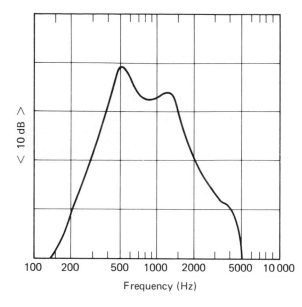

Figure 28.6 The output from a bone conduction vibrator measured in terms of acceleration on an artificial mastoid conforming to BS 4009

earphone to operate it at levels useful to conductively deaf people and has a very limited low and high frequency response (*see Figure 28.6*). A considerable pressure is required to achieve the best conduction of the vibrations to the head from the vibrator and this pressure can cause considerable discomfort to patients. Bone vibrators used with bodyworn aids may be mounted on the side arms of reinforced spectacle frames for less conspicuous use.

Power supply

Personal hearing aids use 'batteries', or to be more precise, primary or secondary cells, a battery being a number of cells joined together. Bodyworn aids can be used with a variety of cells, the most frequently used being the zinc carbon 'penlight' cell. Manganese alkaline and mercury cells are two other possibilities. The characteristics of cells differ very significantly in the way that the voltage across the cell and hence the performance of the aid varies with the hours of use. *Figure 28.7* shows the different characteristics of the three cells. For headworn aids the mercury cell is the most commonly used, followed by the silver oxide cell, which has an operating voltage of 1.5 V as opposed to 1.35 V for the mercury cell. A higher voltage in most cases means a small increase in output from the aid but usually at a considerable increase in battery current, hence a shorter battery life. A prime consideration in choosing an aid is the battery current as this obviously affects the running cost of the aid. Battery capacity is quoted in milliampere hours and indicates the number of hours a given current may be taken from the battery, e.g. an aid taking 2 mA used with a battery having a capacity of 180 mAh will give an average life of 90 h.

Rechargeable or secondary cells are available in all hearing aid sizes and are of the nickel cadmium or silver zinc type. These cells have similar characteristics to the mercury cells and can be recharged for a number of years. The use of rechargeable cells has not been widespread largely due to the need for the user to be trained to have a systematic approach to looking after the cells, i.e. one cell in the aid, one spare with

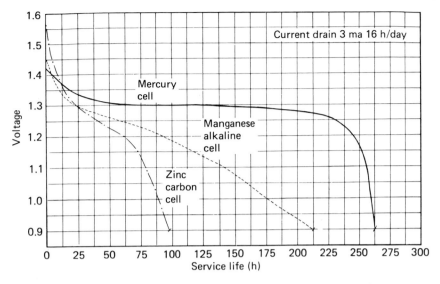

Figure 28.7   Variation of voltage with hours of use for three types of cell

the user and a third being recharged. Considerable financial saving however can be made by recharging and in areas where batteries are difficult to obtain a supply problem can be minimized.

Table 28.1 gives the capacity of a range of widely used cells and the mean current drawn by a range of aids. The maximum acoustic output of the aid is the parameter that largely determines the current taken by the aid; the degree of amplification does not involve any large variation in current drawn from the battery. Most aids take a steady current regardless of output, the exception to this is the push-pull type of aid which takes very little current with no output and a proportionally larger current as the output increases.

Table 28.1   (a) Cell type and capacity

Cell type	Capacity (mAh)
Mallory RM13H	85
Mallory RM401H	800
Mallory RM675H	180
Mallory MP675H	210
Ever Ready HP7	244

(b) Maximum gain and output of typical aids with average current and battery type recommended by manufacturer

	Gain	Output	Current (mA)	Battery type
Bodyworn aids	55	125	4.0	HP7
	80	135	5.0–20.0	RM 401H
Post-aural aids	35	109	0.3	RM 675H
	46	126	1.5	RM 675H
	60	135	1.5–7.0	MP 675H

Earmoulds

The acoustic output from a hearing aid has to be fed into the ear canal and this is achieved by a range of earmoulds (*Figure 28.8*). In most cases the earmould serves two functions:

(a) to hold the earphone in place;
(b) to seal the ear and prevent acoustic feedback (whistling).

A third function may be introduced which then replaces (b), that is to modify the acoustic characteristics of the aid by changing the earmould dimensions.

   Grover (1976) has shown that the diameter of the tube through the mould affects

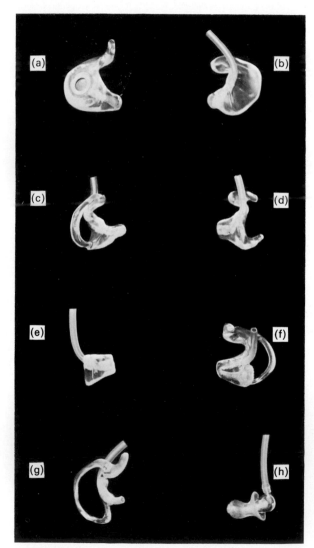

Figure 28.8 A range of earmoulds currently available (from Grover, 1974). (a) Solid mould for body-worn aid. (b) Shell mould for post-aural aid. (c) Skeleton mould for post-aural aid. (d) Three-quarter skeleton mould. (e) Meatal tip. (f) Variable vent in skeleton mould. (g) Open or non-occluding mould. (h) Temporary pip

resonances and low frequencies while the length of the bore moves the resonant peaks in frequency (*Figure 28.9*). There are serious practical problems in attempting to modify the performance by increasing length, but controlling the diameter by inserting a smaller bore tube inside the existing tube is possible. A further method of modifying the response is by inserting acoustic filters in the bore of the tubing.

A widely used technique for obtaining acoustic modifications is to use a vent. A vent is a hole drilled either parallel to the main bore called a lateral vent, or drilled to join the main bore, called a side branch vent. The performance differences in practice between the two positions is small. *Figure 28.10* shows the effect of different sizes of vent. It should be noted that a very large hole is required to affect frequencies up to 700 Hz. To obtain a larger effect an open mould may be used consisting of only a small tube at the entrance to the meatus. The open mould has a considerable effect on frequencies below 2 kHz as shown in *Figure 28.10*. Earmoulds with variable vents are available but tend to have an effect of being open or closed with little practical control between the two extremes (*Figure 28.10*).

A further aspect of a venting mould is that it is claimed to give relief to some patients from the 'blocked up' feeling of the closed mould.

While the above effects are easily measured it has been shown (Grover and Martin, 1978) that they do not necessarily produce the expected effect on hearing-impaired persons that it clearly does on normal hearing people. The effect of sensorineural hearing loss would appear to reduce the ability of the dispenser to predict the likely effect of any acoustic modification.

It should be remembered that leakage occurs on most moulds naturally and this causes a reduction of low frequency sounds heard. If however the leakage is too great, acoustic feedback may start. This is usually the limiting factor with venting and open moulds; Grover and Martin (1974) have shown that some 50 dB of amplification should be obtained with little difficulty in post-aural aids. With open moulds only some 25 dB of amplification may be achieved.

Earmoulds may be produced in a variety of materials, hard acrylic being the most widely used. However, soft materials are claimed to give a better seal in cases where high amplification is required.

Performance figures

The performance of a hearing aid is often specified by a single figure followed by the letters HAIC, i.e. Gain is 50 dB. HAIC stands for the Hearing Aid Industry Conference (1961) which in the USA laid down rules for stating the average gain and maximum acoustic output as well as the bandwidth of the aid. The gain and output figures are obtained from the average of 500, 1000 and 2500 Hz values. More recently an American standard ASA (1976) has used the same procedure but uses the frequencies 1000, 1600 and 2500 Hz. These frequencies are used in preference to the HAIC frequencies as most aids have their maximum gain above 1 kHz. The bandwidth of the aid is obtained by taking a value 20 dB below the average gain and drawing a horizontal line. Where the horizontal line cuts the frequency response is then defined as the bandwidth of the aid.

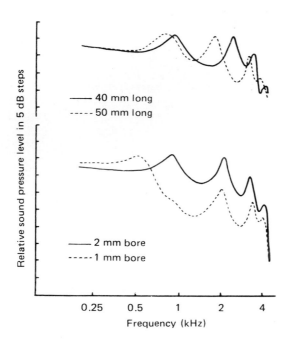

Figure 28.9 (Upper traces) Effect of tube length on the frequency response of a post-aural receiver. (Lower traces) Effect of tube bore on the frequency response of a post-aural receiver. (From Grover, 1976)

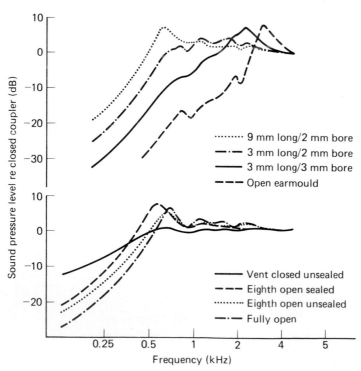

Figure 28.10 (Upper traces) Effects of short lateral vents. (Lower traces) Characteristics of a variable venting valve. (From Grover, 1976)

Current aids

The number of hearing aids on the commercial market is very large, and the Royal National Institute for the Deaf Current List of Hearing Aids (RNID, 1977) lists some 300 different models from 27 manufacturers. This wide range of aids can be grouped into a small number of performance categories on the basis of gain, maximum acoustic output and frequency response.

Table 28.2 indicates the categories that might be used for gain and output while *Table 28.3* covers the range of frequency responses.

Table 28.2

	Gain in dB at 1 kHz	Maximum acoustic output (dB SPL at 1 kHz)
Bodyworn aids		
Low	Under 40	Under 115
Medium	40–55	116–125
High	56–70	126–135
Very high	Over 70	Over 135
Headworn aids		
Low	Under 40	Under 110
Medium	40–55	111–120
High	55–60	120–125
Very high	Over 60	Over 125

Table 28.3

	Aid cut off low frequency	Aid cut off high frequency
Narrow	1 kHz	2 kHz
Medium	500 Hz	3 kHz
Wide	200 Hz	4–5 kHz
Very wide	100 Hz	6 kHz

CROS hearing aids

A person with a unilateral hearing loss is at a serious disadvantage when wishing to hear someone on his deaf side, i.e. a head shadow effect. He also suffers from a loss of directional hearing.

To minimize this problem a microphone is placed on the deaf ear and the signal from that microphone taken to an aid on the 'good' side. In many cases normal hearing will exist on the good side and it would not be desirable to block up the good ear or feed in high levels of sound. Consequently the good ear is provided with an open mould and a low output amplifier. The result of this Contralateral Routing of Signals (CROS) (Harford and Barry, 1965) is for the head shadow effect to be reduced and also, because of the difference in tonal quality of the sound coming from the microphone side, some pseudo-directional hearing ability is restored.

The most convenient manner of wearing a CROS aid is by mounting the microphone in one arm of a pair of spectacles and running the connecting wires through the frame to the other side arm. The amplifier and earphone are housed in the other side arm and the sound conducted via a tube into the ear. Two post-aural aids connected by a wire around the back of the neck can also be used. Where the patient has one severely impaired ear and the other ear also has a loss then a microphone may be used on both sides and the ear sealed with a conventional earmould. This type of fitting is termed a BICROS aid. *Table 28.4* lists the more widely used terms for various types of aid, derived from the basic CROS aid.

Table 28.4   Types of CROS aid (from Dunlavy, 1974)

Classic CROS	Microphone on same side as that of deaf ear: earphone connected to good ear with open earmould
Regular BICROS	Two microphones (one on each side) connected through single amplifier and earphone to closed earmould in better ear
Open BICROS	Same as regular BICROS but with tube (open canal earmould system) in better ear
UNICROS	One microphone feeding two amplifiers and two earphones. Closed mould fitted to poorer ear, tube (open canal earmould system) to better ear
Power CROS	Same as classic CROS but with high gain and output amplifier and closed earmould. Minimizes feedback problems
FROS	Frontal routing of signals. Microphone in front of spectacle frame feeding amplifier and earphone on same side.
BIFROS	A FROS system on each side
BIFROS 270	Same as BIFROS but with an extra microphone on each side set in side arms of spectacle aid

Frequency transposing aid

In cases of severe high frequency deafness and profound deafness where only low frequency hearing remains, frequency transposition (Johansson, 1959, 1966) has been tried. Frequency transposition in hearing aids consists of taking a band, say, 4–8 kHz and transposing it down to a region below 1 kHz and superimposing it on the existing low frequency signal. *Figure 28.11* shows the operation of one commercially available transposing aid. This type of aid however only produces a low frequency noise in place of the high frequency signal. More recent work has attempted to reproduce the high frequency pattern as a low frequency pattern rather than a noise (Velmans, 1974). In using transposing aids it must be remembered that the user probably has to undergo a considerable learning programme to make use of the new information. The ratio of the transposed channel to the direct channel is important and has to be set with care.

Equipment for hearing aid evaluation

In order to evaluate the effectiveness of a hearing aid it is necessary to have a certain minimum of equipment.

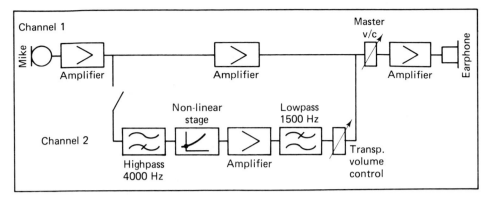

Figure 28.11   Commercially available frequency transposer made as a body-worn hearing aid. (Courtesy Oticon Limited)

Two approaches to the practical fitting of hearing aids may be found. The most widely used is that of presenting speech and other stimuli through a loudspeaker to the patient wearing a chosen aid and controlling the level of sound by means of an audiometer. *Figure 28.12* shows the arrangement used at the RNID where the audiometer is the main control unit. Audiometers for hearing aid evaluation work should have a facility for tape input and an output to drive an external amplifier and loudspeaker. Where an output socket is not available a signal can be taken from the headphone socket provided the output is properly loaded to ensure that the attenuator works correctly.

A second approach to hearing aid fitting is to use a master hearing aid. A master hearing aid is a desk top unit which is basically an amplifier with facilities to adjust gain, output and frequency response. Some master hearing aids do not use hearing aid microphones and earphones worn as a hearing aid and consequently it is very difficult to equate the results obtained with the master hearing aid to a personal aid.

Performance measurements

The performance of hearing aids is measured in a manner recommended by an International Standard, IEC 118 and its supplements (IEC 1959, 1975, 1977). While these measurements of performance are widely quoted it is not often realized how they are obtained and the limitations that exist in applying these measurements to the needs of patients.

Hearing aids are measured in a strictly artificial manner in that no attempt at the present time is made in making the measurements simulate what will happen when the aid is on the user's head and body, or what happens when the earphone is fitted on a real ear. While this may be thought to be a very regrettable situation it can be explained by the fact that the technical information and the standardization necessary have not yet been produced.

The instrumentation required for testing hearing aids is shown in *Figure 28.13*. The major difficulty in making hearing aid measurements is that they require to be carried out in a relatively quiet situation, hence a soundproof enclosure is required to minimize

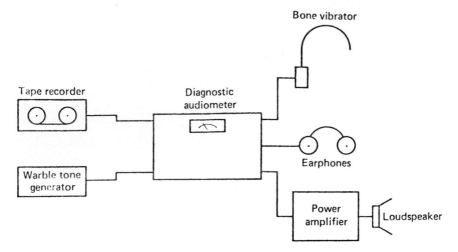

Figure 28.12   A practical arrangement of equipment for hearing aid evaluation. If live voice facilities are required a microphone and amplifier can be plugged in, in place of the tape recorder. The audiometer must have a metering facility to allow for proper calibration of speech and other stimuli

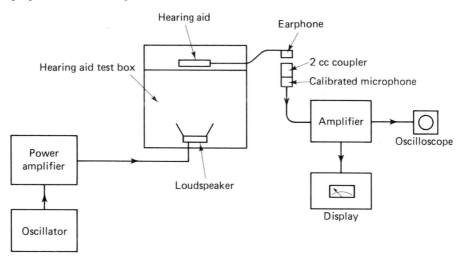

Figure 28.13   Basic instrumentation for measuring the performance of a hearing aid. The oscillator generates pure tones which are fed at predetermined levels to a power amplifier and loudspeaker. The loudspeaker is housed in a test box and the hearing aid placed with the microphone facing it. The sound pressure level at the face of the hearing aid microphone is set to be a known value. The sound output from the aid is measured by the calibrated microphone in the 2 cc coupler. The output from the microphone is amplified, measured by a meter and may also be displayed on an oscilloscope to show distortion

ambient noise. By using automatic testing equipment which sweeps a test tone through a selected frequency range and which records the output of the aid on a chart, testing can be carried out in a few minutes.

The output sound from the hearing aid is measured in a 2 cc acoustic coupler, IEC 126 (1973) (*Figure 28.14*). This is often incorrectly referred to as an artificial ear, the difference between an acoustic coupler and an artificial ear being that the latter simulates the mean acoustic impedance of the adult ear while the former does not. Hence, to determine the sound pressure at the eardrum it is necessary to make corrections to acoustic coupler measurements. In general the corrections are small at frequencies below 1 kHz but large at higher frequencies. It is important to note the following warning that is given in IEC 126.

> The use of this coupler does not allow the actual performance of a hearing aid on a person to be obtained: the IEC recommends its use as a simple and ready means for the exchange of specifications and of physical data on hearing aids.

No standard as yet exists for an insert artificial ear or ear simulator but work based on that of Zwislocki (1970) provides a device that is likely to become standardized in the near future.

Figure 28.15 is typical of the performance that may be obtained with a bodyworn hearing aid and serves as an example of the three main performance parameters of an aid, i.e. frequency response, amplification and maximum acoustic output.

Frequency response

The frequency response of an aid will vary with the degree of amplification, the acoustic output, the control setting of the aid and the earphone used. A basic frequency

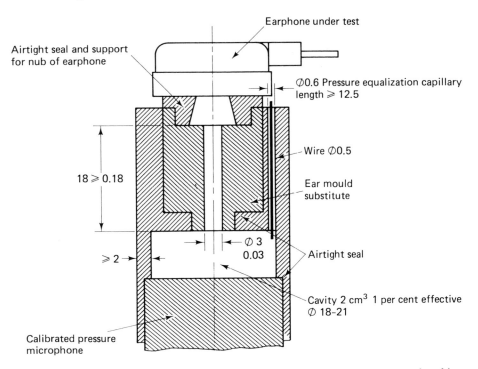

Figure 28.14   Drawing of an IEC 2 cc acoustic coupler. Connection for post-aural and in-the-ear aids is achieved by modifying the connection at the top of the coupler or by removing the ear mould substitute (Dimensions in mm.) (From IEC 126, 1973)

response curve is one taken at an acoustic input which gives an output which varies in a linear manner with the input, with a stated control setting and earphone. However, this may not necessarily relate to the frequency response at a high output level as may be seen in *Figure 28.15*. In practice the frequency response will be further altered by the head and body baffle effects of the user.

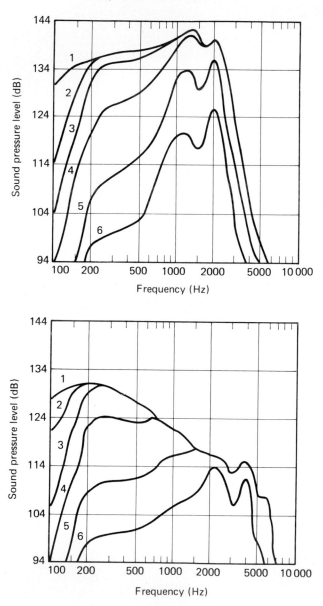

Figure 28.15 Overall acoustic performance of a body-worn hearing aid. Curves 1–6 correspond to input sound pressure levels reducing from 94 to 44 dB SPL in 10 dB steps. The upper set of curves are for the aid fitted with a high power earphone while in the lower set the aid is fitted with a wide range earphone

Amplification

Amplification may be defined as the increase in amplitude between the input and output signals. The frequency response curve normally shows how amplification varies with frequency over a specified range. Amplification can be calculated from *Figure 28.15* by subtracting the input level from the output level and it will be seen that due to limiting, the amplification is not the same at high output levels as it is at low levels.

Maximum acoustic output

When the input signal is high it may attempt to drive the output of the aid beyond the power handling capacity of the output transistor or the earphone. From *Figure 28.16* it can be seen that the type of earphone used dramatically affects the maximum acoustic output and that it is not possible to get high acoustic output at high frequencies, i.e. above 3 kHz, with small earphones. The importance of the maximum acoustic output to the patient is that it is this parameter that will influence whether or not the aid is exceeding his loudness discomfort level. Maximum acoustic output is independent of amplification and hence aids can have high output and low gain and vice versa.

Maximum acoustic output may only be achieved in some cases at abnormally high inputs and therefore a constant high input sound pressure level of 90 dB is now used to achieve a practical measure. This measurement is termed SSPL 90, i.e. Saturation Sound Pressure Level for an input of 90 dB, and is described in ASA (1976).

It has been shown (Martin, 1976) that if the maximum acoustic output is too low for a specific user he will turn the gain control up to maximum in order to hear. A difference in maximum output as small as 2.5 dB can cause the user to go from a realistic degree of amplification to the maximum gain of the aid. This observation is considered to be particularly relevant to the use of aids by profoundly deaf children where acoustic feedback, caused by high amplification, is a continual problem.

Other performance factors are the signal-to-noise ratio and harmonic and intermodulation distortion. The signal-to-noise ratio in most aids will be greater than 40 dB and background electrical noise only appears to be a problem with small hearing losses.

Harmonic distortion is often thought to be a most important factor in determining the efficiency of a hearing aid and it cannot be denied that if distortion becomes gross, i.e. 20 per cent or more then some loss of intelligibility of speech may be introduced. Harmonic distortion in an average domestic radio or television will be about 5 per cent at comfortable listening levels and 1 per cent in a high fidelity system.

In specifying hearing aid performance a curve is often drawn showing percentage distortion against acoustic output as in *Figure 28.16*. From this figure it may be seen that distortion occurs at a significant level only near saturation or the maximum acoustic output. Hence if a user has his aid turned halfway down he will rarely enter the area of severe distortion. It has been shown (Gabrielsson *et al.*, 1977) that hearing-impaired people have significantly poorer discrimination of distortion than normally hearing people, so that the problem is not so crucial as may be first thought.

Other types of distortion such as intermodulation and transient distortion may be

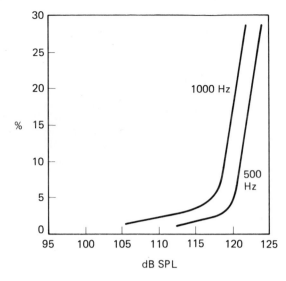

Figure 28.16 The total harmonic distortion present in the acoustic output of a hearing aid is plotted for different output sound pressures at two frequencies. It will be seen that a significant amount of distortion is not introduced until the aid approaches its maximum acoustic output which is 120 dB SPL at 1 kHz and 125 dB SPL at 500 Hz

equally as important as harmonic distortion, but little evidence is yet available as to the subjective effects of these types of distortion.

Output control

As most patients with sensorineural hearing loss will have a reduced dynamic range for sound, it becomes important to consider ways in which the output of the aid may be controlled to restrict the sound to a level below the loudness discomfort level of the patient. Two main methods are used to achieve this, i.e. peak clipping (PC) and automatic gain control (AGC).

Peak clipping as its name implies instantaneously cuts off the peaks of the output at some predetermined level (*Figure 28.17*), hence introducing distortion once the clipping level has been reached. AGC on the other hand takes a finite time to operate and does not introduce significant distortion (*Figure 28.17*).

The effect of output control systems may be shown in the form of an input/output graph (*Figure 28.18*). The input/output curve can be divided into a linear mode, where input and output are proportional and AGC mode where the input range is reduced at the output.

With AGC the time constants of the on and off time are defined in *Figure 28.17*. Modern aids tend to have fast time constants, i.e. 30 ms attack time and 50 ms delay time. A wide range of terms are used to denote some form of compression, i.e. DRC (Dynamic Range Compression), LDC (Linear Dynamic Compression), ALC (Automatic Loudness Control) but the differences are often in name only. One major difference is that caused by the position of the gain control in the AGC circuit (*Figure 28.4*). If the gain control is outside the feedback loop the effect is to maintain the input/output characteristic constant for all positions of the gain control. The advantage of this type of circuit is that the patient can control the output sound

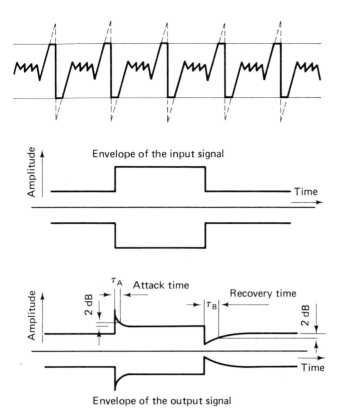

Figure 28.17 The upper drawing indicates a peak clipping action where the high level signals are cut off instantaneously. The dotted portion indicates the waveform that would have been passed through had no clipping action taken place. The lower diagram shows the effect of an AGC system on the envelope of a signal. The waveform of the signal is preserved within the envelope. (From IEC 118-2, 1977)

closely, which is not possible with the gain control inside the AGC loop. With the gain control inside the loop the maximum acoustic output is fixed to some predetermined level and the patient can only alter the gain. In practice most hearing aid users use their aids at a level well below the point where AGC becomes operative hence many users of AGC aids in practice never have AGC operating.

It is often thought that AGC is a means of minimizing the effects of background noise; however, the opposite is probably the case. The AGC circuit in current aids is effectively controlled by the loudest sound reaching the microphone; consequently in a noisy situation the speech that the user wishes to hear may well be suppressed. In a quiet situation AGC will be of benefit and ideally aids should have a switch which will switch in and out the AGC when required.

The type of AGC circuit that is at present available controls the overall gain of the aid, but recruitment does not appear equally at all frequencies and hence there is a requirement to divide the spectrum up into appropriate bands and apply compression appropriately in each band (Barford, 1976). Multichannel master hearing aids are

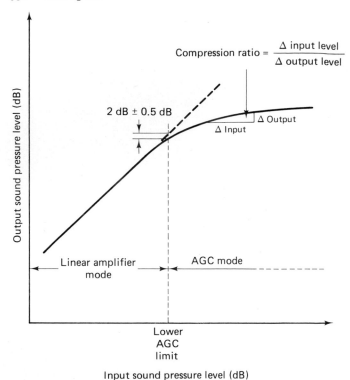

Figure 28.18   Example of an AGC steady state input/output graph (From IEC 118-2, 1977)

becoming available but a question that has to be answered is how many channels are required for optimum performance.

Fitting of hearing aids

The performance of a hearing aid can be measured accurately but, as has been indicated, the technical information provided on an aid does not enable that aid to be fitted without making subjective measurements of the aid on the user. Furthermore, there are a number of other factors which have to be taken into account. To enable a logical approach to be adopted to fitting an aid a flow diagram (*Figure 28.19*) may be of use (Martin, 1978). The flow diagram does not attempt to detail procedures but to structure the approach to the problem.

The fitting of an aid may be considered in five parts:

(1) Pre-fitting considerations.
(2) Basic audiological considerations.
(3) Putting the aid on the patient.
(4) Measurement of aided benefit.
(5) Trial period and after-care.

1. Pre-fitting considerations

The purpose of this part of the procedure is to determine if the patient can physically handle the aid and has the right attitude to the problem. In either case if the patient cannot or will not cope with the aid then there is little point in continuing to supply one. The otologist has to agree that there is no medical reason why an aid should not be used and if there is a problem that precludes the use of an aid then suitable after-care should be arranged.

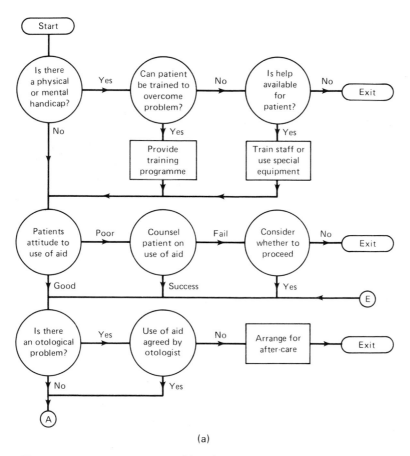

(a)

Figure 28.19   (a) Pre-fitting considerations

2. Basic audiological considerations

Pure-tone air and bone conduction thresholds are useful indicators of the problems likely to be encountered in fitting an aid. If the patient is unable to undertake normal audiometry then objective tests, e.g. post-auricular muscle response, acoustic reflex, give useful information that at least acts as a guide to the dispenser. If it is not possible to make any type of measurement due to lack of equipment one has to resort to experience or guesswork. As well as pure-tone detection threshold a loudness discomfort level test should be undertaken thus giving an indication of the dynamic

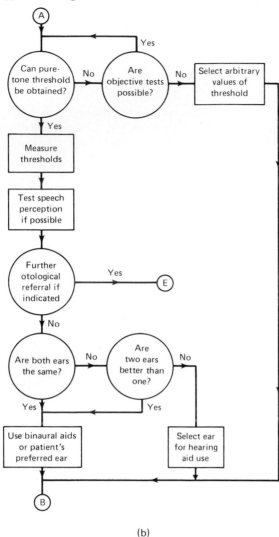

(b)

Figure 28.19   (b) Basic audiological considerations

range of the ear to be aided. Objective tests have yet to be shown to relate to subjective impressions. The acoustic reflex in particular has been shown not to relate well with the subjective correlation of loudness discomfort (Woodford and Holmes, 1977).

The main aim of the hearing aid is to amplify and improve the discrimination of speech and therefore some measure of speech discrimination ability is essential. Speech tests at comfortable listening level and loudness discomfort level give an indication of the dynamic range for speech.

It is possible that as a result of the tests carried out for fitting an aid evidence will arise to suggest that further otological examinations are required.

From the tests above, the pure-tone threshold, the loudness discomfort level for pure tones and speech and the comfortable listening level for speech for each ear will be

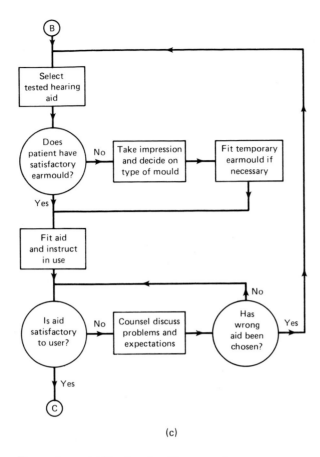

(c)

Figure 28.19 (c) Putting the aid on a patient

known. From this information a decision has to be made whether to fit both ears or one, and if one ear, which one.

As a general guide if the two ears are similar in all respects then a binaural fitting might be used. If the two ears are dissimilar it is still possible that two will function better than one. However if one ear only is to be used the considerations as to which ear might be taken are as follows.

What is the difference in hearing loss between the two ears? If the good ear can make use of normal sound but the poor ear cannot then one should attempt to fit the poor ear. If neither ear can make use of normal sounds then one should choose the ear with the better hearing level or the one which has the better speech discrimination. It must be stressed that ideally no decisions should be made without appropriate measurements.

Suggestions have been made by a number of authors as to how data from pure-tone audiograms may be used to determine aid parameters. Berger (1976) has suggested the following formula for calculating gain and maximum output at different frequencies under the following conditions: Monaural listening, forward facing microphone, close coupled earphone, sensorineural hearing loss.

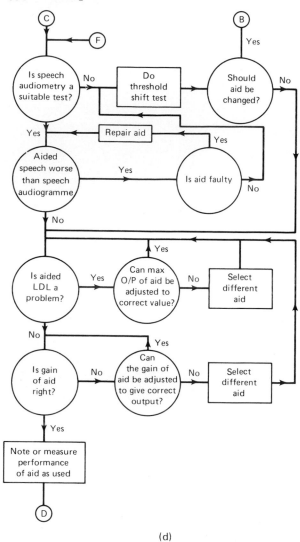

(d)

Figure 28.19　(d) Measurement of aided benefit

CALCULATION OF SATURATION SOUND PRESSURE LEVEL (SSPL)

At each frequency the loudness discomfort level (LDL) is measured and to it is added a correction to give the value of SSPL required from the aid in terms of Sound Pressure Level (SPL), not Hearing Level. The correction value is obtained by taking the standardized value of SPL for audiometric zero and subtracting 3 dB as a safety margin to ensure the LDL is not exceeded, i.e. at 1 kHz audiometric zero, for a

Table 28.5　Values of SSPL for frequency range 0.5–4 kHz

500	SSPL = LDL + 8 dB or 110 dB whichever is lower
1000	SSPL = LDL + 4 dB
2000	SSPL = LDL + 6 dB
3000	SSPL = LDL + 5 dB
4000	SSPL = LDL + 6 dB

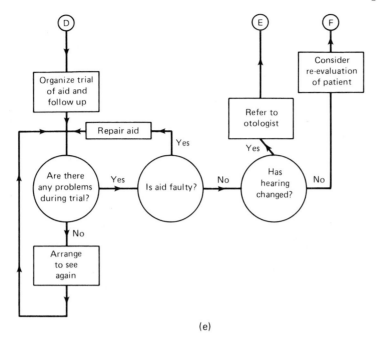

(e)

Figure 28.19   (e) Trial period and after-care

TDH 39 earphone measured on a 6 cc acoustic coupler, is 7 dB; subtracting 3 dB for safety gives a value of 4 dB which is added to the value of LDL measured on the patient to give the saturation sound pressure level required from the aid.

CALCULATION OF MAXIMUM GAIN (dB) AT SPECIFIC FREQUENCIES

The required maximum gain in the hearing aid to be used is calculated on the basis of the patient's hearing level (HL) at a particular frequency plus a correction factor, all divided by a second factor which mirrors the long-term spectrum of speech between 500 and 2000 Hz.

The correction factor to be added is 10 dB which gives a reserve of gain if speech levels fall, etc. The factor used as a divisor is such that it aims to produce an amplification that is approximately half the hearing loss of the patient modified by the long-term spectrum of speech to give greater emphasis to high frequencies.

Example

The measured hearing level at 500 Hz has 10 dB added to it and is then divided by 2 to obtain the maximum gain required at that frequency.

Table 28.6   Calculation of maximum gain (dB) at specific frequencies

$$500 \text{ Hz} = \frac{\text{HL at 500 Hz}}{2} + 10 \text{ dB reserve gain}$$

$$1 \text{ kHz} = \frac{\text{HL at 1000 Hz}}{1.6} + 10 : 2 \text{ kHz gain} = \frac{\text{HL at 2000 Hz}}{1.5} + 10$$

$$3 \text{ kHz} = \frac{\text{HL at 3000 Hz}}{1.7} + 10 : 4 \text{ kHz gain} = \frac{\text{HL at 4000 Hz}}{2} + 10$$

CORRECTIONS TO CALCULATED GAIN FIGURES

Where a conductive component exists in the hearing loss the additional gain of one quarter of the air–bone gap is added, i.e. after the 10 dB conductive factor add

$$\frac{\text{Air Conduction threshold} - \text{Bone Conduction threshold}}{4} \quad \text{or} \quad \frac{\text{AC} - \text{BC}}{4}$$

For bodyworn aids the correction factors at 500 Hz and 2 kHz are changed from 2 to 2.2 and 1.5 to 1.4 respectively to account for body baffle effects.

For in-the-ear aids the correction values at 2 and 3 kHz are changed from 1.5 to 1.6 and 1.7 to 1.9 respectively to account for the effect of the pinna on the aid.

The formulae are not intended to be optimum but to act as a useful guide. Peaks in the frequency response are thought to control the gain used. See Berger, Hagberg and Lane (1977) for a full explanation of the procedures used.

Brooks (1973), Byrne and Fifield (1974) and Martin (1973) have investigated the gain used in practice and found that a gain equal to approximately half the hearing loss acts as a rule of thumb for determining the degree of amplification required. This guide has been disputed by Powell and Tucker (1976) and discussed by Martin, Brooks and Morris (1977). All rules or formulae can be used to check results obtained or guide when measurements are not possible; at no time should they be used in place of measurements.

3. Putting the aid on the patient

In order to test the patient properly it is important to have an appropriate well-fitting earmould. It is also important to know that the aid selected is working properly.

When putting the aid on a patient for the first time it is imperative that the patient knows what to expect and realizes that things will sound different through the aid. Hearing aid users are often led to expect great clarity from hearing aids which they will never achieve and thus become rapidly disillusioned. However if both the advantages and disadvantages of aids are carefully explained many potential users will face the new situation realistically.

4. Measurement of aided benefit

Once a hearing aid is placed upon the patient it is desirable to know in as much detail as possible what benefit it affords him. Where great obvious benefit is obtained it may not appear necessary to undertake any tests but where benefit is not apparent tests are essential.

Speech perception is of prime importance and if speech audiometry can be undertaken then it may be checked that the aided articulation score is at least no worse than that achieved with the audiometer. If however the patient cannot undertake speech audiometry, e.g. foreign speaking, too deaf to achieve any articulation score, then a free field threshold shift test is of value.

The purpose of the threshold shift test is to measure the aided and unaided thresholds for warbled pure tones or bands of noise (Gengel, Pascoe and Shore, 1971), and to thus determine the degree of subjective gain that the user obtains. This technique also allows the threshold level of sound at the face of the microphone to be determined and hence whether or not normal speech sounds are likely to be heard. *Figure 28.20* shows a number of results obtained using this technique.

Having assessed a degree of benefit from the aid it is important to determine if the output power of the aid is too high and likely to cause discomfort. On many aids pre-set controls allow the maximum output to be adjusted in a continuously variable manner.

It is also important that the gain control on the aid is not set near to the upper or lower end of its travel. Either position will cause problems; if the control is up high it is possible that the aid is not powerful enough, if it is too low the patient will have difficulty in setting the correct degree of amplification.

Each of the above adjustments are interactive and therefore making one adjustment will often mean altering others.

The tests described above do not include any tests of the patient's ability to hear in noise or reverberation. For a full evaluation such tests would be required and may well show considerable differences between patients.

5. Trial period and after-care

In spite of making many measurements it is still not possible to be dogmatic that a particular aid will be of optimum benefit to the patient, hence it is necessary for the patient to have the aid on trial prior to deciding whether or not to keep it.

Because of the uncertainties involved in hearing aid fitting an after-care service is essential.

The procedures described above are time-consuming and an initial full fitting of a hearing aid will take at least an hour with a number of further visits of similar length to try and resolve difficult problems. It may rightly be argued that this amount of time cannot be spent on every patient but in difficult cases there is no alternative way of arriving at an answer. The fitting of hearing aids must include measurements on the individual user under free-field (loudspeaker) conditions

Educational aids

Hearing aids used in the education of hearing-impaired children fall into three categories:

(a) personal aids;
(b) group aids and auditory training units;
(c) electromagnetic transmitting and receiving aids, i.e. inductive loop, radio microphone systems, etc.

(a) Personal hearing aids have been largely covered and the additional educational facilities required are the provision of a combined inductive pick-up coil (T) and microphone (M) position on the aid. This combined position allows the teacher's voice to be heard as well as the child's own voice and the sound present around him. A requirement on British National Health Service Medresco aids, i.e. OL57 was that the pick-up coil should be relatively more sensitive than the microphone by some 10 dB, thus ensuring that the teacher's voice was always louder than the other signals from the microphone. Some bodyworn aids have baby locks that allow the controls to be covered as well as covers for the microphone to prevent food and liquid from entering the microphone aperture.

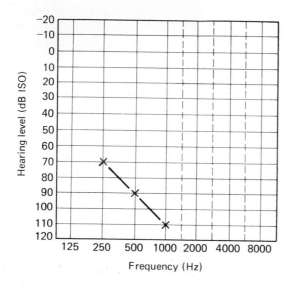

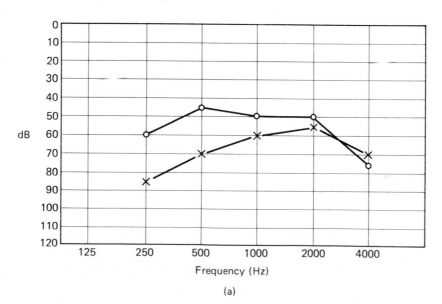

(a)

Figure 28.20   (a) The pure-tone audiogram (top) and the free field threshold shift (bottom) are shown for a profoundly deaf patient. Two different high powered aids have been used with one showing greater benefit at low frequencies. No unaided threshold was possible with this patient. Maximum speech discrimination score was 10 per cent

Maintenance of aids

The maintenance of hearing aids in schools for the deaf has been a constant problem and a number of surveys (Coleman, 1975), have all shown that some 50 per cent of aids used in schools are likely to be faulty in one way or another. The majority of faults in aids tend to be of a simple nature, i.e. broken cords, cases, etc. In order to provide a true aural education the utmost dedication to maintaining aids and ensuring their optimum use must be undertaken. Only daily inspection, or even twice daily by both teachers and children is likely to ensure 100 per cent level of use.

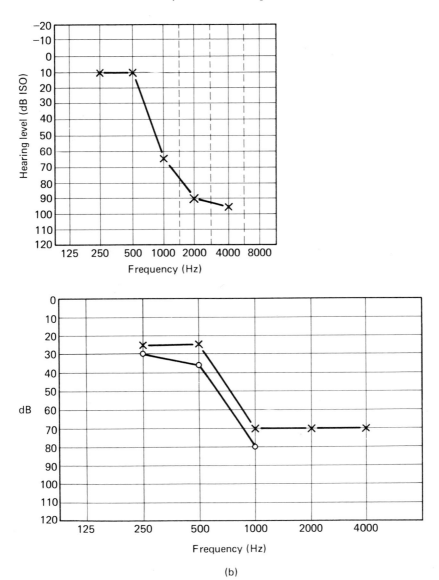

(b)

Figure 28.20 (b) A patient with severe high tone loss. The threshold shift is not great and the degree of benefit obtained at high frequencies is small in spite of high gain at high frequencies. Unaided threshold ○－○; aided threshold ×－×

(b) Group hearing aids today usually consist of a number of independent channels of amplification, one for each child. Each child has a common input from the teacher's microphone and the facility for each child in the group to hear the teacher and every other child. Each channel will have a means of adjusting the frequency response by at least high and low frequency cuts.

In the United Kingdom the group aid has always been fitted with large supra-aural or circum-aural earphones rather than the insert type normally used on bodyworn hearing aids. The reason for this is that the larger type of earphone is capable of reproducing frequencies above 3 kHz, at levels in excess of 130 dB SPL whereas insert earphones are not capable of doing this. However, in many other European countries the insert earphone is used with the philosophy that the child will have to live with an insert earphone and therefore should learn through the same type of device.

The auditory training unit can be considered as a single channel of a group hearing aid.

Recommendations for the measurement of the performance of group hearing aids and auditory training units are specified in IEC 118–3 (1978) 'Methods of measurement of hearing aids not entirely worn on the person'. Performance requirements for the UK are suggested in 'The Teacher of the Deaf' (1977).

(c) A major problem faced by any hearing aid user is the adverse effect of background noise and distance from the person speaking. To minimize this problem systems have been developed which pick up the speaker's voice by means of a microphone close to the mouth and then transmit the speech signal directly to the listener's ear.

The first system to be widely used for this purpose was the inductive loop system which consists of a loop of one or more turns of wire around the room and connected to an audio frequency amplifier (*Figure 28.21*). The amplifier drives an electric current around the loop which generates a magnetic field which varies in the same manner as the input to the amplifier. Hearing aids fitted with a pick-up coil have a switch marked with an 'M' for the normal microphone and 'T' for a pick-up coil which is sensitive to the varying magnetic field. Thus the wearer when using his aid on the 'T' position hears no acoustic signals through the microphone and only hears the signal being fed into the loop. If a microphone is used on the input to the loop amplifier the speaker's voice is connected without loss due to distance and with a minimum of interference from background noise due to the microphone being close to the person speaking. The essential part in using educational amplifying equipment is to ensure good microphone technique, to avoid overloading the amplifier if the microphone is too close or introducing background noise if it is too far away.

The inductive loop system has fallen into disrepute for two reasons. The first is that too much power is put into the loop causing more overspill than is necessary. Overspill is the term used to describe the magnetic field that inevitably goes outside the loop itself and therefore may interfere with another loop user in an adjacent room. Certain loop configurations (*Figure 28.22*) will minimize the overspill.

The second reason for unsatisfactory use of the loop system is the large variation in the sensitivity of pick-up coils in hearing aids; as much as 30 dB difference has been found between different models of aid.

Two recent international standards IEC 118–1 (1975) and IEC 118–4 (1978) have established a recommended field strength and a method of measuring the performance of aids with pick-up coils which has ensured far better use of the loop system than ever

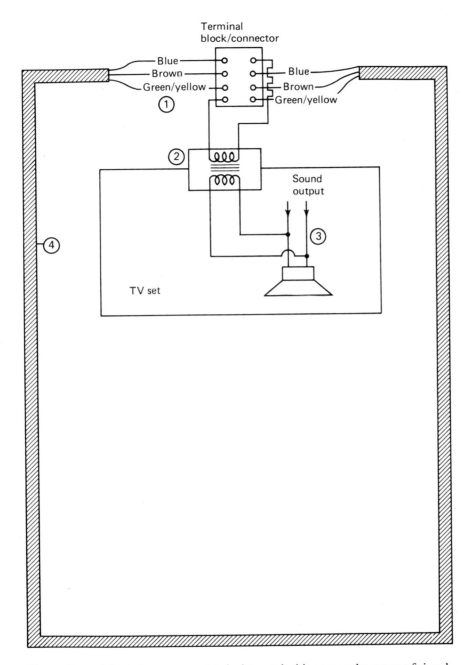

Figure 28.21 A basic loop system attached to a television set as the source of signal. The TV set can be replaced by any audio frequency power amplifier with a low impedance output. (1) Connection of 3-core miniature mains cable to form three turns in series around the room. (2) Isolating transformer or pack, fitted by TV engineer. (3) A parallel connection is shown, but in certain circumstances a series connection may be used. When fitting isolating packs, the suppliers' instructions must be closely followed. (4) TV loop around perimeter of room, consisting of 3-core miniature mains cable

before. In the UK all aids issued under the National Health Service have pick-up coils, and while the use of the loop system in public places is still small, a far greater use is for listening to television with a suitably modified television set.

For educational purposes, having a trailing lead from the microphone to the loop amplifier can cause difficulties. To overcome this, radio microphone systems were introduced; these consisted of a microphone connected to a radio transmitter small enough to be worn around the neck. A radio receiver connected to the loop amplifier receives the transmissions from the radio microphone thus giving freedom of movement to the teacher, as well as to the children who listen through the loop system.

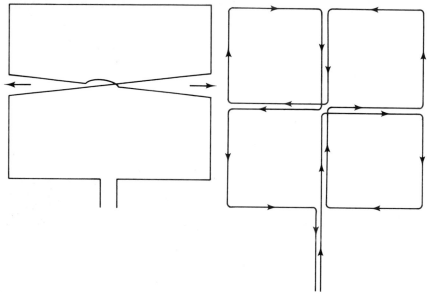

Figure 28.22   Two configurations of loop. The four-square loop (right) minimizes overspill in all directions but does suffer, as do all loops with null points over the top of the loop wires. In the figure-of-eight loop the reduction of overspill is in the direction of the arrows

A further development has been to replace the child's aid with a hearing aid containing a radio receiver thus giving the teacher and child complete freedom of movement with no need for installation of loop equipment. Furthermore, the radio system works on a specific radio frequency and interference from one room to another is negligible if different frequencies are used.

The latest development has been to fit hearing aids with a socket which allows an external electrical signal to be connected as from a separate radio receiver.

An alternative means of connecting an external drive such as a radio receiver is by providing the external device with a small transmitting coil, i.e. a miniature inductive loop, which can then be placed against the aid and used with the pick-up coil in the aid when switched to the 'T' position.

One disadvantage, educationally, of the above systems is that the user of the aid can hear his own voice and that of the teacher but cannot hear directly other children in the group, as can be achieved in a group aid.

Acoustic aids

While the ear trumpet and speaking tube are perhaps considered by many as music hall jokes they do have a considerable use for the geriatric patient. Acoustic aids can have an effective gain of about 20 dB which is sufficient for moderate losses that can occur with age. What is often overlooked with the speaking tube is that when the tube is put close to the mouth the sound pressure is high, i.e. 90–100 dB, and this sound pressure is transmitted directly to the ear of the listener. The acoustic aid does not have any maintenance problems, apart from keeping the earpip clean, and it is available for immediate use. For countries with limited technical resources acoustic aids offer the possibility of amplification with locally produced devices, if the resistance to what is considered old fashioned technology can be overcome.

Conclusion

Today a wide range of aids is available and can provide amplification for losses ranging from very small to profound. A major difficulty exists in knowing how to apply this amplification in the best possible manner. To make the tests necessary to determine optimum amplification takes a considerable time, but without tests the fitting of aids becomes largely guesswork. However, even after making the most comprehensive tests we have to rely on the patient to say if the aid is meeting his needs. After-care for the hearing aid user is of prime importance and must be an integral part of the total hearing aid service.

References

ASA (1976) *Acoustical Society of America* Standard ASA STD 7–1976 specification of hearing aid characteristics. New York; American Institute of Physics

Barford, J. (1976) *Multichannel Compression Hearing Aids*. Report No. 11, Technical University of Denmark; Acoustics Laboratory

Berger, K. W. (1976) 'Prescription of hearing aids. A rationale', *J. American Audiological Soc.*, **3**, 71

Berger K. W., Hagberg E. M. and Lane R. L. (1977) *Prescription of Hearing Aids: Rationale, Procedure and Results*. Ohio; Herald Publishing House

Brooks, D. (1973) 'Gain requirements of hearing aid users', *Scandinavian Audiology*, **2**, 199

Byrne, D. and Fifield, D. (1974) 'Evaluation of hearing aid fittings for infants', *British Journal of Audiology*, **8**, 47

Coleman, R. F. (1975) 'Is anyone listening', *Language, Speech and Hearing Services in Schools*, **6**, 102

Dunlavy, A. R. (1974) 'CROS: A review of applications of fittings utilizing contralateral routing of signals', *National Hearing Aid Journal*, July

Gabrielsson, A., Nyberg, P., Sjogren, H. and Svensson L. (1977) 'Detection of, amplitude distortion by normal hearing and hearing impaired subjects'. Karolinska Institute, Report TA No. 83, Stockholm

Gengel, R. W., Pascoe, D. and Shore, I. (1971) 'A frequency response procedure for evaluating and selecting hearing aids for severely hearing impaired children', *Journal of Speech and Hearing Disorders*, **36**, 341

Grover, B. C. (1974) 'The shape of earmoulds', *Hearing*, **29**, 232

Grover, B. C. (1976) 'Acoustic modifications to earmoulds', *British Journal of Audiology*, **10**, 8

Grover, B. C. and Martin, M. C. (1974) 'On the practical gain limit for post aural hearing aids', *British Journal of Audiology*, **8**, 121

Grover, B. C. and Martin, M. C. (1978) Physical and subjective correlations of earmould occlusion. *Audiology* (In press)

HAIC (1961) *Standard method of Expressing the Performance of Hearing Aids*. Washington D.C.; Hearing Aid Industry Conference Inc.

Harford, E. and Barry, J. (1965) 'A rehabilitative approach to the problems of unilateral hearing impairment: The Contralateral Routing of Signals (CROS)', *Journal of Speech and Hearing Disorders*, **30**, 121

Johannson, B. (1959) 'A new coding amplifier system for the severely hard of hearing'. *Proceedings of Third International Congress of Acoustics, Stuttgart*, Vol. **2**, 655

Johannson, B. (1966) 'The use of the transposer for the management of the deaf child', *Journal of International Society of Audiology*, **5**, 362

IEC Publication 118 (1959) *Recommended Methods for Measurements of the Electro-acoustical Characteristics of Hearing Aids*. Geneva; International Electrotechnical Commission

IEC Publication 118-1 (1975) *Methods of Measurement of Characteristics of Hearing Aids with Induction Pick-up Coil Input*. Geneva; International Electrotechnical Commission

IEC Publication 118-2 (1977) *Hearing Aids with Automatic Gain Control Circuits*. Geneva; International Electrotechnical Commission

IEC 118-3 (1978) *Hearing Aid Equipment not entirely Worn on the Listener*. Geneva; International Electrotechnical Commission

IEC 118-4 (1978) *Magnetic Field Strength in Induction Loops*. Geneva; International Electrotechnical Commission

IEC Publication 126 (1973) *IEC Reference Coupler for the Measurement of Hearing Aids Using Earphones Coupled to the Ear by Means of Ear Inserts*. Geneva; International Electrotechnical Commission.

Martin, M. C. (1973) 'Hearing aid gain requirements in sensorineural hearing loss', *British Journal of Audiology* **7**, 21

Martin, M. C. (1976) 'Hearing aid gain and output requirements in sensorineural hearing loss'. In *Disorders of Auditory Function*, II, pp. 265–272 Ed. by Stephens, S. D. G. London; Academic Press

Martin, M. C. (1978) 'Individual hearing aids: selection and prescription', *Journal of the Royal Society of Medicine*, **71**, 4

Powell, C. A. and Tucker, I. G. (1976) 'A method of predicting the optimum listening levels of hearing impaired children', *Scandinavian Audiology*, **5**, 167

RNID (1977) *A List of Current Hearing Aids*. London; Royal National Institute for the Deaf

Velmans, M. (1974) 'The design of speech recoding devices for the deaf', *British Journal of Audiology*, **8**, 1

Woodford, C. M. and Holmes, D. W. (1977) 'Relationship between loudness discomfort level and acoustic threshold in a clinical population, *Audiology and Hearing Education*, Oct./Nov.

Zwislocki, J. J. (1970) *An Acoustic Coupler for Earphone Calibration*, Report LSC—5–7. Syracuse University; Laboratory of Sensory Communications

29 Rehabilitation of adults with acquired hearing loss
K S Pegg

THE problem of deafness, as with any other aspect of human behaviour is unique to the individual concerned. With most aspects of physical handicap, expectations are apparent and behaviour is determined by the obvious nature of the disability; this is not true of the deaf. The terms 'hearing impairment' or 'deafness' which are used to describe a person's disability give no indication of the degree of impairment, and to define deafness as a malfunction of the auditory mechanism is no more satisfactory, because it tells us nothing about the functional nature of the handicap. Whilst there is no clearly defined and accepted system of classification, it would seem convenient to define the handicap in terms of need and function.

Broadly speaking there are three groups of deaf people. There are those who are deaf from birth; those who become deaf in childhood after hearing normally; and the largest group of all, those with an acquired hearing loss who become hard of hearing in adult life. This chapter is mainly concerned with the problems of the last group; problems which differ little from those described by Beethoven 175 years ago.

'O my fellow men who consider me, or describe me as, unfriendly, peevish or even misanthropic, how greatly do you wrong me. For you do not know the secret reason why I appear to you to be so . . . Though endowed with a passionate and lively temperament and ever fond of the distractions offered by society I was soon obliged to seclude myself and live in solitude. If at times I decided just to ignore my infirmity, alas, how cruelly was I then driven back by the intensified sad experience of my poor hearing. Yet I could not bring myself to say to people: "Speak up, shout, for I am deaf " . . . Moreover my misfortune pains me doubly, for inasmuch as it leads to my being misjudged. For there can be no relaxation in human society, no refined conversation, no mutual confidences. I must live quite alone and may creep into society only as often as sheer necessity demands. I must live like an outcast. If I appear in company I am overcome by a burning anxiety, a fear that I am running the risk of letting people know my condition . . . But how humiliated I have felt if someone standing beside me heard the sound of a flute in the distance and I heard nothing—such experiences almost made me despair, and I was at the point of putting an end to my life—the only thing that held me back was my art. For indeed it seemed to me to be impossible to leave this world before I had produced all the works that I felt the urge to compose . . .' (Marek, 1969.)

The following comments were made, in written form, by a housewife suffering from a sensorineural hearing impairment. She was undertaking a rehabilitation programme at the time.

' "You don't look deaf!" This was said to me last week and led me on to a train of thought. What is a deaf person meant to look like, and if we don't fit into the image, does this cause a breakdown in communication? If one isn't elderly, wears a small post-aural aid and still has a spring in the step, is it too much to expect normal hearing people to cooperate? Do we have to do all the hard work of making sense of what others say, trying not to inconvenience them? Advertisements for hearing aids tell us: "Wear such and such a hearing aid and your friends will never know you are hard of hearing." Why the guilt complex?

Even when your friends know, they aren't much help. An evening spent in their home and you end up feeling like a puppet, nodding and smiling at what you hope are the right moments. If you are dining out it is easier, the range is closer, but if you lip-read everything stops while you tackle your meal! If you are not the type to be constantly demanding, "Speak up, I am deaf", what can you do?

In the past few years, people have said to me, "You manage very well, you don't inflict your handicap on others"—but I have still suffered in the process.

In this enlightened and permissive age, when anything and everything from drugs to sex are frankly discussed, and even have official backing, surely public opinion and imagination could be stimulated to help the deaf, whose only shortcoming is not being able to comprehend their native tongue.

I am very grateful for the loan of the headphones to enable me to listen to radio, TV and records. It was such a successful experiment that we now have bought a set and for the first time in many years I can hear clearly over the various items of equipment and delight in being able to really participate.'

As knowledge and understanding of the problems increase so too does the realization that greater efforts are needed to help the hearing-impaired to achieve a greater degree of adjustment to their disability. As has been said, the problem differs from individual to individual, but most adults with a socially significant hearing loss which cannot be treated medically or surgically could obtain some help from a hearing aid given that follow-up support was available. Yet too often the only treatment offered to the hard-of-hearing person is the issue of a hearing aid, and such treatment, without proper counselling is generally thought to be inadequate.

The problem of the child deaf from birth is different from that of a person who suddenly becomes deaf in adult life. The adult who has become progressively deaf over a number of years is different again, but for all of them difficulties in communication present practical problems. When the time comes for the born-deaf youngster to leave school his language development, speech, educational standards and general knowledge will generally be much below average. This means that he is likely to accept an occupation at a standard considerably below the level of his innate ability, because he is generally unable to compete with his hearing peers in employment. He is unable to follow courses of further education unless given a great deal of assistance, and his social activities may be restricted. The problem of the adult who has become deaf either slowly or suddenly presents quite a different picture. It is true that his handicap is still one of communcication. Whilst he can speak he cannot clearly understand the speech of others. He feels isolated and tends more and more to avoid company unless measures are taken to assist him to overcome his handicap, and to the normal stress of everyday life is added a further strain.

It is almost impossible for those who have been brought up in a hearing and speaking society to imagine what it would be like to be born deaf. We can, however, try to put ourselves in the position of an adult who has an acquired hearing loss. We can imagine passing from the stage when people no longer seem to speak as clearly as they once did, to the stage when we are forced to accept that there is something wrong with our hearing. On seeking medical advice we may find that there is no treatment appropriate in our case, but we can have a hearing aid. Up to this point we may have felt depressed, but are now likely to be less so because we are going to be given an instrument which will restore our hearing. It could be, however, that we will be disappointed. We could well find that whilst sounds generally are made much louder, the sounds of speech are no clearer, and we are quite unprepared for this. If, we are amongst the fortunate ones, we will be given instruction in how to use the instrument to the best advantage. We may also be told that it would be advisable to learn to lip-read and be told where we might go for instruction. However, the chances are that we will not be given this information, but will be left to work out our own salvation, often with tragic social results.

If, however, we are amongst the fortunate few we will be shown comprehensively how to use the hearing aid, told what it will do and what it will not do, where it will work most effectively and where it will not. We will practise lip-reading and find that our ability to communicate is improving, but we may also find that even using hearing and lip-reading combined, we become tired much more quickly than in the past. We may also become aware that lip-reading is ambiguous and that we make mistakes, and whilst some people are easy to lip-read, others are almost impossible.

Practical problems may well be increasing at the same time. We begin to find that our leisure-time activities are curtailed and that we can get little pleasure from the radio or record player, and only a limited amount from television. We try to keep going with visits to friends but are likely to be resentful if we are not helped to take part in conversation and we shall be disinclined to accept an invitation to dinner when we know that our hostess is keen on dining by candlelight. If we get into difficulties with our friends and family what is likely to happen at work? It may have taken us 20 years to reach our present level of employment, but can we still manage? It is imperative that we do so, because if we fail it will almost inevitably mean a financial loss could affect not only our self-esteem but could possibly even change the living standards of our family. There are many things to remember and practise if we are to overcome our handicap. We have to try not to strain to see or hear speech and we must try to remain relaxed, but at the same time alert and 'tuned in'. We know that we are not going to understand every word and that we must be constantly looking for key words. We have to manage every situation to our advantage, but we have also to remember that conversation is a two-way affair, so that in attempting to control it we must not monopolize it.

Irene Ewing described her own experience as a hard-of-hearing person suffering from progressive deafness and the effect it had on hearing speech. She carefully noted the stages of her own deafness which gave an indication of the increase in difficulty in proportion to the degree of deafness. First she found that attentive listening became necessary in order to follow speech in a large room, or where several people were talking simultaneously. She then found that in spite of attentive listening, many words and phrases were inaudible in everyday conversation, and unstressed and unfamiliar words were rarely intelligible. As her hearing deteriorated further she found that concentrated listening was necessary at all times, unstressed syllables were inaudible, and although a speaker's voice was heard, few words were intelligible. Finally with very severe deafness only a few stressed words could be heard and sometimes only the vowels could be identified (Ewing and Ewing, 1947).

Some or all of these difficulties are part of the everyday experience of hard-of-hearing adults. They occur in spite of long-established mental habits that condition and facilitate the comprehension of speech, and the use of words in the expression of thought. 'Why is it so difficult for other people to understand our difficulties?' This question, posed in a variety of ways, is almost inevitably raised by the hard-of-hearing adult who is aware of the care and help which is available for other disabled people, but cannot understand why society is so little concerned with the problem of deafness.

Certainly the effects of deafness are not always easily perceived, but it should be remembered that whilst blindness cuts off a person from things, deafness cuts off a person from other people. The hard-of-hearing person may feel embarrassed, frustrated, irritated or perhaps humiliated when he fails to grasp, even after several repetitions, the meaning of what has been said to him because of the inherent ambiguities of lip-reading. The effects of this long-drawn-out form of mental stress are cumulative over the months and years. We are not suggesting that physically normal people do not suffer from irritation, frustration and embarrassment from time to time for various reasons, but it is obvious that the hard-of-hearing share all these experiences, but with the added frustration caused by their inability to take part easily in normal communication. As was pointed out in the Department of Health and Social Security Report (1973):

> 'However, an acquired hearing loss in adults may also have grave social consequences, with impairment of the ability to understand normal speech. The difficulty normal people have in comprehending this disability may be responsible, in part, for the lack of research work with the exception of surgically remedial deafness.'

A hearing loss inevitably causes some degree of psychological disruption to which a person must become adjusted. Much human interreaction and learning depends to a great extent on what is heard. Psychological problems of the hard-of-hearing seem to manifest themselves in varying degrees of inadequacy due to missing much of what is being said; feelings of being talked about and above all the significantly reduced communication skills. It is little wonder that the adult who has lost his hearing to whatever degree will often become discouraged and depressed, and sometimes will even become suspicious of friends and family.

With hard-of-hearing adults one sometimes observes a subtle personality change, which appears to be more serious than might be expected from the degree of hearing loss, and this suggests that other factors are involved. Some explanation for this can be found in considering the working of normal hearing and the three operational levels of functioning, as Ramsdell (1970) has pointed out. The first on the social level, where hearing is used to comprehend spoken language, and since language is symbolic in nature, this level of auditory function may be called 'the symbolic level'. Sound also serves as a direct signal or sign through which we make adjustments in daily living, and this level can be referred to as a 'warning level'. Thirdly, there is the level at which sound serves neither as a symbol nor a warning but simply as a background to our feeling of being part of a living world and contributing to our sense of being alive. At this level we react to the changing background of sounds of the world around us without being aware that we hear them. Lack of this background of feeling adds greatly to the hard-of-hearing person's sense of isolation. So hearing loss presents obvious problems at the symbolic level, the warning level and the background level. It is small wonder that some hard-of-hearing people suffer from depression, isolation, self-consciousness, unsociability, lack of confidence and sometimes neurotic conditions, and that they are in need of rehabilitative help. It has been argued that acquired deafness, especially if sudden in onset, causes more emotional trauma and adjustment problems than does congenital deafness. It may well be that losing something one has always experienced has adverse consequences, which are worse than not having had it at all. Such arguments, however, are hypothetical and fail to take into account the linguistic and experiential difficulty of those deaf from birth.

The intellectual capacity of the hard-of-hearing adult must be included in any considerations concerning the relationship between hearing impairment and the overall handicap. Often the more able person will be likely to compensate for his hearing impairment more readily than the person with a lesser intellectual ability. It must be borne in mind however that there are numerous cases to which this criterion does not apply. A hearing impairment has many far-reaching implications for the person's life-style. For the hard-of-hearing adult, impairment is bound up with an interaction between intellectual ability, the drive to improve, the onset of the hearing loss and its extent, the type of impairment, the age, and to a large measure the effectiveness of the remedial programmes available. The last 20 years have seen progress in a number of fields which have brought benefit to the hard-of-hearing. In medicine there is the availability of antibiotics and the micro-surgery of the middle ear; there has been improvement in the design of amplifying equipment of all kinds; speech audiometry has been used as a standardized procedure for the prescription of hearing aids; and there has been an expansion of lip-reading facilities, although this form of rehabilitation remains inadequate. The hard-of-hearing individual is forced by the very nature of his handicap to utilize lip-reading as a major suppport for diminished and sometimes distorted auditory information. People with normal hearing utilize visual clues subconsciously, but since they are seldom in a situation in which they are wholly dependent upon them they are generally unaware that they possess this ability, to lesser or greater extent.

Lip-reading

Lip-reading for those who are deaf can be described as the total process of looking at, perceiving and interpreting spoken words. The lip-reader as a person must be concerned with the sensory reception of the movement pattern of spoken words, the perception of the pattern and its association at a conceptual level. He must also have flexibility in order to replace or 'fill in' information he has received.

Most of us have unconsciously learned that if we watch a speaker, we do not have to listen as intently. We get information more readily when we can both see and hear the speaker and in a verbal exchange we watch intently, not only to enhance the verbal message, but to take in the facial expressions, the gestures, the subtle postural changes, as well as the situational clues which can convey so much information. In noisy situations such as are found at large social gatherings, on the underground train or in a factory, people become even more dependent on visual clues, if they are to communicate effectively. A person who becomes deaf is sometimes advised to take a course of lip-reading instruction and there is a tendency towards the idea that if a hearing-impaired person learns to lip-read his ability to communicate will be restored to normal, but there are wide variations in the ability to lip-read. Some are 'born lip-readers', the majority have reasonable facility in utilizing visual clues, but some find it most difficult. Certain factors which make for good lip-reading have been explored, but there is reason to suppose that there may be other factors underlying the process that are not fully understood. Lip-reading skills can be improved with training, determination and practice, but individual differences seem to persist despite training—at least with the kind of training commonly employed to date.

Pauls (1970) considered that language is man's most unique characteristic and can be defined as the mind's use of a common symbol code. It is the core of all aspects of human communication, whether it be the comprehension of oral language through hearing or lip-reading, the comprehension of reading or of the spoken word. Lip-reading is a process similar to reading and, like learning to read, learning to lip-read has two steps. Firstly, one must learn to identify and hold in memory a sequence of visual patterns and secondly, one must comprehend the message that is conveyed by the language code. One must have an adequate command of language in order to read, or to lip-read for comprehension. The adult who has language firmly established before acquiring a hearing loss has a different problem from that of the child who has never heard, or who has never heard well, and so must slowly acquire his language in spite of a defective auditory system. One cannot readily understand language forms that one does not know, either from the lips or from the printed page.

Decoding lip-reading is a more difficult process than reading the printed page. In both processes one is identifying and discriminating fleeting visual events that must be held in short-term memory as the language message unfolds. For the lip-reader however, these patterns are never fixed as they are on the printed page, and he cannot review unless the speaker repeats. To complicate the process further there are wide variations in the phonemes that make up spoken words, phrases and sentences. Similarly there are variations in the visual patterns that are presented by different speakers even when using the same material. All this is further affected by lighting, distance from the speaker and the angle at which the speaker must be read. Although lip-reading involves the same processes as scanning the printed page, it demands more of the lip-reader in terms of visual perception and visual memory.

Jeffers and Barley (1971) refer to certain factors which influence progress in lip-reading.

(1) Perceptual efficiency—which includes the ability to identify speech sounds or elements and perceive them rapidly, and also the ability to gain information from the face when the focus is on the mouth. Associated with these processes are visual acuity, attention, speed of focusing and peripheral vision.

(2) Synthetic ability—which includes the ability to identify parts and patterns (words and phrases) and the overall content of a message.

(3) Flexibility—which fosters the ability to revise tentative identification of a message.

Among secondary factors are the amount and kind of training, language proficiency, motivation, and reaction to frustration and failure. Associated with language proficiency is intelligence and the extent and pattern of the subject's impairment of hearing, its duration and age of onset.

Lip-reading as a skill enables a person, regardless of whether his hearing is normal or impaired, to understand language by attentively observing the speaker.

Spoken language is a rapid succession of meaningful sounds with varying degrees of visibility. These sounds are divided into vowels and consonants and are produced by changing the shape of the mouth and the positions of the tongue, teeth, lips and jaw, and it is these rapidly changing movements that the lip-reader must interpret. Only about one third of speech sounds are clearly visible but the lip-reader must be able to recognize these movements and learn to 'fill-in' those which are invisible. It may seem impossible to lip-read when only one third of the sounds are clearly visible, but we are all accustomed to the same sort of confusion, although to a lesser degree. Two or more words may look alike on the lips, and the lip-reader must decide from context which one is said. This is not so different from what we must all do with words that sound alike, or the words that have different meanings depending on how they are used. However the lip-reader has many more choices to make as well as blanks to fill in and he must learn to hold in mind the visual pattern as it appears on the lips and translate it into meaningful language. The same group of words said with different emphasis and phrasing will have its meaning changed completely. In this way Pauls (1970) suggests that we read aloud the following sentences, stressing the words in capitals, and not the result:

> "GOOD! By God, we're going to Kansas"
> "Goodbye! GOD, We're going to Kansas"
> "Goodbye, God! We're going to KANSAS"

Facial expression, gesture and postural changes are frequently as revealing as the words uttered. Often the object handled, or pointed to, gives a valuable clue, and the place and the particular speaker shed light on the topic under discussion. The deaf and hard-of-hearing must learn to recognize and employ the details of every speech situation. The more limited his hearing, the greater the strain on the lip-reader, for his attention is concentrated on this rapid succession of ever changing movements that vary with each speaker. This rapid flow of speech must be grasped in a fleeting instance, for there is no opportunity for review. Interpretation must be almost instantaneous. Lip-reading is seldom easy, because there are so many factors which cannot be controlled. Attentive observation of all these factors demands such alertness that tension and fatigue are produced in a relatively short time. Then, too, poor lighting, distance, noise and confusion and distracting movements can defeat even the most experienced lip-reader. The secret of successful lip-reading lies in the ability to grasp an idea intuitively and develop its meaning without attempting to follow every word. A too literal person, or one who clings tenaciously to an idea about where the conversation is leading, always has serious difficulties. Whilst it is essential to be on the alert to spot trends and changes in conversation, it is also true that undue tension and fatigue may cause a breakdown in communication. Therefore the lip-reader must strive for the happy medium. From the beginning the lip-reader needs to cultivate a sense of humour to help him to overcome the inevitable failures.

The deafened adult's application and determination are vital factors in achieving success and it should be emphasized that a person with a hearing loss should frankly face the fact. The natural tendency is to ignore the hearing impairment or to attempt to conceal it, but these efforts, even though partially sucessful for a while, lead to an increasing strain. Eventually, social and business life will be affected.

Ballantyne (1960) quotes the words of Kenneth M. Day, himself a severely-deafened otologist:

> 'I wasted from five to ten of what should have been the best years of my life as a selfish, depressed and self-pitying man . . . I was like an ostrich with my head in the sand trying to conceal something which everyone already knew. It was not until I finally accepted my deafness as an unalterable fact and acquired the determination to overcome my handicap, that I really began to enjoy life again . . .'

Since 1900 there have been a number of advocates of specific methods of teaching lip-reading and some have written about their approaches. These include Nitchie (1912), Bruhn (1924), Ewing (1930), Kinzie and Kinzie (1931) and Bunger (1961).

All these lip-reading methods tend to be overtly structured, outlining materials and procedures in detail, but they do contain the distillation of years of experience. Many people have learned to lip-read by each of these methods, but there is no evidence to date that one approach is more effective than another. All stress the need for synthesis, rather than analysis, for successful lip-reading. Also in varying degrees, they stress the value of auditory and kinesthetic clues in enhancing visual clues. The major differences lie in the way the speech positions and movements are presented to the student so that he learns to recognize and discriminate between them on the lips. All systematically employ syllabic drills using the movement or position of the lesson, and then provide practice using them in words, sentences and stories. All but the Jena method—used by Bunger—proceed from the visible to the less visible and from the simple to the complex as the lessons are developed in a course. The Jena method is unique in its presentation of an overall introduction to phonetics in the first few lessons, then relying on rhythmic syllable drills and talking-together exercises to enhance automatic recognition. It is held that this has the advantage of permitting more freedom in the construction of the lesson by not restricting students to a particular sound per lesson. Instead, each lesson is constructed round a topic, such as dining out, shopping, travel and the like. Interest is sustained by the unity of the topic and valuable experience in anticipating the turn of the conversation can be set up, as a wealth of material can be employed round a central theme.

Traditionally, the teaching of lip-reading has been approached like other academic subjects. Teachers planning lessons have stressed starting with certain sounds and movements and progressing through a series of exercises until the work has been covered. In doing so it was hoped that the hearing-impaired student would succeed in the art of lip-reading. There is some merit in formal lip-reading lessons but it is felt that a flexible approach has more to offer. No two hearing-impaired persons are alike and therefore the needs of each differ. Whilst the long-term aim of a teacher of lip-reading will be the same for the number of persons in the class—teaching them all to lip-read—the intermediate aims will vary, and it is with these specific aims that the teacher is concerned daily. The methods used to attain these specific aims are dictated by the hard-of-hearing individual and will depend upon the degree of hearing impairment; to what extent is he prepared to admit to an impairment; his lip-reading ability and how motivated he is to improve this ability; his age, occupation and social life. Each person must be dealt with individually and in terms of his individual needs but this does not mean that all lip-reading training must be carried out on a one-to-one basis. For most students class instruction is preferable to individual instruction but in the class every effort must be made to provide each individual with material and practice he needs by presenting carefully planned lessons.

As an alternative to formal exercises there is a place for the more varied and stimulating approach. All teachers should be aware of the analytical method. There are those whose personalities are more suited to a formal presentation of a lesson whilst others teach more effectively by using a freer approach.

The historical development of lip-reading and research

We will now look briefly at some aspects of the historical development of lip-reading. Records indicate that a few individuals in England from the middle of the seventeenth century had been concerned with the problems of deaf children but not with deafened adults, for example Bulwer, Wallis, Holder, Dalgarno, Baker and Braidwood. The first institution for the education of deaf mutes was firmly established in the Old Kent Road, London by the beginning of the nineteenth century. In the decade which followed schools for the deaf were opened in Birmingham, Manchester, Liverpool, Exeter and Doncaster. As a result of the Education Act 1870, School Boards were set up. The provision for deaf children made by the London School Board was the first occasion in which the education of these children was assisted by public funds. Very soon other areas followed this example and classes for the deaf were opened in Sheffield, Leeds, Nottingham, Bradford, Bristol, Leicester and Oldham.

Most of the early teachers of the deaf were oralists who taught speech to their children. Emphasis in training was usually placed on the development of speech. Speech and lip-reading were not taught directly. Learning to understand through speech-reading was believed to occur as a by-product of the development of articulation skill. Certainly in the process of learning to talk many children also learned to lip-read as they observed their teacher. During the years methods of teaching language and speech, but not of lip-reading as such, emerged and were recorded in the literature. By the last decades of the nineteenth century lip-reading was beginning to be thought of as a separate skill to be taught apart from the teaching of articulation to deaf children. In various parts of the world hard-of-hearing adults had become aware of lip-reading and were asking for classes to be started for them. It apparently did not occur to anyone to consider seriously how the approach to lip-reading instruction might be different if one were dealing with individuals with established speech and language patterns. The early teachers taught lip-reading to the hard-of-hearing almost as though they were teaching articulation, and used a similar approach, working from the part to the whole, that is from the element to the syllable to the word to the phrase.

'The development of a philosophy and methodology of teaching speech-reading as a receptive skill distinct from speech had to wait the time when attention turned to helping the hard-of-hearing adult with established speech and language patterns. This did not occur until near the end of the nineteenth century. And by this time the teaching of speech-reading was inextricably interwoven and confused with the teaching of articulation to deaf children.' (Marek, 1969.)

This confusion between speech- and lip-reading was to continue for a number of years. There were three major errors in this thinking. The first was the assumption that the student must know how the sounds are formed, the second and perhaps major error was the implicit assumption that skill in lip-reading could be developed sound by sound, that is through a cumulative knowledge of lip movements or articulatory positions. It was assumed that all speech sounds were visible at least to some degree. Sounds that were not normally visible were made visible. The third confusion was to do with mirror practice which had stemmed from the teaching of articulation.

'To attempt to learn to speech-read others by watching oneself is comparable to trying to learn to read through reading what one has just written. Such practice can scarcely be considered speech-reading since the student knows what he is saying.' (Jeffers and Barley, 1971.)

It took a number of years to develop the insight that something was wrong with the part-whole method of teaching lip-reading. One of the first teachers of lip-reading to realize this appears to have been Nitchie (1912, 1917) in the USA. Although accepting that the part-whole method of teaching lip-reading is wrong we must not lose sight of the fact that a knowledge of articulation is necessary both to the teacher and the student in the area of speech conservation. Although lip-reading has been taught in England for many years there has been relatively little interest in research in this area. The teachers concerned seem to have been always more concerned with teaching than with research, and with results rather than with theory. Most of the early work was, of course, with born-deaf children and the most significant advances with adults with acquired hearing loss have only taken place during the present century. Even today some of the most skilled teachers of lip-reading find difficulty in analysing exactly what they are doing in the intuitive approaches they use. It is, therefore, not surprising that in Britain today there appears to be no well documented research information concerning lip-reading. On the whole the few articles available are anecdotal and concerned mainly with methodology (Boultbee, 1902; Hewett, 1904; Story, 1910; Boultbee, 1913; Ewing 1930; Clegg, 1953; Wyatt, 1960). Of course the complexity of lip-reading and the factors that are believed to affect the acquisition of this skill may well have daunted many. Lip-reading skill involves visual acuity, memory, synthetic ability, language-handling proficiency and maturation, to name some of these factors. It is extremely difficult, if not impossible, to study one of these variables, while, at the same time controlling the others. Lip-reading is, of course, a skill amenable to training, but it can be a skill for which a person may or may not have natural aptitude. This causes us to ask how good lip-readers differ from poor lip-readers. Can we isolate the physical, intellectual, educational and emotional variables which go to make up success in lip-reading. At this stage of our knowledge, much of our analysis has to be based on experience and intuitive knowledge. This is not meant to disparage either experience or intuitive knowledge but rather to suggest that this is best supported by scientific measurement and research.

Although research in lip-reading has not been productive in our country there has been some considerable work carried out in the USA to which we must now turn.

Probably the first experimental investigation of lip-reading was attempted by Kitson (1915), who carried out a study of the various factors assumed to be related to speech-reading skill. Much of this and other early research was lost sight of in attempts to develop tests of speech-reading for deaf children. Pintner (1929) employed face-to-face lip-reading tests in a study of the lip-reading ability of deaf students enrolled in a residential school for the deaf. No significant correlation was found between lip-reading ability and the scores obtained from the Pintner Non-Language Mental Test. Heider and Heider (1940) using a filmed test of lip-reading performance found no significant relationship between speech-reading proficiency and scholastic achievement.

Reid (1946) also used a filmed lip-reading test with deaf girls and found that there was no significant correlation between speech-reading, and scholastic achievement and intelligence as measured by the Stanford Achievement Tests. Utley (1946 a) produced what is probably the best known and most widely used test of lip-reading ability. This test was based on interests and experiences that were believed to be common to children of secondary-school age. It was not found possible to standardize this test of lip-reading in the sense of establishing norms with respect to age or some common variable. However, the data were organized according to raw scores and percentile ranks from which it was possible to judge the relative proficiency indicated by a given score.

The hypothesis that it should be possible to predict lip-reading skill from measurements of learning or training was repostulated by both Reid (1946) and Utley (1946, a and b), although the previous research of Pintner (1929) and Heider and Heider (1940) had indicated no such predictive relationship. The work of Utley and the test she evolved have been criticized as being excessively difficult by Di Carlo and Kataja (1951) and Heider (1949). More recently Jeffers (1967) attempted to re-evaluate the Utley lip-reading sentence test and she concluded that there was reason to believe that some of the difficulty at least was in the filming and not in the content. This point of view was also confirmed by Jeffers and Barley (1971) who reaffirmed the usefulness of the Utley Sentence Tests for the diagnosis of lip-reading ability provided the test was given 'live' and presented in such a way as to provide optimal viewing conditions.

The idea that a high degree of association should exist between lip-reading and measures of learning has died hard because of its apparent reasonableness. Utley's work is especially important in this respect, for correlations high enough to permit prediction were not found between her test and reading level, scholastic achievement, chronological age, age of onset of deafness or school placement. Her work also points to the fact that lip-reading was not highly correlated with indices of language comprehension or training and that the skill development could not be predicted from such measures. Teachers of lip-reading have always been aware of the marked individual differences in students to master the skill. Experience seems to point to the fact that many lip-readers have marked ability not based in logic. Perhaps this is why many years before, both Kitson (1915) and Nitchie (1917) felt in a rather intuitive way that there was some mental ability or combination of mental abilities at the basis of lip-reading skill. They suggested that there was a possible importance of concentration on visual memory and intuitive reasoning. Since Utley's major contribution the attention of research has moved more in this direction with a consideration of specific visual and mental aptitudes that might account for the wide differences that are found in respect of lip-reading proficiency. In very recent years there have been many moves in research along these broad lines.

Lowell (1961) as a result of the many studies carried out in the John Tracy Clinic, Los Angeles, involving several thousand hearing and deaf people, felt there was evidence to confirm the fact that whilst ability to lip-read varies widely from person to person, on average women are better lip-readers than men. The use of aptitude and personality tests as prognostic instruments concerned with lip-reading efficiency yielded barely significant coefficients of correlation. It was claimed that lip-reading ability was relatively independent of other abilities, or that it is so complex that no test of a single trait or ability will prognosticate lip-reading success.

Black, O'Reilly and Peck (1963) sought to measure the influence of training on lip-reading skill using a self-administered teaching machine approach. In this experiment the lip-reader largely determined his procedure for increasing proficiency in lip-reading a set passage. A study involving only a single training period could of course do little more than suggest that a programmed and self-administered approach to lip-reading instruction should be explored further. The speed of presenting the silent filmed material did not appear critical, at least within a range from normal speed to 15 per cent reduction in speed.

Schwartz and Black (1967) looked at the effect of sentence structure on lip-reading. They used a kernel sentence and a comparison was made of the difficulty in lip-reading various transformations. Six kernel sentences and their transpositions were repeated to normal-hearing students in the presence of masking noise. The results were claimed to indicate that generative grammar with its transformational rules (Chomsky, 1965) related systematically to success in lip-reading. Kernel sentences and passive structures were most easily lip-read, whereas negative and query-type structures were least so.

Jeffers (1969) considered the social adequacy of two selected samples of geriatric presbyacusics with significant hearing loss. She examined clinical records and used a test of social adequacy with these subjects who had been enrolled in adult lip-reading classes. It was estimated that approximately only 15 per cent had serious problems of speech reception when utilizing hearing aids and lip-reading. This was felt to indicate that the presbyacusis population was not more neglected than other populations as is so often assumed. No account appears to have been taken of the motivation factors which had caused the subjects to enrol in the first place, and of course, we know nothing about the much greater number of them who, for one reason or another, did not avail themselves of any rehabilitative help.

Sanders and Coscarelli (1970) conducted a study concerning the relationship of visual synthesis skill to lip-reading. The lip-reading scores they obtained were significantly correlated with the visual synthesis scores. It is of interest to note that the better lip-readers, with or without training, were superior in visual synthesis to the poorer speech-readers. These results argue strongly for a synthetic approach to the teaching of speech-reading and suggest a need for special teaching procedures to develop and enhance visual synthetic skills in students of lip-reading.

Hardick, Oyer and Irion (1970) considered lip-reading performance as related to measurements of vision. They administered the Utley speech-reading test to a group of 53 undergraduates. The eight subjects who obtained the highest scores and the eight who obtained the lowest scores were then given a complete ophthalmic examination. A significant relationship was found between visual acuity and lip-reading performance. Berger (1971) attempted to measure the influence of motivation as related to lip-reading ability but met with little success. Following the attempted motivation the resulting scores differed only slightly and were attributed to guessing rather than actual change in skill. He suggested that areas other than motivation needed to be investigated in attempts to improve lip-reading skills.

Berger, Garner and Sudman (1971) investigated the effect of degree of facial exposure and vertical angle of vision on lip-reading performance. In a study on 30 female university students they failed to find statistically significant test differences.

It was however suggested that lip-reading appeared to be most efficient when the teacher was positioned on the same level as the lip-reader and allowed the entire face to be clearly visible. Berger, Martin and Sakoff (1970) considered the effect of visual distractions on lip-reading. Moving and changing distractions were designed to simulate real-life situations. Unexpectedly, the difference between the two groups of the experiment appeared to have no statistical significance. It was considered that this pointed to a relatively small effect of visual distractions on lip-reading. On the other hand the effect of noise on lip-reading performance of normal hearing young adults carried out by Berger and Lewis (1972) is of interest. Using a test of lip-reading in quiet and in continuous and intermittent noise backgrounds they too found their results were not statistically significant. They hypothesized that the predictable nature of the noises used in their experiment allowed the subjects to adapt more readily to them.

It seems that there has been a considerable contribution to research into lip-reading during the last decade, not the least being the contribution of Jeffers and Barley (1971). This work acts as a guide to skills believed necessary for lip-reading success, and divides the factors which appear to determine lip-reading ability into primary and secondary factors. The primary factors are derived from an analysis of what the speech-reader does and in essence constitute the processes encompassed by the skill. They are visual perceptual proficiency (visual perception, speed of perception, peripheral perception), synthetic ability (perceptual closure, conceptual closure) and flexibility (revision of perceptual closures and revision of conceptual closures). The secondary factors are in reality 'back-up' factors. They include training, knowledge of language and emotional attitudes or sets that facilitate the acquisition of lip-reading skill. There is little doubt that motivation plays an important part in lip-reading, as we have already seen. As yet there has been little other significant work in the area of motivation which has provided 'spin-off' into the teaching of lip-reading skills.

It has been emphasized that areas other than motivation should also be investigated in attempts to improve lip-reading skills. Sudman and Berger (1971) also considered aspects of two-dimensional versus three-dimensional viewing in speech-reading. They examined this by requiring 20 subjects alternatively to lip-read the profile of a speaker as seen by silhouette and as seen normally. The normal profile view produced significantly higher lip-reading scores than the silhouette-profile view. It was speculated that the visual clues available to the lip-reader are greater in a live situation than by film or television, and greater in a filmed or televised view than in a silhouette view.

Auditory training

Auditory training involves a number of steps whereby the severely handicapped person learns to take advantage of all the acoustic clues still available to him. There must first be a development of awareness of sound, then experience and training in differentiating grossly different sounds from one another, making broad discriminations among speech sounds, and finally close discrimination among speech sounds with highly similar characteristics.

Hirsch (1970) felt that, in very early childhood, babies with normal hearing accompanied by normal intelligence learn to respond to and to distinguish between a wide variety of sounds; they seem to differentiate the sounds of different persons approaching, to recognize speech-like sounds from adults and other children, and eventually to control, through hearing, their own production of speech. Through their auditory reception of speech around them they appear to acquire the rules for making words and sentences in their own language.

The normal processes of auditory learning are not followed either by the child with a congenital hearing impairment or by the adventitiously deafened child or adult, and compensatory auditory training should be provided. The subject must have intact perceptual discrimination to enable him to distinguish meaningful sound from background noise, and his short-term memory must be sufficiently good for the sounds perceived to be stored so that they may be fitted into the pattern of phrases and sentences. He must also be capable of understanding the rules of his language so that the patterns become meaningful. Thus equipped, the hearing-impaired person must learn to use his residual hearing to the fullest possible extent. Auditory training should include helping him to notice facial expression, intonation, gesture as well as attending to acoustic clues. Auditory perception is based upon the ability to respond differently to different sound patterns.

The historical development of auditory training and research

Although auditory training has occupied the attention of educators and physicians over the years, as with speech-reading, it had its real beginnings in the early education of deaf children. However, unlike the development of lip-reading in which fairly well-defined and somewhat formal methods were evolved, the development of auditory training has in most instances been generally less formal.

The first real attempt to make use of the hearing of deaf children through auditory training took place in France. Jean Itard, a prominent Paris otologist in 1802 can be regarded as the pioneer in accomplishing auditory training. He found that the regular repetition of loud sounds developed an increased perception of speech in severely-deaf children. Musical tones, the drum and the sonorous tones of a bell were used, and he emphasized that all such stimuli must be consistently and persistently applied.

Many of these ideas were taken up by others. In England, Toynbee and Wilde showed interest in this field. In Germany Beck, Jager, Wolff and Frank were carrying out similar work; in France, Itard's contribution was extended by Blanchet and Deleau; and in the USA at Nebraska there are reports of teachers experimenting along similar lines.

The next great contribution comes from Vienna. In 1892, Urbantschitsch carried out an experiment with a group of deaf children. They had all been classified as totally deaf, having failed to respond to tuning-fork tests by air or bone conduction. They were unable to identify sustained vowels called loudly into their ears, neither could they hear musical tones. In 1893 he demonstrated before the Medical Society of Vienna auditory improvements varying from differentiation of vowels to perception of complete sentences. Urbantschitsch's auditory stimulation was by means of loud voices close to the ear, by conversation tubes and harmonica work with reeds of different pitch. At about the same time Kerr-Love in Scotland had found that less than 5 per cent of the children in the Glasgow Institute for the Deaf were totally deaf and was advocating the benefit of acoustic training using ear-trumpets, speaking-tubes and other devices for amplifying sound.

In 1900 Alt, an assistant at the Politzer Clinic in Vienna, produced the first electrical amplifying device for hard-of-hearing people. It consisted of a small loudspeaker microphone, a telephone receiver and dry-cell batteries linked up together. It was a most significant advance on large hearing-trumpets and other acoustic devices of that time.

With the rapid development of electronics in our lifetime the technological basis of electronic hearing-aid construction was developed. We find group hearing aids being used in the Pennsylvania School for the Deaf in 1928. In England, helped by Littler from the National Physical Laboratory, the Manchester University Department for the Education of the Deaf designed a powerful valve-operated group hearing aid and used it at the Royal Residential Schools for Deaf Children at Manchester in 1932. Audiometric surveys carried out by the 'Manchester Department' confirmed Kerr-Love's earlier findings that only a minority of children are totally deaf. Ewing and Littler (1935) considered the effects of stimulating the ears of normal and partially deaf subjects with sounds of high intensities. They found that neither deaf nor normal listeners were found to suffer any diminution in hearing after listening to speech at very high intensity levels. Normal listeners experienced a temporary loss of hearing when subjected to pure tones of sufficiently loud and prolonged nature, whilst the deaf did not appear to be susceptible to this temporarily-induced deafness. Their work was extended to study the responses of partially deaf patients to amplified speech at controlled intensities. They found that hearing aids capable of very high amplification proved extraordinarily helpful in the development of speech in many deaf children, and in facilitating the general education of children with defects of hearing.

During the period 1912–1919 Irene Ewing, who was at that time in charge of a residential school for young deaf children, had begun to practise ways of making use of any residual hearing capacity that she could discover among her young deaf pupils to promote the development of their speech and language.

In the USA at the Central Institute for the Deaf, St. Louis, Goldstein (1921) retried Urbantschitsch's ideas in a somewhat modified form. He published a book on the acoustic method (1939), and reported that although the audiograms of deaf children showed no improvement and even sometimes a deterioration, the ability to understand speech was greatly improved. His system of auditory training classified the work programme into two types of instruction. Passive education consisted of the child listening to the tones produced by musical instruments or sustained amplified frequencies of the audiometer. Active education was subdivided into analytic exercises, consonants and syllables as actual auditory impressions independent of the association of ideas or word imagery; and synthetic exercises which developed auditory comprehension of speech and language.

On discovering that Urbantschitsch's method was not only applicable to children who had a considerable degree of useful hearing, Barczi (1934) devised an acoustic training programme for profoundly deaf children who gave no response to sound above 2000 cycles/s. His hypothesis was that these children could best perceive speech by the use of both auditory and tactile senses. Oral rhythm exercises were the basis of this hypothesis. He disapproved of the use of isolated phonemes and nonsense syllables, and taught only from meaningful material.

Ewing and Ewing (1936) suggested that with the powerful and reliable apparatus available, 70 per cent of the children who were deaf or who had acquired deafness during infancy could make use of their hearing; although in many instances only to a very limited extent, in learning to talk. In their later work the Ewings full developed these ideas and this led to the hearing lip-reading method (1938). Associated with the principle that hearing and lip-reading should be combined at all times, was the need for listening training to be given often and regularly so that the child could learn to use his hearing to the greatest extent possible. The aim of this ear training was to help the deaf child to interpret and to assimilate the words he was to hear. They rejected Goldstein's analytic exercises because they considered that interpretation of sound is greatly enhanced by context and by lip-reading.

It is evident that the concept of auditory training is not new, but most researchers have been concerned with the needs of children. Carhart (1947) considered that an awareness of sound could best be developed by surrounding the child with loud noises that were related to everyday life. On the other hand to Whitehurst (1949), the term auditory training was synonymous with directed listening. She held that the most effective means of achieving this was through a carefully graded series of listening exercises which began with single words and progressed to a complex pattern of sounds. Ronnei (1951) maintained that listening was a complex function, the habit of which was acquired 'through interest in, concentration on, and repetition of, satisfying (auditory) experiences'. Huizing (1951) recommended training the auditory function and gave consideration to six factors. These factors were the development of discrimination or rhythmic patterns, practice in frequency discrimination, recognition of variations in intensity, raising the level of tolerance to sound, drills in the perception of various speech sounds and the 'unconscious absorption' of all types of sound.

Wedenberg (1954) devised an auditory training scheme for deaf children which gave particular emphasis to the frequencies of speech sounds—especially the vowel formants, and he also considered that hearing words should precede seeing them so that they would become auditorily minded. Hudgins (1954) considered that auditory training was concerned with the development of auditory speech perception, better speech from the point of view of intelligibility, naturalness and rhythm. Ewing and Ewing (1954) appear to be among the first writers to outline comprehensive schemes of auditory training for children, but Watson (1967) indicated that he disapproved of courses of graded listening exercises for deaf children and preferred to speak of auditory 'experience' rather than of auditory 'training'. Kelly (1953) considered auditory training as a system of study leading to greater attention to listening, improved discrimination for the sounds of speech, and improved auditory memory span.

Ingeberg (1967) reviewed the rationale for auditory training and more recently Bode and Oyer (1970) carried out further studies of auditory training and speech discrimination with deafened adults.

Combining lip-reading and auditory training

There are certain adults with an acquired hearing loss for whom the visual clues of lip-reading may not provide enough information for efficient communication. There are similar restrictions for those adults for whom no amount of auditory training will lead to a satisfactory level of speech discrimination. Whilst both of these conditions are generally recognized the implications for rehabilitation have not generally been put into practice.

O'Neill and Oyer (1961) considered that the combined use of visual and auditory modalities was essential but not always applied. They go on to say that many therapists stress only one form of rehabilitative procedure. A great deal of verbal emphasis is placed upon a combined approach, but in actual practice, major attention is directed toward the use of only one of the sensory modalities. Auditory training is neglected, with the result that lip-reading becomes the major therapeutic technique. The existence of residual hearing is accepted but very little auditory training is provided. They also argue that, in some cases, lack of interest may be attributed to a reluctance to manipulate equipment, or to lack of equipment and appropriate materials. In other instances, lack of experience in auditory training contributes to its neglect.

When we combine the two sensory channels provided by lip-reading and auditory training each channel makes a contribution to speech intelligibility not provided by either as a single sensory mode. Hutton, Curry and Armstrong (1959) Hutton (1959, 1960), considered that in lip-reading, no matter how effective the method or teacher, visual clues alone were not likely to provide enough information for efficient communication. They presented a rationale for combining auditory and visual stimuli in aural rehabilitation; a view which was supported by the work of Siegenthaler and Gruber (1969) and an investigation which has been carried out at the 'City Lit', Centre for the Deaf, London (Watts and Pegg, 1977).

In this investigation, it was found that there appeared to be no significant evidence in Britain to indicate the benefits, or otherwise, of courses that do exist to help adults who have acquired a hearing loss. The writer, who carried out this work, designed it to evaluate the effectiveness of lip-reading as a single mode of instruction, and the effectiveness of lip-reading and auditory training as a combined mode of instruction. The results of this investigation indicated that the most effective form of rehabilitation was one where visual and auditory channels were combined to reduce sensory confusion, and to produce a more effective communication ability.

Finally, it should be emphasized that any programme of rehabilitation designed for hearing-impaired adults must take into account individual needs and expectations, and ameliorative techniques should include:

(1) The establishment of rapport and confidence, based upon understanding between pupil and teacher. This is considered to be very important. Patients are concerned about the effects of their hearing impairment and need time to discuss its implications. For example, they may have problems at home, at work or in their social life due to deafness.
(2) Counselling about hearing aids.
(3) Counselling about environmental aids

and the following questions should always be in the mind of the teacher.

(1) Is lip-reading instruction necessary?
(2) Is auditory training required?
(3) Are there indications that speech conservation is required?
(4) Have problems appeared which indicate the need for a referral to other professional workers.

Rehabilitation implies restoring, as far as is possible, functions that were previously normal, but further research is necessary. However, such research should not be expected to yield rapid results, not to provide ready-made answers to the questions we have considered.

References

Ballantyne, J. C. (1960). *Deafness.* London; Churchill

Barczi, G. (1934). Address before the International Congress of Logopedia and Phoneatrics in Budapest—Wedenberg, E. (1951) *Acta Otolaryngologica,* Suppl. **94**, 25 'Horerwecken and Hörenzichen' Salzburg 1933

Berger, K. W. (1971). 'Motivation in speech reading', *Teacher of the Deaf,* **69**, 30

Berger, K. W., Garner, M. and Sudman, J. (1971). 'The effect of degree of facial exposure and the vertical angle of vision on speech reading performance', *Teacher of the Deaf,* **69**, 222

Berger, K. W. and Lewis, M. A. (1972). 'The effect of noise on lipreading', *Sound,* **6**(1), 7

Berger, K. W., Martin, J. and Sakoff, R. (1970). 'The effect of visual distractions on speechreading performance', *Teacher of the Deaf,* **68**, 384

Black, J. W., O'Reilly, P. P. and Peck, L. (1963). 'Self-administered training in lipreading', *Journal of Speech and Hearing Disorders,* **28**, 183

Bode, D. L. and Oyer, H. J. (1970). 'Auditory training and speech discrimination', *Journal of Speech and Hearing Research,* **13**, 839

Boultbee, E. F. (1902). *Practical lipreading for the use of the deaf.* London; Upcott Gill

Boultbee, E. F. (1913). *Help for the deaf: What lipreading is.* London; Hodder and Stoughton

Bruhn, E. (1924). *The Mueller-Walle method of lipreading for the deaf.* Lynn, Massachusetts; Nichols Press

Bunger, A. (1961). *Speechreading—Jena method* Fourth edition. Danville, Illinois; Interstate Press

Carhart, R. (1947). 'Auditory training', In *Hearing and Deafness: A guide for laymen.* Ed. by Davis, H. London; Murray Hill Books

Chomsky, N. (1965). *Aspects of the theory of syntax.* Cambridge, Mass.; M.I.T. Press

Clegg, D. G. (1953). *The listening eye: a simple introduction to the art of lipreading.* London; Methuen

Department of Health and Social Security (1973). 'Deafness: Report of a Departmental Enquiry into the promotion of research', *Reports on Health and Social Subjects No. 4,* London; HMSO

Di Carlo, L. M. and Kataja, R. (1951). 'An analysis of the Utley Lipreading Test', *Journal of Speech and Hearing Disorders,* **16**, 226

Ewing, I. R. (1930). *Lipreading.* Manchester; Manchester University Press

Ewing, I. R. and Ewing, A. W. G. (1936). 'The use of hearing aids in the treatment of defects of hearing in children', *Journal of Laryngology and Otology,* **51**, 213

Ewing, I. R. and Ewing, A. W. G. (1938). *The Handicap of Deafness.* London; Longman Green

Ewing, I. R. and Ewing, A. W. G. (1947). *Opportunity and the deaf child.* London; University of London Press

Ewing, I. R. and Ewing, A. W. G. (1954). *Speech and the Deaf Child.* Manchester; Manchester University Press

Ewing, A. W. G. and Littler, J. B. (1935). 'The responses of partially deaf patients to amplified speech at controlled intensities.' Paper given at the Annual Meeting of the British Medical Association. Norwich, Sept. 5th

Goldstein, M. A. (1921). 'An acoustic method', Report on the proceedings of the Twenty Second meeting of the joint convention of American Instructors of the Deaf. pp. 70-79. Washington; Government Printing Office

Goldstein, M. A. (1939). *The Acoustic Method.* St. Louis; Laryngoscope Press

Hardick, E. J., Oyer, H. J. and Irion, P. E. (1970). 'Lipreading performance as related to measurement of vision'. *Journal of Speech and Hearing Research,* **13**, 92

Heider, G. M. (1949). 'The Utley lipreading test', *Volta Review,* **49**, 457, 480 and 490

Heider, F. and Heider, G. (1940). 'An experimental investigation of lipreading', *Psychology Monographs,* **232**, 1

Hewett, E. K. (1904). *Lipreading for the Deaf or Sight Hearing.* London; Harewood Press

Hirsch, I. J. (1970). 'Auditory Training.' In *Hearing and Deafness.* Ed. by Davis and Silverman, New York; Holt, Rinehart & Winston

Hudgins, C. V. (1954). 'Auditory training: its possibilities and limitations', *Volta Review,* **56**, 339

Huizing, H. C. (1951). 'Auditory Training', *Acta Otologia*, Suppl. 100

Hutton, C. (1959). 'Combining auditory and visual stimuli in aural rehabilitation', *Volta Review*, **61**, 316

Hutton, C. (1960). 'A diagnostic approach to combined techniques in aural rehabilitation', *Journal of Speech Hearing Disorders*, **25**, 267

Hutton, C., Curry, E. T. and Armstrong, M. B. (1959). 'Semi-diagnostic test materials for aural rehabilitation', *Journal of Speech Hearing Disorders*, **24**, 319

Ingeberg, B. O. (1967). 'Rehabiliturung Erwachsener mit Schwerhorigbeit', *Journal of Laryngology, Rhinology and Otology*, **46**, 148–151 (Rehabilitation of adults with hearing loss).

Jeffers, J. (1967). 'A re-evaluation of the Utley Lipreading Sentence Test', Paper presented at the 1967 convention of the American Speech and Hearing Association. Chicago, Illinois

Jeffers, J. (1969). 'The social adequacy of two selected samples of geriatric–presbyacusics with significant hearing losses', *International Audiology*, **8**, 317

Jeffers, J. and Barley, M. (1971). *Speechreading (lipreading)*. Springfield, Illinois; Thomas

Kelly, J. C. (1953). *Clinician's handbook for auditory training*. Dubuque, Iowa; Brown

Kinzie, C. E. and Kinzie, R. (1931). *Lipreading for the Deafened Adult*. Philadelphia; Winston

Kitson, H. D. (1915). 'Psychological tests for lipreading ability', *Volta Review*, **17**, 471

Lowell, E. L. (1961). 'New insight into lipreading', *Rehabilitation Review*, July–August

Marek, J. R. (1969). *Beethoven. Biography of a Genius*. London; Kimber

Nitchie, E. B. (1912). *Lip-reading Principles and Practice*. New York; Stokes

Nitchie, E. B. (1917). 'Tests for determining skill in lip-reading', *Volta Review*, **19**, 222

O'Neill, J. J. and Oyer, H. J. (1961). *Visual Communication for the Hard of Hearing*. Englewood Cliffs; Prentice-Hall

Pauls, M. D. (1970) 'Speech Reading.' In *Hearing & Deafness*. Ed. by Davis and Silverman. New York; Holt, Rinehart & Winston

Pintner, R. (1929). 'Speech and speechreading tests for the deaf', *American Annals of the Deaf*, **74**, 480 also *Journal of Applied Psychology*, **12**, 220

Ramsdell, D. A. (1970). 'The Psychology of the Hard of Hearing and Deafened Adult.' In *Hearing and Deafness*. Ed. by Davis & Silverman New York; Holt, Rinehart & Winston.

Reid, G. A. (1946) 'A preliminary investigation in the testing of lipreading achievement', *American Annals of the Deaf*, **91**, 403

Ronnei, E. C. (1951). *Learning to Look and Listen* New York; Columbia University Teachers' College and New York League for the Hard of Hearing

Sanders, J. W. and Coscarelli, J. E. (1970). 'The relationship of visual synthesis skill to lipreading', *American Annals of the Deaf*, **115**, 23

Schwartz, J. R. and Black, J. W. (1967). 'Some aspects of sentence structure in speechreading', *Central States Speech Journal*, **18**, 86

Siegenthaler, B. M. and Gruber, V. (1969). 'Combining vision and audition for speech reception', *Journal of Speech Hearing Disorders*, **34**, 58

Stroy, A. J. (1910). *Speech-reading*. London; Yellon, Williams

Sudman, J. A. and Berger, K. W. (1971). 'Two-dimension versus three-dimension viewing in specchreading', *Journal of Communication Disorders*, **4**, 195

Utley, J. (1946a). 'A test of lipreading ability', *Journal of Speech Disorders*, **11**, 109

Utley, J. (1946b). 'Factors involved in the teaching and testing of lipreading ability through the use of motion pictures', *Volta Review*, **48**, 657

Watson, T. J. (1967). *The Education of Hearing Handicapped Children*. London; University of London Press

Watts, W. J. and Pegg, K. S. (1977). 'The rehabilitation of adults with acquired hearing loss', *British Journal of Audiology*, **11** No. 4, 103

Wedenberg, E. (1954). 'Auditory Training of Deaf and Hard of Hearing Children', *Acta Otologia*, Suppl. 110

Whitehurst, M. W. (1949). *Auditory Training for Children*. New York; Hearing Rehabilitation Center

Wyatt, O. M. (1961). *Teach yourself lipreading*. London; English Universities Press

30 The cochlear implant
Ellis Douek

It is in the nature of progress in human endeavour that achievement in a particular area directs further research towards the remaining, unresolved aspects. What seemed initially to be a minor, unimportant section of a vast problem unexpectedly becomes the growing point of research.

In this way, it is only when many of the fundamental problems of conductive deafness had been resolved, with the field now in the realm of clinical progress, that attention on a large scale turned toward sensorineural hearing loss.

It had been clear for a long time that the techniques required to treat this type of deafness lay beyond the limits of ear surgery as we know it and even into what can be termed the experimental aspects of medicine. At this stage of any development, application to patients can only be very tentative and applicable to a few highly deprived individuals for whom the ratio of possible benefit to the risk of making them worse is very high.

In the case of sensorineural hearing loss these would be people with complete bilateral deafness. Furthermore, they should be old enough to give their informed consent to the procedure and to have been deafened late enough in life to have developed and retained understanding of spoken means of communication. These individuals are necessarily few, but it is with them that the first steps in this field must be taken.

In 1976 a Medical Research Council Working Party compiled the following very tentative and very conservative figures to aid the Council and the Department of Health and Social Security in their understanding of the question:

Deaf population	*1 750 000*
50 per cent too old	875 000
2 per cent with bilateral loss	17 500
33 per cent with eighth-nerve loss	11 566
40 per cent with suitable intelligence/language	4464
20 per cent available for tests	about 900

In other words, not more than 1000 people would be suitable to undergo tests with possible benefit, in the UK, in these early stages. The case was made that these people, however few, are in greater need than the majority of deaf people and that if the risks were diminished in relation to the benefits, the numbers who may be helped in this way would be greater. The most important point, however, is that these new techniques may well be only the first steps in the treatment of sensorineural deafness, whether total or partial, in which case the advances in this field would carry a much greater potential.

The efforts that have been made and which have taken us to the present point have involved a considerable number of experiments on animals in many laboratories throughout the world. Nevertheless, in this chapter we shall limit our discussion to the work done in man, its clinical implications, and refer to animal experiments only insofar as they are directly relevant to it. The approach may be from a number of different aspects.

(1) An historical and chronological approach is useful so as to record the steps that have been taken over the years and to give due credit. A fact which requires recognition at this stage is that much that could be done is due to availability of a suitable technology. The reason why this subject is coming to prominence at present is the development of cheap micro-processors by the electronic and computer industry, as it is only these advances which make the cochlear implant a practical possibility.

(2) An important discussion should be the question of a single or a multi-channel stimulus unit and this will be dealt with in detail.

(3) In view of the exceptional interest that has been taken by public authorities in these developments it is of interest to note that these have taken place until this moment in three countries only. This is worth mentioning as the approach has to some extent been guided by what is considered acceptable, suitable or appropriate in these different countries. Although some initial historic steps were taken in France, it is in the USA, and specifically in California, that most of the basic work has been done. There is no doubt that this required considerable moral courage and a certain pioneering flair that should rightly be recognized. Whether this is associated with the temperament of the geographical locality or whether other factors were at play is not clear, but it is always valuable to those wishing to promote advances to consider the climate which has given rise to them. Present French work, important and interesting in its findings, could not have been carried out in this country, for instance, as the need for an intracranial approach to the cochlea would, rightly or wrongly, be unacceptable at this early stage. Work in the UK came late in the day, initiated by a group working together at Guy's Hospital and University College, London, and at Cambridge. This group was funded by the Medical Research Council and received encouragement from the Department of Health. This third approach appears to be more cautious from the risk/benefit point of view but possibly more widely applicable. Again it may be that the needs and social conditions influence the direction which a research programme may take.

Finally, the author, while actively participating in this research, is conscious of the fact that his chapter must be quite different from the others in this book. It cannot be based on a body of knowledge added to over the years leading to the most recent advances. It deals, on the contrary, with theoretical considerations which are unproven, pathological conditions which are unknown, clinical material which is too sparse to discuss with confidence and the profound uncertainty of where the next step will lie. There can be few lines in textbooks more likely to be superseded in the immediate future and few comments which are more likely to seem naive and unsophisticated at the end of the next decade. It is this consciousness which has required the placing of today's position in its proper context.

History

It is known that Benjamin Franklin in 1751 had commented on the possibility of using electricity to produce a sensation of hearing in the deaf, but with the limited knowledge of electricity and of the hearing mechanism at the time his suggestion could not properly be applied. He was not the only one, however, to show interest in this field as Le Roy reported various attempts at obtaining cures using electricity, to the French Academie des Sciences in 1755. Volta in 1790 placed metal rods into his own ears and, connecting them to a source producing about 50 volts, experienced a shock associated with a sound of boiling liquid. Many physicians in the nineteenth century, including Ritter (1801) as well as such well-known figures as Politzer and Gradenigo experimented with crude external electrodes both as a form of therapy and diagnosis, and detailed descriptions were given by Roosa (1873) and Scheppegrell (1898).

It was only after it became known that electrical potentials arose in the cochlea as a result of acoustic stimulation that a more quantitative approach took place. The tones which could be heard by a normal ear stimulated by a nearby electrode were termed 'electrophonic hearing' and were studied by Stevens and Jones (1939), Jones, Stevens and Lurie (1940) and Flottorp (1953) in the following years. Electrophonic hearing is not, of course, what is meant by electrical stimulation of a totally deafened patient and it was Djourno and Eyries (1957) who published the results of electrical stimulation of the totally deaf patient by a wire implanted into the cochlea. It is this report which can truly be said to have initiated the work which is now under consideration. Simmons *et al.* (1964) were encouraged following a similar experiment and implanted six electrodes in the modiolar tissue of the auditory nerve of a bilaterally deaf patient (Simmons, 1966). Simmons reported that pitch variations were related to the electrode stimulated and to the frequency, and also that the loudness depended on the amplitude of the stimulus. At the same time House had investigated the effects of single channel electrical stimulation, which he reviewed in 1973 and 1976; also Michelson, who together with Merzenich, Schindler and Petit, reported some of their findings in 1971, 1973 and 1975.

None of these devices produced recognizable speech but the patients claimed closer contact with the environment and an improvement in their lip-reading ability.

More recently Bilger (1977) was able to evaluate independently 13 patients who had working implants placed by House or Michelson.

In 1973 Dobelle *et al.* in Utah reported experiments in direct stimulation of the auditory cortex. Despite encouraging results the dangers of intracranial procedures turned their attention to intra-cochlear multi-channel devices which might take advantage of the cochlea's tonotopic organization. Initially, they investigated a patient of House's, who had been implanted with five electrodes (Mladejovsky *et al,.* 1975) with more sophisticated stimulating equipment. This produced extremely encouraging results.

A multi-channel approach was also reported by Chouard and MacLeod (1973). They subsequently described seven patients who had been implanted with up to eight intra-cochlear electrodes each. These were separately inserted into an electrically isolated compartment of the scala tympani. The surgical approach required a double exposure through the middle ear and through the middle cranial fossa.

It was only much later that work on the cochlear implant began in the UK. While agreeing that it is only through a multi-channel stimulating device that we can hope eventually to offer true speech discrimination, Douek *et al.* (1977) reported a new approach. This was based on simple, extra-cochlear, virtually non-invasive stimulation. Their hope was that this would be applicable to a larger number of people and provide some early benefit on a wider scale.

Theoretical considerations

The cochlear implant, as has been described in the preceding section, involves stimulating the auditory system with electrical impulses rather than auditory ones. Its use is demanded by those patients who are so deaf that their cochlea does not respond to sound stimuli no matter how greatly amplified.

The choice of electrical stimulation as an alternative rather than other possible forms of stimulus, such as chemical or mechanical, is not only because of the ease with which electrical impulses can be applied, but also because the cochlea normally acts as a transducer changing the mechanical energy of sound vibration into electrical impulses. It is these impulses which are transmitted along the nerve.

Transforming sound into electrical energy is a simple act performed every moment of the day by all our means of communication. The difficulty lies in our ignorance of the special code used by the auditory system to recognize the relation between the various sounds and the electrical impulses. It is relatively easy to understand possible methods of coding rhythms or loudness, say by rate of impulses or by their amplitude, but the difficulty lies in the most important piece of coding and that is pitch.

For this there are two basic theories:

1. The place theory

The pitch of a pure tone is determined by the nerve fibres which are most active. This is related to the point of maximum displacement of the travelling wave. According to this theory it is the place along the cochlea where stimulus is initiated which determines the pitch of the tone. Although attractive from the point of view of our knowledge of tone production by instruments such as the piano, this theory does not provide a satisfactory explanation for some of the psycho-acoustic and neurophysiological findings.

2. The temporal theory

It is the time pattern of the neural impulses which determines pitch perception. Temporal information of this type depends on phase-locking, the nerves firing at a particular phase of the stimulating wave-form. For sinusoids the time intervals between firings are approximately integral multiples of the wave-form period. Experiments done on animals showed that phase-locking is limited to frequencies below 4-5 kHz. This is because of a temporal 'jitter' which accompanies phase-locking. At higher frequencies this jitter comes near the period of the wave-form of the stimulus so that the nerve firings become blurred.

In theory, then, if the place concept were working we would have to stimulate the cells of the different parts of the cochlea according to which tone we wished to produce. On the other hand, if the temporal theory were correct for all pitches then we would need only one electrode as all information would be carried by the rate and time pattern of the firing.

In fact, there is evidence that both types of neural information contribute to the perception of pitch but their relative effectiveness differs in different parts of the frequency range, temporal encoding being valid only for the lower frequencies and place for the upper tones. It is the important middle range for which there is considerable doubt regarding the relative importance of the two mechanisms.

When we consider the practical implications for electrical stimulation we see that with a single electrode we can only make use of the temporal mechanism whereas with a multiple channel system we could, at least in theory, make use of the place mechanism.

There is no doubt that speculation on theories can now take us no further. Animal experiments have only a small place as far as perception is concerned so it can only be to patients who have experienced electrical stimulation that we have to turn for the next element of information.

Aural pathology and patient selection

Most types of aural pathology can cause total or very severe hearing loss. Those which have been considered by the author's group have included the following disorders:

(1) Congenital deafness
(2) Trauma—head injury
        —surgical
(3) Labryrinthitis—viral or bacterial
(4) Ototoxic drugs
(5) Menière's disease
(6) Meningitis
(7) Unknown or uncertain aetiology

We should at once draw attention to the defects of such a list which is only superficially plausible. The immediate question must be how certain are we of the diagnosis? The patient would like to have some idea of the cause of his complaint and asks the question. The physician has to give some answer if only for therapeutic reasons. He also knows that in the case of total deafness it will make no difference to the outcome. He will need to classify diseases if only to be able to discuss them in the literature. When we come to experimental and scientific work it seems that we are more uncertain regarding the diagnosis in many more cases and it is the last, (7), which predominates here. Furthermore, whereas we could consider patients' audiograms in great detail and classify their disability according to the hearing level so as to advise on management, this is not the case in total deafness. Here, since amplification does not help, they form one single group of 'unhelpables'. The analogy is similar to when 'deafness' could not be broken up into those who could be helped by surgery and those who could not. Now that we must consider a new form of management altogether, and when we realize that again some will be helped and some not, new information will be necessary, a 'new electrical audiogram' to guide us. It is not enough to give 'trauma' as a diagnosis when we need to know if the nerve is viable and able to conduct our electrical impulses.

In this we face a difficulty as adequate post-mortem material is difficult to obtain. Nevertheless, some is available.

Kerr and Schuknecht (1968) studied 41 temporal bones of individuals with profound hearing loss. Further cases have been reported (Schuknecht *et al.*, 1973 and 1974). A number of post-mortem specimens were of individuals who had suffered profound deafness from inner-ear concussion with or without fracture. Although these showed severe loss of hair-cells, the neuronal population remained good. Patients with unilateral sudden deafness who had come to post mortem showed an unexpected normality in the number of viable neurones compared with the other ear. Patients deafened by ototoxic antibiotics also showed remarkably good neuronal survival as compared with hair-cell loss. On the other hand, patients with a Mondini-type dysplasia showed much greater variability in the state of the neurones as did those with the Scheibe type of cochleo–saccular degeneration.

Meningitis accompanied by profound deafness appears to suffer from a bacterial labyrinthitis producing a fibro–osseus obliteration of the inner ear. Of interest in this context is Schuknecht and Woellner's experiments in animals (1953) which showed that up to 75 per cent of the neurones can be destroyed by nerve section without affecting the pure-tone threshold.

This uncertainty regarding the likely state of the neuronal population obviously creates problems in the selection of suitable patients and these points should be considered.

1. Total deafness by pure-tone audiometry

In all discussion regarding selection of patients it has been a *sine qua non* that these should show no response on pure-tone audiometry. This has never been entirely acceptable to the author and an example is his patient WS as described in a review of the group's work (Fourcin *et al.*, 1978). In one ear there was no auditory response at all and an *extra*-cochlear electrode had been placed against the round window. In the other ear there was a measurable flat audiogram at 100–110 dB. A comparison of usefulness in communication between electrocochlear stimulation and loud amplification showed definite advantage to the former. Amplification in the non-implanted ear turned out to be of no value whatsoever. It should also be noted that amplification of that degree could be relied upon to destroy finally any lingering auditory function, however useful. This is one example only and in the author's opinion it is whether the patient has any *functional* measurable hearing which is relevant.

2. Electrocochleography

It had been hoped that the findings of electrocochleographic examination in these patients might offer a guide to their potential as implant patients (Aran, 1974). The place of ECochG as a diagnostic tool has not yet been fully explored but there is no doubt any information regarding the site of the lesion or the quality of the surviving neurones would be of great value. On the other hand, a suggestion that the ECochG can give a direct indication as to whether a patient may or may not benefit from an implant is too simplistic.

3. Promontory stimulation

This has been extensively used, as if a patient cannot 'hear' an electrical stimulus, then the implant is of no value. Brackmann (1976) describes a technique using the same needle which has been inserted for ECochG recording. A low frequency (30–120 Hz), low voltage (0.3–1.2 V) alternating current is applied. These parameters had been found most effective. It is also possible to record objective brain-stem responses simultaneously.

Although workers in this field had thought initially that these responses were a sufficient indication of likely success the author and his colleagues are now convinced that threshold measurements of this type do not signify that the patient would be able to discriminate speech. They now favour a more chronic if temporary implantation.

4. Test by chronic implant

In the author's cases a single electrode has been placed by tympanotomy into the round window niche and this has been done under local or general anaesthesia. This allows the patient to be tested over the next few days. These tests can now be quite elaborate and carried out and repeated in comfort. Threshold tests may indeed be carried out but there are two more important aspects:

(1) Speech discrimination tests may be carried out with and without lip-reading as well as before and after practising. This has shown that the correlation between threshold measurement and speech comprehension potential is far from close, so that reliance on promontory stimulation alone is not adequate.

(2) The patient now knows exactly what the permanent implant is likely to do and can decide whether he wants to have it or not. This avoids the situation of having to offer the patient a new form of perception of which neither he nor the physician has a true concept.

The conclusion is that as the exact pathology, not to mention the neuronal state, of a particular patient's ear can still not be properly elucidated, it is only trial and error which can decide the indication for an implant. Our efforts at this stage should be to mitigate the likelihood of error as much as possible.

At this stage of development everything is still possible and a number of different approaches not considered now may still emerge. Nevertheless, we will consider a number of possibilities:

(1) Cortical stimulation.
(2) Acoustic nerve stimulation.
(3) Single-channel intra-cochlear stimulation.
(4) Multiple channel intra-cochlear stimulation.
(5) Extra-cochlear stimulation.

1. Cortical stimulation

In theory this would be the most advantageous as virtually the whole of the deaf population could be treated in this way. Furthermore, there may be advantage in approaching the terminal cells of the auditory pathways directly. Some technology has already been developed in transmitting visual impulses in this way (Brindley and Lewin, 1968) for more than ten years and this could no doubt help to establish an auditory dimension to cortical stimulation. The feasibility of such an approach has been studied by Dobelle *et al.* (1973) but they considered a number of disadvantages. The first is the problem of surgical access to the auditory cortex and the second the small number of patients who could be asked to cooperate in the early stages. These would be those patients who require resection of tumours of the insula or the upper margins of the Sylvian fissure; vascular abnormalities such as middle cerebral artery aneurysms; or resections for temporal lobe epilepsy as these operations may allow access to the auditory cortex.

According to Penfield and Perot (1963) the primary auditory cortex is on the most anterior of the tranverse gyri of Heschl and on the superior surface of the temporal lobe inside the Sylvian fissure. The lower lip of the Sylvian fissure also produced auditory sensations but the writers considered these to be alterations and interpretations of sounds being heard rather than new sounds in themselves. In practice, only the lower lip of the Sylvian fissure provides easy access as retraction of the fissure would be necessary to reach Heschl's gyrus. Needle electrodes passed though the brain substance would pose further problems not justified at present.

There are also other anatomical problems which would make a prosthesis more difficult, namely the middle cerebellar artery and its branches create a considerable risk.

Nevertheless, the preliminary work carried out by Dobelle and his co-workers is of prime value at the present stage of our knowledge.

They have chosen to call the subjective sensations of sound which electrical stimulation of the human auditory cortex produces 'audenes' by analogy with the 'phosphenes' of the visual cortex. Different waveforms and polarity do not seem to influence the sensation greatly which is of interest both for general physiological reasons and because it means that waveform may be selected for its efficacy in long-term stimulation. Changes in pulse amplitude produce changes in loudness perceived and the thresholds were around 6 ma. This is about twice as high as the levels obtained from visual cortical stimulation (Brindley and Lewin, 1968). The reason for Dobelle's findings may be that the area he stimulated, the lateral lip of the Sylvian fissure, was not actually the one responding, and that the current may have had to spread to areas within the fissure to produce auditory sensation. The auditory cortex is also thicker than the visual one and the responding cells may well be further from the surface. No changes in the subjective sensation were noted by patients when the frequency varied between 25/s and 100/s, and it should be noted that this is quite different from both nerve and cochlear stimulation. This suggests that in a future implant pitch modulation may have to be obtained by selecting different electrodes from an array rather than by changing the stimulus on a single electrode. In the same way pulse duration does not seem to affect markedly subjective sensation. Descriptions by the patients of the nature of the sounds included 'buzzing', 'humming', 'knocking', 'crickets', 'wavering'. These are singularly like the descriptions obtained from cochlear stimulation.

These findings would suggest that the crucial factor in electrical stimulation which is recognition of pitch variations may possibly require stimulation of different areas over a 'tonotopic map'. Preparation of such a map, if it exists, is made very difficult by what seems to be the anatomical situation of the auditory cortex. The likelihood that this is deep within the Sylvian fissure makes an early approach of this type unlikely.

2. Acoustic nerve stimulation

Direct access to the acoustic nerve itself without greatly disturbing it or its surrounding structures is entirely possible by a middle fossa approach or by a posterior craniotomy. The advantages here appear to be negligible as we have two aspects of pitch. Firstly, rate-pitch which is related to the number of impulses/s and which appears to function well for low tones. An electrode placed directly on the nerve itself would certainly offer this type of perception as it seems to be independent of which nerve fibre is stimulated but there does not appear to be any advantage over the simple type of extracochlear stimulation described below in Section 5. Secondly, place-pitch where the perceived tone is determined by the particular fibres which have been stimulated. Of course, once a stimulus becomes repetitive a rate-pitch type of response will also be obtained so that there will be no clear distinction between the two types. According to Blair Simmons (1974) once a repetitive stimulus occurs at 20–30 pulses/s the high frequency fibres will produce a ringing sound and low frequency ones a roar or vibrating sensation. It is only at rates above 60–80 pulses/s that a steady, continuous sound is produced. Below this rate, therefore, it is place-pitch which has the dominant role, but above 80 pulses/s it is the rate–pitch perception which becomes increasingly dominant. In the latter case, therefore, the effect on the stimulated high frequency fibre will be to produce a low pitch. On the other hand, as the rate continues to rise the pitch heard will appear progressively smoother and higher but eventually the rate–pitch sensation declines and only place remains.

In order to achieve place–pitch sensation by electrode implantation would demand not only extreme precision in the exact location, with limitation in the diffusion of the stimulus, but also stability in the placement.

None of these requirements seem possible as far as the nerve itself is concerned and hence it is to a more peripheral location that we must turn.

3. Single-channel intra-cochlear stimulation

Two techniques have been used here. In the first type, carried out by the House group in Los Angeles and reported by Brackmann (1976), patients had a unipolar electrode placed in the scala tympani with a ground wire in the temporalis muscle area. These leads were connected to an induction coil embedded in the bone of the mastoid cortex. An external unit was made which produced a 16 000-Hz carrier wave. Incoming acoustic stimuli were converted to a signal which produced a 90 per cent amplitude modulation of the carrier wave. This carrier wave and its parameters were arrived at on a basis of trial and error, by allowing the first patient, implanted chronically in May 1972, to select the stimulus mode which gave him most benefit.

These patients perceived periodicity–pitch (rate–pitch) at frequencies up to 800 Hz and gave, broadly speaking, the same results as the patients in the next group.

The second type of electrode is bipolar and also implanted into the scala tympani. This was carried out in San Francisco and reported by Michelson (1971, a, b) and carefully investigated by Merzenich, Michelson and their associates (1973).

The electrode was inserted about 11 mm into the scala tympani via the round window. It derived its input from an implanted radio receiver which in turn was activated by a microphone–amplifier–transmitter package worn externally. The antenna of the transmitter was worn like a bone-conduction hearing aid. The transmission was across the skin and subcutaneous tissue to a receiver embedded in the mastoid cortex. The result was that an electrical analogue of any sound-stimulus could be delivered to the intra-cochlear stimulating electrode. This package was relatively stable and it allowed the San Francisco group to carry out both psycho-acoustic and physiological experiments.

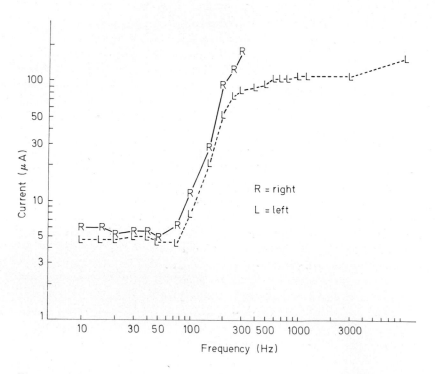

Figure 30.1   Current/frequency threshold detection curve for a patient with a chronic round window implant

Threshold curves were derived using a method of limits (*Figure 30.1*). Sounds were evoked by sinusoidal electrical stimulation from 25 Hz to above 10 000 Hz. These were described as having a tonal quality from 100 Hz up to at least several thousand Hz. The apparent pitch, however, changed as a rapid function of stimulus frequency only up to about 500 Hz.

Pitch-scaling experiments showed that as stimulus frequency rises, the note perceived rises up to about 500 Hz. At higher frequencies an almost constant note is heard. Again, it is only up to 500 Hz that discriminative hearing is possible and even then the range is variable so that at 100 Hz the discriminable difference in pitch was 1–2 Hz; at 300 Hz about 5 Hz, and at 500 Hz it ranged from 7–10 Hz in one subject, to 30 Hz in another. This means that the ability to discriminate is poor even at the low frequency range. Furthermore, the subjects could not hear simultaneously different frequency components of a sound, and loudness increased as a very steep function of stimulus intensity.

4. Multiple channel intra-cochlear stimulation

The fact that single-cochlear stimulation did not lead by itself to the transmission of intelligible speech has led to the development of multi-channel electrode systems. The aim is to take advantage of the cochlea's tonotopic organization to obtain some degree of place-pitch reception. Studies on these patients were undertaken through collaboration between the University of Utah and The Ear Research Institute in Los Angeles (Eddington *et al.*, 1978) as well as a considerable amount of work done in San Francisco (Merzenich *et al.*, 1974, 1976, 1978).

The *scala tympani* has remained the location of choice for these reasons:

(1) The cochlear nerve fibres are suitably distributed.
(2) It is accessible from the external ear.
(3) It is more easily accessible than the scala vestibuli as electrodes can be threaded in though the round window and are guided along by a bony boundary.
(4) The modiolus does produce a place-pitch response (Simmons, 1966) but is not easily accessible.

Chouard and McLeod (1976) approached it by a different technique, fenestrating the cochlea in different places, using Silastic in an attempt at isolation.

Pitch appears to be determined by the location of the electrode so that basal electrodes produce a higher sensation than apical ones up to a limit of around 800 Hz. Loudness sensation increases together with amplitude of current. It seems also that different wave-forms produce only marginal differences in subjective sensations and these may themselves be the result of variations in intensity and current spread.

The particular problem of current spread is a complex one and it is not likely that simple divisions by insulating material such as Silastic could be of much value. The use of bipolar electrodes helps to minimize current spread as opposed to monopolar as the flow is from one to the other rather than to the ground electrode. Merzenich *et al.* (1974, 1975) carried out experiments on cats using bipolar stimulation with 0.4 mm– 1.1 mm spacing. They were able to record single unit responses in the inferior colliculus nucleus and to determine the voltage necessary to stimulate fibres at various distances from the bipolar electrode. Such an electrode pair producing a frequency of about 5.7 Hz required a 10 dB difference of 3.2 times greater voltage than that needed to excite a unit of 10 kHz, directly under the electrode.

The results of the work recently carried out are encouraging from the point of view of both place–pitch and periodicity–pitch but the number of experiments and the number of patients under investigation are still very few.

5. Extra-cochlear stimulation

The author and his colleagues in England deal with this situation by approaching it from a different direction. First, experiments with an electrode placed *on* the round window but not into the scala tympani appeared to produce similar results to those with a single electrode inside the cochlea without its complications. Although these are mainly theoretical, there remains the anxiety that the electrode itself may alter the environment in the inner ear. On the other hand, it was quite clear that no place–pitch responses could be obtained without a multi-channel system. A decision was, therefore, made to develop a simple non-invasive system consisting of an extra-cochlear electrode and to explore its potentialities. The results have been described in 1977 (Douek *et al.*) and by Fourcin *et al.* (1978). The most important difference that this technique has offered is in the nature of the stimulus offered. Previous work has directly used the raw acoustic signal obtained from filtering microphone output. In this case, as it was accepted that little discrimination could be expected from a single electrode, all efforts were directed towards an aid to lip-reading. The lip-reader can make reasonably accurate distinctions between 'bow' and 'doe', for instance, but finds it difficult to discriminate between 'doe' and 'know' or 'Sue' and 'zoo'. The question was whether introducing the low frequency range of sound available from electrical stimulation could contribute anything to the visual clues on which the lip-reader depends. It was noted that there was a very close similarity between that range and the frequency distribution of the human voice (*Figure 30.2*) both male and female or, in other words, there should be little difficulty in making the laryngeal tone of the speaker available to the deaf patient as an auditory sensation. In order to do this use was made of the laryngograph (Fourcin and Abberton, 1971; Fourcin, 1974). This provides an electrical signal from an external electrode which senses closure of the vocal cords, operating immediately, safely and without special preparation (*Figure 30.3*). The signal is nearly sinusoidal and since it has the frequency of the speaker's larynx vibration, provides a direct stimulus to the implanted electrode.

The details of the work and of the speech and psycho-acoustic tests are available in the published work referred to; nevertheless, the findings may here be mentioned from a clinical point of view:

(1) The capacity to discriminate words purely by electrical stimulation without lip-reading was very poor.

(2) Although in some patients there was improvement in distinguishing single words, meaningful or meaningless, when lip-reading was supplemented by the stimulus overall the results were disappointing.

(3) When listening to whole sentences and meaningful speech the results were very satisfactory to the patient as well as to the tester. The reasons for this are only now becoming clear but two points have emerged already. First, the 'voice' sound

allows the patient to distinguish the tone differences between statement, question, etc. This means that certain aspects of communication including emotion can be perceived. Secondly, the patient is able to perceive the rhythm of speech and particularly which word is stressed in a sentence. The amount of information transmitted in this way is considerable.

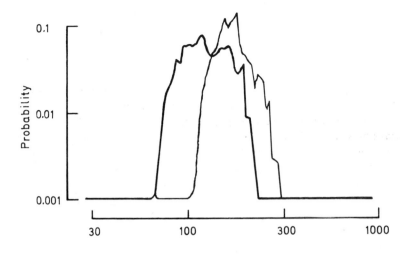

Figure 30.2   Frequency distribution of male (thick line) and female (thin line) voice. (Plotted by Fourcin)

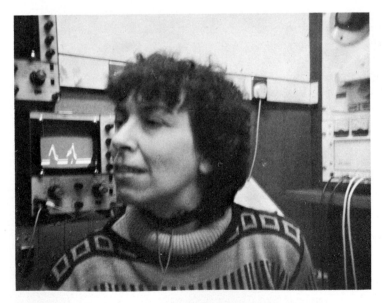

Figure 30.3   Laryngograph apparatus as developed by Fourcin

Conclusion

What then is the position regarding electrical stimulation of the cochlea?

(1) It has now emerged from the purely experimental stage and it can truly offer some help to some patients. These are people who have lost all hearing in both ears and are prepared to cooperate in a rehabilitation process which associates electrical stimulation with lip-reading.

(2) The actual techniques used and the apparatus are still in the process of development and have not yet reached a stable point.

(3) The nature of the operation/rehabilitation process is quite different from previous otological advances. Previous steps have all been made through the efforts of surgeons improving techniques. Here there is a need for a team of workers which includes experts in physics, phonetics, engineering and psycho-acoustics. This need not always be so and when a more standard type of test and equipment is available individual surgeons may be able to make use of it, as with all new prosthetic aids. At present every item will have to be developed for each patient and the results assessed as the process develops. This means that it is limited to centres which are prepared to put together teams of this type.

(4) The team-work situation is one unfamiliar to surgeons even though they may have experience of working with ancillary helpers such as audiometric technicians, speech therapists and teachers. This is because his colleagues would not be ancillaries and because the techniques they will offer may be to a large extent outside his comprehension. This creates a feeling of uncertainty where no one is sure of the limits of his duties. The surgeon, if he wishes to undertake this type of work, would be wise to remember that he retains total clinical and legal responsibility for his patient and that he cannot in any sense devolve it onto colleagues who are not doctors. This means that the primary role of selecting the patient rests entirely on him and it is his role to advise the patient whether he is a suitable candidate and to explain to him the expectations and limitations of what is offered. It is the surgeon's role to decide on clinical grounds whether enough tests have been carried out to make a decision and it is for him to admit, discharge and arrange for rehabilitation. If he offers this framework his scientific colleagues can function without hesitation and without being hindered by responsibilities which make their own appraisal, difficult enough as it is, more complex.

References

Aran, J. M. (1974). *Electrical Stimulation of the Acoustic Nerve in Man*, Ed. by Merzenich, M. M., Schindler, M. D., Sooy, F. A. San Francisco; Velo-bind Inc.

Bilger, R. C. (1977). *Annals of Otology, Rhinology and Laryngology*, Suppl. 38, 86

Brackmann, D. E. (1976). *Laryngoscope*, **86**, 373

Brindley, G. S. and Lewin, W. S. (1968). *Journal of Physiology*, **196**, 479

Chouard, C. H. and MacLeod, P. (1973). *Nouvelle Presse Medical*, **44**, 2953

Chouard, C. H. and MacLeod, P. (1976). *Laryngoscope*, **86**, 1743

Djourno, A. and Eyries, C. (1957). *Presse medical*, **35**, 1417

Dobelle, W. H., Mladejovsky, M. G., Stensaas, S. S. and Smith, J. B. (1973). *Annals of Otology, Rhinology and Laryngology*, **82**, 445

Douek, E., Fourcin, A. J., Moore, B. C. J. and Clarke, G. P. (1977). *Proceedings of the Royal Society of Medicine*, **70**, 379

Eddington, D. K., Dobelle, W. H., Brackmann, D. E., Mladesovsky, M. G. and Parkin, J. L. (1978). In press

Flottorp, G. (1953). *Journal of the Acoustical Society of America*, **25**, 236

Fourcin, A. J. (1974). *Ventilatory and Phonatory Control Systems.* Ed. by Wyke, B. London; Oxford University Press

Fourcin, A. J. and Abberton, E. (1971). *Medical and Biological Illustration*, **21**, 172

Fourcin, A. J., Rosen, S. M., Moore, B. C. J., Douek, E. E., Clarke, G. P., Dodson, H. and Bannister, L. H. (1978)

House, W. F. (1976). *Annals of Otology, Rhinology and Laryngology*, **85**, Suppl. 27

House, W. F. and Urban, J. (1973). *Annals of Otology, Rhinology and Laryngology*, **82**, 504

Jones, R., Stevens, S. and Lurie, M. (1940), *Journal of the Acoustical Society of America*, **12**, 281

Kerr, A. and Schuknecht, H. (1968). *Acta Otolaryngologica*, **65**, 586

Merzenich, M. M., Michelson, R. P., Schindler, R. A., Pettit, C. R. and Reid, M. (1973). *Annals of Otology, Rhinology and Laryngology*, **82**, 456

Merzenich, M. M., Schindler, R. A. and Sooy, F. A. (1974). In *Electrical Stimulation of the Acoustic Nerve in Man.* San Francisco; Velo-bind

Merzenich, M. M., Schindler, D. N. and White, M. W. (1974). *Laryngoscope*, **84**, 1887

Merzenich, M. M. and White, M. W. (1978). *Cochlear Implants: The Interface Problem.* In press

Michelson, R. P. (1971). *Archives of Otolaryngology*, **93**, 317

Mladejovsky, M. G. (1975). *Transactions of the American Society of Artificial Internal Organs*, **21**

Penfield, W. and Perot, P. (1968). *Brain*, **86**, 595

Schuknecht, H. F. (1974). *Electrical Stimulation of the Acoustic Nerve in Man.* San Francisco; Velo-bind Inc.

Schuknecht, H. F. (1974). *Pathology of the Ear.* Cambridge, Mass.; Harvard Press

Schuknecht, H. F. and Woellner, R. C. (1953). *Laryngoscope*, **63**, 441

Simmons, F. B. (1966). *Archives of Otolaryngology*, **84**, 24

Simmons, F. B. (1974). In *Electrical Stimulation of the Acoustic Nerve in Man.* San Francisco; Velo-bind Inc.

Simmons, F. B., Mongeon, C. J., Lewis, W. R. *et al.* (1964). *Archives of Otolaryngology*, **79**, 559

Stevens, S. S. and Jones, R. C. (1939). *Journal of the Acoustical Society of America*, **10**, 261

Index